D1571224

2012

Leonard L. Lance, RPh, BSPharm
Senior Editor
Pharmacist
Lexi-Comp, Inc.
Hudson, Ohio

Charles F. Lacy, RPh, MS, PharmD, FCSHP
Editor
Vice President for Executive Affairs
Professor, Pharmacy Practice
Professor, Business Leadership
University of Southern Nevada
Las Vegas, Nevada

Morton P. Goldman, RPh, PharmD, BCPS, FCCP
Associate Editor
Director of Pharmacotherapy Services
Department of Pharmacy
Cleveland Clinic
Cleveland, Ohio

Lora L. Armstrong, RPh, PharmD, BCPS
Associate Editor
Vice President, Clinical Affairs
Pharmacy & Therapeutics Formulary Process
Clinical Program Oversight
CaremarkRx
Northbrook, Illinois

NOTICE

This data is intended to serve the user as a handy reference and not as a complete drug information resource. It does not include information on every therapeutic agent available. The publication covers over 1800 commonly used drugs and is specifically designed to present important aspects of drug data in a more concise format than is typically found in medical literature or product material supplied by manufacturers.

The nature of drug information is that it is constantly evolving because of ongoing research and clinical experience and is often subject to interpretation. While great care has been taken to ensure the accuracy of the information and recommendations presented, the reader is advised that the authors, editors, reviewers, contributors, and publishers cannot be responsible for the continued currency of the information or for any errors, omissions, or the application of this information, or for any consequences arising therefrom. Therefore, the author(s) and/or the publisher shall have no liability to any person or entity with regard to claims, loss, or damage caused, or alleged to be caused, directly or indirectly, by the use of information contained herein. Because of the dynamic nature of drug information, readers are advised that decisions regarding drug therapy must be based on the independent judgment of the clinician, changing information about a drug (eg, as reflected in the literature and manufacturer's most current product information), and changing medical practices. Therefore, this data is designed to be used in conjunction with other necessary information and is not designed to be solely relied upon by any user. The user of this data hereby and forever releases the authors and publishers of this data from any and all liability of any kind that might arise out of the use of this data. The editors are not responsible for any inaccuracy of quotation or for any false or misleading implication that may arise due to the text or formulas as used or due to the quotation of revisions no longer official.

Certain of the authors, editors, and contributors have written this book in their private capacities. No official support or endorsement by any federal or state agency or pharmaceutical company is intended or inferred.

The publishers have made every effort to trace any third party copyright holders, if any, for borrowed material. If they have inadvertently overlooked any, they will be pleased to make the necessary arrangements at the first opportunity.

Book revisions are available at our website at http://www.lexi.com/home/revisions/.

Copyright © 2012 by Lexi-Comp, Inc. All rights reserved.

Printed in the United States of America. No part of this publication may be reproduced, stored in a retrieval system, used as a source of information for transcription into a hospital information system or electronic health or medical record, or transmitted in any form or by any means, electronic, mechanical, photocopying, recording or otherwise, without the prior written permission of the publisher. Should you or your institution have a need for this information in a format we protect, we have solutions for you. Please contact our office at the number below.

This manual was produced using Lexi-Comp's Information Management System™ (LIMS) — a complete publishing service of Lexi-Comp Inc.

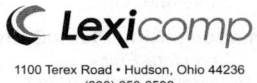

1100 Terex Road • Hudson, Ohio 44236
(330) 650-6506

TABLE OF CONTENTS

Visit thePoint http://thepoint.lww.com/QL2012 for exclusive access to:

    Apothecary/Metric Conversions

    Pounds/Kilograms Conversion

    Temperature Conversion

    Pharmaceutical Manufacturers and Distributors

    Multivitamin Products

Refer to the inside front cover of this book for your online access code.

ABOUT THE EDITORS

Leonard L. Lance, RPh, BSPharm

Leonard L. (Bud) Lance has been directly involved in the pharmaceutical industry since receiving his bachelor's degree in pharmacy from Ohio Northern University in 1970. Upon graduation from ONU, Mr Lance spent four years as a Navy pharmacist in various military assignments and was instrumental in the development and operation of the first whole hospital I.V. admixture program in a military (Portsmouth Naval Hospital) facility.

After completing his military service, he entered the retail pharmacy field and has managed a chain store (Revco), an independent (Klein's), and a home I.V. franchise pharmacy operation (OptionCare). Since the late 1970s, Mr Lance has focused much of his interest on using computers to improve pharmacy service. Klein's Pharmacy was one of the first retail pharmacies in the State of Ohio to computerize (1977) while he served as manager.

His love for computers and pharmacy led him to Lexi-Comp, Inc. in 1988. He was the first pharmacist at Lexi-Comp and helped develop Lexi-Comp's first drug database in 1989 and was involved in the editing and publishing of Lexi-Comp's first *Drug Information Handbook* in 1990.

As a result of his strong publishing interest, he serves in the capacity of pharmacy editor and technical advisor at Lexi-Comp. Mr Lance has assisted over 400 major hospitals in producing their own custom formulary projects through Lexi-Comp's custom publishing service. Mr Lance presently works as a Pharmaceutical Database Specialist in the Dosage Forms Database Department in the Content Division at Lexi-Comp.

Mr Lance has served as president of the Summit Pharmaceutical Association (SPA). He is a member of the Ohio Pharmacists Association (OPA), the American Pharmaceutical Association (APhA), and the American Society of Health-System Pharmacists (ASHP).

Charles F. Lacy, RPh, MS, PharmD, FCSHP

Dr Lacy is the co-founder and the current Vice President of Executive Affairs at the University of Southern Nevada. In this capacity, Dr Lacy fosters, develops, and maintains new opportunities for the university in the areas of business partnerships, foundational development, external programs development, international affiliations, and outreach project design and coordination. Dr Lacy is Professor of Pharmacy Practice in the Nevada College of Pharmacy and Guest Professor in the MBA program and the College of Nursing.

Prior to his promotion to Executive Affairs, Dr Lacy was Vice President for Information Technologies at the University and the Facilitative Officer for Clinical Programs where he managed the clinical curriculum, clinical faculty activities, student experiential programs, pharmacy residency programs, and the college continuing education programs.

Additionally, he spent 20 years at Cedars-Sinai Medical Center, where he was the Department of Pharmacy's Clinical Coordinator. With over 20 years of clinical experience at one of the nation's largest teaching hospitals, he developed a reputation as an acknowledged expert in drug information, pharmacotherapy, and critical care drug interventions.

Dr Lacy received his doctorate from the University of Southern California School of Pharmacy. Presently, Dr Lacy holds teaching affiliations with the Nevada College of Pharmacy, the University of Southern Nevada, Showa University in Tokyo, Japan, the University of Alberta at Edmonton School of Pharmacy and Health Sciences, KLE University in Bangalore, India, and the Hokkaido College of Pharmacy in Sapporo, Japan. He also received his master's degree from Phillips Graduate Institute in Psychology with an emphasis in Marriage and Family Therapy.

Dr Lacy is an active member of numerous professional associations including the American Society of Health-System Pharmacists (ASHP), the American College of Clinical Pharmacy (ACCP), the American Association of Colleges of Pharmacy (AACP), the American Society of Consultant Pharmacists (ASCP), American Pharmaceutical Association (APhA), the Federation of International Pharmacy (FIP), the Japanese Pharmaceutical Association (JPA), the Nevada Pharmacy Alliance (NPA), and the California Society of Hospital Pharmacists (CSHP), through which he has chaired many committees and subcommittees. He is also an active member of the California Association of Marriage and Family Therapists (CAMFT), American Association of Marriage and Family Therapists (AAMFT), the North American Congress of Clinical Toxicology (NACCT) and the European Congress of Clinical Toxicology (ECCT).

Morton P. Goldman, RPh, PharmD, BCPS, FCCP

Dr Goldman received his bachelor's degree in pharmacy from the University of Pittsburgh, College of Pharmacy and his Doctor of Pharmacy degree from the University of Cincinnati, Division of Graduate Studies and Research. He completed his concurrent 2-year hospital pharmacy residency at the VA Medical Center in Cincinnati. Dr Goldman is presently the Director of Pharmacotherapy Services for the Department of Pharmacy at the Cleveland Clinic (CC) after having spent over 4 years at CC as an Infectious Disease pharmacist and 10 years as Clinical Manager/Assistant Director. He holds faculty appointments from The University of Toledo and Ohio Northern University Colleges of Pharmacy, Northeastern Ohio Universities College of Pharmacy, and The Cleveland Clinic Lerner College of Medicine of Case Western Reserve University where he is the Pharmacology Curriculum Director. Dr Goldman is a Board-Certified Pharmacotherapy Specialist (BCPS) with added qualifications in infectious diseases.

In his capacity as Director of Pharmacotherapy Services at CC, Dr Goldman remains actively involved in patient care and clinical research as well as the continuing education of the medical and pharmacy staff. He is an editor of CC's *Guidelines for Antibiotic Use* and participates in their annual Antimicrobial Review retreat. He is a member of the Cleveland Clinic Health System Medical Staff Pharmacy and Therapeutics Committee and many of its specialty panels. Dr Goldman has authored numerous journal articles and lectures locally and nationally on infectious diseases topics, education methods, and current drug therapies.

Dr Goldman is an active member of the Ohio College of Clinical Pharmacy, the Society of Infectious Disease Pharmacists, the American College of Clinical Pharmacy (and is a Fellow of the College), and the American Society of Health-Systems Pharmacists.

Lora L. Armstrong, RPh, PharmD, BCPS

Dr Armstrong received her bachelor's degree in pharmacy from Ferris State University and her Doctor of Pharmacy degree from Midwestern University. Dr Armstrong is a Board-Certified Pharmacotherapy Specialist (BCPS).

In her current position, Dr Armstrong serves as Vice President of Clinical Affairs with responsibility for the National Pharmacy & Therapeutics Committee process, Clinical Program Oversight process, and Pharmaceutical Pipeline Services at CVS Caremark. Prior to joining Caremark, Inc, Dr Armstrong served as the Director of Drug Information Services at the University of Chicago Hospitals. She obtained experience in a variety of clinical settings including critical care, hematology, oncology, infectious diseases, and clinical pharmacokinetics. Dr Armstrong played an active role in the education and training of medical, pharmacy, and nursing staff. She coordinated the Drug Information Center, the medical center's Adverse Drug Reaction Monitoring Program, and the continuing Education Program for pharmacists. She also maintained the hospital's strict formulary program and was the editor of the University of Chicago Hospitals' *Formulary of Accepted Drugs* and the drug information center's monthly newsletter *Topics in Drug Therapy*.

Dr Armstrong is an active member of the Academy of Managed Care Pharmacy (AMCP), the American Society of Health-Systems Pharmacists (ASHP), the American Pharmaceutical Association (APhA), the American College of Clinical Pharmacy (ACCP), and the Pharmacy & Therapeutics Society (P & T Society). Dr Armstrong wrote the chapter entitled "Drugs and Hormones Used in Endocrinology" in the 4th edition of the textbook *Endocrinology*. She is an Adjunct Clinical Instructor of Pharmacy Practice at Midwestern University. Dr Armstrong currently serves on the Drug Information Advisory Board for the American Pharmaceutical Association Scientific Review Panel for Evaluations of Drug Interactions (EDI).

EDITORIAL ADVISORY PANEL

Amanda H. Corbett, PharmD, BCPS, FCCP, AAHIVE
Clinical Assistant Professor
University of North Carolina
Eshelman School of Pharmacy
Chapel Hill, North Carolina

Harold L. Crossley, DDS, PhD
Associate Professor of Pharmacology
Baltimore College of Dental Surgery
Dental School
University of Maryland Baltimore
Baltimore, Maryland

Melanie W. Cucchi, BS, PharmD, RPh
Pharmacotherapy Contributor
Lexi-Comp, Inc
Hudson, Ohio

Laura Cummings, PharmD, BCPS
Clinical Pharmacy Specialist, Pediatrics
The Children's Hospital at MetroHealth
Cleveland, Ohio

William J. Dana, PharmD, FASHP
Pharmacy Quality Assurance
Harris County Hospital District
Houston, Texas

Beth Deen, PharmD, BDNSP
Senior Pediatric Clinical Pharmacy Specialist
Cook Children's Medical Center
Fort Worth, Texas

Julie A. Dopheide, PharmD, BCPP
*Associate Professor of Clinical Pharmacy,
Psychiatry and the Behavioral Sciences*
University of Southern California
Schools of Pharmacy and Medicine
Los Angeles, California

Teri Dunsworth, PharmD, FCCP, BCPS
Pharmacotherapy Specialist
Lexi-Comp, Inc
Hudson, Ohio

Eve Echt, MD
Medical Staff
Department of Radiology
Akron General Medical Center
Akron, Ohio

Michael S. Edwards, PharmD, MBA, BCOP
*Chief, Oncology Pharmacy
Director, Oncology Pharmacy Residency Program*
Walter Reed Army Medical Center
Washington, D.C.

Vicki L. Ellingrod, PharmD, BCPP
*Head, Clinical Pharmacogenomics Laboratory
Associate Professor*
College of Pharmacy
Associate Professor
College of Medicine
Department of Psychiatry
University of Michigan
Ann Arbor, Michigan

Kelley K. Engle, BSPharm
Medical Science Pharmacist
Lexi-Comp, Inc
Hudson, Ohio

Christopher Ensor, PharmD, BCPS (AQ-CV)
Clinical Specialist
Cardiothoracic Transplantation and
Mechanical Circulatory Support
The Johns Hopkins Hospital
Baltimore, Maryland

Erin Fabian, PharmD, RPh
Pharmacotherapy Specialist
Lexi-Comp, Inc
Hudson, Ohio

Elizabeth A. Farrington, PharmD, FCCP, FCCM, FPPAG, BCPS
Pharmacist III - Pediatrics
New Hanover Regional Medical Center
Wilmington, North Carolina

Margaret A. Fitzgerald, MS, APRN, BC, NP-C, FAANP
President
Fitzgerald Health Education Associates, Inc.
North Andover, Massachusetts
Family Nurse Practitioner
Greater Lawrence Family Health Center
Lawrence, Massachusetts

Lawrence A. Frazee, PharmD, BCPS
Pharmacotherapy Specialist in Internal Medicine
Akron General Medical Center
Akron, Ohio

Matthew A. Fuller, PharmD, BCPS, BCPP, FASHP
Clinical Pharmacy Specialist, Psychiatry
Cleveland Department of Veterans Affairs
Medical Center
Brecksville, Ohio
*Associate Clinical Professor of Psychiatry
Clinical Instructor of Psychology*
Case Western Reserve University
Cleveland, Ohio
Adjunct Associate Professor of Clinical Pharmacy
University of Toledo
Toledo, Ohio

Jennifer L. Gardner, PharmD
Neonatal Clinical Pharmacy Specialist
Texas Children's Hospital
Houston, Texas

Meredith D. Girard, MD, FACP
Medical Staff
Department of Internal Medicine
Summa Health Systems
Akron, Ohio
Assistant Professor Internal Medicine
Northeast Ohio Medical University (NEOMED)
Rootstown, Ohio

6

Donna M. Kraus, PharmD, FAPhA, FPPAG
Associate Professor of Pharmacy Practice
Departments of Pharmacy Practice and Pediatrics
Pediatric Clinical Pharmacist
University of Illinois
Chicago, Illinois

Daniel L. Krinsky, RPh, MS
Manager, MTM Services
Giant Eagle Pharmacy
Ravenna, Ohio
Assistant Professor
Department of Pharmacy Practice
Northeast Ohio Medical University (NEOMED)
Rootstown, Ohio

Kay Kyllonen, PharmD
Clinical Specialist
The Cleveland Clinic Children's Hospital
Cleveland, Ohio

Charles Lacy, MS, PharmD, FCSHP
Vice President for Executive Affairs
Professor, Pharmacy Practice
Professor, Business Leadership
University of Southern Nevada
Las Vegas, Nevada

Brenda R. Lance, RN, MSN
Program Development Director
Northcoast HealthCare Management Company
Northcoast Infusion Network
Beachwood, Ohio

Leonard L. Lance, RPh, BSPharm
Pharmacist
Lexi-Comp, Inc
Hudson, Ohio

Tim T.Y. Lau, PharmD, ACPR, FCSHP
Pharmacotherapeutic Specialist
in Infectious Diseases
Pharmaceutical Sciences
Vancouver General Hospital
Clinical Associate Professor
Faculty of Pharmaceutical Sciences
Associate Member
Division of Infectious Diseases
Faculty of Medicine
University of British Columbia
Vancouver, British Columbia, Canada

Mandy C. Leonard, PharmD, BCPS
Assistant Professor
Cleveland Clinic Lerner College of Medicine
of Case Western University
Assistant Director, Drug Information Services
Cleveland Clinic
Cleveland, Ohio

John J. Lewin III, PharmD, BCPS
Clinical Specialist, Neurosciences Critical Care
The Johns Hopkins Hospital
Baltimore, Maryland

Jeffrey D. Lewis, PharmD, MACM
Assistant Dean and
Associate Professor of Pharmacy Practice
Cedarville University School of Pharmacy
Cedarville, Ohio

John Lindsley, PharmD, BCPS
Cardiology Clinical Pharmacy Specialist
The Johns Hopkins Hospital
Baltimore, Maryland

Jennifer Fisher Lowe, PharmD, BCOP
Pharmacotherapy Contributor
Lexi-Comp, Inc
Hudson, Ohio

Sherry Luedtke, PharmD
Associate Professor
Department of Pharmacy Practice
Texas Tech University HSC School of Pharmacy
Amarillo, Texas

Melissa Makii, PharmD, BCPS
Clinical Pharmacy Specialist
Pediatric Oncology
Rainbow Babies & Children's Hospital
Cleveland, Ohio

Vincent F. Mauro, BS, PharmD, FCCP
Professor of Clinical Pharmacy
College of Pharmacy
Adjunct Professor of Medicine
College of Medicine
The University of Toledo
Toledo, Ohio

Barrie McCombs, MD, FCFP
Medical Information Service Coordinator
The Alberta Rural Physician Action Plan
Calgary, Alberta, Canada

Christopher McPherson, PharmD
Clinical Pharmacist
Neonatal Intensive Care Unit
St. Louis Children's Hospital
St. Louis, Missouri

Timothy F. Meiller, DDS, PhD
Professor
Oncology and Diagnostic Sciences
Baltimore College of Dental Surgery
Professor of Oncology
Marlene and Stewart Greenebaum Cancer Center
University of Maryland Medical System
Baltimore, Maryland

Geralyn M. Meny, MD
Medical Director
American Red Cross, Penn-Jersey Region
Philadelphia, Pennsylvania

Charla E. Miller, RPh, PharmD
Neonatal Clinical Pharmacy Specialist
Wolfson Children's Hospital
Jacksonville, Florida

Julie Miller, PharmD
Pharmacy Clinical Specialist, Cardiology
Columbus Children's Hospital
Columbus, Ohio

Katherine Mills, PharmD
Pharmacotherapy Contributor
Lexi-Comp, Inc
Hudson, Ohio

8

Carol K. Taketomo, PharmD
Director of Pharmacy and Nutrition Services
Children's Hospital Los Angeles
Los Angeles, California

Mary Temple-Cooper, PharmD
Pediatric Clinical Research Specialist
Hillcrest Hospital
Mayfield Heights, Ohio

Elizabeth A. Tomsik, PharmD, BCPS
Manager
Adverse Drug Reactions Group
Lexi-Comp, Inc
Hudson, Ohio

Dana Travis, RPh
Pharmacotherapy Specialist
Lexi-Comp, Inc
Hudson, Ohio

Jennifer Trofe-Clark, PharmD
Clinical Transplant Pharmacist
Hospital of The University of Pennsylvania
Philadelphia, Pennsylvania

Beatrice B. Turkoski, RN, PhD
Associate Professor, Graduate Faculty,
Pharmacology for Advanced Practice Nurses
College of Nursing
Kent State University
Kent, Ohio

John N. van den Anker, MD, PhD, FCP, FAAP
Vice Chair of Pediatrics
for Experimental Therapeutics
Evan and Cindy Jones Professor of Pediatric
Clinical Pharmacology
Chief, Division of Pediatric Clinical Pharmacology
Children's National Medical Center
Professor of Pediatrics, Pharmacology & Physiology
George Washington University School of Medicine
and Health Sciences
Washington, D.C.

Heather L. VandenBussche, PharmD
Professor of Pharmacy, Pediatrics
Pharmacy Practice
Ferris State University College of Pharmacy
Kalamazoo, Michigan

Amy Van Orman, PharmD, BCPS
Pharmacotherapy Specialist
Lexi-Comp, Inc
Hudson, Ohio

Kristin Watson, PharmD, BCPS
Assistant Professor, Cardiology
University of Maryland School of Pharmacy
Baltimore, Maryland

David M. Weinstein, PhD, RPh
Manager
Metabolism, Interactions, and Genomics Group
Lexi-Comp, Inc
Hudson, Ohio

Anne Marie Whelan, PharmD
College of Pharmacy
Dalhouise University
Halifax, Nova Scotia, Canada

Sherri J. Willard Argyres, MA, PharmD
Medical Science Pharmacist
Lexi-Comp, Inc
Hudson, Ohio

Nathan Wirick, PharmD
Infectious Disease and Antibiotic Management
Clinical Specialist
Hillcrest Hospital
Cleveland, Ohio

Richard L. Wynn, BSPharm, PhD
Professor of Pharmacology
Baltimore College of Dental Surgery
Dental School
University of Maryland Baltimore
Baltimore, Maryland

Sallie Young, PharmD, BCPS, AQ Cardiology
Clinical Pharmacy Specialist, Cardiology
Penn State Milton S. Hershey Medical Center
Hershey, Pennsylvania

Jennifer Zimmer-Young, PharmD, CCRP
Educator, Clinical Pharmacist
ThedaCare
Appleton, Wisconsin

PREFACE

Working with clinical pharmacists, hospital pharmacy and therapeutics committees, and hospital drug information centers, the editors of this handbook have directly assisted in the development and production of hospital-specific formulary documentation for several hundred major U.S. and International medical institutions. The resultant documentation provides relevant detail concerning use of medications within the hospital and other clinical settings. Current information on medications has been extracted from pertinent sources, reviewed, coalesced, and cross-referenced by the editors to create this *Quick Look Drug Book*.

Designed to meet the unique needs of medical transcription, this handbook gives the user quick access to data on over 1800 medications with cross-referencing to 7855 U.S. and Canadian brand or trade names. Selection of the included medications was based on the analysis of those medications offered in a wide range of hospital formularies. The concise standardized format for data used in this handbook was developed to ensure a consistent presentation of information for all medications.

All generic drug names and synonyms appear in lower case, whereas brand or trade names appear in upper/lower case with the proper trademark information. These three items appear as individual entries in the alphabetical listing of drugs and, thus, there is no requirement for an alphabetical index of drugs names.

Chemotherapy regimens along with an index are provided in the section directly following the alphabetical listing of drugs. The mailing and web site addresses for pharmaceutical manufacturers and drug distributors can be accessed online using the code located on the inside front cover of this book.

The Indication/Therapeutic Category Index is an expedient mechanism for locating the medication of choice along with its classification. This index will help the user, with knowledge of the disease state, to identify medications which are most commonly used in treatment. All disease states are cross-referenced to a varying number of medications with the most frequently used medication(s) noted.
— L.L. Lance

USE OF THE HANDBOOK

The *Quick Look Drug Book* is organized into a drug information section, an appendix, and an indication/therapeutic category index.

The drug information section of the handbook, wherein all drugs are listed alphabetically, details information pertinent to each drug. Extensive cross-referencing is provided by brand name and synonyms.

Drug information is presented in a consistent format and for quick reference will provide the following:

Generic Name	U.S. Adopted Name (USAN) or International Nonproprietary Name (INN)
	If a drug product is only available in Canada, a *(Canada only)* will be attached to that product and will appear with every occurrence of that drug throughout the book
Pronunciation Guide	Subjective aid for pronouncing drug names
Medication Safety Issues	In an effort to promote the safe use of medications, this field is intended to highlight possible sources of medication errors such as sound-alike/look-alike drugs or highly concentrated formulations which require vigilance on the part of healthcare professionals. In addition, medications which have been associated with severe consequences in the event of a medication error are also identified in this field.
Synonyms	Includes names or accepted abbreviations of the generic drug; may include common brand names no longer available; this field is used to create cross-references to monographs
Tall-Man	"Tall-Man" lettering revisions recommended by the FDA
U.S. Brand Names	Trade names (manufacturer-specific) found in the United States. The symbol [DSC] appears after trade names that have been recently discontinued.
Canadian Brand Names	Trade names found in Canada
Therapeutic Category	Lexicomp's own system of logical medication classification
Controlled Substance	Contains controlled substance schedule information as assigned by the United States Drug Enforcement Administration (DEA) or Canadian Controlled Substance Act (CDSA). CDSA information is only provided for drugs available in Canada and not available in the U.S.
Use	Information pertaining to appropriate use of the drug
General Dosage Range	The range of dosing typically used during therapy in children and adults based upon route of administration. The information included is useful for confirming the dose is within the range but should not be used for prescribing purposes. Medications with a variety of indication-specific doses that cannot be encompassed by a range will not have a dose.
Product Availability	Provides availability information on products that have been approved by the FDA, but not yet available for use. Estimates for when a product may be available are included, when this information is known. May also provide any unique or critical drug availability issues.
Dosage Forms	Information with regard to form, strength, and availability of the drug in the United States.
Dosage Forms - Canada	Information with regard to form, strength, and availability of products that are uniquely available in Canada, but currently not available in the United States.

Appendix

The appendix offers a compilation of tables, guidelines, and conversion information that can often be helpful when considering patient care.

Indication/Therapeutic Category Index

This index provides a listing of accepted drugs for various disease states thus focusing attention on selection of medications most frequently prescribed in relation to a clinical diagnosis. Diseases may have other nonofficial drugs for their treatment and this indication/therapeutic category index should not be used by itself to determine the appropriateness of a particular therapy. The listed indications may encompass varying degrees of severity and, since certain medications may not be appropriate for a given degree of severity, it should not be assumed that the agents listed for specific indications are interchangeable. Also included as a valuable reference is each medication's therapeutic category.

FDA NAME DIFFERENTIATION PROJECT: THE USE OF TALL-MAN LETTERS

Confusion between similar drug names is an important cause of medication errors. For years, The Institute For Safe Medication Practices (ISMP), has urged generic manufacturers to use a combination of large and small letters as well as bolding (ie, chlorpro**MAZINE** and chlorpro**PAMIDE**) to help distinguish drugs with look-alike names, especially when they share similar strengths. Recently the FDA's Division of Generic Drugs began to issue recommendation letters to manufacturers suggesting this novel way to label their products to help reduce this drug name confusion. Although this project has had marginal success, the method has successfully eliminated problems with products such as diphenhydr**AMINE** and dimenhy-**DRINATE**. Hospitals should also follow suit by making similar changes in their own labels, preprinted order forms, computer screens and printouts, and drug storage location labels.

Lexi-Comp, Inc. Medical Publishing will use "Tall-Man" letters for the drugs suggested by the FDA or recommended by ISMP.

The following is a list of generic and brand name product names and recommended revisions.

Drug Product	Recommended Revision
acetazolamide	aceta**ZOLAMIDE**
alprazolam	**ALPRAZ**olam
amiloride	a**MIL**oride
amlodipine	am**LODIP**ine
aripiprazole	**ARIP**iprazole
Avinza	**AVIN**za
azacitidine	aza**CITID**ine
azathioprine	aza**THIO**prine
bupropion	bu**PROP**ion
buspirone	bus**PIR**one
carbamazepine	car**BAM**azepine
carboplatin	**CARBO**platin
cefazolin	ce**FAZ**olin
cefotetan	cefo**TE**tan
cefoxitin	cef**OX**itin
ceftazidime	cef**TAZ**idime
ceftriaxone	cef**TRIAX**one
Celebrex	Cele**BREX**
Celexa	Cele**XA**
chlordiazepoxide	chlordiaze**POXIDE**
chlorpromazine	chlorpro**MAZINE**
chlorpropamide	chlorpro**PAMIDE**
cisplatin	**CIS**platin
clomiphene	clomi**PHENE**
clomipramine	clomi**PRAMINE**
clonazepam	clonaze**PAM**
clonidine	clo**NID**ine
clozapine	clo**ZAP**ine
cycloserine	cyclo**SERINE**
cyclosporine	cyclo**SPORINE**
dactinomycin	**DACTIN**omycin
daptomycin	**DAPTO**mycin
daunorubicin	**DAUNO**rubicin
dimenhydrinate	dimenhy**DRINATE**
diphenhydramine	diphenhydr**AMINE**
dobutamine	**DOBUT**amine
docetaxel	**DOCE**taxel
dopamine	**DOP**amine
doxorubicin	**DOXO**rubicin
duloxetine	**DUL**oxetine

Drug Product	Recommended Revision
ephedrine	ePHEDrine
epinephrine	EPINEPHrine
fentanyl	fentaNYL
flavoxate	flavoxATE
fluoxetine	FLUoxetine
fluphenazine	fluPHENAZine
fluvoxamine	fluvoxaMINE
glipizide	glipiZIDE
glyburide	glyBURIDE
guaifenesin	guaiFENesin
guanfacine	guanFACINE
Humalog	HumaLOG
Humulin	HumuLIN
hydralazine	hydrALAZINE
hydrocodone	HYDROcodone
hydromorphone	HYDROmorphone
hydroxyzine	hydrOXYzine
idarubicin	IDArubicin
infliximab	inFLIXimab
Invanz	INVanz
isotretinoin	ISOtretinoin
Klonopin	KlonoPIN
Lamictal	LaMICtal
Lamisil	LamISIL
lamivudine	lamiVUDine
lamotrigine	lamoTRIgine
levetiracetam	LevETIRAcetam
levocarnitine	levOCARNitine
lorazepam	LORazepam
medroxyprogesterone	medroxyPROGESTERone
metformin	metFORMIN
methylprednisolone	methylPREDNISolone
methyltestosterone	methylTESTOSTERone
metronidazole	metroNIDAZOLE
mitomycin	mitoMYcin
mitoxantrone	MitoXANtrone
Nexavar	NexAVAR
Nexium	NexIUM
nicardipine	niCARdipine
nifedipine	NIFEdipine
nimodipine	niMODipine
Novolin	NovoLIN
Novolog	NovoLOG
olanzapine	OLANZapine
oxcarbazepine	OXcarbazepine
oxycodone	oxyCODONE
Oxycontin	OxyCONTIN
paclitaxel	PACLitaxel
paroxetine	PARoxetine
pemetrexed	PEMEtrexed
pentobarbital	PENTobarbital
phenobarbital	PHENobarbital
pralatrexate	PRALAtrexate
prednisolone	prednisoLONE
prednisone	predniSONE
Prilosec	PriLOSEC
Prozac	PROzac

Drug Product	Recommended Revision
quetiapine	QUEtiapine
quinidine	quiNIDine
quinine	quiNINE
rabeprazole	RABEprazole
Risperdal	RisperDAL
risperidone	risperiDONE
rituximab	riTUXimab
romidepsin	romiDEPsin
romiplostim	romiPLOStim
ropinirole	rOPINIRole
Sandimmune	sandIMMUNE
Sandostatin	SandoSTATIN
Seroquel	SEROquel
Sinequan	SINEquan
sitagliptin	sitaGLIPtin
Solu-Cortef	Solu-CORTEF
Solu-Medrol	Solu-MEDROL
sorafenib	SORAfenib
sufentanil	SUFentanil
sulfadiazine	sulfADIAZINE
sulfasalazine	sulfaSALAzine
sumatriptan	SUMAtriptan
sunitinib	SUNItinib
Tegretol	TEGretol
tiagabine	tiaGABine
tizanidine	tiZANidine
tolazamide	TOLAZamide
tolbutamide	TOLBUTamide
tramadol	traMADol
trazodone	traZODone
Trental	TRENtal
valacyclovir	valACYclovir
valganciclovir	valGANciclovir
vinblastine	vinBLAStine
vincristine	vinCRIStine
zolmitriptan	ZOLMitriptan
Zyprexa	ZyPREXA
Zyrtec	ZyrTEC

"FDA and ISMP Lists of Look-Alike Drug Names with Recommended Tall Man Letter." Available at http://www.ismp.org/tools/tallmanletters.pdf. Last accessed January 6, 2011.

"Name Differentiation Project." Available at http://www.fda.gov/Drugs/DrugSafety/MedicationErrors/ucm164587.htm. Last accessed January 6, 2011.

U.S. Pharmacopeia, "USP Quality Review: Use Caution-Avoid Confusion," March 2001, No. 76. Available at http://www.usp.org

PREVENTING PRESCRIBING ERRORS

Prescribing errors account for the majority of reported medication errors and have prompted healthcare professionals to focus on the development of steps to make the prescribing process safer. Prescription legibility has been attributed to a portion of these errors and legislation has been enacted in several states to address prescription legibility. However, eliminating handwritten prescriptions and ordering medications through the use of technology [eg, computerized prescriber order entry (CPOE)] has been the primary recommendation. Whether a prescription is electronic, typed, or hand-printed, additional safe practices should be considered for implementation to maximize the safety of the prescribing process. Listed below are suggestions for safer prescribing:

- Ensure correct patient by using at least 2 patient identifiers on the prescription (eg, full name, birth date, or address). Review prescription with the patient or patient's caregiver.
- If pediatric patient, document patient's birth date or age and most recent weight. If geriatric patient, document patient's birth date or age.
- Prevent drug name confusion:
    - Use TALLman lettering (eg, buPROPion, busPIRone, predniSONE, prednisoLONE). For more information see: http://www.fda.gov/Drugs/DrugSafety/MedicationErrors/ucm164587.htm.
    - Avoid abbreviated drug names (eg, MSO_4, $MgSO_4$, MS, HCT, 6MP, MTX), as they may be misinterpreted and cause error.
    - Avoid investigational names for drugs with FDA approval (eg, FK-506, CBDCA).
    - Avoid chemical names such as 6-mercaptopurine or 6-thioguanine, as sixfold overdoses have been given when these were not recognized as chemical names. The proper names of these drugs are mercaptopurine or thioguanine.
    - Use care when prescribing drugs that look or sound similar (eg, look- alike, sound-alike drugs). Common examples include: Celebrex® vs Celexa®, hydroxyzine vs hydralazine, Zyprexa® vs Zyrtec®.
- Avoid dangerous, error-prone abbreviations (eg, regardless of letter-case: U, IU, QD, QOD, µg, cc, @). Do not use apothecary system or symbols. Additionally, text messaging abbreviations (eg, "2Day") should never be used.
    - For more information see: http://www.ismp.org/Tools/errorproneabbreviations.pdf
- Always use a leading zero for numbers less than 1 (0.5 mg is correct and .5 mg is **incorrect**) and never use a trailing zero for whole numbers (2 mg is correct and 2.0 mg is **incorrect**).
- Always use a space between a number and its units as it is easier to read. There should be no periods after the abbreviations mg or mL (10 mg is correct and 10mg is **incorrect**).
- For doses that are greater than 1,000 dosing units, use properly placed commas to prevent 10-fold errors (100,000 units is correct and 100000 units is **incorrect**).
- Do not prescribe drug dosage by the type of container in which the drug is available (eg, do not prescribe "1 amp", "2 vials", etc).
- Do not write vague or ambiguous orders which have the potential for misinterpretation by other healthcare providers. Examples of vague orders to avoid: "resume pre-op medications," "give drug per protocol," or "continue home medications."
- Review each prescription with patient (or patient's caregiver) including the medication name, indication, and directions for use.
- Take extra precautions when prescribing *high alert drugs* (drugs that can cause significant patient harm when prescribed in error). Common examples of these drugs include: Anticoagulants, chemotherapy, insulins, opiates, and sedatives.
    - For more information see: http://www.ismp.org/Tools/highalertmedications.pdf

To Err is Human: Building a Safer Health System, Kohn LT, Corrigan JM, and Donaldson MS, eds, Washington, D.C.: National Academy Press, 2000.

A Complete Outpatient Prescription[1]

A complete outpatient prescription can prevent the prescriber, the pharmacist, and/or the patient from making a mistake and can eliminate the need for further clarification. The complete outpatient prescription should contain:

- Patient's full name
- Medication indication
- Allergies
- Prescriber name and telephone or pager number
- For pediatric patients: Their birth date or age and current weight
- For geriatric patients: Their birth date or age
- Drug name, dosage form and strength
- For pediatric patients: Intended daily weight-based dose so that calculations can be checked by the pharmacist (ie, mg/kg/day or units/kg/day)
- Number or amount to be dispensed
- Complete instructions for the patient or caregiver, including the purpose of the medication, directions for use (including dose), dosing frequency, route of administration, duration of therapy, and number of refills.
- Dose should be expressed in convenient units of measure.
- When there are recognized contraindications for a prescribed drug, the prescriber should indicate knowledge of this fact to the pharmacist (ie, when prescribing a potassium salt for a patient receiving an ACE inhibitor, the prescriber should write "K serum leveling being monitored").

Upon dispensing of the final product, the pharmacist should ensure that the patient or caregiver can effectively demonstrate the appropriate administration technique. An appropriate measuring device should be provided or recommended. Household teaspoons and tablespoons should not be used to measure liquid medications due to their variability and inaccuracies in measurement; oral medication syringes are recommended.

For additional information see: http://www.ppag.org/attachments/files/111/Guidelines_Peds.pdf
[1]Levine SR, Cohen MR, Blanchard NR, et al, "Guidelines for Preventing Medication Errors in Pediatrics," *J Pediatr Pharmacol Ther*, 2001, 6:426-42.

ALPHABETICAL LISTING OF DRUGS

A-25 [OTC] *see* vitamin A *on page 917*
A200® Lice [OTC] *see* permethrin *on page 691*
A-200® Lice Treatment Kit [OTC] *see* pyrethrins and piperonyl butoxide *on page 756*
A-200® Maximum Strength [OTC] *see* pyrethrins and piperonyl butoxide *on page 756*
A and D® Original [OTC] *see* vitamin A and vitamin D *on page 917*

abacavir (a BAK a veer)
Synonyms abacavir sulfate; ABC
U.S. Brand Names Ziagen®
Canadian Brand Names Ziagen®
Therapeutic Category Antiretroviral Agent, Nucleoside Reverse Transcriptase Inhibitor (NRTI)
Use Treatment of HIV infections in combination with other antiretroviral agents
General Dosage Range Dosage adjustment recommended in patients with hepatic impairment
Oral:
  Children 3 months to 16 years: 8 mg/kg twice daily (maximum: 300 mg twice daily)
  Adults: 600 mg/day in 1-2 divided (maximum: 600 mg/day)
Dosage Forms
  Solution, oral:
  Ziagen®: 20 mg/mL (240 mL)
  Tablet, oral:
  Ziagen®: 300 mg

abacavir and lamivudine (a BAK a veer & la MI vyoo deen)
Synonyms abacavir sulfate and lamivudine; lamivudine and abacavir
U.S. Brand Names Epzicom®
Canadian Brand Names Kivexa™
Therapeutic Category Antiretroviral Agent, Nucleoside Reverse Transcriptase Inhibitor (NRTI)
Use Treatment of HIV infections in combination with other antiretroviral agents
General Dosage Range Oral: *Adults:* One tablet (abacavir 600 mg and lamivudine 300 mg) once daily
Dosage Forms
  Tablet:
  Epzicom®: Abacavir 600 mg and lamivudine 300 mg

abacavir, lamivudine, and zidovudine
(a BAK a veer, la MI vyoo deen, & zye DOE vyoo deen)
Synonyms 3TC, abacavir, and zidovudine; azidothymidine, abacavir, and lamivudine; AZT, abacavir, and lamivudine; compound S, abacavir, and lamivudine; lamivudine, abacavir, and zidovudine; ZDV, abacavir, and lamivudine; zidovudine, abacavir, and lamivudine
U.S. Brand Names Trizivir®
Canadian Brand Names Trizivir®
Therapeutic Category Antiretroviral Agent, Nucleoside Reverse Transcriptase Inhibitor (NRTI)
Use Treatment of HIV infection (either alone or in combination with other antiretroviral agents) in patients whose regimen would otherwise contain the components of Trizivir®
General Dosage Range Oral: *Adolescents ≥40 kg and Adults:* 1 tablet twice daily
Dosage Forms
  Tablet, oral:
  Trizivir®: Abacavir 300 mg, lamivudine 150 mg, and zidovudine 300 mg

abacavir sulfate *see* abacavir *on page 20*
abacavir sulfate and lamivudine *see* abacavir and lamivudine *on page 20*

abatacept (ab a TA sept)
Medication Safety Issues
  Sound-alike/look-alike issues:
  Orencia® may be confused with Oracea®
Synonyms BMS-188667; CTLA-4Ig
U.S. Brand Names Orencia®
Canadian Brand Names Orencia®

Therapeutic Category Antirheumatic, Disease Modifying
Use
Treatment of moderately- to severely-active adult rheumatoid arthritis (RA); may be used as monotherapy or in combination with other DMARDs
Treatment of moderately- to severely-active juvenile idiopathic arthritis (JIA); may be used as monotherapy or in combination with methotrexate
Note: Abatacept should **not** be used in combination with anakinra or TNF-blocking agents
General Dosage Range
I.V.: Repeat dose at 2 weeks and 4 weeks, then every 4 weeks thereafter
Children ≥6 years and <75 kg: 10 mg/kg/dose
Children ≥6 years and 75-100 kg: 750 mg/dose
Children ≥6 years and >100 kg: 1000 mg/dose
Adults <60 kg: 500 mg/dose
Adults 60-100 kg: 750 mg/dose
Adults >100 kg: 1000 mg/dose
SubQ: *Adults:* 125 mg/dose once weekly
Product Availability
Orencia® 125 mg/mL prefilled syringe: FDA approved August 2011; availability expected in September 2011
Orencia® 125 mg/mL prefilled syringe is a subcutaneously administered once-weekly formulation approved for the treatment of adult rheumatoid arthritis.
Dosage Forms
Injection, powder for reconstitution [preservative free]:
Orencia®: 250 mg

abbott-43818 *see* leuprolide *on page 516*
ABC *see* abacavir *on page 20*
ABCD *see* amphotericin B cholesteryl sulfate complex *on page 75*

abciximab (ab SIK si mab)
Medication Safety Issues
High alert medication:
The Institute for Safe Medication Practices (ISMP) includes this medication among its list of drugs which have a heightened risk of causing significant patient harm when used in error.
Synonyms 7E3; C7E3
U.S. Brand Names Reopro®
Canadian Brand Names ReoPro®
Therapeutic Category Platelet Aggregation Inhibitor
Use Prevention of cardiac ischemic complications in patients undergoing percutaneous coronary intervention (PCI); prevention of cardiac ischemic complications in patients with unstable angina not responding to conventional therapy when PCI is scheduled within 24 hours
Note: Intended for use with aspirin and heparin, at a minimum.
General Dosage Range I.V.: *Adults:* Bolus: 0.25 mg/kg; Infusion: 0.125 mcg/kg/minute (maximum: 10 mcg/minute)
Dosage Forms
Injection, solution [preservative free]:
Reopro®: 2 mg/mL (5 mL)

Abelcet® *see* amphotericin B lipid complex *on page 76*
Abenol® (Can) *see* acetaminophen *on page 23*
ABI-007 *see* paclitaxel (protein bound) *on page 667*
Abilify® *see* aripiprazole *on page 93*
Abilify Discmelt® *see* aripiprazole *on page 93*

abiraterone acetate (a bir A ter one AS e tate)
Synonyms CB7630
U.S. Brand Names Zytiga™
Canadian Brand Names Zytiga™
Therapeutic Category Antiandrogen

◀ **Use** Treatment of metastatic, castration-resistant prostate cancer (in combination with prednisone) in patients previously treated with docetaxel

General Dosage Range Dosage adjustment recommended in patients with hepatic impairment or who develop toxicity.

Oral: *Adults:* 1000 mg once daily

Dosage Forms

Tablet, oral:

Zytiga™: 250 mg

Ablavar® *see* gadofosveset *on page 407*

ABLC *see* amphotericin B lipid complex *on page 76*

abobotulinumtoxinA (aye bo BOT yoo lin num TOKS in aye)

Medication Safety Issues

Administration issues:

Botulinum products are not interchangeable; potency differences may exist between the products.

Synonyms botulinum toxin type A

U.S. Brand Names Dysport™

Therapeutic Category Neuromuscular Blocker Agent, Toxin

Use Treatment of cervical dystonia in both toxin-naive and previously treated patients; temporary improvement in the appearance of moderate-severe glabellar lines associated with procerus and corrugator muscle activity

General Dosage Range I.M.:

Adults: Cervical dystonia: Initial: 500 units/treatment; subsequent doses: 250-1000 units

Adults <65 years: Reduction of glabellar lines: 10 units (0.05 mL or 0.08 mL) into each site (total dose: 50 units)

Dosage Forms

Injection, powder for reconstitution:

Dysport™: 500 units

Abraxane® *see* paclitaxel (protein bound) *on page 667*

Abreva® [OTC] *see* docosanol *on page 302*

absorbable cotton *see* cellulose, oxidized regenerated *on page 186*

absorbable gelatin sponge *see* gelatin (absorbable) *on page 412*

Abstral® *see* fentanyl *on page 371*

Abstral™ (Can) *see* fentanyl *on page 371*

ABT-335 *see* fenofibric acid *on page 369*

ABX-EGF *see* panitumumab *on page 672*

AC 2993 *see* exenatide *on page 363*

ACAM2000® *see* smallpox vaccine *on page 817*

acamprosate (a kam PROE sate)

Synonyms acamprosate calcium; calcium acetylhomotaurinate

U.S. Brand Names Campral®

Canadian Brand Names Campral®

Therapeutic Category GABA Agonist/Glutamate Antagonist

Use Maintenance of alcohol abstinence

General Dosage Range Dosage adjustment recommended in patients with renal impairment.

Oral: *Adults:* 666 mg 3 times/day (maximum: 1998 mg/day)

Dosage Forms

Tablet, delayed release, enteric coated, oral:

Campral®: 333 mg

acamprosate calcium *see* acamprosate *on page 22*

Acanya® *see* clindamycin and benzoyl peroxide *on page 219*

acarbose (AY car bose)

Medication Safety Issues
Sound-alike/look-alike issues:
Precose® may be confused with PreCare®
International issues:
Precose® [U.S., Malaysia] may be confused with Precosa brand name for *Saccharomyces boulardii* [Finland, Sweden]
U.S. Brand Names Precose®
Canadian Brand Names Glucobay™
Therapeutic Category Antidiabetic Agent, Oral
Use Adjunct to diet and exercise to lower blood glucose in patients with type 2 diabetes mellitus (noninsulin-dependent, NIDDM)
General Dosage Range Dosage adjustment recommended in patients on concomitant therapy
Oral: *Adults:* Initial: 25 mg 1-3 times/day; Maintenance: 75-300 mg/day in 3 divided doses (maximum: ≤60 kg: 150 mg/day; >60 kg: 300 mg/day)
Dosage Forms
Tablet, oral: 25 mg, 50 mg, 100 mg
Precose®: 25 mg, 50 mg, 100 mg

A-Caro-25 [OTC] *see* beta-carotene *on page 128*
Accel-Amlodipine (Can) *see* amlodipine *on page 69*
Accel-Pioglitazone (Can) *see* pioglitazone *on page 706*
Accolate® *see* zafirlukast *on page 926*
AccuNeb® *see* albuterol *on page 45*
Accupril® *see* quinapril *on page 761*
Accuretic® *see* quinapril and hydrochlorothiazide *on page 761*
Accutane® (Can) *see* isotretinoin *on page 495*
ACE *see* captopril *on page 170*

acebutolol (a se BYOO toe lole)

Medication Safety Issues
Sound-alike/look-alike issues:
Sectral® may be confused with Seconal®, Septra®
Synonyms acebutolol hydrochloride
U.S. Brand Names Sectral®
Canadian Brand Names Apo-Acebutolol®; Mylan-Acebutolol; Mylan-Acebutolol (Type S); Novo-Acebutolol; Nu-Acebutolol; Rhotral; Sandoz-Acebutolol; Sectral®; Teva-Acebutolol
Therapeutic Category Antiarrhythmic Agent, Class II; Beta-Adrenergic Blocker
Use Treatment of hypertension; management of ventricular arrhythmias
General Dosage Range Dosage adjustment recommended in patients with renal impairment
Oral:
Adults: 200-1200 mg/day in 2 divided doses (maximum: 1200 mg/day)
Elderly: 200-800 mg/day in 2 divided doses (maximum: 800 mg/day)
Dosage Forms
Capsule, oral: 200 mg, 400 mg
Sectral®: 200 mg, 400 mg

acebutolol hydrochloride *see* acebutolol *on page 23*
Aceon® *see* perindopril erbumine *on page 690*
Acephen™ [OTC] *see* acetaminophen *on page 23*
Acerola [OTC] *see* ascorbic acid *on page 96*
Acetadote® *see* acetylcysteine *on page 36*
Aceta-Gesic [OTC] *see* acetaminophen and phenyltoloxamine *on page 28*

acetaminophen (a seet a MIN oh fen)

Medication Safety Issues
Sound-alike/look-alike issues:
Acephen® may be confused with AcipHex®

FeverALL® may be confused with Fiberall®

Triaminic™ Children's Fever Reducer Pain Reliever may be confused with Triaminic® cough and cold products

Tylenol® may be confused with atenolol, timolol, Tylenol® PM, Tylox®

Other safety concerns:

Duplicate therapy issues: This product contains acetaminophen, which may be a component of combination products. Do not exceed the maximum recommended daily dose of acetaminophen.

International issues:

Depon [Greece] may be confused with Depen brand name for penicillamine [U.S.]; Depin brand name for nifedipine [India]; Dipen brand name for dilitazem [Greece]

Duorol [Spain] may be confused with Diuril brand name for chlorothiazide [U.S., Canada]

Paralen [Czech Republic] may be confused with Aralen brand name for chloroquine [U.S., Mexico]

Synonyms APAP; n-acetyl-p-aminophenol; paracetamol

U.S. Brand Names Acephen™ [OTC]; APAP 500 [OTC]; Aspirin Free Anacin® Extra Strength [OTC]; Cetafen® Extra [OTC]; Cetafen® [OTC]; Excedrin® Tension Headache [OTC]; Feverall® [OTC]; Infantaire [OTC]; Little Fevers™ [OTC]; Mapap® Arthritis Pain [OTC]; Mapap® Children's [OTC]; Mapap® Extra Strength [OTC]; Mapap® Infant's [OTC]; Mapap® Junior Rapid Tabs [OTC]; Mapap® [OTC]; Nortemp Children's [OTC]; Ofirmev™; Pain & Fever Children's [OTC]; Pain Eze [OTC]; Silapap Children's [OTC]; Silapap Infant's [OTC]; Triaminic™ Children's Fever Reducer Pain Reliever [OTC]; Tylenol® 8 Hour [OTC]; Tylenol® Arthritis Pain Extended Relief [OTC]; Tylenol® Children's Meltaways [OTC]; Tylenol® Children's [OTC]; Tylenol® Extra Strength [OTC]; Tylenol® Infant's Concentrated [OTC]; Tylenol® Jr. Meltaways [OTC]; Tylenol® [OTC]; Valorin Extra [OTC]; Valorin [OTC]

Canadian Brand Names Abenol®; Apo-Acetaminophen®); Atasol®; Novo-Gesic; Pediatrix; Tempra®; Tylenol®

Therapeutic Category Analgesic, Nonnarcotic; Antipyretic

Use Treatment of mild-to-moderate pain and fever (analgesic/antipyretic)

I.V.: Additional indication: Management of moderate-to-severe pain when combined with opioid analgesia

General Dosage Range Dosage adjustment recommended in patients with renal impairment

Oral, rectal:

Children 0-3 months: 10-15 mg/kg/dose **or** 40 mg/dose every 4-6 hours as needed (maximum: 2.6 g/day)

Children 4-11 months: 10-15 mg/kg/dose **or** 80 mg/dose every 4-6 hours as needed (maximum: 2.6 g/day)

Children 1-2 years: 10-15 mg/kg/dose **or** 120 mg/dose every 4-6 hours as needed (maximum: 2.6 g/day)

Children 2-3 years: 10-15 mg/kg/dose **or** 160 mg/dose every 4-6 hours as needed (maximum: 2.6 g/day)

Children 4-5 years: 10-15 mg/kg/dose **or** 240 mg/dose every 4-6 hours as needed (maximum: 2.6 g/day)

Children 6-8 years: 10-15 mg/kg/dose **or** 320 mg/dose every 4-6 hours as needed (maximum: 2.6 g/day)

Children 9-10 years: 10-15 mg/kg/dose **or** 400 mg/dose every 4-6 hours as needed (maximum: 2.6 g/day)

Children 11 years: 10-15 mg/kg/dose **or** 480 mg/dose every 4-6 hours as needed (maximum: 2.6 g/day)

Adults: 325-650 mg every 4-6 hours as needed **or** 1000 mg 3-4 times/day as needed (maximum: 4 g/day)

I.V.:

Children 2-12 years: 15 mg/kg every 6 hours **or** 12.5 mg/kg every 4 hours; maximum single dose: 15 mg/kg/dose; maximum daily dose: 75 mg/kg/day (≤3.75 g/day)

Adolescents >12 years and Adults <50 kg: 15 mg/kg every 6 hours **or** 12.5 mg/kg every 4 hours; maximum daily dose: 75 mg/kg/day (≤3.75 g/day)

Adolescents >12 years and Adults ≥50 kg: 650 mg every 4 hours **or** 1000 mg every 6 hours; maximum daily dose: 4 g/day

Dosage Forms

Caplet, oral: 500 mg

Cetafen® Extra [OTC]: 500 mg

Mapap® Extra Strength [OTC]: 500 mg

Pain Eze [OTC]: 650 mg

Tylenol® [OTC]: 325 mg

Tylenol® Extra Strength [OTC]: 500 mg

Caplet, extended release, oral:
  Mapap® Arthritis Pain [OTC]: 650 mg
  Tylenol® 8 Hour [OTC]: 650 mg
  Tylenol® Arthritis Pain Extended Relief [OTC]: 650 mg
Capsule, oral:
  Mapap® Extra Strength [OTC]: 500 mg
Captab, oral: 500 mg
Elixir, oral:
  Mapap® Children's [OTC]: 160 mg/5 mL (118 mL, 480 mL)
Gelcap, oral:
  Mapap® [OTC]: 500 mg
Gelcap, rapid release, oral:
  Tylenol® Extra Strength [OTC]: 500 mg
Geltab, oral:
  Excedrin® Tension Headache [OTC]: 500 mg
Injection, solution [preservative free]:
  Ofirmev™: 10 mg/mL (100 mL)
Liquid, oral:
  APAP 500 [OTC]: 500 mg/5 mL (237 mL)
  Silapap Children's [OTC]: 160 mg/5 mL (118 mL, 237 mL, 473 mL)
  Tylenol® Extra Strength [OTC]: 500 mg/15 mL (240 mL)
Solution, oral: 160 mg/5 mL (5 mL, 10 mL, 20 mL, 118 mL, 473 mL); 80 mg/0.8 mL (15 mL)
  Infantaire [OTC]: 80 mg/0.8 mL (15 mL, 30 mL)
  Little Fevers™ [OTC]: 80 mg/mL (30 mL)
  Mapap® [OTC]: 80 mg/0.8 mL (15 mL)
  Pain & Fever Children's [OTC]: 160 mg/5 mL (118 mL, 473 mL)
  Silapap Infant's [OTC]: 80 mg/0.8 mL (15 mL, 30 mL)
Suppository, rectal: 120 mg (12s, 50s, 100s); 325 mg (12s); 650 mg (12s, 50s, 100s)
  Acephen™ [OTC]: 120 mg (12s, 50s, 100s); 325 mg (6s, 12s, 50s, 100s); 650 mg (12s, 50s, 100s)
  Feverall® [OTC]: 80 mg (6s, 50s); 120 mg (6s, 50s); 325 mg (6s, 50s); 650 mg (50s)
Suspension, oral: 160 mg/5 mL (5 mL, 10 mL, 10.15 mL, 20 mL, 20.3 mL); 80 mg/0.8 mL (0.8 mL, 2 mL)
  Mapap® Children's [OTC]: 160 mg/5 mL (118 mL)
  Mapap® Infant's [OTC]: 80 mg/0.8 mL (15 mL, 30 mL)
  Nortemp Children's [OTC]: 160 mg/5 mL (118 mL)
  Tylenol® Children's [OTC]: 160 mg/5 mL (60 mL, 120 mL)
  Tylenol® Infant's Concentrated [OTC]: 80 mg/0.8 mL (15 mL, 30 mL)
Syrup, oral:
  Triaminic™ Children's Fever Reducer Pain Reliever [OTC]: 160 mg/5 mL (118 mL)
Tablet, oral: 325 mg, 500 mg
  Aspirin Free Anacin® Extra Strength [OTC]: 500 mg
  Cetafen® [OTC]: 325 mg
  Mapap® [OTC]: 325 mg
  Tylenol® [OTC]: 325 mg
  Valorin [OTC]: 325 mg
  Valorin Extra [OTC]: 500 mg
Tablet, chewable, oral: 80 mg
  Mapap® Children's [OTC]: 80 mg
Tablet, orally disintegrating, oral:
  Mapap® Children's [OTC]: 80 mg
  Mapap® Junior Rapid Tabs [OTC]: 160 mg
  Tylenol® Children's Meltaways [OTC]: 80 mg
  Tylenol® Jr. Meltaways [OTC]: 160 mg

acetaminophen and butalbital *see* butalbital and acetaminophen *on page 153*
acetaminophen and chlorpheniramine *see* chlorpheniramine and acetaminophen *on page 198*

acetaminophen and codeine (a seet a MIN oh fen & KOE deen)

Medication Safety Issues

Sound-alike/look-alike issues:

Tylenol® may be confused with atenolol, timolol, Tylox®

High alert medication:

The Institute for Safe Medication Practices (ISMP) includes this medication among its list of drug classes which have a heightened risk of causing significant patient harm when used in error.

Other safety concerns:

Duplicate therapy issues: This product contains acetaminophen, which may be a component of other combination products. Do not exceed the maximum recommended daily dose of acetaminophen.

T3 is an error-prone abbreviation (mistaken as liothyronine)

International issues:

Codex: Brand name for acetaminophen/codeine [Brazil], but also the brand name for *saccharomyces boulardii* [Italy]

Codex [Brazil] may be confused with Cedax brand name for ceftibuten [U.S. and multiple international markets]

Synonyms codeine and acetaminophen; Tylenol #2; Tylenol #3; Tylenol Codeine

U.S. Brand Names Capital® and Codeine; Tylenol® with Codeine No. 3; Tylenol® with Codeine No. 4

Canadian Brand Names ratio-Emtec; ratio-Lenoltec; Triatec-30; Triatec-8; Triatec-8 Strong; Tylenol Elixir with Codeine; Tylenol No. 1; Tylenol No. 1 Forte; Tylenol No. 2 with Codeine; Tylenol No. 3 with Codeine; Tylenol No. 4 with Codeine

Therapeutic Category Analgesic, Narcotic

Controlled Substance C-III; C-V

Use Relief of mild-to-moderate pain

General Dosage Range Dosage adjustment recommended in patients with renal impairment

Oral:

Acetaminophen:

Children ≤12 years: 10-15 mg/kg/dose every 4-6 hours as needed (maximum: 2.6 g/day)

Children >12 years and Adults: 325-650 mg every 4-6 hours as needed (maximum: 4 g/day)

Codeine:

Children: 0.5-1 mg/kg/dose every 4-6 hours (maximum: 60 mg/dose)

Adults: 15-60 mg/dose every 4-6 hours (maximum: 360 mg/day)

Dosage Forms

Solution, oral [C-V]: Acetaminophen 120 mg and codeine 12 mg per 5 mL

Suspension, oral [C-V]: Acetaminophen 120 mg and codeine 12 mg per 5 mL

Capital® and Codeine [C-V]: Acetaminophen 120 mg and codeine 12 mg per 5 mL

Tablet [C-III]: Acetaminophen 300 mg and codeine 15 mg; acetaminophen 300 mg and codeine 30 mg; acetaminophen 300 mg and codeine 60 mg

Tylenol® with Codeine No. 3: Acetaminophen 300 mg and codeine 30 mg

Tylenol® with Codeine No. 4: Acetaminophen 300 mg and codeine 60 mg

Dosage Forms - Canada Note: In countries outside of the U.S., some formulations of Tylenol® with Codeine include caffeine.

Caplet:

ratio-Lenoltec No. 1, Tylenol No. 1: Acetaminophen 300 mg, codeine 8 mg, and caffeine 15 mg

Tylenol No. 1 Forte: Acetaminophen 500 mg, codeine 8 mg, and caffeine 15 mg

Solution, oral:

Tylenol Elixir with Codeine: Acetaminophen 160 mg and codeine 8 mg per 5 mL

Tablet:

ratio-Emtec, Triatec-30: Acetaminophen 300 mg and codeine 30 mg

ratio-Lenoltec No. 1: Acetaminophen 300 mg, codeine 8 mg, and caffeine 15 mg

ratio-Lenoltec No. 2, Tylenol No. 2 with Codeine: Acetaminophen 300 mg, codeine 15 mg, and caffeine 15 mg

ratio-Lenoltec No. 3, Tylenol No. 3 with Codeine: Acetaminophen 300 mg, codeine 30 mg, and caffeine 15 mg

ratio-Lenoltec No. 4, Tylenol No. 4 with Codeine: Acetaminophen 300 mg and codeine 60 mg

Triatec-8: Acetaminophen 325 mg, codeine 8 mg, and caffeine 30 mg

Triatec-8 Strong: Acetaminophen 500 mg, codeine 8 mg, and caffeine 30 mg

acetaminophen and diphenhydramine (a seet a MIN oh fen & dye fen HYE dra meen)

Medication Safety Issues

Sound-alike/look-alike issues:
Excedrin® may be confused with Dexedrine®
Percogesic® may be confused with paregoric, Percodan®
Tylenol® may be confused with atenolol, timolol, Tylox®
Tylenol® PM may be confused with Tylenol®

Other safety concerns:
Duplicate therapy issues: This product contains acetaminophen, which may be a component of other combination products. Do not exceed the maximum recommended daily dose of acetaminophen.

Synonyms diphenhydramine and acetaminophen

U.S. Brand Names Excedrin PM® [OTC]; Goody's PM® [OTC]; Legatrin PM® [OTC]; Mapap PM [OTC]; Percogesic® Extra Strength [OTC]; TopCare® Pain Relief PM [OTC]; Tylenol® PM [OTC]; Tylenol® Severe Allergy [OTC]

Therapeutic Category Analgesic, Nonnarcotic

Use Aid in the relief of insomnia accompanied by minor pain

General Dosage Range Oral: *Children ≥12 years and Adults:* 50 mg of diphenhydramine HCl (76 mg diphenhydramine citrate) at bedtime

Dosage Forms

Caplet, oral: Acetaminophen 500 mg and diphenhydramine 25 mg
Excedrin PM® [OTC]: Acetaminophen 500 mg and diphenhydramine 38 mg
Legatrin PM® [OTC]: Acetaminophen 500 mg and diphenhydramine 50 mg
Mapap PM [OTC], TopCare® Pain Relif PM [OTC], Tylenol® PM [OTC]: Acetaminophen 500 mg and diphenhydramine 25 mg
Percogesic® Extra Strength [OTC]: Acetaminophen 500 mg and diphenhydramine 12.5 mg
Tylenol® Severe Allergy [OTC]: Acetaminophen 500 mg and diphenhydramine 12.5 mg
Captab, oral: Acetaminophen 500 mg and diphenhydramine 25 mg
Gelcap, rapid release, oral:
Tylenol® PM [OTC]: Acetaminophen 500 mg and diphenhydramine 25 mg
Geltab, oral: Acetaminophen 500 mg and diphenhydramine 25 mg
Excedrin® PM [OTC]: Acetaminophen 500 mg and diphenhydramine 38 mg
Tylenol® PM [OTC]: Acetaminophen 500 mg and diphenhydramine 25 mg
Liquid, oral:
Tylenol® PM [OTC]: Acetaminophen 500 mg and diphenhydramine 25 mg per 15 mL
Powder for solution, oral:
Goody's PM® [OTC]: Acetaminophen 500 mg and diphenhydramine 38 mg
Tablet, oral: Acetaminophen 500 mg and diphenhydramine 25 mg
Excedrin® PM [OTC]: Acetaminophen 500 mg and diphenhydramine 38 mg

acetaminophen and hydrocodone *see* hydrocodone and acetaminophen *on page 446*
acetaminophen and oxycodone *see* oxycodone and acetaminophen *on page 662*

acetaminophen and pamabrom (a seet a MIN oh fen & PAM a brom)

Medication Safety Issues
Other safety concerns:
Duplicate therapy issues: This product contains acetaminophen, which may be a component of other combination products. Do not exceed the maximum recommended daily dose of acetaminophen.

Synonyms pamabrom and acetaminophen

U.S. Brand Names Cramp Tabs [OTC]; Midol® Teen Formula [OTC]; Tylenol® Women's Menstrual Relief [OTC]

Therapeutic Category Analgesic, Miscellaneous; Diuretic, Combination

Use Temporary relief of symptoms associated with premenstrual and menstrual symptoms (eg, cramps, bloating, water-weight gain, headache, backache, muscle aches)

General Dosage Range Oral: *Children ≥12 years and Adults:* Acetaminophen 650-1000 mg and pamabrom 50 mg every 4-6 hours as needed (maximum: 8 caplets/tablets/24 hours)

Dosage Forms
Caplet:
Midol® Teen Formula: Acetaminophen 500 mg and pamabrom 25 mg
Tylenol® Women's Menstrual Relief: Acetaminophen 500 mg and pamabrom 25 mg

◀ **Tablet:**
Cramp Tabs: Acetaminophen 325 mg and pamabrom 25 mg

acetaminophen and pentazocine *see* pentazocine and acetaminophen *on page 687*

acetaminophen and phenylephrine (a seet a MIN oh fen & fen il EF rin)

Medication Safety Issues

Other safety concerns:
Duplicate therapy issues: This product contains acetaminophen, which may be a component of combination products. Do not exceed the maximum recommended daily dose of acetaminophen.

Synonyms phenylephrine hydrochloride and acetaminophen

U.S. Brand Names Alka-Seltzer Plus® Sinus Formula [OTC]; Cetafen Cold® [OTC]; Contac® Cold + Flu Maximum Strength Non-Drowsy [OTC]; Excedrin® Sinus Headache [OTC]; Mapap® Sinus Congestion and Pain Daytime [OTC]; Sinus Pain & Pressure [OTC]; Sinutab® Sinus [OTC]; Sudafed PE® Pressure + Pain [OTC]; Tylenol® Sinus Congestion & Pain Daytime [OTC]; Vicks® DayQuil® Sinus [OTC]

Therapeutic Category Analgesic, Miscellaneous; Decongestant

Use Temporary relief of sinus/nasal congestion and pressure, headache, and minor aches and pains

General Dosage Range Oral: *Children ≥12 years and Adults:* Acetaminophen 325 mg and phenylephrine 5 mg/caplet: Take 2 caplets every 4 hours as needed (maximum: 12 caplets/24 hours; maximum acetaminophen: 4 g/day)

Dosage Forms

Caplet, oral:
Contac® Cold + Flu Maximum Strength Non Drowsy [OTC]: Acetaminophen 500 mg and phenylephrine 5 mg
Excedrin® Sinus Headache [OTC], Mapap® Sinus Congestion and Pain Daytime [OTC], Sinutab® Sinus [OTC], Sudafed PE® Pressure + Pain [OTC]: Acetaminophen 325 mg and phenylephrine 5 mg
Tylenol® Sinus Congestion & Pain Daytime [OTC]: Acetaminophen 325 mg and phenylephrine 5 mg [Cool Burst™ flavor]

Capsule, liquicap, oral:
Vicks® DayQuil® Sinus [OTC]: Acetaminophen 325 mg and phenylephrine 5 mg

Gelcap, oral:
Tylenol® Sinus Congestion & Pain Daytime [OTC]: Acetaminophen 325 mg and phenylephrine 5 mg

Gelcap, rapid release, oral:
Tylenol® Sinus Congestion & Pain Daytime [OTC]: Acetaminophen 325 mg and phenylephrine 5 mg

Tablet for solution, oral [effervescent]:
Alka-Seltzer Plus® Sinus Formula [OTC]: Acetaminophen 250 mg and phenylephrine 5 mg

Tablet, oral:
Cetafen Cold® [OTC], Sinus Pain & Pressure [OTC]: Acetaminophen 500 mg and phenylephrine 5 mg

acetaminophen and phenyltoloxamine (a seet a MIN oh fen & fen il to LOKS a meen)

Medication Safety Issues

Sound-alike/look-alike issues:
Percogesic® may be confused with paregoric, Percodan®

Other safety concerns:
Duplicate therapy issues: This product contains acetaminophen, which may be a component of other combination products. Do not exceed the maximum recommended daily dose of acetaminophen.

Synonyms phenyltoloxamine citrate and acetaminophen

U.S. Brand Names Aceta-Gesic [OTC]; BP Poly 650 [DSC]; Lagesic™ [DSC]; Phenagesic [OTC] [DSC]; RhinoFlex™; RhinoFlex™-650; Zgesic

Therapeutic Category Analgesic, Nonnarcotic

Use Relief of mild-to-moderate pain

General Dosage Range Oral: Based on acetaminophen component:
Children <12 years: 10-15 mg/kg/dose every 4-6 hours as needed (maximum: 2.6 g/day)
Children ≥12 years and Adults: 325-650 mg every 4-6 hours as needed (maximum: 4 g/day)

Dosage Forms

Tablet: Acetaminophen 325 mg and phenyltoloxamine 30 mg
Aceta-Gesic [OTC]: Acetaminophen 325 mg and phenyltoloxamine 30 mg
RhinoFlex™: Acetaminophen 500 mg and phenyltoloxamine 50 mg
RhinoFlex™-650: Acetaminophen 650 mg and phenyltoloxamine 50 mg

Tablet, prolonged release, oral:
Zgesic: Acetaminophen 600 mg and phenyltoloxamine 66 mg

acetaminophen and propoxyphene *see* propoxyphene and acetaminophen *on page 746*

acetaminophen and pseudoephedrine (a seet a MIN oh fen & soo doe e FED rin)
Medication Safety Issues
Sound-alike/look-alike issues:
Ornex® may be confused with Orexin®, Orinase®
Other safety concerns:
Duplicate therapy issues: This product contains acetaminophen, which may be a component of other combination products. Do not exceed the maximum recommended daily dose of acetaminophen.
Synonyms pseudoephedrine and acetaminophen; pseudoephedrine hydrochloride and acetaminophen
U.S. Brand Names Ornex® Maximum Strength [OTC]; Ornex® [OTC]
Canadian Brand Names Contac® Cold and Sore Throat, Non Drowsy, Extra Strength; Dristan® N.D.; Dristan® N.D., Extra Strength; Sinutab® Non Drowsy; Sudafed® Head Cold and Sinus Extra Strength; Tylenol® Decongestant; Tylenol® Sinus
Therapeutic Category Decongestant/Analgesic
Use Temporary relief of nasal congestion, and minor aches and pains associated with colds, flu, sinusitis, or allergies
General Dosage Range Oral:
Children 6-11 years: Acetaminophen 325 mg/pseudoephedrine 30 mg every 4-6 hours (maximum: 120 mg/day pseudoephedrine)
Children ≥12 years and Adults: Acetaminophen 625-1000 mg/pseudoephedrine 60 mg every 4-6 hours (maximum: 240 mg/day pseudoephedrine)
Dosage Forms
Caplet:
Ornex® [OTC]: Acetaminophen 325 mg and pseudoephedrine 30 mg
Ornex® Maximum Strength [OTC]: Acetaminophen 500 mg and pseudoephedrine 30 mg

acetaminophen and tramadol (a seet a MIN oh fen & TRA ma dole)
Medication Safety Issues
Sound-alike/look-alike issues:
Ultracet® may be confused with Ultane®, Ultram®
Other safety concerns:
Duplicate therapy issues: This product contains acetaminophen, which may be a component of other combination products. Do not exceed the maximum recommended daily dose of acetaminophen.
Synonyms APAP and tramadol; tramadol hydrochloride and acetaminophen
U.S. Brand Names Ultracet®
Canadian Brand Names Apo-Tramadol/Acet®; Tramacet
Therapeutic Category Analgesic, Miscellaneous; Analgesic, Nonnarcotic
Use Short-term (≤5 days) management of acute pain
General Dosage Range Dosage adjustment recommended in patients with renal impairment
Oral: *Adults:* Two tablets every 4-6 hours as needed (maximum: 8 tablets/day)
Dosage Forms
Tablet: Acetaminophen 325 mg and tramadol 37.5 mg
Ultracet®: Acetaminophen 325 mg and tramadol 37.5 mg

acetaminophen, aspirin, and caffeine (a seet a MIN oh fen, AS pir in, & KAF een)
Medication Safety Issues
Sound-alike/look-alike issues:
Excedrin® may be confused with Dexedrine®
Other safety concerns:
Duplicate therapy issues: This product contains acetaminophen, which may be a component of other combination products. Do not exceed the maximum recommended daily dose of acetaminophen.
Synonyms aspirin, acetaminophen, and caffeine; aspirin, caffeine, and acetaminophen; caffeine, acetaminophen, and aspirin; caffeine, aspirin, and acetaminophen
U.S. Brand Names Anacin® Advanced Headache Formula [OTC]; Excedrin® Extra Strength [OTC]; Excedrin® Migraine [OTC]; Fem-Prin® [OTC]; Goody's® Extra Strength Headache Powder [OTC]; Goody's® Extra Strength Pain Relief [OTC]; Pain-Off [OTC]; Vanquish® Extra Strength Pain Reliever [OTC]
Therapeutic Category Analgesic, Nonnarcotic

◀ **Use** Relief of mild-to-moderate pain; mild-to-moderate pain associated with migraine headache

General Dosage Range Oral: *Children >12 years and Adults:* 1-2 doses every 4-6 hours as needed (maximum: 4 g/day [based on acetaminophen and aspirin component])

Dosage Forms

Caplet: Acetaminophen 250 mg, aspirin 250 mg, and caffeine 65 mg; acetaminophen 194 mg, aspirin 227 mg, and caffeine 33 mg

Excedrin® Extra Strength [OTC], Excedrin® Migraine [OTC]: Acetaminophen 250 mg, aspirin 250 mg, and caffeine 65 mg

Vanquish® Extra Strength Pain Reliever [OTC]: Acetaminophen 194 mg, aspirin 227 mg, and caffeine 33 mg

Geltab: Acetaminophen 250 mg, aspirin 250 mg, and caffeine 65 mg

Excedrin® Extra Strength [OTC], Excedrin® Migraine [OTC]: Acetaminophen 250 mg, aspirin 250 mg, and caffeine 65 mg

Powder: Acetaminophen 260 mg, aspirin 520 mg, and caffeine 32.5 mg

Goody's® Extra Strength Headache Powder [OTC]: Acetaminophen 260 mg, aspirin 520 mg, and caffeine 32.5 mg

Tablet:

Anacin® Advanced Headache Formula [OTC], Excedrin® Extra Strength [OTC], Excedrin® Migraine [OTC], Pain-Off [OTC]: Acetaminophen 250 mg, aspirin 250 mg, and caffeine 65 mg

Fem-Prin® [OTC]: Acetaminophen 194.4 mg, aspirin 226.8 mg, and caffeine 32.4 mg

Goody's® Extra Strength Pain Relief [OTC]: Acetaminophen 130 mg, aspirin 260 mg, and caffeine 16.25 mg

acetaminophen, butalbital, and caffeine *see* butalbital, acetaminophen, and caffeine *on page 152*

acetaminophen, caffeine, and dihydrocodeine
(a seet a MIN oh fen, KAF een, & dye hye droe KOE deen)

Medication Safety Issues

Sound-alike/look-alike issues:

Panlor® may be confused with Pamelor®

High alert medication:

The Institute for Safe Medication Practices (ISMP) includes this medication among its list of drug classes which have a heightened risk of causing significant patient harm when used in error.

Other safety concerns:

Duplicate therapy issues: This product contains acetaminophen, which may be a component of other combination products. Do not exceed the maximum recommended daily dose of acetaminophen.

Synonyms caffeine, dihydrocodeine, and acetaminophen; dihydrocodeine bitartrate, acetaminophen, and caffeine

U.S. Brand Names Panlor® SS [DSC]; Trezix™; ZerLor™ [DSC]

Therapeutic Category Analgesic Combination (Opioid)

Controlled Substance C-III

Use Relief of moderate- to moderately-severe pain

General Dosage Range Oral: *Adults:* 1 tablet or 2 capsules every 4 hours as needed (maximum: 10 capsules/day or 5 tablets/day)

Dosage Forms

Capsule:

Trezix™: Acetaminophen 356.4 mg, caffeine 30 mg, and dihydrocodeine 16 mg

Tablet: Acetaminophen 712.8 mg, caffeine 60 mg, and dihydrocodeine bitartrate 32 mg

acetaminophen, caffeine, codeine, and butalbital *see* butalbital, acetaminophen, caffeine, and codeine *on page 153*

acetaminophen, chlorpheniramine, and pseudoephedrine
(a seet a MIN oh fen, klor fen IR a meen, & soo doe e FED rin)

Medication Safety Issues

Other safety concerns:

Duplicate therapy issues: This product contains acetaminophen, which may be a component of other combination products. Do not exceed the maximum recommended daily dose of acetaminophen.

Synonyms acetaminophen, chlorpheniramine maleate, and pseudoephedrine hydrochloride; acetamino-phen, pseudoephedrine, and chlorpheniramine; chlorpheniramine, acetaminophen, and pseudoephe-drine; chlorpheniramine, pseudoephedrine, and acetaminophen; pseudoephedrine, acetaminophen, and chlorpheniramine; pseudoephedrine, chlorpheniramine, and acetaminophen

U.S. Brand Names Drinex [OTC] [DSC]; Relief-SF®

Therapeutic Category Antihistamine/Decongestant/Analgesic

Use Temporary relief of cold, allergy, or sinus symptoms

General Dosage Range Oral: *Children ≥12 years and Adults:* Drinex: 1 tablet 3-4 times/day (maximum: 4 tablets/24 hours); Relief-SF®: 1-2 caplets every 6 hours (maximum: 8 caplets/24 hours)

Dosage Forms

Caplet: Acetaminophen 325 mg, chlorpheniramine 2 mg, and pseudoephedrine 30 mg

Relief-SF®: Acetaminophen 500 mg, chlorpheniramine 2 mg, and pseudoephedrine 30 mg

acetaminophen, chlorpheniramine maleate, and pseudoephedrine hydrochloride *see* acetaminophen, chlorpheniramine, and pseudoephedrine *on page 30*

acetaminophen, chlorpheniramine, phenylephrine, and phenyltoloxamine (a seet a MIN oh fen, klor fen IR a meen, fen il EF rin, & fen il tole LOKS a meen)

Synonyms chlorpheniramine maleate, acetaminophen, phenylephrine hydrochloride, and phenyltolox-amine citrate; phenylephrine, chlorpheniramine, acetaminophen, and phenyltoloxamine; phenyltolox-amine, chlorpheniramine, phenylephrine, and acetaminophen

U.S. Brand Names norel® SR

Therapeutic Category Alkylamine Derivative; Alpha/Beta Agonist; Analgesic, Miscellaneous; Decongestant; Ethanolamine Derivative; Histamine H_1 Antagonist; Histamine H_1 Antagonist, First Generation

Use Temporary relief of cold, allergy, or sinus symptoms caused from inhalation of airborne irritants

General Dosage Range Oral: *Children >12 years and Adults:* One tablet every 12 hours

Dosage Forms

Tablet, extended release, oral:

norel® SR: Acetaminophen 325 mg, chlorpheniramine maleate 8 mg, phenylephrine hydrochloride 40 mg, and phenyltoloxamine citrate 50 mg [scored]

acetaminophen, codeine, and doxylamine (Canada only)
(a seet a MIN oh fen, KOE deen, & dox IL a meen)

Medication Safety Issues

High alert medication:

The Institute for Safe Medication Practices (ISMP) includes this medication among its list of drug classes which have a heightened risk of causing significant patient harm when used in error.

Other safety concerns:

Duplicate therapy issues: This product contains acetaminophen, which may be a component of other combination products. Do not exceed the maximum recommended daily dose of acetaminophen.

Synonyms codeine, doxylamine, and acetaminophen; doxylamine succinate, codeine phosphate, and acetaminophen

Canadian Brand Names Mersyndol® With Codeine

Therapeutic Category Analgesic, Opioid; Antihistamine

Controlled Substance CDSA-1

Use Relief of headache, cold symptoms, neuralgia, and muscular aches/pain

General Dosage Range Oral: *Children >12 years and Adults:* 1-2 tablets every 4 hours as needed (maximum: 12 tablets/day)

Product Availability Not available in U.S.

Dosage Forms - Canada

Tablet, oral:

Mersyndol® With Codeine: Acetaminophen 325 mg, codeine 8 mg, and doxylamine 5 mg

acetaminophen, dextromethorphan, and doxylamine

(a seet a MIN oh fen, deks troe meth OR fan, & dox IL a meen)

Medication Safety Issues

Other safety concerns:

Duplicate therapy issues: This product contains acetaminophen, which may be a component of other combination products. Do not exceed the maximum recommended daily dose of acetaminophen.

Synonyms dextromethorphan hydrobromide, acetaminophen, and doxylamine succinate; doxylamine, acetaminophen, and dextromethorphan

U.S. Brand Names All-Nite [OTC]; Tylenol® Cough & Sore Throat Nighttime [OTC]; Vicks® NyQuil® Cold & Flu Multi-Symptom [OTC]

Therapeutic Category Analgesic, Miscellaneous; Antitussive; Histamine H_1 Antagonist; Histamine H_1 Antagonist, First Generation

Use Temporary relief of common cold and flu symptoms (eg, minor aches and pain, fever, cough, runny nose, sneezing, sore throat)

General Dosage Range Oral: *Children ≥12 years and Adults:* Two capsules **or** 30 mL every 6 hours (maximum: 8 capsules **or** 240 mL/24 hours)

Dosage Forms

Capsule, liquicap:

Vicks® NyQuil® Cold & Flu Multi-Symptom [OTC]: Acetaminophen 325 mg, dextromethorphan 15 mg, and doxylamine 6.25 mg

Liquid:

All-Nite [OTC]: Acetaminophen 500 mg, dextromethorphan 15 mg, and doxylamine 6.25 mg per 15 mL

Tylenol® Cough & Sore Throat Nighttime [OTC]: Acetaminophen 500 mg, dextromethorphan 15 mg, and doxylamine 6.25 mg per 15 mL

Vicks® NyQuil® Cold & Flu Multi-Symptom [OTC]: Acetaminophen 500 mg, dextromethorphan hydrobromide 15 mg, and doxylamine succinate 6.25 mg per 15 mL

acetaminophen, dextromethorphan, and phenylephrine

(a seet a MIN oh fen, deks troe meth OR fan, & fen il EF rin)

Medication Safety Issues

Other safety concerns:

Duplicate therapy issues: This product contains acetaminophen, which may be a component of other combination products. Do not exceed the maximum recommended daily dose of acetaminophen.

Synonyms dextromethorphan hydrobromide, acetaminophen, and phenylephrine hydrochloride; phenylephrine, acetaminophen, and dextromethorphan; phenylephrine, dextromethorphan, and acetaminophen

U.S. Brand Names Alka-Seltzer Plus® Day Cold [OTC]; Comtrex® Maximum Strength, Non-Drowsy Cold & Cough [OTC]; Mapap® Multi-Symptom Cold [OTC]; Theraflu Warming Relief® Daytime Multi-Symptom Cold [OTC]; Theraflu Warming Relief® Daytime Severe Cold & Cough [OTC]; Theraflu® Daytime Severe Cold & Cough [OTC]; Tylenol® Cold Head Congestion Daytime [OTC]; Tylenol® Cold Multi-Symptom Daytime [OTC]; Vicks® DayQuil® Cold & Flu Multi-Symptom [OTC]

Therapeutic Category Analgesic, Miscellaneous; Antitussive; Decongestant

Use Temporary relief of common cold and flu symptoms (eg, pain, fever, cough, congestion)

General Dosage Range Oral: *Children ≥6 years and Adults:* Dosage varies greatly depending on product

Dosage Forms

Caplet, oral:

Comtrex® Maximum Strength, Non-Drowsy Cold & Cough [OTC], Mapap® Multi-Symptom Cold [OTC], Theraflu Warming Relief® Daytime Multi-Symptom Cold [OTC], Tylenol® Cold Head Congestion Daytime [OTC], Tylenol® Cold Multi-Symptom Daytime [OTC]: Acetaminophen 325 mg, dextromethorphan 10 mg, and phenylephrine 5 mg

Capsule, liquid gel, oral:

Alka-Seltzer Plus® Day Cold [OTC]: Acetaminophen 325 mg, dextromethorphan 10 mg, and phenylephrine 5 mg

Capsule, liquicap, oral:

Vicks® DayQuil® Cold & Flu Multi-Symptom [OTC], Tylenol® Cold Multi-Symptom Daytime [OTC]: Acetaminophen 325 mg, dextromethorphan 10 mg, and phenylephrine 5 mg

Gelcap, rapid release, oral:

Tylenol® Cold Multi-Symptom Daytime [OTC]: Acetaminophen 325 mg, dextromethorphan 10 mg, and phenylephrine 5 mg

Liquid, oral:
Tylenol® Cold Multi-Symptom Daytime [OTC], Vicks® DayQuil® Cold & Flu Multi-Symptom [OTC]: Acetaminophen 325 mg, dextromethorphan 10 mg, and phenylephrine 5 mg per 15 mL
Powder for solution, oral:
Theraflu® Daytime Severe Cold & Cough [OTC]: Acetaminophen 650 mg, dextromethorphan 20 mg, and phenylephrine 10 mg per packet
Syrup, oral:
Theraflu Warming Relief® Daytime Severe Cold & Cough [OTC]: Acetaminophen 325 mg, dextromethorphan 10 mg, and phenylephrine 5 mg per 15 mL

acetaminophen, dextromethorphan, doxylamine, and pseudoephedrine
(a seet a MIN oh fen, deks troe meth OR fan, dox IL a meen & soo doe e FED rin)

Synonyms dextromethorphan hydrobromide, acetaminophen, doxylamine succinate, and pseudoephedrine hydrochloride; doxylamine, acetaminophen, dextromethorphan, and pseudoephedrine; pseudoephedrine, dextromethorphan, doxylamine, and acetaminophen

U.S. Brand Names All-Nite Multi-Symptom Cold/Flu [OTC]; Vicks® NyQuil® D Cold & Flu Multi-Symptom [OTC]

Therapeutic Category Analgesic, Miscellaneous; Antitussive; Decongestant; Histamine H_1 Antagonist; Histamine H_1 Antagonist, First Generation

Use Temporary relief of common cold and flu symptoms (eg, minor aches and pain, fever, cough, congestion, runny nose, sneezing, sore throat)

General Dosage Range Oral: *Children ≥12 years and Adults:* 30 mL every 6 hours (maximum: 120 mL/24 hours)

Dosage Forms
Liquid:
All-Nite Multi-Symptom Cold/Flu [OTC]: Acetaminophen 500 mg, dextromethorphan hydrobromide 15 mg, doxylamine succinate 6.25 mg and pseudoephedrine hydrochloride 30 mg per 15 mL
Vicks® NyQuil® D Cold & Flu Multi-Symptom [OTC]: Acetaminophen 500 mg, dextromethorphan hydrobromide 15 mg, doxylamine succinate 6.25 mg and pseudoephedrine hydrochloride 30 mg per 15 mL

acetaminophen, dichloralphenazone, and isometheptene *see* acetaminophen, isometheptene, and dichloralphenazone *on page 34*

acetaminophen, diphenhydramine, and phenylephrine
(a seet a MIN oh fen, dye fen HYE dra meen, & fen il EF rin)
Medication Safety Issues
Other safety concerns:
Duplicate therapy issues: This product contains acetaminophen, which may be a component of combination products. Do not exceed the maximum recommended daily dose of acetaminophen.

Synonyms acetaminophen, phenylephrine, and diphenhydramine; diphenhydramine, phenylephrine hydrochloride, and acetaminophen; phenylephrine hydrochloride, acetaminophen, and diphenhydramine

U.S. Brand Names Benadryl® Allergy and Cold [OTC]; Benadryl® Allergy and Sinus Headache [OTC]; Benadry® Maximum Strength Severe Allergy and Sinus Headache [OTC]; Cold Control PE [OTC]; One Tab™ Allergy & Sinus [OTC]; One Tab™ Cold & Flu [OTC]; Sudafed PE® Nighttime Cold [OTC]; Sudafed PE® Severe Cold [OTC]; Theraflu® Nighttime Severe Cold & Cough [OTC]; Theraflu® Sugar-Free Nighttime Severe Cold & Cough [OTC]; Theraflu® Warming Relief ™ Flu & Sore Throat [OTC]; Theraflu® Warming Relief™ Nighttime Severe Cold & Cough [OTC]; Tylenol® Allergy Multi-Symptom Nighttime [OTC]; Tylenol® Children's Plus Cold and Allergy [OTC]

Therapeutic Category Analgesic, Miscellaneous; Decongestant; Histamine H_1 Antagonist

Use Temporary relief of symptoms of hay fever and the common cold, including sinus/nasal congestion and pain/pressure, headache, sneezing, runny nose, itchy/watery eyes, sore throat, fever, cough, and minor aches and pains

General Dosage Range Oral:
Caplet:
Children 6-11 years: One caplet every 4 hours as needed (maximum: 5 doses/caplets)
Children ≥12 years and Adults: Two caplets every 4 hours as needed (maximum: 12 caplets/24 hours)
Liquid: *Children 6-11 years and 48-95 lbs:* 10 mL every 4 hours as needed (maximum: 5 doses/24 hours)
Powder for solution: *Children ≥12 years and Adults:* One packet every 4 hours as needed (maximum: 6 doses/24 hours)
Syrup: *Children ≥12 years and Adults:* 30 mL every 4 hours as needed (maximum: 6 doses/24 hours)

◀ **Dosage Forms**
Caplet, oral:
Benadryl® Allergy and Cold [OTC], Benadryl® Allergy and Sinus Headache [OTC], Sudafed PE® Severe Cold [OTC]: Acetaminophen 325 mg, diphenhydramine 12.5 mg, and phenylephrine 5 mg
Benadry® Maximum Strength Severe Allergy and Sinus Headache [OTC], Sudafed PE® Nighttime Cold [OTC], Tylenol® Allergy Multi-Symptom Nighttime [OTC]: Acetaminophen 325 mg, diphenhydramine 25 mg, and phenylephrine 5 mg
Cold Control PE [OTC]: Acetaminophen 650 mg, diphenhydramine 25 mg, and phenylephrine 10 mg
One Tab™ Allergy & Sinus, One Tab™ Cold and Flu: Acetaminophen 650 mg, diphenhydramine 25 mg, and phenylephrine 10 mg
Liquid, oral:
Tylenol® Children's Plus Cold and Allergy [OTC]: Acetaminophen 160 mg, diphenhydramine 12.5 mg, and phenylephrine 2.5 mg per 5 mL
Powder for solution, oral:
Theraflu® Nighttime Severe Cold & Cough [OTC], Theraflu® Sugar-Free Nighttime Severe Cold & Cough [OTC]: Acetaminophen 650 mg, diphenhydramine 25 mg, and phenylephrine 10 mg per packet (6s)
Syrup, oral:
Theraflu® Warming Relief™ Flu & Sore Throat [OTC], Theraflu® Warming Relief™ Nighttime Severe Cold & Cough [OTC]: Acetaminophen 325 mg, diphenhydramine 12.5 mg, and phenylephrine 5 mg per 15 mL (245.5 mL)

acetaminophen, isometheptene, and dichloralphenazone
(a seet a MIN oh fen, eye soe me THEP teen, & dye KLOR al FEN a zone)
Medication Safety Issues
Sound-alike/look-alike issues:
Midrin® may be confused with midodrine, Mydfrin®
Other safety concerns:
Duplicate therapy issues: This product contains acetaminophen, which may be a component of other combination products. Do not exceed the maximum recommended daily dose of acetaminophen.
Synonyms acetaminophen, dichloralphenazone, and isometheptene; dichloralphenazone, acetaminophen, and isometheptene; dichloralphenazone, isometheptene, and acetaminophen; isometheptene, acetaminophen, and dichloralphenazone; isometheptene, dichloralphenazone, and acetaminophen
U.S. Brand Names Epidrin [DSC]; Midrin® [DSC]
Therapeutic Category Analgesic, Nonnarcotic
Controlled Substance C-IV
Use Relief of migraine and tension headache
General Dosage Range Oral: *Adults:* 2 capsules initially, then 1 capsule every hour until relief; alternatively, 1-2 capsules every 4 hours (maximum: 5 capsules/12 hours or 8 capsules/day)

acetaminophen, phenylephrine, and diphenhydramine *see* acetaminophen, diphenhydramine, and phenylephrine *on page* 33
acetaminophen, pseudoephedrine, and chlorpheniramine *see* acetaminophen, chlorpheniramine, and pseudoephedrine *on page* 30
Acetasol® HC *see* acetic acid, propylene glycol diacetate, and hydrocortisone *on page* 35

acetazolamide (a set a ZOLE a mide)
Medication Safety Issues
International issues:
Diamox [Canada and multiple international markets] may be confused with Diabinese brand name for chlorpropamide [Multiple international markets]; Dobutrex brand name for dobutamine [Multiple international markets]; Trimox brand name for amoxicillin [Brazil]; Zimox brand name for amoxicillin [Italy] and carbidopa/levodopa [Greece]
Tall-Man acetaZOLAMIDE
U.S. Brand Names Diamox® Sequels®
Canadian Brand Names Apo-Acetazolamide®; Diamox®
Therapeutic Category Anticonvulsant; Carbonic Anhydrase Inhibitor

Use Treatment of glaucoma (chronic simple open-angle, secondary glaucoma, preoperatively in acute angle-closure); drug-induced edema or edema due to congestive heart failure (adjunctive therapy); centrencephalic epilepsies (immediate release dosage form); prevention or amelioration of symptoms associated with acute mountain sickness

General Dosage Range Dosage adjustment recommended in patients with renal impairment

I.V.:
Children: 20-40 mg/kg/day divided every 6 hours **or** 5 mg/kg (150 mg/m^2) once daily (maximum: 1 g/day)
Adults: 250-500 mg/day (maximum: 1 g/day)

Oral:
Immediate release:
Children: 5-30 mg/kg/day (150-900 mg/m^2/day) divided in 1-4 doses (maximum: 1 g/day)
Adults: 250-1000 mg/day in 1-4 divided doses (maximum: 1 g/day)
Elderly: Initial: 250 mg once or twice daily
Extended release:
Adults: 500 mg every 12-24 hours (maximum 1 g/day)

Dosage Forms
Capsule, extended release, oral: 500 mg
Capsule, sustained release, oral:
Diamox® Sequels®: 500 mg
Injection, powder for reconstitution: 500 mg
Tablet, oral: 125 mg, 250 mg

acetic acid (a SEE tik AS id)

Medication Safety Issues
Sound-alike/look-alike issues:
Acetic acid for irrigation may be confused with glacial acetic acid
VoSol® may be confused with Vexol®,VoSol® HC

Synonyms ethanoic acid

U.S. Brand Names VoSoL®

Therapeutic Category Antibacterial, Otic; Antibacterial, Topical

Use Irrigation of the bladder; periodic irrigation of indwelling catheters; treatment of superficial bacterial infections of the external auditory canal

General Dosage Range
Irrigation:
Adults: Continuous: 0.25% at a rate approximate to urine flow; usually 500-1500 mL/day; Periodic: 50 mL of 0.25%
Otic:
Children ≥3 years: Instill 3-5 drops 3-4 times/day
Adults: Instill 5 drops 3-4 times/day

Dosage Forms
Solution, for irrigation: 0.25% (1000 mL)
Solution, for irrigation [preservative free]: 0.25% (250 mL, 500 mL, 1000 mL)
Solution, otic: 2% (15 mL, 60 mL)
VoSoL®: 2% (15 mL)

acetic acid, hydrocortisone, and propylene glycol diacetate *see* acetic acid, propylene glycol diacetate, and hydrocortisone *on page 35*

acetic acid, propylene glycol diacetate, and hydrocortisone
(a SEE tik AS id, PRO pa leen GLY kole dye AS e tate, & hye droe KOR ti sone)

Medication Safety Issues
Sound-alike/look-alike issues:
VoSol® may be confused with Vexol®

Synonyms acetic acid, hydrocortisone, and propylene glycol diacetate; hydrocortisone, acetic acid, and propylene glycol diacetate; propylene glycol diacetate, acetic acid, and hydrocortisone

U.S. Brand Names Acetasol® HC; VoSol® HC

Therapeutic Category Antibiotic/Corticosteroid, Otic

Use Treatment of superficial infections of the external auditory canal caused by organisms susceptible to the action of the antimicrobial, complicated by swelling

◀ **General Dosage Range Otic:** *Children ≥3 years and Adults:* Instill 3-5 drops in ear(s) every 4-6 hours
Dosage Forms
    Solution, otic [drops]: Acetic acid 2%, propylene glycol diacetate 3%, and hydrocortisone 1% (10 mL)
    Acetasol® HC, VoSol® HC: Acetic acid 2%, propylene glycol diacetate 3%, and hydrocortisone 1% (10 mL)

acetohydroxamic acid (a SEE toe hye droks am ik AS id)

Medication Safety Issues
    Sound-alike/look-alike issues:
    Lithostat® may be confused with Lithobid®
Synonyms AHA
U.S. Brand Names Lithostat®
Canadian Brand Names Lithostat®
Therapeutic Category Urinary Tract Product
Use Adjunctive therapy in chronic urea-splitting urinary infection
General Dosage Range Oral:
    Children: Initial: 10 mg/kg/day
    Adults: 250 mg 3-4 times/day (maximum: 10-15 mg/kg/day)
Dosage Forms
    Tablet, oral:
    Lithostat®: 250 mg

Acetoxyl® (Can) *see* benzoyl peroxide *on page 124*
acetoxymethylprogesterone *see* medroxyprogesterone *on page 554*

acetylcholine (a se teel KOE leen)

Medication Safety Issues
    Sound-alike/look-alike issues:
    Acetylcholine may be confused with acetylcysteine
Synonyms acetylcholine chloride
U.S. Brand Names Miochol®-E
Canadian Brand Names Miochol®-E
Therapeutic Category Cholinergic Agent
Use Produces complete miosis in cataract surgery, keratoplasty, iridectomy, and other anterior segment surgery where rapid miosis is required
General Dosage Range Intraocular: *Adults:* Instill 0.5-2 mL of 1% injection (5-20 mg)
Dosage Forms
    Powder for solution, intraocular:
    Miochol®-E: 20 mg (2 mL)

acetylcholine chloride *see* acetylcholine *on page 36*

acetylcysteine (a se teel SIS teen)

Medication Safety Issues
    Sound-alike/look-alike issues:
    Acetylcysteine may be confused with acetylcholine
    Mucomyst® may be confused with Mucinex®
Synonyms *N*-acetyl-L-cysteine; *N*-acetylcysteine; acetylcysteine sodium; mercapturic acid; Mucomyst; NAC
U.S. Brand Names Acetadote®
Canadian Brand Names Acetylcysteine Solution; Mucomyst®; Parvolex®
Therapeutic Category Mucolytic Agent
Use Antidote for acute acetaminophen poisoning; repeated supratherapeutic ingestion (RSTI) of acetaminophen; adjunctive mucolytic therapy in patients with abnormal or viscid mucous secretions in acute and chronic bronchopulmonary diseases; pulmonary complications of surgery and cystic fibrosis; diagnostic bronchial studies

General Dosage Range

Inhalation:

Nebulization:

Infants: 1-2 mL of 20% solution or 2-4 mL 10% solution 3-4 times/day

Children and Adults: 1-10 mL of 20% solution or 2-20 mL of 10% solution every 2-6 hours

Direct instillation: *Adults:* 1-4 mL of 10% or 1-2 mL of 20% solution every 1-4 hours

I.V.: Acetadote®:

Children and Adults: 21-hour regimen: Consists of 3 doses; total dose delivered: 300 mg/kg

Loading dose: 150 mg/kg (maximum: 15 g) infused over 60 minutes

Second dose: 50 mg/kg (maximum: 5 g) infused over 4 hours

Third dose: 100 mg/kg (maximum: 10 g) infused over 16 hours

Oral:

Children and Adults: Acetaminophen poisoning: 72-hour regimen: Consists of 18 doses; total dose delivered: 1330 mg/kg

Loading dose: 140 mg/kg

Maintenance dose: 70 mg/kg every 4 hours

Adults: Renal protectant for radiocontrast: 600-1200 mg twice daily for 2 days

Dosage Forms

Injection, solution [preservative free]:

Acetadote®: 20% [200 mg/mL] (30 mL)

Solution, for inhalation/oral: 10% [100 mg/mL] (10 mL, 30 mL); 20% [200 mg/mL] (10 mL, 30 mL)

Solution, for inhalation/oral [preservative free]: 10% [100 mg/mL] (4 mL, 10 mL); 20% [200 mg/mL] (4 mL, 10 mL, 30 mL)

acetylcysteine, methylcobalamin, and methylfolate *see* methylfolate, methylcobalamin, and acetylcysteine *on page 576*

acetylcysteine, methylfolate, and methylcobalamin *see* methylfolate, methylcobalamin, and acetylcysteine *on page 576*

acetylcysteine sodium *see* acetylcysteine *on page 36*

Acetylcysteine Solution (Can) *see* acetylcysteine *on page 36*

acetylsalicylic acid *see* aspirin *on page 98*

achromycin *see* tetracycline *on page 857*

aciclovir *see* acyclovir (systemic) *on page 39*

aciclovir *see* acyclovir (topical) *on page 39*

Acid Control (Can) *see* famotidine *on page 366*

Acid Gone [OTC] *see* aluminum hydroxide and magnesium carbonate *on page 59*

Acid Gone Extra Strength [OTC] *see* aluminum hydroxide and magnesium carbonate *on page 59*

Acid Reducer (Can) *see* ranitidine *on page 767*

acidulated phosphate fluoride *see* fluoride *on page 386*

Acilac (Can) *see* lactulose *on page 507*

AcipHex® *see* rabeprazole *on page 763*

acitretin (a si TRE tin)

Medication Safety Issues

Sound-alike/look-alike issues:

Soriatane® may be confused with Loxitane®, sertraline, Sonata®

U.S. Brand Names Soriatane®

Canadian Brand Names Soriatane®

Therapeutic Category Retinoid-like Compound

Use Treatment of severe psoriasis

General Dosage Range Oral: *Adults:* 25-50 mg/day as a single dose

Dosage Forms

Capsule, oral:

Soriatane®: 10 mg, 17.5 mg, 25 mg

Aclaro® *see* hydroquinone *on page 453*

Aclaro PD® *see* hydroquinone *on page 453*

Aclasta® (Can) *see* zoledronic acid *on page 932*

Aclovate® *see* alclometasone *on page 46*

Acne Clear Maximum Strength [OTC] *see* benzoyl peroxide *on page 124*

acrivastine and pseudoephedrine (AK ri vas teen & soo doe e FED rin)

Synonyms pseudoephedrine hydrochloride and acrivastine

U.S. Brand Names Semprex®-D

Therapeutic Category Antihistamine/Decongestant Combination

Use Relief of symptoms associated with seasonal allergic rhinitis

General Dosage Range Oral: *Children ≥12 years and Adults:* One capsule every 4-6 hours (maximum: 4 doses/24 hours)

Dosage Forms
  Capsule:
    Semprex®-D: Acrivastine 8 mg and pseudoephedrine 60 mg

Act® [OTC] *see* fluoride *on page 386*

ACT-D *see* dactinomycin *on page 249*

Actemra® *see* tocilizumab *on page 874*

ACTH *see* corticotropin *on page 236*

Acthar *see* corticotropin *on page 236*

ActHIB® *see* Haemophilus B conjugate vaccine *on page 432*

Acthrel® *see* corticorelin *on page 236*

Acticin® [DSC] *see* permethrin *on page 691*

Actidose®-Aqua [OTC] *see* charcoal *on page 191*

Actidose® with Sorbitol [OTC] *see* charcoal *on page 191*

Actifed® (Can) *see* triprolidine and pseudoephedrine *on page 893*

Actifed® Cold & Allergy [OTC] *[reformulation]* *see* chlorpheniramine and phenylephrine *on page 198*

Actigall® *see* ursodiol *on page 902*

Actimmune® *see* interferon gamma-1b *on page 482*

actinomycin *see* dactinomycin *on page 249*

actinomycin D *see* dactinomycin *on page 249*

actinomycin CI *see* dactinomycin *on page 249*

Actiq® *see* fentanyl *on page 371*

Activase® *see* alteplase *on page 58*

Activase® rt-PA (Can) *see* alteplase *on page 58*

activated carbon *see* charcoal *on page 191*

activated charcoal *see* charcoal *on page 191*

activated dimethicone *see* simethicone *on page 812*

activated ergosterol *see* ergocalciferol *on page 336*

activated factor XIII *see* factor XIII concentrate (human) *on page 366*

activated methylpolysiloxane *see* simethicone *on page 812*

activated protein C, human, recombinant *see* drotrecogin alfa *on page 315*

Activella® *see* estradiol and norethindrone *on page 345*

Act® Kids [OTC] *see* fluoride *on page 386*

Actonel® *see* risedronate *on page 782*

Actonel® and Calcium *see* risedronate and calcium *on page 783*

Actonel® DR (Can) *see* risedronate *on page 782*

Actonel Plus Calcium (Can) *see* risedronate and calcium *on page 783*

Actoplus Met® *see* pioglitazone and metformin *on page 706*

Actoplus Met® XR *see* pioglitazone and metformin *on page 706*

Actos® *see* pioglitazone *on page 706*

Act® Restoring™ [OTC] *see* fluoride *on page 386*

Act® Total Care™ [OTC] *see* fluoride *on page 386*

Acular® *see* ketorolac (ophthalmic) *on page 502*

Acular LS® *see* ketorolac (ophthalmic) *on page 502*

Acuvail® *see* ketorolac (ophthalmic) *on page 502*

ACV *see* acyclovir (systemic) *on page 39*
ACV *see* acyclovir (topical) *on page 39*
acycloguanosine *see* acyclovir (systemic) *on page 39*
acycloguanosine *see* acyclovir (topical) *on page 39*

acyclovir (systemic) (ay SYE kloe veer)
Medication Safety Issues
Sound-alike/look-alike issues:
Acyclovir may be confused with ganciclovir, Retrovir®, valacyclovir
Zovirax® may be confused with Doribax®, Valtrex®, Zithromax®, Zostrix®, Zyloprim®, Zyvox®
Synonyms aciclovir; ACV; acycloguanosine
U.S. Brand Names Zovirax®
Canadian Brand Names Apo-Acyclovir®; Gen-Acyclovir; Mylan-Acyclovir; Novo-Acyclovir; Nu-Acyclovir; ratio-Acyclovir; Teva-Acyclovir; Zovirax®
Therapeutic Category Antiviral Agent
Use Treatment of genital herpes simplex virus (HSV) and HSV encephalitis
General Dosage Range Dosage adjustment recommended in patients with renal impairment
I.V.:
Children <12 years: 10-20 mg/kg/dose every 8 hours (maximum: 60 mg/kg/day)
Children ≥12 years and Adults: 5-10 mg/kg/dose **or** 500 mg/m^2/dose every 8 hours (maximum: 45 mg/kg/day)
Oral:
Children ≥2 years and ≤40 kg: 20 mg/kg/dose 4 times/day (maximum: 800 mg/dose)
Children ≥2 years and >40 kg: 800 mg/dose 4 times/day
Adults: 200-800 mg/dose 3-5 times/day
Dosage Forms
Capsule, oral: 200 mg
Zovirax®: 200 mg
Injection, powder for reconstitution: 500 mg, 1000 mg
Injection, solution [preservative free]: 50 mg/mL (10 mL, 20 mL)
Suspension, oral: 200 mg/5 mL (473 mL)
Zovirax®: 200 mg/5 mL (473 mL)
Tablet, oral: 400 mg, 800 mg
Zovirax®: 400 mg, 800 mg

acyclovir (topical) (ay SYE kloe veer)
Medication Safety Issues
Sound-alike/look-alike issues:
Acyclovir may be confused with ganciclovir, Retrovir®, valacyclovir
Zovirax® may be confused with Doribax®, Valtrex®, Zithromax®, Zostrix®, Zyloprim®, Zyvox®
International issues:
Opthavir [Mexico] may be confused with Optivar brand name for azelastine [U.S.]
Synonyms aciclovir; ACV; acycloguanosine
U.S. Brand Names Zovirax®
Canadian Brand Names Zovirax®
Therapeutic Category Antiviral Agent, Topical
Use Treatment of herpes labialis (cold sores), mucocutaneous HSV in immunocompromised patients
General Dosage Range Topical:
Children ≥12 years: Cream: Apply 5 times/day
Adults: Cream: Apply 5 times/day; Ointment: 1/2" ribbon for a 4" square surface area 6 times/day
Dosage Forms
Cream, topical:
Zovirax®: 5% (2 g, 5 g)
Ointment, topical:
Zovirax®: 5% (15 g, 30 g)

acyclovir and hydrocortisone (ay SYE kloe veer & hye droe KOR ti sone)
Synonyms hydrocortisone and acyclovir; ME-609; Xerclear
U.S. Brand Names Xerese™

◀ **Therapeutic Category** Antiviral Agent, Topical; Corticosteroid, Topical
Use Treatment of recurrent herpes labialis (cold sores)
General Dosage Range Topical: *Children ≥12 years and Adults:* Apply 5 times/day

ACZ885 *see* canakinumab *on page 167*
Aczone® *see* dapsone (topical) *on page 252*
AD32 *see* valrubicin *on page 905*
Adacel® *see* diphtheria, tetanus toxoids, and acellular pertussis vaccine *on page 296*
Adagen® *see* pegademase (bovine) *on page 678*
Adalat® XL® (Can) *see* nifedipine *on page 626*
Adalat® CC *see* nifedipine *on page 626*

adalimumab (a da LIM yoo mab)

Medication Safety Issues
Sound-alike/look-alike issues:
Humira® may be confused with Humulin®, Humalog®
Humira® Pen may be confused with HumaPen® Memoir®
Synonyms antitumor necrosis factor alpha (human); D2E7; human antitumor necrosis factor alpha
U.S. Brand Names Humira®; Humira® Pen
Canadian Brand Names Humira®
Therapeutic Category Antirheumatic, Disease Modifying; Monoclonal Antibody
Use
Treatment of active rheumatoid arthritis (moderate-to-severe) and active psoriatic arthritis; may be used alone or in combination with disease-modifying antirheumatic drugs (DMARDs); treatment of ankylosing spondylitis
Treatment of moderately- to severely-active Crohn disease in patients with inadequate response to conventional treatment, or patients who have lost response to or are intolerant of infliximab
Treatment of moderate-to-severe plaque psoriasis
Treatment of moderately- to severely-active juvenile idiopathic arthritis
General Dosage Range SubQ:
Children ≥4 years: 15 kg to <30 kg: 20 mg every other week; ≥30 kg: 40 mg every other week
Adults: Initial: 80-160 mg; Maintenance: 40 mg every other week (maximum: 40 mg every week)
Dosage Forms
Injection, solution [preservative free]:
Humira®: 20 mg/0.4 mL (0.4 mL); 40 mg/0.8 mL (0.8 mL)
Humira® Pen: 40 mg/0.8 mL (0.8 mL)

adamantanamine hydrochloride *see* amantadine *on page 62*

adapalene (a DAP a leen)

U.S. Brand Names Differin®
Canadian Brand Names Differin®; Differin® XP
Therapeutic Category Acne Products
Use Treatment of acne vulgaris
General Dosage Range Topical: *Children >12 years and Adults:* Apply once daily at bedtime
Dosage Forms
Cream, topical: 0.1% (45 g)
Differin®: 0.1% (45 g)
Gel, topical: 0.1% (45 g)
Differin®: 0.1% (45 g); 0.3% (45 g)

adapalene and benzoyl peroxide (a DAP a leen & BEN zoe il peer OKS ide)

Synonyms benzoyl peroxide and adapalene
U.S. Brand Names Epiduo®
Canadian Brand Names Tactuo™
Therapeutic Category Acne Products; Topical Skin Product; Topical Skin Product, Acne
Use Topical treatment of acne vulgaris
General Dosage Range Topical: *Children ≥12 years and Adults:* Apply once daily

Dosage Forms
Gel, topical:
Epiduo®: Adapalene 0.1% and benzoyl peroxide 2.5% (45 g)

Adcetris™ *see* brentuximab vedotin *on page 140*
Adcirca® *see* tadalafil *on page 842*
ADD 234037 *see* lacosamide *on page 505*
Addaprin [OTC] *see* ibuprofen *on page 460*
Adderall® [DSC] *see* dextroamphetamine and amphetamine *on page 269*
Adderall XR® *see* dextroamphetamine and amphetamine *on page 269*

adefovir (a DEF o veer)

Synonyms adefovir dipivoxil; bis-POM PMEA
U.S. Brand Names Hepsera®
Canadian Brand Names Hepsera™
Therapeutic Category Antiretroviral Agent, Nonnucleoside Reverse Transcriptase Inhibitor (NNRTI)
Use Treatment of chronic hepatitis B with evidence of active viral replication (based on persistent elevation of ALT/AST or histologic evidence), including patients with lamivudine-resistant hepatitis B
General Dosage Range Dosage adjustment recommended in patients with renal impairment
Oral: *Children ≥12 years and Adults:* 10 mg once daily
Dosage Forms
Tablet, oral:
Hepsera®: 10 mg

adefovir dipivoxil *see* adefovir *on page 41*
ADEKs® [OTC] *see* vitamins (multiple/pediatric) *on page 920*
Adenocard® (Can) *see* adenosine *on page 41*
Adenocard® IV *see* adenosine *on page 41*
Adenoscan® *see* adenosine *on page 41*

adenosine (a DEN oh seen)

Medication Safety Issues
High alert medication:
The Institute for Safe Medication Practices (ISMP) includes this medication among its list of drugs which have a heightened risk of causing significant patient harm when used in error.
Synonyms 9-beta-d-ribofuranosyladenine
U.S. Brand Names Adenocard® IV; Adenoscan®
Canadian Brand Names Adenocard®; Adenoscan®; Adenosine Injection, USP; PMS-Adenosine
Therapeutic Category Antiarrhythmic Agent, Class IV; Diagnostic Agent
Use
Adenocard®: Treatment of paroxysmal supraventricular tachycardia (PSVT) including that associated with accessory bypass tracts (Wolff-Parkinson-White syndrome); when clinically advisable, appropriate vagal maneuvers should be attempted prior to adenosine administration; **not effective for conversion of atrial fibrillation, atrial flutter, or ventricular tachycardia**
Adenoscan®: Pharmacologic stress agent used in myocardial perfusion thallium-201 scintigraphy
General Dosage Range I.V.:
Children <50 kg: Initial: 0.05-0.1 mg/kg/dose (maximum initial dose: 6 mg); repeat: 0.05-0.3 mg/kg/dose (maximum: 0.3 mg/kg/dose or 12 mg/dose)
Children ≥50 kg and Adults: Initial: 6 mg; if not effective, 12 mg may be given; may repeat 12 mg if needed (maximum: 12 mg/dose)
Dosage Forms
Injection, solution [preservative free]: 3 mg/mL (2 mL, 4 mL)
Adenocard® IV: 3 mg/mL (2 mL, 4 mL)
Adenoscan®: 3 mg/mL (20 mL, 30 mL)

Adenosine Injection, USP (Can) *see* adenosine *on page 41*
adenovirus type 4 and type 7 vaccine *see* adenovirus (types 4, 7) vaccine *on page 42*

adenovirus (types 4, 7) vaccine (ad e noh VYE rus typs for SEV en vak SEEN)

Synonyms adenovirus type 4 and type 7 vaccine; adenovirus vaccine; adenovirus vaccine (types 4 and 7); type 4 and type 7 adenovirus vaccine

Therapeutic Category Vaccine, Live (Viral)

Use Prevention of acute febrile respiratory disease caused by adenovirus types 4 and 7 (approved for use in military populations)

General Dosage Range Oral: *Adolescents ≥17 years and Adults ≤50 years:* One tablet each of type 4 and type 7 as a single vaccine dose

Dosage Forms

Tablet, enteric coated, oral [combination package]:
Adenovirus type 4 ≥4.5 $\log_{10}$ TCID$_{50}$ [contains albumin (human); 100 white tablets]
Adenovirus type 7 ≥4.5 $\log_{10}$ TCID$_{50}$ [contains albumin (human); 100 white tablets]

adenovirus vaccine *see* adenovirus (types 4, 7) vaccine *on page 42*

adenovirus vaccine (types 4 and 7) *see* adenovirus (types 4, 7) vaccine *on page 42*

ADH *see* vasopressin *on page 910*

Adipex-P® *see* phentermine *on page 695*

ADL-2698 *see* alvimopan *on page 61*

Adoxa® *see* doxycycline *on page 312*

Adoxa® Pak™ 1/75 *see* doxycycline *on page 312*

Adoxa® Pak™ 1/150 *see* doxycycline *on page 312*

Adrenaclick™ [DSC] *see* epinephrine (systemic, oral inhalation) *on page 331*

Adrenalin® *see* epinephrine (nasal) *on page 332*

Adrenalin® *see* epinephrine (systemic, oral inhalation) *on page 331*

adrenaline *see* epinephrine (nasal) *on page 332*

adrenaline *see* epinephrine (systemic, oral inhalation) *on page 331*

adrenocorticotropic hormone *see* corticotropin *on page 236*

ADR (error-prone abbreviation) *see* doxorubicin *on page 310*

AdreView™ *see* iobenguane I 123 *on page 483*

adria *see* doxorubicin *on page 310*

Adriamycin® *see* doxorubicin *on page 310*

Adrucil® *see* fluorouracil (systemic) *on page 388*

adsorbent charcoal *see* charcoal *on page 191*

Advagraf™ (Can) *see* tacrolimus (systemic) *on page 842*

Advair® (Can) *see* fluticasone and salmeterol *on page 394*

Advair Diskus® *see* fluticasone and salmeterol *on page 394*

Advair® HFA *see* fluticasone and salmeterol *on page 394*

Advate *see* antihemophilic factor (recombinant) *on page 81*

Advicor® *see* niacin and lovastatin *on page 623*

Advil® [OTC] *see* ibuprofen *on page 460*

Advil® (Can) *see* ibuprofen *on page 460*

Advil® Allergy Sinus *see* ibuprofen, pseudoephedrine, and chlorpheniramine *on page 462*

Advil® Children's [OTC] *see* ibuprofen *on page 460*

Advil® Cold and Sinus Nighttime (Can) *see* ibuprofen, pseudoephedrine, and chlorpheniramine *on page 462*

Advil® Cold and Sinus Plus (Can) *see* ibuprofen, pseudoephedrine, and chlorpheniramine *on page 462*

Advil® Cold & Sinus [OTC] *see* pseudoephedrine and ibuprofen *on page 753*

Advil® Cold & Sinus (Can) *see* pseudoephedrine and ibuprofen *on page 753*

Advil® Cold & Sinus Daytime (Can) *see* pseudoephedrine and ibuprofen *on page 753*

Advil® Infants' [OTC] *see* ibuprofen *on page 460*

Advil® Migraine [OTC] *see* ibuprofen *on page 460*

Advil® Multi-Symptom Cold *see* ibuprofen, pseudoephedrine, and chlorpheniramine *on page 462*

Aerius® (Can) *see* desloratadine *on page 261*

Aerius® Kids (Can) *see* desloratadine *on page 261*

aerohist plus™ [DSC] see chlorpheniramine, phenylephrine, and methscopolamine on page 200

aeroKid™ see chlorpheniramine, phenylephrine, and methscopolamine on page 200

Afeditab® CR see nifedipine on page 626

Afinitor® see everolimus on page 362

Afluria® see influenza virus vaccine (inactivated) on page 473

A-Free Prenatal [OTC] see vitamins (multiple/prenatal) on page 920

Afrin® Extra Moisturizing [OTC] see oxymetazoline (nasal) on page 664

Afrin® Original [OTC] see oxymetazoline (nasal) on page 664

Afrin® Severe Congestion [OTC] see oxymetazoline (nasal) on page 664

Afrin® Sinus [OTC] see oxymetazoline (nasal) on page 664

agalsidase alfa *(Canada only)* (aye GAL si days AL fa)

Medication Safety Issues

Sound-alike/look-alike issues:

Agalsidase alfa may be confused with agalsidase beta, alglucerase, alglucosidase alfa

Synonyms agalsidase alpha; alpha-galactosidase-A (gene-activated)

Canadian Brand Names Replagal™

Therapeutic Category Enzyme

Use Replacement therapy for Fabry disease

General Dosage Range I.V.: *Children and Adults:* 0.2 mg/kg every 2 weeks

Product Availability Not available in U.S.

Dosage Forms - Canada

Injection, solution [preservative free]:

Replagal™: 1 mg/1 mL (3.5 mL)

agalsidase alpha see agalsidase alfa *(Canada only)* on page 43

agalsidase beta (aye GAL si days BAY ta)

Medication Safety Issues

Sound-alike/look-alike issues:

Agalsidase beta may be confused with agalsidase alfa, alglucerase, alglucosidase alfa

Synonyms alpha-galactosidase-A (recombinant); r-h α-GAL

U.S. Brand Names Fabrazyme®

Canadian Brand Names Fabrazyme®

Therapeutic Category Enzyme

Use Replacement therapy for Fabry disease

General Dosage Range I.V.: *Children ≥8 years and Adults:* 1 mg/kg every 2 weeks

Dosage Forms

Injection, powder for reconstitution:

Fabrazyme®: 5 mg, 35 mg

Aggrastat® see tirofiban on page 871

Aggrenox® see aspirin and dipyridamole on page 99

AGN 1135 see rasagiline on page 769

AgNO₃ see silver nitrate on page 812

Agrylin® see anagrelide on page 78

AHA see acetohydroxamic acid on page 36

AH-Chew® [DSC] see chlorpheniramine, phenylephrine, and methscopolamine on page 200

AH-Chew™ Ultra [DSC] see chlorpheniramine, phenylephrine, and methscopolamine on page 200

AHF (human) see antihemophilic factor (human) on page 81

AHF (human) see antihemophilic factor/von Willebrand factor complex (human) on page 82

AHF (recombinant) see antihemophilic factor (recombinant) on page 81

Ahist™ see chlorpheniramine on page 197

A-hydroCort see hydrocortisone (systemic) on page 449

A-Hydrocort® see hydrocortisone (systemic) on page 449

A-hydroCort see hydrocortisone (topical) on page 450

AICC *see* antiinhibitor coagulant complex *on page 83*

Airomir (Can) *see* albuterol *on page 45*

AK Cide Oph (Can) *see* sulfacetamide and prednisolone *on page 835*

AK-Con™ *see* naphazoline (ophthalmic) *on page 611*

AK-Dilate™ *see* phenylephrine (ophthalmic) *on page 697*

AK-Fluor® *see* fluorescein *on page 386*

Akne-mycin® *see* erythromycin (topical) *on page 340*

AK-Pentolate™ *see* cyclopentolate *on page 242*

AK-Poly-Bac™ *see* bacitracin and polymyxin B *on page 111*

AK Sulf Liq (Can) *see* sulfacetamide (ophthalmic) *on page 835*

Akten™ *see* lidocaine (ophthalmic) *on page 524*

AK-Tob™ *see* tobramycin (ophthalmic) *on page 873*

Akwa Tears® [OTC] *see* artificial tears *on page 96*

ALA *see* aminolevulinic acid *on page 66*

5-ALA *see* aminolevulinic acid *on page 66*

Ala-Cort *see* hydrocortisone (topical) *on page 450*

Alagesic LQ *see* butalbital, acetaminophen, and caffeine *on page 152*

Alamag [OTC] *see* aluminum hydroxide and magnesium hydroxide *on page 60*

Alamag Plus [OTC] *see* aluminum hydroxide, magnesium hydroxide, and simethicone *on page 60*

Alamast® *see* pemirolast *on page 683*

Ala-Scalp *see* hydrocortisone (topical) *on page 450*

Alavert® Allergy 24 Hour [OTC] *see* loratadine *on page 536*

Alavert™ Allergy and Sinus [OTC] *see* loratadine and pseudoephedrine *on page 537*

Alavert® Children's Allergy [OTC] *see* loratadine *on page 536*

Alaway™ [OTC] *see* ketotifen (ophthalmic) *on page 503*

albendazole (al BEN da zole)

Medication Safety Issues
Sound-alike/look-alike issues:
Albenza® may be confused with Aplenzin™, Relenza®
International issues:
Albenza [U.S.] may be confused with Avanza brand name for mirtazapine [Australia]
U.S. Brand Names Albenza®
Therapeutic Category Anthelmintic
Use Treatment of parenchymal neurocysticercosis caused by *Taenia solium* and cystic hydatid disease of the liver, lung, and peritoneum caused by *Echinococcus granulosus*
General Dosage Range Oral:
Children and Adults <60 kg: 15 mg/kg/day in 2 divided doses (maximum: 800 mg/day)
Children and Adults ≥60 kg: 800 mg/day in 2 divided doses (maximum: 800 mg/day)
Dosage Forms
Tablet, oral:
Albenza®: 200 mg

Albenza® *see* albendazole *on page 44*

Albert® Pentoxifylline (Can) *see* pentoxifylline *on page 689*

albumin (al BYOO min)

Medication Safety Issues
Sound-alike/look-alike issues:
Albutein® may be confused with albuterol
Buminate® may be confused with bumetanide
Synonyms albumin (human); normal human serum albumin; normal serum albumin (human); salt-poor albumin; SPA
U.S. Brand Names Albuminar®-25; Albuminar®-5; AlbuRx® 25; AlbuRx® 5; Albutein®; Buminate; Flexbumin 25%; Human Albumin Grifols® 25%; Plasbumin®-25; Plasbumin®-5
Canadian Brand Names Plasbumin®-25; Plasbumin®-5
Therapeutic Category Blood Product Derivative

Use Plasma volume expansion and maintenance of cardiac output in the treatment of certain types of shock or impending shock; may be useful for burn patients, ARDS, and cardiopulmonary bypass; other uses considered by some investigators (but not proven) are retroperitoneal surgery, peritonitis, and ascites; unless the condition responsible for hypoproteinemia can be corrected, albumin can provide only symptomatic relief or supportive treatment

Note: Nutritional supplementation is not an appropriate indication.

General Dosage Range I.V.:
Children: 0.5-1 g/kg/dose (10-20 mL/kg/dose) as needed
Adults: 0.5-1 g/kg/dose as needed **or** 25 g/dose may repeat in 15-30 minutes if response inadequate (maximum: 250 g/48 hours)

Dosage Forms
Injection, solution [preservative free]: 5% [50 mg/mL] (250 mL, 500 mL); 20% [200 mg/mL] (50 mL, 100 mL); 25% [250 mg/mL] (50 mL, 100 mL)
Albuminar®-5: 5% [50 mg/mL] (250 mL, 500 mL)
Albuminar®-25: 25% [250 mg/mL] (50 mL, 100 mL)
AlbuRx® 5: 5% [50 mg/mL] (250 mL, 500 mL)
AlbuRx® 25: 25% [250 mg/mL] (50 mL, 100 mL)
Albutein®: 5% [50 mg/mL] (250 mL, 500 mL); 25% [250 mg/mL] (50 mL, 100 mL)
Buminate: 5% [50 mg/mL] (250 mL, 500 mL); 25% [250 mg/mL] (20 mL)
Flexbumin 25%: 25% [250 mg/mL] (50 mL, 100 mL)
Human Albumin Grifols® 25%: 25% [250 mg/mL] (50 mL, 100 mL)
Plasbumin®-5: 5% [50 mg/mL] (50 mL, 250 mL)
Plasbumin®-25: 25% [250 mg/mL] (20 mL, 50 mL, 100 mL)

Albuminar®-5 *see albumin on page 44*

Albuminar®-25 *see albumin on page 44*

albumin-bound paclitaxel *see paclitaxel (protein bound) on page 667*

albumin (human) *see albumin on page 44*

albumin-stabilized nanoparticle paclitaxel *see paclitaxel (protein bound) on page 667*

AlbuRx® 5 *see albumin on page 44*

AlbuRx® 25 *see albumin on page 44*

Albutein® *see albumin on page 44*

albuterol (al BYOO ter ole)

Medication Safety Issues
Sound-alike/look-alike issues:
Albuterol may be confused with Albutein®, atenolol
Proventil® may be confused with Bentyl®, PriLOSEC®, Prinivil®
Salbutamol may be confused with salmeterol
Ventolin® may be confused with phentolamine, Benylin®, Vantin

Synonyms albuterol sulfate; salbutamol; salbutamol sulphate

U.S. Brand Names AccuNeb®; ProAir® HFA; Proventil® HFA; Ventolin® HFA; VoSpire ER®

Canadian Brand Names Airomir; Apo-Salvent®; Apo-Salvent® AEM; Apo-Salvent® CFC Free; Apo-Salvent® Sterules; Dom-Salbutamol; Med-Salbutamol; Mylan-Salbutamol Respirator Solution; Mylan-Salbutamol Sterinebs P.F.; Novo-Salbutamol HFA; Nu-Salbutamol; PHL-Salbutamol; PMS-Salbutamol; ratio-Ipra-Sal; ratio-Salbutamol; Sandoz-Salbutamol; Ventolin®; Ventolin® Diskus; Ventolin® HFA; Ventolin® I.V. Infusion; Ventolin® Nebules P.F.

Therapeutic Category Adrenergic Agonist Agent

Use Treatment or prevention of bronchospasm in patients with reversible obstructive airway disease; prevention of exercise-induced bronchospasm

General Dosage Range
Inhalation via metered-dose inhaler (90 mcg/puff): *Children and Adults:* 2 puffs every 4-6 hours **or** 4-8 puffs every 1-4 hours [acute symptoms] **or** 1-2 puffs prior to exercise
Nebulization:
Children <12 years: 0.15-0.3 mg/kg (maximum: 10 mg) every 1-4 hours **or** 0.63-1.25 mg 3-4 times/day **or** 0.5 mg/kg/hour by continuous nebulization
Children ≥12 years: 2.5-10 mg every 1-4 hours **or** 10-15 mg/hour by continuous nebulization
Adults: 2.5-10 mg every 1-4 hours **or** 10-15 mg/hour by continuous nebulization

◄ **Oral:**
  Regular release:
   Children 2-6 years: 0.1-0.2 mg/kg/dose 3 times/day (maximum: 12 mg/day)
   Children 6-12 years: 2 mg/dose 3-4 times/day (maximum: 24 mg/day)
   Children >12 years and Adults: 2-4 mg/dose 3-4 times/day (maximum: 32 mg/day)
  Extended release:
   Children 6-12 years: 4 mg every 12 hours (maximum: 24 mg/day)
   Children >12 years and Adults: 8 mg every 12 hours (maximum: 32 mg/day)

Dosage Forms
  Aerosol, for oral inhalation:
   ProAir® HFA: 90 mcg/inhalation (8.5 g)
   Proventil® HFA: 90 mcg/inhalation (6.7 g)
   Ventolin® HFA: 90 mcg/inhalation (8 g, 18 g)
  Solution, for nebulization: 0.083% [2.5 mg/3 mL] (25s, 30s, 60s); 0.5% [100 mg/20 mL] (1s)
  Solution, for nebulization [preservative free]: 0.021% [0.63 mg/3 mL] (25s); 0.042% [1.25 mg/3 mL]
   (25s, 30s); 0.083% [2.5 mg/3 mL] (3 mL, 10s, 24s, 25s, 30s, 60s); 0.5% [2.5 mg/0.5 mL] (10s, 30s)
   AccuNeb®: 0.021% [0.63 mg/3 mL] (25s); 0.042% [1.25 mg/3 mL] (25s)
  Syrup, oral: 2 mg/5 mL (473 mL, 480 mL)
  Tablet, oral: 2 mg, 4 mg
  Tablet, extended release, oral: 4 mg, 8 mg
   VoSpire ER®: 4 mg, 8 mg

Dosage Forms - Canada
  Injection, solution:
   Ventolin® I.V.: 1 mg/1mL (5 mL)

albuterol and ipratropium *see* ipratropium and albuterol *on page 489*
albuterol sulfate *see* albuterol *on page 45*

alcaftadine (al KAF ta deen)

U.S. Brand Names Lastacaft™
Therapeutic Category Histamine H₁ Antagonist; Mast Cell Stabilizer
Use Prevention of itching associated with allergic conjunctivitis
General Dosage Range Ophthalmic: *Children ≥2 years and Adults:* Instill 1 drop into each eye once daily
Dosage Forms
  Solution, ophthalmic:
   Lastacaft™: 0.25% (3 mL)

Alcaine® *see* proparacaine *on page 745*
Alcalak [OTC] *see* calcium carbonate *on page 161*

alclometasone (al kloe MET a sone)

Medication Safety Issues
  Sound-alike/look-alike issues:
   Aclovate® may be confused with Accolate®
  International issues:
   Cloderm: Brand name for alclometasone [Indonesia], but also brand name for clobetasol [China, India,
    Malaysia, Singapore, Thailand]; clocortolone [U.S., Canada]; clotrimazole [Germany]
Synonyms alclometasone dipropionate
U.S. Brand Names Aclovate®
Therapeutic Category Corticosteroid, Topical
Use Treatment of inflammation of corticosteroid-responsive dermatosis (low-to-medium potency topical
  corticosteroid)
General Dosage Range Topical: *Children ≥1 year and Adults:* Apply a thin film to the affected area 2-3
  times/day
Dosage Forms
  Cream, topical: 0.05% (15 g, 45 g, 60 g)
   Aclovate®: 0.05% (15 g, 60 g)
  Ointment, topical: 0.05% (15 g, 45 g, 60 g)
   Aclovate®: 0.05% (15 g, 60 g)

alclometasone dipropionate *see* alclometasone *on page 46* alcohol, absolute *see* alcohol (ethyl) *on page 47*

alcohol, dehydrated *see* alcohol (ethyl) *on page 47*

alcohol (ethyl) (AL koe hol, ETH il)

Medication Safety Issues
Sound-alike/look-alike issues:
Ethanol may be confused with Ethyol®, Ethamolin®

Synonyms alcohol, absolute; alcohol, dehydrated; ethanol; ethyl alcohol; EtOH

U.S. Brand Names Epi-Clenz™ [OTC]; Gel-Stat™ [OTC]; GelRite™ [OTC]; Isagel® [OTC]; Lavacol® [OTC]; Prevacare® [OTC]; Protection Plus® [OTC]; Purell® 2 in 1 [OTC]; Purell® Lasting Care [OTC]; Purell® Moisture Therapy [OTC]; Purell® with Aloe [OTC]; Purell® [OTC]

Canadian Brand Names Biobase-G™; Biobase™

Therapeutic Category Intravenous Nutritional Therapy; Pharmaceutical Aid

Use Topical antiinfective; pharmaceutical aid; therapeutic neurolysis (nerve or ganglion block); replenishment of carbohydrate calories

General Dosage Range
I.V.:
Infusion: *Adults:* Dosage varies depending on indication
Intraneural: *Adults:* Dosage varies depending on indication
Topical: *Children and Adults:* Apply 1-3 times/day as needed

Dosage Forms
Aerosol, topical:
Epi-Clenz™ [OTC]: 70% (240 mL)
Gel, topical:
Epi-Clenz™ [OTC]: 70% (45 mL, 120 mL, 480 mL)
Gel-Stat™ [OTC]: 62% (120 mL, 480 mL)
GelRite™ [OTC]: 67% (120 mL, 480 mL, 800 mL)
Isagel® [OTC]: 60% (59 mL, 118 mL, 621 mL, 800 mL)
Prevacare® [OTC]: 60% (120 mL, 240 mL, 960 mL, 1200 mL, 1500 mL)
Purell® [OTC]: 62% (15 mL, 30 mL, 59 mL, 60 mL, 120 mL, 236 mL, 240 mL, 250 mL, 360 mL, 500 mL, 800 mL, 1000 mL, 2000 mL)
Purell® Lasting Care [OTC]: 62% (120 mL, 240 mL, 1000 mL)
Purell® Moisture Therapy [OTC]: 62% (75 mL)
Purell® with Aloe [OTC]: 62% (15 mL, 59 mL, 60 mL, 120 mL, 236 mL, 354 mL, 800 mL, 1000 mL, 2000 mL)
Injection, solution [preservative free]: ≥ 98% (1 mL, 5 mL)
Liquid, topical: 70% (480 mL, 3840 mL)
Lavacol® [OTC]: 70% (473 mL)
Lotion, topical:
Purell® 2 in 1 [OTC]: 62% (60 mL, 360 mL, 1000 mL)
Pad, topical:
Isagel® [OTC]: 60% (50s, 300s)
Purell® [OTC]: 62% (24s, 35s, 175s)
Solution, topical:
Protection Plus® [OTC]: 62% (800 mL)

Alcortin® A *see* iodoquinol and hydrocortisone *on page 485*

Aldactazide® *see* hydrochlorothiazide and spironolactone *on page 446*

Aldactazide 25® (Can) *see* hydrochlorothiazide and spironolactone *on page 446*

Aldactazide 50® (Can) *see* hydrochlorothiazide and spironolactone *on page 446*

Aldactone® *see* spironolactone *on page 829*

Aldara® *see* imiquimod *on page 467*

aldesleukin (al des LOO kin)

Medication Safety Issues
Sound-alike/look-alike issues:
Aldesleukin may be confused with oprelvekin

◄ Proleukin® may be confused with oprelvekin

High alert medication:
The Institute for Safe Medication Practices (ISMP) includes this medication among its list of drug classes which have a heightened risk of causing significant patient harm when used in error.

Synonyms IL-2; interleukin 2; interleukin-2; lymphocyte mitogenic factor; recombinant human interleukin-2; T-cell growth factor; TCGF; thymocyte stimulating factor

U.S. Brand Names Proleukin®

Canadian Brand Names Proleukin®

Therapeutic Category Biological Response Modulator

Use Treatment of metastatic renal cell cancer, metastatic melanoma

General Dosage Range Dosage adjustment recommended in patients who develop toxicities
I.V.: *Adults:* 600,000 int. units/kg every 8 hours (maximum: 14 doses); may repeat after 9 days for a total of 28 doses/course

Dosage Forms
Injection, powder for reconstitution:
Proleukin®: 22×10^6 int. units

Aldex® AN *see* doxylamine *on page 313*

Aldex® CT *see* diphenhydramine and phenylephrine *on page 292*

Aldex®D [DSC] *see* phenylephrine and pyrilamine *on page 698*

Aldomet *see* methyldopa *on page 575*

Aldoril *see* methyldopa and hydrochlorothiazide *on page 575*

Aldroxicon I [OTC] *see* aluminum hydroxide, magnesium hydroxide, and simethicone *on page 60*

Aldroxicon II [OTC] *see* aluminum hydroxide, magnesium hydroxide, and simethicone *on page 60*

Aldurazyme® *see* laronidase *on page 512*

alefacept (a LE fa sept)

Synonyms B 9273; BG 9273; human LFA-3/IgG(1) fusion protein; LFA-3/IgG(1) fusion protein, human

U.S. Brand Names Amevive®

Canadian Brand Names Amevive®

Therapeutic Category Monoclonal Antibody

Use Treatment of moderate-to-severe chronic plaque psoriasis in adults who are candidates for systemic therapy or phototherapy

General Dosage Range I.M.: *Adults:* 15 mg once weekly

Dosage Forms
Injection, powder for reconstitution:
Amevive®: 15 mg

alemtuzumab (ay lem TU zoo mab)

Medication Safety Issues
High alert medication:
The Institute for Safe Medication Practices (ISMP) includes this medication among its list of drug classes which have a heightened risk of causing significant patient harm when used in error.

Synonyms anti-CD52 monoclonal antibody; campath-1H; humanized IgG1 anti-CD52 monoclonal antibody; MoAb CD52; monoclonal antibody campath-1H; monoclonal antibody CD52

U.S. Brand Names Campath®

Canadian Brand Names MabCampath®

Therapeutic Category Antineoplastic Agent, Monoclonal Antibody

Use Treatment of B-cell chronic lymphocytic leukemia (B-CLL)

General Dosage Range Dosage adjustment recommended in patients who develop toxicities
I.V. (infusion): *Adults:* Initial: 3 mg/day, then 10 mg/day; Maintenance: 30 mg/day 3 times/week on alternate days; Maximum dose: 30 mg/day; 90 mg/week (cumulative)

Dosage Forms
Injection, solution [preservative free]:
Campath®: 30 mg/mL (1 mL)

alendronate (a LEN droe nate)

Medication Safety Issues
Sound-alike/look-alike issues:
Alendronate may be confused with risedronate
Fosamax® may be confused with Flomax®, Fosamax Plus D®, fosinopril, Zithromax®
International issues:
Fosamax [U.S., Canada, and multiple international markets] may be confused with Fisamox brand name for amoxicillin [Australia]
Synonyms alendronate sodium; alendronic acid monosodium salt trihydrate; MK-217
U.S. Brand Names Fosamax®
Canadian Brand Names Alendronate-FC; Apo-Alendronate®; CO Alendronate; Dom-Alendronate; Fosamax®; Mylan-Alendronate; Novo-Alendronate; PHL-Alendronate; PMS-Alendronate; PMS-Alendronate-FC; ratio-Alendronate; Riva-Alendronate; Sandoz-Alendronate; Teva-Alendronate
Therapeutic Category Bisphosphonate Derivative
Use Treatment and prevention of osteoporosis in postmenopausal females; treatment of osteoporosis in males; Paget disease of the bone in patients who are symptomatic, at risk for future complications, or with alkaline phosphatase ≥2 times the upper limit of normal; treatment of glucocorticoid-induced osteoporosis in males and females with low bone mineral density who are receiving a daily dosage ≥7.5 mg of prednisone (or equivalent)
General Dosage Range Oral: *Adults:* 5-10 mg/day **or** 35-70 mg once weekly (maximum: 70 mg/week) **or** 40 mg once daily [Paget disease]
Dosage Forms
Tablet, oral: 5 mg, 10 mg, 35 mg, 40 mg, 70 mg
Fosamax®: 10 mg, 70 mg

alendronate and cholecalciferol (a LEN droe nate & kole e kal SI fer ole)

Medication Safety Issues
Sound-alike/look-alike issues:
Fosamax Plus D® may be confused with Fosamax®
Synonyms alendronate sodium and cholecalciferol; cholecalciferol and alendronate; vitamin D_3 and alendronate
U.S. Brand Names Fosamax Plus D®
Canadian Brand Names Fosavance
Therapeutic Category Bisphosphonate Derivative; Vitamin D Analog
Use Treatment of osteoporosis in postmenopausal females; increase bone mass in males with osteoporosis
General Dosage Range Oral: *Adults:* One tablet (alendronate 70 mg/cholecalciferol 2800-5600 international units) once weekly
Dosage Forms
Tablet:
Fosamax Plus D® 70/2800: Alendronate 70 mg and cholecalciferol 2800 int. units
Fosamax Plus D® 70/5600: Alendronate 70 mg and cholecalciferol 5600 int. units

Alendronate-FC (Can) *see* alendronate *on page 49*
alendronate sodium *see* alendronate *on page 49*
alendronate sodium and cholecalciferol *see* alendronate and cholecalciferol *on page 49*
alendronic acid monosodium salt trihydrate *see* alendronate *on page 49*
Aler-Cap [OTC] *see* diphenhydramine (systemic) *on page 290*
Aler-Dryl [OTC] *see* diphenhydramine (systemic) *on page 290*
Aler-Tab [OTC] *see* diphenhydramine (systemic) *on page 290*
Alertec® (Can) *see* modafinil *on page 594*
Alesse® (Can) *see* ethinyl estradiol and levonorgestrel *on page 353*
Aleve® [OTC] *see* naproxen *on page 612*
Aleve®-D Sinus & Cold [OTC] *see* naproxen and pseudoephedrine *on page 613*
Aleve®-D Sinus & Headache [OTC] *see* naproxen and pseudoephedrine *on page 613*
1alfacalcidol *see* alfacalcidol *(Canada only) on page 50*

alfacalcidol *(Canada only)* (Al fa CAL ce dol)

Medication Safety Issues
Sound-alike/look-alike issues:
Alfacalcidol may be confused with calcitriol, cholecalciferol, ergocalciferol, paricalcitol

Synonyms 1-α-hydroxycholecalciferol; 1-α-hydroxyvitamin D_3; 1alfacalcidol; $_1$alfa-hydroxyvitamin D3

Canadian Brand Names One-Alpha®

Therapeutic Category Vitamin D Analog

Use Management of hypocalcemia, secondary hyperparathyroidism, and osteodystrophy in patients with chronic renal failure

General Dosage Range Individualize dosage:
Oral: *Adults:* 0.25-3 mcg/day
I.V.: *Adults:* 1-12 mcg/week (with dialysis)

Product Availability Not available in the U.S.

Dosage Forms - Canada
Capsule, softgel, oral:
One-Alpha®: 0.25 mcg, 1 mcg [contains sesame oil]
Injection, solution:
One-Alpha®: 2 mcg/mL
Solution, oral [drops]:
One-Alpha®: 2 mcg/mL

$_1$**alfa-hydroxyvitamin D3** *see* alfacalcidol *(Canada only) on page 50*

Alfenta® *see* alfentanil *on page 50*

alfentanil (al FEN ta nil)

Medication Safety Issues
Sound-alike/look-alike issues:
Alfentanil may be confused with Anafranil®, fentanyl, remifentanil, sufentanil
Alfenta® may be confused with Sufenta®
High alert medication:
The Institute for Safe Medication Practices (ISMP) includes this medication among its list of drug classes which have a heightened risk of causing significant patient harm when used in error.

Synonyms alfentanil hydrochloride

U.S. Brand Names Alfenta®

Canadian Brand Names Alfentanil Injection, USP; Alfenta®

Therapeutic Category Analgesic, Narcotic; General Anesthetic

Controlled Substance C-II

Use Analgesic adjunct for the induction and maintenance of general anesthesia; analgesic component for monitored anesthesia care (MAC)

General Dosage Range I.V.:
Anesthetic induction: *Children ≥12 years and Adults:* Initial: 130-245 mcg/kg; Maintenance: 0.5-1.5 mcg/kg/minute
Continuous infusion: *Children ≥12 years and Adults:* Initial: 50-75 mcg/kg; Maintenance: 0.5-3 mcg/kg/minute
Incremental injection: *Children ≥12 years and Adults:*
≤30 minutes anesthesia: Initial: 8-20 mcg/kg; Maintenance: 3-5 mcg/kg **or** 0.5-1 mcg/kg/minute (maximum: 40 mcg/kg total dose)
≥30 minutes anesthesia: Initial: 20-50 mcg/kg; Maintenance: 5-15 mcg/kg (maximum: 75 mcg/kg total dose)

Dosage Forms
Injection, solution [preservative free]: 500 mcg/mL (2 mL, 5 mL, 10 mL, 20 mL)
Alfenta®: 500 mcg/mL (2 mL, 5 mL)

alfentanil hydrochloride *see* alfentanil *on page 50*
Alfentanil Injection, USP (Can) *see* alfentanil *on page 50*
Alferon® N *see* interferon alfa-n3 *on page 482*

alfuzosin (al FYOO zoe sin)

Synonyms alfuzosin hydrochloride

U.S. Brand Names Uroxatral®
Canadian Brand Names Apo-Alfuzosin®; Sandoz-Alfuzosin; Teva-Alfuzosin PR; Xatral
Therapeutic Category Alpha-Adrenergic Blocking Agent
Use Treatment of the functional symptoms of benign prostatic hyperplasia (BPH)
General Dosage Range Oral: *Adults:* 10 mg once daily
Dosage Forms
 Tablet, extended release, oral: 10 mg
  Uroxatral®: 10 mg

alfuzosin hydrochloride *see* alfuzosin *on page 50*

alglucerase (al GLOO ser ase)

Medication Safety Issues
 Sound-alike/look-alike issues:
  Alglucerase may be confused with agalsidase alfa, agalsidase beta, alglucosidase alfa
  Ceredase® may be confused with Cerezyme®
Synonyms glucocerebrosidase
U.S. Brand Names Ceredase®
Therapeutic Category Enzyme
Use Replacement therapy for Gaucher disease (type 1)
General Dosage Range I.V.: *Children and Adults:* Initial: 30-60 units/kg every 2 weeks; Maintenance (range): 2.5 units/kg 3 times/week to 60 units/kg once weekly to every 4 weeks
Dosage Forms
 Injection, solution [preservative free]:
  Ceredase®: 80 units/mL (5 mL)

alglucosidase *see* alglucosidase alfa *on page 51*

alglucosidase alfa (al gloo KOSE i dase AL fa)

Medication Safety Issues
 Sound-alike/look-alike issues:
  Alglucosidase alfa may be confused with agalsidase alfa, agalsidase beta, alglucerase
Synonyms alglucosidase; GAA; rhGAA
U.S. Brand Names Lumizyme®; Myozyme®
Canadian Brand Names Myozyme®
Therapeutic Category Enzyme
Use
 Lumizyme™: Replacement therapy for late-onset (noninfantile) Pompe disease without evidence of cardiac hypertrophy in patients 8 years and older
 Myozyme®: Replacement therapy for infantile-onset Pompe disease
General Dosage Range I.V.:
 Myozyme®: *Children 1 month to 3.5 years:* 20 mg/kg every 2 weeks
 Lumizyme™: *Children ≥8 years and Adults:* 20 mg/kg every 2 weeks
Dosage Forms
 Injection, powder for reconstitution:
  Lumizyme®: 50 mg
  Myozyme®: 50 mg

Aliclen™ *see* salicylic acid *on page 795*
Alimta® *see* pemetrexed *on page 682*
Alinia® *see* nitazoxanide *on page 628*

aliskiren (a lis KYE ren)

Medication Safety Issues
 Sound-alike/look-alike issues:
  Tekturna® may be confused with Valturna®
Synonyms aliskiren hemifumarate; SPP100
U.S. Brand Names Tekturna®
Canadian Brand Names Rasilez®

◀ **Therapeutic Category** Renin Inhibitor
Use Treatment of hypertension, alone or in combination with other antihypertensive agents
General Dosage Range Oral: *Adults:* 150-300 mg once daily (maximum: 300 mg/day)
Dosage Forms
Tablet, oral:
Tekturna®: 150 mg, 300 mg

aliskiren, amlodipine, and hydrochlorothiazide
(a lis KYE ren, am LOE di peen, & hye droe klor oh THYE a zide)
Medication Safety Issues
Sound-alike/look-alike issues:
Amturnide™ may be confused with AMILoride
Synonyms aliskiren, hydrochlorothiazide, and amlodipine; amlodipine besylate, aliskiren hemifumarate, and hydrochlorothiazide; amlodipine, aliskiren, and hydrochlorothiazide; amlodipine, hydrochlorothiazide, and aliskiren; hydrochlorothiazide, aliskiren, and amlodipine; hydrochlorothiazide, amlodipine, and aliskiren
U.S. Brand Names Amturnide™
Therapeutic Category Calcium Channel Blocker; Calcium Channel Blocker, Dihydropyridine; Diuretic, Thiazide; Renin Inhibitor
Use Treatment of hypertension (not for initial therapy)
General Dosage Range Oral: *Adults:* Aliskiren 150-300 mg and Amlodipine 5-10 mg and Hydrochlorothiazide 12.5-25 mg once daily (maximum recommended daily dose: Aliskiren 300 mg; amlodipine 10 mg; hydrochlorothiazide 25 mg)
Dosage Forms
Tablet, oral:
Amturnide™: Aliskiren 150 mg, amlodipine 5 mg, and hydrochlorothiazide 12.5 mg; Aliskiren 300 mg, amlodipine 5 mg, and hydrochlorothiazide 12.5 mg; Aliskiren 300 mg, amlodipine 5 mg, and hydrochlorothiazide 25 mg; Aliskiren 300 mg, amlodipine 10 mg, and hydrochlorothiazide 12.5 mg; Aliskiren 300 mg, amlodipine 10 mg, and hydrochlorothiazide 25 mg

aliskiren and amlodipine (a lis KYE ren & am LOE di peen)
Synonyms aliskiren hemifumarate and amlodipine besylate; amlodipine and aliskiren
U.S. Brand Names Tekamlo™
Therapeutic Category Calcium Channel Blocker; Calcium Channel Blocker, Dihydropyridine; Renin Inhibitor
Use Treatment of hypertension, alone or in combination with other antihypertensive agents, including use as initial therapy in patients likely to need multiple antihypertensives for adequate control
General Dosage Range Oral: *Adults:* Aliskiren 150-300 mg and amlodipine 5-10 mg once daily (maximum: 300 mg/day [aliskiren]; 10 mg/day [amlodipine])
Dosage Forms
Tablet, oral:
Tekamlo™: 150/5: Aliskiren 150 mg and amlodipine 5 mg, 300/5: Aliskiren 300 mg and amlodipine 5 mg, 150/10: Aliskiren 150 mg and amlodipine 10 mg, 300/10: Aliskiren 300 mg and amlodipine 10 mg

aliskiren and hydrochlorothiazide (a lis KYE ren & hye droe klor oh THYE a zide)
Synonyms aliskiren hemifumarate and hydrochlorothiazide; hydrochlorothiazide and aliskiren
U.S. Brand Names Tekturna HCT®
Canadian Brand Names Rasilez HCT
Therapeutic Category Antihypertensive Agent, Combination; Diuretic, Thiazide; Renin Inhibitor
Use Treatment of hypertension, including use as initial therapy in patients likely to need multiple antihypertensives for adequate control
General Dosage Range Oral: *Adults:* Aliskiren 150-300 mg and hydrochlorothiazide 12.5-25 mg once daily (maximum: 300 mg/day [aliskiren]; 25 mg/day [hydrochlorothiazide])
Dosage Forms
Tablet:
Tekturna HCT®: 150/12.5: Aliskiren 150 mg and hydrochlorothiazide 12.5 mg; 150/25: Aliskiren 150 mg and hydrochlorothiazide 25 mg; 300/12.5: Aliskiren 300 mg and hydrochlorothiazide 12.5 mg; 300/25: Aliskiren 300 mg and hydrochlorothiazide 25 mg

aliskiren and valsartan (a lis KYE ren & val SAR tan)
Medication Safety Issues
Sound-alike/look-alike issues:
Valturna® may be confused with Tekturna®, valsartan
Synonyms aliskiren hemifumarate and valsartan; valsartan and aliskiren
U.S. Brand Names Valturna®
Therapeutic Category Angiotensin II Receptor Blocker; Renin Inhibitor
Use Treatment of hypertension, including use as initial therapy in patients likely to need multiple antihypertensives for adequate control
General Dosage Range Oral: *Adults:* Aliskiren 150-300 mg and valsartan 160-320 mg once daily (maximum: 300 mg/day [aliskiren]; 320 mg/day [valsartan])
Dosage Forms
Tablet:
Valturna®: 150/160: Aliskiren 150 mg and valsartan 160 mg; 300/320: Aliskiren 300 mg and valsartan 320 mg

aliskiren hemifumarate *see* aliskiren *on page 51*
aliskiren hemifumarate and amlodipine besylate *see* aliskiren and amlodipine *on page 52*
aliskiren hemifumarate and hydrochlorothiazide *see* aliskiren and hydrochlorothiazide *on page 52*
aliskiren hemifumarate and valsartan *see* aliskiren and valsartan *on page 53*
aliskiren, hydrochlorothiazide, and amlodipine *see* aliskiren, amlodipine, and hydrochlorothiazide *on page 52*

alitretinoin (a li TRET i noyn)
Medication Safety Issues
Sound-alike/look-alike issues:
Panretin® may be confused with pancreatin
High alert medication:
The Institute for Safe Medication Practices (ISMP) includes this medication among its list of drugs which have a heightened risk of causing significant patient harm when used in error.
U.S. Brand Names Panretin®
Canadian Brand Names Panretin®
Therapeutic Category Antineoplastic Agent; Retinoic Acid Derivative
Use Orphan drug: Topical treatment of cutaneous lesions in AIDS-related Kaposi sarcoma
General Dosage Range Topical: *Adults:* Apply twice daily
Dosage Forms
Gel, topical:
Panretin®: 0.1% (60 g)

Alka-Mints® [OTC] *see* calcium carbonate *on page 161*
Alka-Seltzer Plus® Day Cold [OTC] *see* acetaminophen, dextromethorphan, and phenylephrine *on page 32*
Alka-Seltzer Plus® Sinus Formula [OTC] *see* acetaminophen and phenylephrine *on page 28*
Alkeran® *see* melphalan *on page 556*
All Day Allergy [OTC] *see* cetirizine *on page 189*
Allegra® *see* fexofenadine *on page 375*
Allegra-D® (Can) *see* fexofenadine and pseudoephedrine *on page 375*
Allegra-D® 12 Hour *see* fexofenadine and pseudoephedrine *on page 375*
Allegra-D® 24 Hour *see* fexofenadine and pseudoephedrine *on page 375*
Allegra® Allergy 12 Hour [OTC] *see* fexofenadine *on page 375*
Allegra® Allergy 24 Hour [OTC] *see* fexofenadine *on page 375*
Allegra® Children's Allergy [OTC] *see* fexofenadine *on page 375*
Allegra® Children's Allergy ODT [OTC] *see* fexofenadine *on page 375*
Allegra® ODT [DSC] *see* fexofenadine *on page 375*
Aller-Chlor® [OTC] *see* chlorpheniramine *on page 197*
Allerdryl® (Can) *see* diphenhydramine (systemic) *on page 290*

Allerest *see* chlorpheniramine and pseudoephedrine *on page 199*
Allerfrim [OTC] *see* triprolidine and pseudoephedrine *on page 893*
AllerMax® [OTC] *see* diphenhydramine (systemic) *on page 290*
Allernix (Can) *see* diphenhydramine (systemic) *on page 290*
AlleRx™-D [DSC] *see* pseudoephedrine and methscopolamine *on page 753*
Allfen [OTC] *see* guaifenesin *on page 425*
Allfen CD *see* guaifenesin and codeine *on page 426*
Allfen CDX *see* guaifenesin and codeine *on page 426*
Allfen DM [OTC] [DSC] *see* guaifenesin and dextromethorphan *on page 427*
Alli® [OTC] *see* orlistat *on page 655*
All-Nite [OTC] *see* acetaminophen, dextromethorphan, and doxylamine *on page 32*
All-Nite Multi-Symptom Cold/Flu [OTC] *see* acetaminophen, dextromethorphan, doxylamine, and pseudoephedrine *on page 33*
Alloprin® (Can) *see* allopurinol *on page 54*

allopurinol (al oh PURE i nole)

Medication Safety Issues
Sound-alike/look-alike issues:
Allopurinol may be confused with Apresoline
Zyloprim® may be confused with ZORprin®, Zovirax®
Synonyms allopurinol sodium
U.S. Brand Names Aloprim®; Zyloprim®
Canadian Brand Names Alloprin®; Apo-Allopurinol®; Novo-Purol; Zyloprim®
Therapeutic Category Xanthine Oxidase Inhibitor
Use
Oral: Management of primary or secondary gout (acute attack, tophi, joint destruction, uric acid lithiasis, and/or nephropathy); management of hyperuricemia associated with cancer treatment for leukemia, lymphoma, or solid tumor malignancies; management of recurrent calcium oxalate calculi (with uric acid excretion >800 mg/day in men and >750 mg/day in women)
I.V.: Management of hyperuricemia associated with cancer treatment for leukemia, lymphoma, or solid tumor malignancies
General Dosage Range Dosage adjustment recommended in patients with renal impairment
I.V.:
Children: Initial: 200 mg/m^2/day as a single infusion or in equally divided doses at 6-, 8-, or 12-hour intervals
Adults: 200-400 mg/m^2/day as a single infusion or in equally divided doses at 6-, 8-, or 12-hour intervals (maximum: 600 mg/day)
Oral:
Children <6 years: 150 mg/day
Children 6-10 years: 10 mg/kg/day
Children >10 years and Adults: 100-800 mg/day in 1-3 divided doses (maximum: 800 mg/day)
Dosage Forms
Injection, powder for reconstitution: 500 mg (base)
Aloprim®: 500 mg (base)
Tablet, oral: 100 mg, 300 mg
Zyloprim®: 100 mg, 300 mg

allopurinol sodium *see* allopurinol *on page 54*
all-*trans* retinoic acid *see* tretinoin (systemic) *on page 885*
all-*trans* vitamin A acid *see* tretinoin (systemic) *on page 885*
Almacone® [OTC] *see* aluminum hydroxide, magnesium hydroxide, and simethicone *on page 60*
Almacone Double Strength® [OTC] *see* aluminum hydroxide, magnesium hydroxide, and simethicone *on page 60*

almotriptan (al moh TRIP tan)

Medication Safety Issues
Sound-alike/look-alike issues:
Axert® may be confused with Antivert®

Synonyms almotriptan malate

U.S. Brand Names Axert®

Canadian Brand Names Axert®

Therapeutic Category Serotonin 5-HT$_{1D}$ Receptor Agonist

Use Acute treatment of migraine with or without aura in adults (with a history of migraine) and adolescents (with a history of migraine lasting ≥4 hours when left untreated)

General Dosage Range Dosage adjustment recommended in patients with hepatic or renal impairment and/or on concomitant therapy

Oral: *Children ≥12 years and Adults:* 6.25-12.5 mg in a single dose; may repeat after 2 hours (maximum daily dose: 25 mg)

Dosage Forms
Tablet, oral:
Axert®: 6.25 mg, 12.5 mg

almotriptan malate *see* almotriptan *on page 54*

Alocril® *see* nedocromil *on page 615*

Alodox™ *see* doxycycline *on page 312*

Aloe Vesta® Antifungal [OTC] *see* miconazole (topical) *on page 585*

Alomide® *see* lodoxamide *on page 533*

Alophen® [OTC] *see* bisacodyl *on page 134*

Aloprim® *see* allopurinol *on page 54*

Alora® *see* estradiol (systemic) *on page 343*

alosetron (a LOE se tron)

Medication Safety Issues
Sound-alike/look-alike issues:
Lotronex® may be confused with Lovenox®, Protonix®

U.S. Brand Names Lotronex®

Therapeutic Category 5-HT$_3$ Receptor Antagonist

Use Treatment of women with severe diarrhea-predominant irritable bowel syndrome (IBS) who have failed to respond to conventional therapy

General Dosage Range Oral: *Adults:* Initial: 0.5 mg twice daily; may increase to 1 mg twice daily if needed (maximum: 2 mg/day)

Dosage Forms
Tablet, oral:
Lotronex®: 0.5 mg, 1 mg

Aloxi® *see* palonosetron *on page 669*

alpha₁-antiprotease *see* alpha₁-proteinase inhibitor *on page 55*

alpha₁-antitrypsin *see* alpha₁-proteinase inhibitor *on page 55*

A₁-PI *see* alpha₁-proteinase inhibitor *on page 55*

α₁-PI *see* alpha₁-proteinase inhibitor *on page 55*

alpha₁-PI *see* alpha₁-proteinase inhibitor *on page 55*

alpha₁-proteinase inhibitor, human *see* alpha₁-proteinase inhibitor *on page 55*

alpha₁-proteinase inhibitor (al fa won PRO tee in ase in HI bi tor)

Synonyms A₁-PI; alpha₁-antiprotease; alpha₁-antitrypsin; alpha₁-PI; alpha₁-proteinase inhibitor, human; α₁-PI

U.S. Brand Names Aralast NP; Glassia™; Prolastin®-C; Zemaira®

Canadian Brand Names Prolastin®-C

Therapeutic Category Antitrypsin Deficiency Agent

Use Replacement therapy in congenital alpha₁-proteinase inhibitor (alpha₁-antitrypsin, A₁-PI) deficiency with clinical emphysema

General Dosage Range I.V.: *Adults:* 60 mg/kg once weekly

▶

◄ **Dosage Forms**
  Injection, powder for reconstitution [preservative free]:
    Aralast NP: ~500 mg, ~1000 mg
    Prolastin®-C: ~1000 mg
    Zemaira®: ~1000 mg
  Injection, solution [preservative free]:
    Glassia™: ~1000 mg (50 mL)

alpha-galactosidase (AL fa ga lak TOE si days)

Medication Safety Issues
  Sound-alike/look-alike issues:
    beano® may be confused with B&O (belladonna and opium)
Synonyms *Aspergillus niger*
U.S. Brand Names beano® Meltaways [OTC]; beano® [OTC]
Therapeutic Category Enzyme
Use Prevention of flatulence and bloating attributed to a variety of grains, cereals, nuts, and vegetables
General Dosage Range Oral: *Children ≥12 years and Adults:*
  Tablet, chewable (beano®): Usual dose: 2-3 tablets/meal
  Tablet, orally disintegrating (beano® Meltaways): One tablet per meal
Dosage Forms
  Tablet, chewable, oral:
    beano® [OTC]: 150 Galactosidase units
  Tablet, orally disintegrating, oral:
    beano® Meltaways [OTC]: 300 Galactosidase units

alpha-galactosidase-A (gene-activated) *see* agalsidase alfa *(Canada only) on page 43*
alpha-galactosidase-A (recombinant) *see* agalsidase beta *on page 43*
1α-hydroxyergocalciferol *see* doxercalciferol *on page 310*
Alphagan® (Can) *see* brimonidine *on page 141*
Alphagan® P *see* brimonidine *on page 141*
Alphanate® *see* antihemophilic factor/von Willebrand factor complex (human) *on page 82*
AlphaNine® SD *see* factor IX *on page 365*
Alphaquin HP® *see* hydroquinone *on page 453*
Alph-E [OTC] *see* vitamin E *on page 918*
Alph-E-Mixed [OTC] *see* vitamin E *on page 918*

alprazolam (al PRAY zoe lam)

Medication Safety Issues
  Sound-alike/look-alike issues:
    ALPRAZolam may be confused with alprostadil, LORazepam, triazolam
    Xanax® may be confused with Fanapt®, Lanoxin®, Tenex®, Tylox®, Xopenex®, Zantac®, ZyrTEC®
  BEERS Criteria medication:
    This drug may be inappropriate for use in geriatric patients (high severity risk).
Tall-Man ALPRAZolam
U.S. Brand Names Alprazolam Intensol™; Niravam™; Xanax XR®; Xanax®
Canadian Brand Names Apo-Alpraz®; Apo-Alpraz® TS; Mylan-Alprazolam; Novo-Alprazol; Nu-Alpraz; Teva-Alprazolam; Xanax TS™; Xanax®
Therapeutic Category Benzodiazepine
Controlled Substance C-IV
Use Treatment of anxiety disorder (GAD); panic disorder, with or without agoraphobia; anxiety associated with depression
General Dosage Range Dosage adjustment recommended in patients with hepatic impairment
  Oral:
    Immediate release:
      Adults: 0.5-6 mg/day in divided doses (maximum: 10 mg/day)
      Elderly: Initial: 0.125-0.25 mg 2-3 times/day; Maintenance: Increase by 0.125 mg/day as needed
    Extended release:
      Adults: 0.5-6 once daily (maximum: 6 mg/day)
      Elderly: Initial: 0.5 mg/day

Dosage Forms
  Solution, oral:
    Alprazolam Intensol™: 1 mg/mL (30 mL)
  Tablet, oral: 0.25 mg, 0.5 mg, 1 mg, 2 mg
    Xanax®: 0.25 mg, 0.5 mg, 1 mg, 2 mg
  Tablet, extended release, oral: 0.5 mg, 1 mg, 2 mg, 3 mg
    Xanax XR®: 0.5 mg, 1 mg, 2 mg, 3 mg
  Tablet, orally disintegrating, oral: 0.25 mg, 0.5 mg, 1 mg, 2 mg
    Niravam™: 0.25 mg, 0.5 mg, 1 mg, 2 mg

Alprazolam Intensol™ *see* alprazolam *on page 56*

alprostadil (al PROS ta dill)

Medication Safety Issues
  Sound-alike/look-alike issues:
    Alprostadil may be confused with alPRAZolam
Synonyms PGE₁; prostaglandin E₁
U.S. Brand Names Caverject Impulse®; Caverject®; Edex®; Muse®; Prostin VR Pediatric®
Canadian Brand Names Caverject®; Muse® Pellet; Prostin® VR
Therapeutic Category Prostaglandin
Use
  Prostin VR Pediatric®: Temporary maintenance of patency of ductus arteriosus in neonates with ductal-dependent congenital heart disease until surgery can be performed. These defects include cyanotic (eg, pulmonary atresia, pulmonary stenosis, tricuspid atresia, Fallot tetralogy, transposition of the great vessels) and acyanotic (eg, interruption of aortic arch, coarctation of aorta, hypoplastic left ventricle) heart disease.
  Caverject®: Treatment of erectile dysfunction of vasculogenic, psychogenic, or neurogenic etiology; adjunct in the diagnosis of erectile dysfunction
  Edex®, Muse®: Treatment of erectile dysfunction of vasculogenic, psychogenic, or neurogenic etiology
General Dosage Range
  I.V.: *Neonates:* Initial: 0.05-0.1 mcg/kg/minute; Maintenance: 0.01-0.4 mcg/kg/minute
  Intracavernous: *Adults:* Initial: 1.25-2.5 mcg; Maintenance: Increase to effective dose no more than 3 times/week with at least 24 hours between doses (maximum: 40 mcg/dose [Edex®]; 60 mcg/dose [Caverject®])
  Intraurethral: *Adults:* Initial: 125-250 mcg; Maintenance: As needed (maximum: 2 doses/day)
Dosage Forms
  Injection, powder for reconstitution:
    Caverject Impulse®: 10 mcg, 20 mcg
    Caverject®: 20 mcg, 40 mcg
    Edex®: 10 mcg, 20 mcg, 40 mcg
  Injection, solution: 500 mcg/mL (1 mL)
    Prostin VR Pediatric®: 500 mcg/mL (1 mL)
  Pellet, urethral:
    Muse®: 125 mcg (1s, 6s); 250 mcg (1s, 6s); 500 mcg (1s, 6s); 1000 mcg (1s, 6s)

Alrex® *see* loteprednol *on page 539*

Alsuma™ *see* sumatriptan *on page 839*

Altabax™ *see* retapamulin *on page 775*

Altacaine *see* tetracaine (ophthalmic) *on page 856*

Altace® *see* ramipril *on page 766*

Altace® HCT (Can) *see* ramipril and hydrochlorothiazide *(Canada only) on page 766*

Altace® Plus Felodipine (Can) *see* ramipril and felodipine *(Canada only) on page 766*

Altachlore [OTC] *see* sodium chloride *on page 818*

Altafrin *see* phenylephrine (ophthalmic) *on page 697*

Altamist [OTC] *see* sodium chloride *on page 818*

Altaryl [OTC] *see* diphenhydramine (systemic) *on page 290*

alteplase (AL te plase)

Medication Safety Issues

Sound-alike/look-alike issues:
Activase® may be confused with Cathflo® Activase®, TNKase®
Alteplase may be confused with Altace®
"tPA" abbreviation should not be used when writing orders for this medication; has been misread as TNKase (tenecteplase)

High alert medication:
The Institute for Safe Medication Practices (ISMP) includes this medication (I.V.) among its list of drugs which have a heightened risk of causing significant patient harm when used in error.

Synonyms alteplase, recombinant; alteplase, tissue plasminogen activator, recombinant; tPA

U.S. Brand Names Activase®; Cathflo® Activase®

Canadian Brand Names Activase® rt-PA; Cathflo® Activase®

Therapeutic Category Fibrinolytic Agent

Use Management of ST-elevation myocardial infarction (STEMI) for the lysis of thrombi in coronary arteries; management of acute ischemic stroke (AIS); management of acute pulmonary embolism (PE)
Recommended criteria for treatment:
STEMI: Chest pain ≥20 minutes duration, onset of chest pain within 12 hours of treatment (or within prior 12-24 hours in patients with continuing ischemic symptoms), and ST-segment elevation >0.1 mV in at least two contiguous precordial leads or two adjacent limb leads on ECG or new or presumably new left bundle branch block (LBBB)
AIS: Onset of stroke symptoms within 3 hours of treatment
Acute pulmonary embolism: Age ≤75 years: Documented massive PE (defined as acute PE with sustained hypotension [SBP <90 mm Hg for ≤15 minutes or requiring inotropic support], persistent profound bradycardia [HR <40 bpm with signs or symptoms of shock], or pulselessness); alteplase may be considered for submassive PE with clinical evidence of adverse prognosis (eg, new hemodynamic instability, worsening respiratory insufficiency, severe RV dysfunction, or major myocardial necrosis) and low risk of bleeding complications. **Note:** Not recommended for patients with low-risk PE (eg, normotensive, no RV dysfunction, normal biomarkers) or submassive acute PE with minor RV dysfunction, minor myocardial necrosis, and no clinical worsening (Jaff, 2011).
Cathflo® Activase®: Restoration of central venous catheter function

General Dosage Range

Intracatheter:
Children <30 kg: 110% of the internal lumen volume of the catheter; retain in catheter for 0.5-2 hours; may repeat once (maximum: 2 mg/2 mL/dose)
Children ≥30 kg and Adults: 2 mg (2 mL) retain in catheter for 0.5-2 hours; may repeat once
I.V. infusion: *Adults:* Dosage varies greatly depending on indication

Dosage Forms

Injection, powder for reconstitution:
Activase®: 50 mg [29 million int. units], 100 mg [58 million int. units]
Cathflo® Activase®: 2 mg

altretamine (al TRET a meen)

Medication Safety Issues
High alert medication:
This medication is in a class the Institute for Safe Medication Practices (ISMP) includes among its list of drug classes which have a heightened risk of causing significant patient harm when used in error.
International issues:
Hexalen: Brand name altretamine [U.S., Canada, and Thailand], but also brand name for hexetidine [Greece]
Synonyms hexamethylmelamine; HEXM; HMM; HXM; NSC-13875
U.S. Brand Names Hexalen®
Canadian Brand Names Hexalen®
Therapeutic Category Antineoplastic Agent
Use Palliative treatment of persistent or recurrent ovarian cancer
General Dosage Range Dosage adjustment recommended in patients who develop toxicities
Oral: *Adults:* 260 mg/m^2/day in 4 divided doses for 14 or 21 days of a 28-day cycle
Dosage Forms
Capsule, oral:
Hexalen®: 50 mg

aluminum chloride hexahydrate (a LOO mi num KLOR ide heks a HYE drate)

Medication Safety Issues
Sound-alike/look-alike issues:
Drysol™ may be confused with Drisdol®
U.S. Brand Names Certain Dri® [OTC]; Drysol™; Hypercare™; Xerac™ AC
Therapeutic Category Topical Skin Product
Use Astringent in the management of hyperhidrosis
General Dosage Range Topical: *Adults:* Apply once daily
Dosage Forms
Solution, topical:
Certain Dri® [OTC]: 12% (36 mL)
Drysol™: 20% (35 mL, 37.5 mL, 60 mL)
Hypercare™: 20% (35 mL, 37.5 mL, 60 mL)
Xerac™ AC: 6.25% (35 mL, 60 mL)

aluminum hydroxide (a LOO mi num hye DROKS ide)

U.S. Brand Names ALternaGel® [OTC]; Dermagran® [OTC]
Canadian Brand Names Amphojel®; Basaljel®
Therapeutic Category Antacid
Use Treatment of hyperacidity; hyperphosphatemia; temporary protection of minor cuts, scrapes, and burns
General Dosage Range
Oral:
Children: 50-150 mg/kg/day in divided doses every 4-6 hours
Adults: 300-1200 mg 3-4 times/day
Topical: *Children and Adults:* Apply to affected area as needed; reapply at least every 12 hours
Dosage Forms
Ointment, topical:
Dermagran® [OTC]: 0.275% (113 g)
Suspension, oral: 320 mg/5 mL (30 mL, 355 mL, 473 mL); 600 mg/5 mL (355 mL)
ALternaGel® [OTC]: 600 mg/5 mL (360 mL)

aluminum hydroxide and magnesium carbonate

(a LOO mi num hye DROKS ide & mag NEE zhum KAR bun nate)
Medication Safety Issues
International issues:
Remegel [Netherlands] may be confused with Renagel brand name for sevelamer [U.S., Canada, and multiple international markets]

Remegel: Brand name for aluminum hydroxide and magnesium carbonate [Netherlands], but also the brand name for calcium carbonate [Great Britain, Hungary, and Ireland]

Synonyms magnesium carbonate and aluminum hydroxide

U.S. Brand Names Acid Gone Extra Strength [OTC]; Acid Gone [OTC]; Gaviscon® Extra Strength [OTC]; Gaviscon® Liquid [OTC]; Genaton™ [OTC]

Therapeutic Category Antacid

Use Temporary relief of symptoms associated with gastric acidity

General Dosage Range Oral: *Adults:* 15-30 mL **or** 2-4 tablets 4 times/day

Dosage Forms
Liquid: Aluminum hydroxide 31.7 mg and magnesium carbonate 119.3 mg per 5 mL; aluminum hydroxide 84.6 mg and magnesium carbonate 79.1 mg per 5 mL
Acid Gone [OTC], Gaviscon® [OTC], Genaton™ [OTC]: Aluminum hydroxide 31.7 mg and magnesium carbonate 119.3 mg per 5 mL
Gaviscon® Extra Strength [OTC]: Aluminum hydroxide 84.6 mg and magnesium carbonate 79.1 mg per 5 mL
Tablet, chewable: Aluminum hydroxide 160 mg and magnesium carbonate 105 mg
Acid Gone Extra Strength [OTC], Gaviscon® Extra Strength [OTC]: Aluminum hydroxide 160 mg and magnesium carbonate 105 mg

aluminum hydroxide and magnesium hydroxide
(a LOO mi num hye DROKS ide & mag NEE zhum hye DROK side)

Synonyms magnesium hydroxide and aluminum hydroxide

U.S. Brand Names Alamag [OTC]; Mag-Al Ultimate [OTC]; Mag-Al [OTC]

Canadian Brand Names Diovol®; Diovol® Ex; Gelusil® Extra Strength; Mylanta™

Therapeutic Category Antacid

Use Antacid for symptoms related to hyperacidity associated with heartburn, hiatal hernia, upset stomach, peptic ulcer, peptic esophagitis, or gastritis

General Dosage Range Oral: *Children ≥12 years and Adults:* 10-20 mL 4 times/day (maximum: magnesium hydroxide 4500 mg/day; aluminum hydroxide 4500 mg/day) **or** 1-2 tablets as needed (maximum: 16 tablets)

Dosage Forms
Liquid, oral:
Mag-Al [OTC]: Aluminum hydroxide 200 mg and magnesium hydroxide 200 mg per 5 mL
Suspension, oral:
Mag-Al Ultimate [OTC]: Aluminum hydroxide 500 mg and magnesium hydroxide 500 mg per 5 mL
Tablet, chewable:
Alamag [OTC]: Aluminum hydroxide 300 mg and magnesium hydroxide 150 mg

aluminum hydroxide and magnesium trisilicate
(a LOO mi num hye DROKS ide & mag NEE zhum trye SIL i kate)

Synonyms magnesium trisilicate and aluminum hydroxide

U.S. Brand Names Gaviscon® Tablet [OTC]

Therapeutic Category Antacid

Use Temporary relief of hyperacidity

General Dosage Range Oral: *Adults:* 2-4 tablets 4 times/day

Dosage Forms
Tablet, chewable: Aluminum hydroxide 80 mg and magnesium trisilicate 20 mg
Gaviscon® [OTC]: Aluminum hydroxide 80 mg and magnesium trisilicate 20 mg

aluminum hydroxide, magnesium hydroxide, and simethicone
(a LOO mi num hye DROKS ide, mag NEE zhum hye DROKS ide, & sye METH i kone)

Medication Safety Issues
Sound-alike/look-alike issues:
Maalox® may be confused with Maox®, Monodox®
Mylanta® may be confused with Mynatal®
Other safety concerns:
Liquid Maalox® products contain a different formulation than Maalox® Total Relief® which contains bismuth subsalicylate.

Synonyms magnesium hydroxide, aluminum hydroxide, and simethicone; simethicone, aluminum hydroxide, and magnesium hydroxide

U.S. Brand Names Alamag Plus [OTC]; Aldroxicon I [OTC]; Aldroxicon II [OTC]; Almacone Double Strength® [OTC]; Almacone® [OTC]; Gelusil® [OTC]; Maalox® Advanced Maximum Strength [OTC]; Maalox® Advanced Regular Strength [OTC]; Mi-Acid Maximum Strength [OTC] [DSC]; Mi-Acid [OTC]; Mintox Plus [OTC]; Mylanta® Classic Maximum Strength Liquid [OTC]; Mylanta® Classic Regular Strength Liquid [OTC]; Rulox [OTC]

Canadian Brand Names Diovol Plus®; Gelusil®; Mylanta® Double Strength; Mylanta® Extra Strength; Mylanta® Regular Strength

Therapeutic Category Antacid; Antiflatulent

Use Temporary relief of hyperacidity associated with gas; may also be used for indications associated with other antacids

General Dosage Range Oral: *Adults:* 10-20 mL or 2-4 tablets 4-6 times/day

Dosage Forms

Liquid: Aluminum hydroxide 200 mg, magnesium hydroxide 200 mg, and simethicone 20 mg per 5 mL; aluminum hydroxide 400 mg, magnesium hydroxide 400 mg, and simethicone 40 mg per 5 mL

Aldroxicon I [OTC], Almacone® [OTC], Maalox® Advanced Regular Strength [OTC], Mi-Acid [OTC], Mylanta® Classic Regular Strength [OTC]: Aluminum hydroxide 200 mg, magnesium hydroxide 200 mg, and simethicone 20 mg per 5 mL

Aldroxicon II [OTC], Almacone Double Strength [OTC], Maalox® Advanced Maximum Strength [OTC], Mi-Acid Maximum Strength [OTC], Mylanta® Classic Maximum Strength [OTC]: Aluminum hydroxide 400 mg, magnesium hydroxide 400 mg, and simethicone 40 mg per 5 mL

Suspension: Aluminum hydroxide 225 mg, magnesium hydroxide 200 mg, and simethicone 25 mg per 5 mL

Rulox [OTC]: Aluminum hydroxide 200 mg, magnesium hydroxide 200 mg, and simethicone 25 mg per 5 mL

Tablet, chewable: Aluminum hydroxide 200 mg, magnesium hydroxide 200 mg, and simethicone 25 mg

Alamag Plus [OTC], Gelusil® [OTC], Mintox Plus [OTC]: Aluminum hydroxide 200 mg, magnesium hydroxide 200 mg, and simethicone 25 mg

Almacone® [OTC]: Aluminum hydroxide 200 mg, magnesium hydroxide 200 mg, and simethicone 20 mg

aluminum sucrose sulfate, basic *see* sucralfate *on page 833*

aluminum sulfate and calcium acetate (a LOO mi num SUL fate & KAL see um AS e tate)

Synonyms calcium acetate and aluminum sulfate

U.S. Brand Names Domeboro® [OTC]; Gordon Boro-Packs [OTC]; Pedi-Boro® [OTC]

Therapeutic Category Topical Skin Product

Use Astringent wet dressing for relief of inflammatory conditions of the skin; reduce weeping that may occur in dermatitis

General Dosage Range Topical: *Adults:* Soak affected area or wet dressing in the solution 2-4 times/day

Dosage Forms

Powder, for topical solution:

Domeboro® [OTC]: Aluminum sulfate 1191 mg and calcium acetate 839 mg per packet (12s, 100s)

Gordon Boro-Packs: Aluminum sulfate 49% and calcium acetate 51% per packet (100s)

Pedi-Boro® [OTC]: Aluminum sulfate 1191 mg and calcium acetate 839 mg per packet (12s, 100s)

Alupent *see* metaproterenol *on page 566*

Alvesco® *see* ciclesonide (oral inhalation) *on page 207*

alvimopan (al VI moe pan)

Medication Safety Issues

Sound-alike/look-alike issues:

Alvimopan may be confused with almotriptan

Synonyms ADL-2698; LY246736

U.S. Brand Names Entereg®

Therapeutic Category Gastrointestinal Agent, Miscellaneous; Opioid Antagonist, Peripherally-Acting

Use Accelerate the time to upper and lower GI recovery following partial large or small bowel resection surgery with primary anastomosis

◀ **General Dosage Range Oral:** *Adults:* Initial: 12 mg prior to surgery; Maintenance: 12 mg twice daily (maximum: 15 doses)

Dosage Forms
Capsule, oral:
Entereg®: 12 mg

amantadine (a MAN ta deen)

Medication Safety Issues
Sound-alike/look-alike issues:
Amantadine may be confused with ranitidine, rimantadine
Symmetrel may be confused with Synthroid®

Synonyms adamantanamine hydrochloride; amantadine hydrochloride; Symmetrel

Canadian Brand Names Endantadine®; Mylan-Amantadine; PMS-Amantadine; Symmetrel®

Therapeutic Category Anti-Parkinson Agent (Dopamine Agonist); Antiviral Agent

Use Prophylaxis and treatment of influenza A viral infection (per manufacturer labeling; also refer to current ACIP guidelines for recommendations during current flu season); treatment of parkinsonism; treatment of drug-induced extrapyramidal symptoms

General Dosage Range Dosage adjustment recommended in patients with renal impairment
Oral:
Children 1-9 years: 4.4-8.8 mg/kg/day in 2 divided doses (maximum: 150 mg/day)
Children ≥10 years and <40 kg: 5 mg/kg/day in 2 divided doses
Children ≥10 years and ≥40 kg: 100 mg twice daily (maximum: 200 mg/day)
Adults: 200-400 mg/day in 2 divided doses (maximum: 400 mg/day)
Elderly: 100-400 mg/day in 2 divided doses (maximum: 400 mg/day)

Dosage Forms
Capsule, oral: 100 mg
Capsule, softgel, oral: 100 mg
Solution, oral: 50 mg/5 mL (473 mL)
Syrup, oral: 50 mg/5 mL (10 mL, 473 mL, 480 mL)
Tablet, oral: 100 mg

amantadine hydrochloride *see* amantadine *on page 62*
Amaryl® *see* glimepiride *on page 418*
Amatine® (Can) *see* midodrine *on page 588*

ambenonium (am be NOE nee um)

Synonyms ambenonium chloride
U.S. Brand Names Mytelase®
Canadian Brand Names Mytelase®
Therapeutic Category Cholinergic Agent
Use Treatment of myasthenia gravis
General Dosage Range Oral: *Adults:* 5-25 mg 3-4 times/day
Dosage Forms
Caplet, oral:
Mytelase®: 10 mg

ambenonium chloride *see* ambenonium *on page 62*
Ambi 10PEH/400GFN [OTC] *see* guaifenesin and phenylephrine *on page 428*
Ambien® *see* zolpidem *on page 933*
Ambien CR® *see* zolpidem *on page 933*
Ambifed [OTC] [DSC] *see* guaifenesin and pseudoephedrine *on page 429*
Ambifed DM *see* guaifenesin, pseudoephedrine, and dextromethorphan *on page 430*
Ambifed-G [OTC] *see* guaifenesin and pseudoephedrine *on page 429*
Ambifed-G DM *see* guaifenesin, pseudoephedrine, and dextromethorphan *on page 430*
AmBisome® *see* amphotericin B liposomal *on page 76*

ambrisentan (am bri SEN tan)

Synonyms BSF208075
U.S. Brand Names Letairis®

Canadian Brand Names Volibris®

Therapeutic Category Endothelin Antagonist

Use Treatment of pulmonary artery hypertension (PAH) World Health Organization (WHO) Group I to improve exercise ability and decrease the rate of clinical deterioration

General Dosage Range Dosage adjustment recommended in patients on concomitant therapy.
Oral: *Adults:* Initial: 5 mg once daily (maximum: 10 mg/day)

Dosage Forms
Tablet, oral:
Letairis®: 5 mg, 10 mg

amcinonide (am SIN oh nide)

Canadian Brand Names Amcort®; Cyclocort®; ratio-Amcinonide; Taro-Amcinonide

Therapeutic Category Corticosteroid, Topical

Use Relief of the inflammatory and pruritic manifestations of corticosteroid-responsive dermatoses (high potency corticosteroid)

General Dosage Range Topical: *Adults:* Apply in a thin film 2-3 times/day

Dosage Forms
Cream, topical: 0.1% (15 g, 30 g, 60 g)
Lotion, topical: 0.1% (60 mL)
Ointment, topical: 0.1% (15 g, 30 g, 60 g)

Amcort® (Can) see amcinonide on page 63

AMD3100 see plerixafor on page 710

Amdry-C see chlorpheniramine, pseudoephedrine, and methscopolamine on page 202

Amerge® see naratriptan on page 613

Americaine® Hemorrhoidal [OTC] see benzocaine on page 121

A-Methapred® see methylprednisolone on page 578

Amethia™ see ethinyl estradiol and levonorgestrel on page 353

amethocaine hydrochloride see tetracaine (ophthalmic) on page 856

amethocaine hydrochloride see tetracaine (systemic) on page 856

amethocaine hydrochloride see tetracaine (topical) on page 856

amethopterin see methotrexate on page 571

Amethyst™ see ethinyl estradiol and levonorgestrel on page 353

Ametop™ (Can) see tetracaine (topical) on page 856

Amevive® see alefacept on page 48

amfepramone see diethylpropion on page 281

AMG 073 see cinacalcet on page 209

AMG-162 see denosumab on page 259

AMG 531 see romiplostim on page 789

Amicar® see aminocaproic acid on page 65

Amidate® see etomidate on page 360

amifostine (am i FOS teen)

Medication Safety Issues
Sound-alike/look-alike issues:
Ethyol® may be confused with ethanol

Synonyms ethiofos; gammaphos; WR-2721; YM-08310

U.S. Brand Names Ethyol®

Canadian Brand Names Ethyol®

Therapeutic Category Antidote

Use Reduce the incidence of moderate-to-severe xerostomia in patients undergoing postoperative radiation treatment for head and neck cancer, where the radiation port includes a substantial portion of the parotid glands; reduce the cumulative renal toxicity associated with repeated administration of cisplatin

General Dosage Range I.V.: *Adults:* 910 mg/m^2 once daily 30 minutes prior to cytotoxic therapy **or** 200 mg/m^2/day 15-30 minutes prior to radiation therapy

◀ **Dosage Forms**
Injection, powder for reconstitution: 500 mg
Ethyol®: 500 mg

Amigesic® (Can) see salsalate on page 799
Ami-Hydro (Can) see amiloride and hydrochlorothiazide on page 64

amikacin (am i KAY sin)

Medication Safety Issues
Sound-alike/look-alike issues:
Amikacin may be confused with Amicar®, anakinra
Amikin® may be confused with Amicar®, Kineret®
Synonyms amikacin sulfate
Canadian Brand Names Amikacin Sulfate Injection, USP; Amikin®
Therapeutic Category Aminoglycoside (Antibiotic)
Use Treatment of serious infections (bone infections, respiratory tract infections, endocarditis, and septicemia) due to organisms resistant to gentamicin and tobramycin, including *Pseudomonas*, *Proteus*, *Serratia*, and other gram-negative bacilli; documented infection of mycobacterial organisms susceptible to amikacin
General Dosage Range Dosage adjustment recommended in patients with renal impairment
I.M.: *Infants, Children, and Adults:* 5-7.5 mg/kg/dose every 8 hours (maximum: 20 mg/kg/day)
I.V.:
Infants and Children: 5-7.5 mg/kg/dose every 8 hours (maximum: 20 mg/kg/day)
Adults: 5-7.5 mg/kg/dose every 8 hours **or** 15-20 mg/kg as a single daily dose (maximum: 20 mg/kg/day)
Dosage Forms
Injection, solution: 250 mg/mL (2 mL, 4 mL)

amikacin sulfate see amikacin on page 64
Amikacin Sulfate Injection, USP (Can) see amikacin on page 64
Amikin® (Can) see amikacin on page 64

amiloride (a MIL oh ride)

Medication Safety Issues
Sound-alike/look-alike issues:
AMILoride may be confused with amiodarone, amLODIPine, inamrinone
Synonyms amiloride hydrochloride
Tall-Man aMILoride
Canadian Brand Names Apo-Amiloride®; Midamor
Therapeutic Category Diuretic, Potassium Sparing
Use Counteracts potassium loss induced by other diuretics in the treatment of hypertension or edematous conditions including CHF, hepatic cirrhosis, and hypoaldosteronism; usually used in conjunction with more potent diuretics such as thiazides or loop diuretics
General Dosage Range Dosage adjustment recommended in patients with renal impairment
Oral:
Adults: 5-10 mg/day in 1-2 divided doses (maximum: 20 mg/day)
Elderly: Initial: 5 mg once daily or every other day
Dosage Forms
Tablet, oral: 5 mg

amiloride and hydrochlorothiazide (a MIL oh ride & hye droe klor oh THYE a zide)

Synonyms hydrochlorothiazide and amiloride
Canadian Brand Names Ami-Hydro; Apo-Amilzide®; Gen-Amilazide; Moduret; Novamilor; Nu-Amilzide
Therapeutic Category Diuretic, Combination
Use Potassium-sparing diuretic; antihypertensive
General Dosage Range Dosage adjustment recommended in patients with renal impairment
Oral:
Adults: 1-2 tablets (amiloride 5 mg/HCTZ 50 mg per tablet) once daily (maximum: 2 tablets/day)
Elderly: Initial: 1/2 to 1 tablet/day (maximum: 2 tablets/day)

Dosage Forms
  Tablet: 5/50: Amiloride 5 mg and hydrochlorothiazide 50 mg

amiloride hydrochloride *see* amiloride *on page 64*
2-amino-6-mercaptopurine *see* thioguanine *on page 862*
2-amino-6-methoxypurine arabinoside *see* nelarabine *on page 616*
2-amino-6-trifluoromethoxy-benzothiazole *see* riluzole *on page 781*

amino acid injection (a MEE noe AS id in JEK shun)

Medication Safety Issues
  Sound-alike/look-alike issues:
    TrophAmine® may be confused with tromethamine

U.S. Brand Names Aminosyn®; Aminosyn® II; Aminosyn®-HBC; Aminosyn®-PF; Aminosyn®-RF; BranchAmin®; Clinisol®; FreAmine® HBC; FreAmine® III; HepatAmine®; Hepatasol®; NephrAmine®; PremaSol™; Prosol; Travasol®; TrophAmine®

Canadian Brand Names Aminosyn; Aminosyn-PF; Aminosyn-RF; Primene®

Therapeutic Category Intravenous Nutritional Therapy

Use As part of parenteral nutrition to prevent nitrogen loss or treat negative nitrogen balance when alimentary tract cannot be used (eg, GI absorption is impaired, bowel rest is needed). Specialty amino acid formulas may be considered only in certain instances.

General Dosage Range Dosage adjustment recommended in patients with hepatic or renal impairment
I.V.:
  Children: 1-3.85 g/kg/day
  Adults: 0.8-2 g/kg/day

Dosage Forms
  Injection, solution:
    Aminosyn®: 8.5% (500 mL); 10% (500 mL, 1000 mL)
    Aminosyn® II: 8.5% (500 mL); 10% (500 mL, 1000 mL, 2000 mL); 15% (2000 mL)
    Aminosyn®-HBC: 7% (500 mL)
    Aminosyn®-PF: 7% (500 mL); 10% (1000 mL)
    Aminosyn®-RF: 5.2% (500 mL)
    BranchAmin®: 4% (500 mL)
    Clinisol®: 15% (500 mL, 2000 mL)
    FreAmine® HBC: 6.9% (750 mL)
    FreAmine® III: 3% (1000 mL); 8.5% (500 mL); 10% (500 mL, 1000 mL)
    HepatAmine®: 8% (500 mL)
    Hepatasol®: 8% (500 mL)
    NephrAmine®: 5.4% (250 mL)
    PremaSol™: 6% (500 mL); 10% (500 mL, 1000 mL, 2000 mL)
    Prosol: 20% (2000 mL)
    Travasol®: 10% (500 mL, 1000 mL, 2000 mL)
    TrophAmine®: 6% (500 mL); 10% (500 mL)

aminobenzylpenicillin *see* ampicillin *on page 76*

aminocaproic acid (a mee noe ka PROE ik AS id)

Medication Safety Issues
  Sound-alike/look-alike issues:
    Amicar® may be confused with amikacin, Amikin®
  International issues:
    Amicar [U.S.] may be confused with Omacor brand name for Omega-3-Acid Ethyl Esters [multiple international markets]

Synonyms EACA; epsilon aminocaproic acid

U.S. Brand Names Amicar®

Therapeutic Category Hemostatic Agent

Use To enhance hemostasis when fibrinolysis contributes to bleeding (causes may include cardiac surgery, hematologic disorders, neoplastic disorders, abruption placentae, hepatic cirrhosis, and urinary fibrinolysis)

◀ **General Dosage Range**
I.V.: *Adults:* Dosage varies greatly depending on indication
Oral: *Adults:* Initial: Loading dose: 4-5 g for first hour; Maintenance: 1 g/hour (or 1.25 g/hour using oral solution) for 8 hours or until bleeding controlled (maximum: 30 g/day)
Dosage Forms
Injection, solution: 250 mg/mL (20 mL)
Solution, oral: 1.25 g/5 mL (237 mL, 473 mL)
Syrup, oral:
Amicar®: 1.25 g/5 mL (473 mL)
Tablet, oral: 500 mg
Amicar®: 500 mg, 1000 mg

aminolevulinic acid (a MEE noh lev yoo lin ik AS id)

Medication Safety Issues
Sound-alike/look-alike issues:
Aminolevulinic acid may be confused with methyl aminolevulinate
Synonyms 5-ALA; 5-aminolevulinic acid; ALA; amino levulinic acid; aminolevulinic acid hydrochloride
U.S. Brand Names Levulan® Kerastick®
Canadian Brand Names Levulan® Kerastick®
Therapeutic Category Photosensitizing Agent, Topical; Porphyrin Agent, Topical
Use Treatment of minimally to moderately thick actinic keratoses (grade 1 or 2) of the face or scalp; to be used in conjunction with blue light illumination
General Dosage Range Topical: *Adults:* Apply to actinic keratoses once; may repeat after 8 weeks
Dosage Forms
Powder for solution, topical:
Levulan® Kerastick®: 20% (6s)

amino levulinic acid *see* aminolevulinic acid *on page 66*
5-aminolevulinic acid *see* aminolevulinic acid *on page 66*
aminolevulinic acid hydrochloride *see* aminolevulinic acid *on page 66*

aminophylline (am in OFF i lin)

Medication Safety Issues
Sound-alike/look-alike issues:
Aminophylline may be confused with amitriptyline, ampicillin
Synonyms theophylline ethylenediamine
Canadian Brand Names Phyllocontin®; Phyllocontin®-350
Therapeutic Category Theophylline Derivative
Use Treatment of symptoms and reversible airway obstruction due to asthma or other chronic lung diseases (eg, emphysema, chronic bronchitis)

Note: The National Heart, Lung, and Blood Institute Guidelines (2007) do not recommend aminophylline I.V. for the treatment of asthma exacerbations.
General Dosage Range
I.V.:
Infants to Adults: Loading dose: 5.7 mg/kg
Children 6 weeks to 1 year: Maintenance: Equivalent theophylline dose: mg/kg/hour = (0.008)(age in weeks) + 0.21
Children 1-9 years: Maintenance: 1.01 mg/kg/hour
Children 9-12 years: Maintenance: 0.89 mg/kg/hour
Adolescents 12-16 years (smokers): Maintenance: 0.89 mg/kg/hour
Adolescents 12-16 years (nonsmokers): Maintenance: 0.63 mg/kg/hour
Adolescents >16 years and Adults ≤60 years (nonsmokers): Maintenance: 0.51 mg/kg/hour (maximum: 900 mg/day)
Adults >60 years (nonsmokers): Maintenance: 0.38 mg/kg/hour (maximum: 400 mg/day)
Oral:
Children 1-15 years and <45 kg (without risk factors for impaired clearance): Initial: 15.2-17.7 mg/kg/day divided every 4-6 hours for 3 days (maximum: 380 mg), then increase to 20.3 mg/kg/day divided every 4-6 hours for 3 days (maximum: 400 mg/day); Maintenance: 25.3 mg/kg/day divided every 4-6 hours (maximum: 760 mg/day)

Children ≥45 kg and Adults: Initial: 380 mg/day divided every 6-8 hours for 3 days, then 507 mg/day divided every 6-8 hours for 3 days; Maintenance: 760 mg/day divided every 6-8 hours

Dosage Forms
  Injection, solution: 25 mg/mL (10 mL, 20 mL)
  Injection, solution [preservative free]: 25 mg/mL (10 mL, 20 mL)
  Tablet, oral: 100 mg, 200 mg
Dosage Forms - Canada
  Tablet, oral, sustained release as dihydrate
    Phyllocontin® 225 mg
    Phyllocontin®-350: 350 mg

4-aminopyridine *see* dalfampridine *on page 250*
aminosalicylate sodium *see* aminosalicylic acid *on page 67*

aminosalicylic acid (a mee noe sal i SIL ik AS id)

Synonyms 4-aminosalicylic acid; aminosalicylate sodium; para-aminosalicylate sodium; PAS; sodium PAS
U.S. Brand Names Paser®
Therapeutic Category Nonsteroidal Antiinflammatory Drug (NSAID)
Use Adjunctive treatment of tuberculosis used in combination with other antitubercular agents
General Dosage Range Dosage adjustment recommended in patients with renal impairment
  Oral:
    Children: 200-300 mg/kg/day in 3-4 equally divided doses
    Adults: 150 mg/kg/day in 2-3 equally divided doses
Dosage Forms
  Granules, delayed release, oral:
    Paser®: 4 g/packet (30s)

4-aminosalicylic acid *see* aminosalicylic acid *on page 67*
5-aminosalicylic acid *see* mesalamine *on page 564*
Aminosyn® *see* amino acid injection *on page 65*
Aminosyn (Can) *see* amino acid injection *on page 65*
Aminosyn® II *see* amino acid injection *on page 65*
Aminosyn®-HBC *see* amino acid injection *on page 65*
Aminosyn®-PF *see* amino acid injection *on page 65*
Aminosyn-PF (Can) *see* amino acid injection *on page 65*
Aminosyn®-RF *see* amino acid injection *on page 65*
Aminosyn-RF (Can) *see* amino acid injection *on page 65*
Aminoxin® [OTC] *see* pyridoxine *on page 758*

amiodarone (a MEE oh da rone)

Medication Safety Issues
  Sound-alike/look-alike issues:
    Amiodarone may be confused with aMILoride, inamrinone
    Cordarone® may be confused with Cardura®, Cordran®
  High alert medication:
    The Institute for Safe Medication Practices (ISMP) includes this medication among its list of drugs which have a heightened risk of causing significant patient harm when used in error.
  BEERS Criteria medication:
    This drug may be inappropriate for use in geriatric patients (high severity risk).
Synonyms amiodarone hydrochloride
U.S. Brand Names Cordarone®; Nexterone®; Pacerone®
Canadian Brand Names Apo-Amiodarone®; Cordarone®; Dom-Amiodarone; Mylan-Amiodarone; Novo-Amiodarone; PHL-Amiodarone; PMS-Amiodarone; PRO-Amiodarone; ratio-Amiodarone; ratio-Amiodarone I.V.; Riva-Amiodarone; Sandoz-Amiodarone; Teva-Amiodarone
Therapeutic Category Antiarrhythmic Agent, Class III
Use Management of life-threatening recurrent ventricular fibrillation (VF) or hemodynamically-unstable ventricular tachycardia (VT) refractory to other antiarrhythmic agents or in patients intolerant of other agents used for these conditions

◀ **General Dosage Range**
I.O.: *Children (PALS dosing):* 5 mg/kg (maximum: 300 mg/day); may repeat up to maximum dose of 15 mg/kg/day
I.V.:
Children (PALS dosing): 5 mg/kg (maximum: 300 mg/day); may repeat up to maximum dose of 15 mg/kg/day
Adults: Initial: 150-300 mg bolus **or** 5-7 mg/kg; Maintenance: 1200-1800 mg/day continuous infusion until 10 g total **or** 1 mg/minute infusion for 6 hours, then 0.5 mg/minute infusion for 18 hours (maximum: 2.1 g/day)
Oral: *Adults:* Initial: 600-1600 mg/day until 10 g total; Maintenance: 100-400 mg/day
Dosage Forms
Infusion, premixed iso-osmotic dextrose solution:
Nexterone®: 150 mg (100 mL); 360 mg (200 mL)
Injection, solution: 50 mg/mL (3 mL, 9 mL, 18 mL)
Tablet, oral: 200 mg, 400 mg
Cordarone®: 200 mg
Pacerone®: 100 mg, 200 mg, 400 mg

amiodarone hydrochloride *see* amiodarone *on page 67*
Amitiza® *see* lubiprostone *on page 541*

amitriptyline (a mee TRIP ti leen)
Medication Safety Issues
Sound-alike/look-alike issues:
Amitriptyline may be confused with aminophylline, imipramine, nortriptyline
Elavil® may be confused with Aldoril®, Eldepryl®, enalapril, Equanil®, Plavix®
BEERS Criteria medication:
This drug may be inappropriate for use in geriatric patients (high severity risk).
Synonyms amitriptyline hydrochloride; Elavil
Canadian Brand Names Apo-Amitriptyline®; Bio-Amitriptyline; Dom-Amitriptyline®; Elavil; Levate®; Novo-Triptyn; PMS-Amitriptyline
Therapeutic Category Antidepressant, Tricyclic (Tertiary Amine)
Use Relief of symptoms of depression
General Dosage Range Oral:
Adolescents: Initial: 25-50 mg/day; Maintenance: 25-100 mg/day (maximum: 100 mg/day)
Adults: 50-300 mg/day as a single dose at bedtime or in divided doses (maximum: 300 mg/day)
Elderly: Initial: 10-25 mg at bedtime; Maintenance: 25-150 mg/day (maximum: 150 mg/day)
Dosage Forms
Tablet, oral: 10 mg, 25 mg, 50 mg, 75 mg, 100 mg, 150 mg

amitriptyline and chlordiazepoxide (a mee TRIP ti leen & klor dye az e POKS ide)
Medication Safety Issues
BEERS Criteria medication:
This drug may be inappropriate for use in geriatric patients (high severity risk).
Synonyms chlordiazepoxide and amitriptyline hydrochloride; Limbitrol
Therapeutic Category Antidepressant, Tricyclic (Tertiary Amine)
Controlled Substance C-IV
Use Treatment of moderate-to-severe anxiety and/or agitation and depression
General Dosage Range Oral: *Adults:* 2-6 tablets (amitriptyline 12.5-25 mg/chlordiazepoxide 5-10 mg per tablet)/day (maximum: 6 tablets/day)
Dosage Forms
Tablet: 12.5/5: Amitriptyline 12.5 mg and chlordiazepoxide 5 mg; 25/10: Amitriptyline 25 mg and chlordiazepoxide 10 mg

amitriptyline and perphenazine (a mee TRIP ti leen & per FEN a zeen)
Synonyms perphenazine and amitriptyline hydrochloride
Canadian Brand Names PMS-Levazine
Therapeutic Category Antidepressant/Phenothiazine
Use Treatment of patients with moderate-to-severe anxiety and depression

General Dosage Range Oral: *Adults:* 1 tablet (amitriptyline 10-50 mg/perphenazine 2-4 mg per tablet) 2-4 times/day

Dosage Forms
Tablet: 2-10: Amitriptyline 10 mg and perphenazine 2 mg; 2-25: Amitriptyline 25 mg and perphenazine 2 mg; 4-10: Amitriptyline 10 mg and perphenazine 4 mg; 4-25: Amitriptyline 25 mg and perphenazine 4 mg; 4-50: Amitriptyline 50 mg and perphenazine 4 mg

amitriptyline hydrochloride *see* amitriptyline *on page 68*
AMJ 9701 *see* palifermin *on page 668*
AmLactin® [OTC] *see* lactic acid and ammonium hydroxide *on page 506*

amlexanox (am LEKS an oks)
U.S. Brand Names Aphthasol®
Therapeutic Category Antiinflammatory Agent, Locally Applied
Use Treatment of aphthous ulcers (ie, canker sores)
General Dosage Range Topical: *Adults:* ~1/4 inch (0.5 cm) directly on ulcers 4 times/day
Dosage Forms
Paste, oral:
Aphthasol®: 5% (3 g)

amlodipine (am LOE di peen)
Medication Safety Issues
Sound-alike/look-alike issues:
AmLODIPine may be confused with aMILoride
Norvasc® may be confused with Navane®, Norvir®, Vascor®
International issues:
Norvasc [U.S., Canada, and multiple international markets] may be confused with Vascor brand name for imidapril [Philippines] and simvastatin [Malaysia, Singapore, and Thailand]
Synonyms amlodipine besylate
Tall-Man amLODIPine
U.S. Brand Names Norvasc®
Canadian Brand Names Accel-Amlodipine; Apo-Amlodipine®; CO Amlodipine; Dom-Amlodipine; GD-Amlodipine; JAMP-Amlodipine; Mint-Amlodipine; Mylan-Amlodipine; Norvasc®; PHL-Amlodipine; PMS-Amlodipine; RAN™-Amlodipine; ratio-Amlodipine; Riva-Amlodipine; Sandoz Amlodipine; Septa-Amlodipine; Teva-Amlodipine; ZYM-Amlodipine
Therapeutic Category Calcium Channel Blocker
Use Treatment of hypertension; treatment of symptomatic chronic stable angina, vasospastic (Prinzmetal) angina (confirmed or suspected); prevention of hospitalization due to angina with documented CAD (limited to patients without heart failure or ejection fraction <40%)
General Dosage Range Dosage adjustment recommended in patients with hepatic impairment
Oral:
Children 6-17 years: 2.5-5 mg once daily
Adults: Initial: 5 mg once daily; Maintenance: 2.5-10 mg once daily (maximum: 10 mg/day)
Elderly: 2.5-5 mg once daily
Dosage Forms
Tablet, oral: 2.5 mg, 5 mg, 10 mg
Norvasc®: 2.5 mg, 5 mg, 10 mg

amlodipine, aliskiren, and hydrochlorothiazide *see* aliskiren, amlodipine, and hydrochlorothiazide *on page 52*
amlodipine and aliskiren *see* aliskiren and amlodipine *on page 52*

amlodipine and atorvastatin (am LOW di peen & a TORE va sta tin)
Synonyms atorvastatin and amlodipine; atorvastatin calcium and amlodipine besylate
U.S. Brand Names Caduet®
Canadian Brand Names Caduet®
Therapeutic Category Antilipemic Agent, HMG-CoA Reductase Inhibitor; Calcium Channel Blocker

◀ **Use** For use when treatment with both amlodipine and atorvastatin is appropriate:

Amlodipine: Treatment of hypertension; treatment of chronic stable angina, vasospastic (Prinzmetal) angina (confirmed or suspected); prevention of hospitalization or to decrease coronary revascularization procedure due to angina with documented CAD (limited to patients without heart failure or ejection fraction <40%)

Atorvastatin: Treatment of dyslipidemias or primary prevention of cardiovascular disease (atherosclerotic) as detailed here:

Primary prevention of cardiovascular disease (high-risk for CVD): To reduce the risk of MI or stroke in patients without evidence of coronary heart disease who have multiple CVD risk factors or type 2 diabetes; also reduces the risk for angina or revascularization procedures in patients with multiple CVD risk factors without evidence of coronary heart disease

Secondary prevention of cardiovascular disease: To reduce the risk of MI, stroke, revascularization procedures, angina, and hospitalization for heart failure

Treatment of dyslipidemias: To reduce elevations in total cholesterol, LDL-C, apolipoprotein B, and triglycerides in patients with elevations of one or more components, and/or to increase low HDL-C as present in heterozygous familial/nonfamilial hypercholesterolemia and mixed dyslipidemia (Fredrickson type IIa and IIb hyperlipidemias); treatment of primary dysbetalipoproteinemia (Fredrickson type III), elevated serum TG levels (Fredrickson type IV), and homozygous familial hypercholesterolemia

Treatment of heterozygous familial hypercholesterolemia (HeFH) in adolescent patients (10-17 years of age, females >1 year postmenarche) having LDL-C ≥190 mg/dL or LDL-C ≥160 mg/dL with positive family history of premature cardiovascular disease (CVD) or with two or more CVD risk factors.

General Dosage Range Dosage adjustment recommended in patients on concomitant therapy

Oral:

Children 10-17 years (females >1 year postmenarche): 2.5-5 mg (amlodipine) and 10-20 mg (atorvastatin) once daily (maximum: amlodipine 5 mg/day; atorvastatin 20 mg/day)

Adults: 2.5-10 mg (amlodipine) and 10-80 mg (atorvastatin) once daily (maximum: amlodipine 10 mg/day; atorvastatin 80 mg/day)

Dosage Forms

Tablet:

Caduet®:

2.5/10: Amlodipine 2.5 mg and atorvastatin 10 mg; 2.5/20: Amlodipine 2.5 mg and atorvastatin 20 mg; 2.5/40: Amlodipine 2.5 mg and atorvastatin 40 mg

5/10: Amlodipine 5 mg and atorvastatin 10 mg; 5/20: Amlodipine 5 mg and atorvastatin 20 mg; 5/40: Amlodipine 5 mg and atorvastatin 40 mg; 5/80: Amlodipine 5 mg and atorvastatin 80 mg

10/10: Amlodipine 10 mg and atorvastatin 10 mg; 10/20: Amlodipine 10 mg and atorvastatin 20 mg; 10/40: Amlodipine 10 mg and atorvastatin 40 mg; 10/80: Amlodipine 10 mg and atorvastatin 80 mg

amlodipine and benazepril (am LOE di peen & ben AY ze pril)

Synonyms benazepril hydrochloride and amlodipine besylate

U.S. Brand Names Lotrel®

Therapeutic Category Antihypertensive Agent, Combination

Use Treatment of hypertension

General Dosage Range Dosage adjustment recommended in patients with hepatic impairment

Oral:

Adults: 2.5-10 mg (amlodipine) and 10-40 mg (benazepril) once daily (maximum: amlodipine 10 mg/day; benazepril 80 mg/day)

Elderly: Initial: 2.5 mg/day (based on amlodipine component)

Dosage Forms

Capsule: 2.5/10: Amlodipine 2.5 mg and benazepril 10 mg; 5/10: Amlodipine 5 mg and benazepril 10 mg; 5/20: Amlodipine 5 mg and benazepril 20 mg; 5/40: Amlodipine 5 mg and benazepril hydrochloride 40 mg; 10/20: Amlodipine 10 mg and benazepril 20 mg; 10/40: Amlodipine 10 mg and benazepril hydrochloride 40 mg

Lotrel®: 2.5/10: Amlodipine 2.5 and benazepril 10 mg; 5/10: Amlodipine 5 mg and benazepril 10 mg; 5/20: Amlodipine 5 mg and benazepril 20 mg; 5/40: Amlodipine 5 mg and benazepril 40 mg; 10/20: Amlodipine 10 mg and benazepril 20 mg; 10/40: Amlodipine 10 mg and benazepril 40 mg

amlodipine and olmesartan (am LOE di peen & olme SAR tan)

Synonyms amlodipine besylate and olmesartan medoxomil; olmesartan and amlodipine

U.S. Brand Names Azor™

Therapeutic Category Angiotensin II Receptor Blocker Combination; Antihypertensive Agent, Combination; Calcium Channel Blocker

Use Treatment of hypertension, including initial treatment in patients who will require multiple antihypertensives for adequate control

General Dosage Range Oral: *Adults:* Amlodipine 5-10 mg and olmesartan 20-40 mg once daily (maximum: 10 mg/day [amlodipine]; 40 mg/day [olmesartan])

Dosage Forms

Tablet:

Azor™: 5/20: Amlodipine 5 mg and olmesartan medoxomil 20 mg; 5/40: Amlodipine 5 mg and olmesartan medoxomil 40 mg; 10/20: Amlodipine 10 mg and olmesartan medoxomil 20 mg; 10/40: Amlodipine 10 mg and olmesartan medoxomil 40 mg

amlodipine and telmisartan *see* telmisartan and amlodipine *on page 848*

amlodipine and valsartan (am LOE di peen & val SAR tan)

Synonyms amlodipine besylate and valsartan; valsartan and amlodipine

U.S. Brand Names Exforge®

Therapeutic Category Angiotensin II Receptor Blocker Combination; Antihypertensive Agent, Combination; Calcium Channel Blocker

Use Treatment of hypertension

General Dosage Range Oral: *Adults:* Amlodipine 5-10 mg and valsartan 160-320 mg once daily (maximum: 10 mg/day [amlodipine]; 320 mg/day [valsartan])

Dosage Forms

Tablet:

Exforge®: 5/160: Amlodipine 5 mg and valsartan 160 mg; 5/320 mg: Amlodipine 5 mg and valsartan 320 mg; 10/160: Amlodipine 10 mg and valsartan 160 mg; 10/320: Amlodipine 10 mg and valsartan 320 mg

amlodipine besylate *see* amlodipine *on page 69*

amlodipine besylate, aliskiren hemifumarate, and hydrochlorothiazide *see* aliskiren, amlodipine, and hydrochlorothiazide *on page 52*

amlodipine besylate and olmesartan medoxomil *see* amlodipine and olmesartan *on page 70*

amlodipine besylate and telmisartan *see* telmisartan and amlodipine *on page 848*

amlodipine besylate and valsartan *see* amlodipine and valsartan *on page 71*

amlodipine besylate, olmesartan medoxomil, and hydrochlorothiazide *see* olmesartan, amlodipine, and hydrochlorothiazide *on page 646*

amlodipine besylate, valsartan, and hydrochlorothiazide *see* amlodipine, valsartan, and hydrochlorothiazide *on page 71*

amlodipine, hydrochlorothiazide, and aliskiren *see* aliskiren, amlodipine, and hydrochlorothiazide *on page 52*

amlodipine, hydrochlorothiazide, and olmesartan *see* olmesartan, amlodipine, and hydro-chlorothiazide *on page 646*

amlodipine, hydrochlorothiazide, and valsartan *see* amlodipine, valsartan, and hydrochlorothia-zide *on page 71*

amlodipine, valsartan, and hydrochlorothiazide
(am LOE di peen, val SAR tan, & hye droe klor oh THYE a zide)

Synonyms amlodipine besylate, valsartan, and hydrochlorothiazide; amlodipine, hydrochlorothiazide, and valsartan; hydrochlorothiazide, amlodipine, and valsartan; valsartan, hydrochlorothiazide, and amlodipine

U.S. Brand Names Exforge HCT®

Therapeutic Category Angiotensin II Receptor Blocker; Calcium Channel Blocker; Diuretic, Thiazide

Use Treatment of hypertension (not for initial therapy)

General Dosage Range Oral: *Adults:* Amlodipine 5-10 mg and valsartan 160-320 mg and hydro-chlorothiazide 12.5-25 mg once daily (maximum: 10 mg/day [amlodipine]; 25 mg/day [hydrochlorothia-zide]; 320 mg/day [valsartan])

◀ **Dosage Forms**
Tablet, oral:
  Exforge HCT®: Amlodipine 5 mg, valsartan 160 mg, and hydrochlorothiazide 12.5 mg; Amlodipine 5 mg, valsartan 160 mg, and hydrochlorothiazide 25 mg; Amlodipine 10 mg, valsartan 160 mg, and hydrochlorothiazide 12.5 mg; Amlodipine 10 mg, valsartan 160 mg, and hydrochlorothiazide 25 mg; Amlodipine 10 mg, valsartan 320 mg, and hydrochlorothiazide 25 mg

Ammens® Original Medicated [OTC] *see* zinc oxide *on page 930*
Ammens® Shower Fresh [OTC] *see* zinc oxide *on page 930*
ammonapse *see* sodium phenylbutyrate *on page 822*

ammonia spirit (aromatic) (a MOE nee ah SPEAR it, air oh MAT ik)
Synonyms smelling salts
Therapeutic Category Respiratory Stimulant
Use Prevention or treatment of fainting
General Dosage Range Inhalation: *Children >12 years and Adults:* Slowly inhale the vapors of one crushed ampul or opened bottle of solution until fainting resolves
Dosage Forms
  Solution, for inhalation: 1.7% to 2.1% (0.33 mL, 60 mL)

ammonium chloride (a MOE nee um KLOR ide)
Therapeutic Category Electrolyte Supplement, Oral
Use Treatment of hypochloremic states or metabolic alkalosis
General Dosage Range Metabolic alkalosis: The following equations represent different methods of correction utilizing either the serum HCO_3^-, the serum chloride, or the base excess
  Dosing of mEq NH_4 Cl via the chloride-deficit method (hypochloremia):
    Dose of mEq NH_4Cl = [0.2 L/kg x body weight (kg)] x [103 - observed serum chloride]; administer 50% of dose over 12 hours, then re-evaluate
    Note: 0.2 L/kg is the estimated chloride volume of distribution and 103 is the average normal serum chloride concentration (mEq/L)
  Dosing of mEq NH_4 Cl via the bicarbonate-excess method (refractory hypochloremic metabolic alkalosis):
    Dose of NH_4Cl = [0.5 L/kg x body weight (kg)] x (observed serum HCO_3^- - 24); administer 50% of dose over 12 hours, then re-evaluate
    Note: 0.5 L/kg is the estimated bicarbonate volume of distribution and 24 is the average normal serum bicarbonate concentration (mEq/L)
  These equations will yield different requirements of ammonium chloride
Dosage Forms
  Injection, solution: Ammonium 5 mEq/mL and chloride 5 mEq/mL (20 mL)

ammonium hydroxide and lactic acid *see* lactic acid and ammonium hydroxide *on page 506*
ammonium lactate *see* lactic acid and ammonium hydroxide *on page 506*
Ammonul® *see* sodium phenylacetate and sodium benzoate *on page 822*
AMN107 *see* nilotinib *on page 626*
Amnesteem® *see* isotretinoin *on page 495*

amobarbital (am oh BAR bi tal)
Synonyms amobarbital sodium; amylobarbitone
U.S. Brand Names Amytal®
Canadian Brand Names Amytal®
Therapeutic Category Barbiturate
Controlled Substance C-II
Use Hypnotic in short-term treatment of insomnia; reduce anxiety and provide sedation preoperatively
General Dosage Range Dosage adjustment recommended in patients with hepatic or renal impairment
I.M., I.V.:
  Children 6-12 years: Sedative: 65-500 mg/dose
  Adults:
    Hypnotic: 65-200 mg at bedtime (maximum single dose: 1000 mg)
    Sedative: 30-50 mg 2-3 times/day (maximum single dose: 1000 mg)

Dosage Forms
Injection, powder for reconstitution:
Amytal®: 0.5 g

amobarbital sodium *see amobarbital on page 72*
Amoclan *see amoxicillin and clavulanate potassium on page 74*

amoxapine (a MOKS a peen)

Medication Safety Issues
Sound-alike/look-alike issues:
Amoxapine may be confused with amoxicillin, Amoxil
Asendin may be confused with aspirin

Synonyms Asendin [DSC]

Therapeutic Category Antidepressant, Tricyclic (Secondary Amine)

Use Treatment of depression, psychotic depression, depression accompanied by anxiety or agitation

General Dosage Range Oral:
Adolescents: Initial: 25-50 mg/day as a single dose or in divided doses; Maintenance: 25-100 mg/day as a single dose at bedtime or in divided doses (maximum: 100 mg/day)
Adults: Initial: 50-75 mg/day in 2-3 divided doses; Maintenance 50-300 mg/day in 2-3 divided doses (maximum: 600 mg/day [inpatient]; 400 mg/day [outpatient])

Dosage Forms
Tablet, oral: 25 mg, 50 mg, 100 mg, 150 mg

amoxicillin (a moks i SIL in)

Medication Safety Issues
Sound-alike/look-alike issues:
Amoxicillin may be confused with amoxapine, Augmentin®
Amoxil may be confused with amoxapine

International issues:
Fisamox [Australia] may be confused with Fosamax brand name for alendronate [U.S., Canada, and multiple international markets] and Vigamox brand name for moxifloxacin [U.S., Canada, and multiple international markets]
Limoxin [Mexico] may be confused with Lanoxin brand name for digoxin [U.S., Canada, and multiple international markets]; Lincocin brand name for lincomycin [U.S., Canada, and multiple international markets]
Zimox: Brand name for amoxicillin [Italy], but also the brand name for carbidopa/levodopa [Greece]
Zimox [Italy] may be confused with Diamox which is the brand name for acetazolamide [Canada and multiple international markets]

Synonyms *p*-hydroxyampicillin; amoxicillin trihydrate; Amoxil; amoxycillin

U.S. Brand Names Moxatag™

Canadian Brand Names Apo-Amoxi®; Gen-Amoxicillin; Lin-Amox; Mylan-Amoxicillin; Novamoxin®; Nu-Amoxi; PHL-Amoxicillin; PMS-Amoxicillin

Therapeutic Category Penicillin

Use Treatment of otitis media, sinusitis, and infections caused by susceptible organisms involving the upper and lower respiratory tract, skin, and urinary tract; prophylaxis of infective endocarditis in patients undergoing surgical or dental procedures; as part of a multidrug regimen for *H. pylori* eradication

General Dosage Range Dosage adjustment recommended in patients with renal impairment
Oral:
Immediate release:
Infants ≤3 months: 20-30 mg/kg/day divided every 12 hours
Children >3 months and <40 kg: 20-90 mg/kg/day divided every 8-12 hours
Children ≥4 months: 20-100 mg/kg/day divided every 8 hours
Adults: 250-500 mg every 8 hours **or** 500-875 mg twice daily (maximum: 875 mg/dose)
Extended release: *Children ≥12 years and Adults:* 775 mg once daily

Dosage Forms
Capsule, oral: 250 mg, 500 mg
Powder for suspension, oral: 125 mg/5 mL (80 mL, 100 mL, 150 mL); 200 mg/5 mL (50 mL, 75 mL, 100 mL); 250 mg/5 mL (80 mL, 100 mL, 150 mL); 400 mg/5 mL (50 mL, 75 mL, 100 mL)

◀ **Tablet, oral**: 500 mg, 875 mg
Tablet, chewable, oral: 125 mg, 200 mg, 250 mg, 400 mg
Tablet, extended release, oral:
Moxatag™: 775 mg

amoxicillin and clavulanate potassium
(a moks i SiL in & klav yoo LAN ate poe TASS ee um)
Medication Safety Issues
Sound-alike/look-alike issues:
Augmentin® may be confused with amoxicillin, Azulfidine®
Synonyms amoxicillin and clavulanic acid; clavulanic acid and amoxicillin
U.S. Brand Names Amoclan; Augmentin ES-600® [DSC]; Augmentin XR®; Augmentin®
Canadian Brand Names Amoxi-Clav; Apo-Amoxi-Clav®; Clavulin®; Novo-Clavamoxin; ratio-Aclavulanate
Therapeutic Category Penicillin
Use Treatment of otitis media, sinusitis, and infections caused by susceptible organisms involving the lower respiratory tract, skin and skin structure, and urinary tract; spectrum same as amoxicillin with additional coverage of beta-lactamase producing *B. catarrhalis, H. influenzae, N. gonorrhoeae*, and *S. aureus* (not MRSA). The expanded coverage of this combination makes it a useful alternative when amoxicillin resistance is present and patients cannot tolerate alternative treatments.
General Dosage Range Dosage adjustment recommended in patients with renal impairment
Oral:
Immediate release:
Infants <3 months: 30 mg/kg/day divided every 12 hours
Children ≥3 months and <40 kg: 25-90 mg/kg/day divided every 12 hours **or** 20-40 mg/kg/day divided every 8 hours
Children >40 kg and Adults: 250-500 mg every 8 hours **or** 875 mg every 12 hours
Extended release: *Children ≥16 years and Adults:* 2000 mg every 12 hours (maximum: 2000 mg/dose)
Dosage Forms
Powder for oral suspension: 200: Amoxicillin 200 mg and clavulanate potassium 28.5 mg per 5 mL; 250: Amoxicillin 250 mg and clavulanate potassium 62.5 mg per 5 mL; 400: Amoxicillin 400 mg and clavulanate potassium 57 mg per 5 mL; 600: Amoxicillin 600 mg and clavulanate potassium 42.9 mg per 5 mL
Amoclan:
200: Amoxicillin 200 mg and clavulanate potassium 28.5 mg per 5 mL
400: Amoxicillin 400 mg and clavulanate potassium 57 mg per 5 mL
600: Amoxicillin 600 mg and clavulanate potassium 42.9 mg per 5 mL
Augmentin®:
125: Amoxicillin 125 mg and clavulanate potassium 31.25 mg per 5 mL
250: Amoxicillin 250 mg and clavulanate potassium 62.5 mg per 5 mL
Tablet: 250: Amoxicillin 250 mg and clavulanate potassium 125 mg; 500: Amoxicillin 500 mg and clavulanate potassium 125 mg; 875: Amoxicillin 875 mg and clavulanate potassium 125 mg
Augmentin®:
500: Amoxicillin 500 mg and clavulanate potassium 125 mg
875: Amoxicillin 875 mg and clavulanate potassium 125 mg
Tablet, chewable: 200: Amoxicillin 200 mg and clavulanate potassium 28.5 mg; 400: Amoxicillin 400 mg and clavulanate potassium 57 mg
Tablet, extended release: Amoxicillin 1000 mg and clavulanate acid 62.5 mg
Augmentin XR®: 1000: Amoxicillin 1000 mg and clavulanate acid 62.5 mg

amoxicillin and clavulanic acid *see* amoxicillin and clavulanate potassium *on page 74*
amoxicillin, clarithromycin, and lansoprazole *see* lansoprazole, amoxicillin, and clarithromycin *on page 511*
amoxicillin trihydrate *see* amoxicillin *on page 73*
Amoxi-Clav (Can) *see* amoxicillin and clavulanate potassium *on page 74*
Amoxil *see* amoxicillin *on page 73*
amoxycillin *see* amoxicillin *on page 73*
Amphadase™ *see* hyaluronidase *on page 443*
amphetamine and dextroamphetamine *see* dextroamphetamine and amphetamine *on page 269*
Amphojel® (Can) *see* aluminum hydroxide *on page 59*

Amphotec® *see* amphotericin B cholesteryl sulfate complex *on page* 75

amphotericin B cholesteryl sulfate complex
(am foe TER i sin bee kole LES te ril SUL fate KOM plecks)

Medication Safety Issues
High alert medication:
The Institute for Safe Medication Practices (ISMP) includes this medication among its list of drugs which have a heightened risk of causing significant patient harm when used in error.
Other safety concerns:
Lipid-based amphotericin formulations (Amphotec®) may be confused with conventional formulations (Amphocin®, Fungizone®)

Large overdoses have occurred when conventional formulations were dispensed inadvertently for lipid-based products. Single daily doses of conventional amphotericin formulation never exceed 1.5 mg/kg.

Synonyms ABCD; amphotericin B colloidal dispersion

U.S. Brand Names Amphotec®

Canadian Brand Names Amphotec®

Therapeutic Category Antifungal Agent

Use Treatment of invasive aspergillosis in patients who have failed amphotericin B deoxycholate treatment, or who have renal impairment or experience unacceptable toxicity which precludes treatment with amphotericin B deoxycholate in effective doses.

General Dosage Range I.V.: *Children and Adults:* 3-4 mg/kg/day (maximum: 7.5 mg/kg/day)

Dosage Forms
Injection, powder for reconstitution:
Amphotec®: 50 mg, 100 mg

amphotericin B colloidal dispersion *see* amphotericin B cholesteryl sulfate complex *on page* 75

amphotericin B (conventional) (am foe TER i sin bee con VEN sha nal)

Medication Safety Issues
High alert medication:
The Institute for Safe Medication Practices (ISMP) includes this medication (intrathecal administration) among its list of drugs which have a heightened risk of causing significant patient harm when used in error.
Other safety concerns:
Conventional amphotericin formulations (Amphocin®, Fungizone®) may be confused with lipid-based formulations (AmBisome®, Abelcet®, Amphotec®).

Large overdoses have occurred when conventional formulations were dispensed inadvertently for lipid-based products. Single daily doses of conventional amphotericin formulation never exceed 1.5 mg/kg.

Synonyms amphotericin B deoxycholate; amphotericin B desoxycholate

Canadian Brand Names Fungizone®

Therapeutic Category Antifungal Agent

Use Treatment of severe systemic and central nervous system infections caused by susceptible fungi such as *Candida* species, *Histoplasma capsulatum*, *Cryptococcus neoformans*, *Aspergillus* species, *Blastomyces dermatitidis*, *Torulopsis glabrata*, and *Coccidioides immitis*; fungal peritonitis; irrigant for bladder fungal infections; used in fungal infection in patients with bone marrow transplantation, amebic meningoencephalitis, ocular aspergillosis (intraocular injection), candidal cystitis (bladder irrigation), chemoprophylaxis (low-dose I.V.), immunocompromised patients at risk of aspergillosis (intranasal/nebulized), refractory meningitis (intrathecal), coccidioidal arthritis (intraarticular/I.M.).

Low-dose amphotericin B has been administered after bone marrow transplantation to reduce the risk of invasive fungal disease.

General Dosage Range Dosage adjustment recommended in patients who develop toxicities
I.V.:
Infants and Children: Test dose: 0.1 mg/kg/dose (maximum: 1 mg); Maintenance: 0.25-1 mg/kg/day given once daily; 1-1.5 mg/kg every other day may be given once therapy is established (maximum: 1.5-4 g cumulative dose)
Adults: Test dose: 1 mg infused; Maintenance: 0.3-1.5 mg/kg/day given once daily; 1-1.5 mg/kg every other day may be given once therapy is established (maximum: 1.5 mg/kg/day)
Dosage Forms
Injection, powder for reconstitution: 50 mg

amphotericin B deoxycholate *see* amphotericin B (conventional) *on page 75*

amphotericin B desoxycholate *see* amphotericin B (conventional) *on page 75*

amphotericin B lipid complex (am foe TER i sin bee LIP id KOM pleks)

Medication Safety Issues

High alert medication:
The Institute for Safe Medication Practices (ISMP) includes this medication among its list of drugs which have a heightened risk of causing significant patient harm when used in error.

Other safety concerns:
Lipid-based amphotericin formulations (Abelcet®) may be confused with conventional formulations (Amphocin®, Fungizone®)

Large overdoses have occurred when conventional formulations were dispensed inadvertently for lipid-based products. Single daily doses of conventional amphotericin formulation never exceed 1.5 mg/kg.

Synonyms ABLC

U.S. Brand Names Abelcet®

Canadian Brand Names Abelcet®

Therapeutic Category Antifungal Agent

Use Treatment of aspergillosis or any type of progressive fungal infection in patients who are refractory to or intolerant of conventional amphotericin B therapy

General Dosage Range Dosage adjustment recommended in patients who develop toxicities
I.V.: *Children and Adults:* 2.5-5 mg/kg/day as a single daily dose (maximum: 5 mg/kg/day)

Dosage Forms

Injection, suspension [preservative free]:
Abelcet®: 5 mg/mL (20 mL)

amphotericin B liposomal (am foe TER i sin bee lye po SO mal)

Medication Safety Issues

High alert medication:
The Institute for Safe Medication Practices (ISMP) includes this medication among its list of drugs which have a heightened risk of causing significant patient harm when used in error.

Other safety concerns:
Lipid-based amphotericin formulations (AmBisome®) may be confused with conventional formulations (Amphocin®, Fungizone®) or with other lipid-based amphotericin formulations (Abelcet®, Amphotec®)

Large overdoses have occurred when conventional formulations were dispensed inadvertently for lipid-based products. Single daily doses of conventional amphotericin formulation never exceed 1.5 mg/kg.

Synonyms L-AmB

U.S. Brand Names AmBisome®

Canadian Brand Names AmBisome®

Therapeutic Category Antifungal Agent, Systemic

Use Empirical therapy for presumed fungal infection in febrile, neutropenic patients; treatment of patients with *Aspergillus* species, *Candida* species, and/or *Cryptococcus* species infections refractory to amphotericin B desoxycholate (conventional amphotericin), or in patients where renal impairment or unacceptable toxicity precludes the use of amphotericin B desoxycholate; treatment of cryptococcal meningitis in HIV-infected patients; treatment of visceral leishmaniasis

General Dosage Range I.V.: *Children and Adults:* 3-6 mg/kg/day as a single daily dose (maximum: 6 mg/kg/day)

Dosage Forms

Injection, powder for reconstitution:
AmBisome®: 50 mg

ampicillin (am pi SIL in)

Medication Safety Issues

Sound-alike/look-alike issues:
Ampicillin may be confused with aminophylline

Synonyms aminobenzylpenicillin; ampicillin sodium; ampicillin trihydrate

Canadian Brand Names Apo-Ampi®; Novo-Ampicillin; Nu-Ampi

Therapeutic Category Penicillin

Use Treatment of susceptible bacterial infections (nonbeta-lactamase-producing organisms); treatment or prophylaxis of infective endocarditis; susceptible bacterial infections caused by streptococci, pneumococci, nonpenicillinase-producing staphylococci, *Listeria*, meningococci; some strains of *H. influenzae*, *Salmonella*, *Shigella*, *E. coli*, *Enterobacter*, and *Klebsiella*

General Dosage Range Dosage adjustment recommended in patients with renal impairment
I.M., I.V.:
  Infants and Children: 100-400 mg/kg/day divided every 6 hours (maximum: 12 g/day)
  Adults: 250-500 mg every 6 hours or up to 150-250 mg/kg/day divided every 3-4 hours (maximum: 12 g/day)
Oral:
  Infants and Children: 50-100 mg/kg/day divided every 6 hours (maximum: 4 g/day)
  Adults: 250-500 mg every 6 hours

Dosage Forms
  Capsule, oral: 250 mg, 500 mg
  Injection, powder for reconstitution: 125 mg, 250 mg, 500 mg, 1 g, 2 g, 10 g
  Powder for suspension, oral: 125 mg/5 mL (100 mL, 200 mL); 250 mg/5 mL (100 mL, 200 mL)

ampicillin and sulbactam (am pi SIL in & SUL bak tam)

Synonyms sulbactam and ampicillin
U.S. Brand Names Unasyn®
Canadian Brand Names Unasyn®
Therapeutic Category Penicillin
Use Treatment of susceptible bacterial infections involved with skin and skin structure, intraabdominal infections, gynecological infections; spectrum is that of ampicillin plus organisms producing beta-lactamases such as *S. aureus*, *H. influenzae*, *E. coli*, *Klebsiella*, *Acinetobacter*, *Enterobacter*, and anaerobes

General Dosage Range Dosage adjustment recommended in patients with renal impairment
I.M.: *Adults:* 1-2 g (1.5-3 g Unasyn®) ampicillin every 6 hours (maximum: 8 g ampicillin/day)
I.V.:
  Children ≥1 year: 100-400 mg ampicillin/kg/day divided every 6 hours (maximum: 8 g ampicillin/day)
  Adults: 1-2 g (1.5-3 g Unasyn®) ampicillin every 6 hours (maximum: 8 g ampicillin/day)

Dosage Forms
  Injection, powder for reconstitution: 1.5 g [ampicillin 1 g and sulbactam 0.5 g]; 3 g [ampicillin 2 g and sulbactam 1 g]; 15 g [ampicillin 10 g and sulbactam 5 g]
    Unasyn®: 1.5 g [ampicillin 1 g and sulbactam 0.5 g]; 3 g [ampicillin 2 g and sulbactam 1 g]; 15 g [ampicillin 10 g and sulbactam 5 g]; 15 g [ampicillin 10 g and sulbactam 5 g

ampicillin sodium *see* ampicillin *on page 76*
ampicillin trihydrate *see* ampicillin *on page 76*
AMPT *see* metyrosine *on page 584*
Ampyra™ *see* dalfampridine *on page 250*
amrinone lactate *see* inamrinone *on page 469*
Amrix® *see* cyclobenzaprine *on page 241*
Amturnide™ *see* aliskiren, amlodipine, and hydrochlorothiazide *on page 52*
Amvisc® *see* hyaluronate and derivatives *on page 443*
Amvisc® Plus *see* hyaluronate and derivatives *on page 443*
amylase, lipase, and protease *see* pancrelipase *on page 670*

amyl nitrite (AM il NYE trite)

Synonyms isoamyl nitrite
Therapeutic Category Vasodilator
Use Coronary vasodilator in angina pectoris; adjunct in treatment of cyanide poisoning; produce changes in the intensity of heart murmurs
General Dosage Range Nasal inhalation: *Adults:* 1-6 inhalations from 1 crushed ampul; may repeat in 3-5 minutes
Dosage Forms
  Liquid, for inhalation: USP: 85% to 103% (0.3 mL)

amyl nitrite, sodium nitrite, and sodium thiosulfate *see* sodium nitrite, sodium thiosulfate, and amyl nitrite *on page 821*

amylobarbitone *see* amobarbital *on page 72*

Amytal® *see* amobarbital *on page 72*

AN100226 *see* natalizumab *on page 614*

Anacin® Advanced Headache Formula [OTC] *see* acetaminophen, aspirin, and caffeine *on page 29*

Anadrol®-50 *see* oxymetholone *on page 665*

Anafranil® *see* clomipramine *on page 222*

anagrelide (an AG gre lide)

Medication Safety Issues
Sound-alike/look-alike issues:
Anagrelide may be confused with anastrozole

Synonyms anagrelide hydrochloride; BL4162A

U.S. Brand Names Agrylin®

Canadian Brand Names Agrylin®; Dom-Anagrelide; Mylan-Anagrelide; PMS-Anagrelide; Sandoz-Anagrelide

Therapeutic Category Platelet Reducing Agent

Use Treatment of thrombocythemia associated with myeloproliferative disorders (eg, chronic myelogenous leukemia, essential thrombocythemia, polycythemia vera, myeloid metaplasia with myelofibrosis, or other myeloproliferative disorder)

General Dosage Range Dosage adjustment recommended in patients with hepatic impairment
Oral:
Children: Initial: 0.5 mg/day; Maintenance: 0.5 mg 1-4 times/day (maximum: 10 mg/day; 2.5 mg/dose)
Adults: Initial: 0.5 mg 4 times/day **or** 1 mg twice daily (maximum: 10 mg/day; 2.5 mg/dose)

Dosage Forms
Capsule, oral: 0.5 mg, 1 mg
Agrylin®: 0.5 mg

anagrelide hydrochloride *see* anagrelide *on page 78*

anakinra (an a KIN ra)

Medication Safety Issues
Sound-alike/look-alike issues:
Anakinra may be confused with amikacin, Ampyra™
Kineret® may be confused with Amikin®

Synonyms IL-1Ra; interleukin-1 receptor antagonist

U.S. Brand Names Kineret®

Canadian Brand Names Kineret®

Therapeutic Category Antirheumatic, Disease Modifying

Use Treatment of moderately- to severely-active rheumatoid arthritis in adult patients who have failed one or more disease-modifying antirheumatic drugs (DMARDs); may be used alone or in combination with DMARDs (other than tumor necrosis factor-blocking agents)

General Dosage Range Dosage adjustment recommended in patients with renal impairment
SubQ: *Adults:* 100 mg once daily

Dosage Forms
Injection, solution [preservative free]:
Kineret®: 100 mg/0.67 mL (0.67 mL)

Ana-Kit® *see* epinephrine and chlorpheniramine *on page 332*

Analpram E™ *see* pramoxine and hydrocortisone *on page 731*

Analpram HC® *see* pramoxine and hydrocortisone *on page 731*

AnaMantle HC® Cream *see* lidocaine and hydrocortisone *on page 526*

AnaMantle HC® Forte *see* lidocaine and hydrocortisone *on page 526*

AnaMantle HC® Gel *see* lidocaine and hydrocortisone *on page 526*

Anandron® (Can) *see* nilutamide *on page 627*

Anaplex® DM *see* brompheniramine, pseudoephedrine, and dextromethorphan *on page 144*

Anaprox® *see* naproxen *on page 612*
Anaprox® DS *see* naproxen *on page 612*
Anascorp® *see* Centruroides immune F(ab')$_2$ (equine) *on page 187*
Anaspaz® *see* hyoscyamine *on page 457*

anastrozole (an AS troe zole)

Medication Safety Issues
Sound-alike/look-alike issues:
  Anastrozole may be confused with anagrelide, letrozole
  Arimidex® may be confused with Aromasin®
Synonyms ICI-D1033; ZD1033
U.S. Brand Names Arimidex®
Canadian Brand Names Arimidex®
Therapeutic Category Antineoplastic Agent
Use First-line treatment of locally-advanced or metastatic breast cancer (hormone receptor-positive or unknown) in postmenopausal women; treatment of advanced breast cancer in postmenopausal women with disease progression following tamoxifen therapy; adjuvant treatment of early hormone receptor-positive breast cancer in postmenopausal women
General Dosage Range Oral: *Adults:* 1 mg once daily
Dosage Forms
  Tablet, oral: 1 mg
    Arimidex®: 1 mg

A-Natural [OTC] *see* vitamin A *on page 917*
A-Natural-25 [OTC] *see* vitamin A *on page 917*
Anbesol® [OTC] *see* benzocaine *on page 121*
Anbesol® Baby [OTC] *see* benzocaine *on page 121*
Anbesol® Baby (Can) *see* benzocaine *on page 121*
Anbesol® Cold Sore Therapy [OTC] *see* benzocaine *on page 121*
Anbesol® Jr. [OTC] *see* benzocaine *on page 121*
Anbesol® Maximum Strength [OTC] *see* benzocaine *on page 121*
ancef *see* cefazolin *on page 180*
Ancobon® *see* flucytosine *on page 382*
Andriol® (Can) *see* testosterone *on page 854*
Androcur® (Can) *see* cyproterone *(Canada only) on page 245*
Androcur® Depot (Can) *see* cyproterone *(Canada only) on page 245*
Androderm® *see* testosterone *on page 854*
AndroGel® *see* testosterone *on page 854*
Android® *see* methyltestosterone *on page 579*
Andropository (Can) *see* testosterone *on page 854*
Androvite® [OTC] *see* vitamins (multiple/oral) *on page 919*
Androxy™ *see* fluoxymesterone *on page 389*
AneCream™ [OTC] *see* lidocaine (topical) *on page 524*
Anectine® *see* succinylcholine *on page 832*
Anestafoam™ [OTC] *see* lidocaine (topical) *on page 524*
aneurine hydrochloride *see* thiamine *on page 862*
Anexate® (Can) *see* flumazenil *on page 383*
Angeliq® *see* drospirenone and estradiol *on page 315*
Angiofluor™ [DSC] *see* fluorescein *on page 386*
Angiofluor™ Lite [DSC] *see* fluorescein *on page 386*
Angiomax® *see* bivalirudin *on page 137*
anhydrous glucose *see* dextrose *on page 273*

anidulafungin (ay nid yoo la FUN jin)

Synonyms LY303366
U.S. Brand Names Eraxis™

◀ **Canadian Brand Names** Eraxis™

Therapeutic Category Antifungal Agent, Parenteral; Echinocandin

Use Treatment of candidemia and other forms of *Candida* infections (including those of intraabdominal, peritoneal, and esophageal locus)

General Dosage Range I.V.: *Adults:* Loading dose: 100-200 mg as a single dose; Maintenance: 50-100 mg daily

Dosage Forms

Injection, powder for reconstitution:
  Eraxis™: 50 mg, 100 mg

Anolor 300 *see* butalbital, acetaminophen, and caffeine *on page 152*

Ansaid® (Can) *see* flurbiprofen (systemic) *on page 391*

ansamycin *see* rifabutin *on page 779*

Antabuse® *see* disulfiram *on page 299*

antagon *see* ganirelix *on page 411*

Antara® *see* fenofibrate *on page 369*

Anthraforte® (Can) *see* anthralin *on page 80*

anthralin (AN thra lin)

Synonyms dithranol

U.S. Brand Names Dritho-Creme®; Dritho-Scalp®; Zithranol®-RR

Canadian Brand Names Anthraforte®; Anthranol®; Anthrascalp®; Micanol®

Therapeutic Category Keratolytic Agent

Use Treatment of psoriasis (quiescent or chronic psoriasis)

General Dosage Range Topical: *Adults:* Generally, apply once a day or as directed

Dosage Forms

Cream, topical:
  Dritho-Creme®: 1% (50 g)
  Dritho-Scalp®: 0.5% (50 g)
  Zithranol®-RR: 1.2% (45 g)

Anthranol® (Can) *see* anthralin *on page 80*

Anthrascalp® (Can) *see* anthralin *on page 80*

anthrax vaccine, adsorbed (AN thraks vak SEEN ad SORBED)

Synonyms AVA

U.S. Brand Names BioThrax®

Therapeutic Category Vaccine

Use Immunization against *Bacillus anthracis* in persons at high risk for exposure.

The Advisory Committee on Immunization Practices (ACIP) recommends routine vaccination (pre-exposure vaccination) for the following:
  • Persons who work directly with the organism in the laboratory
  • Persons who handle animals or animal products only when
    - potentially infected in research settings;
    - in areas of high incidence of enzootic anthrax; or
    - where standards and restrictions are not sufficient to prevent exposure
  • Military personnel deployed to areas with high risk of exposure as recommended by the Department of Defense (DoD)
  • Persons engaged in environmental investigations or remediation efforts

Routine immunization for the general population is not recommended. Routine vaccination may be offered to emergency and other responders (police and fire departments, the National Guard, etc) on a voluntary basis under the direction of a comprehensive occupational health and safety program.

The ACIP recommends postexposure prophylaxis for the following (in the absence of completing a pre-exposure, routine vaccination schedule):
  • The general public, including pregnant and breast-feeding women
  • Medical professionals
  • Children ages 0-18 years as determined on an event-by-event basis
  • Persons engaged in handling certain animals or animal products

- Persons who work directly with the organism in the laboratory (postexposure vaccination dependant upon pre-event vaccination status)
- Military personnel as recommended by the DoD
- Persons engaged in environmental investigations or remediation efforts (postexposure vaccination dependent upon pre-event vaccination status)
- Emergency and other responders (police and fire departments, the National Guard, etc)
- Persons working in postal facilities

General Dosage Range
I.M.: *Adults ≤65 years:* 0.5 mL
SubQ: *Adults:* 0.5 mL

Dosage Forms
Injection, suspension:
BioThrax®: *Bacillus anthracis* proteins (5 mL)

anti-4 alpha integrin *see* natalizumab *on page 614*

131 I anti-B1 antibody *see* tositumomab and iodine I 131 tositumomab *on page 879*

131 I-anti-B1 monoclonal antibody *see* tositumomab and iodine I 131 tositumomab *on page 879*

antibody-drug conjugate SGN-35 *see* brentuximab vedotin *on page 140*

anti-CD20 monoclonal antibody *see* rituximab *on page 784*

anti-CD20-murine monoclonal antibody I-131 *see* tositumomab and iodine I 131 tositumomab *on page 879*

anti-CD30 ADC SGN-35 *see* brentuximab vedotin *on page 140*

anti-CD30 antibody-drug conjugate SGN-35 *see* brentuximab vedotin *on page 140*

anti-CD52 monoclonal antibody *see* alemtuzumab *on page 48*

anti-c-erB-2 *see* trastuzumab *on page 882*

Anti-Diarrheal [OTC] *see* loperamide *on page 535*

antidigoxin fab fragments, ovine *see* digoxin immune Fab *on page 284*

antidiuretic hormone *see* vasopressin *on page 910*

anti-ERB-2 *see* trastuzumab *on page 882*

Anti-Fungal™ [OTC] *see* clotrimazole (topical) *on page 226*

antihemophilic factor (human) (an tee hee moe FIL ik FAK tor HYU man)

Medication Safety Issues
Sound-alike/look-alike issues:
Factor VIII may be confused with Factor XIII
Other safety concerns:
Confusion may occur due to the omitting of "Factor VIII" from some product labeling. Review product contents carefully prior to dispensing any antihemophilic factor.

Synonyms AHF (human); factor VIII (human)

U.S. Brand Names Hemofil M; Koāte®-DVI; Monoclate-P®

Canadian Brand Names Hemofil M

Therapeutic Category Blood Product Derivative

Use Prevention and treatment of hemorrhagic episodes in patients with hemophilia A (classic hemophilia); perioperative management of hemophilia A; can be of significant therapeutic value in patients with acquired factor VIII inhibitors not exceeding 10 Bethesda units/mL

General Dosage Range I.V.: *Children and Adults:* Dosage varies greatly depending on indication

Dosage Forms
Injection, powder for reconstitution:
Hemofil M: Vial labeled with international units
Koāte®-DVI: ~250 int. units, ~500 int. units, ~1000 int. units
Monoclate-P®: ~250 int. units, ~500 int. units, ~1000 int. units, ~1500 int. units

antihemophilic factor (recombinant) (an tee hee moe FIL ik FAK tor ree KOM be nant)

Medication Safety Issues
Sound-alike/look-alike issues:
Factor VIII may be confused with Factor XIII
Other safety concerns:
Confusion may occur due to the omitting of "Factor VIII" from some product labeling. Review product contents carefully prior to dispensing any antihemophilic factor.

◀ **Synonyms** AHF (recombinant); factor VIII (recombinant); rAHF

U.S. Brand Names Advate; Helixate® FS; Kogenate® FS; Recombinate; Xyntha®; Xyntha® Solofuse™

Canadian Brand Names Advate; Helixate® FS; Kogenate® FS; Xyntha®

Therapeutic Category Blood Product Derivative

Use Prevention and treatment of hemorrhagic episodes in patients with hemophilia A (classic hemophilia or congenital factor VIII deficiency); perioperative management of hemophilia A; prophylaxis of joint bleeding and to reduce risk of joint damage in children with hemophilia A with no pre-existing joint damage (Helixate® FS, Kogenate® FS); can be of therapeutic value in patients with acquired factor VIII inhibitors ≤10 Bethesda units/mL (Recombinate)

General Dosage Range I.V.: *Children and Adults:* Dosage varies greatly depending on indication

Dosage Forms

Injection, powder for reconstitution:
Recombinate: 2000 int. units

Injection, powder for reconstitution [preservative free]:
Advate: 250 int. units, 500 int. units, 1000 int. units, 1500 int. units, 2000 int. units, 3000 int. units
Helixate® FS: 250 int. units, 500 int. units, 1000 int. units, 2000 int. units, 3000 int. units
Kogenate® FS: 250 int. units, 500 int. units, 1000 int. units, 2000 int. units, 3000 int. units
Recombinate: 250 int. units, 500 int. units, 1000 int. units, 1500 int. units
Xyntha®: 250 int. units, 500 int. units, 1000 int. units, 2000 int. units
Xyntha® Solofuse™: 1000 int. units, 2000 int. units, 3000 int. units

antihemophilic factor/von Willebrand factor complex (human)
(an tee hee moe FIL ik FAK tor von WILL le brand FAK tor KOM plex HYU man)

Medication Safety Issues

Sound-alike/look-alike issues:
Factor VIII may be confused with Factor XIII

Synonyms AHF (human); factor VIII (human); factor VIII concentrate; FVIII/vWF; von willebrand factor/ factor VIII complex; VWF/FVIII concentrate; VWF:RCo; vWF:RCof

U.S. Brand Names Alphanate®; Humate-P®; Wilate®

Canadian Brand Names Humate-P®

Therapeutic Category Antihemophilic Agent; Blood Product Derivative

Use

Factor VIII deficiency: Alphanate®, Humate-P®: Prevention and treatment of hemorrhagic episodes in patients with hemophilia A (classical hemophilia) or acquired factor VIII deficiency (Alphanate® only); **Note:** Wilate® is not approved for use in patients with hemophilia A or acquired factor VIII deficiency

von Willebrand disease (VWD):
Alphanate®: Prophylaxis with surgical and/or invasive procedures in patients with VWD when desmopressin is either ineffective or contraindicated; **Note:** Not indicated for patients with severe VWD undergoing major surgery

Humate-P®: Treatment of spontaneous or trauma-induced bleeding, as well as prevention of excessive bleeding during and after surgery in patients with severe VWD, including mild or moderate disease where use of desmopressin is known or suspected to be inadequate; **Note:** Not indicated for the prophylaxis of spontaneous bleeding episodes

Wilate®: Treatment of spontaneous and trauma-induced bleeding in patients with severe VWD, including mild or moderate disease where use of desmopressin is known or suspected to be inadequate or contraindicated; **Note:** Not indicated for prophylaxis of spontaneous bleeding or prevention of excessive bleeding during and after surgery)

General Dosage Range I.V.: *Children and Adults:* Dosage varies greatly depending on indication

Dosage Forms

Injection, powder for reconstitution [human derived]:
Alphanate®:
250 int. units [Factor VIII and VWF:RCo ratio varies by lot]
500 int. units [Factor VIII and VWF:RCo ratio varies by lot]
1000 int. units [Factor VIII and VWF:RCo ratio varies by lot]
1500 int. units [Factor VIII and VWF:RCo ratio varies by lot]
Humate-P®:
FVIII 250 int. units and VWF:RCo 600 int. units
FVIII 500 int. units and VWF:RCo 1200 int. units
FVIII 1000 int. units and VWF:RCo 2400 int. units

Anti-Hist [OTC] *see* diphenhydramine (systemic) *on page 290*

antiinhibitor coagulant complex (an TEE in HI bi tor coe AG yoo lant KOM pleks)

Synonyms AICC; aPCC; coagulant complex inhibitor
U.S. Brand Names Feiba NF; Feiba VH [DSC]
Canadian Brand Names Feiba NF
Therapeutic Category Hemophilic Agent
Use Hemophilia A & B patients with inhibitors who are to undergo surgery or those who are bleeding
General Dosage Range I.V.: *Children and Adults:* 50-100 units/kg every 6-12 hours (maximum: 200 units/kg/day)
Dosage Forms
Injection, powder for reconstitution:
Feiba NF: ~500 units, ~1000 units, ~2500 units

Antiphlogistine Rub A-535 No Odour (Can) *see* trolamine *on page 894*

antipyrine and benzocaine (an tee PYE reen & BEN zoe kane)

Synonyms benzocaine and antipyrine
Canadian Brand Names Auralgan®
Therapeutic Category Otic Agent, Analgesic; Otic Agent, Ceruminolytic
Use Temporary relief of pain and reduction of swelling associated with acute congestive and serous otitis media, swimmer's ear, otitis externa; facilitates ear wax removal
General Dosage Range Otic: *Children and Adults:* Instill drops 3-4 times/day (ear wax removal) or fill ear canal every 1-2 hours (otitis media)
Dosage Forms
Solution, otic [drops]: Antipyrine 5.4% and benzocaine 1.4% (10 mL, 15 mL)

anti-tac monoclonal antibody *see* daclizumab *on page 249*
antithrombin III *see* antithrombin III *on page 83*
antithrombin alfa *see* antithrombin III *on page 83*

antithrombin III (an tee THROM bin)

Synonyms antithrombin alfa; antithrombin III; AT; AT-III; hpAT; rhAT; rhATIII
U.S. Brand Names Atryn®; Thrombate III®
Canadian Brand Names Thrombate III®
Therapeutic Category Blood Product Derivative
Use Prophylaxis (ATryn®, Thrombate III®) of thromboembolic events in patients with hereditary antithrombin (AT or AT-III) deficiency undergoing surgical or obstetrical procedures (eg, childbirth); treatment (Thrombate III®) of thromboembolism in patients with hereditary AT deficiency
General Dosage Range I.V.: *Adults:* Dosage varies greatly depending on indication
Dosage Forms
Injection, powder for reconstitution [preservative free]:
Atryn®: ~1750 int. units
Thrombate III®: ~500 int. units

antithymocyte globulin (equine) (an te THY moe site GLOB yu lin, E kwine)

Medication Safety Issues
Sound-alike/look-alike issues:
Antithymocyte globulin equine (Atgam®) may be confused with antithymocyte globulin rabbit (Thymoglobulin®)
Atgam® may be confused with Ativan®
Synonyms antithymocyte immunoglobulin; ATG; horse antihuman thymocyte gamma globulin; lymphocyte immune globulin
U.S. Brand Names Atgam®
Canadian Brand Names Atgam®
Therapeutic Category Immunosuppressant Agent
Use Prevention and treatment of acute renal allograft rejection; treatment of moderate-to-severe aplastic anemia in patients not considered suitable candidates for bone marrow transplantation

◀ **General Dosage Range I.V.:**
Children: Initial: 5-25 mg/kg/day administered daily for 8-14 days; may be followed by administration every other day (maximum: 21 doses in 28 days)
Adults: Initial: 10-20 mg/kg/day administered daily; may be followed by administration every other day (maximum: 21 doses in 28 days)
Dosage Forms
Injection, solution:
Atgam®: 50 mg/mL (5 mL)

antithymocyte globulin (rabbit) (an te THY moe site GLOB yu lin RAB bit)

Medication Safety Issues
Sound-alike/look-alike issues:
Antithymocyte globulin rabbit (Thymoglobulin®) may be confused with antithymocyte globulin equine (Atgam®)
Synonyms antithymocyte immunoglobulin; rATG
U.S. Brand Names Thymoglobulin®
Therapeutic Category Immunosuppressant Agent
Use Treatment of acute rejection of renal transplant; used in conjunction with concomitant immunosuppression
General Dosage Range I.V.: *Children and Adults:* 1.5 mg/kg/day as a single daily dose
Dosage Forms
Injection, powder for reconstitution:
Thymoglobulin®: 25 mg

antithymocyte immunoglobulin *see* antithymocyte globulin (equine) *on page 83*
antithymocyte immunoglobulin *see* antithymocyte globulin (rabbit) *on page 84*
antitumor necrosis factor alpha (human) *see* adalimumab *on page 40*
anti-VEGF monoclonal antibody *see* bevacizumab *on page 132*
anti-VEGF rhuMAb *see* bevacizumab *on page 132*
antivenin (*Centruroides*) immune F(ab')$_2$ (equine) *see* Centruroides immune F(ab')$_2$ (equine) *on page 187*
antivenin (crotalidae) polyvalent, FAB (ovine) *see* crotalidae polyvalent immune FAB (ovine) *on page 239*

antivenin *(Latrodectus mactans)* (an tee VEN in lak tro DUK tus MAK tans)

Synonyms *Latrodectus mactans* antivenin; *Latrodectus* antivenin; black widow spider species antivenin
Therapeutic Category Antivenin
Use Treatment of patients with moderate-to-severe symptoms (eg, cramping, intractable pain, hypertension) due to black widow spider bites
General Dosage Range
I.M.: *Children ≥12 years:* 1-2 vials (2.5-5 mL)
I.V.: *Children and Adults:* 1-2 vials (2.5-5 mL)
Dosage Forms
Injection, powder for reconstitution: 6000 Antivenin units

antivenin *(Micrurus fulvius)* (an tee VEN in mye KRU rus FUL vee us)

Synonyms *Micrurus fulvius* antivenin; North American coral snake antivenin
Therapeutic Category Antivenin
Use Neutralization of venoms of Eastern coral snake and Texas coral snake
General Dosage Range I.V.: *Children and Adults:* 3-5 vials; some patients may need more than 10 vials

antivenin scorpion *see* Centruroides immune F(ab')$_2$ (equine) *on page 187*
Antivert® *see* meclizine *on page 552*
Antizol® *see* fomepizole *on page 398*
Anucort-HC™ *see* hydrocortisone (topical) *on page 450*
Anu-Med [OTC] *see* phenylephrine (topical) *on page 698*
Anu-med HC *see* hydrocortisone (topical) *on page 450*
Anusol-HC® *see* hydrocortisone (topical) *on page 450*

Anuzinc (Can) *see* zinc sulfate *on page 931*
Anzemet® *see* dolasetron *on page 303*
4-AP *see* dalfampridine *on page 250*
APAP *see* acetaminophen *on page 23*
APAP 500 [OTC] *see* acetaminophen *on page 23*
APAP and tramadol *see* acetaminophen and tramadol *on page 29*
APC8015 *see* sipuleucel-T *on page 815*
aPCC *see* antiinhibitor coagulant complex *on page 83*
ApexiCon™ *see* diflorasone *on page 282*
ApexiCon® E *see* diflorasone *on page 282*
Aphthasol® *see* amlexanox *on page 69*
Apidra® *see* insulin glulisine *on page 477*
Apidra® SoloStar® *see* insulin glulisine *on page 477*
Aplenzin™ *see* bupropion *on page 150*
Aplisol® *see* tuberculin tests *on page 896*
aplonidine *see* apraclonidine *on page 91*
Apo-Acebutolol® (Can) *see* acebutolol *on page 23*
Apo-Acetaminophen® (Can) *see* acetaminophen *on page 23*
Apo-Acetazolamide® (Can) *see* acetazolamide *on page 34*
Apo-Acyclovir® (Can) *see* acyclovir (systemic) *on page 39*
Apo-Alendronate® (Can) *see* alendronate *on page 49*
Apo-Alfuzosin® (Can) *see* alfuzosin *on page 50*
Apo-Allopurinol® (Can) *see* allopurinol *on page 54*
Apo-Alpraz® (Can) *see* alprazolam *on page 56*
Apo-Alpraz® TS (Can) *see* alprazolam *on page 56*
Apo-Amiloride® (Can) *see* amiloride *on page 64*
Apo-Amilzide® (Can) *see* amiloride and hydrochlorothiazide *on page 64*
Apo-Amiodarone® (Can) *see* amiodarone *on page 67*
Apo-Amitriptyline® (Can) *see* amitriptyline *on page 68*
Apo-Amlodipine® (Can) *see* amlodipine *on page 69*
Apo-Amoxi® (Can) *see* amoxicillin *on page 73*
Apo-Amoxi-Clav® (Can) *see* amoxicillin and clavulanate potassium *on page 74*
Apo-Ampi® (Can) *see* ampicillin *on page 76*
Apo-Atenidone® (Can) *see* atenolol and chlorthalidone *on page 101*
Apo-Atenol® (Can) *see* atenolol *on page 101*
Apo-Atorvastatin® (Can) *see* atorvastatin *on page 102*
Apo-Azathioprine® (Can) *see* azathioprine *on page 107*
Apo-Azithromycin® (Can) *see* azithromycin (systemic) *on page 108*
Apo-Baclofen® (Can) *see* baclofen *on page 112*
Apo-Beclomethasone® (Can) *see* beclomethasone (nasal) *on page 117*
Apo-Benztropine® (Can) *see* benztropine *on page 126*
Apo-Benzydamine® (Can) *see* benzydamine *(Canada only) on page 126*
Apo-Bicalutamide® (Can) *see* bicalutamide *on page 133*
Apo-Bisacodyl® (Can) *see* bisacodyl *on page 134*
Apo-Bisoprolol® (Can) *see* bisoprolol *on page 136*
Apo-Brimonidine® (Can) *see* brimonidine *on page 141*
Apo-Brimonidine P® (Can) *see* brimonidine *on page 141*
Apo-Bromazepam® (Can) *see* bromazepam *(Canada only) on page 142*
Apo-Bromocriptine® (Can) *see* bromocriptine *on page 142*
Apo-Buspirone® (Can) *see* buspirone *on page 151*
Apo-Butorphanol® (Can) *see* butorphanol *on page 155*
Apo-Cal® (Can) *see* calcium carbonate *on page 161*
Apo-Calcitonin® (Can) *see* calcitonin *on page 159*

Apo-Candesartan (Can) *see* candesartan *on page 167*
Apo-Capto® (Can) *see* captopril *on page 170*
Apo-Carbamazepine® (Can) *see* carbamazepine *on page 171*
Apo-Carvedilol® (Can) *see* carvedilol *on page 178*
Apo-Cefaclor® (Can) *see* cefaclor *on page 180*
Apo-Cefadroxil® (Can) *see* cefadroxil *on page 180*
Apo-Cefoxitin® (Can) *see* cefoxitin *on page 182*
Apo-Cefprozil® (Can) *see* cefprozil *on page 183*
Apo-Cefuroxime® (Can) *see* cefuroxime *on page 185*
Apo-Cephalex® (Can) *see* cephalexin *on page 188*
Apo-Cetirizine® (Can) *see* cetirizine *on page 189*
Apo-Chlorax® (Can) *see* clidinium and chlordiazepoxide *on page 217*
Apo-Chlordiazepoxide® (Can) *see* chlordiazepoxide *on page 194*
Apo-Chlorpropamide® (Can) *see* chlorpropamide *on page 203*
Apo-Chlorthalidone® (Can) *see* chlorthalidone *on page 204*
Apo-Cilazapril® (Can) *see* cilazapril *(Canada only) on page 208*
Apo-Cilazapril®/Hctz (Can) *see* cilazapril and hydrochlorothiazide *(Canada only) on page 208*
Apo-Cimetidine® (Can) *see* cimetidine *on page 209*
Apo-Ciproflox® (Can) *see* ciprofloxacin (systemic) *on page 210*
Apo-Citalopram® (Can) *see* citalopram *on page 213*
Apo-Clarithromycin® (Can) *see* clarithromycin *on page 215*
Apo-Clindamycin® (Can) *see* clindamycin (systemic) *on page 217*
Apo-Clobazam® (Can) *see* clobazam *(Canada only) on page 220*
Apo-Clomipramine® (Can) *see* clomipramine *on page 222*
Apo-Clonazepam® (Can) *see* clonazepam *on page 222*
Apo-Clonidine® (Can) *see* clonidine *on page 223*
Apo-Clorazepate® (Can) *see* clorazepate *on page 225*
Apo-Cloxi® (Can) *see* cloxacillin *(Canada only) on page 226*
Apo-Clozapine® (Can) *see* clozapine *on page 227*
Apo-Cyclobenzaprine® (Can) *see* cyclobenzaprine *on page 241*
Apo-Cyclosporine® (Can) *see* cyclosporine (systemic) *on page 243*
Apo-Desipramine® (Can) *see* desipramine *on page 260*
Apo-Desmopressin® (Can) *see* desmopressin *on page 262*
Apo-Dexamethasone® (Can) *see* dexamethasone (systemic) *on page 264*
Apo-Diazepam® (Can) *see* diazepam *on page 276*
Apo-Diclo® (Can) *see* diclofenac (systemic) *on page 277*
Apo-Diclo Rapide® (Can) *see* diclofenac (systemic) *on page 277*
Apo-Diclo® SR® (Can) *see* diclofenac (systemic) *on page 277*
Apo-Diflunisal® (Can) *see* diflunisal *on page 282*
Apo-Digoxin® (Can) *see* digoxin *on page 283*
Apo-Diltiaz® (Can) *see* diltiazem *on page 286*
Apo-Diltiaz CD® (Can) *see* diltiazem *on page 286*
Apo-Diltiaz® Injectable (Can) *see* diltiazem *on page 286*
Apo-Diltiaz SR® (Can) *see* diltiazem *on page 286*
Apo-Diltiaz TZ® (Can) *see* diltiazem *on page 286*
Apo-Dimenhydrinate® (Can) *see* dimenhydrinate *on page 288*
Apo-Dipyridamole FC® (Can) *see* dipyridamole *on page 298*
Apo-Divalproex® (Can) *see* divalproex *on page 300*
Apo-Docusate-Sodium® (Can) *see* docusate *on page 302*
Apo-Domperidone® (Can) *see* domperidone *(Canada only) on page 305*
Apo-Dorzo-Timop (Can) *see* dorzolamide and timolol *on page 308*
Apo-Doxazosin® (Can) *see* doxazosin *on page 308*
Apo-Doxepin® (Can) *see* doxepin (systemic) *on page 309*

Apo-Doxy® (Can) *see* doxycycline *on page 312*
Apo-Doxy Tabs® (Can) *see* doxycycline *on page 312*
Apo-Enalapril® (Can) *see* enalapril *on page 326*
Apo-Erythro Base® (Can) *see* erythromycin (systemic) *on page 339*
Apo-Erythro E-C® (Can) *see* erythromycin (systemic) *on page 339*
Apo-Erythro-ES® (Can) *see* erythromycin (systemic) *on page 339*
Apo-Erythro-S® (Can) *see* erythromycin (systemic) *on page 339*
Apo-Esomeprazole® (Can) *see* esomeprazole *on page 342*
Apo-Etodolac® (Can) *see* etodolac *on page 360*
Apo-Famciclovir® (Can) *see* famciclovir *on page 366*
Apo-Famotidine® (Can) *see* famotidine *on page 366*
Apo-Famotidine® Injectable (Can) *see* famotidine *on page 366*
Apo-Fenofibrate® (Can) *see* fenofibrate *on page 369*
Apo-Feno-Micro® (Can) *see* fenofibrate *on page 369*
Apo-Feno-Super® (Can) *see* fenofibrate *on page 369*
Apo-Ferrous Gluconate® (Can) *see* ferrous gluconate *on page 373*
Apo-Ferrous Sulfate® (Can) *see* ferrous sulfate *on page 374*
Apo-Flavoxate® (Can) *see* flavoxate *on page 379*
Apo-Flecainide® (Can) *see* flecainide *on page 379*
Apo-Floctafenine® (Can) *see* floctafenine *(Canada only) on page 380*
Apo-Fluconazole® (Can) *see* fluconazole *on page 381*
Apo-Flunarizine® (Can) *see* flunarizine *(Canada only) on page 383*
Apo-Flunisolide® (Can) *see* flunisolide (nasal) *on page 384*
Apo-Fluoxetine® (Can) *see* fluoxetine *on page 389*
Apo-Fluphenazine® (Can) *see* fluphenazine *on page 390*
Apo-Fluphenazine Decanoate® (Can) *see* fluphenazine *on page 390*
Apo-Flurazepam® (Can) *see* flurazepam *on page 391*
Apo-Flurbiprofen® (Can) *see* flurbiprofen (systemic) *on page 391*
Apo-Flutamide® (Can) *see* flutamide *on page 392*
Apo-Fluticasone® (Can) *see* fluticasone (nasal) *on page 393*
Apo-Fluvoxamine® (Can) *see* fluvoxamine *on page 395*
Apo-Folic® (Can) *see* folic acid *on page 396*
Apo-Fosinopril® (Can) *see* fosinopril *on page 401*
Apo-Furosemide® (Can) *see* furosemide *on page 404*
Apo-Gabapentin® (Can) *see* gabapentin *on page 405*
Apo-Gain® (Can) *see* minoxidil (topical) *on page 591*
Apo-Gemfibrozil® (Can) *see* gemfibrozil *on page 414*
Apo-Gliclazide® (Can) *see* gliclazide *(Canada only) on page 417*
Apo-Gliclazide® MR (Can) *see* gliclazide *(Canada only) on page 417*
Apo-Glimepiride® (Can) *see* glimepiride *on page 418*
Apo-Glyburide® (Can) *see* glyburide *on page 420*
Apo-Haloperidol® (Can) *see* haloperidol *on page 434*
Apo-Haloperidol LA® (Can) *see* haloperidol *on page 434*
Apo-Hydralazine® (Can) *see* hydralazine *on page 444*
Apo-Hydro® (Can) *see* hydrochlorothiazide *on page 445*
Apo-Hydroxyquine® (Can) *see* hydroxychloroquine *on page 454*
Apo-Hydroxyurea® (Can) *see* hydroxyurea *on page 456*
Apo-Hydroxyzine® (Can) *see* hydroxyzine *on page 456*
Apo-Ibuprofen® (Can) *see* ibuprofen *on page 460*
Apo-Imipramine® (Can) *see* imipramine *on page 467*
Apo-Indapamide® (Can) *see* indapamide *on page 470*
Apo-Indomethacin® (Can) *see* indomethacin *on page 471*
Apo-Ipravent® (Can) *see* ipratropium (nasal) *on page 489*

Apo-ISMN® (Can) *see* isosorbide mononitrate *on page 495*
Apo-K® (Can) *see* potassium chloride *on page 724*
Apo-Keto® (Can) *see* ketoprofen *on page 501*
Apo-Ketoconazole® (Can) *see* ketoconazole (systemic) *on page 500*
Apo-Keto-E® (Can) *see* ketoprofen *on page 501*
Apo-Ketorolac® (Can) *see* ketorolac (systemic) *on page 501*
Apo-Ketorolac Injectable® (Can) *see* ketorolac (systemic) *on page 501*
Apo-Keto SR® (Can) *see* ketoprofen *on page 501*
Apokyn® *see* apomorphine *on page 89*
Apo-Labetalol® (Can) *see* labetalol *on page 504*
Apo-Lactulose® (Can) *see* lactulose *on page 507*
Apo-Lamotrigine® (Can) *see* lamotrigine *on page 509*
Apo-Lansoprazole® (Can) *see* lansoprazole *on page 511*
Apo-Leflunomide® (Can) *see* leflunomide *on page 514*
Apo-Levetiracetam® (Can) *see* levetiracetam *on page 517*
Apo-Levobunolol® (Can) *see* levobunolol *on page 517*
Apo-Levocarb® (Can) *see* carbidopa and levodopa *on page 174*
Apo-Levocarb® CR (Can) *see* carbidopa and levodopa *on page 174*
Apo-Lisinopril® (Can) *see* lisinopril *on page 531*
Apo-Lisinopril®/Hctz (Can) *see* lisinopril and hydrochlorothiazide *on page 532*
Apo-Lithium® Carbonate (Can) *see* lithium *on page 532*
Apo-Lithium® Carbonate SR (Can) *see* lithium *on page 532*
Apo-Loperamide® (Can) *see* loperamide *on page 535*
Apo-Loratadine® (Can) *see* loratadine *on page 536*
Apo-Lorazepam® (Can) *see* lorazepam *on page 537*
Apo-Lovastatin® (Can) *see* lovastatin *on page 540*
Apo-Loxapine® (Can) *see* loxapine *on page 541*
Apo-Medroxy® (Can) *see* medroxyprogesterone *on page 554*
Apo-Mefenamic® (Can) *see* mefenamic acid *on page 555*
Apo-Mefloquine® (Can) *see* mefloquine *on page 555*
Apo-Megestrol® (Can) *see* megestrol *on page 555*
Apo-Meloxicam® (Can) *see* meloxicam *on page 556*
Apo-Memantine (Can) *see* memantine *on page 556*
Apo-Metformin® (Can) *see* metformin *on page 566*
Apo-Methazide® (Can) *see* methyldopa and hydrochlorothiazide *on page 575*
Apo-Methazolamide® (Can) *see* methazolamide *on page 568*
Apo-Methoprazine® (Can) *see* methotrimeprazine *(Canada only) on page 572*
Apo-Methotrexate® (Can) *see* methotrexate *on page 571*
Apo-Methyldopa® (Can) *see* methyldopa *on page 575*
Apo-Methylphenidate® (Can) *see* methylphenidate *on page 577*
Apo-Methylphenidate® SR (Can) *see* methylphenidate *on page 577*
Apo-Metoclop® (Can) *see* metoclopramide *on page 580*
Apo-Metoprolol® (Can) *see* metoprolol *on page 581*
Apo-Metoprolol SR® (Can) *see* metoprolol *on page 581*
Apo-Metoprolol (Type L®) (Can) *see* metoprolol *on page 581*
Apo-Metronidazole® (Can) *see* metronidazole (systemic) *on page 582*
Apo-Midazolam® (Can) *see* midazolam *on page 587*
Apo-Midodrine® (Can) *see* midodrine *on page 588*
Apo-Minocycline® (Can) *see* minocycline *on page 590*
Apo-Mirtazapine® (Can) *see* mirtazapine *on page 592*
Apo-Misoprostol® (Can) *see* misoprostol *on page 592*
Apo-Moclobemide® (Can) *see* moclobemide *(Canada only) on page 594*
Apo-Modafinil® (Can) *see* modafinil *on page 594*

apomorphine (a poe MOR feen)

Synonyms apomorphine hydrochloride; apomorphine hydrochloride hemihydrate
U.S. Brand Names Apokyn®
Therapeutic Category Anti-Parkinson Agent (Dopamine Agonist)
Use Treatment of hypomobility, "off" episodes with Parkinson disease
General Dosage Range Dosage adjustment recommended in patients with renal impairment
  SubQ: *Adults:* Initial test dose: 2 mg; Starting dose: 2-3 mg/dose at time of "off" episode; Maintenance dose: 2-6 mg/dose at time of "off" episode (maximum: 20 mg/day; 6 mg/dose; 5 doses/day)
Dosage Forms
  Injection, solution:
    Apokyn®: 10 mg/mL (3 mL)

apomorphine hydrochloride *see* apomorphine *on page 89*
apomorphine hydrochloride hemihydrate *see* apomorphine *on page 89*
Apo-Nabumetone® (Can) *see* nabumetone *on page 607*
Apo-Nadol® (Can) *see* nadolol *on page 607*
Apo-Napro-Na® (Can) *see* naproxen *on page 612*
Apo-Napro-Na DS® (Can) *see* naproxen *on page 612*
Apo-Naproxen® (Can) *see* naproxen *on page 612*
Apo-Naproxen EC® (Can) *see* naproxen *on page 612*
Apo-Naproxen SR® (Can) *see* naproxen *on page 612*
Apo-Nifed PA® (Can) *see* nifedipine *on page 626*
Apo-Nitrazepam® (Can) *see* nitrazepam *(Canada only) on page 628*
Apo-Nitrofurantoin® (Can) *see* nitrofurantoin *on page 629*
Apo-Nizatidine® (Can) *see* nizatidine *on page 631*
Apo-Norflox® (Can) *see* norfloxacin *on page 633*
Apo-Nortriptyline® (Can) *see* nortriptyline *on page 634*
Apo-Oflox® (Can) *see* ofloxacin (systemic) *on page 644*
Apo-Olanzapine® (Can) *see* olanzapine *on page 645*
Apo-Omeprazole® (Can) *see* omeprazole *on page 649*
Apo-Ondansetron® (Can) *see* ondansetron *on page 651*
Apo-Orciprenaline® (Can) *see* metaproterenol *on page 566*
Apo-Oxaprozin® (Can) *see* oxaprozin *on page 659*
Apo-Oxazepam® (Can) *see* oxazepam *on page 659*
Apo-Oxcarbazepine® (Can) *see* oxcarbazepine *on page 660*
Apo-Oxybutynin® (Can) *see* oxybutynin *on page 661*
Apo-Paclitaxel® (Can) *see* paclitaxel *on page 667*
Apo-Pantoprazole® (Can) *see* pantoprazole *on page 672*
Apo-Paroxetine® (Can) *see* paroxetine *on page 676*
Apo-Pentoxifylline SR® (Can) *see* pentoxifylline *on page 689*
Apo-Pen VK® (Can) *see* penicillin V potassium *on page 686*
Apo-Perindopril® (Can) *see* perindopril erbumine *on page 690*
Apo-Perphenazine® (Can) *see* perphenazine *on page 692*
Apo-Pimozide® (Can) *see* pimozide *on page 704*
Apo-Pindol® (Can) *see* pindolol *on page 705*
Apo-Pioglitazone® (Can) *see* pioglitazone *on page 706*
Apo-Piroxicam® (Can) *see* piroxicam *on page 708*
Apo-Pramipexole® (Can) *see* pramipexole *on page 729*
Apo-Pravastatin® (Can) *see* pravastatin *on page 732*
Apo-Prazo® (Can) *see* prazosin *on page 733*
Apo-Prednisone® (Can) *see* prednisone *on page 735*
Apo-Primidone® (Can) *see* primidone *on page 737*
Apo-Procainamide® (Can) *see* procainamide *on page 739*
Apo-Prochlorperazine® (Can) *see* prochlorperazine *on page 740*

Apo-Propafenone® (Can) *see* propafenone *on page 744*
Apo-Propranolol® (Can) *see* propranolol *on page 747*
Apo-Quetiapine® (Can) *see* quetiapine *on page 760*
Apo-Quinidine® (Can) *see* quinidine *on page 762*
Apo-Quinine® (Can) *see* quinine *on page 762*
Apo-Raloxifene® (Can) *see* raloxifene *on page 765*
Apo-Ramipril® (Can) *see* ramipril *on page 766*
Apo-Ranitidine® (Can) *see* ranitidine *on page 767*
Apo-Risedronate® (Can) *see* risedronate *on page 782*
Apo-Risperidone® (Can) *see* risperidone *on page 783*
Apo-Salvent® (Can) *see* albuterol *on page 45*
Apo-Salvent® AEM (Can) *see* albuterol *on page 45*
Apo-Salvent® CFC Free (Can) *see* albuterol *on page 45*
Apo-Salvent® Sterules (Can) *see* albuterol *on page 45*
Apo-Selegiline® (Can) *see* selegiline *on page 806*
Apo-Sertraline® (Can) *see* sertraline *on page 809*
Apo-Sibutramine® (Can) *see* sibutramine *on page 810*
Apo-Simvastatin® (Can) *see* simvastatin *on page 813*
Apo-Sotalol® (Can) *see* sotalol *on page 828*
Apo-Sucralfate (Can) *see* sucralfate *on page 833*
Apo-Sulfatrim® (Can) *see* sulfamethoxazole and trimethoprim *on page 836*
Apo-Sulfatrim® DS (Can) *see* sulfamethoxazole and trimethoprim *on page 836*
Apo-Sulfatrim® Pediatric (Can) *see* sulfamethoxazole and trimethoprim *on page 836*
Apo-Sulin® (Can) *see* sulindac *on page 839*
Apo-Sumatriptan® (Can) *see* sumatriptan *on page 839*
Apo-Tamox® (Can) *see* tamoxifen *on page 843*
Apo-Temazepam® (Can) *see* temazepam *on page 848*
Apo-Terazosin® (Can) *see* terazosin *on page 851*
Apo-Terbinafine® (Can) *see* terbinafine (systemic) *on page 851*
Apo-Tetra® (Can) *see* tetracycline *on page 857*
Apo-Theo LA® (Can) *see* theophylline *on page 860*
Apo-Tiaprofenic® (Can) *see* tiaprofenic acid *(Canada only) on page 867*
Apo-Ticlopidine® (Can) *see* ticlopidine *on page 868*
Apo-Timol® (Can) *see* timolol (systemic) *on page 868*
Apo-Timop® (Can) *see* timolol (ophthalmic) *on page 869*
Apo-Tizanidine® (Can) *see* tizanidine *on page 872*
Apo-Tolbutamide® (Can) *see* tolbutamide *on page 875*
Apo-Topiramate® (Can) *see* topiramate *on page 877*
Apo-Tramadol/Acet® (Can) *see* acetaminophen and tramadol *on page 29*
Apo-Trazodone® (Can) *see* trazodone *on page 884*
Apo-Trazodone D® (Can) *see* trazodone *on page 884*
Apo-Triazide® (Can) *see* hydrochlorothiazide and triamterene *on page 446*
Apo-Triazo® (Can) *see* triazolam *on page 888*
Apo-Trifluoperazine® (Can) *see* trifluoperazine *on page 890*
Apo-Trimethoprim® (Can) *see* trimethoprim *on page 892*
Apo-Trimip® (Can) *see* trimipramine *on page 892*
Apo-Valacyclovir® (Can) *see* valacyclovir *on page 903*
Apo-Valproic® (Can) *see* valproic acid *on page 904*
Apo-Verap® (Can) *see* verapamil *on page 912*
Apo-Verap® SR (Can) *see* verapamil *on page 912*
Apo-Warfarin® (Can) *see* warfarin *on page 922*
Apo-Zidovudine® (Can) *see* zidovudine *on page 929*
Apo-Zopiclone® (Can) *see* zopiclone *(Canada only) on page 934*

APPG *see* penicillin G procaine *on page 685*

apraclonidine (a pra KLOE ni deen)

Medication Safety Issues
  Sound-alike/look-alike issues:
    Iopidine® may be confused with indapamide, iodine, Lodine®
Synonyms aplonidine; apraclonidine hydrochloride; p-aminoclonidine
U.S. Brand Names Iopidine®
Canadian Brand Names Iopidine®
Therapeutic Category Alpha$_2$ Agonist, Ophthalmic
Use Prevention and treatment of postsurgical intraocular pressure (IOP) elevation; short-term, adjunctive therapy in patients who require additional reduction of IOP
General Dosage Range Ophthalmic: *Adults:* 0.5%: Instill 1-2 drops in the affected eye(s) 3 times/day; 1%: Instill 1 drop in operative eye 1 hour prior to and upon completion of surgery
Dosage Forms
  Solution, ophthalmic: 0.5% (5 mL, 10 mL)
    Iopidine®: 0.5% (5 mL, 10 mL); 1% (0.1 mL)

apraclonidine hydrochloride *see* apraclonidine *on page 91*

aprepitant (ap RE pi tant)

Medication Safety Issues
  Sound-alike/look-alike issues:
    Aprepitant may be confused with fosaprepitant
    Emend® (aprepitant) oral capsule formulation may be confused with Emend® for injection (fosaprepitant)
Synonyms L 754030; MK 869
U.S. Brand Names Emend®
Canadian Brand Names Emend®
Therapeutic Category Antiemetic
Use Prevention of acute and delayed nausea and vomiting associated with moderately- and highly-emetogenic chemotherapy (in combination with other antiemetics); prevention of postoperative nausea and vomiting (PONV)
General Dosage Range Oral: *Adults:* 125 mg on day 1, followed by 80 mg on days 2 and 3 **or** 40 mg within 3 hours prior to induction with anesthesia
Dosage Forms
  Capsule, oral:
    Emend®: 40 mg, 80 mg, 125 mg
  Combination package, oral:
    Emend®: Capsule: 80 mg (2s) and Capsule: 125 mg (1s)

aprepitant injection *see* fosaprepitant *on page 400*
Apresoline [DSC] *see* hydralazine *on page 444*
Apresoline® (Can) *see* hydralazine *on page 444*
Apri® *see* ethinyl estradiol and desogestrel *on page 351*
Apriso™ *see* mesalamine *on page 564*
Aprodine [OTC] *see* triprolidine and pseudoephedrine *on page 893*

aprotinin (a proe TYE nin)

Canadian Brand Names Trasylol®
Therapeutic Category Hemostatic Agent
Use Prevention of perioperative blood loss in patients who are at increased risk for blood loss and blood transfusions in association with cardiopulmonary bypass in coronary artery bypass graft (CABG) surgery

Note: Aprotinin has been withdrawn from the worldwide market due to evidence demonstrating an increased risk of renal dysfunction, myocardial infarction, and mortality in patients undergoing cardiac surgery (Canada has lifted this suspension); use limited to investigational use in the U.S. only according to a special treatment protocol allowing for treatment in select patients at increased risk of blood loss and transfusion during CABG surgery when alternative therapies are unacceptable.

◄ **General Dosage Range I.V.:** *Adults:* Test dose: 1 mL (1.4 mg) 10 minutes prior to loading dose; Loading dose: 1-2 million KIU (140-280 mg; 100-200 mL); Pump prime volume: 1-2 million KIU (140-280 mg, 100-200 mL); Infusion: 250,000-500,000 KIU/hour (35-70 mg/hour; 25-50 mL/hour)

Dosage Forms
Injection, solution:
Trasylol®: 1.4 mg/mL [10,000 KIU/mL] (100 mL, 200 mL)

Aptivus® *see* tipranavir *on page 871*
Aqua-Ban® Maximum Strength [OTC] *see* pamabrom *on page 669*
Aqua Care® [OTC] *see* urea *on page 900*
Aquacort® (Can) *see* hydrocortisone (topical) *on page 450*
AquADEKs™ [OTC] *see* vitamins (multiple/pediatric) *on page 920*
Aqua Gem-E™ [OTC] *see* vitamin E *on page 918*
AquaLase® *see* balanced salt solution *on page 113*
AquaMEPHYTON® (Can) *see* phytonadione *on page 703*
Aquanil HC® [OTC] *see* hydrocortisone (topical) *on page 450*
Aquaphilic® with Carbamide [OTC] *see* urea *on page 900*
Aquasol A® *see* vitamin A *on page 917*
Aquasol E® [OTC] *see* vitamin E *on page 918*
aquavan *see* fospropofol *on page 402*
aqueous procaine penicillin G *see* penicillin G procaine *on page 685*
Aquoral™ *see* saliva substitute *on page 798*
ara-C *see* cytarabine *on page 246*
arabinosylcytosine *see* cytarabine *on page 246*
Aralast NP *see* alpha$_1$-proteinase inhibitor *on page 55*
Aralen® *see* chloroquine *on page 196*
Aranelle® *see* ethinyl estradiol and norethindrone *on page 355*
Aranesp® *see* darbepoetin alfa *on page 253*
Aranesp® SingleJect® *see* darbepoetin alfa *on page 253*
Arava® *see* leflunomide *on page 514*
Arbinoxa™ *see* carbinoxamine *on page 174*
Arcalyst™ *see* rilonacept *on page 781*
Arcapta™ Neohaler™ *see* indacaterol *on page 470*
Aredia® *see* pamidronate *on page 670*
Arestin Microspheres (Can) *see* minocycline *on page 590*

arformoterol (ar for MOE ter ol)

Synonyms (R,R)-formoterol L-tartrate; arformoterol tartrate
U.S. Brand Names Brovana®
Therapeutic Category Beta$_2$-Adrenergic Agonist
Use Long-term maintenance treatment of bronchoconstriction in chronic obstructive pulmonary disease (COPD), including chronic bronchitis and emphysema
General Dosage Range Nebulization: *Adults:* 5 mcg twice daily (maximum: 30 mcg/day)
Dosage Forms
Solution, for nebulization:
Brovana®: 15 mcg/2 mL (30s, 60s)

arformoterol tartrate *see* arformoterol *on page 92*

argatroban (ar GA troh ban)

Medication Safety Issues
Sound-alike/look-alike issues:
Argatroban may be confused with Aggrastat®, Orgaran®
High alert medication:
The Institute for Safe Medication Practices (ISMP) includes this medication among its list of drugs which have a heightened risk of causing significant patient harm when used in error.
Therapeutic Category Anticoagulant, Thrombin Inhibitor

Use Prophylaxis or treatment of thrombosis in patients with heparin-induced thrombocytopenia (HIT); adjunct to percutaneous coronary intervention (PCI) in patients who have or are at risk of thrombosis associated with HIT

General Dosage Range Dosage adjustment recommended in patients with hepatic impairment

I.V.:

Children: Initial dose: 0.75 mcg/kg/minute; dosage may be adjusted in increments of 0.1-0.25 mcg/kg/minute

Adults: Bolus dose: 150-350 mcg/kg during procedure; Infusion: Initial: 2 mcg/kg/minute **or** 25 mcg/kg/minute during procedure; Maintenance: 0.5-10 mcg/kg/minute (maximum: 10 mcg/kg/minute) **or** 25-40 mcg/kg/minute during procedure

Adults (critically-ill): Initial: 0.2 mcg/kg/minute; Maintenance: 0.5-1.3 mcg/kg/minute

Dosage Forms

Infusion, premixed in NS: 125 mg (125 mL)

Injection, solution: 100 mg/mL (2.5 mL)

arginine (AR ji neen)

Medication Safety Issues

Administration issues:

The Food and Drug Administration (FDA) has identified several cases of fatal arginine overdose in children and has recommended that healthcare professionals always recheck dosing calculations prior to administration of arginine. Doses used in children should not exceed usual adult doses.

Synonyms arginine HCl; arginine hydrochloride; L-arginine; L-arginine hydrochloride

U.S. Brand Names R-Gene® 10

Therapeutic Category Diagnostic Agent

Use Pituitary function test (growth hormone)

General Dosage Range I.V.:

Children: 0.5 g/kg/dose as a single dose

Adults: 30 g (300 mL) as a single dose

Dosage Forms

Injection, solution:

R-Gene® 10: 10% [100 mg/mL] (300 mL)

arginine HCl *see arginine on page 93*

arginine hydrochloride *see arginine on page 93*

8-arginine vasopressin *see vasopressin on page 910*

Aricept® *see donepezil on page 306*

Aricept® ODT *see donepezil on page 306*

Aricept® RDT (Can) *see donepezil on page 306*

Aridol™ *see mannitol on page 548*

Arimidex® *see anastrozole on page 79*

aripiprazole (ay ri PIP ray zole)

Medication Safety Issues

Sound-alike/look-alike issues:

Abilify® may be confused with Ambien®

ARIPiprazole may be confused with proton pump inhibitors (dexlansoprazole, esomeprazole, lansoprazole, omeprazole, pantoprazole, RABEprazole)

Synonyms BMS 337039; OPC-14597

Tall-Man ARIPiprazole

U.S. Brand Names Abilify Discmelt®; Abilify®

Canadian Brand Names Abilify®

Therapeutic Category Antipsychotic Agent, Quinolone

Use

Oral: Acute and maintenance treatment of schizophrenia; acute (manic and mixed episodes) and maintenance treatment of bipolar I disorder as monotherapy or as an adjunct to lithium or valproic acid; adjunctive treatment of major depressive disorder; treatment of irritability associated with autistic disorder

Injection: Agitation associated with schizophrenia or bipolar I disorder

▶

◀ **General Dosage Range** Dosage adjustment recommended in patients on concomitant therapy
  Oral:
    Children 6-9 years: 5-15 mg once daily (maximum: 15 mg/day)
    Children ≥10 years: 5-30 mg once daily (maximum: 30 mg/day)
    Adults: 10-30 mg once daily (maximum: 30 mg/day)
  I.M.: *Adults:* 9.75 mg as a single dose (maximum: 30 mg/day)
Dosage Forms
  Injection, solution:
    Abilify®: 7.5 mg/mL (1.3 mL)
  Solution, oral:
    Abilify®: 1 mg/mL (150 mL)
  Tablet, oral:
    Abilify®: 2 mg, 5 mg, 10 mg, 15 mg, 20 mg, 30 mg
  Tablet, orally disintegrating, oral:
    Abilify Discmelt®: 10 mg, 15 mg

Aristospan® *see* triamcinolone (systemic) *on page 886*
Arixtra® *see* fondaparinux *on page 398*

armodafinil (ar moe DAF i nil)
Synonyms R-modafinil
U.S. Brand Names Nuvigil®
Therapeutic Category Stimulant
Controlled Substance C-IV
Use Improve wakefulness in patients with excessive daytime sleepiness associated with narcolepsy and shift work sleep disorder (SWSD); adjunctive therapy for obstructive sleep apnea/hypopnea syndrome (OSAHS)
General Dosage Range Dosage adjustment recommended in patients with hepatic impairment
  Oral: *Adults:* 150-250 mg once daily
Dosage Forms
  Tablet, oral:
    Nuvigil®: 50 mg, 150 mg, 250 mg

Armour® Thyroid *see* thyroid, desiccated *on page 865*
Aromasin® *see* exemestane *on page 363*
Arranon® *see* nelarabine *on page 616*

arsenic trioxide (AR se nik tri OKS id)
Medication Safety Issues
  High alert medication:
    This medication is in a class the Institute for Safe Medication Practices (ISMP) includes among its list of drugs which have a heightened risk of causing significant patient harm when used in error.
Synonyms As_2O_3
U.S. Brand Names Trisenox®
Therapeutic Category Antineoplastic Agent, Miscellaneous
Use Remission induction and consolidation in patients with relapsed or refractory acute promyelocytic leukemia (APL) characterized by t(15;17) translocation or PML/RAR-alpha gene expression
General Dosage Range Dosage adjustment recommended for renal impairment.
  I.V.: *Children ≥4 years and Adults:* Induction: 0.15 mg/kg/day (maximum: 60 doses); Consolidation: 0.15 mg/kg/day (maximum: 25 doses over a period of up to 5 weeks)
Dosage Forms
  Injection, solution [preservative free]:
    Trisenox®: 1 mg/mL (10 mL)

Artane *see* trihexyphenidyl *on page 891*
artemether and benflumetol *see* artemether and lumefantrine *on page 94*

artemether and lumefantrine (ar TEM e ther & loo me FAN treen)
Synonyms artemether and benflumetol; benflumetol and artemether; lumefantrine and artemether
U.S. Brand Names Coartem®

Therapeutic Category Antimalarial Agent

Use Treatment of acute, uncomplicated malaria infections due to *Plasmodium falciparum*, including geographical regions where chloroquine resistance has been reported

General Dosage Range Oral:

Children 2 months to ≤16 years:

5 to <15 kg: Artemether 20 mg/lumefantrine 120 mg twice daily (maximum: 6 tablets per treatment course)

15 to <25 kg: Artemether 40 mg/lumefantrine 240 mg twice daily (maximum: 12 tablets per treatment course)

25 to <35 kg: Artemether 60 mg/lumefantrine 360 mg twice daily (maximum: 18 tablets per treatment course)

≥35 kg: Artemether 80 mg/lumefantrine 480 mg twice daily (maximum: 24 tablets per treatment course)

Children >16 years and Adults:

25 to <35 kg: Artemether 60 mg/lumefantrine 360 mg twice daily (maximum: 18 tablets per treatment course)

≥35 kg: Artemether 80 mg/lumefantrine 480 mg twice daily (maximum: 24 tablets per treatment course)

Dosage Forms

Tablet:

Coartem®: Artemether 20 mg and lumefantrine 120 mg

Arthrotec® *see* diclofenac and misoprostol *on page 279*

articaine and epinephrine (AR ti kane & ep i NEF rin)

Synonyms epinephrine and articaine hydrochloride

U.S. Brand Names Septocaine® with epinephrine 1:100,000; Septocaine® with epinephrine 1:200,000; Zorcaine™

Canadian Brand Names Astracaine® with epinephrine 1:200,000; Astracaine® with epinephrine forte 1:100,000; Septanest® N; Septanest® SP; Ultracaine® DS; Ultracaine® DS Forte; Zorcaine™

Therapeutic Category Local Anesthetic

Use Local, infiltrative, or conductive anesthesia during simple and complex dental procedures

General Dosage Range Local injection:

Children 4-16 years: Maximum: 7 mg/kg (0.175 mL/kg)

Complex procedures: 0.37-7.48 mg/kg (0.7-3.9 mL)

Simple procedures: 0.76-5.65 mg/kg (0.9-5.1 mL)

Adults: Maximum: 7 mg/kg (0.175 mL/kg)

Infiltration: 0.5-2.5 mL of 4% solution; Total dose: 20-100 mg

Nerve block: 0.5-3.4 mL of 4% solution; Total dose: 20-136 mg

Oral surgery: 1-5.1 mL of 4% solution; Total dose: 40-204 mg

Elderly 65-75 years:

Complex procedures: 1.05-4.27 mg/kg (1.3-6.8 mL)

Simple procedures: 0.43-4.76 mg/kg (0.9-11.9 mL)

Elderly ≥75 years:

Complex procedures: 1.12-2.17 mg/kg (1.3-5.1 mL)

Simple procedures: 0.78-4.76 mg/kg (1.3-11.9 mL)

Dosage Forms

Injection, solution [for dental use]:

Septocaine® with epinephrine 1:100,000: Articaine 4% and epinephrine 1:100,000 (1.7 mL)

Septocaine® with epinephrine 1:200,000: Articaine 4% and epinephrine 1:200,000 (1.7 mL)

Zorcaine™: Articaine 4% and epinephrine 1:100,000 (1.7 mL) [contains sodium metabisulfite]

Dosage Forms - Canada

Injection, solution [for dental use]:

Astracaine® with epinephrine 1:200,000: Articaine 4% and epinephrine 1:200,000 (1.8 mL)

Astracaine® Forte with epinephrine forte 1:100,000: Articaine 4% and epinephrine 1:100,000 (1.8 mL)

Septanest® N: Articaine 4% and epinephrine 1:200,000 (1.7 mL)

Septanest® SP: Articaine 4% and epinephrine 1:100,000 (1.7 mL)

Ultracaine® DS: Articaine 4% and epinephrine 1:200,000 (1.7 mL)

Ultracaine® DS Forte: Articaine 4% and epinephrine 1:100,000 (1.7 mL)

artificial saliva *see* saliva substitute *on page 798*

artificial tears (ar ti FISH il tears)

Medication Safety Issues

Sound-alike/look-alike issues:
Isopto® Tears may be confused with Isoptin®

Synonyms hydroxyethylcellulose; polyvinyl alcohol

U.S. Brand Names Akwa Tears® [OTC]; Bion® Tears [OTC]; HypoTears PF [OTC]; HypoTears [OTC]; Liquifilm® Tears [OTC]; Moisture® Eyes PM [OTC]; Moisture® Eyes [OTC]; Murine Tears® [OTC]; Murocel® [OTC]; Nature's Tears® [OTC]; Nu-Tears® II [OTC]; Nu-Tears® [OTC]; Refresh Plus® [OTC]; Refresh Tears® [OTC]; Refresh® [OTC]; Soothe® [OTC]; Systane® Free [OTC]; Systane® [OTC]; Teargen® II [OTC]; Teargen® [OTC]; Tearisol® [OTC]; Tears Again® [OTC]; Tears Naturale® Free [OTC]; Tears Naturale® II [OTC]; Tears Naturale® [OTC]; Tears Plus® [OTC]; Tears Renewed® [OTC]; Ultra Tears® [OTC]; Viva-Drops® [OTC]

Canadian Brand Names Teardrops®

Therapeutic Category Ophthalmic Agent, Miscellaneous

Use Ophthalmic lubricant; for relief of dry eyes and eye irritation

General Dosage Range Ophthalmic: *Children and Adults:* 1-2 drops into eye(s) 3-4 times/day as needed

Dosage Forms

Solution, ophthalmic: 15 mL and 30 mL dropper bottles

Artiss *see* fibrin sealant *on page 376*

Arzerra™ *see* ofatumumab *on page 643*

As$_2$O$_3$ *see* arsenic trioxide *on page 94*

ASA *see* aspirin *on page 98*

5-ASA *see* mesalamine *on page 564*

ASA and diphenhydramine *see* aspirin and diphenhydramine *on page 99*

Asacol® *see* mesalamine *on page 564*

Asacol® 800 (Can) *see* mesalamine *on page 564*

Asacol® HD *see* mesalamine *on page 564*

Asaphen (Can) *see* aspirin *on page 98*

Asaphen E.C. (Can) *see* aspirin *on page 98*

Asclera™ *see* polidocanol *on page 716*

Asco-Caps-500 [OTC] *see* ascorbic acid *on page 96*

Asco-Caps-1000 [OTC] *see* ascorbic acid *on page 96*

Ascocid® [OTC] *see* ascorbic acid *on page 96*

Ascocid®-500 [OTC] *see* ascorbic acid *on page 96*

Ascomp® with Codeine *see* butalbital, aspirin, caffeine, and codeine *on page 154*

Ascor L 500® *see* ascorbic acid *on page 96*

Ascor L NC® *see* ascorbic acid *on page 96*

ascorbic acid (a SKOR bik AS id)

Medication Safety Issues

International issues:
Rubex [Ireland] may be confused with Brivex brand name for brivudine [Switzerland]
Rubex: Brand name for ascorbic acid [Ireland], but also the brand name for doxorubicin [Brazil]

Synonyms vitamin C

U.S. Brand Names Acerola [OTC]; Asco-Caps-1000 [OTC]; Asco-Caps-500 [OTC]; Asco-Tabs-1000 [OTC]; Ascocid® [OTC]; Ascocid®-500 [OTC]; Ascor L 500®; Ascor L NC®; C-Gel [OTC]; C-Gram [OTC]; C-Time [OTC]; Cemill 1000 [OTC]; Cemill 500 [OTC]; Chew-C [OTC]; Dull-C® [OTC]; Mild-C® [OTC]; One Gram C [OTC]; Time-C® [OTC]; Vicks® Vitamin C [OTC]; Vita-C® [OTC]

Canadian Brand Names Proflavanol C™; Revitalose C-1000®

Therapeutic Category Vitamin, Water Soluble

Use Prevention and treatment of scurvy; acidify the urine

General Dosage Range

I.M., SubQ:
Children: 100-300 mg/day in divided doses
Adults: 100-250 mg 1-2 times/day

I.V., Oral:
  Children: 100-300 mg/day in divided doses (maximum: 500 mg every 6-8 hours)
  Adults: 100-250 mg 1-2 times/day (maximum: 4-12 g/day in 3-4 divided doses)
Dosage Forms
  Caplet, oral: 1000 mg
  Caplet, timed release, oral: 500 mg, 1000 mg
  Capsule, oral:
    Mild-C® [OTC]: 500 mg
  Capsule, softgel, oral:
    C-Gel [OTC]: 1000 mg
  Capsule, sustained release, oral:
    C-Time [OTC]: 500 mg
  Capsule, timed release, oral: 500 mg
    Asco-Caps-500 [OTC]: 500 mg
    Asco-Caps-1000 [OTC]: 1000 mg
    Time-C® [OTC]: 500 mg
  Crystals for solution, oral: (170 g, 1000 g)
    Mild-C® [OTC]: (170 g, 1000 g)
    Vita-C® [OTC]: (113 g, 454 g)
  Injection, solution: 500 mg/mL (50 mL)
    Ascor L 500®: 500 mg/mL (50 mL)
  Injection, solution [preservative free]: 500 mg/mL (50 mL)
    Ascor L NC®: 500 mg/mL (50 mL)
  Liquid, oral: 500 mg/5 mL (118 mL, 473 mL)
  Lozenge, oral:
    Vicks® Vitamin C [OTC]: 25 mg (20s)
  Powder for solution, oral:
    Ascocid® [OTC]: (227 g, 454 g)
    Dull-C® [OTC]: (113 g, 454 g)
  Tablet, oral: 100 mg, 250 mg, 500 mg, 1000 mg
    Asco-Tabs-1000 [OTC]: 1000 mg
    Ascocid®-500 [OTC]: 500 mg
    C-Gram [OTC]: 1000 mg
    One Gram C [OTC]: 1000 mg
  Tablet, chewable, oral: 250 mg, 500 mg
    Acerola [OTC]: 500 mg
    Chew-C [OTC]: 500 mg
    Mild-C® [OTC]: 250 mg
  Tablet, timed release, oral: 500 mg, 1000 mg
    Cemill 500 [OTC]: 500 mg
    Cemill 1000 [OTC]: 1000 mg
    Mild-C® [OTC]: 1000 mg

Asco-Tabs-1000 [OTC] *see* ascorbic acid *on page 96*
Ascriptin® Maximum Strength [OTC] *see* aspirin *on page 98*
Ascriptin® Regular Strength [OTC] *see* aspirin *on page 98*

asenapine (a SEN a peen)

U.S. Brand Names Saphris®
Therapeutic Category Antimanic Agent; Antipsychotic Agent, Atypical
Use Acute and maintenance treatment of schizophrenia; treatment of acute mania or mixed episodes associated with bipolar I disorder (as monotherapy or in combination with lithium or valproate)
General Dosage Range Oral: *Adults:* 5-10 mg twice daily
Dosage Forms
  Tablet, sublingual:
    Saphris®: 5 mg, 10 mg

Asendin [DSC] *see* amoxapine *on page 73*
Asmanex® Twisthaler® *see* mometasone (oral inhalation) *on page 595*

asparaginase (a SPEAR a ji nase)

Medication Safety Issues
Sound-alike/look-alike issues:
Asparaginase may be confused with pegaspargase
Elspar® may be confused with Elaprase®, Oncaspar®
High alert medication:
This medication is in a class the Institute for Safe Medication Practices (ISMP) includes among its list of drug classes which have a heightened risk of causing significant patient harm when used in error.
Synonyms *E. coli* asparaginase; *Erwinia* asparaginase; L-asparaginase
U.S. Brand Names Elspar®
Canadian Brand Names Kidrolase®
Therapeutic Category Antineoplastic Agent
Use Treatment (in combination with other chemotherapy) of acute lymphoblastic leukemia (ALL)
General Dosage Range
I.M.: *Children and Adults:* 6000 units/m^2/dose 3 times/week **or** 6000 units/m^2 every ~3 days
I.V.: *Children and Adults:* Dosage varies greatly depending on indication
Intradermal: *Children and Adults:* Test dose: 0.1-0.2 mL of a 20-250 units/mL concentration
Dosage Forms
Injection, powder for reconstitution:
Elspar®: 10,000 int. units

aspart insulin *see* insulin aspart *on page 475*
Aspercin [OTC] *see* aspirin *on page 98*
Aspercreme® [OTC] *see* trolamine *on page 894*
Aspergillus niger *see* alpha-galactosidase *on page 56*
Aspergum® [OTC] *see* aspirin *on page 98*

aspirin (AS pir in)

Medication Safety Issues
Sound-alike/look-alike issues:
Aspirin may be confused with Afrin®
Ascriptin® may be confused with Aricept®
Ecotrin® may be confused with Edecrin®, Epogen®
Halfprin® may be confused with Haltran®
ZORprin® may be confused with Zyloprim®
International issues:
Cartia [multiple international markets] may be confused with Cartia XT brand name for diltiazem [U.S.]
Synonyms acetylsalicylic acid; ASA; baby aspirin
U.S. Brand Names Ascriptin® Maximum Strength [OTC]; Ascriptin® Regular Strength [OTC]; Aspercin [OTC]; Aspergum® [OTC]; Aspir-low [OTC]; Aspirtab [OTC]; Bayer® Aspirin Extra Strength [OTC]; Bayer® Aspirin Regimen Adult Low Strength [OTC]; Bayer® Aspirin Regimen Children's [OTC]; Bayer® Aspirin Regimen Regular Strength [OTC]; Bayer® Genuine Aspirin [OTC]; Bayer® Plus Extra Strength [OTC]; Bayer® Women's Low Dose Aspirin [OTC]; Buffasal [OTC]; Bufferin® Extra Strength [OTC]; Bufferin® [OTC]; Buffinol [OTC]; Ecotrin® Arthritis Strength [OTC]; Ecotrin® Low Strength [OTC]; Ecotrin® [OTC]; Halfprin® [OTC]; St Joseph® Adult Aspirin [OTC]; Tri-Buffered Aspirin [OTC]
Canadian Brand Names Asaphen; Asaphen E.C.; Entrophen®; Novasen; Praxis ASA EC 81 Mg Daily Dose
Therapeutic Category Analgesic, Nonnarcotic; Antiplatelet Agent; Antipyretic; Nonsteroidal Antiinflammatory Drug (NSAID)
Use Treatment of mild-to-moderate pain, inflammation, and fever; prevention and treatment of myocardial infarction (MI), acute ischemic stroke, and transient ischemic episodes; management of rheumatoid arthritis, rheumatic fever, osteoarthritis; adjunctive therapy in revascularization procedures (coronary artery bypass graft [CABG], percutaneous transluminal coronary angioplasty [PTCA], carotid endarterectomy), stent implantation
General Dosage Range
Oral:
Children: 10-15 mg/kg/dose every 4-6 hours (maximum: 4 g/day) **or** 60-100 mg/kg/day divided every 4-8 hours **or** 1-20 mg/kg/day as a single dose

Adults: 325-650 mg every 4-6 hours (maximum: 4 g/day) **or** 2.4-5.4 g/day in divided doses **or** 40-325 mg/day as a single dose

Rectal:
  Children: 10-15 mg/kg/dose every 4-6 hours (maximum: 4 g/day)
  Adults: 300-600 mg every 4-6 hours (maximum: 4 g/day)

Dosage Forms
  Caplet, oral:
    Ascriptin® Maximum Strength [OTC]: 500 mg
    Bayer® Aspirin Extra Strength [OTC]: 500 mg
    Bayer® Genuine Aspirin [OTC]: 325 mg
    Bayer® Plus Extra Strength [OTC]: 500 mg
    Bayer® Women's Low Dose Aspirin [OTC]: 81 mg
  Caplet, enteric coated, oral:
    Bayer® Aspirin Regimen Regular Strength [OTC]: 325 mg
  Gum, chewing, oral:
    Aspergum® [OTC]: 227 mg (12s)
  Suppository, rectal: 300 mg (12s); 600 mg (12s)
  Tablet, oral: 325 mg
    Ascriptin® Regular Strength [OTC]: 325 mg
    Aspercin [OTC]: 325 mg
    Aspirtab [OTC]: 325 mg
    Bayer® Genuine Aspirin [OTC]: 325 mg
    Buffasal [OTC]: 325 mg
    Bufferin® [OTC]: 325 mg
    Bufferin® Extra Strength [OTC]: 500 mg
    Buffinol [OTC]: 324 mg
    Tri-Buffered Aspirin [OTC]: 325 mg
  Tablet, chewable, oral: 81 mg
    Bayer® Aspirin Regimen Children's [OTC]: 81 mg
    St Joseph® Adult Aspirin [OTC]: 81 mg
  Tablet, enteric coated, oral: 81 mg, 325 mg, 650 mg
    Aspir-low [OTC]: 81 mg
    Bayer® Aspirin Regimen Adult Low Strength [OTC]: 81 mg
    Ecotrin® [OTC]: 325 mg
    Ecotrin® Arthritis Strength [OTC]: 500 mg
    Ecotrin® Low Strength [OTC]: 81 mg
    Halfprin® [OTC]: 81 mg, 162 mg
    St Joseph® Adult Aspirin [OTC]: 81 mg

aspirin, acetaminophen, and caffeine *see* acetaminophen, aspirin, and caffeine *on page 29*

aspirin and carisoprodol *see* carisoprodol and aspirin *on page 177*

aspirin and diphenhydramine (AS pir in & dye fen HYE dra meen)

Synonyms ASA and diphenhydramine; aspirin and diphenhydramine citrate; diphenhydramine and ASA; diphenhydramine and aspirin; diphenhydramine citrate and aspirin

U.S. Brand Names Bayer® PM [OTC]

Therapeutic Category Analgesic, Miscellaneous

Use Aid in the relief of insomnia accompanied by minor pain or headache

General Dosage Range Oral: *Children ≥12 years and Adults:* Two caplets (1000 mg aspirin/77 mg diphenhydramine citrate) at bedtime

Dosage Forms
  Caplet, oral:
    Bayer® PM [OTC]: Aspirin 500 mg and diphenhydramine 38.3 mg

aspirin and diphenhydramine citrate *see* aspirin and diphenhydramine *on page 99*

aspirin and dipyridamole (AS pir in & dye peer ID a mole)

Medication Safety Issues
  Sound-alike/look-alike issues:
    Aggrenox® may be confused with Aggrastat®

Synonyms aspirin and extended-release dipyridamole; dipyridamole and aspirin

U.S. Brand Names Aggrenox®

▶

◀ **Canadian Brand Names** Aggrenox®
Therapeutic Category Antiplatelet Agent
Use Reduction in the risk of stroke in patients who have had transient ischemia of the brain or ischemic stroke due to thrombosis
General Dosage Range Oral: *Adults:* 1 capsule (200 mg dipyridamole, 25 mg aspirin) twice daily
Dosage Forms
  Capsule:
    Aggrenox®: Aspirin 25 mg [immediate release] and dipyridamole 200 mg [extended release]

aspirin and extended-release dipyridamole *see* aspirin and dipyridamole *on page 99*
aspirin and oxycodone *see* oxycodone and aspirin *on page 664*
aspirin, caffeine, and acetaminophen *see* acetaminophen, aspirin, and caffeine *on page 29*
aspirin, caffeine, and butalbital *see* butalbital, aspirin, and caffeine *on page 154*
aspirin, caffeine, and orphenadrine *see* orphenadrine, aspirin, and caffeine *on page 655*
aspirin, caffeine, codeine, and butalbital *see* butalbital, aspirin, caffeine, and codeine *on page 154*
aspirin, carisoprodol, and codeine *see* carisoprodol, aspirin, and codeine *on page 177*
Aspirin Free Anacin® Extra Strength [OTC] *see* acetaminophen *on page 23*
aspirin, orphenadrine, and caffeine *see* orphenadrine, aspirin, and caffeine *on page 655*
Aspir-low [OTC] *see* aspirin *on page 98*
Aspirtab [OTC] *see* aspirin *on page 98*
Astelin® *see* azelastine (nasal) *on page 107*
Astepro® *see* azelastine (nasal) *on page 107*
Astracaine® with epinephrine 1:200,000 (Can) *see* articaine and epinephrine *on page 95*
Astracaine® with epinephrine forte 1:100,000 (Can) *see* articaine and epinephrine *on page 95*
Astramorph®/PF *see* morphine (systemic) *on page 598*
AT *see* antithrombin III *on page 83*
AT-III *see* antithrombin III *on page 83*
Atacand® *see* candesartan *on page 167*
Atacand HCT® *see* candesartan and hydrochlorothiazide *on page 167*
Atacand® Plus (Can) *see* candesartan and hydrochlorothiazide *on page 167*
Atarax® (Can) *see* hydroxyzine *on page 456*
Atasol® (Can) *see* acetaminophen *on page 23*

atazanavir (at a za NA veer)
Synonyms atazanavir sulfate; ATV; BMS-232632
U.S. Brand Names Reyataz®
Canadian Brand Names Reyataz®
Therapeutic Category Antiretroviral Agent, Protease Inhibitor
Use Treatment of HIV-1 infections in combination with at least two other antiretroviral agents
General Dosage Range Dosage adjustment recommended in patients with hepatic or renal impairment or on concomitant therapy
  Oral:
    Children 6-17 years:
      15-24 kg (antiretroviral-naive patients): Atazanavir 150 mg once daily
      25-31 kg: Atazanavir 200 mg once daily
      32-38 kg: Atazanavir 250 mg once daily
      ≥39 kg: Atazanavir 300 mg once daily
      or
      15-19 kg: Atazanavir 8.5 mg/kg/dose once daily (rounded to available capsule strengths)
      ≥20 kg: Atazanavir 7 mg/kg/dose once daily (round to available capsule strengths) (maximum: 300 mg)
    Children ≥13 years (≥39 kg) and Adults: 400 mg once daily (antiretroviral-naive) **or** atazanavir 300 mg once daily
Dosage Forms
  Capsule, oral:
    Reyataz®: 100 mg, 150 mg, 200 mg, 300 mg

atazanavir sulfate *see* atazanavir *on page 100*

Atelvia™ *see* risedronate *on page 782*

atenolol (a TEN oh lole)
Medication Safety Issues
Sound-alike/look-alike issues:
Atenolol may be confused with albuterol, Altenol®, timolol, Tylenol®
Tenormin® may be confused with Imuran®, Norpramin®, thiamine, Trovan®
U.S. Brand Names Tenormin®
Canadian Brand Names Apo-Atenol®; CO Atenolol; Dom-Atenolol; JAMP-Atenolol; Mint-Atenolol; Mylan-Atenolol; Nu-Atenol; PHL-Atenolol; PMS-Atenolol; RAN™-Atenolol; ratio-Atenolol; Riva-Atenolol; Sandoz-Atenolol; Septa-Atenolol; Tenormin®; Teva-Atenolol
Therapeutic Category Beta-Adrenergic Blocker
Use Treatment of hypertension, alone or in combination with other agents; management of angina pectoris; secondary prevention postmyocardial infarction
General Dosage Range Dosage adjustment recommended in patients with renal impairment
Oral:
Children: 0.5-1 mg/kg/dose given daily; range of 0.5-1.5 mg/kg/day (maximum dose: 2 mg/kg/day up to 100 mg/day)
Adults: 25-100 mg/day as a single daily dose (maximum dose: 100 mg/day)
Dosage Forms
Tablet, oral: 25 mg, 50 mg, 100 mg
Tenormin®: 25 mg, 50 mg, 100 mg

atenolol and chlorthalidone (a TEN oh lole & klor THAL i done)
Synonyms chlorthalidone and atenolol
U.S. Brand Names Tenoretic®
Canadian Brand Names Apo-Atenidone®; Novo-Atenolthalidone; Tenoretic®; Teva-Atenolol Chlorthalidone
Therapeutic Category Antihypertensive Agent, Combination
Use Treatment of hypertension with a cardioselective beta-blocker and a diuretic
General Dosage Range Dosage adjustment recommended in patients with renal impairment
Oral: *Adults:* Initial: 50 mg (atenolol) and 25 mg (chlorthalidone) once daily; Maintenance: 50-100 mg (atenolol) and 25 mg (chlorthalidone) once daily (maximum: Atenolol 100 mg/day; chlorthalidone 25 mg/day)
Dosage Forms
Tablet, oral: Atenolol 50 mg and chlorthalidone 25 mg; atenolol 100 mg and chlorthalidone 25 mg
Tenoretic®: Atenolol 50 mg and chlorthalidone 25 mg; atenolol 100 mg and chlorthalidone 25 mg

ATG *see* antithymocyte globulin (equine) *on page 83*
Atgam® *see* antithymocyte globulin (equine) *on page 83*
Ativan® *see* lorazepam *on page 537*
atlizumab *see* tocilizumab *on page 874*
ATNAA *see* atropine and pralidoxime *on page 104*

atomoxetine (AT oh mox e teen)
Medication Safety Issues
Sound-alike/look-alike issues:
Atomoxetine may be confused with atorvastatin
Synonyms atomoxetine hydrochloride; LY139603; methylphenoxy-benzene propanamine; tomoxetine
U.S. Brand Names Strattera®
Canadian Brand Names Strattera®
Therapeutic Category Norepinephrine Reuptake Inhibitor, Selective
Use Treatment of attention-deficit/hyperactivity disorder (ADHD)
General Dosage Range Dosage adjustment recommended in patients with hepatic impairment
Oral:
Children ≥6 years and ≤70 kg: Initial: 0.5 mg/kg/day in 1-2 divided doses; Maintenance: 0.5-1.4 mg/kg/day as a single daily dose or 2 evenly divided doses (maximum: 1.4 mg/kg/day **or** 100 mg/day whichever is less)

Children ≥6 years and >70 kg and Adults: Initial: 40 mg/day in 1-2 divided doses; Maintenance: 40-100 mg/day in 1-2 divided doses (maximum: 100 mg/day)

Dosage Forms
Capsule, oral:
Strattera®: 10 mg, 18 mg, 25 mg, 40 mg, 60 mg, 80 mg, 100 mg

atomoxetine hydrochloride *see* atomoxetine *on page 101*
Atopiclair® *see* emollients *on page 325*

atorvastatin (a TORE va sta tin)

Medication Safety Issues
Sound-alike/look-alike issues:
Atorvastatin may be confused with atomoxetine, lovastatin, nystatin, pitavastatin, pravastatin, rosuvastatin, simvastatin
Lipitor® may be confused with labetalol, Levatol®, lisinopril, Loniten®, Lopid®, Mevacor®, Zocor®, ZyrTEC®

Synonyms atorvastatin calcium
U.S. Brand Names Lipitor®
Canadian Brand Names Apo-Atorvastatin®; CO Atorvastatin; GD-Atorvastatin; Lipitor®; Novo-Atorvastatin; PMS-Atorvastatin; RAN™-Atorvastatin; ratio-Atorvastatin; Sandoz-Atorvastatin
Therapeutic Category HMG-CoA Reductase Inhibitor
Use Treatment of dyslipidemias or primary prevention of cardiovascular disease (atherosclerotic) as detailed below:

Primary prevention of cardiovascular disease (high-risk for CVD): To reduce the risk of MI or stroke in patients without evidence of heart disease who have multiple CVD risk factors or type 2 diabetes. Treatment reduces the risk for angina or revascularization procedures in patients with multiple risk factors.
Secondary prevention of cardiovascular disease: To reduce the risk of nonfatal MI, nonfatal stroke, revascularization procedures, hospitalization for heart failure, and angina in patients with evidence of coronary heart disease.
Treatment of dyslipidemias: To reduce elevations in total cholesterol (C), LDL-C, apolipoprotein B, and triglycerides in patients with elevations of one or more components, and/or to increase low HDL-C as present in Fredrickson type IIa, IIb, III, and IV hyperlipidemias, heterozygous familial and nonfamilial hypercholesterolemia, and homozygous familial hypercholesterolemia
Treatment of heterozygous familial hypercholesterolemia (HeFH) in adolescent patients (10-17 years of age, females >1 year postmenarche) having LDL-C ≥190 mg/dL or LDL-C ≥160 mg/dL with positive family history of premature cardiovascular disease (CVD) or with two or more CVD risk factors.

General Dosage Range Dosage adjustment recommended in patients on concomitant therapy
Oral:
Children 10-17 years (females >1 year postmenarche): 10-20 mg/day (maximum: 20 mg/day)
Adults: Maintenance: 10-80 mg once daily (maximum: 80 mg/day)
Dosage Forms
Tablet, oral:
Lipitor®: 10 mg, 20 mg, 40 mg, 80 mg

atorvastatin and amlodipine *see* amlodipine and atorvastatin *on page 69*
atorvastatin calcium *see* atorvastatin *on page 102*
atorvastatin calcium and amlodipine besylate *see* amlodipine and atorvastatin *on page 69*

atovaquone (a TOE va kwone)

U.S. Brand Names Mepron®
Canadian Brand Names Mepron®
Therapeutic Category Antiprotozoal
Use Acute oral treatment of mild-to-moderate *Pneumocystis jirovecii* pneumonia (PCP) in patients who are intolerant to co-trimoxazole; prophylaxis of PCP in patients who are intolerant to co-trimoxazole
General Dosage Range Oral: *Children 13-16 years and Adults:* 1500 mg/day in 1-2 divided doses
Dosage Forms
Suspension, oral:
Mepron®: 750 mg/5 mL (5 mL, 210 mL)

atovaquone and proguanil (a TOE va kwone & pro GWA nil)

Synonyms atovaquone and proguanil hydrochloride; proguanil and atovaquone; proguanil hydrochloride and atovaquone

U.S. Brand Names Malarone®

Canadian Brand Names Malarone®; Malarone® Pediatric

Therapeutic Category Antimalarial Agent

Use Prevention or treatment of acute, uncomplicated *P. falciparum* malaria

General Dosage Range Oral:
Children 5-8 kg: Treatment: 125 mg/50 mg as a single daily dose
Children 9-10 kg: Treatment: 187.5 mg/75 mg as a single daily dose
Children 11-20 kg: Prophylaxis: 62.5 mg/25 mg; Treatment: 250 mg/100 mg as a single daily dose
Children 21-30 kg: Prophylaxis: 125 mg/50 mg; Treatment: 500 mg/200 mg as a single daily dose
Children 31-40 kg: Prophylaxis: 187.5 mg/75 mg; Treatment: 750 mg/300 mg as a single daily dose
Children >40 kg and Adults: Prophylaxis: 250 mg/100 mg; Treatment: 1 g/400 mg as a single daily dose

Dosage Forms
Tablet:
Malarone®: Atovaquone 250 mg and proguanil 100 mg
Tablet [pediatric]:
Malarone®: Atovaquone 62.5 mg and proguanil 25 mg

atovaquone and proguanil hydrochloride *see* atovaquone and proguanil *on page 103*
ATRA *see* tretinoin (systemic) *on page 885*

atracurium (a tra KYOO ree um)

Medication Safety Issues
High alert medication:
The Institute for Safe Medication Practices (ISMP) includes this medication among its list of drugs which have a heightened risk of causing significant patient harm when used in error.
Other safety concerns:
United States Pharmacopeia (USP) 2006: The Interdisciplinary Safe Medication Use Expert Committee of the USP has recommended the following:
- Hospitals, clinics, and other practice sites should institute special safeguards in the storage, labeling, and use of these agents and should include these safeguards in staff orientation and competency training.
- Healthcare professionals should be on **high alert** (especially vigilant) whenever a neuromuscular-blocking agent (NMBA) is stocked, ordered, prepared, or administered.

Synonyms atracurium besylate

Canadian Brand Names Atracurium Besylate Injection

Therapeutic Category Skeletal Muscle Relaxant

Use Adjunct to general anesthesia to facilitate endotracheal intubation and to relax skeletal muscles during surgery; to facilitate mechanical ventilation in ICU patients; does not relieve pain or produce sedation

General Dosage Range I.V.:
Children 1 month to 2 years: Initial: 0.3-0.4 mg/kg; Maintenance: Doses as needed to maintain neuromuscular blockade; Infusion: 10-20 mcg/kg/minute
Children >2 years and Adults: Initial: 0.4-0.5 mg/kg; Maintenance: 0.08-1 mg/kg at 15- to 25-minute intervals; Infusion: 5-13 mcg/kg/minute

Dosage Forms
Injection, solution: 10 mg/mL (10 mL)
Injection, solution [preservative free]: 10 mg/mL (5 mL)

atracurium besylate *see* atracurium *on page 103*
Atracurium Besylate Injection (Can) *see* atracurium *on page 103*
Atralin™ *see* tretinoin (topical) *on page 885*
Atriance™ (Can) *see* nelarabine *on page 616*
Atripla® *see* efavirenz, emtricitabine, and tenofovir *on page 321*
AtroPen® *see* atropine *on page 103*

atropine (A troe peen)

Synonyms atropine sulfate

◄ **U.S. Brand Names** AtroPen®; Atropine Care™; Isopto® Atropine; Sal-Tropine™ [DSC]
Canadian Brand Names Dioptic's Atropine Solution; Isopto® Atropine
Therapeutic Category Anticholinergic Agent
Use
Injection: Preoperative medication to inhibit salivation and secretions; treatment of symptomatic sinus bradycardia, AV block (nodal level); antidote for acetylcholinesterase inhibitor poisoning (carbamate insecticides, nerve agents, organophosphate insecticides); adjuvant use with anticholinesterases (eg, edrophonium, neostigmine) to decrease their side effects during reversal of neuromuscular blockade
Note: Use is no longer recommended in the management of asystole or pulseless electrical activity (PEA) (ACLS, 2010).
Ophthalmic: Produce mydriasis and cycloplegia for examination of the retina and optic disc and accurate measurement of refractive errors; uveitis
Oral: Inhibit salivation and secretions
General Dosage Range
I.M.; SubQ:
Children ≤5 kg: 0.02 mg/kg/dose every 4-6 hours as needed
Children >5 kg: 0.01-0.2 mg/kg/dose every 4-6 hours as needed (maximum: 0.4 mg/dose; minimum: 0.1 mg/dose)
Adults: 0.4-0.6 mg every 4-6 hours as needed
AtroPen® (I.M.):
Children 6.8-18 kg: 0.5 mg/dose (maximum: 3 doses)
Children >41 kg and Adults: 2 mg/dose (maximum: 3 doses)
I.V.: *Children and Adults:* Dosage varies greatly depending on indication
Ophthalmic: *Adults:* Ointment: Apply a small amount in the conjunctival sac up to 3 times/day; Solution (1%): Instill 1-2 drops 4 times/day
Oral:
Children ≤5 kg: 0.02 mg/kg/dose every 4-6 hours as needed
Children >5 kg: 0.01-0.2 mg/kg/dose every 4-6 hours as needed (maximum: 0.4 mg/dose)
Adults: 0.4 mg every 4-6 hours
Dosage Forms
Injection, solution: 0.05 mg/mL (5 mL); 0.1 mg/mL (5 mL, 10 mL)
AtroPen®: 0.25 mg/0.3 mL (0.3 mL); 0.5 mg/0.7 mL (0.7 mL); 1 mg/0.7 mL (0.7 mL); 2 mg/0.7 mL (0.7 mL)
Injection, solution [preservative free]: 0.4 mg/0.5 mL (0.5 mL); 0.4 mg/mL (1 mL); 1 mg/mL (1 mL)
Ointment, ophthalmic: 1% (3.5 g)
Solution, ophthalmic: 1% (2 mL, 5 mL, 15 mL)
Atropine Care™: 1% (2 mL, 5 mL, 15 mL)
Isopto® Atropine: 1% (5 mL, 15 mL)

atropine and difenoxin *see* difenoxin and atropine *on page 282*
atropine and diphenoxylate *see* diphenoxylate and atropine *on page 293*

atropine and pralidoxime (A troe peen & pra li DOKS eem)

Synonyms atropine and pralidoxime chloride; Mark 1™; NAAK; nerve agent antidote kit; pralidoxime and atropine
U.S. Brand Names ATNAA; Duodote™
Therapeutic Category Anticholinergic Agent; Antidote
Use
ATNAA: Treatment of poisoning by susceptible organophosphorous nerve agents having acetylcholinesterase-inhibiting activity for self- or buddy-administration by military personnel
Duodote™: Treatment of poisoning by organophosphorous nerve agents (eg, tabun, sarin, soman) or organophosphorous insecticide for use by trained emergency medical services personnel
General Dosage Range I.M.: *Adults:* 1-3 injections (maximum: 3 injections)
Dosage Forms
Injection, solution:
ATNAA, Duodote™: Atropine 2.1 mg/0.7 mL and pralidoxime chloride 600 mg/2 mL [contains benzyl alcohol; prefilled auto-injector]

atropine and pralidoxime chloride *see* atropine and pralidoxime *on page 104*
Atropine Care™ *see* atropine *on page 103*

atropine, hyoscyamine, phenobarbital, and scopolamine *see* hyoscyamine, atropine, scopolamine, and phenobarbital *on page 459*

atropine sulfate *see* atropine *on page 103*

atropine sulfate and edrophonium chloride *see* edrophonium and atropine *on page 321*

Atrovent® *see* ipratropium (nasal) *on page 489*

Atrovent® HFA *see* ipratropium (oral inhalation) *on page 489*

Atryn® *see* antithrombin III *on page 83*

ATV *see* atazanavir *on page 100*

Augmentin® *see* amoxicillin and clavulanate potassium *on page 74*

Augmentin ES-600® [DSC] *see* amoxicillin and clavulanate potassium *on page 74*

Augmentin XR® *see* amoxicillin and clavulanate potassium *on page 74*

Auralgan® (Can) *see* antipyrine and benzocaine *on page 83*

auranofin (au RANE oh fin)

Medication Safety Issues
Sound-alike/look-alike issues:
Ridaura® may be confused with Cardura®

U.S. Brand Names Ridaura®

Canadian Brand Names Ridaura®

Therapeutic Category Gold Compound

Use Management of active stage of classic or definite rheumatoid arthritis in patients who do not respond to or tolerate other agents; psoriatic arthritis; adjunctive or alternative therapy for pemphigus

General Dosage Range Dosage adjustment recommended in patients with renal impairment
Oral:
Children: Initial: 0.1 mg/kg/day; Maintenance: 0.1-0.2 mg/kg/day in 1-2 divided doses (maximum: 0.2 mg/kg/day)
Adults: Initial: 6 mg/day; Maintenance: 6-9 mg/day (maximum: 9 mg/day)

Dosage Forms
Capsule, oral:
Ridaura®: 3 mg

Auraphene B® [OTC] *see* carbamide peroxide *on page 172*

Auro® [OTC] *see* carbamide peroxide *on page 172*

Auro-Nevirapine (Can) *see* nevirapine *on page 621*

Auro-Terbinafine (Can) *see* terbinafine (systemic) *on page 851*

AVA *see* anthrax vaccine, adsorbed *on page 80*

Avagard™ [OTC] *see* chlorhexidine gluconate *on page 194*

Avage® *see* tazarotene *on page 845*

avakine *see* infliximab *on page 472*

Avalide® *see* irbesartan and hydrochlorothiazide *on page 490*

Avamys® (Can) *see* fluticasone (nasal) *on page 393*

Avandamet® *see* rosiglitazone and metformin *on page 791*

Avandaryl® *see* rosiglitazone and glimepiride *on page 791*

Avandia® *see* rosiglitazone *on page 791*

Avapro® *see* irbesartan *on page 490*

Avapro® HCT *see* irbesartan and hydrochlorothiazide *on page 490*

AVAR™ *see* sulfur and sulfacetamide *on page 838*

AVAR™-e *see* sulfur and sulfacetamide *on page 838*

AVAR™-e Green *see* sulfur and sulfacetamide *on page 838*

AVAR™-e LS *see* sulfur and sulfacetamide *on page 838*

AVAR™ LS *see* sulfur and sulfacetamide *on page 838*

Avastin® *see* bevacizumab *on page 132*

Avaxim® (Can) *see* hepatitis A vaccine *on page 437*

Avaxim®-Pediatric (Can) *see* hepatitis A vaccine *on page 437*

AVC™ *see* sulfanilamide *on page 837*

Avelox® *see* moxifloxacin (systemic) *on page 600*

Avelox® ABC Pack *see* moxifloxacin (systemic) *on page 600*

Avelox® I.V. *see* moxifloxacin (systemic) *on page 600*

Aventyl® (Can) *see* nortriptyline *on page 634*

Aviane™ *see* ethinyl estradiol and levonorgestrel *on page 353*

Aviane® (Can) *see* ethinyl estradiol and levonorgestrel *on page 353*

avian influenza virus vaccine *see* influenza virus vaccine (H5N1) *on page 473*

AVINza® *see* morphine (systemic) *on page 598*

Avita® *see* tretinoin (topical) *on page 885*

Avitene® *see* collagen hemostat *on page 233*

Avitene® Flour *see* collagen hemostat *on page 233*

Avitene® Ultrafoam™ *see* collagen hemostat *on page 233*

Avodart® *see* dutasteride *on page 317*

Avonex® *see* interferon beta-1a *on page 482*

AVP *see* vasopressin *on page 910*

Axert® *see* almotriptan *on page 54*

Axid® *see* nizatidine *on page 631*

Axiron® *see* testosterone *on page 854*

AY-25650 *see* triptorelin *on page 894*

Aygestin® *see* norethindrone *on page 633*

Ayr® Allergy Sinus [OTC] *see* sodium chloride *on page 818*

Ayr® Baby Saline [OTC] *see* sodium chloride *on page 818*

Ayr® Saline [OTC] *see* sodium chloride *on page 818*

Ayr® Saline No-Drip [OTC] *see* sodium chloride *on page 818*

5-Aza-2'-deoxycytidine *see* decitabine *on page 256*

azacitidine (ay za SYE ti deen)

Medication Safety Issues

Sound-alike/look-alike issues:

AzaCITIDine may be confused with azaTHIOprine

High alert medication:

This medication is in a class the Institute for Safe Medication Practices (ISMP) includes among its list of drug classes which have a heightened risk of causing significant patient harm when used in error.

Synonyms 5-azacytidine; 5-AZC; AZA-CR; azacytidine; ladakamycin

Tall-Man azaCITIDine

U.S. Brand Names Vidaza®

Therapeutic Category Antineoplastic Agent, Antimetabolite (Pyrimidine)

Use Treatment of myelodysplastic syndrome (MDS)

General Dosage Range Dosage adjustment recommended in patients who develop toxicities

I.V., SubQ: *Adults:* 75-100 mg/m^2/day for 7 days/28-day treatment cycle

Dosage Forms

Injection, powder for suspension:

Vidaza®: 100 mg

AZA-CR *see* azacitidine *on page 106*

Azactam® *see* aztreonam *on page 110*

azacytidine *see* azacitidine *on page 106*

5-azacytidine *see* azacitidine *on page 106*

5-Aza-dCyd *see* decitabine *on page 256*

azaepothilone B *see* ixabepilone *on page 497*

Azarga™ (Can) *see* brinzolamide and timolol *(Canada only) on page 141*

Azasan® *see* azathioprine *on page 107*

AzaSite® *see* azithromycin (ophthalmic) *on page 109*

azathioprine (ay za THYE oh preen)

Medication Safety Issues
Sound-alike/look-alike issues:
AzaTHIOprine may be confused with azaCITIDine, azidothymidine, azithromycin, Azulfidine®
Imuran® may be confused with Elmiron®, Enduron, Imdur®, Inderal®, Tenormin®
Other safety concerns:
Azathioprine is metabolized to mercaptopurine; concurrent use of these commercially-available products has resulted in profound myelosuppression.

Synonyms azathioprine sodium
Tall-Man azaTHIOprine
U.S. Brand Names Azasan®; Imuran®
Canadian Brand Names Apo-Azathioprine®; Imuran®; Mylan-Azathioprine; Teva-Azathioprine
Therapeutic Category Immunosuppressant Agent
Use Adjunctive therapy in prevention of rejection of kidney transplants; management of active rheumatoid arthritis (RA)
General Dosage Range Dosage adjustment recommended in patients with renal impairment, on concomitant therapy, or who develop toxicities
I.V.: *Adults:* Transplant immunosuppression: Initial: 3-5 mg/kg/day as a single daily dose; Maintenance: 1-3 mg/kg/day as a single daily dose
Oral: *Adults:*
Transplant immunosuppression: Initial: 3-5 mg/kg/day in 1-2 divided doses; Maintenance: 1-3 mg/kg/day in 1-2 divided doses
Rheumatoid arthritis: Initial: 1 mg/kg/day (50-100 mg) in 1-2 divided doses; Maintenance: 0.5-2.5 mg/kg/day in 1-2 divided doses
Dosage Forms
Injection, powder for reconstitution: 100 mg
Tablet, oral: 50 mg
Azasan®: 75 mg, 100 mg
Imuran®: 50 mg

azathioprine sodium *see* azathioprine *on page 107*
5-AZC *see* azacitidine *on page 106*
AZD6140 *see* ticagrelor *on page 867*
AZD6474 *see* vandetanib *on page 907*

azelaic acid (a zeh LAY ik AS id)

U.S. Brand Names Azelex®; Finacea®; Finacea® Plus™
Canadian Brand Names Finacea®
Therapeutic Category Topical Skin Product
Use Topical treatment of inflammatory papules and pustules of mild-to-moderate rosacea; mild-to-moderate inflammatory acne vulgaris
Finacea®: Not FDA-approved for the treatment of acne
General Dosage Range
Topical: *Children ≥12 years and Adults:* Massage gently into affected areas twice daily.
Dosage Forms
Cream, topical:
Azelex®: 20% (30 g, 50 g)
Gel, topical:
Finacea®: 15% (50 g)
Finacea® Plus™: 15% (50 g)

azelastine (nasal) (a ZEL as teen)

Medication Safety Issues
Sound-alike/look-alike issues:
Astelin® may be confused with Astepro®
Synonyms azelastine hydrochloride
U.S. Brand Names Astelin®; Astepro®
Canadian Brand Names Astelin®
Therapeutic Category Histamine H_1 Antagonist; Histamine H_1 Antagonist, Second Generation

◀ **Use** Treatment of the symptoms of seasonal allergic rhinitis such as rhinorrhea, sneezing, and nasal pruritus; treatment of the symptoms of vasomotor rhinitis

General Dosage Range Intranasal:
Children 5-11 years: 1 spray in each nostril twice daily
Children ≥12 years and Adults: 1-2 sprays in each nostril twice daily

Dosage Forms
Solution, intranasal: 0.1% [137 mcg/spray] (30 mL)
Astelin®: 0.1% [137 mcg/spray] (30 mL)
Astepro®: 0.15% [205.5 mcg/spray] (30 mL)

azelastine (ophthalmic) (a ZEL as teen)

Medication Safety Issues
Sound-alike/look-alike issues:
Optivar® may be confused with Optiray®, Optive™
International issues:
Optivar [U.S.] may be confused with Opthavir brand name for acyclovir [Mexico]
Synonyms azelastine hydrochloride
U.S. Brand Names Optivar®
Therapeutic Category Histamine H₁ Antagonist; Histamine H₁ Antagonist, Second Generation
Use Treatment of itching of the eye associated with seasonal allergic conjunctivitis
General Dosage Range Ophthalmic: *Children ≥3 years and Adults:* Instill 1 drop into affected eye(s) twice daily
Dosage Forms
Solution, ophthalmic: 0.05% (6 mL)
Optivar®: 0.05% (6 mL)

azelastine hydrochloride *see* azelastine (nasal) *on page 107*
azelastine hydrochloride *see* azelastine (ophthalmic) *on page 108*
Azelex® *see* azelaic acid *on page 107*
azidothymidine *see* zidovudine *on page 929*
azidothymidine, abacavir, and lamivudine *see* abacavir, lamivudine, and zidovudine *on page 20*
Azilect® *see* rasagiline *on page 769*

azilsartan (ay zil SAR tan)

Synonyms azilsartan medoxomil; AZL-M
U.S. Brand Names Edarbi™
Therapeutic Category Angiotensin II Receptor Blocker
Use Treatment of hypertension; may be used alone or in combination with other antihypertensives
General Dosage Range Oral: *Adults:* 40-80 mg once daily
Dosage Forms
Tablet, oral:
Edarbi™: 40 mg, 80 mg

azilsartan medoxomil *see* azilsartan *on page 108*

azithromycin (systemic) (az ith roe MYE sin)

Medication Safety Issues
Sound-alike/look-alike issues:
Azithromycin may be confused with azathioprine, erythromycin
Zithromax® may be confused with Fosamax®, Zinacef®, Zovirax®
Synonyms azithromycin dihydrate; azithromycin hydrogencitrate; azithromycin monohydrate; Z-Pak
U.S. Brand Names Zithromax®; Zithromax® TRI-PAK™; Zithromax® Z-PAK®; Zmax®
Canadian Brand Names Apo-Azithromycin®; CO Azithromycin; Dom-Azithromycin; Mylan-Azithromycin; Novo-Azithromycin; PHL-Azithromycin; PMS-Azithromycin; PRO-Azithromycin; ratio-Azithromycin; Riva-Azithromycin; Sandoz-Azithromycin; Zithromax®
Therapeutic Category Antibiotic, Macrolide
Use Oral, I.V.: Treatment of acute otitis media due to *H. influenzae*, *M. catarrhalis*, or *S. pneumoniae*; pharyngitis/tonsillitis due to *S. pyogenes*; treatment of mild-to-moderate upper and lower respiratory tract infections, infections of the skin and skin structure, community-acquired pneumonia, pelvic inflammatory

disease (PID), sexually-transmitted diseases (urethritis/cervicitis), and genital ulcer disease (chancroid) due to susceptible strains of *Chlamydophila pneumoniae, C. trachomatis, M. catarrhalis, H. influenzae, S. aureus, S. pneumoniae, Mycoplasma genitalium, Mycoplasma pneumoniae*, and *C. psittaci*; acute bacterial exacerbations of chronic obstructive pulmonary disease (COPD) due to *H. influenzae, M. catarrhalis*, or *S. pneumoniae*; acute bacterial sinusitis; prevention, alone or in combination with rifabutin, of MAC in patients with advanced HIV infection; treatment, in combination with ethambutol, of disseminated MAC in patients with advanced HIV infection

General Dosage Range
I.V.: *Adults:* 500 mg as a single daily dose
Oral:
Immediate release:
Children ≥6 months to 2 years: 5-10 mg/kg as a single daily dose (maximum: 500 mg/dose) **or** 30 mg/kg as a single dose (maximum: 1500 mg/dose)
Children ≥2 years: 5-12 mg/kg as single daily dose (maximum: 500 mg/dose) **or** 30 mg/kg as a single dose (maximum: 1500 mg/dose)
Adults: 250-500 mg as a single daily dose **or** 1-2 g as a single dose
Extended release (suspension):
Children ≥6 months and <34 kg: 60 mg/kg as a single dose
Children ≥6 months and ≥34 kg and Adults: 2 g as a single dose

Dosage Forms
Injection, powder for reconstitution: 500 mg
Zithromax®: 500 mg
Microspheres for suspension, extended release, oral:
Zmax®: 2 g/bottle (60 mL)
Powder for suspension, oral: 100 mg/5 mL (15 mL); 200 mg/5 mL (15 mL, 22.5 mL, 30 mL); 1 g/packet (3s, 10s)
Zithromax®: 100 mg/5 mL (15 mL); 200 mg/5 mL (15 mL, 22.5 mL, 30 mL); 1 g/packet (3s, 10s)
Tablet, oral: 250 mg, 500 mg, 600 mg
Zithromax®: 250 mg, 500 mg, 600 mg
Zithromax® TRI-PAK™: 500 mg
Zithromax® Z-PAK®: 250 mg

azithromycin (ophthalmic) (az ith roe MYE sin)

Medication Safety Issues
Sound-alike/look-alike issues:
Azithromycin may be confused with azathioprine, erythromycin
U.S. Brand Names AzaSite®
Therapeutic Category Antibiotic, Macrolide; Antibiotic, Ophthalmic
Use Bacterial conjunctivitis
General Dosage Range Ophthalmic: *Children ≥1 year and Adults:* Days 1 and 2: 1 drop into affected eye(s) twice daily; Days 3-7: 1 drop into affected eye(s) once daily
Dosage Forms
Solution, ophthalmic:
AzaSite®: 1% (2.5 mL)

aztreonam (AZ tree oh nam)

Medication Safety Issues
Sound-alike/look-alike issues:
Aztreonam may be confused with azidothymidine

Synonyms azthreonam

U.S. Brand Names Azactam®; Cayston®

Therapeutic Category Antibiotic, Miscellaneous

Use
Injection: Treatment of patients with urinary tract infections, lower respiratory tract infections, septicemia, skin/skin structure infections, intraabdominal infections, and gynecological infections caused by susceptible gram-negative bacilli
Inhalation: Improve respiratory symptoms in cystic fibrosis (CF) patients with *Pseudomonas aeruginosa*

General Dosage Range Dosage adjustment recommended in patients with renal impairment
I.M.:
Children >1 month: 30-50 mg/kg/dose every 6-8 hours (maximum: 8 g/day)
Adults: 500 mg to 1 g every 8-12 hours
I.V.:
Children >1 month: 30-50 mg/kg/dose every 6-8 hours (maximum: 8 g/day)
Adults: 1-2 g every 6-12 hours (maximum: 8 g/day)
Oral inhalation: *Children ≥7 years and Adults:* 75 mg 3 times/day

Dosage Forms
Infusion, premixed iso-osmotic solution:
Azactam®: 1 g (50 mL); 2 g (50 mL)
Injection, powder for reconstitution: 1 g, 2 g
Azactam®: 1 g, 2 g
Powder for reconstitution, for oral inhalation [preservative free]:
Cayston®: 75 mg

Azulfidine® *see* sulfasalazine *on page 837*

Azulfidine EN-tabs® *see* sulfasalazine *on page 837*

Azurette™ *see* ethinyl estradiol and desogestrel *on page 351*

B6 *see* pyridoxine *on page 758*

B1939 *see* eribulin *on page 337*

B2036-PEG *see* pegvisomant *on page 682*

B 9273 *see* alefacept *on page 48*

baby aspirin *see* aspirin *on page 98*

BabyBIG® *see* botulism immune globulin (intravenous-human) *on page 139*

Bacid® [OTC] *see* Lactobacillus *on page 506*

Bacid® (Can) *see* Lactobacillus *on page 506*

Baciguent® [OTC] *see* bacitracin *on page 110*

Baciguent® (Can) *see* bacitracin *on page 110*

BACiiM™ *see* bacitracin *on page 110*

Baciject® (Can) *see* bacitracin *on page 110*

bacillus Calmette-Guérin (BCG) live *see* BCG *on page 115*

Baci-Rx [DSC] *see* bacitracin *on page 110*

bacitracin (bas i TRAY sin)

Medication Safety Issues
Sound-alike/look-alike issues:
Bacitracin may be confused with Bactrim™, Bactroban®

U.S. Brand Names Baci-Rx [DSC]; Baciguent® [OTC]; BACiiM™

Canadian Brand Names Baciguent®; Baciject®

Therapeutic Category Antibiotic, Miscellaneous; Antibiotic, Ophthalmic; Antibiotic, Topical

Use Treatment of susceptible bacterial infections mainly (has activity against gram-positive bacilli); due to toxicity risks, systemic and irrigant uses of bacitracin should be limited to situations where less toxic alternatives would not be effective

General Dosage Range
I.M.:
Infants ≤2.5 kg: 900 units/kg/day in 2-3 divided doses
Infants >2.5 kg: 1000 units/kg/day in 2-3 divided doses
Ophthalmic: *Children and Adults:* Instill 1/4" to 1/2" ribbon every 3-4 hours (acute infections) or 2-3 times/day (mild-to-moderate infections)
Oral: *Adults:* 25,000 units 4 times/day
Topical: *Children and Adults:* Apply 1-3 times/day
Dosage Forms
Injection, powder for reconstitution: 50,000 units
BACiiM™: 50,000 units
Ointment, ophthalmic: 500 units/g (3.5 g)
Ointment, topical: 500 units/g (0.9 g, 15 g, 30 g, 120 g, 454 g)
Baciguent® [OTC]: 500 units/g (30 g)

bacitracin and polymyxin B (bas i TRAY sin & pol i MIKS in bee)

Medication Safety Issues
Sound-alike/look-alike issues:
Betadine® may be confused with Betagan®, betaine
Synonyms polymyxin B and bacitracin
U.S. Brand Names AK-Poly-Bac™; Polycin™; Polysporin® [OTC]
Canadian Brand Names LID-Pack®; Optimyxin®
Therapeutic Category Antibiotic, Ophthalmic; Antibiotic, Topical
Use Treatment of superficial infections caused by susceptible organisms
General Dosage Range
Ophthalmic: *Children and Adults:* Instill 1/2" ribbon in the affected eye(s) every 3-4 hours (acute infections) **or** 2-3 times/day (mild-to-moderate infections)
Topical: *Children and Adults:* Apply to affected area 1-4 times/day
Dosage Forms
Ointment, ophthalmic: Bacitracin 500 units and polymyxin B 10,000 units per g (3.5 g)
AK-Poly-Bac™: Bacitracin 500 units and polymyxin B 10,000 units per g (3.5 g)
Polycin™: Bacitracin 500 units and polymyxin B 10,000 units per g (3.5 g)
Ointment, topical: Bacitracin 500 units and polymyxin B 10,000 units per g in white petrolatum (15 g, 30 g)
Polysporin®: Bacitracin 500 units and polymyxin B 10,000 units per g (0.9 g, 15 g, 30 g)
Powder, topical:
Polysporin®: Bacitracin 500 units and polymyxin B 10,000 units per g (10 g)

bacitracin, neomycin, and polymyxin B
(bas i TRAY sin, nee oh MYE sin, & pol i MIKS in bee)

Synonyms neomycin, bacitracin, and polymyxin B; polymyxin B, bacitracin, and neomycin; triple antibiotic
U.S. Brand Names Neo-Polycin™; Neosporin® Neo To Go® [OTC]; Neosporin® Topical [OTC]
Therapeutic Category Antibiotic, Ophthalmic; Antibiotic, Topical
Use Helps prevent infection in minor cuts, scrapes, and burns; short-term treatment of superficial external ocular infections caused by susceptible organisms
General Dosage Range
Ophthalmic: *Children and Adults:* Instill 1/2" every 3-4 hours
Topical: *Children and Adults:* Apply 1-3 times/day
Dosage Forms
Ointment, ophthalmic: Bacitracin 400 units, neomycin 3.5 mg, and polymyxin B 10,000 units per g (3.5 g)
Neo-Polycin™: Bacitracin 400 units, neomycin 3.5 mg, and polymyxin B 10,000 units per g (3.5 g)
Ointment, topical: Bacitracin 400 units, neomycin 3.5 mg, and polymyxin B 5000 units per g (0.9 g, 15 g, 30 g, 454 g)
Neosporin® [OTC]: Bacitracin 400 units, neomycin 3.5 mg, and polymyxin B 5000 units per g (15 g, 30 g)
Neosporin® Neo To Go® [OTC]: Bacitracin 400 units, neomycin 3.5 mg, and polymyxin B 5000 units per g (0.9 g)

bacitracin, neomycin, polymyxin B, and hydrocortisone
(bas i TRAY sin, nee oh MYE sin, pol i MIKS in bee, & hye droe KOR ti sone)

Synonyms hydrocortisone, bacitracin, neomycin, and polymyxin B; neomycin, bacitracin, polymyxin B, and hydrocortisone; polymyxin B, bacitracin, neomycin, and hydrocortisone

U.S. Brand Names Cortisporin® Ointment; Neo-Polycin™ HC

Canadian Brand Names Cortisporin® Topical Ointment

Therapeutic Category Antibiotic/Corticosteroid, Ophthalmic; Antibiotic/Corticosteroid, Topical

Use Prevention and treatment of susceptible inflammatory conditions where bacterial infection (or risk of infection) is present

General Dosage Range
Ophthalmic: *Children and Adults:* Instill 1/2 inch every 3-4 hours
Topical: *Children and Adults:* Apply sparingly 2-4 times/day

Dosage Forms
Ointment, ophthalmic: Bacitracin 400 units, neomycin sulfate 3.5 mg, polymyxin B 10,000 units, and hydrocortisone 10 mg per g (3.5 g)
Neo-Polycin™ HC: Bacitracin 400 units, neomycin 3.5 mg, polymyxin B 10,000 units, and hydrocortisone 10 mg per g (3.5 g)
Ointment, topical:
Cortisporin®: Bacitracin 400 units, neomycin 3.5 mg, polymyxin B 5000 units, and hydrocortisone 10 mg per g (15 g)

bacitracin, neomycin, polymyxin B, and pramoxine
(bas i TRAY sin, nee oh MYE sin, pol i MIKS in bee, & pra MOKS een)

Synonyms neomycin, bacitracin, polymyxin B, and pramoxine; polymyxin B, neomycin, bacitracin, and pramoxine; pramoxine, neomycin, bacitracin, and polymyxin B

U.S. Brand Names Neosporin® + Pain Relief Ointment [OTC]; Tri Biozene [OTC]

Therapeutic Category Antibiotic, Topical

Use Prevention and treatment of susceptible superficial topical infections and provide temporary relief of pain or discomfort

General Dosage Range Topical: *Children ≥2 years and Adults:* Apply 1-3 times/day to infected areas

Dosage Forms
Ointment, topical: Bacitracin 500 units, neomycin 3.5 mg, polymyxin B 10,000 units, and pramoxine 10 mg (15 g, 30 g)
Neosporin® + Pain Relief Ointment [OTC]: Bacitracin 500 units, neomycin 3.5 mg, polymyxin B 10,000 units, and pramoxine 10 mg (15 g, 30 g)
Tri Biozene [OTC]: Bacitracin 500 units, neomycin 3.5 mg, polymyxin B 10,000 units, and pramoxine 10 mg (15 g)

baclofen (BAK loe fen)

Medication Safety Issues
Sound-alike/look-alike issues:
Baclofen may be confused with Bactroban®
Lioresal® may be confused with lisinopril, Lotensin®
High alert medication:
The Institute for Safe Medication Practices (ISMP) includes this medication (intrathecal administration) among its list of drugs which have a heightened risk of causing significant patient harm when used in error.

U.S. Brand Names Gablofen®; Lioresal®

Canadian Brand Names Apo-Baclofen®; Dom-Baclofen; Lioresal®; Liotec; Med-Baclofen; Mylan-Baclofen; Novo-Baclofen; Nu-Baclo; PHL-Baclofen; PMS-Baclofen; ratio-Baclofen; Riva-Baclofen

Therapeutic Category Skeletal Muscle Relaxant

Use Treatment of reversible spasticity associated with multiple sclerosis or spinal cord lesions
Orphan drug: Intrathecal: Treatment of intractable spasticity caused by spinal cord injury, multiple sclerosis, and other spinal disease (spinal ischemia or tumor, transverse myelitis, cervical spondylosis, degenerative myelopathy)

General Dosage Range
Intrathecal:
Children: Test dose: 25-100 mcg; Initial infusion: Infuse at a 24-hourly rate dosed at twice the test dose
Adults: Test dose: 50-100 mcg; Initial infusion: Infuse at a 24-hourly rate dosed at twice the test dose

Oral:
Adults: Initial: 5 mg 3 times/day; Maintenance: Up to 80 mg/day in 2-3 divided doses
Elderly: Initial: 5 mg 2-3 times/day, increasing gradually as needed
Dosage Forms
Injection, solution, intrathecal [preservative free]:
Gablofen®: 50 mcg/mL (1 mL); 500 mcg/mL (20 mL); 2000 mcg/mL (20 mL)
Lioresal®: 50 mcg/mL (1 mL); 500 mcg/mL (20 mL); 2000 mcg/mL (5 mL, 20 mL)
Tablet, oral: 10 mg, 20 mg

Bactoshield® CHG [OTC] *see* chlorhexidine gluconate *on page 194*
Bactrim™ *see* sulfamethoxazole and trimethoprim *on page 836*
Bactrim™ DS *see* sulfamethoxazole and trimethoprim *on page 836*
Bactroban® *see* mupirocin *on page 603*
Bactroban Cream® *see* mupirocin *on page 603*
Bactroban Nasal® *see* mupirocin *on page 603*
baking soda *see* sodium bicarbonate *on page 818*
BAL *see* dimercaprol *on page 288*
Balacet 325™ [DSC] *see* propoxyphene and acetaminophen *on page 746*

balanced salt solution (BAL anced salt soe LOO shun)

U.S. Brand Names AquaLase®; BSS Plus®; BSS®
Canadian Brand Names BSS Plus®; BSS®; Eye-Stream®
Therapeutic Category Ophthalmic Agent, Miscellaneous
Use
Irrigation solution for ophthalmic surgery:
AquaLase®, BSS®: Intraocular or extraocular irrigating solution
BSS Plus®: Intraocular irrigating solution
Irrigation solution for eyes, ears, nose, or throat
General Dosage Range Irrigation: *Children and Adults:* Based on standard for each surgical procedure
Dosage Forms
Solution, ophthalmic [irrigation; preservative free]: Sodium chloride 0.64%, potassium chloride 0.075%, calcium chloride 0.048%, magnesium chloride 0.03%, sodium acetate 0.39%, sodium citrate 0.17% (18 mL, 500 mL)
AquaLase®: Sodium chloride 0.64%, potassium chloride 0.075%, calcium chloride 0.048%, magnesium chloride 0.03%, sodium acetate 0.39%, sodium citrate 0.17% (90 mL)
BSS®: Sodium chloride 0.64%, potassium chloride 0.075%, calcium chloride 0.048%, magnesium chloride 0.03%, sodium acetate 0.39%, sodium citrate 0.17% (15 mL, 30 mL, 250 mL, 500 mL)
BSS Plus®: Sodium chloride 0.71%, potassium chloride 0.038%, calcium chloride 0.015%, magnesium chloride 0.02%, sodium phosphate 0.042%, sodium bicarbonate 0.21%, dextrose 0.092%, glutathione 0.018% (250 mL, 500 mL)

BAL in Oil® *see* dimercaprol *on page 288*
Balmex® [OTC] *see* zinc oxide *on page 930*
Balminil Decongestant (Can) *see* pseudoephedrine *on page 751*
Balminil DM D (Can) *see* pseudoephedrine and dextromethorphan *on page 752*
Balminil DM + Decongestant + Expectorant (Can) *see* guaifenesin, pseudoephedrine, and dextromethorphan *on page 430*
Balminil DM E (Can) *see* guaifenesin and dextromethorphan *on page 427*
Balminil Expectorant (Can) *see* guaifenesin *on page 425*
Balnetar® [OTC] *see* coal tar *on page 227*
Balnetar® (Can) *see* coal tar *on page 227*

balsalazide (bal SAL a zide)

Medication Safety Issues
Sound-alike/look-alike issues:
Colazal® may be confused with Clozaril®
Synonyms balsalazide disodium
U.S. Brand Names Colazal®
Therapeutic Category 5-Aminosalicylic Acid Derivative; Antiinflammatory Agent

◀ **Use** Treatment of mild-to-moderate active ulcerative colitis
General Dosage Range Oral:
Children ≥5 years: 750 mg **or** 2.25 g 3 times/day
Adults: 2.25 g 3 times/day
Dosage Forms
Capsule, oral: 750 mg
Colazal®: 750 mg

balsalazide disodium *see* balsalazide *on page 113*
balsam Peru, castor oil, and trypsin *see* trypsin, balsam Peru, and castor oil *on page 896*
Balziva™ *see* ethinyl estradiol and norethindrone *on page 355*
Band-Aid® Hurt Free™ Antiseptic Wash [OTC] *see* lidocaine (topical) *on page 524*
Banophen™ [OTC] *see* diphenhydramine (systemic) *on page 290*
Banophen™ Anti-Itch [OTC] *see* diphenhydramine (topical) *on page 291*
Banzel® *see* rufinamide *on page 793*
Banzel™ (Can) *see* rufinamide *on page 793*
Baraclude® *see* entecavir *on page 329*
Baridium [OTC] *see* phenazopyridine *on page 692*

barium (BA ree um)

Synonyms barium sulfate
U.S. Brand Names Digibar™ 190; E-Z Cat® Dry; E-Z-Cat®; E-Z-Disk™; E-Z-Dose™ with Liquid Polibar Plus®; E-Z-HD™; E-Z-Paque®; E-Z-Paste®; Entero Vu™; Entero VU™ 24%; Entero-H™; Esopho-Cat®; Liquid Entero Vu™; Liquid Polibar Plus®; Liquid Polibar®; Maxibar™; Polibar® ACB; Readi-Cat®; Readi-Cat® 2; Sensatrast™; Tagitol™ V; Ultra-R®; Varibar® Honey; Varibar® Nectar; Varibar® Pudding; Varibar® Thin Honey; Varibar® Thin Liquid; VoLumen®
Therapeutic Category Radiopaque Agents
Use Diagnostic aid for computed tomography or x-ray examinations of the GI tract
Dosage Forms
Cream, oral:
E-Z-Paste®: 60% w/w (454 g)
Esopho-Cat®: 3% w/w (30 g)
Paste, oral:
Varibar® Pudding: 40% w/v (230 mL)
Powder for suspension, oral:
Digibar™ 190: 190% w/v after reconstitution (232 g)
E-Z Cat® Dry: 2% w/w after reconstitution (23 g)
E-Z-HD™: 98% w/w before reconstitution (340 g)
E-Z-Paque®: 96% w/w before reconstitution (176 g, 1200 g)
Entero Vu™: 13% w/v after reconstitution (100 g)
Ultra-R®: 95% w/w before reconstitution (170 g)
Varibar® Thin Liquid: 40% w/v after reconstitution (148 g)
Powder for suspension, oral/rectal:
Sensatrast™: 100% before reconstitution (120 g)
Powder for suspension, rectal:
Polibar® ACB: 96% w/w before reconstitution (397 g, 454 g)
Suspension, oral:
E-Z-Cat®: 4.9% w/v (255 mL)
Entero VU™ 24%: 24% w/v (600 mL)
Entero-H™: 80% w/v (1900 mL)
Liquid Entero Vu™: 13% w/v (600 mL)
Maxibar™: 210% w/v (120 mL)
Readi-Cat® 2: 2.1% w/v (250 mL, 450 mL)
Tagitol™ V: 40% w/v (20 mL)
Varibar® Honey: 40% w/v (250 mL)
Varibar® Nectar: 40% w/v (240 mL)
Varibar® Thin Honey: 40% w/v (250 mL)
VoLumen®: 0.1% w/v (450 mL)

Suspension, oral/rectal:
Liquid Polibar Plus®: 105% w/v (1900 mL)
Liquid Polibar®: 100% w/v (1900 mL)
Readi-Cat®: 1.3% w/v (450 mL, 900 mL, 1900 mL)
Readi-Cat® 2: 2.1% w/v (450 mL, 900 mL, 1900 mL)
Suspension, rectal:
E-Z-Dose™ with Liquid Polibar Plus®: 105% w/v (650 mL)
Tablet, oral:
E-Z-Disk™: 648 mg

barium sulfate see barium on page 114
Basaljel® (Can) see aluminum hydroxide on page 59
base ointment see zinc oxide on page 930

basiliximab (ba si LIK si mab)

U.S. Brand Names Simulect®
Canadian Brand Names Simulect®
Therapeutic Category Immunosuppressant Agent
Use Prophylaxis of acute organ rejection in renal transplantation (in combination with cyclosporine and corticosteroids)
General Dosage Range I.V.:
Children <35 kg: 10 mg within 2 hours prior to transplant surgery, followed by a second 10 mg dose 4 days after transplantation
Children ≥35 kg and Adults: 20 mg within 2 hours prior to transplant surgery, followed by a second 20 mg dose 4 days after transplantation
Dosage Forms
Injection, powder for reconstitution:
Simulect®: 10 mg, 20 mg

BAY 43-9006 see sorafenib on page 827
BAY 59-7939 see rivaroxaban on page 786
Baycadron™ see dexamethasone (systemic) on page 264
Bayer® Aspirin Extra Strength [OTC] see aspirin on page 98
Bayer® Aspirin Regimen Adult Low Strength [OTC] see aspirin on page 98
Bayer® Aspirin Regimen Children's [OTC] see aspirin on page 98
Bayer® Aspirin Regimen Regular Strength [OTC] see aspirin on page 98
Bayer® Genuine Aspirin [OTC] see aspirin on page 98
Bayer® Plus Extra Strength [OTC] see aspirin on page 98
Bayer® PM [OTC] see aspirin and diphenhydramine on page 99
Bayer® Women's Low Dose Aspirin [OTC] see aspirin on page 98
BayGam® (Can) see immune globulin on page 468
Baza® Antifungal [OTC] see miconazole (topical) on page 585
Baza® Clear [OTC] see vitamin A and vitamin D on page 917
B-Caro-T™ [OTC] see beta-carotene on page 128

BCG (bee see jee)

Medication Safety Issues
Sound-alike/look-alike issues:
BCG (intravesical) may be confused with BCG for immunization
High alert medication:
The Institute for Safe Medication Practices (ISMP) includes this medication among its list of drugs which have a heightened risk of causing significant patient harm when used in error.
Synonyms bacillus Calmette-Guérin (BCG) live; BCG vaccine U.S.P. *(percutaneous use product)*; BCG, live
U.S. Brand Names BCG Vaccine; TheraCys®; TICE® BCG
Canadian Brand Names ImmuCyst®; Oncotice™; Pacis™
Therapeutic Category Biological Response Modulator

◀ **Use**

BCG intravesical: Treatment and prophylaxis of carcinoma *in situ* of the bladder; prophylaxis of primary or recurrent superficial papillary tumors following transurethral resection

BCG vaccine: Immunization against *Mycobacterium tuberculosis* in persons not previously infected and who are at high risk for exposure

BCG vaccine is not routinely administered for the prevention of *M. tuberculosis* in the United States. The Advisory Committee on Immunization Practices (ACIP) recommends vaccination be considered for the following:

- Children with a negative tuberculin skin test who are continually exposed to (and cannot be separated from) adults who are untreated or ineffectively treated for TB disease when the child cannot be given long-term treatment for infection **or** if the adult has TB caused by strains resistant to isoniazid and rifampin.

- Healthcare workers with a high percentage of patients with *M. tuberculosis* strains resistant to both isoniazid and rifampin, if there is ongoing transmission of the resistant strains and subsequent infection is likely, or if comprehensive infection-control precautions have not been successful. In addition, healthcare workers should be counseled on the risks and benefits of vaccination and treatment of latent TB infection

General Dosage Range

Percutaneous:

Children <1 month: 0.2-0.3 mL (half-strength dilution)

Children >1 month and Adults: 0.2-0.3 mL (full-strength dilution)

Intravesicular: *Adults:*

TheraCys®: 1 dose instilled into bladder (for 2 hours) once weekly for 6 weeks followed by 1 treatment at 3, 6, 12, 18, and 24 months after initial treatment

TICE® BCG: 1 dose instilled into bladder (for 2 hours) once weekly for 6 weeks (may repeat cycle 1 time), followed by once monthly for 6-12 months

Dosage Forms

Injection, powder for reconstitution, intravesical:

TICE® BCG: 50 mg

Injection, powder for reconstitution, intravesical [preservative free]:

TheraCys®: 81 mg

Injection, powder for reconstitution, percutaneous:

BCG Vaccine: 50 mg

BCG, live *see BCG on page 115*

BCG Vaccine *see BCG on page 115*

BCG vaccine U.S.P. (percutaneous use product) *see BCG on page 115*

BCNU *see carmustine on page 177*

B complex combinations *see vitamin B complex combinations on page 918*

BD™ Glucose [OTC] *see dextrose on page 273*

beano® [OTC] *see alpha-galactosidase on page 56*

beano® Meltaways [OTC] *see alpha-galactosidase on page 56*

Bebulin® VH *see factor IX complex (human) on page 365*

becaplermin (be KAP ler min)

Medication Safety Issues

Sound-alike/look-alike issues:

Regranex® may be confused with Granulex®, Repronex®

Synonyms recombinant human platelet-derived growth factor B; rPDGF-BB

U.S. Brand Names Regranex®

Canadian Brand Names Regranex®

Therapeutic Category Topical Skin Product

Use Adjunctive treatment of diabetic neuropathic ulcers occurring on the lower limbs and feet that extend into subcutaneous tissue (or beyond) and have adequate blood supply

General Dosage Range Topical: *Adults:* Apply once daily; to determine the length of gel to apply to the ulcer, measure the greatest length of the ulcer by the greatest width of the ulcer. Tube size and unit of measure will determine the formula used in the calculation. Recalculate amount of gel needed every 1-2 weeks, depending on the rate of change in ulcer area.

Centimeters: 15 g tube: [ulcer length (cm) x width (cm)] divided by 4 = length of gel (cm); 2 g tube: [ulcer length (cm) x width (cm)] divided by 2 = length of gel (cm)

Inches: 15 g tube: [length (in) x width (in)] x 0.6 = length of gel (in); 2 g tube: [length (in) x width (in)] x 1.3 = length of gel (in)

Dosage Forms
  Gel, topical:
    Regranex®: 0.01% (15 g)

beclomethasone (oral inhalation) (be kloe METH a sone)

Medication Safety Issues
  Sound-alike/look-alike issues:
    Vanceril® may be confused with Vancenase

Synonyms Vancenase

U.S. Brand Names QVAR®

Canadian Brand Names QVAR®; Vanceril® AEM

Therapeutic Category Corticosteroid, Inhalant (Oral)

Use Oral inhalation: Maintenance and prophylactic treatment of asthma; includes those who require corticosteroids and those who may benefit from a dose reduction/elimination of systemically-administered corticosteroids. Not for relief of acute bronchospasm.

General Dosage Range Inhalation:
  Children 5-11 years: Initial: 40 mcg twice daily; Maintenance: 80->320 mcg/day in 2 divided doses
  Children ≥12 years and Adults: Initial: 40-160 mcg twice daily; Maintenance: 80->480 mcg/day in 2 divided doses

Dosage Forms
  Aerosol, for oral inhalation:
    QVAR®: 40 mcg/inhalation (8.7 g); 80 mcg/inhalation (8.7 g)

beclomethasone (nasal) (be kloe METH a sone)

Synonyms beclomethasone dipropionate

U.S. Brand Names Beconase AQ®

Canadian Brand Names Apo-Beclomethasone®; Gen-Beclo; Nu-Beclomethasone; Rivanase AQ

Therapeutic Category Corticosteroid, Nasal

Use Symptomatic treatment of seasonal or perennial rhinitis; prevent recurrence of nasal polyps following surgery.

General Dosage Range Intranasal: *Children ≥6 years and Adults:* 1-2 inhalations each nostril twice daily (maximum: 336 mcg/day)

Dosage Forms
  Suspension, intranasal:
    Beconase AQ®: 42 mcg/inhalation (25 g)

beclomethasone dipropionate see beclomethasone (nasal) *on page 117*
Beconase AQ® see beclomethasone (nasal) *on page 117*
behenyl alcohol see docosanol *on page 302*

belatacept (bel AT a sept)

Synonyms BMS-224818; LEA29Y

U.S. Brand Names Nulojix®

Therapeutic Category Selective T-Cell Costimulation Blocker

Use Prophylaxis of organ rejection concomitantly with basiliximab, mycophenolate, and corticosteroids in Epstein-Barr virus (EBV) seropositive kidney transplant recipients

General Dosage Range I.V.: *Adults:* Initial phase: 10 mg/kg/dose; maintenance phase: 5 mg/kg/dose

Dosage Forms
  Injection, powder for reconstitution:
    Nulojix®: 250 mg

belimumab (be LIM yoo mab)

U.S. Brand Names Benlysta®

Canadian Brand Names Benlysta™

Therapeutic Category Monoclonal Antibody

Use Treatment of autoantibody-positive (antinuclear antibody [ANA] and/or anti-double-stranded DNA [anti-ds-DNA]) systemic lupus erythematosus (SLE) in addition to standard therapy

General Dosage Range I.V.: *Adults:* 10 mg/kg every 2 weeks for 3 doses; Maintenance: 10 mg/kg every 4 weeks

Dosage Forms

Injection, powder for reconstitution:
  Benlysta®: 120 mg, 400 mg

belladonna alkaloids with phenobarbital *see* hyoscyamine, atropine, scopolamine, and phenobarbital *on page 459*

belladonna and opium (bel a DON a & OH pee um)

Medication Safety Issues

Sound-alike/look-alike issues:
  B&O may be confused with beano®

BEERS Criteria medication:
  This drug may be inappropriate for use in geriatric patients (high severity risk).

Synonyms B&O; opium and belladonna

Therapeutic Category Analgesic, Narcotic

Controlled Substance C-II

Use Relief of moderate-to-severe pain associated with ureteral spasms not responsive to nonopioid analgesics and to space intervals between injections of opiates

General Dosage Range Rectal: *Children >12 years and Adults:* 1 suppository 1-2 times/day (maximum: 4 doses/day)

Dosage Forms

Suppository: Belladonna extract 16.2 mg and opium 30 mg; belladonna extract 16.2 mg and opium 60 mg

Benadryl® (Can) *see* diphenhydramine (systemic) *on page 290*

Benadryl-D® Allergy & Sinus [OTC] *see* diphenhydramine and phenylephrine *on page 292*

Benadryl-D® Children's Allergy & Sinus [OTC] *see* diphenhydramine and phenylephrine *on page 292*

Benadryl® Allergy [OTC] *see* diphenhydramine (systemic) *on page 290*

Benadryl® Allergy and Cold [OTC] *see* acetaminophen, diphenhydramine, and phenylephrine *on page 33*

Benadryl® Allergy and Sinus Headache [OTC] *see* acetaminophen, diphenhydramine, and phenylephrine *on page 33*

Benadryl® Allergy Quick Dissolve [OTC] *see* diphenhydramine (systemic) *on page 290*

Benadryl® Children's Allergy [OTC] *see* diphenhydramine (systemic) *on page 290*

Benadryl® Children's Allergy FastMelt® [OTC] *see* diphenhydramine (systemic) *on page 290*

Benadryl® Children's Allergy Perfect Measure™ [OTC] *see* diphenhydramine (systemic) *on page 290*

Benadryl® Children's Dye Free Allergy [OTC] *see* diphenhydramine (systemic) *on page 290*

Benadryl® Cream (Can) *see* diphenhydramine (topical) *on page 291*

Benadryl® Dye-Free Allergy [OTC] *see* diphenhydramine (systemic) *on page 290*

Benadryl® Extra Strength Itch Stopping [OTC] *see* diphenhydramine (topical) *on page 291*

Benadryl® Itch Relief Extra Strength [OTC] *see* diphenhydramine (topical) *on page 291*

Benadryl® Itch Relief Stick (Can) *see* diphenhydramine (topical) *on page 291*

Benadryl® Itch Stopping [OTC] *see* diphenhydramine (topical) *on page 291*

Benadryl® Itch Stopping Extra Strength [OTC] *see* diphenhydramine (topical) *on page 291*

Benadryl® Spray (Can) *see* diphenhydramine (topical) *on page 291*

Benadry® Maximum Strength Severe Allergy and Sinus Headache [OTC] *see* acetaminophen, diphenhydramine, and phenylephrine *on page 33*

benazepril (ben AY ze pril)

Medication Safety Issues
Sound-alike/look-alike issues:
Benazepril may be confused with Benadryl®
Lotensin® may be confused with Lioresal®, lovastatin
Synonyms benazepril hydrochloride
U.S. Brand Names Lotensin®
Canadian Brand Names Lotensin®
Therapeutic Category Angiotensin-Converting Enzyme (ACE) Inhibitor
Use Treatment of hypertension, either alone or in combination with other antihypertensive agents
General Dosage Range Dosage adjustment recommended in patients with renal impairment
Oral:
Children ≥6 years: Initial: 0.2 mg/kg/day (up to 10 mg/day); Maintenance: 0.1-0.6 mg/kg/day (maximum: 40 mg/day)
Adults: Initial: 5-10 mg/day; Maintenance: 20-80 mg/day in 1-2 divided doses
Dosage Forms
Tablet, oral: 5 mg, 10 mg, 20 mg, 40 mg
Lotensin®: 10 mg, 20 mg, 40 mg

benazepril and hydrochlorothiazide (ben AY ze pril & hye droe klor oh THYE a zide)

Synonyms benazepril hydrochloride and hydrochlorothiazide; hydrochlorothiazide and benazepril
U.S. Brand Names Lotensin HCT®
Therapeutic Category Antihypertensive Agent, Combination
Use Treatment of hypertension
General Dosage Range Oral: *Adults:* Benazepril 5-20 mg and hydrochlorothiazide 6.25-25 mg daily
Dosage Forms
Tablet:
Generics:
5/6.25: Benazepril 5 mg and hydrochlorothiazide 6.25 mg
10/12.5: Benazepril 10 mg and hydrochlorothiazide 12.5 mg
20/12.5: Benazepril 20 mg and hydrochlorothiazide 12.5 mg
20/25: Benazepril 20 mg and hydrochlorothiazide 25 mg
Brands:
Lotensin HCT® 10/12.5: Benazepril 10 mg and hydrochlorothiazide 12.5 mg
Lotensin HCT® 20/12.5: Benazepril 20 mg and hydrochlorothiazide 12.5 mg
Lotensin HCT® 20/25: Benazepril 20 mg and hydrochlorothiazide 25 mg

benazepril hydrochloride *see* benazepril *on page 119*
benazepril hydrochloride and amlodipine besylate *see* amlodipine and benazepril *on page 70*
benazepril hydrochloride and hydrochlorothiazide *see* benazepril and hydrochlorothiazide *on page 119*

bendamustine (ben da MUS teen)

Medication Safety Issues
Sound-alike/look-alike issues:
Bendamustine may be confused with brentuximab, carmustine, lomustine
High alert medication:
This medication is in a class the Institute for Safe Medication Practices (ISMP) includes among its list of drug classes which have a heightened risk of causing significant patient harm when used in error.
Synonyms bendamustine hydrochloride; cytostasan; SDX-105
U.S. Brand Names Treanda®
Therapeutic Category Antineoplastic Agent, Alkylating Agent
Use Treatment of chronic lymphocytic leukemia (CLL); treatment of progressed indolent B-cell non-Hodgkin lymphoma (NHL)
General Dosage Range Dosage adjustment recommended in patients who develop toxicities
I.V.: *Adults:* 100 mg/m^2 on days 1 and 2 of a 28-day treatment cycle **or** 120 mg/m^2 on days 1 and 2 of a 21-day treatment cycle

◄ **Dosage Forms**
Injection, powder for reconstitution:
Treanda®: 25 mg, 100 mg

bendamustine hydrochloride see bendamustine on page 119
bendroflumethiazide and nadolol see nadolol and bendroflumethiazide on page 608
Benefiber® [OTC] see wheat dextrin on page 923
Benefiber® Plus Calcium [OTC] see wheat dextrin on page 923
BeneFix® see factor IX on page 365
Benemid [DSC] see probenecid on page 738
benflumetol and artemether see artemether and lumefantrine on page 94
BenGay® [OTC] see methyl salicylate and menthol on page 579
Benicar® see olmesartan on page 646
Benicar HCT® see olmesartan and hydrochlorothiazide on page 647
Benlysta® see belimumab on page 118
Benlysta™ (Can) see belimumab on page 118
Benoxyl® (Can) see benzoyl peroxide on page 124

benserazide and levodopa *(Canada only)* (ben SER a zide & lee voe DOE pa)

Synonyms levodopa and benserazide
Canadian Brand Names Prolopa®
Therapeutic Category Anti-Parkinson Agent (Dopamine Agonist)
Use Treatment of Parkinson disease (except drug-induced parkinsonism)
General Dosage Range Oral: *Adults:* Initial: Levodopa 100 mg/benserazide 25 mg 1-2 times/day; Maintenance: Levodopa 400-800 mg/benserazide 100-200 mg daily in 4-6 divided doses (maximum: Levodopa/benserazide 1200/300 mg/day)
Product Availability Not available in U.S.
Dosage Forms - Canada
Capsule:
Prolopa®: 50-12.5: Levodopa 50 mg and benserazide 12.5 mg; 100-25: Levodopa 100 mg and benserazide 25 mg; 200-50: Levodopa 200 mg and benserazide 50 mg

bentoquatam (BEN toe kwa tam)

Synonyms quaternium-18 bentonite
U.S. Brand Names Ivy Block® [OTC]
Therapeutic Category Protectant, Topical
Use Skin protectant for the prevention of allergic contact dermatitis to poison oak, ivy, and sumac
General Dosage Range Topical: *Children >6 years and Adults:* Apply to skin 15 minutes prior to potential exposure to poison ivy, poison oak, or poison sumac, and reapply every 4 hours
Dosage Forms
Lotion, topical:
Ivy Block® [OTC]: 5% (120 mL)

Bentyl® see dicyclomine on page 280
Bentylol® (Can) see dicyclomine on page 280
Benuryl™ (Can) see probenecid on page 738
Benylin® 3.3 mg-D-E (Can) see guaifenesin, pseudoephedrine, and codeine on page 430
Benylin® D for Infants (Can) see pseudoephedrine on page 751
Benylin® DM-D (Can) see pseudoephedrine and dextromethorphan on page 752
Benylin® DM-D-E (Can) see guaifenesin, pseudoephedrine, and dextromethorphan on page 430
Benylin® DM-E (Can) see guaifenesin and dextromethorphan on page 427
Benylin® E Extra Strength (Can) see guaifenesin on page 425
Benzac® AC see benzoyl peroxide on page 124
Benzac AC® (Can) see benzoyl peroxide on page 124
BenzaClin® see clindamycin and benzoyl peroxide on page 219
Benzac® W see benzoyl peroxide on page 124
Benzac W® Gel (Can) see benzoyl peroxide on page 124

Benzac W® Wash (Can) *see* benzoyl peroxide *on page 124*

5 Benzagel® *see* benzoyl peroxide *on page 124*

10 Benzagel® *see* benzoyl peroxide *on page 124*

Benzamycin® *see* erythromycin and benzoyl peroxide *on page 340*

Benzamycin® Pak *see* erythromycin and benzoyl peroxide *on page 340*

BenzaShave® *see* benzoyl peroxide *on page 124*

benzathine benzylpenicillin *see* penicillin G benzathine *on page 684*

benzathine penicillin G *see* penicillin G benzathine *on page 684*

Benzedrex® [OTC] *see* propylhexedrine *on page 748*

BenzEFoam™ *see* benzoyl peroxide *on page 124*

benzene hexachloride *see* lindane *on page 528*

benzhexol hydrochloride *see* trihexyphenidyl *on page 891*

Benziq™ *see* benzoyl peroxide *on page 124*

benzmethyzin *see* procarbazine *on page 739*

benzocaine (BEN zoe kane)

Medication Safety Issues
  Sound-alike/look-alike issues:
  Orabase® may be confused with Orinase

Synonyms ethyl aminobenzoate

U.S. Brand Names Americaine® Hemorrhoidal [OTC]; Anbesol® Baby [OTC]; Anbesol® Cold Sore Therapy [OTC]; Anbesol® Jr. [OTC]; Anbesol® Maximum Strength [OTC]; Anbesol® [OTC]; Benzodent® [OTC]; Bi-Zets [OTC]; Boil-Ease® Pain Relieving [OTC]; Cepacol® Fizzlers™ [OTC]; Cepacol® Sore Throat Pain Relief [OTC]; Cepacol® Sore Throat Plus Coating Relief [OTC]; Chiggerex® Plus [OTC]; ChiggerTox® [OTC]; Dent's Extra Strength Toothache Gum [OTC]; Dentapaine [OTC]; Dermoplast® Antibacterial [OTC]; Dermoplast® Pain Relieving [OTC]; Detane® [OTC]; Foille® [OTC]; HDA® Toothache [OTC]; Hurricaine® [OTC]; Ivy-Rid® [OTC]; Kank-A® Soft Brush [OTC]; Lanacane® Maximum Strength [OTC]; Lanacane® [OTC]; Little Teethers® [OTC]; Medicone® Hemorrhoidal [OTC]; Mycinettes® [OTC]; Orabase® with Benzocaine [OTC]; Orajel® Baby Daytime and Nighttime [OTC]; Orajel® Baby Teething Nighttime [OTC]; Orajel® Baby Teething [OTC]; Orajel® Cold Sore [OTC]; Orajel® Denture Plus [OTC]; Orajel® Maximum Strength [OTC]; Orajel® Medicated Mouth Sore [OTC]; Orajel® Medicated Toothache [OTC]; Orajel® Mouth Sore [OTC]; Orajel® Multi-Action Cold Sore [OTC]; Orajel® PM Maximum Strength [OTC]; Orajel® Ultra Mouth Sore [OTC]; Orajel® [OTC]; Outgro® [OTC]; Red Cross™ Canker Sore [OTC]; Rid-A-Pain Dental [OTC]; Sepasoothe® [OTC]; Skeeter Stik® [OTC]; Sore Throat Relief [OTC]; Sting-Kill® [OTC]; Tanac® [OTC]; Thorets [OTC]; Trocaine® [OTC]; Zilactin® Tooth & Gum Pain [OTC]; Zilactin®-B [OTC]

Canadian Brand Names Anbesol® Baby; Zilactin Baby®; Zilactin-B®

Therapeutic Category Local Anesthetic

Use Temporary relief of pain associated with pruritic dermatosis, pruritus, minor burns, acute congestive, bee stings, and insect bites; mouth and gum irritations (toothache, minor sore throat pain, canker sores, dentures, orthodontia, teething, mucositis, stomatitis); sunburn; hemorrhoids; anesthetic lubricant for passage of catheters and endoscopic tubes

General Dosage Range
  Oral: *Children ≥5 years and Adults:* 1 lozenge (10-15 mg) every 2 hours as needed
  Rectal: *Children ≥12 years and Adults:* Apply externally to affected area up to 6 times/day
  Topical: *Children ≥2 years and Adults:* Apply to affected area 3-4 times/day as needed
  Topical (oral): *Children ≥4 months and Adults:* Apply thin layer to affected area up to 4 times/day

Dosage Forms
  Aerosol, oral:
  Hurricaine® [OTC]: 20% (60 mL)
  Aerosol, topical:
  Dermoplast® Antibacterial [OTC]: 20% (82.5 mL)
  Dermoplast® Pain Relieving [OTC]: 20% (60 mL, 82.5 mL)
  Ivy-Rid® [OTC]: 2% (85 g)
  Lanacane® Maximum Strength [OTC]: 20% (120 mL)
  Combination package, oral:
  Orajel® Baby Daytime and Nighttime [OTC]: gel, oral (Daytime Regular formula): benzocaine 7.5% (5.3 g) [1 tube] and gel, oral (Nighttime formula): benzocaine 10% (5.3 g) [1 tube]

◄ **Cream, oral**:
  Benzodent® [OTC]: 20% (7.5 g, 30 g)
  Orajel® PM Maximum Strength [OTC]: 20% (5.3 g, 7 g)
Cream, topical:
  Lanacane® [OTC]: 6% (28 g, 60 g)
  Lanacane® Maximum Strength [OTC]: 20% (28 g)
Gel, oral: 20% (15 g)
  Anbesol® [OTC]: 10% (7.1 g)
  Anbesol® Baby [OTC]: 7.5% (7.1 g)
  Anbesol® Jr. [OTC]: 10% (7.1 g)
  Anbesol® Maximum Strength [OTC]: 20% (7.1 g, 10 g)
  Dentapaine [OTC]: 20% (11 g)
  HDA® Toothache [OTC]: 6.5% (15 mL)
  Hurricaine® [OTC]: 20% (30 g); 20% (5.25 g, 30 g)
  Kank-A® Soft Brush [OTC]: 20% (2 g)
  Little Teethers® [OTC]: 7.5% (9.4 g)
  Orabase® with Benzocaine [OTC]: 20% (7 g)
  Orajel® [OTC]: 10% (5.3 g, 7 g, 9.4 g)
  Orajel® Baby Teething [OTC]: 7.5% (11.9 g); 7.5% (9.4 g)
  Orajel® Baby Teething Nighttime [OTC]: 10% (5.3 g)
  Orajel® Denture Plus [OTC]: 15% (9 g)
  Orajel® Maximum Strength [OTC]: 20% (5.4 g, 7 g, 9.4 g, 11.9 g)
  Orajel® Mouth Sore [OTC]: 20% (5.3 g, 9.4 g, 11.9 g)
  Orajel® Multi-Action Cold Sore [OTC]: 20% (9.4 g)
  Orajel® Ultra Mouth Sore [OTC]: 15% (9.4 g)
  Zilactin®-B [OTC]: 10% (7.5 g)
Gel, topical:
  Detane® [OTC]: 7.5% (15 g)
Liquid, oral: 20% (15 mL)
  Anbesol® [OTC]: 10% (9.3 mL)
  Anbesol® Maximum Strength [OTC]: 20% (9.3 mL)
  Hurricaine® [OTC]: 20% (30 mL)
  Orajel® Baby Teething [OTC]: 7.5% (13.3 mL)
  Orajel® Maximum Strength [OTC]: 20% (13.5 mL)
  Rid-A-Pain Dental [OTC]: 6.3% (30 mL)
  Tanac® [OTC]: 10% (13 mL)
Liquid, topical:
  ChiggerTox® [OTC]: 2% (30 mL)
  Outgro® [OTC]: 20% (9.3 mL)
  Skeeter Stik® [OTC]: 5% (14 mL)
Lozenge, oral: 6 mg (18s)
  Bi-Zets [OTC]: 15 mg (10s)
  Cepacol® Sore Throat Pain Relief [OTC]: 15 mg (16s, 18s)
  Cepacol® Sore Throat Plus Coating Relief [OTC]: 15 mg (18s)
  Mycinettes® [OTC]: 15 mg (12s)
  Sepasoothe® [OTC]: 10 mg (6s, 24s, 100s, 250s, 500s)
  Sore Throat Relief [OTC]: 10 mg (100s, 250s, 500s)
  Thorets [OTC]: 18 mg (300s)
  Trocaine® [OTC]: 10 mg (50s, 300s)
Ointment, oral:
  Anbesol® Cold Sore Therapy [OTC]: 20% (7.1 g)
  Red Cross™ Canker Sore [OTC]: 20% (7.5 g)
Ointment, rectal:
  Americaine® Hemorrhoidal [OTC]: 20% (30 g)
  Medicone® Hemorrhoidal [OTC]: 20% (28.4 g)
Ointment, topical:
  Boil-Ease® Pain Relieving [OTC]: 20% (30 g)
  Chiggerex® Plus [OTC]: 6% (50 g)
  Foille® [OTC]: 5% (3.5 g, 14 g, 28 g)
Pad, topical:
  Sting-Kill® [OTC]: 20% (8s)

Paste, oral:
Orabase® with Benzocaine [OTC]: 20% (6 g)
Solution, oral:
Hurricaine® [OTC]: 20% (30 mL)
Swab, oral:
Hurricaine® [OTC]: 20% (8s, 72s)
Orajel® Baby Teething [OTC]: 7.5% (12s)
Orajel® Cold Sore [OTC]: 20% (12s)
Orajel® Medicated Mouth Sore [OTC]: 20% (8s, 12s)
Orajel® Medicated Toothache [OTC]: 20% (8s, 12s)
Zilactin® Tooth & Gum Pain [OTC]: 20% (8s)
Swab, topical:
Boil-Ease® Pain Relieving [OTC]: 20% (12s)
Sting-Kill® [OTC]: 20% (5s)
Tablet, orally dissolving, oral:
Cepacol® Fizzlers™ [OTC]: 6 mg (12s)
Wax, oral:
Dent's Extra Strength Toothache Gum [OTC]: 20% (1 g)

benzocaine and antipyrine *see* antipyrine and benzocaine *on page 83*

benzocaine, butamben, and tetracaine (BEN zoe kane, byoo TAM ben, & TET ra kane)

Synonyms benzocaine, butamben, and tetracaine hydrochloride; benzocaine, butyl aminobenzoate, and tetracaine; butamben, tetracaine, and benzocaine; tetracaine, benzocaine, and butamben

U.S. Brand Names Cetacaine®; Exactacain®

Therapeutic Category Local Anesthetic

Use Topical anesthetic to control pain in surgical or endoscopic procedures; anesthetic for accessible mucous membranes except for the eyes

General Dosage Range Topical: *Adults:*
Cetacaine®: Aerosol: Apply for ≤1 second (maximum: 2 seconds); Gel: Apply ~1/2" (13 mm) x 3/16" (5 mm) (maximum: 1" [26 cm] x 3/16" [5 mm]); Liquid: Apply 6-7 drops (0.2 mL) (maximum: 12 drops)
Exactacain™: 3 metered sprays (maximum: 6 metered sprays)

Dosage Forms
Aerosol, topical [kit, spray]:
Cetacaine®: Benzocaine 14%, butamben 2%, and tetracaine 2% (56 g)
Aerosol, topical [spray]:
Cetacaine®: Benzocaine 14%, butamben 2%, and tetracaine 2% (56 g)
Exactacain®: Benzocaine 14%, butamben 2%, and tetracaine 2% (60 g)
Gel, topical:
Cetacaine®: Benzocaine 14%, butamben 2%, and tetracaine 2% (32 g)
Liquid, topical, kit:
Cetacaine®: Benzocaine 14%, butamben 2%, and tetracaine 2% (14 g)
Liquid, topical:
Cetacaine®: Benzocaine 14%, butamben 2%, and tetracaine 2% (14 g, 30 g)

benzocaine, butamben, and tetracaine hydrochloride *see* benzocaine, butamben, and tetracaine *on page 123*

benzocaine, butyl aminobenzoate, and tetracaine *see* benzocaine, butamben, and tetracaine *on page 123*

Benzodent® [OTC] *see* benzocaine *on page 121*

benzoic acid, hyoscyamine, methenamine, methylene blue, and phenyl salicylate *see* methenamine, phenyl salicylate, methylene blue, benzoic acid, and hyoscyamine *on page 569*

benzoic acid, methenamine, methylene blue, phenyl salicylate, and hyoscyamine *see* methenamine, phenyl salicylate, methylene blue, benzoic acid, and hyoscyamine *on page 569*

benzoin (BEN zoin)

Synonyms gum benjamin

U.S. Brand Names Benz-Protect Swabs™ [OTC]; Sprayzoin™ [OTC]

Therapeutic Category Pharmaceutical Aid; Protectant, Topical

Use Protective application for irritations of the skin; sometimes used in boiling water as steam inhalants for its expectorant and soothing action

◀ **General Dosage Range Topical:** *Children and Adults:* Apply 1-2 times/day
Dosage Forms
  Tincture, topical: Benzoin Compound USP: Benzoin 10% (30 mL, 59 mL, 60 mL, 120 mL, 473 mL); Benzoin NFXI (59 mL)
  Benz-Protect Swabs™: Benzoin Compound USP: Benzoin 10% (3 mL)
  Tincture, topical [spray]:
  Sprayzoin™: Benzoin Compound USP: Benzoin 10% (120 mL)

benzonatate (ben ZOE na tate)

Synonyms tessalon perles
U.S. Brand Names Tessalon®; Zonatuss™
Therapeutic Category Antitussive
Use Symptomatic relief of nonproductive cough
General Dosage Range Oral: *Children >10 years and Adults:* 100-200 mg 3 times/day as needed (maximum: 600 mg/day)
Dosage Forms
  Capsule, oral:
  Zonatuss™: 150 mg
  Capsule, softgel, oral: 100 mg, 200 mg
  Tessalon®: 100 mg, 200 mg

benzoyl peroxide (BEN zoe il peer OKS ide)

Medication Safety Issues
  Sound-alike/look-alike issues:
  Benzoyl peroxide may be confused with benzyl alcohol
  Benoxyl® may be confused with Brevoxyl®, Peroxyl®
  Benzac® may be confused with Benza®
  Brevoxyl® may be confused with Benoxyl®
  Fostex® may be confused with pHisoHex®
U.S. Brand Names 10 Benzagel®; 5 Benzagel®; Acne Clear Maximum Strength [OTC]; Benzac® AC; Benzac® W; BenzaShave®; BenzEFoam™; Benziq™; BPO; Brevoxyl®-4 [DSC]; Brevoxyl®-8 [DSC]; Clearskin [OTC]; Clinac® BPO; Desquam-X® 10 [OTC]; Desquam-X® 5 [OTC]; Inova™; Lavoclen® Acne Wash Kit; Lavoclen™-4; Lavoclen™-8; Neutrogena® Clear Pore™ [OTC]; Neutrogena® On The Spot® Acne Treatment [OTC]; OXY® Chill Factor® [OTC]; OXY® [OTC]; Pacnex™; Palmer's® Skin Success Invisible Acne [OTC]; PanOxyl® Aqua Gel [OTC] [DSC]; PanOxyl® Bar [OTC]; PanOxyl® [OTC]; PanOxyl®-4 [OTC]; PanOxyl®-8 [OTC]; Triaz®; Zapzyt® [OTC]; ZoDerm®; ZoDerm® Hydrating Wash™; ZoDerm® Redi-Pads™
Canadian Brand Names Acetoxyl®; Benoxyl®; Benzac AC®; Benzac W® Gel; Benzac W® Wash; Desquam-X®; Oxyderm™; PanOxyl®; Solugel®
Therapeutic Category Acne Products
Use Treatment of mild-to-moderate acne vulgaris and acne rosacea
General Dosage Range Topical: *Adolescents and Adults:*
  Cleanser: Wash once or twice daily
  Topical formulations: Apply sparingly once daily; gradually increase to 2-3 times/day if needed
Dosage Forms
  Aerosol, topical:
  BenzEFoam™: 5.3% (60 g)
  Bar, topical:
  PanOxyl® Bar [OTC]: 10% (113 g)
  Zapzyt® [OTC]: 10% (113 g)
  Cloth, topical:
  Triaz®: 3% (60s); 6% (60s)
  Cream, topical:
  BenzaShave®: 5% (113.4 g); 10% (113.4 g)
  Clearskin [OTC]: 10% (28 g)
  Neutrogena® Clear Pore™ [OTC]: 3.5% (125 mL)
  Neutrogena® On The Spot® Acne Treatment [OTC]: 2.5% (22.5 g)
  ZoDerm®: 4.5% (125 mL); 6.5% (125 mL); 8.5% (125 mL)

Gel, topical: 2.5% (60 g); 3% (170 g, 340 g); 5% (45 g, 60 g, 90 g, 150 g, 240 g); 6% (170 g, 340 g); 9% (170 g, 340 g); 10% (45 g, 60 g, 90 g, 150 g, 240 g)
  5 Benzagel®: 5% (45 g)
  10 Benzagel®: 10% (45 g)
  Acne Clear Maximum Strength [OTC]: 10% (42.5 g)
  Benzac® AC: 5% (60 g); 10% (60 g)
  Benziq™: 5.25% (50 g)
  BPO: 4% (42.5 g); 8% (42.5 g)
  Clinac® BPO: 7% (45 g)
  Triaz®: 3% (170 g, 340 g); 6% (170 g, 340 g); 9% (170 g, 340 g)
  Zapzyt® [OTC]: 10% (30 g)
  ZoDerm®: 4.5% (125 mL); 6.5% (125 mL); 8.5% (125 mL)
Liquid, topical: 2.5% (240 mL); 5% (120 mL, 150 mL, 240 mL)
  Benzac® AC: 5% (240 mL); 10% (240 mL)
  Benzac® W: 5% (240 mL); 10% (240 mL)
  Benziq™: 5.25% (175 g)
  Desquam-X® 5 [OTC]: 5% (140 mL)
  Desquam-X® 10 [OTC]: 10% (150 mL)
  OXY® [OTC]: 10% (177 mL)
  OXY® Chill Factor® [OTC]: 10% (177 mL)
  ZoDerm® Hydrating Wash™: 5.75% (473 mL)
Lotion, topical: 5% (30 mL); 10% (30 mL); 5% (227 g); 10% (227 g)
  OXY® [OTC]: 5% (28 g); 10% (28 g)
  Pacnex™: 7% (480 mL)
  Palmer's® Skin Success Invisible Acne [OTC]: 10% (30 mL)
Pad, topical: 3% (30s); 4.5% (30s); 6% (30s); 6.5% (30s); 8.5% (30s); 9% (30s)
  Inova™: 4% (30s); 8% (30s)
  Triaz®: 3% (30s, 60s); 6% (30s, 60s); 9% (30s, 60s)
  ZoDerm® Redi-Pads™: 4.5% (30s); 6.5% (30s); 8.5% (30s)
Soap, topical: 4.5% (400 mL); 6.5% (400 mL); 8.5% (400 mL)
  ZoDerm®: 4.5% (400 mL); 6.5% (400 mL); 8.5% (400 mL)
Wash, topical: 2.5% (227 g); 5% (113 g, 142 g, 227 g); 10% (142 g, 227 g)
  Lavoclen® Acne Wash Kit: 4% (1s); 8% (1s)
  Lavoclen™-4: 4% (170 g)
  Lavoclen™-8: 8% (170 g)
  PanOxyl®-4 [OTC]: 4% (170 g)
  PanOxyl®-8 [OTC]: 8% (170 g)
  PanOxyl® [OTC]: 10% (156 g)

benzoyl peroxide and adapalene *see* adapalene and benzoyl peroxide *on page 40*
benzoyl peroxide and clindamycin *see* clindamycin and benzoyl peroxide *on page 219*
benzoyl peroxide and erythromycin *see* erythromycin and benzoyl peroxide *on page 340*

benzoyl peroxide and hydrocortisone (BEN zoe il peer OKS ide & hye droe KOR ti sone)

Synonyms hydrocortisone and benzoyl peroxide
U.S. Brand Names Vanoxide-HC®
Canadian Brand Names Vanoxide-HC®
Therapeutic Category Acne Products
Use Treatment of acne vulgaris and oily skin
General Dosage Range Topical: *Adolescents ≥12 years and Adults:* Apply thin film 1-3 times/day
Dosage Forms
  Lotion, topical:
    Vanoxide-HC®: Benzoyl peroxide 5% and hydrocortisone 0.5% (25 mL)
  Lotion, topical [kit]:
    Vanoxide-HC®: Benzoyl peroxide 5% and hydrocortisone 0.5% (25 g) packaged with cleanser

benzphetamine (benz FET a meen)

Medication Safety Issues
  BEERS Criteria medication:
    This drug may be inappropriate for use in geriatric patients (high severity risk).
Synonyms benzphetamine hydrochloride

◀ **U.S. Brand Names** Didrex®
Therapeutic Category Anorexiant
Controlled Substance C-III
Use Short-term (few weeks) adjunct to caloric restriction in exogenous obesity

Pharmacotherapy for weight loss is recommended only for obese patients with a body mass index ≥30 kg/m^2, or ≥27 kg/m^2 in the presence of other risk factors such as hypertension, diabetes, and/or dyslipidemia or a high waist circumference; therapy should be used in conjunction with a comprehensive weight management program.

General Dosage Range Oral: *Children ≥12 years and Adults:* Initial: 25-50 mg once daily; Maintenance: 25-50 mg 1-3 times/day (maximum: 150 mg/day)

Dosage Forms
  Tablet, oral: 50 mg
  Didrex®: 50 mg

benzphetamine hydrochloride *see benzphetamine on page 125*
Benz-Protect Swabs™ [OTC] *see benzoin on page 123*

benztropine (BENZ troe peen)

Medication Safety Issues
  Sound-alike/look-alike issues:
  Benztropine may be confused with bromocriptine
Synonyms benztropine mesylate
U.S. Brand Names Cogentin®
Canadian Brand Names Apo-Benztropine®
Therapeutic Category Anti-Parkinson Agent; Anticholinergic Agent
Use Adjunctive treatment of Parkinson disease; treatment of drug-induced extrapyramidal symptoms (except tardive dyskinesia)
General Dosage Range I.M., I.V., Oral: *Adults:* Range: 0.5-8 mg/day
Dosage Forms
  Injection, solution: 1 mg/mL
  Cogentin®: 1 mg/mL
  Tablet, oral: 0.5 mg, 1 mg, 2 mg

benztropine mesylate *see benztropine on page 126*

benzydamine *(Canada only)* (ben ZID a meen)

Synonyms benzydamine hydrochloride
Canadian Brand Names Apo-Benzydamine®; Dom-Benzydamine; Novo-Benzydamine; PMS-Benzydamine; ratio-Benzydamine; Sun-Benz®; Tantum®
Therapeutic Category Analgesic, Topical
Use Symptomatic treatment of pain associated with acute pharyngitis; treatment of pain associated with radiation-induced oropharyngeal mucositis
General Dosage Range Oral rinse: *Adults:* Gargle with 15 mL every 1¹/₂-3 hours until symptoms resolve or 3-4 times/day
Product Availability Not available in U.S.
Dosage Forms - Canada
  Oral rinse: 0.15% (100 mL, 250 mL)

benzydamine hydrochloride *see benzydamine (Canada only) on page 126*

benzyl alcohol (BEN zill AL koe hol)

Medication Safety Issues
  Sound-alike/look-alike issues:
  Benzyl alcohol may be confused with benzoyl peroxide
U.S. Brand Names Ulesfia®; Zilactin®-L [OTC]
Therapeutic Category Antiparasitic Agent, Topical; Pediculocide
Use
  Liquid (Zilactin®-L): Temporary relief of pain from cold sores/fever blisters
  Lotion (Ulesfia™): Treatment of head lice infestation

General Dosage Range Topical:
Liquid: *Children ≥2 years and Adults:* Apply to affected area up to 4 times/day
Lotion: *Children ≥6 months and Adults:* 4-48 ounces per application based upon hair length; repeat in 7 days
Dosage Forms
Liquid, topical:
Zilactin®-L [OTC]: 10% (5.9 mL)
Lotion, topical:
Ulesfia®: 5% (227 g)

benzylpenicillin benzathine *see* penicillin G benzathine *on page 684*
benzylpenicillin potassium *see* penicillin G (parenteral/aqueous) *on page 685*
benzylpenicillin sodium *see* penicillin G (parenteral/aqueous) *on page 685*

benzylpenicilloyl polylysine (BEN zil pen i SIL oyl pol i LIE seen)
Synonyms benzylpenicilloyl-polylysine; penicilloyl-polylysine; PPL
U.S. Brand Names Pre-Pen®
Therapeutic Category Diagnostic Agent
Use Adjunct in assessing the risk of administering penicillin (penicillin G or benzylpenicillin) in patients suspected of clinical penicillin hypersensitivity
General Dosage Range
Intradermal: *Children and Adults:* Inject a volume of skin test solution sufficient to raise a small intradermal bleb ~3 mm in diameter, in duplicate
Puncture test (first step): *Children and Adults:* Apply a small drop of solution to make a single shallow puncture of the epidermis
Dosage Forms
Injection, solution:
Pre-Pen®: 6 x 10⁻⁵ M (0.25 mL)

benzylpenicilloyl-polylysine *see* benzylpenicilloyl polylysine *on page 127*

bepotastine (be poe TAS teen)
Synonyms bepotastine besilate
U.S. Brand Names Bepreve®
Therapeutic Category Histamine H₁ Antagonist; Histamine H₁ Antagonist, Second Generation; Mast Cell Stabilizer
Use Treatment of itching associated with allergic conjunctivitis
General Dosage Range Ophthalmic: *Children ≥2 years and Adults:* Instill 1 drop into the affected eye(s) twice daily
Dosage Forms
Solution, ophthalmic:
Bepreve®: 1.5% (5 mL, 10 mL)

bepotastine besilate *see* bepotastine *on page 127*
Bepreve® *see* bepotastine *on page 127*

beractant (ber AKT ant)
Medication Safety Issues
Sound-alike/look-alike issues:
Survanta® may be confused with Sufenta®
Synonyms bovine lung surfactant; natural lung surfactant
U.S. Brand Names Survanta®
Canadian Brand Names Survanta®
Therapeutic Category Lung Surfactant
Use Prevention and treatment of respiratory distress syndrome (RDS) in premature infants

Prophylactic therapy: Body weight <1250 g in infants at risk for developing, or with evidence of, surfactant deficiency (administer within 15 minutes of birth)
Rescue therapy: Treatment of infants with RDS confirmed by x-ray and requiring mechanical ventilation (administer as soon as possible - within 8 hours of age)

◀ **General Dosage Range Intratracheal:** *Premature infants:* Administer 100 mg phospholipids (4 mL/kg); may repeat if needed, no more frequently than every 6 hours to a maximum of 4 doses/48 hours for prophylactic treatment (maximum: 4 doses/24 hours for rescue treatment)

Dosage Forms
Suspension, intratracheal [preservative free]:
Survanta®: Phospholipids 25 mg/mL (4 mL, 8 mL)

Berinert® *see* C1 inhibitor (human) *on page 156*

besifloxacin (be si FLOX a sin)

Synonyms besifloxacin hydrochloride; BOL-303224-A; SS734
U.S. Brand Names Besivance™
Therapeutic Category Antibiotic, Ophthalmic; Antibiotic, Quinolone
Use Treatment of bacterial conjunctivitis
General Dosage Range Ophthalmic: *Children ≥1 year and Adults:* 1 drop into affected eye(s) 3 times/day (4-12 hours apart)
Dosage Forms
Suspension, ophthalmic:
Besivance™: 0.6% (5 mL)

besifloxacin hydrochloride *see* besifloxacin *on page 128*
Besivance™ *see* besifloxacin *on page 128*
β,β-dimethylcysteine *see* penicillamine *on page 683*
Betacaine® (Can) *see* lidocaine (topical) *on page 524*

beta-carotene (BAY ta KARE oh teen)

U.S. Brand Names A-Caro-25 [OTC]; B-Caro-T™ [OTC]; Lumitene™ [OTC]
Therapeutic Category Vitamin, Fat Soluble
General Dosage Range
Oral:
Children <14 years: 30-150 mg/day
Adults: 30-300 mg/day
Dosage Forms
Capsule, oral:
Lumitene™ [OTC]: 50,000 int. units
Capsule, softgel, oral: 10,000 int. units, 25,000 int. units
A-Caro-25 [OTC]: 25,000 int. units
B-Caro-T™ [OTC]: 25,000 int. units
Tablet, oral: 10,000 int. units

Betaderm (Can) *see* betamethasone *on page 129*
Betadine® *see* povidone-iodine (ophthalmic) *on page 727*
Betadine® [OTC] *see* povidone-iodine (topical) *on page 727*
Betadine® (Can) *see* povidone-iodine (topical) *on page 727*
Betadine® Swab Aids [OTC] *see* povidone-iodine (topical) *on page 727*
9-beta-d-ribofuranosyladenine *see* adenosine *on page 41*
Betagan® *see* levobunolol *on page 517*
Beta-HC® [OTC] *see* hydrocortisone (topical) *on page 450*

betahistine *(Canada only)* (bay ta HISS teen)

Synonyms betahistine dihydrochloride
Canadian Brand Names Novo-Betahistine; Serc®
Therapeutic Category Antihistamine
Use Treatment of Ménière disease (to decrease episodes of vertigo)
General Dosage Range Oral: *Adults:* 8-16 mg 3 times/day or 24 mg twice daily
Product Availability Not available in U.S.

Dosage Forms - Canada
Tablet, oral:
Novo-Betahistine: 8 mg, 16 mg, 24 mg
Serc®: 16 mg, 24 mg

betahistine dihydrochloride *see* betahistine *(Canada only) on page 128*

betaine (BAY ta een)

Medication Safety Issues
Sound-alike/look-alike issues:
Betaine may be confused with Betadine®
Cystadane® may be confused with cysteamine, cysteine
Synonyms betaine anhydrous
U.S. Brand Names Cystadane®
Canadian Brand Names Cystadane®
Therapeutic Category Homocystinuria Agent
Use Treatment of homocystinuria (eg, deficiencies or defects in cystathionine beta-synthase [CBS], 5,10-methylene tetrahydrofolate reductase [MTHFR], and cobalamin cofactor metabolism [CBL])
General Dosage Range Oral:
Children <3 years: Initial: 100 mg/kg/day, then increase weekly by 50 mg/kg increments, as needed
Children ≥3 years and Adults: 3 g twice daily (maximum: 20 g/day)
Dosage Forms
Powder for solution, oral:
Cystadane®: 1 g/scoop (180 g)

betaine anhydrous *see* betaine *on page 129*
Betaject™ (Can) *see* betamethasone *on page 129*
Betaloc® (Can) *see* metoprolol *on page 581*
BetaMed™ [OTC] *see* pyrithione zinc *on page 759*

betamethasone (bay ta METH a sone)

Medication Safety Issues
Sound-alike/look-alike issues:
Luxiq® may be confused with Lasix®
International issues:
Beta-Val [U.S.] may be confused with Betanol brand name for metipranolol [Monaco]
Synonyms betamethasone dipropionate; betamethasone dipropionate, augmented; betamethasone sodium phosphate; betamethasone valerate; flubenisolone
U.S. Brand Names Beta-Val® [DSC]; Celestone®; Celestone® Soluspan®; Diprolene®; Diprolene® AF; Luxiq®
Canadian Brand Names Betaderm; Betaject™; Betnesol®; Betnovate®; Celestone® Soluspan®; Diprolene®; Diprolene® Glycol; Diprosone®; Ectosone; Prevex® B; ratio-Ectosone; ratio-Topilene; ratio-Topisone; Rivasone; Rolene; Rosone; Taro-Sone; Topilene®; Topisone®; Valisone® Scalp Lotion
Therapeutic Category Adrenal Corticosteroid; Corticosteroid, Topical
Use Inflammatory dermatoses such as seborrheic or atopic dermatitis, neurodermatitis, anogenital pruritus, psoriasis, inflammatory phase of xerosis
General Dosage Range
I.M.:
Children ≤12 years: 0.0175-0.125 mg base/kg/day **or** 0.5-7.5 mg base/m^2/day divided every 6-12 hours
Children ≥13 years and Adults: 0.6-9 mg/day divided every 12-24 hours
Intrabursal, intraarticular, intradermal: *Adults:* 0.25-2 mL
Intralesional: *Adults:* Very large joints: 1-2 mL; Large joints: 1 mL; Medium joints: 0.5-1 mL; Small joints: 0.25-0.5 mL
Oral:
Children ≤12 years: 0.0175-0.25 mg/kg/day **or** 0.5-7.5 mg/m^2/day divided every 6-8 hours
Children ≥13 years and Adults: 0.6-7.2 mg/day in 2-4 divided doses
Topical: *Children ≥13 years and Adults:* Apply once or twice daily (maximum: 45-50 g/week; 50 mL/week)

◄ **Dosage Forms**
  Aerosol, topical:
    Luxiq®: 0.12% (50 g, 100 g)
  Cream, topical: 0.05% (15 g, 45 g, 50 g); 0.1% (15 g, 45 g)
    Diprolene® AF: 0.05% (15 g, 50 g)
  Gel, topical: 0.05% (15 g, 50 g)
  Injection, suspension: Betamethasone sodium phosphate 3 mg and betamethasone acetate 3 mg per 1 mL (5 mL)
    Celestone® Soluspan®: Betamethasone sodium phosphate 3 mg and betamethasone acetate 3 mg per 1 mL (5 mL)
  Lotion, topical: 0.05% (30 mL, 60 mL); 0.1% (60 mL)
    Diprolene®: 0.05% (30 mL, 60 mL)
  Ointment, topical: 0.05% (15 g, 45 g, 50 g); 0.1% (15 g, 45 g)
    Diprolene®: 0.05% (15 g, 50 g)
  Solution, oral:
    Celestone®: 0.6 mg/5 mL (118 mL)

betamethasone and clotrimazole (bay ta METH a sone & kloe TRIM a zole)

Medication Safety Issues
Sound-alike/look-alike issues:
  Clotrimazole may be confused with co-trimoxazole
  Lotrisone® may be confused with Lotrimin®

Synonyms clotrimazole and betamethasone

U.S. Brand Names Lotrisone®

Canadian Brand Names Lotriderm®

Therapeutic Category Antifungal/Corticosteroid

Use Topical treatment of various dermal fungal infections (including tinea pedis, cruris, and corpora in patients ≥17 years of age)

General Dosage Range Topical: *Adults:* Apply to affected area twice daily (maximum: 45 g cream/week; 45 mL lotion/week)

Dosage Forms
  Cream: Betamethasone 0.05% and clotrimazole 1% (15 g, 45 g)
    Lotrisone®: Betamethasone 0.05% and clotrimazole 1% (15 g, 45 g)
  Lotion: Betamethasone 0.05% and clotrimazole 1% (30 mL)
    Lotrisone®: Betamethasone 0.05% and clotrimazole 1% (30 mL)

betamethasone dipropionate *see* betamethasone *on page 129*

betamethasone dipropionate and calcipotriene hydrate *see* calcipotriene and betamethasone *on page 158*

betamethasone dipropionate, augmented *see* betamethasone *on page 129*

betamethasone sodium phosphate *see* betamethasone *on page 129*

betamethasone valerate *see* betamethasone *on page 129*

Betapace® *see* sotalol *on page 828*

Betapace AF® *see* sotalol *on page 828*

Beta Sal® [OTC] *see* salicylic acid *on page 795*

Betasept® [OTC] *see* chlorhexidine gluconate *on page 194*

Betaseron® *see* interferon beta-1b *on page 482*

Betatar Gel® [OTC] *see* coal tar *on page 227*

Beta-Val® [DSC] *see* betamethasone *on page 129*

Betaxin® (Can) *see* thiamine *on page 862*

betaxolol (systemic) (be TAKS oh lol)

Medication Safety Issues
Sound-alike/look-alike issues:
  Betaxolol may be confused with bethanechol, labetalol

Synonyms betaxolol hydrochloride

U.S. Brand Names Kerlone®

Canadian Brand Names Sandoz-Betaxolol

Therapeutic Category Beta Blocker, Beta-1 Selective

Use Management of hypertension
General Dosage Range Dosage adjustment recommended in patients with renal impairment
Oral:
  Adults: 5-20 mg/day
  Elderly: Initial dose: 5 mg/day
Dosage Forms
  Tablet, oral: 10 mg, 20 mg
  Kerlone®: 10 mg, 20 mg

betaxolol (ophthalmic) (be TAKS oh lol)
Medication Safety Issues
  Sound-alike/look-alike issues:
  Betoptic® S may be confused with Betagan®, Timoptic®
Synonyms betaxolol hydrochloride
U.S. Brand Names Betoptic S®
Canadian Brand Names Betoptic® S
Therapeutic Category Ophthalmic Agent, Antiglaucoma
Use Treatment of chronic open-angle glaucoma or ocular hypertension
General Dosage Range Ophthalmic:
  Children: Suspension: Instill 1 drop twice daily
  Adults:
    Solution: Instill 1-2 drops twice daily
    Suspension: Instill 1 drop twice daily
Dosage Forms
  Solution, ophthalmic: 0.5% (5 mL, 10 mL, 15 mL)
  Suspension, ophthalmic:
  Betoptic S®: 0.25% (10 mL, 15 mL)

betaxolol hydrochloride *see* betaxolol (ophthalmic) *on page 131*
betaxolol hydrochloride *see* betaxolol (systemic) *on page 130*

bethanechol (be THAN e kole)
Medication Safety Issues
  Sound-alike/look-alike issues:
  Bethanechol may be confused with betaxolol
Synonyms bethanechol chloride
U.S. Brand Names Urecholine®
Canadian Brand Names Duvoid®; PMS-Bethanechol
Therapeutic Category Cholinergic Agent
Use Treatment of acute postoperative and postpartum nonobstructive (functional) urinary retention; treatment of neurogenic atony of the urinary bladder with retention
General Dosage Range Oral: *Adults:* 10-100 mg 2-4 times/day
Dosage Forms
  Tablet, oral: 5 mg, 10 mg, 25 mg, 50 mg
  Urecholine®: 5 mg, 10 mg, 25 mg, 50 mg
Dosage Forms - Canada
  Tablet:
  Duvoid®: 10 mg, 25 mg, 50 mg

bethanechol chloride *see* bethanechol *on page 131*
Betimol® *see* timolol (ophthalmic) *on page 869*
Betnesol® (Can) *see* betamethasone *on page 129*
Betnovate® (Can) *see* betamethasone *on page 129*
Betoptic S® *see* betaxolol (ophthalmic) *on page 131*
Betoptic® S (Can) *see* betaxolol (ophthalmic) *on page 131*

bevacizumab (be vuh SIZ uh mab)

Medication Safety Issues

Sound-alike/look-alike issues:

Avastin® may be confused with Astelin®

Bevacizumab may be confused with brentuximab, cetuximab, riTUXimab

High alert medication:

This medication is in a class the Institute for Safe Medication Practices (ISMP) includes among its list of drug classes which have a heightened risk of causing significant patient harm when used in error.

International issues:

Avastin [U.S., Canada, and multiple international markets] may be confused with Avaxim, a brand name for hepatitis A vaccine [Canada and multiple international markets]

Synonyms anti-VEGF monoclonal antibody; anti-VEGF rhuMAb; rhuMAb-VEGF

U.S. Brand Names Avastin®

Canadian Brand Names Avastin®

Therapeutic Category Antineoplastic Agent, Monoclonal Antibody; Vaccine, Recombinant

Use Treatment of metastatic colorectal cancer; treatment of unresectable, locally advanced, recurrent or metastatic nonsquamous, nonsmall cell lung cancer; treatment of metastatic HER-2 negative breast cancer (who have not received chemotherapy for metastatic disease); treatment of progressive glioblastoma; treatment of metastatic renal cell cancer (not an approved use in Canada)

Note: For the treatment of metastatic breast cancer, effectiveness is based on improvement in progression-free survival; not indicated for the treatment of breast cancer with metastatic disease that has progressed following anthracycline and taxane treatment. For the treatment of glioblastoma, effectiveness is based on improvement in objective response rate.

General Dosage Range I.V.: *Adults:* 5 or 10 mg/kg every 2 weeks **or** 15 mg/kg every 3 weeks

Dosage Forms

Injection, solution [preservative free]:

Avastin®: 25 mg/mL (4 mL, 16 mL)

bexarotene (systemic) (beks AIR oh teen)

Medication Safety Issues

High alert medication:

The Institute for Safe Medication Practices (ISMP) includes this medication among its list of drugs which have a heightened risk of causing significant patient harm when used in error.

U.S. Brand Names Targretin®

Canadian Brand Names Targretin®

Therapeutic Category Antineoplastic Agent, Miscellaneous

Use Treatment of cutaneous manifestations of cutaneous T-cell lymphoma in patients who are refractory to at least one prior systemic therapy

General Dosage Range Oral: *Adults:* 300-400 mg/m^2 once daily

Dosage Forms

Capsule, oral:

Targretin®: 75 mg

bexarotene (topical) (beks AIR oh teen)

Medication Safety Issues

High alert medication:

The Institute for Safe Medication Practices (ISMP) includes this medication among its list of drugs which have a heightened risk of causing significant patient harm when used in error.

U.S. Brand Names Targretin®

Canadian Brand Names Targretin®

Therapeutic Category Antineoplastic Agent, Miscellaneous

Use Treatment of cutaneous lesions in patients with refractory cutaneous T-cell lymphoma (stage 1A and 1B) or who have not tolerated other therapies

General Dosage Range Topical: *Adults:* Initial: Apply once every other day for first week; Maintenance: Apply 1-4 times/day

Dosage Forms

Gel, topical:

Targretin®: 1% (60 g)

Bexxar® *see* tositumomab and iodine I 131 tositumomab *on page 879*
Beyaz™ *see* ethinyl estradiol, drospirenone, and levomefolate *on page 358*

bezafibrate *(Canada only)* (be za FYE brate)
Canadian Brand Names Bezalip® SR
Therapeutic Category Antihyperlipidemic Agent, Miscellaneous
Use Adjunct to diet and other therapeutic measures for treatment of type IIa and IIb mixed hyperlipidemia, to regulate lipid and apoprotein levels (reduce serum TG, LDL-cholesterol, and apolipoprotein B, increase HDL-cholesterol and apolipoprotein A); treatment of adult patients with high to very high triglyceride levels (Fredrickson classification type IV and V hyperlipidemias) who are at high risk of sequelae and complications from their dyslipidemia
General Dosage Range
Oral:
 Children: 10-20 mg/kg/day (maximum: 400 mg)
 Adults: 400 mg once daily
Product Availability Not available in U.S.
Dosage Forms - Canada
Tablet, sustained release, oral:
 Bezalip® SR: 400 mg

Bezalip® SR (Can) *see* bezafibrate *(Canada only) on page 133*
BG 9273 *see* alefacept *on page 48*
BI-1356 *see* linagliptin *on page 528*
Biafine® *see* emollients *on page 325*
Biaxin® *see* clarithromycin *on page 215*
Biaxin® XL *see* clarithromycin *on page 215*

bicalutamide (bye ka LOO ta mide)
Medication Safety Issues
Sound-alike/look-alike issues:
 Casodex® may be confused with Kapidex [DSC]
International issues:
 Casodex [U.S., Canada, and multiple international markets] may be confused with Capadex brand name for propoxyphene/acetaminophen [Australia, New Zealand]
Synonyms CDX; ICI-176334
U.S. Brand Names Casodex®
Canadian Brand Names Apo-Bicalutamide®; Casodex®; CO Bicalutamide; Dom-Bicalutamide; JAMP-Bicalutamide; Mylan-Bicalutamide; Novo-Bicalutamide; PHL-Bicalutamide; PMS-Bicalutamide; PRO-Bicalutamide; ratio-Bicalutamide; Sandoz-Bicalutamide
Therapeutic Category Androgen
Use Treatment of metastatic prostate cancer (in combination with an LHRH agonist)
General Dosage Range Oral: *Adults:* 50 mg once daily
Dosage Forms
Tablet, oral: 50 mg
 Casodex®: 50 mg

Bicillin® L-A *see* penicillin G benzathine *on page 684*
Bicillin® C-R *see* penicillin G benzathine and penicillin G procaine *on page 684*
Bicillin® C-R 900/300 *see* penicillin G benzathine and penicillin G procaine *on page 684*
BiCNU® *see* carmustine *on page 177*
Bidex®-400 [OTC] *see* guaifenesin *on page 425*
BiDil® *see* isosorbide dinitrate and hydralazine *on page 494*
BIG-IV *see* botulism immune globulin (intravenous-human) *on page 139*
Biltricide® *see* praziquantel *on page 733*

bimatoprost (bi MAT oh prost)
U.S. Brand Names Latisse®; Lumigan®
Canadian Brand Names Lumigan®; Lumigan® RC

◀ **Therapeutic Category** Ophthalmic Agent, Miscellaneous

Use Reduction of intraocular pressure (IOP) in patients with open-angle glaucoma or ocular hypertension; hypotrichosis treatment of the eyelashes

General Dosage Range

Ophthalmic: *Adults:* Instill 1 drop into affected eye(s) once daily

Ophthalmic, topical: *Adults:* Place 1 drop on applicator and apply evenly along the skin of the upper eyelid at base of eyelashes once daily

Dosage Forms

Solution, ophthalmic:

Latisse®: 0.03% (3 mL)

Lumigan®: 0.01% (2.5 mL, 5 mL, 7.5 mL); 0.03% (2.5 mL, 5 mL, 7.5 mL)

Bio-D-Mulsion® [OTC] *see* cholecalciferol *on page 204*

Bio-D-Mulsion Forte® [OTC] *see* cholecalciferol *on page 204*

Bio-Amitriptyline (Can) *see* amitriptyline *on page 68*

Biobase™ (Can) *see* alcohol (ethyl) *on page 47*

Biobase-G™ (Can) *see* alcohol (ethyl) *on page 47*

Bio-Furosemide (Can) *see* furosemide *on page 404*

BioGlo™ *see* fluorescein *on page 386*

Bio-Hydrochlorothiazide (Can) *see* hydrochlorothiazide *on page 445*

Bionect® *see* hyaluronate and derivatives *on page 443*

Bioniche Promethazine (Can) *see* promethazine *on page 742*

Bion® Tears [OTC] *see* artificial tears *on page 96*

Bio-Oxazepam (Can) *see* oxazepam *on page 659*

BioQuin® Durules™ (Can) *see* quinidine *on page 762*

BioThrax® *see* anthrax vaccine, adsorbed *on page 80*

Biphentin® (Can) *see* methylphenidate *on page 577*

bird flu vaccine *see* influenza virus vaccine (H5N1) *on page 473*

Bisac-Evac™ [OTC] *see* bisacodyl *on page 134*

bisacodyl (bis a KOE dil)

Medication Safety Issues

Sound-alike/look-alike issues:

Doxidan® may be confused with doxepin

Dulcolax® (bisacodyl) may be confused with Dulcolax® (docusate)

BEERS Criteria medication:

This drug may be inappropriate for use in geriatric patients (high severity risk).

U.S. Brand Names Alophen® [OTC]; Bisac-Evac™ [OTC]; Biscolax™ [OTC]; Correctol® Tablets [OTC]; Dacodyl™ [OTC]; Doxidan® [OTC]; Dulcolax® [OTC]; ex-lax® Ultra [OTC]; Femilax™ [OTC]; Fleet® Bisacodyl [OTC]; Fleet® Stimulant Laxative [OTC]; Veracolate® [OTC]

Canadian Brand Names Apo-Bisacodyl®; Carter's Little Pills®; Dulcolax®; Gentlax®

Therapeutic Category Laxative

Use Treatment of constipation; colonic evacuation prior to procedures or examination

General Dosage Range

Oral:

Children >6 years: 5-10 mg (0.3 mg/kg) once daily

Adults: 5-15 mg as a single dose (maximum: 30 mg)

Rectal:

Children <2 years: 5 mg as a single dose

Children ≥2 years and Adults: 10 mg as a single dose

Dosage Forms

Solution, rectal:

Fleet® Bisacodyl [OTC]: 10 mg/30 mL (37 mL)

Suppository, rectal: 10 mg (12s, 50s, 100s, 500s)

Bisac-Evac™ [OTC]: 10 mg (8s, 12s, 50s, 100s, 500s, 1000s)

Biscolax™ [OTC]: 10 mg (12s, 100s)

Dulcolax® [OTC]: 10 mg (4s, 8s, 16s, 28s, 50s)

Tablet, delayed release, oral: 5 mg
  Doxidan® [OTC]: 5 mg
  Fleet® Stimulant Laxative [OTC]: 5 mg
Tablet, enteric coated, oral: 5 mg
  Alophen® [OTC]: 5 mg
  Bisac-Evac™ [OTC]: 5 mg
  Correctol® Tablets [OTC]: 5 mg
  Dacodyl™ [OTC]: 5 mg
  Dulcolax® [OTC]: 5 mg
  ex-lax® Ultra [OTC]: 5 mg
  Femilax™ [OTC]: 5 mg
  Veracolate® [OTC]: 5 mg

bisacodyl and polyethylene glycol-electrolyte solution *see* polyethylene glycol-electrolyte solution and bisacodyl *on page 719*
bis(chloroethyl) nitrosourea *see* carmustine *on page 177*
bis-chloronitrosourea *see* carmustine *on page 177*
Biscolax™ [OTC] *see* bisacodyl *on page 134*
bismatrol *see* bismuth *on page 135*
Bismatrol [OTC] *see* bismuth *on page 135*
Bismatrol Maximum Strength [OTC] *see* bismuth *on page 135*

bismuth (BIZ muth)

Medication Safety Issues
Sound-alike/look-alike issues:
  Kaopectate® may be confused with Kayexalate®
Other safety concerns:
  Maalox® Total Relief® is a different formulation than other Maalox® liquid antacid products which contain aluminum hydroxide, magnesium hydroxide, and simethicone.
  Canadian formulation of Kaopectate® does not contain bismuth; the active ingredient in the Canadian formulation is attapulgite.

Synonyms bismatrol; bismuth subsalicylate; pink bismuth

U.S. Brand Names Bismatrol Maximum Strength [OTC]; Bismatrol [OTC]; Diotame [OTC]; Kao-Tin [OTC]; Kaopectate® Extra Strength [OTC]; Kaopectate® [OTC]; Maalox® Total Relief® [OTC] [DSC]; Peptic Relief [OTC]; Pepto Relief [OTC]; Pepto-Bismol® Maximum Strength [OTC]; Pepto-Bismol® [OTC]

Therapeutic Category Antidiarrheal

Use Subsalicylate formulation: Symptomatic treatment of mild, nonspecific diarrhea; control of traveler's diarrhea (enterotoxigenic *Escherichia coli*); as part of a multidrug regimen for *H. pylori* eradication to reduce the risk of duodenal ulcer recurrence

General Dosage Range Oral:
Subsalicylate based on 262 mg/5 mL liquid or 262 mg tablet (diarrhea):
  Children 3-6 years: 1/3 tablet **or** 5 mL every 30 minutes to 1 hour as needed (maximum: 8 doses/day)
  Children 6-9 years: 2/3 tablet **or** 10 mL every 30 minutes to 1 hour as needed (maximum: 8 doses/day)
  Children 9-12 years: 1 tablet **or** 15 mL every 30 minutes to 1 hour as needed (maximum: 8 doses/day)
Subsalicylate based on 262 mg/15 mL liquid or 262 mg tablet:
  Children >12 years: Diarrhea: 2 tablets **or** 30 mL every 30 minutes to 1 hour as needed (maximum: 8 doses/day)
  Adults:
    Diarrhea: 2 tablets **or** 30 mL every 30 minutes to 1 hour as needed (maximum: 8 doses/day)
    H. pylori eradication: 524 mg 4 times/day

Dosage Forms
Caplet, oral:
  Pepto-Bismol® [OTC]: 262 mg
Liquid, oral: 262 mg/15 mL (237 mL, 240 mL)
  Bismatrol [OTC]: 262 mg/15 mL (240 mL)
  Bismatrol Maximum Strength [OTC]: 525 mg/15 mL (240 mL)
  Diotame [OTC]: 262 mg/15 mL (30 mL)
  Kao-Tin [OTC]: 262 mg/15 mL (240 mL, 473 mL)
  Kaopectate® [OTC]: 262 mg/15 mL (177 mL, 236 mL, 354 mL)
  Kaopectate® Extra Strength [OTC]: 525 mg/15 mL (236 mL)
  Peptic Relief [OTC]: 262 mg/15 mL (237 mL)

◄ Pepto-Bismol® [OTC]: 262 mg/15 mL (120 mL, 240 mL, 360 mL, 480 mL)
Pepto-Bismol® Maximum Strength [OTC]: 525 mg/15 mL (120 mL, 240 mL, 360 mL)
Suspension, oral: 262 mg/15 mL (30 mL)
Tablet, chewable, oral:
Bismatrol [OTC]: 262 mg
Diotame [OTC]: 262 mg
Peptic Relief [OTC]: 262 mg
Pepto Relief [OTC]: 262 mg
Pepto-Bismol® [OTC]: 262 mg

bismuth, metronidazole, and tetracycline
(BIZ muth, me troe NI da zole, & tet ra SYE kleen)

Synonyms bismuth subcitrate potassium, tetracycline, and metronidazole; bismuth subsalicylate, tetracycline, and metronidazole; metronidazole, bismuth subcitrate potassium, and tetracycline; metronidazole, bismuth subsalicylate, and tetracycline; tetracycline, metronidazole, and bismuth subcitrate potassium; tetracycline, metronidazole, and bismuth subsalicylate

U.S. Brand Names Helidac®; Pylera™

Therapeutic Category Antidiarrheal

Use As part of a multidrug regimen for *H. pylori* eradication to reduce the risk of duodenal ulcer recurrence in combination with an H_2 agonist (Helidac®) or omeprazole (Pylera™)

General Dosage Range Oral: *Adults:*
Helidac®: 2 bismuth subsalicylate 262.4 mg tablets, 1 metronidazole 250 mg tablet, and 1 tetracycline 500 mg capsule 4 times/day at meals and bedtime
Pylera™: 3 capsules 4 times/day after meals and at bedtime

Dosage Forms
Capsule:
Pylera™: Bismuth subcitrate potassium 140 mg, metronidazole 125 mg, and tetracycline hydrochloride 125 mg
Combination package:
Helidac® [each package contains 14 blister cards (2-week supply); each card contains the following]:
Tablet, chewable: Bismuth subsalicylate]: 262.4 mg (8)
Tablet: Metronidazole: 250 mg (4)
Capsule: Tetracycline: 500 mg (4)

bismuth subcitrate potassium, tetracycline, and metronidazole *see* bismuth, metronidazole, and tetracycline *on page 136*

bismuth subsalicylate *see* bismuth *on page 135*

bismuth subsalicylate, tetracycline, and metronidazole *see* bismuth, metronidazole, and tetracycline *on page 136*

bisoprolol (bis OH proe lol)
Medication Safety Issues
Sound-alike/look-alike issues:
Zebeta® may be confused with DiaBeta®, Zetia®

Synonyms bisoprolol fumarate

U.S. Brand Names Zebeta®

Canadian Brand Names Apo-Bisoprolol®; Novo-Bisoprolol; PHL-Bisoprolol; PMS-Bisoprolol; PRO-Bisoprolol; Sandoz-Bisoprolol; ZYM-Bisoprolol

Therapeutic Category Beta-Adrenergic Blocker

Use Treatment of hypertension, alone or in combination with other agents

General Dosage Range Dosage adjustment recommended in patients with renal impairment
Oral: *Adults and Elderly:* Initial: 2.5-5 mg once daily; Maintenance: 2.5-20 mg once daily

Dosage Forms
Tablet, oral: 5 mg, 10 mg
Zebeta®: 5 mg, 10 mg

bisoprolol and hydrochlorothiazide (bis OH proe lol & hye droe klor oh THYE a zide)
Medication Safety Issues
Sound-alike/look-alike issues:
Ziac® may be confused with Tiazac®, Zerit®

Synonyms bisoprolol fumarate and hydrochlorothiazide; hydrochlorothiazide and bisoprolol

U.S. Brand Names Ziac®

Canadian Brand Names Ziac®

Therapeutic Category Antihypertensive Agent, Combination

Use Treatment of hypertension

General Dosage Range Oral: *Adults:* Initial: Bisoprolol 2.5 mg and hydrochlorothiazide 6.25 mg once daily; Maintenance: Bisoprolol 2.5-20 mg and hydrochlorothiazide 6.25-12.5 mg once daily; Maximum dose (manufacturer recommended): Bisoprolol 20 mg and hydrochlorothiazide 12.5 mg once daily

Dosage Forms

Tablet, oral: 2.5/6.25: Bisoprolol 2.5 mg and hydrochlorothiazide 6.25 mg; 5/6.25: Bisoprolol 5 mg and hydrochlorothiazide 6.25 mg; 10/6.25: Bisoprolol 10 mg and hydrochlorothiazide 6.25 mg

Ziac®: 2.5/6.25: Bisoprolol 2.5 mg and hydrochlorothiazide 6.25 mg; 5/6.25: Bisoprolol 5 mg and hydrochlorothiazide 6.25 mg; 10/6.25: Bisoprolol 10 mg and hydrochlorothiazide 6.25 mg

bisoprolol fumarate *see* bisoprolol *on page 136*

bisoprolol fumarate and hydrochlorothiazide *see* bisoprolol and hydrochlorothiazide *on page 136*

bis-POM PMEA *see* adefovir *on page 41*

bistropamide *see* tropicamide *on page 895*

bivalent human papillomavirus vaccine *see* papillomavirus (types 16, 18) vaccine (human, recombinant) *on page 673*

bivalirudin (bye VAL i roo din)

Medication Safety Issues

High alert medication:

The Institute for Safe Medication Practices (ISMP) includes this medication among its list of drugs which have a heightened risk of causing significant patient harm when used in error.

Synonyms hirulog

U.S. Brand Names Angiomax®

Canadian Brand Names Angiomax®

Therapeutic Category Anticoagulant (Other)

Use Anticoagulant used in conjunction with aspirin for patients with unstable angina undergoing percutaneous transluminal coronary angioplasty (PTCA) or percutaneous coronary intervention (PCI) with provisional glycoprotein IIb/IIIa inhibitor; anticoagulant used in conjunction with aspirin for patients undergoing PCI with (or at risk of) heparin-induced thrombocytopenia (HIT) / thrombosis syndrome (HITTS)

General Dosage Range

I.V.: *Adults:* Bolus: 0.75 mg/kg; may repeat at 0.3 mg/kg if necessary; Infusion: 1.75 mg/kg/hour for duration of procedure and up to 4 hours postprocedure if needed; after 4 hours may continue 0.2 mg/kg/minute for up to 20 hours if needed

Dosage adjustment recommended in patients with renal impairment

Dosage Forms

Injection, powder for reconstitution:

Angiomax®: 250 mg

Bi-Zets [OTC] *see* benzocaine *on page 121*

BL4162A *see* anagrelide *on page 78*

Black Draught® [OTC] *see* senna *on page 807*

black widow spider species antivenin *see* antivenin *(Latrodectus mactans) on page 84*

Blenoxane *see* bleomycin *on page 137*

Blenoxane® (Can) *see* bleomycin *on page 137*

bleo *see* bleomycin *on page 137*

bleomycin (blee oh MYE sin)

Medication Safety Issues

Sound-alike/look-alike issues:

Bleomycin may be confused with Cleocin®

High alert medication:

This medication is in a class the Institute for Safe Medication Practices (ISMP) includes among its list of drugs which have a heightened risk of causing significant patient harm when used in error.

◀ **Synonyms** Blenoxane; bleo; bleomycin sulfate; BLM

Canadian Brand Names Blenoxane®; Bleomycin Injection, USP

Therapeutic Category Antineoplastic Agent

Use Treatment of squamous cell carcinomas of the head and neck, penis, cervix, or vulva, testicular carcinoma, Hodgkin lymphoma, and non-Hodgkin lymphoma; sclerosing agent for malignant pleural effusion

General Dosage Range Dosage adjustment recommended in patients with renal impairment

I.V.: *Adults:* Dosage varies greatly depending on indication

Intrapleural: *Adults:* 60 units as a single instillation

Dosage Forms

Injection, powder for reconstitution: 15 units, 30 units

Bleomycin Injection, USP (Can) *see bleomycin on page 137*

bleomycin sulfate *see bleomycin on page 137*

Bleph®-10 *see sulfacetamide (ophthalmic) on page 835*

Bleph 10 DPS (Can) *see sulfacetamide (ophthalmic) on page 835*

Blephamide® *see sulfacetamide and prednisolone on page 835*

BLES (Can) *see bovine lipid extract surfactant (Canada only) on page 140*

Blis-To-Sol® [OTC] *see tolnaftate on page 876*

BLM *see bleomycin on page 137*

BMS-188667 *see abatacept on page 20*

BMS-224818 *see belatacept on page 117*

BMS-232632 *see atazanavir on page 100*

BMS-247550 *see ixabepilone on page 497*

BMS 337039 *see aripiprazole on page 93*

BMS-354825 *see dasatinib on page 254*

BMS-477118 *see saxagliptin on page 803*

B&O *see belladonna and opium on page 118*

boceprevir (boe SE pre vir)

Synonyms SCH503034

U.S. Brand Names Victrelis™

Canadian Brand Names Victrelis™

Therapeutic Category Antiviral Agent; Protease Inhibitor

Use Treatment of chronic hepatitis C (CHC) genotype 1 (in combination with peginterferon alfa and ribavirin) in adult patients with compensated liver disease (including cirrhosis) who were previously untreated or have failed prior therapy with peginterferon alfa and ribavirin therapy

General Dosage Range Oral: *Adults:* 800 mg 3 times/day

Dosage Forms

Capsule, oral:

Victrelis™: 200 mg

Boil-Ease® Pain Relieving [OTC] *see benzocaine on page 121*

BOL-303224-A *see besifloxacin on page 128*

Bonamine™ (Can) *see meclizine on page 552*

Bonefos® (Can) *see clodronate (Canada only) on page 221*

Bonine® [OTC] *see meclizine on page 552*

Bonine® (Can) *see meclizine on page 552*

Boniva® *see ibandronate on page 460*

Bontril® (Can) *see phendimetrazine on page 693*

Bontril® PDM *see phendimetrazine on page 693*

Bontril® Slow-Release *see phendimetrazine on page 693*

Boostrix® *see diphtheria, tetanus toxoids, and acellular pertussis vaccine on page 296*

bortezomib (bore TEZ oh mib)

Medication Safety Issues
High alert medication:
This medication is in a class the Institute for Safe Medication Practices (ISMP) includes among its list of drug classes which have a heightened risk of causing significant patient harm when used in error.

Synonyms LDP-341; MLN341; PS-341

U.S. Brand Names Velcade®

Canadian Brand Names Velcade®

Therapeutic Category Proteasome Inhibitor

Use Treatment of multiple myeloma; treatment of relapsed or refractory mantle cell lymphoma

General Dosage Range Dosage adjustment recommended in patients with hepatic impairment or who develop toxicities.
I.V.: *Adults:* Dosage varies greatly depending on indication

Dosage Forms
Injection, powder for reconstitution:
Velcade®: 3.5 mg

bosentan (boe SEN tan)

Medication Safety Issues
Sound-alike/look-alike issues:
Tracleer® may be confused with TriCor®

U.S. Brand Names Tracleer®

Canadian Brand Names Tracleer®

Therapeutic Category Endothelin Antagonist

Use Treatment of pulmonary artery hypertension (PAH) (WHO Group I) in patients with NYHA Class II, III, or IV symptoms to improve exercise capacity and decrease the rate of clinical deterioration

General Dosage Range Dosage adjustment recommended in patients with hepatic impairment or on concomitant therapy
Oral:
Children >12 years and Adults <40 kg: Initial: 62.5 mg twice daily; Maintenance: 62.5 mg twice daily
Children >12 years and Adults ≥40 kg: Initial: 62.5 mg twice daily; Maintenance: 125 mg twice daily

Dosage Forms
Tablet, oral:
Tracleer®: 62.5 mg, 125 mg

Botox® *see* onabotulinumtoxinA *on page 650*

Botox® Cosmetic *see* onabotulinumtoxinA *on page 650*

botulinum toxin type A *see* abobotulinumtoxinA *on page 22*

botulinum toxin type A *see* incobotulinumtoxinA *on page 470*

botulinum toxin type A *see* onabotulinumtoxinA *on page 650*

botulinum toxin type B *see* rimabotulinumtoxinB *on page 781*

botulism immune globulin (intravenous-human)
(BOT yoo lism i MYUN GLOB you lin, in tra VEE nus, YU man)

Medication Safety Issues
Sound-alike/look-alike issues:
BabyBIG® may be confused with HBIG

Synonyms BIG-IV

U.S. Brand Names BabyBIG®

Therapeutic Category Immune Globulin

Use Treatment of infant botulism caused by toxin type A or B

General Dosage Range I.V.: *Children <1 year:* 100 mg/kg as a single dose

Dosage Forms
Injection, powder for reconstitution [preservative free]:
BabyBIG®: ~100 mg

Boudreaux's® Butt Paste [OTC] *see* zinc oxide *on page 930*

bovine lipid extract surfactant *(Canada only)* (BOH vine LIP id EK strakt ser FAK tunt)
Canadian Brand Names BLES
Therapeutic Category Lung Surfactant
Use Treatment of neonatal respiratory distress syndrome (NRDS)
General Dosage Range Intratracheal: *Infants:* 5 mL/kg/dose (equals phospholipids 135 mg/kg/dose); may repeat if needed (maximum: 4 doses)
Product Availability Not available in U.S.
Dosage Forms - Canada
Suspension, intratracheal [preservative free]:
BLES®: Phospholipids 27 mg/mL (3 mL, 4 mL, 5 mL)

bovine lung surfactant *see* beractant *on page 127*
BP10-1 *see* sulfur and sulfacetamide *on page 838*
BP 50% *see* urea *on page 900*
BP Cleansing Wash *see* sulfur and sulfacetamide *on page 838*
BPM PE *see* brompheniramine and phenylephrine *on page 143*
BPO *see* benzoyl peroxide *on page 124*
BP Poly 650 [DSC] *see* acetaminophen and phenyltoloxamine *on page 28*
BRAF(V600E) kinase inhibitor RO5185426 *see* vemurafenib *on page 911*
BranchAmin® *see* amino acid injection *on page 65*
Bravelle® *see* urofollitropin *on page 902*
Breathe Free® [OTC] *see* sodium chloride *on page 818*

brentuximab vedotin (bren TUX i mab ve DOE tin)
Medication Safety Issues
Sound-alike/look-alike issues:
Brentuximab may be confused with bendamustine, bevacizumab, rituximab
High alert medication:
This medication is in a class the Institute for Safe Medication Practices (ISMP) includes among its list of drug classes which have a heightened risk of causing significant patient harm when used in error.
Synonyms anti-CD30 ADC SGN-35; anti-CD30 antibody-drug conjugate SGN-35; antibody-drug conjugate SGN-35; SGN-35
U.S. Brand Names Adcetris™
Use
Treatment of Hodgkin lymphoma after failure of at least 2 prior chemotherapy regimens (in patients ineligible for transplant) or after stem cell transplant failure; treatment of systemic anaplastic large cell lymphoma (sALCL) after failure of at least 1 prior chemotherapy regimen
General Dosage Range Dosage adjustment recommended in patients who develop toxicities.
I.V.: *Adults:* 1.8 mg/kg every 3 weeks (maximum dose: 180 mg)
Dosage Forms
Injection, powder for reconstitution:
Adcetris™: 50 mg

Brethaire [DSC] *see* terbutaline *on page 852*
brethine *see* terbutaline *on page 852*
Brevibloc *see* esmolol *on page 341*
Brevibloc® (Can) *see* esmolol *on page 341*
Brevicon® *see* ethinyl estradiol and norethindrone *on page 355*
Brevicon® 0.5/35 (Can) *see* ethinyl estradiol and norethindrone *on page 355*
Brevicon® 1/35 (Can) *see* ethinyl estradiol and norethindrone *on page 355*
Brevital® (Can) *see* methohexital *on page 570*
Brevital® Sodium *see* methohexital *on page 570*
Brevoxyl®-4 [DSC] *see* benzoyl peroxide *on page 124*
Brevoxyl®-8 [DSC] *see* benzoyl peroxide *on page 124*
Bricanyl [DSC] *see* terbutaline *on page 852*
Bricanyl® (Can) *see* terbutaline *on page 852*
Brilinta™ *see* ticagrelor *on page 867*

brimonidine (bri MOE ni deen)

Medication Safety Issues
Sound-alike/look-alike issues:
Brimonidine may be confused with bromocriptine
Synonyms brimonidine tartrate
U.S. Brand Names Alphagan® P
Canadian Brand Names Alphagan®; Apo-Brimonidine P®; Apo-Brimonidine®; PMS-Brimonidine Tartrate; ratio-Brimonidine; Sandoz-Brimonidine
Therapeutic Category Alpha$_2$ Agonist, Ophthalmic
Use Lowering of intraocular pressure (IOP) in patients with open-angle glaucoma or ocular hypertension
General Dosage Range Ophthalmic: *Children ≥2 years and Adults:* Instill 1 drop in affected eye(s) 3 times/day
Dosage Forms
Solution, ophthalmic: 0.15% (5 mL, 10 mL, 15 mL); 0.2% (5 mL, 10 mL, 15 mL)
Alphagan® P: 0.1% (5 mL, 10 mL, 15 mL); 0.15% (5 mL, 10 mL, 15 mL)

brimonidine and timolol (bri MOE ni deen & TIM oh lol)

Medication Safety Issues
Sound-alike/look-alike issues:
Combigan® may be confused with Combivent®, Comtan®
Synonyms brimonidine tartrate and timolol maleate; timolol and brimonidine
U.S. Brand Names Combigan®
Canadian Brand Names Combigan®
Therapeutic Category Alpha$_2$ Agonist, Ophthalmic; Beta Blocker, Nonselective; Ophthalmic Agent, Antiglaucoma
Use Reduction of intraocular pressure (IOP) in patients with glaucoma or ocular hypertension
General Dosage Range Ophthalmic: *Children ≥2 years and Adults:* Instill 1 drop into affected eye(s) twice daily
Dosage Forms
Solution, ophthalmic [drops]:
Combigan®: Brimonidine 0.2% and timolol 0.5% (5 mL,10 mL)
Dosage Forms - Canada
Solution, ophthalmic [drops]:
Combigan®: Brimonidine 0.2% and timolol 0.5% (2.5 mL, 5 mL,10 mL)

brimonidine tartrate *see brimonidine on page 141*
brimonidine tartrate and timolol maleate *see brimonidine and timolol on page 141*

brinzolamide (brin ZOH la mide)

U.S. Brand Names Azopt®
Canadian Brand Names Azopt®
Therapeutic Category Carbonic Anhydrase Inhibitor
Use Lowers intraocular pressure in patients with ocular hypertension or open-angle glaucoma
General Dosage Range Ophthalmic: *Adults:* Instill 1 drop in affected eye(s) 3 times/day
Dosage Forms
Suspension, ophthalmic:
Azopt®: 1% (10 mL, 15 mL)

brinzolamide and timolol *(Canada only)* (brin ZOH la mide & TIM oh lol)

Synonyms brinzolamide and timolol maleate; timolol maleate and brinzolamide
Canadian Brand Names Azarga™
Therapeutic Category Beta-Adrenergic Blocker, Nonselective; Carbonic Anhydrase Inhibitor; Ophthalmic Agent, Antiglaucoma
Use Treatment of elevated intraocular pressure in patients with ocular hypertension or open-angle glaucoma
General Dosage Range Ophthalmic: *Adults:* Instill 1 drop twice daily
Product Availability Not available in U.S.

◀ **Dosage Forms - Canada**
Solution, ophthalmic [drops]:
Azarga™: Brinzolamide 1% and timolol maleate 0.5% (5 mL)

brinzolamide and timolol maleate *see* brinzolamide and timolol *(Canada only) on page 141*

Brioschi® [OTC] *see* sodium bicarbonate *on page 818*

British anti-lewisite *see* dimercaprol *on page 288*

BRL 43694 *see* granisetron *on page 424*

Bromaline® [OTC] *see* brompheniramine and pseudoephedrine *on page 144*

Bromaline® DM [OTC] *see* brompheniramine, pseudoephedrine, and dextromethorphan *on page 144*

Bromax *see* brompheniramine *on page 143*

bromazepam *(Canada only)* (broe MA ze pam)

Medication Safety Issues
International issues:
Lexotan [multiple international markets] may be confused with Loxitane brand name for loxapine [U.S.]

Canadian Brand Names Apo-Bromazepam®; Lectopam®; Mylan-Bromazepam; Novo-Bromazepam; Nu-Bromazepam; PRO-Doc Limitee Bromazepam

Therapeutic Category Benzodiazepine; Sedative

Use Short-term, symptomatic treatment of anxiety

General Dosage Range Oral:
Adults: Initial: 6-18 mg/day in divided doses; Maintenance: 6-30 mg/day in divided doses
Elderly: Initial: 3 mg/day in divided doses

Product Availability Not available in U.S.

Dosage Forms - Canada
Tablet: 1.5 mg, 3 mg, 6 mg
Lectopam®: 3 mg, 6 mg

Bromday™ *see* bromfenac *on page 142*

Bromdex D *see* brompheniramine, pseudoephedrine, and dextromethorphan *on page 144*

Bromfed® *see* brompheniramine and phenylephrine *on page 143*

Bromfed® DM *see* brompheniramine, pseudoephedrine, and dextromethorphan *on page 144*

Bromfed®-PD *see* brompheniramine and phenylephrine *on page 143*

bromfenac (BROME fen ak)

Synonyms bromfenac sodium

U.S. Brand Names Bromday™; Xibrom® [DSC]

Therapeutic Category Analgesic, Nonnarcotic; Nonsteroidal Antiinflammatory Drug (NSAID), Ophthalmic

Use Treatment of postoperative inflammation and reduction in ocular pain following cataract removal

General Dosage Range Ophthalmic: *Adults:*
Bromday™: Instill 1 drop into affected eye(s) once daily
Xibrom®: Instill 1 drop into affected eye(s) twice daily

Dosage Forms
Solution, ophthalmic: 0.09% (2.5 mL)
Bromday™: 0.09% (1.7 mL)

bromfenac sodium *see* bromfenac *on page 142*

bromocriptine (broe moe KRIP teen)

Medication Safety Issues
Sound-alike/look-alike issues:
Bromocriptine may be confused with benztropine, brimonidine
Cycloset® may be confused with Glyset®
Parlodel® may be confused with pindolol, Provera®

Synonyms bromocriptine mesylate

U.S. Brand Names Cycloset®; Parlodel®; Parlodel® SnapTabs®

Canadian Brand Names Apo-Bromocriptine®; Dom-Bromocriptine; PMS-Bromocriptine

Therapeutic Category Anti-Parkinson Agent (Dopamine Agonist); Ergot Alkaloid and Derivative

Use Treatment of hyperprolactinemia associated with amenorrhea with or without galactorrhea, infertility, or hypogonadism; treatment of prolactin-secreting adenomas; treatment of acromegaly; treatment of Parkinson disease

Cycloset®: Management of type 2 diabetes mellitus (noninsulin-dependent, NIDDM) as an adjunct to diet and exercise

General Dosage Range Oral:
Children 11-15 years: Initial: 1.25-2.5 mg daily; Maintenance: 2.5-10 mg/day
Children ≥16 years: Initial: 1.25-2.5 mg daily; Maintenance: 2.5-15 mg/day
Adults: Dosage varies greatly depending on indication

Dosage Forms
Capsule, oral: 5 mg
  Parlodel®: 5 mg
Tablet, oral: 2.5 mg
  Cycloset®: 0.8 mg
  Parlodel® SnapTabs®: 2.5 mg

bromocriptine mesylate *see bromocriptine on page 142*
Bromphenex™ DM [OTC] *see brompheniramine, pseudoephedrine, and dextromethorphan on page 144*

brompheniramine (brome fen IR a meen)

Synonyms brompheniramine maleate; brompheniramine tannate
U.S. Brand Names Bromax; Lodrane® 24 [DSC]; LoHist-12; Respa®-BR [DSC]; TanaCof-XR [DSC]
Therapeutic Category Antihistamine
Use Symptomatic relief of perennial and seasonal allergic rhinitis, vasomotor rhinitis, and other respiratory allergies

General Dosage Range Oral:
Children 6-12 years:
  Lodrane® 24: One capsule once daily
  LoHist-12: One tablet every 12 hours (maximum: 2 tablets/day)
Children >12 years and Adults:
  Bromax, Respa®-BR: One tablet twice daily
  Lodrane® 24: 1-2 capsules once daily
  LoHist-12: 1-2 tablets every 12 hours (maximum: 4 tablets/day)

Dosage Forms
Tablet, extended release, oral:
  Bromax: 11 mg
  LoHist-12: 6 mg

brompheniramine and phenylephrine (brome fen IR a meen & fen il EF rin)

Medication Safety Issues
Sound-alike/look-alike issues:
  Bromfed® may be confused with Bromphen®
Synonyms brompheniramine maleate and phenylephrine hydrochloride; brompheniramine tannate and phenylephrine tannate; phenylephrine and brompheniramine
U.S. Brand Names B-Vex D [DSC]; BPM PE; Bromfed®; Bromfed®-PD; C-Tan D; C-Tan D Plus; Dimaphen Cold & Allergy [OTC]; Dimetapp® Children's Cold & Allergy [OTC]
Therapeutic Category Alpha/Beta Agonist; Histamine H$_1$ Antagonist; Histamine H$_1$ Antagonist, First Generation
Use Temporary relief of upper respiratory conditions such as nasal congestion, runny nose, itchy/watery eyes, and sneezing due to the common cold, hay fever, or upper respiratory allergies

General Dosage Range Oral:
Children 2-6 years: B-Vex D: 2.5 mL every 12 hours (maximum: 5 mL/24 hours)
Children 6-11 years:
  B-Vex D, C-Tann D, C-Tann D Plus: 5 mL every 12 hours (maximum: 10 mL/24 hours)
  BPM PE: 2.5 mL every 6 hours as needed (maximum: 15 mL/24 hours)
  Bromfed®-PD: 1 capsule every 12 hours
  Dimaphen Cold & Allergy: 10 mL every 4-6 hours as needed (maximum: 60 mL/24 hours)
  Dimetapp® chewable tablet: 2 tablets every 4 hours as needed (maximum: 12 tablets/24 hours)
  Dimetapp® syrup: 10 mL every 4 hours as needed (maximum: 60 mL/24 hours)

Children ≥12 years and Adults:
B-Vex, C-Tann D, C-Tann D Plus: 5-10 mL every 12 hours (maximum: 20 mL/24 hours)
BPM PE: 5 mL every 6 hours as needed (maximum: 30 mL/24 hours)
Bromfed®: 1 capsule every 12 hours
Bromfed®-PD: 1-2 capsules every 12 hours
Dimaphen Cold & Allergy: 20 mL every 4-6 hours as needed (maximum: 120 mL/24 hours)
Dimetapp® syrup: 20 mL every 4 hours as needed (maximum: 120 mL/24 hours)

Dosage Forms
Capsule, extended release: Brompheniramine 6 mg and phenylephrine 7.5 mg; Brompheniramine 12 mg and phenylephrine 15 mg
Bromfed®: Brompheniramine 12 mg and phenylephrine 15 mg
Bromfed®-PD: Brompheniramine 6 mg and phenylephrine 7.5 mg
Elixir, oral:
Dimaphen Cold & Allergy [OTC]: Brompheniramine 1 mg and phenylephrine 2. 5 mg per 5 mL
Liquid, oral:
BPM PE: Brompheniramine 4 mg and phenylephrine 7.5 mg per 5 mL
Suspension, oral: Brompheniramine 12 mg and phenylephrine 20 mg per 5 mL
C-Tann D: Brompheniramine 4 mg and phenylephrine 5 mg per 5 mL
C-Tann D Plus: Brompheniramine 5 mg and phenylephrine 5 mg per 5 mL
Syrup:
Dimetapp® Children's Cold & Allergy [OTC]: Brompheniramine 1 mg and phenylephrine 2.5 mg per 5 mL
Tablet, chewable:
Dimetapp® Children's Cold & Allergy [OTC]: Brompheniramine 1 mg and phenylephrine 2.5 mg

brompheniramine and pseudoephedrine (brome fen IR a meen & soo doe e FED rin)

Synonyms brompheniramine maleate and pseudoephedrine hydrochloride; brompheniramine maleate and pseudoephedrine sulfate; pseudoephedrine and brompheniramine
U.S. Brand Names Bromaline® [OTC]; Brotapp [OTC]
Therapeutic Category Antihistamine/Decongestant Combination
Use Temporary relief of symptoms associated with seasonal and perennial allergic rhinitis, the common cold, or sinusitis
General Dosage Range
Oral: Liquid:
Children 6-11 years: Brompheniramine 2 mg/pseudoephedrine 30 mg every 6 hours (maximum: 4 doses/day)
Children ≥12 years and Adults: Brompheniramine 4 mg/pseudoephedrine 60 mg every 6 hours (maximum: 4 doses/day)
Dosage Forms
Liquid, oral:
Brotapp [OTC]: Brompheniramine 1 mg and pseudoephedrine 15 mg per 5 mL
Solution, oral:
Bromaline® [OTC]: Brompheniramine 1 mg and pseudoephedrine 15 mg per 5 mL

brompheniramine maleate *see brompheniramine on page 143*
brompheniramine maleate and phenylephrine hydrochloride *see brompheniramine and phenylephrine on page 143*
brompheniramine maleate and pseudoephedrine hydrochloride *see brompheniramine and pseudoephedrine on page 144*
brompheniramine maleate and pseudoephedrine sulfate *see brompheniramine and pseudoephedrine on page 144*

brompheniramine, pseudoephedrine, and dextromethorphan
(brome fen IR a meen, soo doe e FED rin, & deks troe meth OR fan)

Synonyms dextromethorphan hydrobromide, brompheniramine maleate, and pseudoephedrine hydrochloride; pseudoephedrine tannate, dextromethorphan tannate, and brompheniramine tannate
U.S. Brand Names Anaplex® DM; Bromaline® DM [OTC]; Bromdex D; Bromfed® DM; Bromphenex™ DM [OTC]; Bromplex DM [DSC]; Brotapp-DM; EndaCof-DM; EndaCof-PD; Histacol™ BD [DSC]; Myphetane DX [DSC]; Neo DM; PediaHist DM; Resperal-DM
Therapeutic Category Antihistamine; Cough Preparation; Decongestant

Use Relief of cough and upper respiratory symptoms (including nasal congestion) associated with allergy or the common cold

General Dosage Range Oral:
Children 1-3 months: EndaCof-PD: 0.25 mL 4 times/day
Children 3-6 months: EndaCof-PD: 0.5 mL 4 times/day
Children 6-12 months: EndaCof-PD: 0.75 mL 4 times/day
Children 12-24 months: EndaCof-PD: 1 mL 4 times/day
Children 2-6 years: Anaplex® DM, EndaCof-DM: 1.25 mL every 4-6 hours (maximum: 4 doses/day)
Children 6-12 years:
    Anaplex® DM, EndaCof-DM: 2.5 mL every 4-6 hours (maximum: 4 doses/day)
    Bromaline® DM: 10 mL every 4-6 hours (maximum: 4 doses/day)
Children >12 years and Adults:
    Anaplex® DM: 5 mL every 4-6 hours (maximum: 4 doses/day)
    Bromaline® DM: 20 mL every 4-6 hours (maximum: 4 doses/day)

Dosage Forms
Elixir, oral:
    Bromaline® DM [OTC]: Brompheniramine 1 mg, pseudoephedrine 15 mg, and dextromethorphan 5 mg per 5 mL
Liquid, oral:
    Bromphenex™ DM [OTC]: Brompheniramine 4 mg, pseudoephedrine 60 mg, and dextromethorphan 30 mg per 5 mL
    Brotapp-DM: Brompheniramine 1 mg, pseudoephedrine 15 mg, and dextromethorphan 5 mg per 5 mL
Solution, oral [drops]:
    EndaCof-PD: Brompheniramine 1 mg, pseudoephedrine 12.5 mg, and dextromethorphan 3 mg per 1 mL
    PediaHist DM: Brompheniramine 1 mg, pseudoephedrine 15 mg, and dextromethorphan 4 mg per 1 mL
    Resperal-DM: Brompheniramine 1 mg, pseudoephedrine 12 mg, and dextromethorphan 5 mg per 1 mL
Suspension, oral: Brompheniramine 8 mg, pseudoephedrine 90 mg, and dextromethorphan 60 mg per 5 mL
Syrup, oral:
    Anaplex® DM, EndaCof-DM: Brompheniramine 4 mg, pseudoephedrine 60 mg, and dextromethorphan 30 mg per 5 mL
    Bromatane DX, Neo DM: Brompheniramine 2 mg, pseudoephedrine 30 mg, and dextromethorphan 10 mg per 5 mL
    Bromdex D: Brompheniramine 3 mg, pseudoephedrine 50 mg, and dextromethorphan 30 mg per 5 mL

brompheniramine tannate *see brompheniramine on page 143*
brompheniramine tannate and phenylephrine tannate *see brompheniramine and phenylephrine on page 143*
Bromplex DM [DSC] *see brompheniramine, pseudoephedrine, and dextromethorphan on page 144*
Brotapp [OTC] *see brompheniramine and pseudoephedrine on page 144*
Brotapp-DM *see brompheniramine, pseudoephedrine, and dextromethorphan on page 144*
Brovana® *see arformoterol on page 92*
BSF208075 *see ambrisentan on page 62*
BSS® *see balanced salt solution on page 113*
BSS Plus® *see balanced salt solution on page 113*
BTX-A *see onabotulinumtoxinA on page 650*
B-type natriuretic peptide (human) *see nesiritide on page 620*
Budeprion XL® *see bupropion on page 150*
Budeprion SR® *see bupropion on page 150*

budesonide (systemic, oral inhalation) (byoo DES oh nide)

U.S. Brand Names Entocort® EC; Pulmicort Flexhaler®; Pulmicort Respules®
Canadian Brand Names Entocort®; Pulmicort®
Therapeutic Category Corticosteroid, Inhalant (Oral); Corticosteroid, Systemic
Use
Nebulization: Maintenance and prophylactic treatment of asthma
Oral capsule: Treatment of active Crohn disease (mild-to-moderate) involving the ileum and/or ascending colon; maintenance of remission (for up to 3 months) of Crohn disease (mild-to-moderate) involving the ileum and/or ascending colon

◀ Oral inhalation: Maintenance and prophylactic treatment of asthma; includes patients who require oral corticosteroids and those who may benefit from systemic dose reduction/elimination

General Dosage Range
Inhalation:
Children ≥6 years: Initial: 180-360 mcg twice daily; Maintenance: 180->800 mcg/day in 2 divided doses
Adults: Initial: 180-720 mcg twice daily; Maintenance: 180->1200 mcg/day in 2 divided doses
Nebulization: *Children 12 months to 8 years:* 0.25-1 mg in 1-2 divided doses
Oral: *Adults:* Initial: 9 mg once daily; Maintenance: 6 mg once daily

Dosage Forms
Capsule, enteric coated, oral: 3 mg
 Entocort® EC: 3 mg
Powder, for oral inhalation:
 Pulmicort Flexhaler®: 90 mcg/inhalation (165 mg); 180 mcg/inhalation (225 mg)
Suspension, for nebulization: 0.25 mg/2 mL (30s); 0.5 mg/2 mL (30s)
 Pulmicort Respules®: 0.25 mg/2 mL (30s); 0.5 mg/2 mL (30s); 1 mg/2 mL (30s)

Dosage Forms - Canada
Powder for oral inhalation:
 Pulmicort Turbuhaler®: 100 mcg/inhalation, 200 mcg/inhalation, 400 mcg/inhalation

budesonide (nasal) (byoo DES oh nide)

U.S. Brand Names Rhinocort Aqua®
Canadian Brand Names Gen-Budesonide AQ; Mylan-Budesonide AQ; Rhinocort® Aqua™; Rhinocort® Turbuhaler®
Therapeutic Category Corticosteroid, Nasal
Use Management of symptoms of seasonal or perennial rhinitis

 Canadian labeling: Additional use (not in U.S. labeling): Prevention and treatment of nasal polyps
General Dosage Range Intranasal inhalation: *Children ≥6 years and Adults:* 64 mcg/day as a single 32 mcg spray in each nostril (maximum: 128 mcg/day [children <12 years]; 256 mcg/day [children ≥12 years and adults])

Dosage Forms
Suspension, intranasal:
 Rhinocort Aqua®: 32 mcg/inhalation (8.6 g)
Dosage Forms - Canada
Powder for nasal inhalation:
 Rhinocort® Turbuhaler®: 100 mcg/inhalation
Suspension, intranasal [spray]:
 Rhinocort® Aqua®: 64 mcg/inhalation

budesonide and eformoterol *see* budesonide and formoterol *on page 146*

budesonide and formoterol (byoo DES oh nide & for MOH te rol)

Synonyms budesonide and eformoterol; eformoterol and budesonide; formoterol and budesonide; formoterol fumarate dihydrate and budesonide
U.S. Brand Names Symbicort®
Canadian Brand Names Symbicort®
Therapeutic Category Beta$_2$-Adrenergic Agonist Agent; Corticosteroid, Inhalant (Oral)
Use Treatment of asthma in patients ≥12 years of age where combination therapy is indicated; maintenance treatment of airflow obstruction associated with chronic obstructive pulmonary disease (COPD; including chronic bronchitis and emphysema)
General Dosage Range Inhalation:
Children 5-11 years: Symbicort® 80/4.5: Two inhalations twice daily (maximum: 4 inhalations/day)
Children ≥12 years: 2 inhalations once or twice daily (maximum: 4 inhalations/day)
Adults: 2 inhalations twice daily (maximum: 4 inhalations/day)
Dosage Forms
Aerosol for oral inhalation:
 Symbicort® 80/4.5: Budesonide 80 mcg and formoterol fumarate dihydrate 4.5 mcg per actuation (6.9 g) [60 metered inhalations]; budesonide 80 mcg and formoterol fumarate dihydrate 4.5 mcg per actuation (10.2 g) [120 metered inhalations]

Symbicort® 160/4.5: Budesonide 160 mcg and formoterol fumarate dihydrate 4.5 mcg per actuation (6 g) [60 metered inhalations]; budesonide 160 mcg and formoterol fumarate dihydrate 4.5 mcg per actuation (10.2 g) [120 metered inhalations]

Dosage Forms - Canada
Powder for oral inhalation:
Symbicort® 100 Turbuhaler®: Budesonide 100 mcg and formoterol dihydrate 6 mcg per inhalation (available in 60 or 120 metered doses) [delivers ~80 mcg budesonide and 4.5 mcg formoterol per inhalation]
Symbicort® 200 Turbuhaler®: Budesonide 200 mcg and formoterol dihydrate 6 mcg per inhalation (available in 60 or 120 metered doses) [delivers ~160 mcg budesonide and 4.5 mcg formoterol per inhalation]

Buffasal [OTC] *see* aspirin *on page 98*
Bufferin® [OTC] *see* aspirin *on page 98*
Bufferin® Extra Strength [OTC] *see* aspirin *on page 98*
Buffinol [OTC] *see* aspirin *on page 98*
Bulk-K [OTC] *see* psyllium *on page 755*

bumetanide (byoo MET a nide)

Medication Safety Issues
Sound-alike/look-alike issues:
Bumetanide may be confused with Buminate®
Bumex® may be confused with Brevibloc®, Buprenex®
International issues:
Bumex [U.S.] may be confused with Permax brand name for pergolide [multiple international markets]
Synonyms Bumex
Canadian Brand Names Burinex®
Therapeutic Category Diuretic, Loop
Use Management of edema secondary to heart failure or hepatic or renal disease (including nephrotic syndrome)
General Dosage Range
I.M., I.V.:
Infants and Children: 0.015-0.1 mg/kg/dose every 6-24 hours (maximum: 10 mg/day)
Adults: 0.5-1 mg/dose; may repeat in 2-3 hours for up to 2 doses (maximum: 10 mg/day)
Oral:
Infants and Children: 0.015-0.1 mg/kg/dose every 6-24 hours (maximum: 10 mg/day)
Adults: 0.5-2 mg 1-2 times/day; may repeat in 4-5 hours for up to 2 doses (maximum: 10 mg/day)
Dosage Forms
Injection, solution: 0.25 mg/mL (2 mL, 4 mL, 5 mL, 10 mL)
Tablet, oral: 0.5 mg, 1 mg, 2 mg

Bumex *see* bumetanide *on page 147*
Buminate *see* albumin *on page 44*
Bupap *see* butalbital and acetaminophen *on page 153*
Buphenyl® *see* sodium phenylbutyrate *on page 822*

bupivacaine (byoo PIV a kane)

Medication Safety Issues
Sound-alike/look-alike issues:
Bupivacaine may be confused with mepivacaine, ropivacaine
Marcaine® may be confused with Narcan®
High alert medication:
The Institute for Safe Medication Practices (ISMP) includes this medication (epidural administration) among its list of drug classes which have a heightened risk of causing significant patient harm when used in error.
Synonyms bupivacaine hydrochloride
U.S. Brand Names Bupivacaine Spinal; Marcaine®; Marcaine® Spinal; Sensorcaine®; Sensorcaine®-MPF; Sensorcaine®-MPF Spinal
Canadian Brand Names Marcaine®; Sensorcaine®
Therapeutic Category Local Anesthetic

◀ **Use** Local or regional anesthesia; spinal anesthesia; diagnostic and therapeutic procedures; obstetrical procedures (only 0.25% and 0.5% concentrations)

0.25%: Local infiltration, peripheral nerve block, sympathetic block, caudal or epidural block

0.5%: Peripheral nerve block, caudal and epidural block

0.75% **(not for obstetrical anesthesia)**: Retrobulbar block, epidural block. **Note:** Reserve for surgical procedures where a high degree of muscle relaxation and prolonged effect are necessary

General Dosage Range

Caudal block: *Children >12 years and Adults:* 15-30 mL of 0.25% or 0.5%

Epidural block: *Children >12 years and Adults:* 10-20 mL of 0.25% or 0.5% in 3-5 mL increments **or** 10-20 mL of 0.75% if high degree of muscle relaxation and prolonged effects needed

Infiltration (local): *Children >12 years and Adults:* 0.25% (maximum: 175 mg)

Nerve block: *Children >12 years and Adults:*

Peripheral: 5 mL of 0.25% or 0.5% (maximum: 400 mg/day)

Sympathetic: 20-50 mL of 0.25%

Retrobulbar anesthesia: *Children >12 years and Adults:* 2-4 mL of 0.75%

Spinal: *Adults:* Preservative free solution of 0.75% bupivacaine in 8.25% dextrose:

Cesarean section: 1-1.4 mL

Lower abdominal procedures: 1.6 mL

Lower extremity and perineal procedures: 1 mL

Normal vaginal delivery: 0.8 mL (higher doses may be required in some patients)

Dosage Forms

Injection, solution: 0.25% [2.5 mg/mL] (20 mL, 50 mL); 0.5% [5 mg/mL] (20 mL, 50 mL)

Marcaine®: 0.5% [5 mg/mL] (50 mL)

Sensorcaine®: 0.25% [2.5 mg/mL] (50 mL); 0.5% [5 mg/mL] (50 mL)

Injection, solution [preservative free]: 0.25% [2.5 mg/mL] (10 mL, 20 mL, 30 mL, 50 mL); 0.5% [5 mg/mL] (10 mL, 20 mL, 30 mL); 0.75% [7.5 mg/mL] (10 mL, 20 mL, 30 mL)

Marcaine®: 0.25% [2.5 mg/mL] (10 mL, 30 mL, 50 mL); 0.5% [5 mg/mL] (10 mL, 30 mL); 0.75% [7.5 mg/mL] (10 mL, 30 mL)

Sensorcaine®-MPF: 0.25% [2.5 mg/mL] (10 mL, 30 mL); 0.5% [5 mg/mL] (10 mL, 30 mL); 0.75% [7.5 mg/mL] (10 mL, 30 mL)

Injection, solution, premixed in D$_{8.25}$W [preservative free]:

Bupivacaine Spinal: 0.75% [7.5 mg/mL] (2 mL)

Marcaine® Spinal: 0.75% [7.5 mg/mL] (2 mL)

Sensorcaine®-MPF Spinal: 0.75% [7.5 mg/mL] (2 mL)

bupivacaine and epinephrine (byoo PIV a kane & ep i NEF rin)

Medication Safety Issues

High alert medication:

The Institute for Safe Medication Practices (ISMP) includes this medication (epidural administration) among its list of drug classes which have a heightened risk of causing significant patient harm when used in error.

Synonyms epinephrine bitartrate and bupivacaine hydrochloride

U.S. Brand Names Marcaine® with Epinephrine; Sensorcaine® with Epinephrine; Sensorcaine®-MPF with Epinephrine; Vivacaine™

Canadian Brand Names Sensorcaine® with Epinephrine

Therapeutic Category Local Anesthetic

Use Local anesthetic (injectable) for peripheral nerve block, infiltration, sympathetic block, caudal or epidural block, retrobulbar block

General Dosage Range

Caudal block (preservative free): *Children >12 years and Adults:* 15-30 mL of 0.25% or 0.5%

Epidural block (preservative free): *Children >12 years and Adults:* 10-20 mL of 0.25% or 0.5% in 3-5 mL increments **or** 10-20 mL of 0.75% if high degree of muscle relaxation or prolonged effects needed

Infiltration (local): *Children >12 years and Adults:* 0.25% (maximum: 175 mg [bupivacaine])

Infiltration and nerve block (maxillary, mandibular): *Children >12 years and Adults:* 9 mg (1.8 mL) of bupivacaine as a 0.5% solution with epinephrine 1:200,000 per injection site; may repeat after 10 minutes if needed (maximum: 90 mg bupivacaine/appointment)

Nerve block: *Children >12 years and Adults:*

Peripheral: 5 mL of 0.25 or 0.5% (maximum: 400 mg/day [bupivacaine])

Sympathetic: 20-50 mL of 0.25%

Retrobulbar anesthesia: *Children >12 years and Adults:* 2-4 mL of 0.75%

Dosage Forms
Injection, solution [preservative free]: Bupivacaine 0.25% and epinephrine 1:200,000 (10 mL, 30 mL); bupivacaine 0.5% and epinephrine 1:200,000 (10 mL, 30 mL)
  Marcaine® with Epinephrine: Bupivacaine 0.25% and epinephrine 1:200,000 (10 mL, 30 mL); bupivacaine 0.5% and epinephrine 1:200,000 (10 mL, 30 mL)
  Sensorcaine® MPF with Epinephrine: Bupivacaine 0.25% and epinephrine 1:200,000 (10 mL, 30 mL); bupivacaine 0.5% and epinephrine 1:200,000 (10 mL, 30 mL); bupivacaine 0.75% and epinephrine 1:200,000 (30 mL)
Injection, solution: Bupivacaine 0.25% and epinephrine 1:200,000 (50 mL); bupivacaine 0.5% and epinephrine 1:200,000 (50 mL)
  Marcaine® with Epinephrine, Sensorcaine® with Epinephrine: Bupivacaine 0.25% and epinephrine 1:200,000 (50 mL); bupivacaine 0.5% and epinephrine 1:200,000 (50 mL)
Injection, solution [for dental use]:
  Marcaine® with Epinephrine, Vivacaine™: Bupivacaine 0.5% and epinephrine 1:200,000 (1.8 mL)

bupivacaine hydrochloride *see* bupivacaine *on page 147*
Bupivacaine Spinal *see* bupivacaine *on page 147*
Buprenex® *see* buprenorphine *on page 149*

buprenorphine (byoo pre NOR feen)

Medication Safety Issues
Sound-alike/look-alike issues:
  Buprenex® may be confused with Brevibloc®, Bumex®
High alert medication:
  The Institute for Safe Medication Practices (ISMP) includes this medication among its list of drug classes which have a heightened risk of causing significant patient harm when used in error.
Synonyms buprenorphine hydrochloride
U.S. Brand Names Buprenex®; Butrans™; Subutex®
Canadian Brand Names Buprenex®; Subutex®
Therapeutic Category Analgesic, Narcotic
Controlled Substance C-III
Use
  Injection: Management of moderate-to-severe pain
  Sublingual tablet: Treatment of opioid dependence
  Transdermal patch: Management of moderate-to-severe chronic pain in patients requiring an around-the-clock opioid analgesic for an extended period of time
General Dosage Range Dosage adjustment recommended in patients with hepatic impairment.
I.M., I.V.:
  Children 2-12 years: 2-6 mcg/kg every 4-6 hours
  Children ≥13 years and Adults: Initial: 0.3 mg, may repeat once in 30-60 minutes then every 6-8 hours as needed; Maintenance: 0.15-0.6 mg every 4-8 hours as needed
  Elderly: 0.15 mg every 6 hours
Sublingual: *Children ≥16 years and Adults:* Induction: 12-16 mg/day; Maintenance: 12-16 mg/day (target dose: 16 mg/day)
Transdermal: *Adults:* 5-20 mcg/hour applied once every 7 days
Dosage Forms
Injection, solution: 0.3 mg/mL (1 mL)
  Buprenex®: 0.3 mg/mL (1 mL)
Patch, transdermal:
  Butrans™: 5 mcg/hr (4s); 10 mcg/hr (4s); 20 mcg/hr (4s)
Tablet, sublingual: 2 mg, 8 mg
  Subutex®: 2 mg, 8 mg

buprenorphine and naloxone (byoo pre NOR feen & nal OKS one)

Medication Safety Issues
High alert medication:
  The Institute for Safe Medication Practices (ISMP) includes this medication among its list of drug classes which have a heightened risk of causing significant patient harm when used in error.
Synonyms buprenorphine hydrochloride and naloxone hydrochloride dihydrate; naloxone and buprenorphine; naloxone hydrochloride dihydrate and buprenorphine hydrochloride

◀ **U.S. Brand Names** Suboxone®
Canadian Brand Names Suboxone®
Therapeutic Category Analgesic, Narcotic
Controlled Substance C-III
Use Maintenance treatment for opioid dependence
General Dosage Range Sublingual: *Children ≥16 years and Adults:* 4-24 mg/day (target dose: 16 mg/day)
Dosage Forms
Film, sublingual:
Suboxone®: Buprenorphine 2 mg and naloxone 0.5 mg; buprenorphine 8 mg and naloxone 2 mg
Tablet, sublingual:
Suboxone®: Buprenorphine 2 mg and naloxone 0.5 mg; buprenorphine 8 mg and naloxone 2 mg

buprenorphine hydrochloride *see buprenorphine on page* 149
buprenorphine hydrochloride and naloxone hydrochloride dihydrate *see buprenorphine and naloxone on page* 149
Buproban® *see bupropion on page* 150

bupropion (byoo PROE pee on)
Medication Safety Issues
Sound-alike/look-alike issues:
Aplenzin™ may be confused with Albenza®, Relenza®
BuPROPion may be confused with busPIRone
Wellbutrin SR® may be confused with Wellbutrin XL®
Wellbutrin XL® may be confused with Wellbutrin SR®
Zyban® may be confused with Diovan®
Synonyms bupropion hydrobromide; bupropion hydrochloride
Tall-Man buPROPion
U.S. Brand Names Aplenzin™; Budeprion SR®; Budeprion XL®; Buproban®; Wellbutrin SR®; Wellbutrin XL®; Wellbutrin®; Zyban®
Canadian Brand Names Bupropion SR®; Novo-Bupropion SR; PMS-Bupropion SR; ratio-Bupropion SR; Sandoz-Bupropion SR; Wellbutrin® SR; Wellbutrin® XL; Zyban®
Therapeutic Category Antidepressant, Aminoketone
Use Treatment of major depressive disorder, including seasonal affective disorder (SAD); adjunct in smoking cessation
General Dosage Range Dosage adjustment recommended in patients with hepatic impairment
Oral:
Extended release: *Adults:*
Initial: Hydrochloride salt: 150 mg once daily; Maintenance: 300 mg once daily (maximum: 450 mg/day); Hydrobromide salt: 174-522 mg/day
Immediate release hydrochloride salt:
Adults: Initial: 100 mg twice daily; Maintenance: 100 mg 3 times/day (maximum: 450 mg/day)
Elderly: Initial: 37.5 mg twice daily, increase by 37.5-100 mg every 3-4 days as tolerated
Sustained release hydrochloride salt:
Adults: Initial: 150 mg once daily; Maintenance: 150 mg twice daily (maximum: 400 mg/day)
Elderly: Initial: 100 mg/day, increase by 37.5-100 mg every 3-4 days as tolerated
Dosage Forms
Tablet, oral: 75 mg, 100 mg
Wellbutrin®: 75 mg, 100 mg
Tablet, extended release, oral: 100 mg, 150 mg, 200 mg, 300 mg
Aplenzin™: 174 mg, 348 mg, 522 mg
Budeprion SR®: 100 mg, 150 mg
Budeprion XL®: 150 mg, 300 mg
Buproban®: 150 mg
Wellbutrin XL®: 150 mg, 300 mg
Tablet, sustained release, oral:
Wellbutrin SR®: 100 mg, 150 mg, 200 mg
Zyban®: 150 mg

bupropion hydrobromide *see bupropion on page* 150

bupropion hydrochloride *see* bupropion *on page 150*
Bupropion SR® (Can) *see* bupropion *on page 150*
Burinex® (Can) *see* bumetanide *on page 147*
Burn Jel® [OTC] *see* lidocaine (topical) *on page 524*
Burn Jel Plus [OTC] *see* lidocaine (topical) *on page 524*
Buscopan® (Can) *see* scopolamine (systemic) *on page 804*
buserelin acetate *see* buserelin *(Canada only) on page 151*

buserelin *(Canada only)* (BYOO se rel in)
Medication Safety Issues
 Sound-alike/look-alike issues:
   Suprefact® may be confused with Suprane®
Synonyms buserelin acetate
Canadian Brand Names Suprefact®; Suprefact® Depot
Therapeutic Category Luteinizing Hormone-Releasing Hormone Analog
Use Palliative treatment in patients with hormone-dependent advanced prostate cancer (stage D); treatment of endometriosis in women who do not require surgical intervention as first-line therapy (length of therapy is usually 6 months, but no longer than 9 months)
General Dosage Range
 Intranasal: *Adults:* 400 mcg (200 mcg into each nostril) 3 times/day
 SubQ: *Adults:*
   Implants: 6.3 mg every 8 weeks **or** 9.45 mg every 12 weeks
   Injection: Initial: 500 mcg every 8 hours for 7 days; maintenance: 200 mcg once daily
Product Availability Not available in U.S.
Dosage Forms - Canada
 Implant, subcutaneous:
   Suprefact® Depot: 6.3 mg, 9.45 mg
 Injection, solution:
   Suprefact®: 1 mg/mL (5.5 mL, 10 mL)
 Solution, intranasal:
   Suprefact®: 1mg/1mL (10 mL)

BuSpar *see* buspirone *on page 151*
BuSpar® (Can) *see* buspirone *on page 151*
Buspirex (Can) *see* buspirone *on page 151*

buspirone (byoo SPYE rone)
Medication Safety Issues
 Sound-alike/look-alike issues:
   BusPIRone may be confused with buPROPion
Synonyms BuSpar; buspirone hydrochloride
Tall-Man busPIRone
Canadian Brand Names Apo-Buspirone®; BuSpar®; Buspirex; Bustab®; CO Buspirone; Dom-Buspirone; Gen-Buspirone; Lin-Buspirone; Mylan-Buspirone; Novo-Buspirone; Nu-Buspirone; PMS-Buspirone; ratio-Buspirone; Riva-Buspirone
Therapeutic Category Antianxiety Agent
Use Management of generalized anxiety disorder (GAD)
General Dosage Range Oral:
 Children ≥6 years: Initial: 5 mg daily; Maintenance: Up to 60 mg/day in 2-3 divided doses
 Adults: Initial: 7.5 mg twice daily; Maintenance: Up to 60 mg/day in 2 divided doses (target dose: 10-15 mg twice daily)
 Elderly: Initial: 5 mg twice daily; Maintenance: 20-30 mg/day (maximum: 60 mg/day)
Dosage Forms
 Tablet, oral: 5 mg, 7.5 mg, 10 mg, 15 mg, 30 mg

buspirone hydrochloride *see* buspirone *on page 151*
Bustab® (Can) *see* buspirone *on page 151*

busulfan (byoo SUL fan)

Medication Safety Issues
Sound-alike/look-alike issues:
Myleran® may be confused with Alkeran®, Leukeran®, melphalan, Mylicon®
High alert medication:
This medication is in a class the Institute for Safe Medication Practices (ISMP) includes among its list of drug classes which have a heightened risk of causing significant patient harm when used in error.

Synonyms NSC-750
U.S. Brand Names Busulfex®; Myleran®
Canadian Brand Names Busulfex®; Myleran®
Therapeutic Category Antineoplastic Agent
Use
Oral: Chronic myelogenous leukemia (CML); conditioning regimens for bone marrow transplantation
I.V.: Combination therapy with cyclophosphamide as a conditioning regimen prior to allogeneic hematopoietic progenitor cell transplantation for chronic myelogenous leukemia

General Dosage Range
I.V.:
Children ≤12 kg: **BMT:** 1.1 mg/kg (ideal body weight) every 6 hours for 16 doses
Children >12 kg: **BMT:** 0.8 mg/kg (ideal body weight) every 6 hours for 16 doses
Adults: **BMT:** 0.8 mg/kg (ideal body weight or actual body weight, whichever is lower) every 6 hours for 16 doses
Oral:
Children: Induction: 0.06-0.12 mg/kg/day **or** 1.8-4.6 mg/m^2/day; Maintenance: Titrate to maintain leukocyte counts above 40,000/mm^3; **BMT:** 1 mg/kg (ideal body weight) every 6 hours for 16 doses
Adults: Induction: 60 mcg/kg/day or 1.8 mg/m^2/day; usual range: 4-12 mg/day; Maintenance: 1-4 mg/day to 2 mg/week; **BMT:** 1 mg/kg (ideal body weight) every 6 hours for 16 doses

Dosage Forms
Injection, solution:
Busulfex®: 6 mg/mL (10 mL)
Tablet, oral:
Myleran®: 2 mg

Busulfex® *see busulfan on page 152*

butabarbital (byoo ta BAR bi tal)

Medication Safety Issues
Sound-alike/look-alike issues:
Butabarbital may be confused with butalbital
BEERS Criteria medication:
This drug may be inappropriate for use in geriatric patients (high severity risk).

U.S. Brand Names Butisol Sodium®
Therapeutic Category Barbiturate
Controlled Substance C-III
Use Sedative; hypnotic
General Dosage Range Oral:
Children: 2-6 mg/kg preoperatively (maximum: 100 mg)
Adults: 15-30 mg 3-4 times/day **or** 50-100 mg as a single dose

Dosage Forms
Elixir, oral:
Butisol Sodium®: 30 mg/5 mL (480 mL)
Tablet, oral:
Butisol Sodium®: 30 mg, 50 mg

butalbital, acetaminophen, and caffeine
(byoo TAL bi tal, a seet a MIN oh fen, & KAF een)

Medication Safety Issues
Sound-alike/look-alike issues:
Fioricet® may be confused with Fiorinal®, Florinef®, Lorcet®, Percocet®

Repan® may be confused with Riopan®

Other safety concerns:
Duplicate therapy issues: This product contains acetaminophen, which may be a component of other combination products. Do not exceed the maximum recommended daily dose of acetaminophen.

Synonyms acetaminophen, butalbital, and caffeine

U.S. Brand Names Alagesic LQ; Anolor 300; Dolgic® Plus; Esgic-Plus™; Esgic®; Fioricet®; Margesic; Orbivan™; Repan®; Zebutal®

Therapeutic Category Barbiturate/Analgesic

Use Relief of the symptomatic complex of tension or muscle contraction headache

General Dosage Range Oral: *Adults:* 1-2 tablets/capsules or 15-30 mL every 4 hours (maximum: 6 tablets/capsules daily; 180 mL/day)

Dosage Forms
Capsule, oral:
Anolor 300, Esgic®, Margesic: Butalbital 50 mg, acetaminophen 325 mg, and caffeine 40 mg
Esgic-Plus™, Zebutal®: Butalbital 50 mg, acetaminophen 500 mg, and caffeine 40 mg
Orbivan™: Butalbital 50 mg, acetaminophen 300 mg, and caffeine 40 mg
Liquid, oral:
Alagesic LQ: Butalbital 50 mg, acetaminophen 325 mg, and caffeine 40 mg per 15 mL
Tablet, oral: Butalbital 50 mg, acetaminophen 325 mg, and caffeine 40 mg; butalbital 50 mg, acetaminophen 500 mg, and caffeine 40 mg
Dolgic® Plus: Butalbital 50 mg, acetaminophen 750 mg, and caffeine 40 mg
Esgic®, Fioricet®, Repan®: Butalbital 50 mg, acetaminophen 325 mg, and caffeine 40 mg
Esgic-Plus™: Butalbital 50 mg, acetaminophen 500 mg, and caffeine 40 mg

butalbital, acetaminophen, caffeine, and codeine
(byoo TAL bi tal, a seet a MIN oh fen, KAF een, & KOE deen)

Medication Safety Issues
Sound-alike/look-alike issues:
Fioricet® may be confused with Fiorinal®, Florinef®, Lorcet®, Percocet®
Phrenilin may be confused with Phenergan®
High alert medication:
The Institute for Safe Medication Practices (ISMP) includes this medication among its list of drug classes which have a heightened risk of causing significant patient harm when used in error.
Other safety concerns:
Duplicate therapy issues: This product contains acetaminophen, which may be a component of other combination products. Do not exceed the maximum recommended daily dose of acetaminophen.

Synonyms acetaminophen, caffeine, codeine, and butalbital; caffeine, acetaminophen, butalbital, and codeine; codeine, acetaminophen, butalbital, and caffeine

U.S. Brand Names Fioricet® with Codeine

Therapeutic Category Analgesic Combination (Opioid); Barbiturate

Controlled Substance C-III

Use Relief of symptoms of complex tension (muscle contraction) headache

General Dosage Range Oral: *Adults:* 1-2 capsules every 4 hours (maximum: 6 capsules/day)

Dosage Forms
Capsule: Butalbital 50 mg, acetaminophen 325 mg, caffeine 40 mg, and codeine 30 mg
Fioricet® with Codeine: Butalbital 50 mg, acetaminophen 325 mg, caffeine 40 mg, and codeine 30 mg

butalbital and acetaminophen (byoo TAL bi tal & a seet a MIN oh fen)

Medication Safety Issues
Other safety concerns:
Duplicate therapy issues: This product contains acetaminophen, which may be a component of other combination products. Do not exceed the maximum recommended daily dose of acetaminophen.

Synonyms acetaminophen and butalbital

U.S. Brand Names Bupap; Cephadyn; Phrenilin®; Phrenilin® Forte; Promacet; Sedapap®

Therapeutic Category Analgesic, Miscellaneous; Barbiturate

Use Relief of the symptomatic complex of tension or muscle contraction headache

General Dosage Range Oral: *Adults:* 1 tablet/capsule every 4 hours as needed (maximum: 6 doses/day) **or** Phrenilin®: 1-2 tablets every 4 hours as needed (maximum: 6 tablets/day)

◀ **Dosage Forms**
Tablet:
Phrenilin®: Butalbital 50 mg and acetaminophen 325 mg
Bupap, Cephadyn, Promacet, Sedapap®: Butalbital 50 mg and acetaminophen 650 mg
Capsule:
Phrenilin® Forte: Butalbital 50 mg and acetaminophen 650 mg

butalbital, aspirin, and caffeine (byoo TAL bi tal, AS pir in, & KAF een)

Medication Safety Issues
Sound-alike/look-alike issues:
Fiorinal® may be confused with Fioricet®, Florical®, Florinef®
Synonyms aspirin, caffeine, and butalbital; butalbital compound
U.S. Brand Names Fiorinal®
Canadian Brand Names Fiorinal®
Therapeutic Category Barbiturate/Analgesic
Controlled Substance C-III
Use Relief of the symptomatic complex of tension or muscle contraction headache
General Dosage Range Oral: *Adults:* 1-2 tablets/capsules every 4 hours (maximum: 6 tablets/capsules daily)
Dosage Forms
Capsule: Butalbital 50 mg, aspirin 325 mg, and caffeine 40 mg
Fiorinal®: Butalbital 50 mg, aspirin 325 mg, and caffeine 40 mg
Tablet: Butalbital 50 mg, aspirin 325 mg, and caffeine 40 mg

butalbital, aspirin, caffeine, and codeine
(byoo TAL bi tal, AS pir in, KAF een, & KOE deen)

Medication Safety Issues
Sound-alike/look-alike issues:
Fiorinal® may be confused with Fioricet®, Florical®, Florinef®
High alert medication:
The Institute for Safe Medication Practices (ISMP) includes this medication among its list of drug classes which have a heightened risk of causing significant patient harm when used in error.
Synonyms aspirin, caffeine, codeine, and butalbital; butalbital compound and codeine; codeine and butalbital compound; codeine, butalbital, aspirin, and caffeine
U.S. Brand Names Ascomp® with Codeine; Fiorinal® with Codeine
Canadian Brand Names Fiorinal®-C 1/2; Fiorinal®-C 1/4; Tecnal C 1/2; Tecnal C 1/4
Therapeutic Category Analgesic, Narcotic; Barbiturate
Controlled Substance C-III
Use Relief of symptoms of complex tension (muscle contraction) headache
General Dosage Range Oral: *Adults:* 1-2 capsules every 4 hours as needed (maximum: 6 capsules/day)
Dosage Forms
Capsule: Butalbital 50 mg, aspirin 325 mg, caffeine 40 mg, and codeine 30 mg
Ascomp® with Codeine, Fiorinal® with Codeine: Butalbital 50 mg, aspirin 325 mg, caffeine 40 mg, and codeine 30 mg

butalbital compound *see* butalbital, aspirin, and caffeine *on page 154*
butalbital compound and codeine *see* butalbital, aspirin, caffeine, and codeine *on page 154*
butamben, tetracaine, and benzocaine *see* benzocaine, butamben, and tetracaine *on page 123*

butenafine (byoo TEN a feen)

Medication Safety Issues
Sound-alike/look-alike issues:
Lotrimin may be confused with Lotrisone®
Synonyms butenafine hydrochloride
U.S. Brand Names Lotrimin® ultra™ [OTC]; Mentax®
Therapeutic Category Antifungal Agent
Use Topical treatment of tinea pedis (athlete's foot), tinea cruris (jock itch), tinea corporis (ringworm), and tinea versicolor

General Dosage Range Topical: *Children >12 years and Adults:* Apply to affected area once or twice daily

Dosage Forms
  Cream, topical:
    Lotrimin® ultra™ [OTC]: 1% (12 g, 24 g)
    Mentax®: 1% (15 g, 30 g)

butenafine hydrochloride *see* butenafine *on page 154*
Butisol Sodium® *see* butabarbital *on page 152*

butoconazole (byoo toe KOE na zole)
Synonyms butoconazole nitrate
U.S. Brand Names Gynazole-1®
Canadian Brand Names Femstat® One; Gynazole-1®
Therapeutic Category Antifungal Agent
Use Local treatment of vulvovaginal candidiasis
General Dosage Range Intravaginal: *Adults:* Insert 1 applicatorful at bedtime
Dosage Forms
  Cream, vaginal:
    Gynazole-1®: 2% (5 g)

butoconazole nitrate *see* butoconazole *on page 155*

butorphanol (byoo TOR fa nole)
Medication Safety Issues
  Sound-alike/look-alike issues:
    Stadol may be confused with Haldol®, sotalol
  High alert medication:
    The Institute for Safe Medication Practices (ISMP) includes this medication among its list of drug classes which have a heightened risk of causing significant patient harm when used in error.
Synonyms butorphanol tartrate; Stadol
Canadian Brand Names Apo-Butorphanol®; PMS-Butorphanol
Therapeutic Category Analgesic, Narcotic
Controlled Substance C-IV
Use
  Parenteral: Management of moderate-to-severe pain; preoperative medication; supplement to balanced anesthesia; management of pain during labor
  Nasal spray: Management of moderate-to-severe pain, including migraine headache pain
General Dosage Range Dosage adjustment recommended in patients with hepatic or renal impairment
  I.M.:
    Adults: Initial: 2 mg, may repeat every 3-4 hours as needed; Usual range: 1-4 mg every 3-4 hours as needed **or** 2 mg prior to surgery
    Elderly: Initial: 1/2 of the recommended dose, repeated dosing generally should be at least 6 hours apart
  I.V.:
    Adults: Initial: 1 mg, may repeat every 3-4 hours as needed; Usual range: 0.5-2 mg every 3-4 hours as needed **or** 2 mg and/or an incremental dose of 0.5-1 mg (up to 0.06 mg/kg) as supplement to surgery
    Elderly: Initial: 1/2 of the recommended dose, repeated dosing generally should be at least 6 hours apart
  Intranasal:
    Adults: Initial: 1 spray (~1 mg) in 1 nostril, may repeat in 60-90 minutes, then repeat initial dose sequence in 3-4 hours after last dose as needed; may use initial dose of 1 spray in each nostril (2 mg) in patients who will remain recumbent
    Elderly: Initial: Should not exceed 1 mg, may repeat after 90-120 minutes
Dosage Forms
  Injection, solution: 1 mg/mL (1 mL); 2 mg/mL (1 mL, 2 mL, 10 mL)
  Injection, solution [preservative free]: 1 mg/mL (1 mL); 2 mg/mL (1 mL, 2 mL)
  Solution, intranasal: 10 mg/mL (2.5 mL)

butorphanol tartrate *see* butorphanol *on page 155*
Butrans™ *see* buprenorphine *on page 149*
B-Vex D [DSC] *see* brompheniramine and phenylephrine *on page 143*

B vitamin combinations *see* vitamin B complex combinations *on page 918*
BW-430C *see* lamotrigine *on page 509*
BW524W91 *see* emtricitabine *on page 325*
Byetta® *see* exenatide *on page 363*
Bystolic® *see* nebivolol *on page 615*
C1 esterase inhibitor *see* C1 inhibitor (human) *on page 156*
C1-INH *see* C1 inhibitor (human) *on page 156*
C1-inhibitor *see* C1 inhibitor (human) *on page 156*
C1INHRP *see* C1 inhibitor (human) *on page 156*
C2B8 monoclonal antibody *see* rituximab *on page 784*
C7E3 *see* abciximab *on page 21*
C8-CCK *see* sincalide *on page 814*
311C90 *see* zolmitriptan *on page 933*
C225 *see* cetuximab *on page 190*

C1 inhibitor (human) (cee won in HIB i ter HYU man)

Synonyms C1 esterase inhibitor; C1-INH; C1-inhibitor; C1INHRP; human C1 inhibitor
U.S. Brand Names Berinert®; Cinryze™
Canadian Brand Names Berinert®
Therapeutic Category Blood Product Derivative
Use
Berinert®: Treatment of acute abdominal or facial attacks of hereditary angioedema (HAE)
Cinryze™: Routine prophylaxis against angioedema attacks in patients with HAE or inherited C1 inhibitor deficiency
General Dosage Range Oral: *Adolescents and Adults:* 1000 units every 3-4 days **or** 20 units/kg
Dosage Forms
Injection, powder for reconstitution:
Berinert®: 500 units
Cinryze™: 500 units

cabazitaxel (ca baz i TAKS el)

Medication Safety Issues
High alert medication:
This medication is in a class the Institute for Safe Medication Practices (ISMP) includes among its list of drugs which have a heightened risk of causing significant patient harm when used in error.
Administration issues:
Cabazitaxel requires a two-step dilution process prior to administration.
Synonyms RPR-116258A; XRP6258
U.S. Brand Names Jevtana®
Canadian Brand Names Jevtana®
Use Treatment of hormone-refractory metastatic prostate cancer (in patients previously treated with a docetaxel-containing regimen)
General Dosage Range Dosage adjustment recommended in patients with hepatic impairment or who develop toxicities
I.V.: *Adults:* 25 mg/m^2 once every 3 weeks
Dosage Forms
Injection, solution:
Jevtana®: 40 mg/mL (1.5 mL)

cabergoline (ca BER goe leen)

Canadian Brand Names CO Cabergoline; Dostinex®
Therapeutic Category Ergot-like Derivative
Use Treatment of hyperprolactinemic disorders, either idiopathic or due to pituitary adenomas
General Dosage Range Oral: *Adults:* Initial: 0.25 mg twice weekly; Maintenance: Up to 1 mg twice weekly
Dosage Forms
Tablet, oral: 0.5 mg

Ca-DTPA *see* diethylene triamine penta-acetic acid *on page 281*
Caduet® *see* amlodipine and atorvastatin *on page 69*
CaEDTA *see* edetate CALCIUM disodium *on page 320*
Caelyx® (Can) *see* doxorubicin (liposomal) *on page 311*
Cafcit® *see* caffeine *on page 157*
CAFdA *see* clofarabine *on page 221*
Cafergor® (Can) *see* ergotamine and caffeine *on page 337*
Cafergot® *see* ergotamine and caffeine *on page 337*

caffeine (KAF een)

Synonyms caffeine and sodium benzoate; caffeine citrate; caffeine sodium benzoate; sodium benzoate and caffeine
U.S. Brand Names Cafcit®; Enerjets [OTC]; No Doz® Maximum Strength [OTC]; Vivarin® [OTC]
Therapeutic Category Stimulant
Use
Caffeine citrate: Treatment of idiopathic apnea of prematurity
Caffeine and sodium benzoate: Treatment of acute respiratory depression (not a preferred agent)
Caffeine [OTC labeling]: Restore mental alertness or wakefulness when experiencing fatigue
General Dosage Range
I.M. (caffeine and sodium benzoate):
Children: 8 mg/kg every 4 hours as needed
Adults: 250 mg as a single dose; may repeat as needed (maximum: 500 mg/dose; 2500 mg/day)
I.V.:
Neonates (caffeine citrate): Loading dose: 10-20 mg/kg; Maintenance: 5 mg/kg once daily
Children (caffeine and sodium benzoate): 8 mg/kg every 4 hours as needed
Adults (caffeine and sodium benzoate): 250 mg as a single dose; may repeat as needed (maximum: 500 mg/dose; 2500 mg/day) **or** 300-2000 mg (electroconvulsive therapy)
Oral:
Neonates (caffeine citrate): Loading dose: 10-20 mg/kg; Maintenance: 5 mg/kg once daily
Children ≥12 years and Adults: 100-200 mg every 3-4 hours as needed (OTC labeling)
SubQ (caffeine and sodium benzoate): *Children:* 8 mg/kg every 4 hours as needed
Dosage Forms
Caplet:
No Doz® Maximum Strength [OTC], Vivarin® [OTC]: 200 mg
Injection, solution [preservative free]: 20 mg/mL (3 mL)
Cafcit®: 20 mg/mL (3 mL)
Lozenge:
Enerjets® [OTC]: 75 mg
Solution, oral [preservative free]: 20 mg/mL (3 mL)
Cafcit®: 20 mg/mL
Tablet: 200 mg
Vivarin® [OTC]: 200 mg

caffeine, acetaminophen, and aspirin *see* acetaminophen, aspirin, and caffeine *on page 29*
caffeine, acetaminophen, butalbital, and codeine *see* butalbital, acetaminophen, caffeine, and codeine *on page 153*
caffeine and ergotamine *see* ergotamine and caffeine *on page 337*
caffeine and sodium benzoate *see* caffeine *on page 157*
caffeine, aspirin, and acetaminophen *see* acetaminophen, aspirin, and caffeine *on page 29*
caffeine citrate *see* caffeine *on page 157*
caffeine, dihydrocodeine, and acetaminophen *see* acetaminophen, caffeine, and dihydrocodeine *on page 30*
caffeine, orphenadrine, and aspirin *see* orphenadrine, aspirin, and caffeine *on page 655*
caffeine sodium benzoate *see* caffeine *on page 157*
Cal-C-Caps [OTC] *see* calcium citrate *on page 163*
Caladryl® Clear™ [OTC] *see* pramoxine *on page 730*

calamine (KAL a meen)

Synonyms calamine lotion

◀ **Therapeutic Category** Topical Skin Product

Use Employed primarily as an astringent, protectant, and soothing agent for conditions such as poison ivy, poison oak, poison sumac, sunburn, insect bites, or minor skin irritations

General Dosage Range Topical: *Children and Adults:* Apply to affected area as often as needed

Dosage Forms

Suspension, topical: 8% (118 mL, 177 mL, 240 mL)

calamine lotion *see* calamine *on page 157*

Calan® *see* verapamil *on page 912*

Calan® SR *see* verapamil *on page 912*

Calcarb 600 [OTC] [DSC] *see* calcium carbonate *on page 161*

Cal-Cee [OTC] *see* calcium citrate *on page 163*

Calci-Chew® [OTC] *see* calcium carbonate *on page 161*

Calciferol™ [OTC] *see* ergocalciferol *on page 336*

CalciFolic-D™ *see* vitamins (multiple/oral) *on page 919*

Calcijex® *see* calcitriol *on page 159*

Calcimar® (Can) *see* calcitonin *on page 159*

Calci-Mix® [OTC] *see* calcium carbonate *on page 161*

Calcionate [OTC] *see* calcium glubionate *on page 164*

calcipotriene (kal si POE try een)

U.S. Brand Names Calcitrene™; Dovonex®

Canadian Brand Names Dovonex®

Therapeutic Category Antipsoriatic Agent

Use Treatment of plaque psoriasis; chronic, moderate-to-severe psoriasis of the scalp

General Dosage Range Topical: *Adults:* Cream, solution: Apply a thin film to affected area 2 times/day; Ointment: Apply a thin film to affected area 1-2 times/day

Dosage Forms

Cream, topical:

Dovonex®: 0.005% (60 g, 120 g)

Ointment, topical:

Calcitrene™: 0.005% (60 g)

Solution, topical: 0.005% (60 mL)

Dovonex®: 0.005% (60 mL)

calcipotriene and betamethasone (kal si POE try een & bay ta METH a sone)

Synonyms betamethasone dipropionate and calcipotriene hydrate; calcipotriol and betamethasone dipropionate

U.S. Brand Names Taclonex Scalp®; Taclonex®

Canadian Brand Names Dovobet®; Xamiol®

Therapeutic Category Corticosteroid, Topical; Vitamin D Analog

Use Treatment of psoriasis vulgaris

General Dosage Range Topical: *Adults:* Apply to affected area once daily (maximum: 100 g/week)

Dosage Forms

Ointment, topical:

Taclonex®: Calcipotriene 0.005% and betamethasone 0.064% (60 g, 100 g)

Suspension, topical:

Taclonex Scalp®: Calcipotriene 0.005% and betamethasone 0.064%

Dosage Forms - Canada

Gel, topical:

Xamiol®: Calcipotriol 50 mcg/g and betamethasone 0.5 mg/g (30 g, 60 g, 2 x 60 g)

Ointment, topical:

Dovobet®: Calcipotriol 50 mcg/g and betamethasone 0.5 mg/g (30 g, 60 g, 120 g)

calcipotriol and betamethasone dipropionate *see* calcipotriene and betamethasone *on page 158*

Calcite-500 (Can) *see* calcium carbonate *on page 161*

calcitonin (kal si TOE nin)

Medication Safety Issues
Sound-alike/look-alike issues:
Calcitonin may be confused with calcitriol
Miacalcin® may be confused with Micatin®
Administration issues:
Calcitonin nasal spray is administered as a single spray into **one** nostril daily, using alternate nostrils each day.
Synonyms calcitonin (salmon)
U.S. Brand Names Fortical®; Miacalcin®
Canadian Brand Names Apo-Calcitonin®; Calcimar®; Caltine®; Miacalcin® NS; PRO-Calcitonin; Sandoz-Calcitonin
Therapeutic Category Polypeptide Hormone
Use Treatment of Paget disease of bone (osteitis deformans); adjunctive therapy for hypercalcemia; treatment of osteoporosis in women >5 years postmenopause
General Dosage Range
I.M., SubQ: *Adults:* Paget disease/osteoporosis: 50-100 units every 1-3 days; Hypercalcemia: 4-8 units/kg every 12 hours (maximum: 8 units/kg every 6 hours)
Intranasal: *Adults:* 200 units (1 spray) in one nostril daily
Dosage Forms
Injection, solution:
Miacalcin®: 200 int. units/mL (2 mL)
Solution, intranasal: 200 int. units/actuation (3.7 mL)
Fortical®: 200 int. units/actuation (3.7 mL)
Miacalcin®: 200 int. units/actuation (3.7 mL)

calcitonin (salmon) *see calcitonin on page 159*
Calcitrate [OTC] *see calcium citrate on page 163*
Cal-Citrate™ 225 [OTC] *see calcium citrate on page 163*
Calcitrene™ *see calcipotriene on page 158*

calcitriol (kal si TRYE ole)

Medication Safety Issues
Sound-alike/look-alike issues:
Calcitriol may be confused with alfacalcidol, Calciferol™, calcitonin, calcium carbonate, captopril, colestipol, paricalcitol, ropinirole
Administration issues:
Dosage is expressed in mcg (micrograms), **not** mg (milligrams); rare cases of acute overdose have been reported
Synonyms 1,25 dihydroxycholecalciferol
U.S. Brand Names Calcijex®; Rocaltrol®; Vectical™
Canadian Brand Names Calcijex®; Rocaltrol®
Therapeutic Category Vitamin D Analog
Use
Oral, injection: Management of hypocalcemia in patients on chronic renal dialysis; management of secondary hyperparathyroidism in patients with chronic kidney disease (CKD); management of hypocalcemia in hypoparathyroidism and pseudohypoparathyroidism
Topical: Management of mild-to-moderate plaque psoriasis
General Dosage Range Dosage adjustment recommended in patients who develop toxicities
I.V.: *Adults:* 0.5-4 mcg 3 times/week
Oral:
Children: 0.25-0.2 mcg/day **or** 0.01-0.015 mcg/kg/day (maximum: 0.5 mcg/day)
Adults: 0.25 mcg every other day to 2 mcg once daily
Topical: *Adults:* Apply to affected areas twice daily (maximum: 200 g/week)
Dosage Forms
Capsule, softgel, oral: 0.25 mcg, 0.5 mcg
Rocaltrol®: 0.25 mcg, 0.5 mcg
Injection, solution: 1 mcg/mL (1 mL, 2 mL)
Calcijex®: 1 mcg/mL (1 mL)

◄ **Ointment, topical**:
Vectical™: 3 mcg/g (100 g)
Solution, oral: 1 mcg/mL (15 mL)
Rocaltrol®: 1 mcg/mL (15 mL)

calcium acetate (KAL see um AS e tate)

Medication Safety Issues
Sound-alike/look-alike issues:
PhosLo® may be confused with Phos-Flur®, ProSom
U.S. Brand Names Eliphos™; PhosLo®; Phoslyra™
Canadian Brand Names PhosLo®
Therapeutic Category Electrolyte Supplement, Oral
Use Control of hyperphosphatemia in end-stage renal failure; does not promote aluminum absorption
General Dosage Range Oral: *Adults:* Initial: 1334 mg with each meal; Maintenance: 2001-2668 mg with each meal
Dosage Forms
Gelcap, oral: 667 mg
PhosLo®: 667 mg
Solution, oral:
Phoslyra™: 667 mg/5 mL (473 mL)
Tablet, oral:
Eliphos™: 667 mg

calcium acetate and aluminum sulfate *see* aluminum sulfate and calcium acetate *on page 61*
calcium acetylhomotaurinate *see* acamprosate *on page 22*
calcium and risedronate *see* risedronate and calcium *on page 783*

calcium and vitamin D (KAL see um & VYE ta min dee)

Medication Safety Issues
Sound-alike/look-alike issues:
Os-Cal® may be confused with Asacol®
Synonyms vitamin D and calcium carbonate
U.S. Brand Names Cal-CYUM [OTC]; Caltrate® 600+D [OTC]; Caltrate® 600+Soy™ [OTC]; Caltrate® ColonHealth™ [OTC]; Chew-Cal [OTC]; Citracal® Maximum [OTC]; Citracal® Petites [OTC]; Citracal® Regular [OTC]; Liqua-Cal [OTC]; Os-Cal® 500+D [OTC]; Oysco 500+D [OTC]; Oysco D [OTC]; Oyst-Cal-D 500 [OTC]; Oyst-Cal-D [OTC]
Therapeutic Category Calcium Salt; Electrolyte Supplement, Oral; Vitamin, Fat Soluble
Use Dietary supplement, antacid
Dosage Forms
Caplet, oral:
Citracal® Maximum [OTC]: Calcium 315 mg and vitamin D 250 int. units
Capsule, softgel, oral: Calcium 500 mg and vitamin D 500 int. units; calcium 600 mg and vitamin D 100 int. units; calcium 600 mg and vitamin D 200 int. units
Liqua-Cal [OTC]: Calcium 600 mg and vitamin D 200 int. units
Tablet, oral: Calcium 250 mg and vitamin D 125 int. units; calcium 500 mg and vitamin D 125 int. units; calcium 500 mg and vitamin D 200 int. units; calcium 600 mg and vitamin D 125 int. units; calcium 600 mg and vitamin D 200 int. units
Caltrate® 600+D [OTC]: Calcium 600 mg and vitamin D 200 int. units
Caltrate® 600+Soy™ [OTC]: Calcium 600 mg and vitamin D 200 int. units
Caltrate® ColonHealth™ [OTC]: Calcium 600 mg and vitamin D 200 int. units
Citracal® Petites [OTC]: Calcium 200 mg and vitamin D 250 int. units
Citracal® Regular [OTC]: Calcium 250 mg and vitamin D 200 int. units
Oysco D [OTC]: Calcium 250 mg and vitamin D 125 int. units
Oysco 500+D [OTC]: Calcium 500 mg and vitamin D 200 int. units
Oyst-Cal-D [OTC]: Calcium 250 mg and vitamin D 125 int. units
Oyst-Cal-D 500 [OTC]: Calcium 500 mg and vitamin D 200 int. units
Tablet, chewable: Calcium 500 mg and vitamin D 100 int. units; calcium 600 mg and vitamin D 400 int. units
Os-Cal® 500+D [OTC]: Calcium 500 mg and vitamin D 400 int. units

Wafer, chewable:
Cal-CYUM [OTC]: Calcium 519 mg and vitamin D 150 int. units (50s)
Chew-Cal [OTC]: Calcium 333 mg and vitamin D 40 int. units (100s, 250s)

calcium carbonate (KAL see um KAR bun ate)
Medication Safety Issues
Sound-alike/look-alike issues:
Calcium carbonate may be confused with calcitriol
Florical® may be confused with Fiorinal®
Mylanta® may be confused with Mynatal®
Nephro-Calci® may be confused with Nephrocaps®
International issues:
Remegel [Hungary, Great Britain, and Ireland] may be confused with Renagel brand name for sevelamer [U.S., Canada, and multiple international markets]
Remegel: Brand name for calcium carbonate [Hungary, Great Britain, and Ireland], but also the brand name for aluminum hydroxide and magnesium carbonate [Netherlands]

Synonyms oscal

U.S. Brand Names Alcalak [OTC]; Alka-Mints® [OTC]; Cal-Gest [OTC]; Cal-Mint [OTC]; Calcarb 600 [OTC] [DSC]; Calci-Chew® [OTC]; Calci-Mix® [OTC]; Caltrate® 600 [OTC]; Children's Pepto [OTC]; Chooz® [OTC]; Florical® [OTC]; Maalox® Children's [OTC]; Maalox® Regular Strength [OTC]; Nephro-Calci® [OTC]; Nutralox® [OTC]; Oysco 500 [OTC]; Oystercal™ 500 [OTC]; Rolaids® Extra Strength [OTC]; Super Calcium 600 [OTC]; Titralac™ [OTC]; Tums® E-X [OTC]; Tums® Extra Strength Sugar Free [OTC]; Tums® Quickpak [OTC]; Tums® Smoothies™ [OTC]; Tums® Ultra [OTC]; Tums® [OTC]

Canadian Brand Names Apo-Cal®; Calcite-500; Caltrate®; Caltrate® Select; Os-Cal®

Therapeutic Category Antacid; Electrolyte Supplement, Oral

Use As an antacid; treatment and prevention of calcium deficiency or hyperphosphatemia (eg, osteoporosis, osteomalacia, mild/moderate renal insufficiency, hypoparathyroidism, postmenopausal osteoporosis, rickets); has been used to bind phosphate

General Dosage Range Oral:
Children <2 years: 45-65 mg/kg/day in 4 divided doses
Children 0-6 months: Adequate intake: 200 mg/day
Children 7-12 months: Adequate intake: 260 mg/day
Children 1-3 years: RDA: 700 mg/day
Children 2-5 years (24-47 lbs): Antacid: 161 mg (elemental calcium) as needed (maximum: 483 mg/day); Hypocalcemia: 45-65 mg/kg/day in 4 divided doses
Children 4-8 years: RDA: 1000 mg/day
Children 6-11 years (48-95 lbs): Antacid: 322 mg (elemental calcium) as needed (maximum: 966 mg/day); Hypocalcemia: 45-65 mg/kg/day in 4 divided doses
Children 9-18 years: RDA: 1300 mg/day
Children >11 years: 45-65 mg/kg/day in 4 divided doses
Adults 19-50 years: RDA: 1000 mg/day
Adults ≤51 years: Antacid: 1-2 tablets or 5-10 mL every 2 hours (maximum: 7000 mg/day); Hypocalcemia/dietary: 500-2000 mg/day in 2-4 divided doses
Adults ≥51 years, females: RDA: 1200 mg/day
Adults >51 years: Antacid: 1-2 tablets or 5-10 mL every 2 hours (maximum: 7000 mg/day); Hypocalcemia/dietary: 500-2000 mg/day in 2-4 divided doses; Osteoporosis: 1200 mg/day
Adults 51-70 years, males: RDA: 1000 mg/day
Adults >70 years, males: RDA: 1200 mg/day

Dosage Forms
Capsule, oral:
Calci-Mix® [OTC]: 1250 mg
Florical® [OTC]: 364 mg
Gum, chewing, oral:
Chooz® [OTC]: 500 mg (12s)
Powder, oral: (480 g)
Tums® Quickpak [OTC]: 1000 mg/packet (24s)
Suspension, oral: 1250 mg/5 mL (5 mL, 500 mL, 16 oz)
Tablet, oral: 648 mg, 650 mg, 1250 mg, 1500 mg
Caltrate® 600 [OTC]: 1500 mg
Florical® [OTC]: 364 mg
Nephro-Calci® [OTC]: 1500 mg

◀ Oysco 500 [OTC]: 1250 mg
Oystercal™ 500 [OTC]: 1250 mg
Super Calcium 600 [OTC]: 1500 mg
Tablet, chewable, oral: 420 mg, 500 mg, 600 mg, 650 mg, 750 mg, 1250 mg
Alcalak [OTC]: 420 mg
Alka-Mints® [OTC]: 850 mg
Cal-Gest [OTC]: 500 mg
Cal-Mint [OTC]: 650 mg
Calci-Chew® [OTC]: 1250 mg
Children's Pepto [OTC]: 400 mg
Maalox® Children's [OTC]: 400 mg
Maalox® Regular Strength [OTC]: 600 mg
Nutralox® [OTC]: 420 mg
Titralac™ [OTC]: 420 mg
Tums® [OTC]: 500 mg
Tums® E-X [OTC]: 750 mg
Tums® Extra Strength Sugar Free [OTC]: 750 mg
Tums® Smoothies™ [OTC]: 750 mg
Tums® Ultra [OTC]: 1000 mg
Tablet, softchew, oral:
Rolaids® Extra Strength [OTC]: 1177 mg

calcium carbonate and etidronate disodium *see* etidronate and calcium carbonate *(Canada only)* on page 360

calcium carbonate and magnesium hydroxide
(KAL see um KAR bun ate & mag NEE zhum hye DROKS ide)
Medication Safety Issues
Sound-alike/look-alike issues:
Mylanta® may be confused with Mynatal®
Synonyms magnesium hydroxide and calcium carbonate
U.S. Brand Names Mi-Acid™ Double Strength [OTC]; Mylanta® Gelcaps® [OTC]; Mylanta® Supreme [OTC]; Mylanta® Ultra [OTC]; Rolaids® Extra Strength [OTC]; Rolaids® [OTC]
Therapeutic Category Antacid
Use Hyperacidity
General Dosage Range Oral: *Adults:* 2-4 tablets between meals and at bedtime
Dosage Forms
Gelcap:
Mylanta® Gelcaps® [OTC]: Calcium carbonate 550 mg and magnesium hydroxide 125 mg
Liquid:
Mylanta® Supreme [OTC]: Calcium carbonate 400 mg and magnesium hydroxide 135 mg per 5 mL
Tablet, chewable: Calcium carbonate 550 mg and magnesium hydroxide 110 mg; calcium carbonate 675 mg and magnesium hydroxide 135 mg; calcium carbonate 700 mg and magnesium hydroxide 300 mg
Mi-Acid™ Double Strength [OTC], Mylanta® Ultra [OTC]: Calcium carbonate 700 mg and magnesium hydroxide 300 mg
Rolaids® [OTC]: Calcium carbonate 550 mg and magnesium hydroxide 110 mg
Rolaids® Extra Strength [OTC]: Calcium carbonate 675 mg and magnesium hydroxide 135 mg

calcium carbonate and simethicone (KAL see um KAR bun ate & sye METH i kone)
Medication Safety Issues
International issues:
Remegel Wind Relief [Great Britain] may be confused with Renagel brand name for sevelamer [U.S., Canada, and multiple international markets]
Synonyms simethicone and calcium carbonate
U.S. Brand Names Gas Ban™ [OTC]; Maalox® Advanced Maximum Strength [OTC]; Maalox® Junior Plus Antigas [OTC]; Titralac® Plus [OTC]
Therapeutic Category Antacid; Antiflatulent
Use Relief of acid indigestion, heartburn, bloating, pressure, and discomfort of gas

General Dosage Range Oral:
Children 6-11 years: Maalox® Junior Plus Antigas: Two tablets as symptoms occur or as directed by healthcare provider (maximum: 6 tablets/24 hours)
Children ≥12 years; Maalox® Advanced Maximum Strength: 1-2 tablets as symptoms occur or as directed by healthcare provider (maximum: 8 tablets/24 hours)
Adults: Maalox® Advanced Maximum Strength: 1-2 tablets as symptoms occur or as directed by healthcare provider (maximum: 8 tablets/24 hours); Titralac® Plus: Two tablets every 2-3 hours as needed (maximum: 19 tablets/24 hours)

Dosage Forms
Tablet, chewable:
Gas Ban™ [OTC]: Calcium carbonate 300 mg and simethicone 40 mg
Maalox® Advanced Maximum Strength [OTC]: Calcium carbonate 1000 mg and simethicone 60 mg
Maalox® Junior Plus Antigas [OTC]: Calcium carbonate 400 mg and simethicone 24 mg
Titralac® Plus [OTC]: Calcium carbonate 420 mg and simethicone 21 mg

calcium carbonate, folic acid, and magnesium carbonate *see* magnesium carbonate, calcium carbonate, and folic acid *on page 544*

calcium carbonate, magnesium hydroxide, and famotidine *see* famotidine, calcium carbonate, and magnesium hydroxide *on page 367*

calcium chloride (KAL see um KLOR ide)

Medication Safety Issues
Sound-alike/look-alike issues:
Calcium chloride may be confused with calcium gluconate
Administration issues:
Calcium chloride may be confused with calcium gluconate.
Confusion with the different intravenous salt forms of calcium has occurred. There is a threefold difference in the primary cation concentration between calcium chloride (in which 1g = 13.6 mEq [270 mg] of elemental Ca++) and calcium gluconate (in which 1g = 4.65 mEq [90 mg] of elemental Ca++).
Prescribers should specify which salt form is desired. Dosages should be expressed either as mEq, mg, or grams of the salt form.

Therapeutic Category Electrolyte Supplement, Oral
Use Treatment of acute symptomatic hypocalcemia; cardiac disturbances of hyperkalemia or hypocalcemia; emergent treatment of hypocalcemic tetany; treatment of severe hypermagnesemia

General Dosage Range I.V.:
Infants and Children: 10-20 mg/kg **or** 35-50 mg/kg every 6-8 hours **or** 32 mg for each 100 mL of citrated blood infused
Adults: 500-1000 mg; repeat as appropriate **or** 20-50 mg/kg/hour **or** 200-500 mg per 500 mL of citrated blood

Dosage Forms
Injection, solution: 10% (10 mL)
Injection, solution [preservative free]: 10% (10 mL)

calcium citrate (KAL see um SIT rate)

Medication Safety Issues
Sound-alike/look-alike issues:
Citracal® may be confused with Citrucel®
U.S. Brand Names Cal-C-Caps [OTC]; Cal-Cee [OTC]; Cal-Citrate™ 225 [OTC]; Calcitrate [OTC]
Canadian Brand Names Osteocit®
Therapeutic Category Electrolyte Supplement, Oral
Use Antacid; treatment and prevention of calcium deficiency or hyperphosphatemia (eg, osteoporosis, osteomalacia, mild/moderate renal insufficiency, hypoparathyroidism, postmenopausal osteoporosis, rickets)

General Dosage Range Oral:
Children 0-6 months: Adequate intake: 200 mg/day
Children 7-12 months: Adequate intake: 260 mg/day
Children 1-3 years: RDA: 700 mg/day
Children 4-8 years: RDA: 1000 mg/day
Children 9-18 years: RDA: 1300 mg/day
Adults: 500-2000 mg divided 2-4 times/day

Adults 19-50 years: RDA: 1000 mg/day
Adults ≥51 years, females: RDA: 1200 mg/day
Adults 51-70 years, males: RDA: 1000 mg/day
Adults >70 years, males: RDA: 1200 mg/day

Dosage Forms
Capsule, oral:
  Cal-C-Caps [OTC]: Elemental calcium 180 mg
  Cal-Citrate™ 225 [OTC]: Elemental calcium 225 mg
Granules, oral: (480 g)
Tablet, oral: Elemental calcium 250 mg
  Cal-Cee [OTC]: Elemental calcium 250 mg
  Calcitrate [OTC]: Elemental calcium 200 mg

calcium disodium edetate *see* edetate CALCIUM disodium *on page 320*
Calcium Disodium Versenate® *see* edetate CALCIUM disodium *on page 320*
calcium folinate *see* leucovorin calcium *on page 515*

calcium glubionate (KAL see um gloo BYE oh nate)

Medication Safety Issues
Sound-alike/look-alike issues:
  Calcium glubionate may be confused with calcium gluconate
U.S. Brand Names Calcionate [OTC]
Therapeutic Category Electrolyte Supplement, Oral
Use Dietary supplement
General Dosage Range Oral:
  Children 0-6 months: Adequate intake: 200 mg/day
  Children 7-12 months: Adequate intake: 260 mg/day
  Children 1-3 years: RDA: 700 mg/day
  Children 4-8 years: RDA: 1000 mg/day
  Children 9-18 years: RDA: 1300 mg/day
  Adults 19-50 years: RDA: 1000 mg/day
  Adults ≥51 years, females: RDA: 1200 mg/day
  Adults 51-70 years, males: RDA: 1000 mg/day
  Adults >70 years, males: RDA: 1200 mg/day
Dosage Forms
Syrup, oral:
  Calcionate [OTC]: 1.8 g/5 mL (473 mL)

calcium gluconate (KAL see um GLOO koe nate)

Medication Safety Issues
Sound-alike/look-alike issues:
  Calcium gluconate may be confused with calcium glubionate
Administration issues:
  Calcium gluconate may be confused with calcium chloride.
  Confusion with the different intravenous salt forms of calcium has occurred. There is a threefold difference in the primary cation concentration between calcium gluconate (in which 1g = 4.65 mEq [90 mg] of elemental Ca++) and calcium chloride (in which 1g = 13.6 mEq [270 mg] of elemental Ca++).
  Prescribers should specify which salt form is desired. Dosages should be expressed either as mEq, mg, or grams of the salt form.
U.S. Brand Names Cal-G [OTC]; Cal-GLU™ [OTC]
Therapeutic Category Electrolyte Supplement, Oral
Use Treatment and prevention of hypocalcemia; treatment of tetany, cardiac disturbances of hyperkalemia, cardiac resuscitation when epinephrine fails to improve myocardial contractions, hypocalcemia; calcium supplementation; hydrofluoric acid (HF) burns
General Dosage Range
I.V.: *Children and Adults:* Dosage varies greatly depending on indication
Oral:
  Children 0-6 months: Adequate intake: 200 mg/day
  Children 7-12 months: Adequate intake: 260 mg/day

Children 1-3 years: RDA: 700 mg/day
Children 4-8 years: RDA: 1000 mg/day
Children 9-18 years: RDA: 1300 mg/day
Children: 200-500 mg/kg/day (calcium gluconate salt containing 0.465 mEq [9.3 mg]/mL elemental calcium) divided every 6 hours
Adults: 500 mg to 2 g 2-4 times/day (calcium gluconate salt containing 0.465 mEq [9.3 mg]/mL elemental calcium)
Adults 19-50 years: RDA: 1000 mg/day
Adults ≥51 years, females: RDA: 1200 mg/day
Adults 51-70 years, males: RDA: 1000 mg/day
Adults >70 years, males: RDA: 1200 mg/day

Dosage Forms
Capsule, oral:
Cal-G [OTC]: 700 mg
Cal-GLU™ [OTC]: 515 mg
Injection, solution [preservative free]: 10% (10 mL, 50 mL, 100 mL)
Powder, oral: (480 g)
Tablet, oral: 500 mg, 648 mg

calcium lactate (KAL see um LAK tate)

Therapeutic Category Electrolyte Supplement, Oral
Use Adjunct in prevention of postmenopausal osteoporosis; treatment and prevention of calcium depletion
General Dosage Range Oral:
Children 0-6 months: Adequate intake: 200 mg/day
Children 7-12 months: Adequate intake: 260 mg/day
Children 1-3 years: RDA: 700 mg/day
Children 4-8 years: RDA: 1000 mg/day
Children 9-18 years: RDA: 1300 mg/day
Adults 19-50 years: RDA: 1000 mg/day
Adults ≥51 years, females: RDA: 1200 mg/day
Adults 51-70 years, males: RDA: 1000 mg/day
Adults >70 years, males: RDA: 1200 mg/day

Dosage Forms
Tablet, oral: 648 mg, 650 mg

calcium leucovorin *see* leucovorin calcium *on page 515*
calcium levoleucovorin *see* LEVOleucovorin *on page 521*
calcium pantothenate *see* pantothenic acid *on page 673*

calcium phosphate (tribasic) (KAL see um FOS fate tri BAY sik)

Synonyms tricalcium phosphate
U.S. Brand Names Posture® [OTC]
Therapeutic Category Electrolyte Supplement, Oral
Use Dietary supplement
General Dosage Range Oral:
Children 0-6 months: Adequate intake: 200 mg/day
Children 7-12 months: Adequate intake: 260 mg/day
Children 1-3 years: RDA: 700 mg/day
Children 4-8 years: RDA: 1000 mg/day
Children 9-18 years: RDA: 1300 mg/day
Adults: 2 tablets daily
Adults 19-50 years: RDA: 1000 mg/day
Adults ≥51 years, females: RDA: 1200 mg/day
Adults 51-70 years, males: RDA: 1000 mg/day
Adults >70 years, males: RDA: 1200 mg/day

Dosage Forms
Caplet:
Posture® [OTC]: Calcium 600 mg and phosphorus 280 mg

calcium polystyrene sulfonate *(Canada only)* (KAL see um pol i STI reen sul fo NATE)
Medication Safety Issues
Sound-alike/look-alike issues:
Calcium polystyrene sulfonate may be confused with sodium polystyrene sulfonate
Synonyms calcium polystyrene sulphonate
Canadian Brand Names Resonium Calcium®
Therapeutic Category Antidote
Use Treatment of hyperkalemia
General Dosage Range
Oral:
Children: 0.5-1 g/kg/day
Adults: 15 g 3-4 times/day
Rectal:
Children: 0.5-1 g/kg/day
Adults: 30 g once daily
Product Availability Not available in U.S.
Dosage Forms - Canada
Powder for suspension, oral/rectal:
Resonium Calcium®: 300 g

calcium polystyrene sulphonate *see* calcium polystyrene sulfonate *(Canada only) on page 166*
Cal-CYUM [OTC] *see* calcium and vitamin D *on page 160*
Caldecort® [OTC] *see* hydrocortisone (topical) *on page 450*
Caldolor™ *see* ibuprofen *on page 460*

calfactant (kaf AKT ant)
U.S. Brand Names Infasurf®
Therapeutic Category Lung Surfactant
Use Prevention of respiratory distress syndrome (RDS) in premature infants at high risk for RDS and for the treatment ("rescue") of premature infants who develop RDS

Prophylaxis: Therapy at birth with calfactant is indicated for premature infants <29 weeks of gestational age at significant risk for RDS. Should be administered as soon as possible, preferably within 30 minutes after birth.
Treatment: For infants ≤72 hours of age with RDS (confirmed by clinical and radiologic findings) and requiring endotracheal intubation.
General Dosage Range Intratracheal: *Premature infants:* 3 mL/kg (body weight at birth) every 12 hours for a total of 3 doses
Dosage Forms
Suspension, intratracheal [preservative free]:
Infasurf®: 35 mg/mL (3 mL, 6 mL)

Cal-G [OTC] *see* calcium gluconate *on page 164*
Cal-Gest [OTC] *see* calcium carbonate *on page 161*
Cal-GLU™ [OTC] *see* calcium gluconate *on page 164*
Callergy Clear [OTC] *see* pramoxine *on page 730*
Cal-Mint [OTC] *see* calcium carbonate *on page 161*
Calmoseptine® [OTC] *see* menthol and zinc oxide (topical) *on page 560*
Calmylin with Codeine (Can) *see* guaifenesin, pseudoephedrine, and codeine *on page 430*
CaloMist™ *see* cyanocobalamin *on page 241*
Caltine® (Can) *see* calcitonin *on page 159*
Caltrate® (Can) *see* calcium carbonate *on page 161*
Caltrate® 600 [OTC] *see* calcium carbonate *on page 161*
Caltrate® 600+D [OTC] *see* calcium and vitamin D *on page 160*
Caltrate® 600+Soy™ [OTC] *see* calcium and vitamin D *on page 160*
Caltrate® ColonHealth™ [OTC] *see* calcium and vitamin D *on page 160*
Caltrate® Select (Can) *see* calcium carbonate *on page 161*
Cambia™ *see* diclofenac (systemic) *on page 277*

Camila® *see* norethindrone *on page 633*
Campath® *see* alemtuzumab *on page 48*
campath-1H *see* alemtuzumab *on page 48*
Campho-Phenique® [OTC] *see* camphor and phenol *on page 167*

camphor and phenol (KAM for & FEE nole)

Synonyms phenol and camphor
U.S. Brand Names Campho-Phenique® [OTC]
Therapeutic Category Topical Skin Product
Use Relief of pain and itching associated with minor burns, sunburn, minor cuts, insect bites, minor skin irritation; temporary relief of pain from cold sores
General Dosage Range Topical: *Adults:* Apply 1-3 times/day
Dosage Forms
  Gel, topical:
    Campho-Phenique® [OTC]: Camphor 10.8% and phenol 4.7% (7 g, 14 g)
  Liquid, topical: Camphor 10.8% and phenol 4.7% (45 mL)
    Campho-Phenique® [OTC]: Camphor 10.8% and phenol 4.7% (22.5 mL, 45 mL)

camphorated tincture of opium (error-prone synonym) *see* paregoric *on page 675*
Campral® *see* acamprosate *on page 22*
Camptosar® *see* irinotecan *on page 491*
camptothecin-11 *see* irinotecan *on page 491*
Camrese™ *see* ethinyl estradiol and levonorgestrel *on page 353*

canakinumab (can a KIN ue mab)

Synonyms ACZ885
U.S. Brand Names Ilaris®
Therapeutic Category Interleukin-1 Beta Inhibitor; Interleukin-1 Inhibitor; Monoclonal Antibody
Use Treatment of cryopyrin-associated periodic syndromes (CAPS), including familial cold auto-inflammatory syndrome (FCAS) and Muckle-Wells syndrome (MWS)
General Dosage Range SubQ:
  Children ≥4 years and 15-40 kg: 2-3 mg/kg every 8 weeks
  Children ≥4 years and Adults >40 kg: 150 mg every 8 weeks
Dosage Forms
  Injection, powder for reconstitution:
    Ilaris®: 180 mg

Canasa® *see* mesalamine *on page 564*
Cancidas® *see* caspofungin *on page 178*

candesartan (kan de SAR tan)

Medication Safety Issues
  Sound-alike/look-alike issues:
    Atacand® may be confused with antacid
Synonyms candesartan cilexetil
U.S. Brand Names Atacand®
Canadian Brand Names Apo-Candesartan; Atacand®; Sandoz-Candesartan
Therapeutic Category Angiotensin II Receptor Antagonist
Use Alone or in combination with other antihypertensive agents in treating essential hypertension; treatment of heart failure (NYHA class II-IV)
General Dosage Range Oral: *Adults:* Initial: 4-16 mg once daily; Maintenance: 4-32 mg/day in 1-2 divided doses
Dosage Forms
  Tablet, oral:
    Atacand®: 4 mg, 8 mg, 16 mg, 32 mg

candesartan and hydrochlorothiazide (kan de SAR tan & hye droe klor oh THYE a zide)

Synonyms candesartan cilexetil and hydrochlorothiazide; hydrochlorothiazide and candesartan

◀ **U.S. Brand Names** Atacand HCT®
Canadian Brand Names Atacand® Plus
Therapeutic Category Antihypertensive Agent, Combination
Use Treatment of hypertension; combination product should not be used for initial therapy
General Dosage Range Oral: *Adults:* Candesartan 16-32 mg/day in 1-2 divided doses and hydrochlorothiazide 12.5-25 mg once daily
Dosage Forms
Tablet:
Atacand HCT®: 16/12.5: Candesartan 16 mg and hydrochlorothiazide 12.5 mg; 32/12.5: Candesartan 32 mg and hydrochlorothiazide 12.5 mg; 32/25: Candesartan 32 mg and hydrochlorothiazide 25 mg

candesartan cilexetil *see* candesartan *on page 167*
candesartan cilexetil and hydrochlorothiazide *see* candesartan and hydrochlorothiazide *on page 167*

Candida albicans (Monilia) (KAN dee da AL bi kans mo NIL ya)
Synonyms *Monilia* skin test
U.S. Brand Names Candin®
Therapeutic Category Diagnostic Agent
Use Screen for detection of nonresponsiveness to antigens in immunocompromised individuals
General Dosage Range Intradermal: *Children and Adults:* 0.1 mL
Dosage Forms
Injection, solution:
Candin®: 0.1 mL/dose (1 mL)

Candin® *see Candida albicans (Monilia) on page 168*
Candistatin® (Can) *see* nystatin (topical) *on page 642*
CanesOral® (Can) *see* fluconazole *on page 381*
Canesten® Topical (Can) *see* clotrimazole (topical) *on page 226*
Canesten® Vaginal (Can) *see* clotrimazole (topical) *on page 226*
Cankaid® [OTC] *see* carbamide peroxide *on page 172*
cannabidiol and tetrahydrocannabinol *see* tetrahydrocannabinol and cannabidiol *(Canada only) on page 857*
Cantil® *see* mepenzolate *on page 560*
Capastat® Sulfate *see* capreomycin *on page 169*
CAPE *see* capecitabine *on page 168*

capecitabine (ka pe SITE a been)
Medication Safety Issues
Sound-alike/look-alike issues:
Xeloda® may be confused with Xenical®
High alert medication:
This medication is in a class the Institute for Safe Medication Practices (ISMP) includes among its list of drug classes which have a heightened risk of causing significant patient harm when used in error.
Synonyms CAPE
U.S. Brand Names Xeloda®
Canadian Brand Names Xeloda®
Therapeutic Category Antineoplastic Agent, Antimetabolite
Use Treatment of metastatic colorectal cancer; adjuvant therapy of Dukes C colon cancer; treatment of metastatic breast cancer
General Dosage Range Dosage adjustment recommended in patients with renal impairment or who develop toxicities
Oral: *Adults:* 1250 mg/m^2 twice daily for 2 weeks, every 21 days
Dosage Forms
Tablet, oral:
Xeloda®: 150 mg, 500 mg

Capex® *see* fluocinolone (topical) *on page 384*
Caphosol® *see* saliva substitute *on page 798*

Capital® and Codeine *see* acetaminophen and codeine *on page 26*
Capoten® (Can) *see* captopril *on page 170*
Caprelsa® *see* vandetanib *on page 907*

capreomycin (kap ree oh MYE sin)

Medication Safety Issues
Sound-alike/look-alike issues:
Capastat® may be confused with Cepastat®

Synonyms capreomycin sulfate

U.S. Brand Names Capastat® Sulfate

Therapeutic Category Antibiotic, Miscellaneous

Use Treatment of tuberculosis in conjunction with at least one other antituberculosis agent

General Dosage Range Dosage adjustment recommended in patients with renal impairment
I.M., I.V.: *Adults:* 1 g/day (maximum: 20 mg/kg/day) for 60-120 days, followed by 1 g 2-3 times/week

Dosage Forms
Injection, powder for reconstitution:
Capastat® Sulfate: 1 g

capreomycin sulfate *see* capreomycin *on page 169*

capsaicin (kap SAY sin)

Medication Safety Issues
Sound-alike/look-alike issues:
Zostrix® may be confused with Zestril®, Zovirax®

Synonyms NGX-4010

U.S. Brand Names Capzasin-HP® [OTC]; Capzasin-P® [OTC]; DiabetAid® Pain and Tingling Relief [OTC]; Qutenza™; Salonpas® Hot [OTC]; Zostrix® Diabetic Foot Pain [OTC]; Zostrix® [OTC]; Zostrix®-HP [OTC]

Canadian Brand Names Zostrix®; Zostrix® H.P.

Therapeutic Category Analgesic, Topical

Use
Topical patch (Qutenza™): Management of postherpetic neuralgia (PHN)
OTC labeling: Temporary treatment of minor pain associated with muscles and joints due to backache, strains, sprains, bruises, cramps or arthritis; temporary relief of pain associated with diabetic neuropathy

General Dosage Range Topical:
Children ≥12 years: OTC labeling: Patch (Salonpas®-Hot): Apply patch to affected area up to 3-4 times/day
Adults: Patch (Qutenza™[capsaicin 8%]): Apply patch to most painful area for 60 minutes (maximum: 4 patches in a single application); OTC products: Apply to affected area 3-4 times/day

Dosage Forms
Cream, topical: 0.025% (60 g)
Capzasin-HP® [OTC]: 0.1% (42.5 g)
Capzasin-P® [OTC]: 0.035% (42.5 g)
Zostrix® [OTC]: 0.025% (60 g)
Zostrix® Diabetic Foot Pain [OTC]: 0.075% (60 g)
Zostrix®-HP [OTC]: 0.075% (60 g)
Gel, topical:
Capzasin-P® [OTC]: 0.025% (42.5 g)
Liquid, topical:
Capzasin-P® [OTC]: 0.15% (29.5 mL)
Lotion, topical:
DiabetAid® Pain and Tingling Relief [OTC]: 0.025% (120 mL)
Patch, topical:
Qutenza™: 8% (1s, 2s)
Salonpas® Hot [OTC]: 0.025% (1s)

captopril (KAP toe pril)

Medication Safety Issues
Sound-alike/look-alike issues:
Captopril may be confused with calcitriol, Capitrol®, carvedilol
International issues:
Acepril [Great Britain] may be confused with Accupril which is a brand name for quinapril in the U.S.
Acepril: Brand name for captopril [Great Britain], but also the brand name for enalapril [Hungary, Switzerland]; lisinopril [Malaysia]
Synonyms ACE
Canadian Brand Names Apo-Capto®; Capoten®; Dom-Captopril; Mylan-Captopril; Nu-Capto; PMS-Captopril; Teva-Captopril
Therapeutic Category Angiotensin-Converting Enzyme (ACE) Inhibitor
Use Management of hypertension; treatment of heart failure, left ventricular dysfunction after myocardial infarction, diabetic nephropathy
General Dosage Range Dosage adjustment recommended in patients with renal impairment
Oral:
Infants: Initial: 0.15-0.3 mg/kg/dose; Maintenance: 2.5-6 mg/kg/day in 1-4 divided doses
Children: Initial: 0.5 mg/kg/dose; Maintenance: Up to 6 mg/kg/day in 2-4 divided doses
Older Children: Initial: 6.25-12.5 mg every 12-24 hours; Maintenance: Up to 6 mg/kg/day
Adolescents: Initial: 12.5-25 mg every 8-12 hours; Maintenance: Up to 450 mg/day divided every 8-12 hours
Adults: Initial: 6.25-25 mg 2-3 times/day; Maintenance: 25-450 mg/day in 2-3 divided doses
Dosage Forms
Tablet, oral: 12.5 mg, 25 mg, 50 mg, 100 mg

captopril and hydrochlorothiazide (KAP toe pril & hye droe klor oh THYE a zide)

Synonyms hydrochlorothiazide and captopril
Therapeutic Category Antihypertensive Agent, Combination
Use Management of hypertension
General Dosage Range Oral: *Adults:* Captopril 25-150 mg and hydrochlorothiazide 15-50 mg once daily
Dosage Forms
Tablet: 25/15: Captopril 25 mg and hydrochlorothiazide 15 mg; 25/25: Captopril 25 mg and hydrochlorothiazide 25 mg; 50/15: Captopril 50 mg and hydrochlorothiazide 15 mg; 50/25: Captopril 50 mg and hydrochlorothiazide 25 mg

Capzasin-HP® [OTC] *see* capsaicin *on page 169*
Capzasin-P® [OTC] *see* capsaicin *on page 169*
Carac® *see* fluorouracil (topical) *on page 388*
Carafate® *see* sucralfate *on page 833*
Carapres® (Can) *see* clonidine *on page 223*

carbachol (KAR ba kole)

Medication Safety Issues
Sound-alike/look-alike issues:
Isopto® Carbachol may be confused with Isopto® Carpine
Synonyms carbacholine; carbamylcholine chloride
U.S. Brand Names Isopto® Carbachol; Miostat®
Canadian Brand Names Isopto® Carbachol; Miostat®
Therapeutic Category Cholinergic Agent
Use Lowers intraocular pressure in the treatment of glaucoma; cause miosis during surgery
General Dosage Range Ophthalmic: *Adults:* Instill 1-2 drops up to 3 times/day **or** 0.5 mL as a single dose
Dosage Forms
Solution, intraocular:
Miostat®: 0.01% (1.5 mL)
Solution, ophthalmic:
Isopto® Carbachol: 1.5% (15 mL); 3% (15 mL)
carbacholine *see* carbachol *on page 170*

Carbaglu® *see* carglumic acid *on page 176*

carbamazepine (kar ba MAZ e peen)

Medication Safety Issues

Sound-alike/look-alike issues:
CarBAMazepine may be confused with OXcarbazepine
Epitol® may be confused with Epinal®
TEGretol®, TEGretol®-XR may be confused with Mebaral®, Toprol-XL®, Toradol®, TRENtal®

Synonyms CBZ; SPD417

Tall-Man carBAMazepine

U.S. Brand Names Carbatrol®; Epitol®; Equetro®; TEGretol®; TEGretol®-XR

Canadian Brand Names Apo-Carbamazepine®; Dom-Carbamazepine; Mapezine®; Mylan-Carbamazepine CR; Nu-Carbamazepine; PMS-Carbamazepine; Sandoz-Carbamazepine; Taro-Carbamazepine Chewable; Tegretol®; Teva-Carbamazepine

Therapeutic Category Anticonvulsant

Use

Carbatrol®, Tegretol®, Tegretol®-XR: Partial seizures with complex symptomatology (psychomotor, temporal lobe), generalized tonic-clonic seizures (grand mal), mixed seizure patterns, trigeminal neuralgia
Equetro®: Acute manic and mixed episodes associated with bipolar 1 disorder

General Dosage Range Dosage adjustment recommended in patients with renal impairment.

Oral:

Extended release:

Capsules:

Children <12 years: Receiving ≥400 mg/day of carbamazepine may be converted to extended release capsules (Carbatrol®) using the same total daily dosage divided twice daily

Children 12-15 years: Initial: 400 mg/day; Maintenance: 800-1000 mg/day in 2 divided doses (maximum: 1000 mg/day)

Adolescents >15 years: Initial: 400 mg/day; Maintenance: 800-1200 mg/day in 2 divided doses (maximum: 1200 mg/day)

Adults: Bipolar disorder (Equetro®): Initial: 400 mg/day in 2 divided doses: Maintenance: Adjust by 200 mg daily increments (maximum: 1600 mg/day); Epilepsy: Initial: 400 mg/day; Maintenance: 800-1200 mg/day in 2 divided doses (maximum: 2400 mg/day)

Tablets:

Children 6-12 years: Initial: 200 mg/day; Maintenance: 400-800 mg/day in 2 divided doses (maximum: 1000 mg/day)

Children 12-15 years: Initial: 400 mg/day; Maintenance: 800-1000 mg/day in 2 divided doses (maximum: 1000 mg/day)

Adolescents >15 years and Adults: Initial: 400 mg/day; Maintenance: 800-1200 mg/day in 2 divided doses (maximum: 1200 mg/day)

Immediate release:

Children <6 years: Initial: 10-20 mg/kg/day in 2-3 divided doses (tablets) **or** 4 divided doses (suspension); Maintenance: Up to 35 mg/kg/day in 3-4 divided doses

Children 6-12 years: Initial: 200 mg/day in 2 divided doses (tablets) **or** 4 divided doses (suspension); Maintenance: 400-800 mg/day in 2-4 divided doses (maximum: 1000 mg/day)

Children 12-15 years: Initial: 400 mg/day in 2 divided doses (tablets) **or** 4 divided doses (suspension); Maintenance: 800-1000 mg/day in 3-4 divided doses (maximum: 1000 mg/day)

Adolescents >15 years: Initial: 400 mg/day in 2 divided doses (tablets) **or** 4 divided doses (suspension); Maintenance: 800-1200 mg/day in 3-4 divided doses (maximum: 1200 mg/day)

Adults: Epilepsy: Initial: 400 mg/day in 2 divided doses (tablets) **or** 4 divided doses (suspension); Maintenance: 800-1200 mg/day in 3-4 divided doses (maximum: 2400 mg/day); Trigeminal or glossopharyngeal neuralgia: Initial: 200 mg/day in 2 divided doses; Maintenance: 400-800 mg/day in 2 divided doses (maximum: 1200 mg/day)

Dosage Forms

Capsule, extended release, oral:
Carbatrol®: 100 mg, 200 mg, 300 mg
Equetro®: 100 mg, 200 mg, 300 mg

Suspension, oral: 100 mg/5 mL (5 mL, 10 mL, 450 mL)
TEGretol®: 100 mg/5 mL (450 mL)

Tablet, oral: 200 mg
  Epitol®: 200 mg
  TEGretol®: 200 mg
Tablet, chewable, oral: 100 mg
  TEGretol®: 100 mg
Tablet, extended release, oral: 200 mg, 400 mg
  TEGretol®-XR: 100 mg, 200 mg, 400 mg

carbamide see urea on page 900

carbamide peroxide (KAR ba mide per OKS ide)

Synonyms urea peroxide
U.S. Brand Names Auraphene B® [OTC]; Auro® [OTC]; Cankaid® [OTC]; Debrox® [OTC]; E-R-O® [OTC]; Gly-Oxide® [OTC]; Murine® Ear Wax Removal Kit [OTC]; Murine® Ear [OTC]; Otix® [OTC]
Therapeutic Category Antiinfective Agent, Oral; Otic Agent, Ceruminolytic
Use Relief of minor inflammation of gums, oral mucosal surfaces, and lips including canker sores and dental irritation; emulsify and disperse ear wax
General Dosage Range
Otic:
  Children <12 years: Instill 1-5 drops twice daily
  Children ≥12 years and Adults: Instill 5-10 drops twice daily
Topical (oral): *Children ≥2 years and Adults:* Apply several drops on affected area, expectorate after 2-3 minutes 4 times/day **or** place 10 drops on tongue, swish for several minutes, expectorate
Dosage Forms
Liquid, oral: 10% (60 mL)
  Cankaid® [OTC]: 10% (15 mL)
  Gly-Oxide® [OTC]: 10% (15 mL, 60 mL)
Solution, otic: 6.5% (15 mL)
  Auraphene B® [OTC]: 6.5% (15 mL)
  Auro® [OTC]: 6.5% (22.2 mL)
  Debrox® [OTC]: 6.5% (15 mL, 30 mL)
  E-R-O® [OTC]: 6.5% (15 mL)
  Murine® Ear [OTC]: 6.5% (15 mL)
  Murine® Ear Wax Removal Kit [OTC]: 6.5% (15 mL)
  Otix® [OTC]: 6.5% (15 mL)

carbamylcholine chloride see carbachol on page 170
Carbatrol® see carbamazepine on page 171

carbetapentane and chlorpheniramine (kar bay ta PEN tane & klor fen IR a meen)

Synonyms carbetapentane tannate and chlorpheniramine tannate; chlorpheniramine and carbetapentane
U.S. Brand Names C-Tanna 12 [DSC]; Tussi-12 S™; Tussi-12®; Tussizone-12 RF™
Therapeutic Category Antihistamine/Antitussive
Use Symptomatic relief of cough associated with upper respiratory tract conditions, such as the common cold, bronchitis, bronchial asthma
General Dosage Range Oral:
  Children 2-6 years: Carbetapentane 15-30 mg and chlorpheniramine 2-4 mg every 12 hours
  Children >6 years: Carbetapentane 30-60 mg and chlorpheniramine 4-8 mg every 12 hours
  Adults: Carbetapentane 60-120 mg and chlorpheniramine 5-10 mg every 12 hours
Dosage Forms
Tablet:
  Tussi-12®, Tussizone-12 RF™: Carbetapentane 60 mg and chlorpheniramine 5 mg

carbetapentane and pseudoephedrine (kar bay ta PEN tane & soo doe e FED rin)

Synonyms carbetapentane tannate and pseudoephedrine tannate; pseudoephedrine and carbetapentane
U.S. Brand Names Corzall™ Liquid [DSC]
Therapeutic Category Antitussive/Decongestant
Use Relief of cough and congestion due to the common cold, influenza, sinusitis, or bronchitis

General Dosage Range Oral:
Children 6-12 years: 2.5-5 mL every 4-6 hours (maximum: 30 mL/24 hours)
Children >12 years and Adults: 5-10 mL every 4-6 hours (maximum: 60 mL/24 hours)

carbetapentane, ephedrine, phenylephrine, and chlorpheniramine *see* chlorpheniramine, ephedrine, phenylephrine, and carbetapentane *on page 199*

carbetapentane, phenylephrine, and pyrilamine
(kar bay ta PEN tane, fen il EF rin, & peer II a meen)

Synonyms phenylephrine tannate, carbetapentane tannate, and pyrilamine tannate; pyrilamine, phenylephrine, and carbetapentane

U.S. Brand Names C-Tanna 12D [DSC]; Tussi-12® D [DSC]; Tussi-12® DS [DSC]

Therapeutic Category Antihistamine; Antihistamine/Decongestant/Antitussive; Antitussive; Decongestant

Use Symptomatic relief of cough associated with respiratory tract conditions such as the common cold, bronchial asthma, acute and chronic bronchitis

General Dosage Range Oral:
Children 2-6 years: Tussi-12® DS: 2.5-5 mL every 12 hours
Children 6-11 years: Tussi-12® D: 1/2 to 1 tablet every 12 hours; Tussi-12® DS: 5-10 mL every 12 hours
Children ≥12 years and Adults: Tussi-12® D: 1-2 tablets every 12 hours

carbetapentane tannate and chlorpheniramine tannate *see* carbetapentane and chlorpheniramine *on page 172*

carbetapentane tannate and pseudoephedrine tannate *see* carbetapentane and pseudoephedrine *on page 172*

carbetocin *(Canada only)* (kar BE toe sin)

Medication Safety Issues
High alert medication:
The Institute for Safe Medication Practices (ISMP) includes oxytocin (carbetocin analog) among its list of drugs which have a heightened risk of causing significant patient harm when used in error.

Canadian Brand Names Duratocin™

Therapeutic Category Oxytocic Agent

Use Prevention of uterine atony and postpartum hemorrhage following elective cesarean section under anesthesia (epidural or spinal)

General Dosage Range I.V.: *Adults:* 100 mcg (single dose)

Product Availability Not available in U.S.

Dosage Forms - Canada
Injection, solution:
Duratocin™: 100 mcg/mL (1 mL)

carbidopa (kar bi DOE pa)

Medication Safety Issues
International issues:
Lodosyn [U.S.] may be confused with Lidosen brand name for lidocaine [Italy]

U.S. Brand Names Lodosyn®

Therapeutic Category Anti-Parkinson Agent (Dopamine Agonist)

Use Given with levodopa in the treatment of parkinsonism to enable a lower dosage of levodopa to be used and a more rapid response to be obtained and to decrease side effects; for details of administration and dosage, see Levodopa; has no effect without levodopa

General Dosage Range Oral: *Adults:* 70-100 mg/day (maximum: 200 mg/day)

Dosage Forms
Tablet, oral:
Lodosyn®: 25 mg

carbidopa and levodopa (kar bi DOE pa & lee voe DOE pa)

Medication Safety Issues

Sound-alike/look-alike issues:
Sinemet® may be confused with Serevent®

International issues:
Zimox: Brand name for carbidopa and levodopa [Greece], but also the brand name for amoxicillin [Italy]

Zimox [Greece] may be confused with Diamox which is a brand name for acetazolamide [Canada and multiple international markets]

Synonyms levodopa and carbidopa

U.S. Brand Names Parcopa®; Sinemet®; Sinemet® CR

Canadian Brand Names Apo-Levocarb®; Apo-Levocarb® CR; Dom-Levo-Carbidopa; Duodopa™; Endo®-Levodopa/Carbidopa; Levocarb CR; Novo-Levocarbidopa; Nu-Levocarb; PRO-Levocarb; Sinemet®; Sinemet® CR

Therapeutic Category Anti-Parkinson Agent (Dopamine Agonist)

Use Idiopathic Parkinson disease; postencephalitic parkinsonism; symptomatic parkinsonism

Duodopa™ intestinal gel: Canadian labeling (not available in U.S.): Treatment of advanced levodopa-responsive Parkinson disease in which severe motor symptoms are not controlled by other Parkinson agents

General Dosage Range Oral: *Adults:* Immediate release: Initial: Carbidopa 25 mg/levodopa 100 mg 3 times/day (maximum: 8 tablets of any strength/day **or** 200 mg of carbidopa and 2000 mg of levodopa); Controlled release: *Adults:* Initial: Carbidopa 50 mg/levodopa 200 mg 2 times/day, at intervals not <6 hours (maximum: 8 tablets/day)

Dosage Forms

Tablet: 10/100: Carbidopa 10 mg and levodopa 100 mg; 25/100: Carbidopa 25 mg and levodopa 100 mg; 25/250: Carbidopa 25 mg and levodopa 250 mg

Sinemet®:

10/100: Carbidopa 10 mg and levodopa 100 mg

25/100: Carbidopa 25 mg and levodopa 100 mg

25/250: Carbidopa 25 mg and levodopa 250 mg

Tablet, extended release: 25/100: Carbidopa 25 mg and levodopa 100 mg; 50/200: Carbidopa 50 mg and levodopa 200 mg

Tablet, orally disintegrating: 10/100: Carbidopa 10 mg and levodopa 100 mg; 25/100: Carbidopa 25 mg and levodopa 100 mg; 25/250: Carbidopa 25 mg and levodopa 250 mg

Parcopa®:

10/100: Carbidopa 10 mg and levodopa 100 mg [contains phenylalanine 3.4 mg/tablet; mint flavor]

25/100: Carbidopa 25 mg and levodopa 100 mg [contains phenylalanine 3.4 mg/tablet; mint flavor]

25/250: Carbidopa 25 mg and levodopa 250 mg [contains phenylalanine 8.4 mg/tablet; mint flavor]

Tablet, sustained release: 25/100: Carbidopa 25 mg and levodopa 100 mg; 50/200: Carbidopa 50 mg and levodopa 200 mg

Sinemet® CR:

25/100: Carbidopa 25 mg and levodopa 100 mg

50/200: Carbidopa 50 mg and levodopa 200 mg

Dosage Forms - Canada

Intestinal gel:

Duodopa™: Carbidopa 5 mg and levodopa 20 mg/1 mL (100 mL)

carbidopa, entacapone, and levodopa *see* levodopa, carbidopa, and entacapone *on page 519*

carbidopa, levodopa, and entacapone *see* levodopa, carbidopa, and entacapone *on page 519*

carbinoxamine (kar bi NOKS a meen)

Synonyms carbinoxamine maleate

U.S. Brand Names Arbinoxa™; Palgic®

Therapeutic Category Antihistamine

Use Seasonal and perennial allergic rhinitis; vasomotor rhinitis; allergic conjunctivitis; mild manifestations of urticaria and angioedema; dermatographism; adjunct therapy for anaphylactic reactions (after acute manifestations controlled)

General Dosage Range Oral:
Children 2-5 years: 0.2-0.4 mg/kg/day divided into 3-4 doses **or** 1-2 mg 3-4 times/day
Children 6-11 years: 2-4 mg 3-4 times/day
Adults: 4-8 mg 3-4 times/day
Dosage Forms
Solution, oral:
Arbinoxa™: 4 mg/5 mL (480 mL)
Palgic®: 4 mg/5 mL (480 mL)
Tablet, oral:
Arbinoxa™: 4 mg
Palgic®: 4 mg

carbinoxamine maleate *see* carbinoxamine *on page 174*
Carbocaine® *see* mepivacaine *on page 561*
Carbocaine® 2% with Neo-Cobefrin® *see* mepivacaine and levonordefrin *on page 562*
carbolic acid *see* phenol *on page 694*
Carbolith™ (Can) *see* lithium *on page 532*

carboplatin (KAR boe pla tin)
Medication Safety Issues
Sound-alike/look-alike issues:
CARBOplatin may be confused with CISplatin, oxaliplatin
Paraplatin® may be confused with Platinol®
High alert medication:
This medication is in a class the Institute for Safe Medication Practices (ISMP) includes among its list of drugs which have a heightened risk of causing significant patient harm when used in error.
Synonyms CBDCA; Paraplatin
Tall-Man CARBOplatin
Canadian Brand Names Carboplatin Injection; Paraplatin-AQ
Therapeutic Category Antineoplastic Agent
Use Treatment of advanced ovarian cancer
General Dosage Range Dosage adjustment recommended in renal impairment or who develop toxicities
I.V.: *Adults:* 300-360 mg/m^2 every 4 weeks **or** AUC of 4-6 (using Calvert formula)
Dosage Forms
Injection, solution: 10 mg/mL (5 mL, 15 mL, 45 mL, 60 mL)
Injection, solution [preservative free]: 10 mg/mL (5 mL, 15 mL, 45 mL, 60 mL)

Carboplatin Injection (Can) *see* carboplatin *on page 175*
carboprost *see* carboprost tromethamine *on page 175*

carboprost tromethamine (KAR boe prost tro METH a meen)
Synonyms carboprost; prostaglandin F$_2$
U.S. Brand Names Hemabate®
Canadian Brand Names Hemabate®
Therapeutic Category Prostaglandin
Use Termination of pregnancy; treatment of refractory postpartum uterine bleeding
General Dosage Range I.M.: *Adults (females):* Abortion: 250 mcg at 1.5- to 3.5-hour intervals, a 500 mcg dose may be given if uterine response is not adequate after several 250 mcg doses (maximum total dose: 12 mg); Postpartum bleeding: 250 mcg; may repeat if needed (maximum total dose: 2 mg [8 doses])
Dosage Forms
Injection, solution:
Hemabate®: 250 mcg/mL (1 mL)

carbose D *see* carboxymethylcellulose *on page 175*

carboxymethylcellulose (kar boks ee meth il SEL yoo lose)
Medication Safety Issues
Sound-alike/look-alike issues:
Optive™ may be confused with Optivar®
Synonyms carbose D; carboxymethylcellulose sodium

◄ **U.S. Brand Names** Optive™ [OTC]; Refresh Liquigel™ [OTC]; Refresh Plus® [OTC]; Refresh Tears® [OTC]; Tears Again® Gel Drops™ [OTC] [DSC]; Tears Again® Night & Day™ [OTC]; Theratears® [OTC]

Canadian Brand Names Celluvisc™; Refresh Plus®; Refresh Tears®

Therapeutic Category Ophthalmic Agent, Miscellaneous

Use Artificial tear substitute

General Dosage Range Ophthalmic: *Adults:* Instill 1-2 drops into eye(s) 3-4 times/day

Dosage Forms
 Gel, ophthalmic:
  Tears Again® Night & Day™ [OTC]: 1.5% (3.5 g)
 Liquid, ophthalmic:
  Refresh Liquigel™ [OTC]: 1% (15 mL)
 Solution, ophthalmic:
  Optive™ [OTC]: 0.5% (15 mL, 30 mL)
  Refresh Tears® [OTC]: 0.5% (15 mL)
 Solution, ophthalmic [preservative free]:
  Refresh Plus® [OTC]: 0.5% (0.4 mL)
  Theratears® [OTC]: 0.25% (0.6 mL, 15 mL)

carboxymethylcellulose sodium *see carboxymethylcellulose on page 175*

Cardene® I.V. *see nicardipine on page 624*

Cardene® SR *see nicardipine on page 624*

Cardizem® *see diltiazem on page 286*

Cardizem® CD *see diltiazem on page 286*

Cardizem® LA *see diltiazem on page 286*

Cardura® *see doxazosin on page 308*

Cardura-1™ (Can) *see doxazosin on page 308*

Cardura-2™ (Can) *see doxazosin on page 308*

Cardura-4™ (Can) *see doxazosin on page 308*

Cardura® XL *see doxazosin on page 308*

carglumic acid (kar GLU mik AS id)

Synonyms N-carbamoyl-L-glutamic acid; N-carbamylglutamate

U.S. Brand Names Carbaglu®

Therapeutic Category Antidote; Metabolic Alkalosis Agent; Urea Cycle Disorder (UCD) Treatment Agent

Use Adjunctive treatment of acute hyperammonemia and maintenance therapy of chronic hyperammonemia due to the deficiency of the hepatic enzyme N-acetylglutamate synthase (NAGS)

General Dosage Range Oral: *Children and Adults:* <100-250 mg/kg/day given in 2 or 4 divided doses

Dosage Forms
 Tablet for solution, oral:
  Carbaglu®: 200 mg

Carimune® NF *see immune globulin on page 468*

carisoprodate *see carisoprodol on page 176*

carisoprodol (kar eye soe PROE dole)

Medication Safety Issues
 BEERS Criteria medication:
  This drug may be inappropriate for use in geriatric patients (high severity risk).

Synonyms carisoprodate; isobamate

U.S. Brand Names Soma®

Therapeutic Category Skeletal Muscle Relaxant

Use Short-term (2-3 weeks) treatment of acute musculoskeletal pain

General Dosage Range Oral: *Children ≥16 years and Adults:* 250-350 mg 3 times/day and at bedtime

Dosage Forms
 Tablet, oral: 350 mg
  Soma®: 250 mg, 350 mg

carisoprodol and aspirin (kar eye soe PROE dole & AS pir in)

Medication Safety Issues
BEERS Criteria medication:
This drug (carisoprodol) may be inappropriate for use in geriatric patients (high severity risk).
Synonyms aspirin and carisoprodol
U.S. Brand Names Soma® Compound
Therapeutic Category Skeletal Muscle Relaxant
Use Relief of discomfort associated with acute, painful skeletal muscle conditions
General Dosage Range Oral: *Children ≥16 years and Adults:* 1-2 tablets 4 times/day (maximum: 8 tablets/24 hours)
Dosage Forms
Tablet: Carisoprodol 200 mg and aspirin 325 mg
Soma® Compound: Carisoprodol 200 mg and aspirin 325 mg

carisoprodol, aspirin, and codeine (kar eye soe PROE dole, AS pir in, and KOE deen)

Synonyms aspirin, carisoprodol, and codeine; codeine, aspirin, and carisoprodol; soma compound w/ codeine
Therapeutic Category Skeletal Muscle Relaxant
Controlled Substance C-III
Use Skeletal muscle relaxant
General Dosage Range Oral: *Adults:* 1-2 tablets 4 times/day (maximum: 8 tablets/day)
Dosage Forms
Tablet: Carisoprodol 200 mg, aspirin 325 mg, and codeine 16 mg

Carmol® 10 [OTC] *see* urea *on page 900*
Carmol® 20 [OTC] *see* urea *on page 900*
Carmol® 40 *see* urea *on page 900*
Carmol® Deep Cleansing [OTC] *see* urea *on page 900*
Carmol-HC® *see* urea and hydrocortisone *on page 901*
Carmol® Scalp Treatment *see* sulfacetamide (topical) *on page 835*

carmustine (kar MUS teen)

Medication Safety Issues
Sound-alike/look-alike issues:
Carmustine may be confused with bendamustine, lomustine
High alert medication:
This medication is in a class the Institute for Safe Medication Practices (ISMP) includes among its list of drug classes which have a heightened risk of causing significant patient harm when used in error.
Synonyms BCNU; bis(chloroethyl) nitrosourea; bis-chloronitrosourea; carmustine polymer wafer; carmustinum; WR-139021
U.S. Brand Names BiCNU®; Gliadel®
Canadian Brand Names BiCNU®; Gliadel Wafer®
Therapeutic Category Antineoplastic Agent
Use
Injection: Treatment of brain tumors (glioblastoma, brainstem glioma, medulloblastoma, astrocytoma, ependymoma, and metastatic brain tumors), multiple myeloma, Hodgkin lymphoma (relapsed or refractory), non-Hodgkin lymphomas (relapsed or refractory)
Wafer (implant): Adjunct to surgery in patients with recurrent glioblastoma multiforme; adjunct to surgery and radiation in patients with newly-diagnosed high-grade malignant glioma
General Dosage Range Dosage adjustment recommended in patients with renal impairment or who develop toxicity.
I.V.: *Adults:* 150-200 mg/m^2 every 6-8 weeks **or** 75-100 mg/m^2/day for 2 days every 6-8 weeks
Implantation: *Adults:* 8 wafers placed in the resection cavity (total dose: 61.6 mg)
Dosage Forms
Injection, powder for reconstitution:
BiCNU®: 100 mg
Wafer, for implantation:
Gliadel®: 7.7 mg (8s)

carmustine polymer wafer *see* carmustine *on page 177*
carmustinum *see* carmustine *on page 177*
Carnitine-300 [OTC] *see* levocarnitine *on page 518*
Carnitor® *see* levocarnitine *on page 518*
Carnitor® SF *see* levocarnitine *on page 518*
Carrington® Antifungal [OTC] *see* miconazole (topical) *on page 585*
Carrington® Oral Wound Rinse [OTC] *see* maltodextrin *on page 548*

carteolol (ophthalmic) (KAR tee oh lole)

Medication Safety Issues
Sound-alike/look-alike issues:
 Carteolol may be confused with carvedilol
Synonyms carteolol hydrochloride
Therapeutic Category Ophthalmic Agent, Antiglaucoma
Use Treatment of chronic open-angle glaucoma and intraocular hypertension
General Dosage Range Ophthalmic: *Adults:* Instill 1 drop in affected eye(s) twice daily
Dosage Forms
 Solution, ophthalmic: 1% (5 mL, 10 mL, 15 mL)

carteolol hydrochloride *see* carteolol (ophthalmic) *on page 178*
Carter's Little Pills® (Can) *see* bisacodyl *on page 134*
Cartia XT® *see* diltiazem *on page 286*

carvedilol (KAR ve dil ole)

Medication Safety Issues
Sound-alike/look-alike issues:
 Carvedilol may be confused with atenolol, captopril, carbidopa, carteolol
 Coreg® may be confused with Corgard®, Cortef®, Cozaar®
U.S. Brand Names Coreg CR®; Coreg®
Canadian Brand Names Apo-Carvedilol®; Coreg®; Dom-Carvedilol; JAMP-Carvedilol; Mylan-Carvedilol; Novo-Carvedilol; PHL-Carvedilol; PMS-Carvedilol; RAN™-Carvedilol; ratio-Carvedilol; ZYM-Carvedilol
Therapeutic Category Beta-Adrenergic Blocker
Use Mild-to-severe heart failure of ischemic or cardiomyopathic origin (usually in addition to standard therapy); left ventricular dysfunction following myocardial infarction (MI) (clinically stable with LVEF ≤40%); management of hypertension
General Dosage Range Oral: *Adults:* Immediate release: Initial: 3.125-6.25 mg twice daily; Maintenance: 6.25-50 mg twice daily (maximum: 50 mg/day [<85 kg]; 100 mg/day [>85 kg]); Extended release: Initial: 10 mg once daily; range: 10-80 mg once daily
Dosage Forms
 Capsule, extended release, oral:
  Coreg CR®: 10 mg, 20 mg, 40 mg, 80 mg
 Tablet, oral: 3.125 mg, 6.25 mg, 12.5 mg, 25 mg
  Coreg®: 3.125 mg, 6.25 mg, 12.5 mg, 25 mg

Casodex® *see* bicalutamide *on page 133*

caspofungin (kas poe FUN jin)

Synonyms caspofungin acetate
U.S. Brand Names Cancidas®
Canadian Brand Names Cancidas®
Therapeutic Category Antifungal Agent, Systemic
Use Treatment of invasive *Aspergillus* infections in patients who are refractory or intolerant of other therapy; treatment of candidemia and other *Candida* infections (intraabdominal abscesses, esophageal, peritonitis, pleural space); empirical treatment for presumed fungal infections in febrile neutropenic patient

General Dosage Range Dosage adjustment recommended in patients with hepatic impairment or on concomitant therapy
I.V.:
  Children 3 months to 17 years: 70 mg/m^2 on day 1, subsequent dosing: 50-70 mg/m^2 once daily (maximum dose: 70 mg/day)
  Adults: Initial: 70 mg on day 1; Subsequent dose: 50-70 mg once daily
Dosage Forms
  Injection, powder for reconstitution:
  Cancidas®: 50 mg, 70 mg

caspofungin acetate *see* caspofungin *on page 178*
Castellani Paint Modified [OTC] *see* phenol *on page 694*

castor oil (KAS tor oyl)
Synonyms oleum ricini
Therapeutic Category Laxative
Use Preparation for rectal or bowel examination or surgery; rarely used to relieve constipation; also applied to skin as emollient and protectant
General Dosage Range Oral:
  Children 2-11 years: 5-15 mL as a single dose
  Children ≥12 years and Adults: 15-60 mL as a single dose
Dosage Forms
  Oil, oral: 100% (60 mL, 120 mL, 180 mL, 480 mL, 3840 mL)

castor oil, trypsin, and balsam Peru *see* trypsin, balsam Peru, and castor oil *on page 896*
Cataflam® *see* diclofenac (systemic) *on page 277*
Catapres® *see* clonidine *on page 223*
Catapres-TTS®-1 *see* clonidine *on page 223*
Catapres-TTS®-2 *see* clonidine *on page 223*
Catapres-TTS®-3 *see* clonidine *on page 223*
catechins *see* sinecatechins *on page 814*
Cathflo® Activase® *see* alteplase *on page 58*
Caverject® *see* alprostadil *on page 57*
Caverject Impulse® *see* alprostadil *on page 57*
CaviRinse™ *see* fluoride *on page 386*
Cayston® *see* aztreonam *on page 110*
Caziant® *see* ethinyl estradiol and desogestrel *on page 351*
CB-1348 *see* chlorambucil *on page 193*
CB7630 *see* abiraterone acetate *on page 21*
CBDCA *see* carboplatin *on page 175*
CBZ *see* carbamazepine *on page 171*
CC-5013 *see* lenalidomide *on page 514*
CCI-779 *see* temsirolimus *on page 849*
CCNU *see* lomustine *on page 534*
2-CdA *see* cladribine *on page 214*
CDCA *see* chenodiol *on page 192*
CDDP *see* cisplatin *on page 213*
CDP870 *see* certolizumab pegol *on page 188*
CDX *see* bicalutamide *on page 133*
CE *see* estrogens (conjugated/equine, systemic) *on page 347*
CE *see* estrogens (conjugated/equine, topical) *on page 348*
Ceclor® (Can) *see* cefaclor *on page 180*
Cedax® *see* ceftibuten *on page 184*
CEE *see* estrogens (conjugated/equine, systemic) *on page 347*
CEE *see* estrogens (conjugated/equine, topical) *on page 348*
CeeNU® *see* lomustine *on page 534*

cefaclor (SEF a klor)

Medication Safety Issues
Sound-alike/look-alike issues:
Cefaclor may be confused with cephalexin

Canadian Brand Names Apo-Cefaclor®; Ceclor®; Novo-Cefaclor; Nu-Cefaclor; PMS-Cefaclor

Therapeutic Category Cephalosporin (Second Generation)

Use Treatment of susceptible bacterial infections including otitis media, lower respiratory tract infections, acute exacerbations of chronic bronchitis, pharyngitis and tonsillitis, urinary tract infections, skin and skin structure infections

General Dosage Range Dosage adjustment recommended in patients with renal impairment
Oral:
Children >1 month: 20-40 mg/kg/day divided every 8-12 hours (maximum: 1 g/day)
Adults: 250-500 mg every 8 hours

Dosage Forms
Capsule, oral: 250 mg, 500 mg
Powder for suspension, oral: 125 mg/5 mL (75 mL, 150 mL); 250 mg/5 mL (75 mL, 150 mL); 375 mg/5 mL (50 mL, 100 mL)
Tablet, extended release, oral: 500 mg

cefadroxil (sef a DROKS il)

Synonyms cefadroxil monohydrate; Duricef

Canadian Brand Names Apo-Cefadroxil®; Novo-Cefadroxil; PRO-Cefadroxil

Therapeutic Category Cephalosporin (First Generation)

Use Treatment of susceptible bacterial infections, including those caused by group A beta-hemolytic *Streptococcus*

General Dosage Range Dosage adjustment recommended in patients with renal impairment
Oral:
Children: 30 mg/kg/day in 2 divided doses (maximum: 2 g/day)
Adults: 1-2 g/day in 2 divided doses

Dosage Forms
Capsule, oral: 500 mg
Powder for suspension, oral: 250 mg/5 mL (50 mL, 100 mL); 500 mg/5 mL (75 mL, 100 mL)
Tablet, oral: 1 g

cefadroxil monohydrate *see cefadroxil on page 180*

cefazolin (sef A zoe lin)

Medication Safety Issues
Sound-alike/look-alike issues:
CeFAZolin may be confused with cefoTEtan, cefOXitin, cefprozil, cefTAZidime, cefTRIAXone, cephalexin

Synonyms ancef; cefazolin sodium

Tall-Man ceFAZolin

Therapeutic Category Cephalosporin (First Generation)

Use Treatment of respiratory tract, skin, genital, urinary tract, biliary tract, bone and joint infections, and septicemia due to susceptible gram-positive cocci (except *Enterococcus*); some gram-negative bacilli including *E. coli*, *Proteus*, and *Klebsiella* may be susceptible; surgical prophylaxis

General Dosage Range Dosage adjustment recommended in patients with renal impairment
I.M., I.V.:
Children >1 month: 25-100 mg/kg/day divided every 6-8 hours (maximum: 6 g/day)
Adults: 250 mg to 1.5 g every 6-12 hours (maximum: 12 g/day)

Dosage Forms
Infusion, premixed iso-osmotic dextrose solution: 1 g (50 mL)
Injection, powder for reconstitution: 500 mg, 1 g, 10 g, 20 g, 100 g, 300 g

cefazolin sodium *see cefazolin on page 180*

cefdinir (SEF di ner)

Synonyms CFDN

U.S. Brand Names Omnicef®

Canadian Brand Names Omnicef®

Therapeutic Category Cephalosporin (Third Generation)

Use Treatment of community-acquired pneumonia, acute exacerbations of chronic bronchitis, acute bacterial otitis media, acute maxillary sinusitis, pharyngitis/tonsillitis, and uncomplicated skin and skin structure infections.

General Dosage Range Dosage adjustment recommended in patients with renal impairment

Oral:

Children 6 months to 12 years: 14 mg/kg/day in 1-2 divided doses (maximum: 600 mg/day)

Children >12 years and Adults: 600 mg/day in 1-2 divided doses

Dosage Forms

Capsule, oral: 300 mg

Omnicef®: 300 mg

Powder for suspension, oral: 125 mg/5 mL (60 mL, 100 mL); 250 mg/5 mL (60 mL, 100 mL)

Omnicef®: 125 mg/5 mL (60 mL, 100 mL); 250 mg/5 mL (60 mL, 100 mL)

cefditoren (sef de TOR en)

Medication Safety Issues

International issues:

Spectracef [U.S., Great Britain, Mexico, Portugal, Spain] may be confused with Spectrocef brand name for cefotaxime [Italy]

Synonyms cefditoren pivoxil

U.S. Brand Names Spectracef®

Therapeutic Category Antibiotic, Cephalosporin

Use Treatment of acute bacterial exacerbation of chronic bronchitis or community-acquired pneumonia (due to susceptible organisms including *Haemophilus influenzae*, *Haemophilus parainfluenzae*, *Streptococcus pneumoniae*-penicillin susceptible only, *Moraxella catarrhalis*); pharyngitis or tonsillitis (*Streptococcus pyogenes*); and uncomplicated skin and skin-structure infections (*Staphylococcus aureus* - not MRSA, *Streptococcus pyogenes*)

General Dosage Range Dosage adjustment recommended in patients with renal impairment

Oral: *Children ≥12 years and Adults:* 200-400 mg twice daily

Dosage Forms

Tablet, oral: 200 mg, 400 mg

Spectracef®: 200 mg, 400 mg

cefditoren pivoxil *see cefditoren on page 181*

cefepime (SEF e pim)

Medication Safety Issues

Sound-alike/look-alike issues:

Cefepime may be confused with cefixime, cefTAZidime

Synonyms cefepime hydrochloride

U.S. Brand Names Maxipime®

Canadian Brand Names Maxipime®

Therapeutic Category Cephalosporin (Fourth Generation)

Use Treatment of uncomplicated and complicated urinary tract infections, including pyelonephritis caused by *Escherichia coli, Klebsiella pneumoniae*, or *Proteus mirabilis*; monotherapy for febrile neutropenia; uncomplicated skin and skin structure infections caused by *Streptococcus pyogenes* or methicillin-susceptible staphylococci; moderate-to-severe pneumonia caused by *Streptococcus pneumoniae, Pseudomonas aeruginosa, Klebsiella pneumoniae*, or *Enterobacter* species; complicated intraabdominal infections (in combination with metronidazole) caused by *E. coli, P. aeruginosa, K. pneumoniae, Enterobacter* species, or *Bacteroides fragilis* against methicillin-susceptible staphylococci, *Enterobacter* sp, and many other gram-negative bacilli.

Children 2 months to 16 years: Empiric therapy of febrile neutropenia patients, uncomplicated skin/soft tissue infections, pneumonia, and uncomplicated/complicated urinary tract infections, including pyelonephritis.

◀ **General Dosage Range** Dosage adjustment recommended in patients with renal impairment
I.M.:
Children ≥2 months: 50 mg/kg/dose every 12 hours
Adults: 500-1000 mg every 12 hours
I.V.:
Children ≥2 months: 50 mg/kg/dose every 8-12 hours
Adults: 1-2 g every 8-12 hours
Dosage Forms
Infusion, premixed iso-osmotic dextrose solution: 1 g (50 mL); 2 g (100 mL)
Injection, powder for reconstitution: 1 g, 2 g
Maxipime®: 500 mg, 1 g, 2 g

cefepime hydrochloride *see* cefepime *on page 181*

cefotaxime (sef oh TAKS eem)

Medication Safety Issues
Sound-alike/look-alike issues:
Cefotaxime may be confused with cefOXitin, cefuroxime
International issues:
Spectrocef [Italy] may be confused with Spectracef brand name for cefditoren [U.S., Great Britain, Mexico, Portugal, Spain]
Synonyms cefotaxime sodium
U.S. Brand Names Claforan®
Canadian Brand Names Claforan®
Therapeutic Category Cephalosporin (Third Generation)
Use Treatment of susceptible infection in respiratory tract, skin and skin structure, bone and joint, urinary tract, gynecologic as well as septicemia, and documented or suspected meningitis. Active against most gram-negative bacilli (not *Pseudomonas*) and gram-positive cocci (not enterococcus). Active against many penicillin-resistant pneumococci.
General Dosage Range Dosage adjustment recommended in patients with hepatic or renal impairment
I.M.:
Children 1 month to 12 years and <50 kg: 50-200 mg/kg/day in divided doses every 6-8 hours (maximum: 12 g/day)
Children >12 years and ≥50 kg and Adults: 1-2 g every 8-12 hours **or** as a single dose
I.V.:
Children 1 month to 12 years and <50 kg: 50-200 mg/kg/day in divided doses every 6-8 hours (maximum: 12 g/day)
Children >12 years and ≥50 kg and Adults: 1-2 g every 4-12 hours
Dosage Forms
Infusion, premixed iso-osmotic solution:
Claforan®: 1 g (50 mL); 2 g (50 mL)
Injection, powder for reconstitution: 500 mg, 1 g, 2 g, 10 g, 20 g
Claforan®: 500 mg, 1 g, 2 g, 10 g

cefotaxime sodium *see* cefotaxime *on page 182*

cefoxitin (se FOKS i tin)

Medication Safety Issues
Sound-alike/look-alike issues:
CefOXitin may be confused with ceFAZolin, cefotaxime, cefoTEtan, cefTAZidime, cefTRIAXone, Cytoxan
Mefoxin® may be confused with Lanoxin®
Synonyms cefoxitin sodium
Tall-Man cefOXitin
U.S. Brand Names Mefoxin®
Canadian Brand Names Apo-Cefoxitin®
Therapeutic Category Cephalosporin (Second Generation)
Use Less active against staphylococci and streptococci than first generation cephalosporins, but active against anaerobes including *Bacteroides fragilis*; active against gram-negative enteric bacilli including *E. coli*, *Klebsiella*, and *Proteus*; used predominantly for respiratory tract, skin, bone and joint, urinary tract

and gynecologic as well as septicemia; surgical prophylaxis; intraabdominal infections and other mixed infections; indicated for bacterial *Eikenella corrodens* infections

General Dosage Range Dosage adjustment recommended in patients with renal impairment
I.M.:
  Children >3 months: 80-160 mg/kg/day divided every 4-6 hours (maximum: 12 g/day)
  Adolescents: 80-160 mg/kg/day divided every 4-6 hours (maximum: 12 g/day) **or** 1-2 g prior to surgery
  Adults: 1-2 g every 4-8 hours (maximum: 12 g/day) **or** 1-2 g prior to surgery
I.V.:
  Children >3 months: 80-160 mg/kg/day divided every 4-6 hours (maximum: 12 g/day) **or** 30-40 mg/kg prior to surgery
  Adolescents: 80-160 mg/kg/day divided every 4-6 hours (maximum: 12 g/day) **or** 1-2 g prior to surgery
  Adults: 1-2 g every 4-8 hours (maximum: 12 g/day) **or** 1-2 g prior to surgery
Dosage Forms
Infusion, premixed iso-osmotic dextrose solution:
  Mefoxin®: 1 g (50 mL); 2 g (50 mL)
Injection, powder for reconstitution: 1 g, 2 g, 10 g

cefoxitin sodium *see cefoxitin on page 182*

cefpodoxime (sef pode OKS eem)
Medication Safety Issues
Sound-alike/look-alike issues:
  Vantin may be confused with Ventolin®
Synonyms cefpodoxime proxetil; Vantin
Therapeutic Category Cephalosporin (Second Generation)
Use Treatment of susceptible acute, community-acquired pneumonia caused by *S. pneumoniae* or nonbeta-lactamase producing *H. influenzae*; acute uncomplicated gonorrhea caused by *N. gonorrhoeae*; uncomplicated skin and skin structure infections caused by *S. aureus* or *S. pyogenes*; acute otitis media caused by *S. pneumoniae, H. influenzae,* or *M. catarrhalis*; pharyngitis or tonsillitis; and uncomplicated urinary tract infections caused by *E. coli, Klebsiella,* and *Proteus*
General Dosage Range Dosage adjustment recommended in patients with renal impairment
Oral:
  Children 2 months to 12 years: 10 mg/kg/day divided every 12 hours (maximum: 400 mg/day)
  Children ≥12 years and Adults: 100-400 mg every 12 hours **or** 200 mg as a single dose
Dosage Forms
Granules for suspension, oral: 50 mg/5 mL (50 mL, 100 mL); 100 mg/5 mL (50 mL, 100 mL)
Tablet, oral: 100 mg, 200 mg

cefpodoxime proxetil *see cefpodoxime on page 183*

cefprozil (sef PROE zil)
Medication Safety Issues
Sound-alike/look-alike issues:
  Cefprozil may be confused with ceFAZolin, cefuroxime
  Cefzil may be confused with Ceftin®
Synonyms Cefzil
Canadian Brand Names Apo-Cefprozil®; Cefzil®; Mint-Cefprozil; RAN™-Cefprozil; Sandoz-Cefprozil
Therapeutic Category Cephalosporin (Second Generation)
Use Treatment of otitis media and infections involving the respiratory tract and skin and skin structure; active against methicillin-sensitive staphylococci, many streptococci, and various gram-negative bacilli including *E. coli*, some *Klebsiella, P. mirabilis, H. influenzae,* and *Moraxella.*
General Dosage Range Dosage adjustment recommended in patients with renal impairment
Oral:
  Children 6 months to 2 years: 7.5-30 mg/kg/day divided every 12 hours
  Children 2-12 years: 7.5-30 mg/kg/day divided every 12 hours **or** 20 mg/kg every 24 hours (maximum: 1 g/day)
  Adolescents >12 years and Adults: 250-500 mg every 12 hours **or** 500 mg every 24 hours
Dosage Forms
Powder for suspension, oral: 125 mg/5 mL (50 mL, 75 mL, 100 mL); 250 mg/5 mL (50 mL, 75 mL, 100 mL)
Tablet, oral: 250 mg, 500 mg

ceftaroline fosamil (sef TAR oh leen FOS a mil)

Synonyms PPI-0903; PPI-0903M; T-91825; TAK-599

U.S. Brand Names Teflaro™

Therapeutic Category Antibiotic, Cephalosporin (Fifth Generation)

Use Treatment of acute bacterial skin and skin structure infections (ABSSSI) caused by susceptible isolates of *Staphylococcus aureus* (including methicillin-susceptible and –resistant isolates), *Streptococcus pyogenes, Streptococcus agalactiae, Escherichia coli, Klebsiella pneumoniae,* and *Klebsiella oxytoca,* and community-acquired pneumonia (CAP) caused by *Streptococcus pneumoniae* (including cases with concurrent bacteremia), *Staphylococcus aureus* (methicillin-susceptible isolates only), *Haemophilus influenzae, Klebsiella pneumoniae, Klebsiella oxytoca,* and *Escherichia coli*

General Dosage Range Dosage adjustment recommended in patients with renal impairment.

I.V.: *Adults:* 600 mg every 12 hours

Dosage Forms

Injection, powder for reconstitution:
Teflaro™: 600 mg

ceftazidime (SEF tay zi deem)

Medication Safety Issues

Sound-alike/look-alike issues:
CefTAZidime may be confused with ceFAZolin, cefepime, cefoTEtan, cefOXitin, cefTRIAXone
Ceptaz® may be confused with Septra®
Tazicef® may be confused with Tazidime®
Tazidime® may be confused with Tazicef®

International issues:
Ceftim [Portugal] and Ceftime [Thailand] brand names for ceftazidime may be confused with Ceftin brand name for cefuroxime [U.S., Canada]; Cefiton brand name for cefixime [Portugal]

Tall-Man cefTAZidime

U.S. Brand Names Fortaz®; Tazicef®

Canadian Brand Names Fortaz®

Therapeutic Category Cephalosporin (Third Generation)

Use Treatment of documented susceptible *Pseudomonas aeruginosa* infection and infections due to other susceptible aerobic gram-negative organisms; empiric therapy of a febrile, granulocytopenic patient

General Dosage Range Dosage adjustment recommended in patients with renal impairment

I.M.: *Adults:* 500 mg to 2 g every 8-12 hours

I.V.:
Children 1 month to 12 years: 30-50 mg/kg every 8 hours (maximum: 6 g/day)
Children ≥12 years and Adults: 500 mg to 2 g every 8-12 hours (maximum: 6 g/day)

Dosage Forms

Infusion, premixed iso-osmotic solution:
Fortaz®: 1 g (50 mL); 2 g (50 mL)

Injection, powder for reconstitution: 500 mg, 1 g, 2 g, 6 g
Fortaz®: 500 mg, 1 g, 2 g, 6 g
Tazicef®: 1 g, 2 g, 6 g

ceftibuten (sef TYE byoo ten)

Medication Safety Issues

Sound-alike/look-alike issues:
Cedax® may be confused with Cidex®

International issues:
Cedax [U.S. and multiple international markets] may be confused with Codex brand name for acetaminophen/codeine [Brazil] and *Saccharomyces boulardii* [Italy]

U.S. Brand Names Cedax®

Therapeutic Category Cephalosporin (Third Generation)

Use Treatment of acute exacerbations of chronic bronchitis, acute bacterial otitis media, and pharyngitis/tonsillitis

General Dosage Range Dosage adjustment recommended in patients with renal impairment

Oral:
Children 6 months to <12 years: 9 mg/kg/day (maximum: 400 mg/day)
Children ≥12 years and Adults: 400 mg once daily

Dosage Forms
Capsule, oral:
Cedax®: 400 mg
Powder for suspension, oral:
Cedax®: 90 mg/5 mL (60 mL, 90 mL, 120 mL); 180 mg/5 mL (30 mL, 60 mL)

Ceftin® *see* cefuroxime *on page 185*

ceftriaxone (sef trye AKS one)

Medication Safety Issues
Sound-alike/look-alike issues:
CefTRIAXone may be confused with CeFAZolin, cefoTEtan, cefOXitin, cefTAZidime, Cetraxal®
Rocephin® may be confused with Roferon®

Synonyms ceftriaxone sodium

Tall-Man cefTRIAXone

U.S. Brand Names Rocephin®

Canadian Brand Names Ceftriaxone for Injection; Ceftriaxone Sodium for Injection BP; Rocephin®

Therapeutic Category Cephalosporin (Third Generation)

Use Treatment of lower respiratory tract infections, acute bacterial otitis media, skin and skin structure infections, bone and joint infections, intraabdominal and urinary tract infections, pelvic inflammatory disease (PID), uncomplicated gonorrhea, bacterial septicemia, and meningitis; used in surgical prophylaxis

General Dosage Range Dosage adjustment recommended in patients with hepatic and renal impairment
I.M.:
Children: 50-100 mg/kg/day divided every 12-24 hours (maximum: 4 g/day) **or** 125 mg or 50 mg/kg as a single dose
Adults: 1-2 g every 12-24 hours **or** 125-250 mg as a single dose
I.V.:
Children: 50-100 mg/kg/day divided every 12-24 hours (maximum: 4 g/day)
Adults: 1-2 g every 12-24 hours

Dosage Forms
Infusion, premixed in D$_5$W: 1 g (50 mL); 2 g (50 mL)
Injection, powder for reconstitution: 250 mg, 500 mg, 1 g, 2 g, 10 g
Rocephin®: 500 mg, 1 g

Ceftriaxone for Injection (Can) *see* ceftriaxone *on page 185*
ceftriaxone sodium *see* ceftriaxone *on page 185*
Ceftriaxone Sodium for Injection BP (Can) *see* ceftriaxone *on page 185*

cefuroxime (se fyoor OKS eem)

Medication Safety Issues
Sound-alike/look-alike issues:
Cefuroxime may be confused with cefotaxime, cefprozil, deferoxamine
Ceftin® may be confused with Cefzil®, Cipro®
Zinacef® may be confused with Zithromax®
International issues:
Ceftin [U.S., Canada] may be confused with Cefiton brand name for cefixime [Portugal]; Ceftim brand name for ceftazidime [Portugal]; Ceftime brand name for ceftazidime [Thailand]

Synonyms cefuroxime axetil; cefuroxime sodium

U.S. Brand Names Ceftin®; Zinacef®

Canadian Brand Names Apo-Cefuroxime®; Ceftin®; Cefuroxime For Injection; PRO-Cefuroxime; ratio-Cefuroxime

Therapeutic Category Cephalosporin (Second Generation)

Use Treatment of infections caused by staphylococci, group B streptococci, *H. influenzae* (type A and B), *E. coli*, *Enterobacter*, *Salmonella*, and *Klebsiella*; treatment of susceptible infections of the upper and lower respiratory tract, otitis media, urinary tract, uncomplicated skin and soft tissue, bone and joint, sepsis, uncomplicated gonorrhea, and early Lyme disease; surgical prophylaxis

◀ **General Dosage Range** Dosage adjustment recommended in patients with renal impairment
I.M., I.V.:
Children 3 months to 12 years: 75-150 mg/kg/day divided every 8 hours (maximum: 6 g/day)
Adolescents >12 years and Adults: 750 mg to 1.5 g every 6-8 hours (maximum: 6 g/day) **or** 1.5 g as a single dose
Oral:
Children 3 months to 12 years: 20-30 mg/kg/day in 2 divided doses **or** 125-250 mg every 12 hours (maximum: 1 g/day)
Adolescents >12 years and Adults: 125-500 mg every 12 hours **or** 1 g as a single dose
Dosage Forms
Infusion, premixed iso-osmotic solution:
Zinacef®: 750 mg (50 mL); 1.5 g (50 mL)
Injection, powder for reconstitution: 750 mg, 1.5 g, 7.5 g, 75 g
Zinacef®: 750 mg, 1.5 g, 7.5 g
Powder for suspension, oral: 125 mg/5 mL (100 mL); 250 mg/5 mL (50 mL, 100 mL)
Ceftin®: 125 mg/5 mL (100 mL); 250 mg/5 mL (50 mL, 100 mL)
Tablet, oral: 250 mg, 500 mg
Ceftin®: 250 mg, 500 mg

cefuroxime axetil *see* cefuroxime *on page 185*
Cefuroxime For Injection (Can) *see* cefuroxime *on page 185*
cefuroxime sodium *see* cefuroxime *on page 185*
Cefzil *see* cefprozil *on page 183*
Cefzil® (Can) *see* cefprozil *on page 183*
CeleBREX® *see* celecoxib *on page 186*
Celebrex® (Can) *see* celecoxib *on page 186*

celecoxib (se le KOKS ib)
Medication Safety Issues
Sound-alike/look-alike issues:
CeleBREX® may be confused with CeleXA®, Cerebyx®, Cervarix®, Clarinex®
U.S. Brand Names CeleBREX®
Canadian Brand Names Celebrex®
Therapeutic Category Nonsteroidal Antiinflammatory Drug (NSAID), COX-2 Selective
Use Relief of the signs and symptoms of osteoarthritis, ankylosing spondylitis, juvenile idiopathic arthritis (JIA), and rheumatoid arthritis; management of acute pain; treatment of primary dysmenorrhea
General Dosage Range Dosage adjustment recommended in patients with hepatic impairment
Oral:
Children ≥2 years and ≥10 kg to ≤25 kg: 50 mg twice daily
Children ≥2 years and >25 kg: 100 mg twice daily
Adults: 100-400 mg/day in 1-2 divided doses
Dosage Forms
Capsule, oral:
CeleBREX®: 50 mg, 100 mg, 200 mg, 400 mg

Celestone® *see* betamethasone *on page 129*
Celestone® Soluspan® *see* betamethasone *on page 129*
CeleXA® *see* citalopram *on page 213*
Celexa® (Can) *see* citalopram *on page 213*
CellCept® *see* mycophenolate *on page 604*
Cellugel® *see* hydroxypropyl methylcellulose *on page 455*

cellulose, oxidized regenerated (SEL yoo lose, OKS i dyzed re JEN er aye ted)
Synonyms absorbable cotton; oxidized regenerated cellulose
U.S. Brand Names Surgicel®; Surgicel® Fibrillar; Surgicel® NuKnit
Therapeutic Category Hemostatic Agent
Use Hemostatic; temporary packing for the control of capillary, venous, or small arterial hemorrhage
General Dosage Range Topical: *Adults:* Lay or hold firmly minimal amounts of the fabric strip on the bleeding site

Dosage Forms
  Fabric, fibrous:
   Surgicel® Fibrillar:
    1" x 2" (10s)
    2" x 4" (10s)
    4" x 4" (10s)
  Fabric, knitted:
   Surgicel® NuKnit:
    1" x 1" (24s)
    1" x 3¹/₂" (10s)
    3" x 4" (24s)
    6" x 9" (10s)
  Fabric, sheer weave:
   Surgicel®:
    ¹/₂" x 2" (24s)
    2" x 3" (24s)
    2" x 14" (24s)
    4" x 8" (24s)

Celluvisc™ (Can) *see* carboxymethylcellulose *on page 175*
Celontin® *see* methsuximide *on page 573*
Celsentri™ (Can) *see* maraviroc *on page 549*
Cemill 500 [OTC] *see* ascorbic acid *on page 96*
Cemill 1000 [OTC] *see* ascorbic acid *on page 96*
Cenestin® *see* estrogens (conjugated A/synthetic) *on page 347*
Cenestin (Can) *see* estrogens (conjugated A/synthetic) *on page 347*
Centamin [OTC] *see* vitamins (multiple/oral) *on page 919*
Centany® *see* mupirocin *on page 603*
Centany® AT *see* mupirocin *on page 603*
Centrum® [OTC] *see* vitamins (multiple/oral) *on page 919*
Centrum Cardio® [OTC] *see* vitamins (multiple/oral) *on page 919*
Centrum Kids® [OTC] *see* vitamins (multiple/pediatric) *on page 920*
Centrum Performance® [OTC] *see* vitamins (multiple/oral) *on page 919*
Centrum® Silver® [OTC] *see* vitamins (multiple/oral) *on page 919*
Centrum® Silver® Ultra Men's [OTC] *see* vitamins (multiple/oral) *on page 919*
Centrum® Silver® Ultra Women's [OTC] *see* vitamins (multiple/oral) *on page 919*
Centrum® Ultra Men's [OTC] *see* vitamins (multiple/oral) *on page 919*
Centrum® Ultra Women's [OTC] *see* vitamins (multiple/oral) *on page 919*
Centruroides **immune FAB2 (equine)** *see Centruroides* immune F(ab')₂ (equine) *on page 187*

Centruroides immune F(ab')₂ (equine) (sen tra ROY dez i MYUN fab too E kwine)

Synonyms *Centruroides* immune FAB2 (equine); antivenin (*Centruroides*) immune F(ab')₂ (equine); antivenin scorpion; scorpion antivenin
U.S. Brand Names Anascorp®
Therapeutic Category Antivenin
Use Treatment of scorpion envenomation
General Dosage Range
  I.V.: *Children and Adults:* Initial: 3 vials; may administer additional vials in 1-vial increments every 30-60 minutes as needed.
Dosage Forms
  Injection, powder for reconstitution:
   Anascorp®: ≤120 mg total protein

Cepacol® [OTC] *see* cetylpyridinium *on page 190*
Cepacol® Fizzlers™ [OTC] *see* benzocaine *on page 121*
Cepacol® Sore Throat Pain Relief [OTC] *see* benzocaine *on page 121*
Cepacol® Sore Throat Plus Coating Relief [OTC] *see* benzocaine *on page 121*
Cepastat® [OTC] *see* phenol *on page 694*

Cepastat® Extra Strength [OTC] *see* phenol *on page 694*
Cephadyn *see* butalbital and acetaminophen *on page 153*

cephalexin (sef a LEKS in)

Medication Safety Issues
Sound-alike/look-alike issues:
Cephalexin may be confused with cefaclor, ceFAZolin, ciprofloxacin
Keflex® may be confused with Keppra®, Valtrex®
Synonyms cephalexin monohydrate
U.S. Brand Names Keflex®
Canadian Brand Names Apo-Cephalex®; Dom-Cephalexin; Keflex®; Keftab®; Novo-Lexin; Nu-Cephalex; PMS-Cephalexin
Therapeutic Category Cephalosporin (First Generation)
Use Treatment of susceptible bacterial infections including respiratory tract infections, otitis media, skin and skin structure infections, bone infections, and genitourinary tract infections, including acute prostatitis; alternative therapy for acute infective endocarditis prophylaxis
General Dosage Range Dosage adjustment recommended in patients with renal impairment
Oral:
Children >1-15 years: 25-100 mg/kg/day divided every 6-12 hours (maximum: 4 g/day) **or** 50 mg/kg prior to procedure (maximum: 2 g)
Adolescents >15 years: 25-100 mg/kg/day divided every 6-12 hours (maximum: 4 g/day) **or** 50 mg/kg prior to procedure (maximum: 2 g) **or** 500 mg every 12 hours
Adults: 250-1000 mg every 6 hours **or** 500 mg every 12 hours (maximum: 4 g/day) **or** 2 g prior to procedure
Dosage Forms
Capsule, oral: 250 mg, 500 mg
Keflex®: 250 mg, 500 mg, 750 mg
Powder for suspension, oral: 125 mg/5 mL (100 mL, 200 mL); 250 mg/5 mL (100 mL, 200 mL)
Tablet, oral: 250 mg, 500 mg

cephalexin monohydrate *see* cephalexin *on page 188*
Ceprotin *see* protein C concentrate (human) *on page 750*
Cerebyx® *see* fosphenytoin *on page 401*
Ceredase® *see* alglucerase *on page 51*
Cerefolin® NAC *see* methylfolate, methylcobalamin, and acetylcysteine *on page 576*
Cerezyme® *see* imiglucerase *on page 466*
Ceron [DSC] *see* chlorpheniramine and phenylephrine *on page 198*
Ceron-DM [DSC] *see* chlorpheniramine, phenylephrine, and dextromethorphan *on page 200*
Certain Dri® [OTC] *see* aluminum chloride hexahydrate *on page 59*

certolizumab pegol (cer to LIZ u mab PEG ol)

Synonyms CDP870
U.S. Brand Names Cimzia®
Canadian Brand Names Cimzia®
Therapeutic Category Gastrointestinal Agent, Miscellaneous; Tumor Necrosis Factor (TNF) Blocking Agent
Use Treatment of moderately- to severely-active Crohn disease in patients who have inadequate response to conventional therapy; moderately- to severely-active rheumatoid arthritis (as monotherapy or in combination with nonbiological disease-modifying antirheumatic drugs [DMARDS])
General Dosage Range SubQ: Adults: Initial: 400 mg, repeat dose 2 and 4 weeks after initial dose; Maintenance: 400 mg every 4 weeks **or** 200 mg every other week
Dosage Forms
Injection, powder for reconstitution [preservative free]:
Cimzia®: 200 mg
Injection, solution [preservative free]:
Cimzia®: 200 mg/mL (1 mL)

Certuss-D® [DSC] *see* guaifenesin, dextromethorphan, and phenylephrine *on page 429*
Cerubidine® *see* daunorubicin hydrochloride *on page 255*

Cervarix® *see* papillomavirus (types 16, 18) vaccine (human, recombinant) *on page 673*
Cervidil® *see* dinoprostone *on page 289*
C.E.S. *see* estrogens (conjugated/equine, systemic) *on page 347*
C.E.S. *see* estrogens (conjugated/equine, topical) *on page 348*
C.E.S.® (Can) *see* estrogens (conjugated/equine, systemic) *on page 347*
Cesia® [DSC] *see* ethinyl estradiol and desogestrel *on page 351*
Cetacaine® *see* benzocaine, butamben, and tetracaine *on page 123*
Cetafen® [OTC] *see* acetaminophen *on page 23*
Cetafen Cold® [OTC] *see* acetaminophen and phenylephrine *on page 28*
Cetafen® Extra [OTC] *see* acetaminophen *on page 23*

cetirizine (se TI ra zeen)

Medication Safety Issues
Sound-alike/look-alike issues:
ZyrTEC® may be confused with Lipitor®, Serax, Xanax®, Zantac®, Zerit®, Zocor®, ZyPREXA®, ZyrTEC-D®
ZyrTEC® (cetirizine) may be confused with ZyrTEC® Itchy Eye (ketotifen)
Synonyms cetirizine hydrochloride; P-071; UCB-P071
U.S. Brand Names All Day Allergy [OTC]; ZyrTEC® Allergy [OTC]; ZyrTEC® Children's Allergy [OTC]; ZyrTEC® Children's Hives Relief [OTC]
Canadian Brand Names Apo-Cetirizine®; PMS-Cetirizine; Reactine™
Therapeutic Category Antihistamine
Use Perennial and seasonal allergic rhinitis and other allergic symptoms including urticaria; chronic idiopathic urticaria
General Dosage Range Dosage adjustment recommended in patients with hepatic or renal impairment
Oral:
Children 6-12 months: 2.5 mg once daily
Children 12 months to <2 years: 2.5 mg once or twice daily
Children 2-5 years: 2.5-5 mg/day in 1-2 divided doses
Children ≥6 years and Adults: 5-10 mg once daily
Elderly: Initial: 5 mg once daily
Dosage Forms
Capsule, liquid gel, oral:
ZyrTEC® Allergy [OTC]: 10 mg
Solution, oral: 5 mg/5 mL (5 mL)
Syrup, oral: 5 mg/5 mL (5 mL, 118 mL, 120 mL, 473 mL, 480 mL)
ZyrTEC® Children's Allergy [OTC]: 5 mg/5 mL (118 mL)
ZyrTEC® Children's Hives Relief [OTC]: 5 mg/5 mL (118 mL)
Tablet, oral: 5 mg, 10 mg
All Day Allergy [OTC]: 10 mg
ZyrTEC® Allergy [OTC]: 10 mg
Tablet, chewable, oral: 5 mg, 10 mg
All Day Allergy [OTC]: 5 mg
ZyrTEC® Children's Allergy [OTC]: 5 mg, 10 mg

cetirizine and pseudoephedrine (se TI ra zeen & soo doe e FED rin)

Medication Safety Issues
Sound-alike/look-alike issues:
ZyrTEC® may be confused with Lipitor®, Serax, Xanax®, Zantac®, Zocor®, Zyprexa®, Zyrtec-D®
ZyrTEC-D® may be confused with ZyrTEC®
Synonyms cetirizine hydrochloride and pseudoephedrine hydrochloride; pseudoephedrine hydrochloride and cetirizine hydrochloride
U.S. Brand Names ZyrTEC-D® Allergy & Congestion [OTC]
Canadian Brand Names Reactine® Allergy and Sinus
Therapeutic Category Antihistamine/Decongestant Combination
Use Treatment of symptoms of seasonal or perennial allergic rhinitis
General Dosage Range Dosage adjustment recommended in patients with hepatic or renal impairment
Oral: *Children ≥12 years:* 1 tablet twice daily (maximum: 2 tablets/day)

◄ **Dosage Forms**
Tablet, extended release: Cetirizine hydrochloride 5 mg and pseudoephedrine hydrochloride 120 mg
ZyrTEC-D® Allergy & Congestion [OTC]: Cetirizine 5 mg and pseudoephedrine 120 mg

cetirizine hydrochloride *see cetirizine on page 189*

cetirizine hydrochloride and pseudoephedrine hydrochloride *see cetirizine and pseudoephedrine on page 189*

Cetraxal® *see ciprofloxacin (otic) on page 211*

cetrorelix (set roe REL iks)

Synonyms cetrorelix acetate
U.S. Brand Names Cetrotide®
Canadian Brand Names Cetrotide®
Therapeutic Category Antigonadotropic Agent
Use Inhibits premature luteinizing hormone (LH) surges in women undergoing controlled ovarian stimulation
General Dosage Range SubQ: *Adults (females):* 0.25 mg once daily **or** 3 mg as a single dose
Dosage Forms
Injection, powder for reconstitution:
Cetrotide®: 0.25 mg, 3 mg

cetrorelix acetate *see cetrorelix on page 190*
Cetrotide® *see cetrorelix on page 190*

cetuximab (se TUK see mab)

Medication Safety Issues
Sound-alike/look-alike issues:
Cetuximab may be confused with bevacizumab
Synonyms C225; IMC-C225; MOAB C225
U.S. Brand Names Erbitux®
Canadian Brand Names Erbitux®
Therapeutic Category Antineoplastic Agent, Monoclonal Antibody; Epidermal Growth Factor Receptor (EGFR) Inhibitor
Use Treatment of metastatic colorectal cancer; treatment of squamous cell cancer of the head and neck

Note: Subset analyses (retrospective) in metastatic colorectal cancer trials have not shown a benefit with EGFR inhibitor treatment in patients whose tumors have codon 12 or 13 *KRAS* mutations; use is not recommended in these patients.
General Dosage Range Dosage adjustment recommended in patients who develop toxicities
I.V.: *Adults:* Loading dose: 400 mg/m^2; Maintenance: 250 mg/m^2 weekly
Dosage Forms
Injection, solution [preservative free]:
Erbitux®: 2 mg/mL (50 mL, 100 mL)

cetyl alcohol, glycerin, lanolin, mineral oil, and petrolatum *see lanolin, cetyl alcohol, glycerin, petrolatum, and mineral oil on page 510*

cetylpyridinium (SEE til peer i DI nee um)

Synonyms cetylpyridinium chloride; CPC
U.S. Brand Names Cepacol® [OTC]; DiabetAid Therapeutic Gingivitis Mouth Rinse [OTC]
Therapeutic Category Local Anesthetic
Use Antiseptic to aid in the prevention and reduction of plaque and gingivitis, and to freshen breath
General Dosage Range Oral: *Children ≥6 years and Adults:* Rinse or gargle in mouth
Dosage Forms
Liquid, oral:
Cepacol® [OTC]: 0.05% (360 mL, 720 mL)
DiabetAid Therapeutic Gingivitis Mouth Rinse [OTC]: 0.1% (480 mL)

cetylpyridinium chloride *see cetylpyridinium on page 190*

cevimeline (se vi ME leen)

Medication Safety Issues
  Sound-alike/look-alike issues:
    Cevimeline may be confused with Savella®
    Evoxac® may be confused with Eurax®
Synonyms cevimeline hydrochloride
U.S. Brand Names Evoxac®
Canadian Brand Names Evoxac®
Therapeutic Category Cholinergic Agent
Use Treatment of symptoms of dry mouth in patients with Sjögren syndrome
General Dosage Range Oral: *Adults:* 30 mg 3 times/day
Dosage Forms
  Capsule, oral:
    Evoxac®: 30 mg

cevimeline hydrochloride *see* cevimeline *on page 191*
CFDN *see* cefdinir *on page 180*
CG *see* chorionic gonadotropin (human) *on page 206*
CG5503 *see* tapentadol *on page 844*
C-Gel [OTC] *see* ascorbic acid *on page 96*
CGP 33101 *see* rufinamide *on page 793*
CGP-39393 *see* desirudin *on page 261*
CGP-42446 *see* zoledronic acid *on page 932*
CGP-57148B *see* imatinib *on page 465*
C-Gram [OTC] *see* ascorbic acid *on page 96*
CGS-20267 *see* letrozole *on page 515*
Champix® (Can) *see* varenicline *on page 908*
Chantix® *see* varenicline *on page 908*
Charcadole® (Can) *see* charcoal *on page 191*
Charcadole®, Aqueous (Can) *see* charcoal *on page 191*
Charcadole® TFS (Can) *see* charcoal *on page 191*
Char-Caps [OTC] *see* charcoal *on page 191*

charcoal (CHAR kole)

Medication Safety Issues
  Sound-alike/look-alike issues:
    Actidose® may be confused with Actos®
Synonyms activated carbon; activated charcoal; adsorbent charcoal; liquid antidote; medicinal carbon; medicinal charcoal
U.S. Brand Names Actidose® with Sorbitol [OTC]; Actidose®-Aqua [OTC]; Char-Caps [OTC]; Charcoal Plus® DS [OTC]; CharcoCaps® [OTC]; EZ-Char® [OTC]; Kerr Insta-Char® [OTC]; Requa® Activated Charcoal [OTC]
Canadian Brand Names Charcadole®; Charcadole® TFS; Charcadole®, Aqueous
Therapeutic Category Antidote
Use Emergency treatment in poisoning by drugs and chemicals; aids the elimination of certain drugs and improves decontamination of excessive ingestions of sustained-release products or in the presence of bezoars; repetitive doses have proven useful to enhance the elimination of certain drugs (eg, carbamazepine, dapsone, phenobarbital, quinine, or theophylline); repetitive doses for gastric dialysis in uremia to adsorb various waste products; dietary supplement (digestive aid)
General Dosage Range Oral:
  Children <1 year: 10-25 g **or** 0.5-1 g/kg as a single dose; additional doses can be given as 0.25 g/kg/hour or equivalent
  Children 1-12 years: 25-50 g **or** 0.5-1 g/kg as a single dose; additional doses can be given as 0.25 g/kg/hour or equivalent
  Children >12 years: 25-100 g **or** 1 g/kg as a single dose; additional doses can be given as 12.5 g/hour (0.25 g/kg/hour) or equivalent

◄ *Adults:* Acute poisoning: 25-100 mg as a single dose; additional doses can be given as 12.5 g/hour or equivalent; Dietary supplement: 500-520 mg after meals, may repeat in 2 hours (maximum: 10 g/day)

Dosage Forms
Capsule, oral:
Char-Caps [OTC]: 260 mg
CharcoCaps® [OTC]: 260 mg
Pellets for suspension, oral:
EZ-Char® [OTC]: 25 g/bottle (1s)
Powder for suspension, oral: USP: 100% (30 g, 240 g)
Suspension, oral:
Actidose® with Sorbitol [OTC]: 25 g (120 mL); 50 g (240 mL)
Actidose®-Aqua [OTC]: 15 g (72 mL); 25 g (120 mL); 50 g (240 mL)
Kerr Insta-Char® [OTC]: 25 g (120 mL); 50 g (240 mL)
Tablet, oral:
Requa® Activated Charcoal [OTC]: 250 mg
Tablet, enteric coated, oral:
Charcoal Plus® DS [OTC]: 250 mg

Charcoal Plus® DS [OTC] *see* charcoal *on page 191*
CharcoCaps® [OTC] *see* charcoal *on page 191*
Chemet® *see* succimer *on page 832*
Chenodal™ *see* chenodiol *on page 192*
chenodeoxycholic acid *see* chenodiol *on page 192*

chenodiol (kee noe DYE ole)

Synonyms CDCA; chenodeoxycholic acid
U.S. Brand Names Chenodal™
Therapeutic Category Bile Acid
Use Oral dissolution of radiolucent cholesterol gallstones in selected patients as an alternative to surgery
General Dosage Range Oral: *Adults:* Initial: 250 mg twice daily; Maintenance: 13-16 mg/kg/day in 2 divided doses
Dosage Forms
Tablet, oral:
Chenodal™: 250 mg

Cheracol® D [OTC] *see* guaifenesin and dextromethorphan *on page 427*
Cheracol® Plus [OTC] *see* guaifenesin and dextromethorphan *on page 427*
Cheracol® Spray [OTC] *see* phenol *on page 694*
cheratussin *see* guaifenesin *on page 425*
Chew-C [OTC] *see* ascorbic acid *on page 96*
Chew-Cal [OTC] *see* calcium and vitamin D *on page 160*
CHG *see* chlorhexidine gluconate *on page 194*
chickenpox vaccine *see* varicella virus vaccine *on page 908*
Chiggerex® Plus [OTC] *see* benzocaine *on page 121*
ChiggerTox® [OTC] *see* benzocaine *on page 121*
Children's Advil® Cold (Can) *see* pseudoephedrine and ibuprofen *on page 753*
Children's Advil® Cold and Flu Multi-Symptom (Can) *see* ibuprofen, pseudoephedrine, and chlorpheniramine *on page 462*
Children's Nasal Decongestant [OTC] *see* pseudoephedrine *on page 751*
Children's Pepto [OTC] *see* calcium carbonate *on page 161*
children's vitamins *see* vitamins (multiple/pediatric) *on page 920*
Children's Motion Sickness Liquid (Can) *see* dimenhydrinate *on page 288*
ChiRhoStim® *see* secretin *on page 806*
chloditan *see* mitotane *on page 593*
chlodithane *see* mitotane *on page 593*
chloral *see* chloral hydrate *on page 193*

chloral hydrate (KLOR al HYE drate)

Medication Safety Issues
High alert medication:
The Institute for Safe Medication Practices (ISMP) includes this medication among its list of drugs which have a heightened risk of causing significant patient harm when used in error.
Synonyms chloral; hydrated chloral; trichloroacetaldehyde monohydrate
U.S. Brand Names Somnote®
Canadian Brand Names PMS-Chloral Hydrate
Therapeutic Category Hypnotic, Nonbarbiturate
Controlled Substance C-IV
Use Short-term sedative and hypnotic (<2 weeks); sedative/hypnotic for diagnostic procedures; sedative prior to EEG evaluations
General Dosage Range Oral:
Children: Dosage varies greatly depending on indication
Adults: 250 mg 3 times/day **or** 500-1000 mg at bedtime or prior to procedure (maximum: 2 g/day)
Elderly: Hypnotic (oral): Initial: 250 mg at bedtime
Dosage Forms
Capsule, oral:
Somnote®: 500 mg
Syrup, oral: 500 mg/5 mL (5 mL, 473 mL, 480 mL)

chlorambucil (klor AM byoo sil)

Medication Safety Issues
Sound-alike/look-alike issues:
Chlorambucil may be confused with Chloromycetin®
Leukeran® may be confused with Alkeran®, leucovorin, Leukine®, Myleran®
High alert medication:
The Institute for Safe Medication Practices (ISMP) includes this medication among its list of drugs which have a heightened risk of causing significant patient harm when used in error.
Synonyms CB-1348; chlorambucilum; chloraminophene; chlorbutinum; WR-139013
U.S. Brand Names Leukeran®
Canadian Brand Names Leukeran®
Therapeutic Category Antineoplastic Agent
Use Management of chronic lymphocytic leukemia (CLL), Hodgkin lymphoma, non-Hodgkin lymphoma (NHL)
General Dosage Range Dosage adjustment recommended in patients with renal impairment or who develop toxicities
Oral:
Adults: 0.1-0.2 mg/kg/day for 3-6 weeks **or** 0.4 mg/kg biweekly or monthly (may increase by 0.1 mg/kg/ dose) **or** 0.03-0.1 mg/kg/day
Elderly: Usual dose: 2-4 mg/day
Dosage Forms
Tablet, oral:
Leukeran®: 2 mg

chlorambucilum *see* chlorambucil *on page 193*
chloraminophene *see* chlorambucil *on page 193*

chloramphenicol (klor am FEN i kole)

Medication Safety Issues
Sound-alike/look-alike issues:
Chloromycetin® may be confused with chlorambucil, Chlor-Trimeton®
Canadian Brand Names Chloromycetin®; Chloromycetin® Succinate; Diochloram®; Pentamycetin®
Therapeutic Category Antibiotic, Miscellaneous
Use Treatment of serious infections due to organisms resistant to other less toxic antibiotics or when its penetrability into the site of infection is clinically superior to other antibiotics to which the organism is sensitive; useful in infections caused by *Bacteroides, H. influenzae, Neisseria meningitidis, Salmonella,* and *Rickettsia;* active against many vancomycin-resistant enterococci

◀ **General Dosage Range I.V.:**
Infants >30 days, Children, and Adults: 50-100 mg/kg/day divided every 6 hours (maximum: 4 g/day)
Dosage Forms
Injection, powder for reconstitution: 1 g

ChloraPrep® [OTC] *see* chlorhexidine gluconate *on page 194*
ChloraPrep® Frepp® [OTC] *see* chlorhexidine gluconate *on page 194*
ChloraPrep® Sepp® [OTC] *see* chlorhexidine gluconate *on page 194*
Chlorascrub™ [OTC] *see* chlorhexidine gluconate *on page 194*
Chlorascrub™ Maxi [OTC] *see* chlorhexidine gluconate *on page 194*
Chloraseptic® Kids Sore Throat Spray [OTC] *see* phenol *on page 694*
Chloraseptic® Mouth Pain [OTC] *see* phenol *on page 694*
Chloraseptic® Sore Throat Gargle [OTC] *see* phenol *on page 694*
Chloraseptic® Sore Throat Spray [OTC] *see* phenol *on page 694*
chlorbutinum *see* chlorambucil *on page 193*
Chlordex GP [DSC] *see* dextromethorphan, chlorpheniramine, phenylephrine, and guaifenesin *on page 272*

chlordiazepoxide (klor dye az e POKS ide)

Medication Safety Issues
Sound-alike/look-alike issues:
ChlordiazePOXIDE may be confused with chlorproMAZINE
Librium may be confused with Librax®
BEERS Criteria medication:
This drug may be inappropriate for use in geriatric patients (high severity risk).
Synonyms Librium; methaminodiazepoxide hydrochloride
Tall-Man chlordiazePOXIDE
Canadian Brand Names Apo-Chlordiazepoxide®
Therapeutic Category Benzodiazepine
Controlled Substance C-IV
Use Management of anxiety disorder or for the short-term relief of symptoms of anxiety; withdrawal symptoms of acute alcoholism; preoperative apprehension and anxiety
General Dosage Range Dosage adjustment recommended in patients with renal or hepatic impairment.
Oral:
Children ≥6 years: 10-30 mg/day in 2-4 divided doses
Adults: 15-100 mg/day in 3-4 divided doses **or** 50-100 mg to start, may repeat as needed (maximum: 300 mg/day)
Elderly: 10-20 mg/day in 2-4 divided doses
Dosage Forms
Capsule, oral: 5 mg, 10 mg, 25 mg

chlordiazepoxide and amitriptyline hydrochloride *see* amitriptyline and chlordiazepoxide *on page 68*
chlordiazepoxide and clidinium *see* clidinium and chlordiazepoxide *on page 217*
chlorethazine *see* mechlorethamine *on page 552*
chlorethazine mustard *see* mechlorethamine *on page 552*

chlorhexidine gluconate (klor HEKS i deen GLOO koe nate)

Medication Safety Issues
Sound-alike/look-alike issues:
Peridex® may be confused with Precedex®
Synonyms 3M™ Avagard™ [OTC]; CHG
U.S. Brand Names Avagard™ [OTC]; Bactoshield® CHG [OTC]; Betasept® [OTC]; ChloraPrep® Frepp® [OTC]; ChloraPrep® Sepp® [OTC]; ChloraPrep® [OTC]; Chlorascrub™ Maxi [OTC]; Chlorascrub™ [OTC]; Dyna-Hex® [OTC]; Hibiclens® [OTC]; Hibistat® [OTC]; Operand® Chlorhexidine Gluconate [OTC]; Peridex®; periochip®; PerioGard® [OTC]
Canadian Brand Names Hibidil® 1:2000; ORO-Clense; Peridex® Oral Rinse
Therapeutic Category Antibiotic, Oral Rinse; Antibiotic, Topical

Use Skin cleanser for line placement, skin wounds, preoperative skin preparation; germicidal hand rinse; antibacterial dental rinse. Chlorhexidine is active against gram-positive and gram-negative organisms, facultative anaerobes, aerobes, and yeast. Chip, for periodontal pocket insertion: Reduces pocket depth in patients with adult periodontitis

Orphan drug: Peridex®: Oral mucositis with cytoreductive therapy when used for patients undergoing bone marrow transplant

General Dosage Range
Oral:
Periodontal chip: *Adults:* 1 chip is inserted into a periodontal pocket, repeat every 3 months in pockets with depth ≥5 mm (maximum: 8 chips/visit)
Rinse: *Adults:* Swish 15 mL in mouth, then expectorate twice daily
Topical:
Rinse/wash: *Adults:* Apply for 15 seconds and rinse
Sanitizer: *Adults:* Dispense 1 pumpful in each palm; repeat once
Scrub: *Adults:* Scrub 3 minutes and rinse, then wash for additional 3 minutes

Dosage Forms
Chip, for periodontal pocket insertion:
periochip®: 2.5 mg (20s)
Liquid, oral: 0.12% (15 mL, 473 mL, 475 mL, 480 mL)
Peridex®: 0.12% (118 mL, 473 mL, 1893 mL)
PerioGard® [OTC]: 0.12% (480 mL)
Liquid, topical:
Betasept® [OTC]: 4% (118 mL, 237 mL, 473 mL, 946 mL, 3840 mL)
Dyna-Hex® [OTC]: 2% (120 mL, 480 mL, 960 mL, 3840 mL); 4% (120 mL, 240 mL, 480 mL, 960 mL, 3840 mL)
Hibiclens® [OTC]: 4% (15 mL, 118 mL, 236 mL, 473 mL, 946 mL, 3840 mL)
Operand® Chlorhexidine Gluconate [OTC]: 2% (118 mL); 4% (118 mL, 237 mL, 472 mL, 946 mL, 3785 mL)
Lotion, topical:
Avagard™ [OTC]: 1% (500 mL)
Solution, topical:
Bactoshield® CHG [OTC]: 2% (120 mL, 480 mL, 750 mL, 960 mL, 3840 mL); 4% (120 mL, 473 mL, 960 mL, 3840 mL)
Sponge, topical:
ChloraPrep® [OTC]: 2% (25s); 2% (25s); 2% (25s); 2% (25s); 2% (25s); 2% (25s); 2% (25s); 2% (25s)
ChloraPrep® Frepp® [OTC]: 2% (20s)
ChloraPrep® Sepp® [OTC]: 2% (200s)
Sponge/Brush, topical:
Bactoshield® CHG [OTC]: 4% (300s)
Swab, topical:
Chlorascrub™ [OTC]: 3.15% (100s)
Swabsticks, topical:
ChloraPrep® [OTC]: 2% (48s, 120s)
Chlorascrub™ [OTC]: 3.15% (50s)
Chlorascrub™ Maxi [OTC]: 3.15% (30s)
Wipe, topical:
Hibistat® [OTC]: 0.5% (50s)

Chlor Hist [OTC] *see chlorpheniramine on page 197*
chlormeprazine *see prochlorperazine on page 740*
Chlor-Mes-D [DSC] *see chlorpheniramine, phenylephrine, and methscopolamine on page 200*
2-chlorodeoxyadenosine *see cladribine on page 214*
chloroethane *see ethyl chloride on page 359*
Chloromag® *see magnesium chloride on page 544*
Chloromycetin® (Can) *see chloramphenicol on page 193*
Chloromycetin® Succinate (Can) *see chloramphenicol on page 193*

chlorophyll (KLOR oh fil)
Synonyms chlorophyllin
U.S. Brand Names Nullo® [OTC]
Therapeutic Category Gastrointestinal Agent, Miscellaneous

◀ **Use** Control fecal odors in colostomy or ileostomy

General Dosage Range
Oral: *Children >12 years and Adults:* 100-200 mg/day in divided doses (maximum: 300 mg/day)
Ostomy: *Children >12 years and Adults:* Place 1-2 tablets in empty pouch each time it is reused or changed

Dosage Forms
Caplet, oral:
Nullo® [OTC]: Chlorophyllin copper complex 100 mg

chlorophyllin *see* chlorophyll *on page 195*

chloroprocaine (klor oh PROE kane)

Medication Safety Issues
Sound-alike/look-alike issues:
Nesacaine® may be confused with Neptazane™
High alert medication:
The Institute for Safe Medication Practices (ISMP) includes this medication (epidural administration) among its list of drug classes which have a heightened risk of causing significant patient harm when used in error.

Synonyms chloroprocaine hydrochloride

U.S. Brand Names Nesacaine®; Nesacaine®-MPF

Canadian Brand Names Nesacaine®-CE

Therapeutic Category Local Anesthetic

Use Infiltration anesthesia, peripheral nerve block, epidural anesthesia

General Dosage Range
Caudal block: *Adults:* Preservative-free: 2% or 3%: 15-25 mL; may repeat at 40-60 minute intervals
Infiltration and peripheral nerve block:
Children >3 years: Infiltration: Concentrations of 0.5-1% (maximum without epinephrine: 11 mg/kg); Nerve block: Concentrations of 1% to 1.5% (maximum without epinephrine: 11 mg/kg)
Adults: Dosage varies greatly depending on indication
Lumbar epidural block: *Adults:* Preservative-free: 2% or 3%: 2-2.5 mL per segment; Usual total volume: 15-25 mL, may repeat with doses that are 2-6 mL less than total initial dose every 40-50 minutes

Dosage Forms
Injection, solution: 2% [20 mg/mL] (30 mL); 3% [30 mg/mL] (30 mL)
Nesacaine®: 1% [10 mg/mL] (30 mL); 2% [20 mg/mL] (30 mL)
Injection, solution [preservative free]: 2% [20 mg/mL] (20 mL); 3% [30 mg/mL] (20 mL)
Nesacaine®-MPF: 2% [20 mg/mL] (20 mL); 3% [30 mg/mL] (20 mL)

chloroprocaine hydrochloride *see* chloroprocaine *on page 196*

chloroquine (KLOR oh kwin)

Medication Safety Issues
International issues:
Aralen [U.S., Mexico] may be confused with Paralen brand name for acetaminophen [Czech Republic]

Synonyms chloroquine phosphate

U.S. Brand Names Aralen®

Canadian Brand Names Aralen®; Novo-Chloroquine

Therapeutic Category Aminoquinoline (Antimalarial)

Use Suppression/chemoprophylaxis or treatment of acute malaria due to susceptible *Plasmodium malariae, P. vivax, P. ovale, P. falciparum*; extraintestinal amebiasis

General Dosage Range Dosage adjustment recommended in patients with renal impairment
Oral: *Children and Adults:* Dosage varies greatly depending on indication

Dosage Forms
Tablet, oral: 250 mg, 500 mg
Aralen®: 500 mg

chloroquine phosphate *see* chloroquine *on page 196*

chlorothiazide (klor oh THYE a zide)

Medication Safety Issues
International issues:
Diuril [U.S., Canada] may be confused with Duorol brand name for acetaminophen [Spain]
U.S. Brand Names Diuril®; Sodium Diuril®
Canadian Brand Names Diuril®
Therapeutic Category Diuretic, Thiazide
Use Management of mild-to-moderate hypertension; adjunctive treatment of edema
General Dosage Range
I.V.: *Adults:* 250-1000 mg once or twice daily (maximum: 1000 mg/day)
Oral:
Children <6 months: 10-30 mg/kg/day in 2 divided doses (maximum: 375 mg/day)
Children ≥6 months: 10-20 mg/kg/day in 1-2 divided doses (maximum: 375 mg/day)
Adults: 250-2000 mg/day in 1-2 divided doses (maximum: 1000 mg/day [CHF])
Dosage Forms
Injection, powder for reconstitution: 500 mg
Sodium Diuril®: 0.5 g
Suspension, oral:
Diuril®: 250 mg/5 mL (237 mL)
Tablet, oral: 250 mg, 500 mg

Chlorphen [OTC] *see* chlorpheniramine *on page 197*

chlorpheniramine (klor fen IR a meen)

Medication Safety Issues
Sound-alike/look-alike issues:
Chlor-Trimeton® may be confused with Chloromycetin®
BEERS Criteria medication:
This drug may be inappropriate for use in geriatric patients (high severity risk).
Synonyms chlorpheniramine maleate; CTM
U.S. Brand Names Ahist™; Aller-Chlor® [OTC]; Chlor Hist [OTC]; Chlor-Trimeton® Allergy [OTC]; Chlorphen [OTC]; Diabetic Tussin® for Children Allergy Relief [OTC]; Ed Chlorped [DSC]; Ed-Chlortan; P-Tann [DSC]; Teldrin® HBP [OTC]
Canadian Brand Names Chlor-Tripolon®; Novo-Pheniram
Therapeutic Category Antihistamine
Use Perennial and seasonal allergic rhinitis and other allergic symptoms including urticaria
General Dosage Range Oral:
Immediate release:
Children <2 years: 0.35 mg/kg/day divided every 4-6 hours
Children 2-6 years: 1 mg every 4-6 hours **or** 0.35 mg/kg/day divided every 4-6 hours (maximum: 6 mg/day)
Children 6-12 years: 2 mg every 4-6 hours **or** 0.35 mg/kg/day divided every 4-6 hours (maximum: 12 mg/day)
Children >12 years and Adults: 4 mg every 4-6 hours (maximum: 24 mg/day)
Elderly: 4 mg once or twice daily
Sustained release:
Children 6-12 years: 8 mg at bedtime
Children >12 years and Adults: 8-12 mg every 8-12 hours (maximum: 24 mg/day)
Elderly: 8 mg at bedtime
Dosage Forms
Syrup, oral:
Aller-Chlor® [OTC]: 2 mg/5 mL (118 mL)
Diabetic Tussin® for Children Allergy Relief [OTC]: 2 mg/5 mL (118 mL)
Tablet, oral: 4 mg
Aller-Chlor® [OTC]: 4 mg
Chlor Hist [OTC]: 4 mg
Chlor-Trimeton® Allergy [OTC]: 4 mg
Chlorphen [OTC]: 4 mg
Ed-Chlortan: 4 mg
Teldrin® HBP [OTC]: 4 mg

Tablet, extended release, oral:
Chlor-Trimeton® Allergy [OTC]: 12 mg
Tablet, long acting, oral:
Ahist™: 12 mg

chlorpheniramine, acetaminophen, and pseudoephedrine *see* acetaminophen, chlorpheniramine, and pseudoephedrine *on page 30*

chlorpheniramine and acetaminophen (klor fen IR a meen & a seet a MIN oh fen)

Medication Safety Issues
Other safety concerns:
Duplicate therapy issues: This product contains acetaminophen, which may be a component of other combination products. Do not exceed the maximum recommended daily dose of acetaminophen.
Synonyms acetaminophen and chlorpheniramine
U.S. Brand Names Coricidin HBP® Cold and Flu [OTC]
Therapeutic Category Antihistamine/Analgesic
Use Symptomatic relief of congestion, headache, aches and pains of colds and flu
General Dosage Range Oral: *Adults:* 2 tablets every 4 hours
Dosage Forms
Tablet:
Coricidin HBP® Cold and Flu [OTC]: Chlorpheniramine 2 mg and acetaminophen 325 mg

chlorpheniramine and carbetapentane *see* carbetapentane and chlorpheniramine *on page 172*
chlorpheniramine and dextromethorphan *see* dextromethorphan and chlorpheniramine *on page 271*

chlorpheniramine and phenylephrine (klor fen IR a meen & fen il EF rin)

Medication Safety Issues
Sound-alike/look-alike issues:
Rynatan® may be confused with Rynatuss®
Synonyms chlorpheniramine maleate and phenylephrine hydrochloride; chlorpheniramine tannate and phenylephrine tannate; phenylephrine and chlorpheniramine
U.S. Brand Names Actifed® Cold & Allergy [OTC] *[reformulation]*; C-Phen [DSC]; Ceron [DSC]; Dallergy Drops [DSC]; Dallergy®-JR [DSC]; Dec-Chlorphen [DSC]; Ed A-Hist™ [DSC]; Ed ChlorPed D; NoHist [DSC]; PD-Hist-D; Phenabid® [DSC]; R-Tanna; R-Tanna Pediatric; Rynatan®; Rynatan® Pediatric; Sildec PE [DSC]; Sudafed PE® Sinus + Allergy [OTC]; Triaminic® Cold and Allergy [OTC]
Therapeutic Category Antihistamine/Decongestant Combination
Use Temporary relief of upper respiratory conditions such as nasal congestion, runny nose, and sneezing due to the common cold, hay fever, or allergic or vasomotor rhinitis
General Dosage Range Oral: *Children ≥2 years and Adults:* Dosage varies greatly depending on product
Dosage Forms
Liquid:
Triaminic® Cold and Allergy [OTC]: Chlorpheniramine 1 mg and phenylephrine 2.5 mg per 5 mL
Solution, oral [drops]:
PD-Hist-D: Chlorpheniramine 1 mg and phenylephrine 3.5 mg per 1 mL
Suspension, oral: Chlorpheniramine 4 mg and phenylephrine 20 mg per 5 mL
Dallergy®-JR: Chlorpheniramine 4 mg and phenylephrine 20 mg per 5 mL
R-Tanna Pediatric, Rynatan® Pediatric: Chlorpheniramine 4.5 mg and phenylephrine 5 mg per 5 mL
Suspension, oral [drops]:
Ed ChlorPed D: Chlorpheniramine 2 mg and phenylephrine 6 mg per 1 mL
Syrup:
PD-Hist-D: Chlorpheniramine 4 mg and phenylephrine 12.5 mg per 5 mL
Tablet:
Actifed® Cold & Allergy [OTC], Sudafed PE® Sinus + Allergy [OTC]: Chlorpheniramine 4 mg and phenylephrine 10 mg
R-Tanna, Rynatan®: Chlorpheniramine 9 mg and phenylephrine 25 mg
Tablet, chewable:
Rynatan®: Chlorpheniramine 4.5 mg and phenylephrine 5 mg

chlorpheniramine and pseudoephedrine (klor fen IR a meen & soo doe e FED rin)

Medication Safety Issues
Sound-alike/look-alike issues:
Chlor-Trimeton® may be confused with Chloromycetin®
Sudafed® may be confused with Sufenta®

Synonyms Allerest; chlorpheniramine maleate and pseudoephedrine hydrochloride; chlorpheniramine tannate and pseudoephedrine tannate; pseudoephedrine and chlorpheniramine

U.S. Brand Names Dicel® Chewable [OTC]; Dicel® Suspension; LoHist-D; Neutrahist Pediatric [OTC] [DSC]; Suclor™ [DSC]; SudaHist® [DSC]

Canadian Brand Names Triaminic® Cold & Allergy

Therapeutic Category Antihistamine/Decongestant Combination

Use Relief of nasal congestion associated with the common cold, hay fever, and other allergies, sinusitis, eustachian tube blockage, and vasomotor and allergic rhinitis

General Dosage Range Oral:
Immediate release: *Children ≥2 years and Adults:* Dosage varies greatly depending on product
Sustained release: *Children ≥12 years and Adults:* Deconamine® SR: Chlorpheniramine maleate 8 mg and pseudoephedrine hydrochloride 120 mg every 12 hours

Dosage Forms
Capsule, extended release, oral: Chlorpheniramine 8 mg and pseudoephedrine 120 mg; chlorpheniramine 12 mg and pseudoephedrine 100 mg
Liquid, oral:
LoHist-D: Chlorpheniramine 2 mg and pseudoephedrine 30 mg per 5 mL
Suspension, oral:
Dicel®: Chlorpheniramine 5 mg and pseudoephedrine 75 mg per 5 mL
Syrup, oral: Chlorpheniramine 2 mg and pseudoephedrine 30 mg per 5 mL
Tablet, oral: Chlorpheniramine 4 mg and pseudoephedrine 60 mg
Tablet, chewable, oral:
Dicel® [OTC]: Chlorpheniramine 2 mg and pseudoephedrine 30 mg

chlorpheniramine, dextromethorphan, and pseudoephedrine *see* chlorpheniramine, pseudoephedrine, and dextromethorphan *on page 201*

chlorpheniramine, dextromethorphan, phenylephrine, and guaifenesin *see* dextromethorphan, chlorpheniramine, phenylephrine, and guaifenesin *on page 272*

chlorpheniramine, dihydrocodeine, and pseudoephedrine *see* pseudoephedrine, dihydrocodeine, and chlorpheniramine *on page 754*

chlorpheniramine, ephedrine, phenylephrine, and carbetapentane
(klor fen IR a meen, e FED rin, fen il EF rin, & kar bay ta PEN tane)

Medication Safety Issues
Sound-alike/look-alike issues:
Rynatuss® may be confused with Rynatan®

Synonyms carbetapentane, ephedrine, phenylephrine, and chlorpheniramine; ephedrine, chlorpheniramine, phenylephrine, and carbetapentane; phenylephrine, ephedrine, chlorpheniramine, and carbetapentane

U.S. Brand Names Rynatuss®; Tetra Tannate Pediatric [DSC]

Therapeutic Category Antihistamine/Decongestant/Antitussive

Use Symptomatic relief of cough with a decongestant and an antihistamine

General Dosage Range Oral:
Children 2-6 years: 2.5-5 mL every 12 hours
Children >6 years: 5-10 mL every 12 hours
Adults: 1-2 tablets every 12 hours

Dosage Forms
Tablet:
Rynatuss®: Chlorpheniramine 5 mg, ephedrine 10 mg, phenylephrine 10 mg, and carbetapentane 50 mg

chlorpheniramine maleate *see* chlorpheniramine *on page 197*

chlorpheniramine maleate, acetaminophen, phenylephrine hydrochloride, and phenyltoloxamine citrate *see* acetaminophen, chlorpheniramine, phenylephrine, and phenyltoloxamine *on page 31*

chlorpheniramine maleate and dextromethorphan hydrobromide *see* dextromethorphan and chlorpheniramine *on page 271*

chlorpheniramine maleate and hydrocodone bitartrate *see* hydrocodone and chlorpheniramine *on page 448*

chlorpheniramine maleate and phenylephrine hydrochloride *see* chlorpheniramine and phenylephrine *on page 198*

chlorpheniramine maleate and pseudoephedrine hydrochloride *see* chlorpheniramine and pseudoephedrine *on page 199*

chlorpheniramine maleate, dihydrocodeine bitartrate, and phenylephrine hydrochloride *see* dihydrocodeine, chlorpheniramine, and phenylephrine *on page 285*

chlorpheniramine maleate, ibuprofen, and pseudoephedrine *see* ibuprofen, pseudoephedrine, and chlorpheniramine *on page 462*

chlorpheniramine maleate, phenylephrine hydrochloride, and guaifenesin *see* chlorpheniramine, phenylephrine, and guaifenesin *on page 200*

chlorpheniramine maleate, pseudoephedrine hydrochloride, and dextromethorphan hydrobromide *see* chlorpheniramine, pseudoephedrine, and dextromethorphan *on page 201*

chlorpheniramine, phenylephrine, and dextromethorphan
(klor fen IR a meen, fen il EF rin, & deks troe meth OR fan)

Synonyms dextromethorphan, chlorpheniramine, and phenylephrine; phenylephrine, chlorpheniramine, and dextromethorphan

U.S. Brand Names Ceron-DM [DSC]; Corfen DM [DSC]; De-Chlor DM [DSC]; De-Chlor DR [DSC]; Donatussin DM; Ed A-Hist DM [DSC]; Father John's® Plus [OTC]; Neo DM [DSC]; NoHist-DMX [DSC]; PD-Cof [DSC]; PE-Hist DM [DSC]; Sildec PE-DM [DSC]

Therapeutic Category Antihistamine/Decongestant/Antitussive

Use Temporary relief of cough and upper respiratory symptoms associated with allergies or the common cold

General Dosage Range Oral: *Children ≥6 years and Adults:* Dosage varies greatly depending on product

Dosage Forms
Liquid, oral:
Norel DM™: Chlorpheniramine 4 mg, phenylephrine 10 mg, and dextromethorphan 15 mg per 5 mL
Father John's® Plus [OTC]: Chlorpheniramine 2 mg, phenylephrine 5 mg, and dextromethorphan 5 mg per 15 mL
Liquid, oral [drops]:
Donatussin DM: Chlorpheniramine 1 mg, phenylephrine 1.5 mg, and dextromethorphan 3 mg per 1 mL

chlorpheniramine, phenylephrine, and guaifenesin
(klor fen IR a meen, fen il EF rin, & gwye FEN e sin)

Synonyms chlorpheniramine maleate, phenylephrine hydrochloride, and guaifenesin; chlorpheniramine tannate, phenylephrine tannate, and guaifenesin; guaifenesin, phenylephrine, and chlorpheniramine; phenylephrine, chlorpheniramine, and guaifenesin

U.S. Brand Names P Chlor GG [DSC]

Therapeutic Category Cough and Cold Combination

Use Symptomatic relief of upper respiratory symptoms associated with infections such as the common cold or allergies

General Dosage Range Oral:
Children <3 months: 2-3 2-3 drops per month of age every 4-6 hours as needed (maximum: 4 doses/day)
Children 3-6 months: 0.3-0.6 mL every 4-6 hours as needed (maximum: 4 doses/day)
Children 6 months to 1 year: 0.6-1 mL every 4-6 hours as needed (maximum: 4 doses/day)
Children 1-2 years: 1-2 mL every 4-6 hours as needed (maximum: 4 doses/day)

chlorpheniramine, phenylephrine, and methscopolamine
(klor fen IR a meen, fen il EF rin, & meth skoe POL a meen)

Synonyms methscopolamine nitrate, chlorpheniramine maleate, and phenylephrine hydrochloride; phenylephrine tannate, chlorpheniramine tannate, and methscopolamine nitrate

U.S. Brand Names aerohist plus™ [DSC]; aeroKid™; AH-Chew® [DSC]; AH-Chew™ Ultra [DSC]; Chlor-Mes-D [DSC]; Dallergy® [DSC]; Dehistine [DSC]; DryMax; Duradryl®; Histatab PH [DSC]; OMNIhist® II L.A. [DSC]; Rescon®; Triall™ [DSC]

Therapeutic Category Antihistamine/Decongestant/Anticholinergic

Use Treatment of upper respiratory symptoms such as respiratory congestion, allergic rhinitis, vasomotor rhinitis, sinusitis, and allergic skin reactions of urticaria and angioedema

General Dosage Range Oral: *Children ≥6 years and Adults:* Dosage varies greatly depending on product

Dosage Forms
Syrup:
aeroKid™: Chlorpheniramine 4 mg, phenylephrine 10 mg, and methscopolamine 1.25 mg per 5 mL
Duradryl®: Chlorpheniramine 2 mg, phenylephrine 10 mg, and methscopolamine 1.25 mg per 5 mL
DryMax: Chlorpheniramine 4 mg, phenylephrine 15 mg, and methscopolamine 1.25 mg per 5 mL
Tablet, variable release:
Rescon®: Chlorpheniramine 12 mg and phenylephrine 40 mg [sustained release] and methscopolamine 2 mg [immediate release] [MaxRelent release]

chlorpheniramine, phenylephrine, and phenyltoloxamine
(klor fen IR a meen, fen il EF rin, & fen il tole LOKS a meen)

Synonyms phenylephrine, chlorpheniramine, and phenyltoloxamine; phenyltoloxamine, chlorpheniramine, and phenylephrine

U.S. Brand Names Nalex®-A; NoHist-A; Rhinacon A

Therapeutic Category Antihistamine/Decongestant Combination

Use Symptomatic relief of rhinitis and nasal congestion due to colds or allergy

General Dosage Range Oral:
Children 2-6 years: Nalex®-A: 1.25-2.5 mL every 4-6 hours
Children 6-12 years: Nalex®-A: 5 mL every 4-6 hours **or** one-half tablet 2-3 times/day
Children >12 years and Adults: Nalex®-A: 10 mL every 4-6 hours **or** 1 tablet 2-3 times/day

Dosage Forms
Liquid: Chlorpheniramine 2.5 mg, phenylephrine 5 mg, and phenyltoloxamine 7.5 mg per 5 mL
Nalex®-A, NoHist-A: Chlorpheniramine 2.5 mg, phenylephrine 5 mg, and phenyltoloxamine 7.5 mg per 5 mL
Tablet, extended release:
Rhinacon A: Chlorpheniramine 4 mg, phenylephrine 20 mg, and phenyltoloxamine 40 mg
Tablet, prolonged release:
Nalex®-A: Chlorpheniramine 4 mg, phenylephrine 20 mg, and phenyltoloxamine 40 mg

chlorpheniramine, phenylephrine, and pyrilamine *see* chlorpheniramine, pyrilamine, and phenylephrine *on page 202*

chlorpheniramine, pseudoephedrine, and acetaminophen *see* acetaminophen, chlorpheniramine, and pseudoephedrine *on page 30*

chlorpheniramine, pseudoephedrine, and codeine
(klor fen IR a meen, soo doe e FED rin, & KOE deen)

Synonyms codeine, chlorpheniramine, and pseudoephedrine; pseudoephedrine, chlorpheniramine, and codeine

U.S. Brand Names Phenylhistine DH

Therapeutic Category Antihistamine/Decongestant/Antitussive

Controlled Substance C-V

Use Temporary relief of cough associated with minor throat or bronchial irritation or nasal congestion due to common cold, allergic rhinitis, or sinusitis

General Dosage Range Oral:
Children 6-11 years: 5 mL every 4 hours (maximum: 20 mL/24 hours)
Children ≥12 years and Adults: 10 mL every 4 hours (maximum: 40 mL/24 hours)

Dosage Forms
Elixir:
Phenylhistine DH: Chlorpheniramine 2 mg, pseudoephedrine 30 mg, and codeine 10 mg per 5 mL (120 mL, 480 mL)

chlorpheniramine, pseudoephedrine, and dextromethorphan
(klor fen IR a meen, soo doe e FED rin, & deks troe meth OR fan)

Synonyms chlorpheniramine maleate, pseudoephedrine hydrochloride, and dextromethorphan hydrobromide; chlorpheniramine tannate, pseudoephedrine tannate, and dextromethorphan tannate; chlorpheniramine, dextromethorphan, and pseudoephedrine; dexchlorpheniramine tannate,

◀ pseudoephedrine tannate, and dextromethorphan tannate; dextromethorphan, chlorpheniramine, and pseudoephedrine; pseudoephedrine, chlorpheniramine, and dextromethorphan

U.S. Brand Names Dicel® DM Chewable [OTC]; Dicel® DM Suspension; Entre-S; Kidkare Children's Cough/Cold [OTC]; Neutrahist PDX; Pedia Relief™ Cough-Cold [OTC]; Rescon DM [OTC]; Tanafed DMX™

Therapeutic Category Antihistamine/Decongestant/Antitussive

Use Temporarily relieves nasal congestion, runny nose, cough, and sneezing due to the common cold, hay fever, or allergic rhinitis

General Dosage Range Oral: *Children ≥2 years:* Dosage varies greatly depending on product

Dosage Forms

Liquid, oral: Chlorpheniramine 1 mg, pseudoephedrine 15 mg, and dextromethorphan 5 mg per 5 mL
Kidkare Children's Cough/Cold [OTC], Pedia Relief™ [OTC]: Chlorpheniramine 1 mg, pseudoephedrine 15 mg, and dextromethorphan 5 mg per 5 mL
Rescon DM [OTC]: Chlorpheniramine 2 mg, pseudoephedrine 30 mg, and dextromethorphan 10 mg per 5 mL

Liquid, oral [drops]:
Neutrahist PDX: Chlorpheniramine 0.8 mg, pseudoephedrine 9 mg, and dextromethorphan 3 mg per 1 mL

Suspension, oral:
Dicel® DM: Chlorpheniramine 5 mg, pseudoephedrine 75 mg, and dextromethorphan 25 mg per 5 mL
Entre-S: Chlorpheniramine maleate 4 mg, pseudoephedrine 30 mg, and dextromethorphan 30 mg per 5 mL
Tanafed DMX™: Dexchlorpheniramine 2.5 mg, pseudoephedrine 75 mg, and dextromethorphan 25 mg per 5 mL

Tablet, chewable, oral:
Dicel® DM [OTC]: Chlorpheniramine 2 mg, pseudoephedrine 30 mg, and dextromethorphan 10 mg

chlorpheniramine, pseudoephedrine, and hydrocodone *see* hydrocodone, chlorpheniramine, and pseudoephedrine *on page* 449

chlorpheniramine, pseudoephedrine, and methscopolamine
(klor fen IR a meen, soo doe e FED rin, & meth skoe POL a meen)

Synonyms methscopolamine, chlorpheniramine, and pseudoephedrine; methscopolamine, pseudoephedrine, and chlorpheniramine; pseudoephedrine hydrochloride, methscopolamine nitrate, and chlorpheniramine maleate; pseudoephedrine, methscopolamine, and chlorpheniramine

U.S. Brand Names Amdry-C; Coldamine; Durahist™ [DSC]; Hista-Vent® PSE [DSC]

Therapeutic Category Antihistamine/Decongestant/Anticholinergic

Use Relief of symptoms of allergic rhinitis, vasomotor rhinitis, sinusitis, and the common cold

General Dosage Range Oral:
Children 6-11 years: Durahist™, Hista-Vent® PSE: One-half tablet every 12 hours (maximum: 1 tablet/day)
Children ≥12 years and Adults: Durahist™, Hista-Vent® PSE: 1 tablet every 12 hours (maximum: 2 tablets/day)

Dosage Forms

Tablet, extended release:
Coldamine: Chlorpheniramine 8 mg, pseudoephedrine 90 mg, and methscopolamine 2.5 mg

Tablet, sustained release: Chlorpheniramine maleate 8 mg, pseudoephedrine hydrochloride 60 mg, and methscopolamine nitrate 1.25 mg; chlorpheniramine maleate 8 mg, pseudoephedrine hydrochloride 90 mg, and methscopolamine nitrate 2.5 mg
Amdry-C: Chlorpheniramine 8 mg, pseudoephedrine 120 mg, and methscopolamine 2.5 mg [scored]

chlorpheniramine, pyrilamine, and phenylephrine
(klor fen IR a meen, pye RIL a meen, & fen il EF rin)

Synonyms chlorpheniramine, phenylephrine, and pyrilamine; phenylephrine, chlorpheniramine, and pyrilamine; pyrilamine, chlorpheniramine, and phenylephrine

U.S. Brand Names MyHist-PD; Nalex A 12; Pyrichlor PE™; Ru-Hist Forte; Triplex™ AD [DSC]

Therapeutic Category Alpha/Beta Agonist; Histamine H$_1$ Antagonist; Histamine H$_1$ Antagonist, First Generation

Use Symptomatic relief of rhinitis and nasal congestion due to colds or allergy

General Dosage Range Oral: *Children ≥2 years and Adults:* Dosage varies greatly depending on product

Dosage Forms

Liquid, oral:
MyHist-PD: Chlorpheniramine 2 mg, pyrilamine 12.5 mg, and phenylephrine 7.5 mg per 5 mL
Pyrichlor PE™: Chlorpheniramine 2 mg, pyrilamine 10 mg, and phenylephrine 10 mg per 5 mL

Suspension, oral:
Nalex A 12: Chlorpheniramine 2 mg, pyrilamine 12.5 mg, and phenylephrine 5 mg per 5 mL

Tablet, time-released, oral: Chlorpheniramine 4 mg, pyrilamine 25 mg, and phenylephrine 10 mg
Ru-Hist Forte: Chlorpheniramine 4 mg, pyrilamine 25 mg, and phenylephrine 10 mg

chlorpheniramine tannate and phenylephrine tannate *see* chlorpheniramine and phenylephrine *on page 198*

chlorpheniramine tannate and pseudoephedrine tannate *see* chlorpheniramine and pseudoephedrine *on page 199*

chlorpheniramine tannate, phenylephrine tannate, and guaifenesin *see* chlorpheniramine, phenylephrine, and guaifenesin *on page 200*

chlorpheniramine tannate, pseudoephedrine tannate, and dextromethorphan tannate *see* chlorpheniramine, pseudoephedrine, and dextromethorphan *on page 201*

chlorpromazine (klor PROE ma zeen)

Medication Safety Issues

Sound-alike/look-alike issues:
ChlorproMAZINE may be confused with chlordiazePOXIDE, chlorproPAMIDE, clomiPRAMINE, prochlorperazine, promethazine
Thorazine may be confused with thiamine, thioridazine

Synonyms chlorpromazine hydrochloride; CPZ; Thorazine

Tall-Man chlorproMAZINE

Canadian Brand Names Largactil®; Novo-Chlorpromazine

Therapeutic Category Phenothiazine Derivative

Use Management of psychotic disorders (control of mania, treatment of schizophrenia); control of nausea and vomiting; relief of restlessness and apprehension before surgery; acute intermittent porphyria; adjunct in the treatment of tetanus; intractable hiccups; combativeness and/or explosive hyperexcitable behavior in children 1-12 years of age and in short-term treatment of hyperactive children

General Dosage Range

I.M., I.V.:
Children ≥6 months: 0.5-1 mg/kg every 6-8 hours (maximum: <5 years [<22.7 kg]: 40 mg/day; 5-12 years [22.7-45.5 kg]: 75 mg/day)
Adults: Initial: 25 mg; may repeat (25-50 mg) in 1-4 hours; Usual dose: 300-800 mg/day (maximum: 400 mg every 4-6 hours)

Oral:
Children ≥6 months: 0.5-1 mg/ kg every 4-6 hours as needed
Adults: Dosage varies greatly depending on indication

Dosage Forms

Injection, solution: 25 mg/mL (1 mL, 2 mL)
Tablet, oral: 10 mg, 25 mg, 50 mg, 100 mg, 200 mg

chlorpromazine hydrochloride *see* chlorpromazine *on page 203*

chlorpropamide (klor PROE pa mide)

Medication Safety Issues

Sound-alike/look-alike issues:
ChlorproPAMIDE may be confused with chlorproMAZINE
Diabinese may be confused with DiaBeta®, Diamox®

High alert medication:
The Institute for Safe Medication Practices (ISMP) includes this medication among its list of drugs which have a heightened risk of causing significant patient harm when used in error.

BEERS Criteria medication:
This drug may be inappropriate for use in geriatric patients (high severity risk).

Tall-Man chlorproPAMIDE

Canadian Brand Names Apo-Chlorpropamide®; Novo-Propamide

Therapeutic Category Antidiabetic Agent, Oral

◀ **Use** Management of blood sugar in type 2 diabetes mellitus (noninsulin-dependent, NIDDM)
General Dosage Range Oral:
Adults: Initial: 250 mg/day; Maintenance: 100-500 mg/day (maximum: 750 mg/day)
Elderly: Initial: 100-125 mg/day
Dosage Forms
Tablet, oral: 100 mg, 250 mg

chlorthalidone (klor THAL i done)

Synonyms Hygroton
U.S. Brand Names Thalitone®
Canadian Brand Names Apo-Chlorthalidone®
Therapeutic Category Diuretic, Miscellaneous
Use Management of mild-to-moderate hypertension when used alone or in combination with other agents; treatment of edema associated with heart failure or nephrotic syndrome. Recent studies have found chlorthalidone effective in the treatment of isolated systolic hypertension in the elderly.
General Dosage Range Oral:
Adults: 12.5-100 mg/day **or** 100 mg 3 times/week (maximum: 200 mg/day)
Elderly: Initial: 12.5-25 mg/day or every other day
Dosage Forms
Tablet, oral: 25 mg, 50 mg
Thalitone®: 15 mg

chlorthalidone and atenolol *see* atenolol and chlorthalidone *on page 101*
chlorthalidone and clonidine *see* clonidine and chlorthalidone *on page 224*
Chlor-Trimeton® Allergy [OTC] *see* chlorpheniramine *on page 197*
Chlor-Tripolon® (Can) *see* chlorpheniramine *on page 197*
Chlor-Tripolon ND® (Can) *see* loratadine and pseudoephedrine *on page 537*

chlorzoxazone (klor ZOKS a zone)

Medication Safety Issues
BEERS Criteria medication:
This drug may be inappropriate for use in geriatric patients (high severity risk).
U.S. Brand Names Parafon Forte® DSC
Canadian Brand Names Parafon Forte®; Strifon Forte®
Therapeutic Category Skeletal Muscle Relaxant
Use Symptomatic treatment of muscle spasm and pain associated with acute musculoskeletal conditions
General Dosage Range Oral:
Children: 20 mg/kg/day **or** 600 mg/m^2/day in 3-4 divided doses
Adults: 250-750 mg 3-4 times/day
Elderly: Initial: 250 mg 2-4 times/day
Dosage Forms
Caplet, oral:
Parafon Forte® DSC: 500 mg
Tablet, oral: 500 mg

cholecalciferol (kole e kal SI fer ole)

Medication Safety Issues
Sound-alike/look-alike issues:
Cholecalciferol may be confused with alfacalcidol, ergocalciferol
Administration issues:
Liquid vitamin D preparations have the potential for dosing errors when administered to infants. Droppers should be clearly marked to easily provide 400 international units. For products intended for infants, the FDA recommends that accompanying droppers deliver no more than 400 international units per dose.
Synonyms D_3
U.S. Brand Names Bio-D-Mulsion Forte® [OTC]; Bio-D-Mulsion® [OTC]; D-3 [OTC]; D3-50™ [OTC]; D3-5™ [OTC]; DDrops®; DDrops® Baby [OTC]; DDrops® Kids [OTC]; DDrops® [OTC]; Delta® D3 [OTC]; Enfamil® D-Vi-Sol™ [OTC]; Maximum D3® [OTC]; Vitamin D3 [OTC]
Canadian Brand Names D-Vi-Sol®

Therapeutic Category Vitamin D Analog

Use Dietary supplement, treatment of vitamin D deficiency, or prophylaxis of deficiency

General Dosage Range Oral:
  Children 0-12 months: Adequate intake: 400 int. units/day
  Children 1 year to Adults ≤70 years: RDA: 600 int. units/day
  Elderly >70 years: RDA: 800 int. units/day

Dosage Forms
  Capsule, oral: 5000 int. units
  D-3 [OTC]: 1000 int. units
  D3-50™ [OTC]: 50,000 int. units
  D3-5™ [OTC]: 5000 int. units
  Maximum D3® [OTC]: 10,000 int. units
  Capsule, softgel, oral:
  D-3 [OTC]: 2000 int. units
  Solution, oral:
  Bio-D-Mulsion Forte® [OTC]: 2000 int. units/drop (30 mL)
  Bio-D-Mulsion® [OTC]: 400 int. units/drop (30 mL)
  DDrops® [OTC]: 2000 int. units/drop (10 mL); 1000 units/drop (10 mL)
  DDrops® Baby [OTC]: 400 int. units/drop (10 mL)
  DDrops® Kids [OTC]: 400 int. units/drop (10 mL)
  Enfamil® D-Vi-Sol™ [OTC]: 400 int. units/mL (50 mL)
  Tablet, oral: 400 int. units, 1000 int. units
  Delta® D3 [OTC]: 400 int. units
  Vitamin D3 [OTC]: 1000 int. units

cholecalciferol and alendronate *see* alendronate and cholecalciferol *on page 49*

cholera and traveler's diarrhea vaccine *see* traveler's diarrhea and cholera vaccine *(Canada only) on page 883*

cholera vaccine *see* traveler's diarrhea and cholera vaccine *(Canada only) on page 883*

cholestyramine resin (koe LES teer a meen REZ in)

U.S. Brand Names Prevalite®; Questran®; Questran® Light

Canadian Brand Names Novo-Cholamine; Novo-Cholamine Light; Olestyr; PMS-Cholestyramine; Questran®; Questran® Light Sugar Free; ZYM-Cholestyramine-Light; ZYM-Cholestyramine-Regular

Therapeutic Category Bile Acid Sequestrant

Use Adjunct in the management of primary hypercholesterolemia; pruritus associated with elevated levels of bile acids; diarrhea associated with excess fecal bile acids; binding toxicologic agents; pseudomembranous colitis

General Dosage Range Oral:
  Children: 240 mg/kg/day in 3 divided doses
  Adults: 4-24 g/day in 1-6 divided doses

Dosage Forms
  Powder for suspension, oral: Cholestyramine resin 4 g/5 g of powder (210 g); Cholestyramine resin 4 g/5.7 g of powder (239.4 g); Cholestyramine resin 4 g/9 g of powder (378 g); Cholestyramine resin 4 g/5 g packet (60s); Cholestyramine resin 4 g/5.7 g packet (60s); Cholestyramine resin 4 g/9 g packet (60s)
  Prevalite®: Cholestyramine resin 4 g/5.5 g of powder (231 g); Cholestyramine resin 4 g/5.5 g packet (42s, 60s)
  Questran®: Cholestyramine resin 4 g/9 g of powder (378 g); Cholestyramine resin 4 g/9 g packet (60s)
  Questran® Light: Cholestyramine resin 4 g/5 g of powder (210 g); Cholestyramine resin 4 g/5 g packet (60s)

choline fenofibrate *see* fenofibric acid *on page 369*

choline magnesium trisalicylate (KOE leen mag NEE zhum trye sa LIS i late)

Synonyms tricosal; Trilisate

Therapeutic Category Analgesic, Nonnarcotic; Nonsteroidal Antiinflammatory Drug (NSAID)

Use Management of osteoarthritis, rheumatoid arthritis, and other arthritis; acute painful shoulder

General Dosage Range Oral:
  Children <37 kg: 50 mg/kg/day in 2 divided doses
  Children ≥37 kg: 2250 mg/day in divided doses

▶

◀ *Adults:* 500 mg to 1.5 g 2-3 times/day **or** 3 g at bedtime
Elderly: 750 mg 3 times/day
Dosage Forms
Liquid, oral: 500 mg/5 mL (240 mL)

Cholografin® Meglumine *see* iodipamide meglumine *on page 484*
chondroitin sulfate and sodium hyaluronate *see* sodium chondroitin sulfate and sodium hyaluronate *on page 820*
Chooz® [OTC] *see* calcium carbonate *on page 161*
choriogonadotropin alfa *see* chorionic gonadotropin (recombinant) *on page 206*
Chorionic Gonadotropin for Injection (Can) *see* chorionic gonadotropin (human) *on page 206*

chorionic gonadotropin (human) (kor ee ON ik goe NAD oh troe pin, HYU man)
Synonyms CG; hCG
U.S. Brand Names Novarel®; Pregnyl®
Canadian Brand Names Chorionic Gonadotropin for Injection; Pregnyl®
Therapeutic Category Gonadotropin
Use Induces ovulation and pregnancy in anovulatory, infertile females; treatment of hypogonadotropic hypogonadism, prepubertal cryptorchidism; spermatogenesis induction with follitropin alfa
General Dosage Range I.M.:
Children: Dosage varies greatly depending on indication
Adults (females): 5000-10,000 units 1 day following last dose of menotropins
Adults (males): 1000-2000 units 2-3 times/week
Dosage Forms
Injection, powder for reconstitution: 10,000 units
  Novarel®: 10,000 units
  Pregnyl®: 10,000 units

chorionic gonadotropin (recombinant)
(kor ee ON ik goe NAD oh troe pin ree KOM be nant)
Synonyms choriogonadotropin alfa; r-hCG
U.S. Brand Names Ovidrel®
Canadian Brand Names Ovidrel®
Therapeutic Category Gonadotropin; Ovulation Stimulator
Use As part of an assisted reproductive technology (ART) program, induces ovulation in infertile females who have been pretreated with follicle-stimulating hormones (FSH); induces ovulation and pregnancy in infertile females when the cause of infertility is functional
General Dosage Range SubQ: *Adults (female):* 250 mcg given 1 day following last dose of follicle stimulating agent
Dosage Forms
Injection, solution:
  Ovidrel®: 257.5 mcg/0.515 mL (0.515 mL)

chromic phosphate P 32 (KROME ik FOS fate pe THUR tee too)
Synonyms P32; phosphorus p32
U.S. Brand Names Phosphocol® P 32
Therapeutic Category Radiopharmaceutical
Use Treatment of peritoneal or pleural effusions caused by metastatic disease by intracavitary instillation; may be injected interstitially for the treatment of cancer
General Dosage Range Based on 70 kg patient:
  Intraperitoneal instillation: *Adults:* 370-740 megabecquerels (10-20 millicuries)
  Intrapleural instillation: *Adults:* 222-444 megabecquerels (6-12 millicuries)
  Interstitial instillation: *Adults:* ~3.7-18.5 megabecquerels/g of tumor weight (0.1-0.5 millicuries/g)
Dosage Forms
Injection, suspension:
  Phosphocol® P 32: 185 MBq (5mCi) per mL

chromium *see* trace metals *on page 880*
CI-1008 *see* pregabalin *on page 735*

Cialis® *see* tadalafil *on page 842*

ciclesonide (oral inhalation) (sye KLES oh nide)

U.S. Brand Names Alvesco®

Canadian Brand Names Alvesco®

Therapeutic Category Corticosteroid, Inhalant (Oral)

Use Prophylactic management of bronchial asthma

General Dosage Range Oral inhalation: *Children ≥12 years and Adults:* 100-800 mcg/day (1-2 puffs once or twice daily) (maximum: 640 mcg/day)

Dosage Forms

Aerosol, for oral inhalation:

Alvesco®: 80 mcg/inhalation (6.1 g); 160 mcg/inhalation (6.1 g)

Dosage Forms - Canada

Aerosol for oral inhalation:

Alvesco®: 50 mcg/inhalation; 100 mcg/inhalation; 200 mcg/inhalation

ciclesonide (nasal) (sye KLES oh nide)

U.S. Brand Names Omnaris™

Canadian Brand Names Omnaris™

Therapeutic Category Corticosteroid, Nasal

Use Management of seasonal and perennial allergic rhinitis

General Dosage Range Intranasal: *Children ≥6 years and Adults:* 2 sprays (50 mcg/spray) per nostril once daily (maximum: 200 mcg/day)

Dosage Forms

Suspension, intranasal:

Omnaris™: 50 mcg/inhalation (12.5 g)

Ciclodan™ *see* ciclopirox *on page 207*

Ciclodan™ Kit *see* ciclopirox *on page 207*

ciclopirox (sye kloe PEER oks)

Synonyms ciclopirox olamine

U.S. Brand Names Ciclodan™; Ciclodan™ Kit; Loprox®; Penlac®

Canadian Brand Names Loprox®; Penlac®; Stieprox®

Therapeutic Category Antifungal Agent

Use

Cream/suspension: Treatment of tinea pedis (athlete's foot), tinea cruris (jock itch), tinea corporis (ringworm), cutaneous candidiasis, and tinea versicolor (pityriasis)

Gel: Treatment of tinea pedis (athlete's foot), tinea corporis (ringworm); seborrheic dermatitis of the scalp

Lacquer (solution): Topical treatment of mild-to-moderate onychomycosis of the fingernails and toenails due to *Trichophyton rubrum* (not involving the lunula) and the immediately-adjacent skin

Shampoo: Treatment of seborrheic dermatitis of the scalp

General Dosage Range Topical:

Cream/suspension: *Children >10 years and Adults:* Apply twice daily

Gel: *Children >16 years and Adults:* Apply twice daily

Lacquer: *Children ≥12 years and Adults:* Apply to adjacent skin and affected nails daily; remove with alcohol every 7 days

Shampoo: *Children >16 years and Adults:* Apply 5-10 mL to wet hair, lather, and leave in place ~3 minutes, rinse; repeat twice weekly (allow minimum of 3 days between applications)

Dosage Forms

Cream, topical: 0.77% (15 g, 30 g, 90 g)

Gel, topical: 0.77% (30 g, 45 g, 100 g)

Loprox®: 0.77% (30 g, 45 g, 100 g)

Shampoo, topical: 1% (120 mL)

Loprox®: 1% (120 mL)

◀ **Solution, topical**: 8% (6.6 mL)
Ciclodan™: 8% (6.6 mL)
Ciclodan™ Kit: 8% (6.6 mL)
Penlac®: 8% (6.6 mL)
Suspension, topical: 0.77% (30 mL, 60 mL)

ciclopirox olamine see ciclopirox on page 207
cidecin see daptomycin on page 252

cidofovir (si DOF o veer)
U.S. Brand Names Vistide®
Therapeutic Category Antiviral Agent
Use Treatment of cytomegalovirus (CMV) retinitis in patients with acquired immunodeficiency syndrome (AIDS). **Note:** Should be administered with probenecid.
General Dosage Range Dosage adjustment recommended in patients with renal impairment
I.V.: *Adults:* Induction: 5 mg/kg once weekly for 2 consecutive weeks; Maintenance: 5 mg/kg once every 2 weeks
Dosage Forms
Injection, solution [preservative free]:
Vistide®: 75 mg/mL (5 mL)

cilazapril *(Canada only)* (sye LAY za pril)
Synonyms cilazapril monohydrate
Canadian Brand Names Apo-Cilazapril®; CO Cilazapril; Inhibace®; Mylan-Cilazapril; Novo-Cilazapril; PHL-Cilazapril; PMS-Cilazapril
Therapeutic Category Angiotensin-Converting Enzyme (ACE) Inhibitor
Use Management of hypertension; treatment of heart failure
General Dosage Range Dosage adjustment recommended in patients with hepatic or renal impairment
Oral:
Adults: Initial: 0.5-2.5 mg once daily (maximum: 5 mg/day [CHF]; 10 mg/day [HTN])
Elderly: Initial: 0.5-1.25 mg once daily (maximum: 2.5 mg/day [CHF]; 10 mg/day [HTN])
Product Availability Not available in U.S.
Dosage Forms - Canada
Tablet:
Inhibace®, Novo-Cilazapril: 1 mg, 2.5 mg, 5 mg

cilazapril and hydrochlorothiazide *(Canada only)*
(sye LAY za pril & hye droe klor oh THYE a zide)
Synonyms cilazapril monohydrate and hydrochlorothiazide; hydrochlorothiazide and cilazapril
Canadian Brand Names Apo-Cilazapril®/Hctz; Inhibace® Plus; Novo-Cilazapril/HCTZ
Therapeutic Category Angiotensin-Converting Enzyme (ACE) Inhibitor
Use Treatment of mild-to-moderate hypertension; not indicated for initial treatment of hypertension
General Dosage Range Dosage adjustment recommended in hepatic impairment.
Oral: *Adults:* Dose is individualized; range: Cilazapril 2.5-10 mg/hydrochlorothiazide 6.25-25 mg/day
Product Availability Not available in U.S.
Dosage Forms - Canada
Tablet: 5/12.5: Cilazapril 5 mg and hydrochlorothiazide 12.5 mg
Inhibace® Plus 5/12.5: Cilazapril 5 mg and hydrochlorothiazide 12.5 mg

cilazapril monohydrate see cilazapril *(Canada only)* on page 208
cilazapril monohydrate and hydrochlorothiazide see cilazapril and hydrochlorothiazide *(Canada only)* on page 208

cilostazol (sil OH sta zol)
Medication Safety Issues
Sound-alike/look-alike issues:
Pletal® may be confused with Plendil®
Synonyms OPC-13013
U.S. Brand Names Pletal®

Therapeutic Category Platelet Aggregation Inhibitor

Use Symptomatic management of peripheral vascular disease, primarily intermittent claudication

General Dosage Range Dosage adjustment recommended in patients on concomitant therapy
Oral: *Adults:* 100 mg twice daily

Dosage Forms
Tablet, oral: 50 mg, 100 mg
Pletal®: 50 mg, 100 mg

Ciloxan® *see* ciprofloxacin (ophthalmic) *on page 210*

cimetidine (sye MET i deen)

Medication Safety Issues
Sound-alike/look-alike issues:
Cimetidine may be confused with simethicone
BEERS Criteria medication:
This drug may be inappropriate for use in geriatric patients (low severity risk).

U.S. Brand Names Tagamet HB 200® [OTC]

Canadian Brand Names Apo-Cimetidine®; Dom-Cimetidine; Mylan-Cimetidine; Novo-Cimetidine; Nu-Cimet; PMS-Cimetidine; Tagamet® HB

Therapeutic Category Histamine H$_2$ Antagonist

Use Short-term treatment of active duodenal ulcers and benign gastric ulcers; maintenance therapy of duodenal ulcer; treatment of gastric hypersecretory states; treatment of gastroesophageal reflux disease (GERD)

OTC labeling: Prevention or relief of heartburn, acid indigestion, or sour stomach

General Dosage Range Dosage adjustment recommended in patients with renal impaiment
Oral:
Children <12 years: 20-40 mg/kg/day divided every 6 hours
Children ≥12 years: 20-40 mg/kg/day divided every 6 hours **or** 200 mg 1-2 times/day [OTC]
Adults: 300-600 mg 4 times/day **or** 400-800 mg 1-2 times/day **or** 200 mg 1-2 times/day [OTC]

Dosage Forms
Solution, oral: 300 mg/5 mL (237 mL, 240 mL, 250 mL, 473 mL, 480 mL)
Tablet, oral: 200 mg, 300 mg, 400 mg, 800 mg
Tagamet HB 200® [OTC]: 200 mg

Cimzia® *see* certolizumab pegol *on page 188*

cinacalcet (sin a KAL cet)

Synonyms AMG 073; cinacalcet hydrochloride
U.S. Brand Names Sensipar®
Canadian Brand Names Sensipar®
Therapeutic Category Calcimimetic

Use Treatment of secondary hyperparathyroidism in patients with chronic kidney disease (CKD) on dialysis; treatment of hypercalcemia in patients with parathyroid carcinoma; treatment of severe hypercalcemia in patients with primary hyperparathyroidism who are unable to undergo parathyroidectomy

General Dosage Range Dosage adjustment recommended in patients on concomitant therapy or who develop toxicities
Oral: *Adults:* Initial: 30 mg once or twice daily; Maintenance: Increase dose incrementally every 2-4 weeks to normalize calcium levels or maintain iPTH level (maximum: 360 mg/day [parathyroid cancer, primary hyperparathyroidism]; 180 mg/day [secondary hyperparathyroidism])

Dosage Forms
Tablet, oral:
Sensipar®: 30 mg, 60 mg, 90 mg

cinacalcet hydrochloride *see* cinacalcet *on page 209*
Cinryze™ *see* C1 inhibitor (human) *on page 156*
Cipralex® (Can) *see* escitalopram *on page 341*
Cipro® *see* ciprofloxacin (systemic) *on page 210*
Cipro® XL (Can) *see* ciprofloxacin (systemic) *on page 210*
Ciprodex® *see* ciprofloxacin and dexamethasone *on page 211*

ciprofloxacin (systemic) (sip roe FLOKS a sin)

Medication Safety Issues
Sound-alike/look-alike issues:
Ciprofloxacin may be confused with cephalexin
Cipro® may be confused with Ceftin®

Synonyms ciprofloxacin hydrochloride

U.S. Brand Names Cipro®; Cipro® I.V.; Cipro® XR

Canadian Brand Names Apo-CiprofloxⓇ; CiproⓇ; CiproⓇ XL; CO Ciprofloxacin; Dom-Ciprofloxacin; Mint-Ciprofloxacin; Mylan-Ciprofloxacin; Novo-Ciprofloxacin; PHL-Ciprofloxacin; PMS-Ciprofloxacin; PRO-Ciprofloxacin; RAN™-Ciprofloxacin; ratio-Ciprofloxacin; Riva-Ciprofloxacin; Sandoz-Ciprofloxacin; Taro-Ciprofloxacin

Therapeutic Category Antibiotic, Quinolone

Use
Children: Complicated urinary tract infections and pyelonephritis due to *E. coli*. **Note:** Although effective, ciprofloxacin is not the drug of first choice in children.
Children and Adults: To reduce incidence or progression of disease following exposure to aerolized *Bacillus anthracis*.
Adults: Treatment of the following infections when caused by susceptible bacteria: Urinary tract infections; acute uncomplicated cystitis in females; chronic bacterial prostatitis; lower respiratory tract infections (including acute exacerbations of chronic bronchitis); acute sinusitis; skin and skin structure infections; bone and joint infections; complicated intraabdominal infections (in combination with metronidazole); infectious diarrhea; typhoid fever due to *Salmonella typhi* (eradication of chronic typhoid carrier state has not been proven); uncomplicated cervical and urethra gonorrhea (due to *N. gonorrhoeae*); nosocomial pneumonia; empirical therapy for febrile neutropenic patients (in combination with piperacillin)
Note: As of April 2007, the CDC no longer recommends the use of fluoroquinolones for the treatment of gonococcal disease.

General Dosage Range Dosage adjustment recommended in patients with renal impairment
I.V.:
Children: 20-30 mg/kg/day divided every 12 hours (maximum: 800 mg/day)
Adults: 200-400 mg every 8-12 hours
Oral:
Extended release: *Adults:* 500-1000 mg every 24 hours
Immediate release:
Children: 20-30 mg/kg/day in 2 divided doses (maximum: 1.5 g/day)
Adults: 250-750 mg every 12 hours or 250 mg to 1 g as a single dose

Dosage Forms
Infusion, premixed in D_5W: 200 mg (100 mL); 400 mg (200 mL)
Cipro® I.V.: 200 mg (100 mL); 400 mg (200 mL)
Infusion, premixed in D_5W [preservative free]: 200 mg (100 mL); 400 mg (200 mL)
Injection, solution: 10 mg/mL (20 mL, 40 mL, 120 mL)
Injection, solution [preservative free]: 10 mg/mL (20 mL, 40 mL)
Microcapsules for suspension, oral:
Cipro®: 250 mg/5 mL (100 mL); 500 mg/5 mL (100 mL)
Tablet, oral: 100 mg, 250 mg, 500 mg, 750 mg
Cipro®: 250 mg, 500 mg
Tablet, extended release, oral: 500 mg, 1000 mg
Cipro® XR: 500 mg, 1000 mg

ciprofloxacin (ophthalmic) (sip roe FLOKS a sin)

Medication Safety Issues
Sound-alike/look-alike issues:
Ciprofloxacin may be confused with cephalexin
Ciloxan® may be confused with Cytoxan

Synonyms ciprofloxacin hydrochloride

U.S. Brand Names Ciloxan®

Canadian Brand Names Ciloxan®

Therapeutic Category Antibiotic, Ophthalmic; Antibiotic, Quinolone

Use Treatment of superficial ocular infections (corneal ulcers, conjunctivitis) due to susceptible strains

General Dosage Range Ophthalmic:
  Ointment: *Children >2 years and Adults:* Apply a ¹/₂" ribbon into the conjunctival sac 3 times/day for the first 2 days, followed by a ¹/₂" ribbon applied twice daily
  Solution: *Children >1 year and Adults:* Conjunctivitis: Instill 1-2 drops in eye(s) every 2 hours while awake for 2 days, then 1-2 drops every 4 hours while awake; Corneal ulcer: Instill 2 drops into affected eye every 15 minutes for the first 6 hours, then 2 drops every 30 minutes for the remainder of the first day; on day 2 instill 2 drops into the affected eye hourly; on days 3-14 instill 2 drops every 4 hours
Dosage Forms
  Ointment, ophthalmic:
  Ciloxan®: 3.33 mg/g (3.5 g)
  Solution, ophthalmic: 3.5 mg/mL (2.5 mL, 5 mL, 10 mL)
  Ciloxan®: 3.5 mg/mL (5 mL)

ciprofloxacin (otic) (sip roe FLOKS a sin)
Medication Safety Issues
  Sound-alike/look-alike issues:
  Cetraxal® may be confused with cefTRIAXone
  Ciprofloxacin may be confused with cephalexin
Synonyms ciprofloxacin hydrochloride
U.S. Brand Names Cetraxal®
Therapeutic Category Antibiotic, Otic; Antibiotic, Quinolone
Use Treatment of acute otitis externa due to susceptible strains of *Pseudomonas aeruginosa* or *Staphylococcus aureus*
General Dosage Range Otic: *Children ≥1 year and Adults:* 0.5 mg (0.25 mL) every 12 hours
Dosage Forms
  Solution, otic [preservative free]:
  Cetraxal®: 0.5 mg/0.25 mL (14s)

ciprofloxacin and dexamethasone (sip roe FLOKS a sin & deks a METH a sone)
Synonyms ciprofloxacin hydrochloride and dexamethasone; dexamethasone and ciprofloxacin
U.S. Brand Names Ciprodex®
Canadian Brand Names Ciprodex®
Therapeutic Category Antibiotic/Corticosteroid, Otic
Use Treatment of acute otitis media in pediatric patients with tympanostomy tubes or acute otitis externa in children and adults
General Dosage Range Otic: *Children and Adults:* Instill 4 drops into affected ear(s) twice daily
Dosage Forms
  Suspension, otic:
  Ciprodex®: Ciprofloxacin 0.3% and dexamethasone 0.1% (7.5 mL)

ciprofloxacin and hydrocortisone (sip roe FLOKS a sin & hye droe KOR ti sone)
Synonyms ciprofloxacin hydrochloride and hydrocortisone; hydrocortisone and ciprofloxacin
U.S. Brand Names Cipro® HC
Canadian Brand Names Cipro® HC
Therapeutic Category Antibiotic/Corticosteroid, Otic
Use Treatment of acute otitis externa, sometimes known as "swimmer's ear"
General Dosage Range Otic: *Children >1 year and Adults:* 3 drops into affected ear(s) twice daily
Dosage Forms
  Suspension, otic:
  Cipro® HC: Ciprofloxacin 0.2% and hydrocortisone 1% (10 mL)

ciprofloxacin hydrochloride *see* ciprofloxacin (ophthalmic) *on page 210*
ciprofloxacin hydrochloride *see* ciprofloxacin (otic) *on page 211*
ciprofloxacin hydrochloride *see* ciprofloxacin (systemic) *on page 210*
ciprofloxacin hydrochloride and dexamethasone *see* ciprofloxacin and dexamethasone *on page 211*
ciprofloxacin hydrochloride and hydrocortisone *see* ciprofloxacin and hydrocortisone *on page 211*

Cipro® HC *see* ciprofloxacin and hydrocortisone *on page 211*

Cipro® I.V. *see* ciprofloxacin (systemic) *on page 210*

Cipro® XR *see* ciprofloxacin (systemic) *on page 210*

cisapride (SIS a pride)

Medication Safety Issues

Sound-alike/look-alike issues:
Propulsid® may be confused with propranolol

U.S. Brand Names Propulsid®

Therapeutic Category Gastrointestinal Agent, Prokinetic

Use Treatment of nocturnal symptoms of gastroesophageal reflux disease (GERD); has demonstrated effectiveness for gastroparesis, refractory constipation, and nonulcer dyspepsia

General Dosage Range

Oral:
Children: 0.15-0.3 mg/kg 3-4 times/day (maximum: 10 mg/dose)
Adults: Initial: 5-10 mg 4 times/day, may increase to 20 mg 4 times/day if needed

cisatracurium (sis a tra KYOO ree um)

Medication Safety Issues

Sound-alike/look-alike issues:
Nimbex® may be confused with Revex®

High alert medication:
The Institute for Safe Medication Practices (ISMP) includes this medication among its list of drugs which have a heightened risk of causing significant patient harm when used in error.

Other safety concerns:
United States Pharmacopeia (USP) 2006: The Interdisciplinary Safe Medication Use Expert Committee of the USP has recommended the following:
- Hospitals, clinics, and other practice sites should institute special safeguards in the storage, labeling, and use of these agents and should include these safeguards in staff orientation and competency training.
- Healthcare professionals should be on high alert (especially vigilant) whenever a neuromuscular-blocking agent (NMBA) is stocked, ordered, prepared, or administered.

Synonyms cisatracurium besylate

U.S. Brand Names Nimbex®

Canadian Brand Names Nimbex®

Therapeutic Category Skeletal Muscle Relaxant

Use Adjunct to general anesthesia to facilitate endotracheal intubation and to relax skeletal muscles during surgery; to facilitate mechanical ventilation in ICU patients; does not relieve pain or produce sedation

General Dosage Range I.V.:
Children 1-23 months: Intubating dose: 0.15 mg/kg
Children 2-12 years: Intubating dose: 0.1-0.15 mg/kg over 5-15 seconds; Infusion: Initial: 3 mcg/kg/minute; Maintenance: 1-2 mcg/kg/minute (surgery) **or** 0.5-10 mcg/kg/minute (ICU)
Children >12 years: Infusion: Initial: 3 mcg/kg/minute; Maintenance: 1-2 mcg/kg/minute (surgery) **or** 0.5-10 mcg/kg/minute (ICU)
Adults: Intubating dose: 0.1-0.2 mg/kg; Infusion: Initial: 3 mcg/kg/minute; Maintenance: 1-2 mcg/kg/minute (surgery) **or** 0.5-10 mcg/kg/minute (ICU)

Dosage Forms

Injection, solution:
Nimbex®: 2 mg/mL (5 mL, 10 mL); 10 mg/mL (20 mL)

cisatracurium besylate *see* cisatracurium *on page 212*

cisplatin (SIS pla tin)

Medication Safety Issues
Sound-alike/look-alike issues:
CISplatin may be confused with CARBOplatin, oxaliplatin
High alert medication:
This medication is in a class the Institute for Safe Medication Practices (ISMP) includes among its list of drugs which have a heightened risk of causing significant patient harm when used in error.
Administration issues:
Doses >100 mg/m^2 once every 3-4 weeks are rarely used and should be verified with the prescriber.
Synonyms CDDP; Platinol; Platinol-AQ
Tall-Man CISplatin
Therapeutic Category Antineoplastic Agent
Use Treatment of advanced bladder cancer, metastatic testicular cancer, and metastatic ovarian cancer
General Dosage Range Dosage adjustment recommended in patients with renal impairment
I.V.: *Adults:* 50-70 mg/m^2 every 3-4 weeks **or** 75-100 mg/m^2/day every 4 weeks **or** 20 mg/m^2/day for 5 days every 3 weeks
Dosage Forms
Injection, solution [preservative free]: 1 mg/mL (50 mL, 100 mL, 200 mL)

13-*cis*-retinoic acid *see* isotretinoin *on page 495*

citalopram (sye TAL oh pram)

Medication Safety Issues
Sound-alike/look-alike issues:
CeleXA® may be confused with CeleBREX®, Cerebyx®, Ranexa™, ZyPREXA®
Synonyms citalopram hydrobromide; nitalapram
U.S. Brand Names CeleXA®
Canadian Brand Names Apo-Citalopram®; Celexa®; Citalopram-Odan; CO Citalopram; CTP 30; Dom-Citalopram; JAMP-Citalopram; Mint-Citalopram; Mylan-Citalopram; NG-Citalopram; Novo-Citalopram; PHL-Citalopram; PMS-Citalopram; RAN™-Citalo; ratio-Citalopram; Riva-Citalopram; Sandoz-Citalopram; Septa-Citalopram; Teva-Citalopram
Therapeutic Category Antidepressant
Use Treatment of depression
General Dosage Range Dosage adjustment recommended in patients with hepatic impairment
Oral:
Adults: Initial: 20 mg/day; Maintenance: 20-40 mg/day
Elderly: 20 mg/day
Dosage Forms
Solution, oral: 10 mg/5 mL (240 mL)
Tablet, oral: 10 mg, 20 mg, 40 mg
CeleXA®: 10 mg, 20 mg, 40 mg

citalopram hydrobromide *see* citalopram *on page 213*
Citalopram-Odan (Can) *see* citalopram *on page 213*
Citanest® Plain (Can) *see* prilocaine *on page 737*
Citanest® Plain Dental *see* prilocaine *on page 737*
Citracal® Maximum [OTC] *see* calcium and vitamin D *on page 160*
Citracal® Petites [OTC] *see* calcium and vitamin D *on page 160*
Citracal® Regular [OTC] *see* calcium and vitamin D *on page 160*
CitraNatal™ 90 DHA *see* vitamins (multiple/prenatal) *on page 920*
CitraNatal™ Assure *see* vitamins (multiple/prenatal) *on page 920*
CitraNatal™ B-Calm *see* vitamins (multiple/prenatal) *on page 920*
CitraNatal™ DHA *see* vitamins (multiple/prenatal) *on page 920*
CitraNatal® Harmony™ *see* vitamins (multiple/prenatal) *on page 920*
CitraNatal™ Rx *see* vitamins (multiple/prenatal) *on page 920*
citrate of magnesia *see* magnesium citrate *on page 544*
citric acid and D-gluconic acid irrigant *see* citric acid, magnesium carbonate, and glucono-delta-lactone *on page 214*

citric acid and potassium citrate *see* potassium citrate and citric acid *on page 725*

citric acid bladder mixture *see* citric acid, magnesium carbonate, and glucono-delta-lactone *on page 214*

citric acid, magnesium carbonate, and glucono-delta-lactone
(SI trik AS id, mag NEE see um KAR bo nate, and GLOO kon o DEL ta LAK tone)

Medication Safety Issues
Sound-alike/look-alike issues:
Renacidin® may be confused with Remicade®

Synonyms citric acid and D-gluconic acid irrigant; citric acid bladder mixture; citric acid, magnesium hydroxycarbonate, D-gluconic acid, magnesium acid citrate, and calcium carbonate; hemiacidrin

U.S. Brand Names Renacidin®

Therapeutic Category Irrigating Solution

Use Prevention of formation of calcifications of indwelling urinary tract catheters; treatment of renal and bladder calculi of the apatite or struvite type

General Dosage Range Irrigation: *Adults:* 30-60 mL into catheter 2-3 times/day **or** 30 mL into bladder, retained for 30-60 minutes then drained 4-6 times **or** 60-120 mL/hour

Dosage Forms
Solution, irrigation:
Renacidin®: Citric acid 6.602 g, magnesium carbonate 3.177 g, glucono-delta-lactone 0.198 g per 100 mL (500 mL)

citric acid, magnesium hydroxycarbonate, D-gluconic acid, magnesium acid citrate, and calcium carbonate *see* citric acid, magnesium carbonate, and glucono-delta-lactone *on page 214*

citric acid, sodium citrate, and potassium citrate
(SIT rik AS id, SOW dee um SIT rate, & poe TASS ee um SIT rate)

Medication Safety Issues
Sound-alike/look-alike issues:
Polycitra may be confused with Bicitra

Synonyms Polycitra; potassium citrate, citric acid, and sodium citrate; sodium citrate, citric acid, and potassium citrate

U.S. Brand Names Cytra-3; Tricitrates

Therapeutic Category Alkalinizing Agent

Use Conditions where long-term maintenance of an alkaline urine is desirable as in control and dissolution of uric acid and cystine calculi of the urinary tract

General Dosage Range Oral:
Children: 5-15 mL after meals and at bedtime
Adults: 15-30 mL after meals and at bedtime

Dosage Forms
Solution, oral:
Cytra-3, Tricitrates: Citric acid 334 mg, sodium citrate 500 mg, and potassium citrate 550 mg per 5 mL

Citroma® [OTC] *see* magnesium citrate *on page 544*

Citro-Mag® (Can) *see* magnesium citrate *on page 544*

citrovorum factor *see* leucovorin calcium *on page 515*

Citrucel® [OTC] *see* methylcellulose *on page 574*

CL-118,532 *see* triptorelin *on page 894*

Cl-719 *see* gemfibrozil *on page 414*

CL-184116 *see* porfimer *on page 722*

CL-232315 *see* mitoxantrone *on page 593*

cladribine (KLA dri been)

Medication Safety Issues
Sound-alike/look-alike issues:
Cladribine may be confused with clevidipine, clofarabine, fludarabine
Leustatin® may be confused with lovastatin
High alert medication:
This medication is in a class the Institute for Safe Medication Practices (ISMP) includes among its list of drug classes which have a heightened risk of causing significant patient harm when used in error.

Synonyms 2-CdA; 2-chlorodeoxyadenosine; NSC-105014
U.S. Brand Names Leustatin®
Canadian Brand Names Leustatin®
Therapeutic Category Antineoplastic Agent
Use Treatment of hairy cell leukemia
General Dosage Range Dosage adjustment recommended in patients with renal impairment
I.V.: *Adults:* Continuous infusion: 0.09 mg/kg/day for 7 days
Dosage Forms
Injection, solution [preservative free]: 1 mg/mL (10 mL)
Leustatin®: 1 mg/mL (10 mL)

Claforan® *see* cefotaxime *on page 182*
Claravis™ *see* isotretinoin *on page 495*
Clarifoam™ EF *see* sulfur and sulfacetamide *on page 838*
Clarinex® *see* desloratadine *on page 261*
Clarinex-D® 12 Hour *see* desloratadine and pseudoephedrine *on page 261*
Clarinex-D® 24 Hour *see* desloratadine and pseudoephedrine *on page 261*

clarithromycin (kla RITH roe mye sin)

Medication Safety Issues
Sound-alike/look-alike issues:
Clarithromycin may be confused with Claritin®, clindamycin, erythromycin
U.S. Brand Names Biaxin®; Biaxin® XL
Canadian Brand Names Apo-Clarithromycin®; Biaxin®; Biaxin® XL; Dom-Clarithromycin; Mylan-Clarithromycin; PMS-Clarithromycin; RAN™-Clarithromycin; ratio-Clarithromycin; Riva-Clarithromycin; Sandoz-Clarithromycin
Therapeutic Category Macrolide (Antibiotic)
Use
Children:
Acute otitis media (*H. influenzae*, *M. catarrhalis*, or *S. pneumoniae*)
Community-acquired pneumonia due to susceptible *Mycoplasma pneumoniae*, *S. pneumoniae*, or *Chlamydia pneumoniae* (TWAR)
Pharyngitis/tonsillitis due to susceptible *S. pyogenes*, acute maxillary sinusitis due to susceptible *H. influenzae*, *S. pneumoniae,* or *Moraxella catarrhalis*, uncomplicated skin/skin structure infections due to susceptible *S. aureus, S. pyogenes,* and mycobacterial infections
Prevention of disseminated mycobacterial infections due to MAC disease in patients with advanced HIV infection
Adults:
Pharyngitis/tonsillitis due to susceptible *S. pyogenes*
Acute maxillary sinusitis due to susceptible *H. influenzae, M. catarrhalis,* or *S. pneumoniae*
Acute exacerbation of chronic bronchitis due to susceptible *H. influenzae, H. parainfluenzae, M. catarrhalis,* or *S. pneumoniae*
Community-acquired pneumonia due to susceptible *H. influenzae, H. parainfluenzae, Mycoplasma pneumoniae, S. pneumoniae,* or *Chlamydia pneumoniae* (TWAR), *Moraxella catarrhalis*
Uncomplicated skin/skin structure infections due to susceptible *S. aureus, S. pyogenes*
Disseminated mycobacterial infections due to *M. avium* or *M. intracellulare*
Prevention of disseminated mycobacterial infections due to *M. avium* complex (MAC) disease (eg, patients with advanced HIV infection)
Duodenal ulcer disease due to *H. pylori* in regimens with other drugs including amoxicillin and lansoprazole or omeprazole, ranitidine bismuth citrate, bismuth subsalicylate, tetracycline, and/or an H_2 antagonist
General Dosage Range Dosage adjustment recommended in patients with renal impairment
Oral:
Extended release: *Adults:* 1000 mg once daily
Immediate release:
Children: 15 mg/kg/day divided every 12 hours (maximum: 1 g/day) **or** 15 mg/kg prior to procedure (maximum: 500 mg)
Adults: 250-500 mg every 8-12 hours **or** 500 mg prior to procedure

◄ **Dosage Forms**
  Granules for suspension, oral: 125 mg/5 mL (50 mL, 100 mL); 250 mg/5 mL (50 mL, 100 mL)
    Biaxin®: 125 mg/5 mL (50 mL, 100 mL); 250 mg/5 mL (50 mL, 100 mL)
  Tablet, oral: 250 mg, 500 mg
    Biaxin®: 250 mg, 500 mg
  Tablet, extended release, oral: 500 mg
    Biaxin® XL: 500 mg

clarithromycin, lansoprazole, and amoxicillin *see* lansoprazole, amoxicillin, and clarithromycin *on page 511*
Claritin® (Can) *see* loratadine *on page 536*
Claritin® 24 Hour Allergy [OTC] *see* loratadine *on page 536*
Claritin-D® 12 Hour Allergy & Congestion [OTC] *see* loratadine and pseudoephedrine *on page 537*
Claritin-D® 24 Hour Allergy & Congestion [OTC] *see* loratadine and pseudoephedrine *on page 537*
Claritin® Allergic Decongestant (Can) *see* oxymetazoline (nasal) *on page 664*
Claritin® Children's Allergy [OTC] *see* loratadine *on page 536*
Claritin® Extra (Can) *see* loratadine and pseudoephedrine *on page 537*
Claritin™ Eye [OTC] *see* ketotifen (ophthalmic) *on page 503*
Claritin® Kids (Can) *see* loratadine *on page 536*
Claritin® Liberator (Can) *see* loratadine and pseudoephedrine *on page 537*
Claritin® Liqui-Gels® 24 Hour Allergy [OTC] *see* loratadine *on page 536*
Claritin® RediTabs® 24 Hour Allergy [OTC] *see* loratadine *on page 536*
Clarus™ (Can) *see* isotretinoin *on page 495*
Clasteon® (Can) *see* clodronate *(Canada only) on page 221*
clavulanic acid and amoxicillin *see* amoxicillin and clavulanate potassium *on page 74*
Clavulin® (Can) *see* amoxicillin and clavulanate potassium *on page 74*
Clean & Clear® Advantage® Acne Cleanser [OTC] *see* salicylic acid *on page 795*
Clean & Clear® Advantage® Acne Spot Treatment [OTC] *see* salicylic acid *on page 795*
Clean & Clear® Advantage® Invisible Acne Patch [OTC] *see* salicylic acid *on page 795*
Clean & Clear® Advantage® Oil-Free Acne [OTC] *see* salicylic acid *on page 795*
Clean & Clear® Blackhead Clearing Daily Cleansing [OTC] *see* salicylic acid *on page 795*
Clean & Clear® Blackhead Clearing Scrub [OTC] *see* salicylic acid *on page 795*
Clean & Clear® Continuous Control® Acne Wash [OTC] *see* salicylic acid *on page 795*
Clean & Clear® Deep Cleaning [OTC] *see* salicylic acid *on page 795*
Clean & Clear® Dual Action Moisturizer [OTC] *see* salicylic acid *on page 795*
Clean & Clear® Invisible Blemish Treatment [OTC] *see* salicylic acid *on page 795*
Clear eyes® for Dry Eyes Plus ACR Relief [OTC] *see* naphazoline (ophthalmic) *on page 611*
Clear eyes® for Dry Eyes plus Redness Relief [OTC] *see* naphazoline (ophthalmic) *on page 611*
Clear eyes® Redness Relief [OTC] *see* naphazoline (ophthalmic) *on page 611*
Clear eyes® Seasonal Relief [OTC] *see* naphazoline (ophthalmic) *on page 611*
Clearskin [OTC] *see* benzoyl peroxide *on page 124*

clemastine (KLEM as teen)

Synonyms clemastine fumarate
U.S. Brand Names Tavist® Allergy [OTC]
Therapeutic Category Antihistamine
Use Perennial and seasonal allergic rhinitis and other allergic symptoms including urticaria
General Dosage Range Oral:
  Children <6 years: 0.05 mg/kg/day (base) **or** 0.335-0.67 mg/day (fumarate) in 2-3 divided doses (maximum: 1.34 mg/day [fumarate] or 1 mg/day [base])
  Children 6-12 years: 0.67-1.34 mg fumarate (0.5-1 mg base) twice daily (maximum: 4.02 mg/day [3 mg base])
  Children ≥12 years and Adults: 1.34-2.68 mg fumarate (1-2 mg base) 2-3 times/day (maximum: 8.04 mg/day [6 mg base])

Dosage Forms
  Syrup, oral: 0.67 mg/5 mL (120 mL, 473 mL)
  Tablet, oral: 1.34 mg, 2.68 mg
    Tavist® Allergy [OTC]: 1.34 mg

clemastine fumarate see clemastine on page 216
Clenia™ see sulfur and sulfacetamide on page 838
Cleocin® see clindamycin (topical) on page 218
Cleocin HCl® see clindamycin (systemic) on page 217
Cleocin Pediatric® see clindamycin (systemic) on page 217
Cleocin Phosphate® see clindamycin (systemic) on page 217
Cleocin T® see clindamycin (topical) on page 218
Cleocin® Vaginal Ovule see clindamycin (topical) on page 218

clevidipine (klev ID i peen)

Medication Safety Issues
  Sound-alike/look-alike issues:
    Clevidipine may be confused with cladribine, clofarabine, clomiPRAMINE
    Cleviprex™ may be confused with Claravis™
Synonyms clevidipine butyrate
U.S. Brand Names Cleviprex™
Therapeutic Category Calcium Channel Blocker
Use Management of hypertension
General Dosage Range I.V.: Adults: Initial: 1-2 mg/hour; Usual maintenance: 4-6 mg/hour; Maximum: 21 mg/hour (1000 mL/24 hours)
Dosage Forms
  Injection, emulsion:
    Cleviprex™: 0.5 mg/mL (50 mL, 100 mL)

clevidipine butyrate see clevidipine on page 217
Cleviprex™ see clevidipine on page 217

clidinium and chlordiazepoxide (kli DI nee um & klor dye az e POKS ide)

Medication Safety Issues
  Sound-alike/look-alike issues:
    Librax® may be confused with Librium
  BEERS Criteria medication:
    This drug may be inappropriate for use in geriatric patients (high severity risk).
Synonyms chlordiazepoxide and clidinium
U.S. Brand Names Librax® [original formulation]
Canadian Brand Names Apo-Chlorax®; Librax®
Therapeutic Category Anticholinergic Agent
Use Adjunct treatment of peptic ulcer; treatment of irritable bowel syndrome
General Dosage Range Oral: Adults: 1-2 capsules 3-4 times/day
Dosage Forms
  Capsule: Clidinium 2.5 mg and chlordiazepoxide 5 mg
  Librax® [original formulation]: Clidinium 2.5 mg and chlordiazepoxide 5 mg

Climara® see estradiol (systemic) on page 343
ClimaraPro® see estradiol and levonorgestrel on page 345
Clinac® BPO see benzoyl peroxide on page 124
Clindagel® see clindamycin (topical) on page 218
ClindaMax® see clindamycin (topical) on page 218

clindamycin (systemic) (klin da MYE sin)

Medication Safety Issues
  Sound-alike/look-alike issues:
    Cleocin® may be confused with bleomycin, Clinoril®, Cubicin®, Lincocin®
    Clindamycin may be confused with clarithromycin, Claritin®, vancomycin

▶

◀ **Synonyms** clindamycin hydrochloride; clindamycin palmitate

U.S. Brand Names Cleocin HCl®; Cleocin Pediatric®; Cleocin Phosphate®

Canadian Brand Names Alti-Clindamycin; Apo-Clindamycin®; Clindamycin Injection, USP; Clindamycine; Gen-Clindamycin; Mylan-Clindamycin; Novo-Clindamycin; NV-Clindamycin; PMS-Clindamycin; ratio-Clindamycin; Riva-Clindamycin; Teva-Clindamycin

Therapeutic Category Antibiotic, Lincosamide

Use Treatment of susceptible bacterial infections, mainly those caused by anaerobes, streptococci, pneumococci, and staphylococci; pelvic inflammatory disease (I.V.)

General Dosage Range

I.M., I.V.:
Children >1 month: 20-40 mg/kg/day in 3-4 divided doses
Adults: 1.2-2.7 g/day in 2-4 divided doses (maximum: 4.8 g/day)

Oral:
Children: 8-20 mg/kg/day as hydrochloride or 8-25 mg/kg/day as palmitate in 3-4 divided doses (minimum dose of palmitate: 37.5 mg 3 times/day)
Adults: 150-450 mg every 6-8 hours (maximum: 1.8 g/day)

Dosage Forms

Capsule, oral: 75 mg, 150 mg, 300 mg
  Cleocin HCl®: 75 mg, 150 mg, 300 mg
Granules for solution, oral: 75 mg/5 mL (100 mL)
  Cleocin Pediatric®: 75 mg/5 mL (100 mL)
Infusion, premixed in D₅W:
  Cleocin Phosphate®: 300 mg (50 mL); 600 mg (50 mL); 900 mg (50 mL)
Injection, solution: 150 mg/mL (2 mL, 4 mL, 6 mL, 60 mL)
  Cleocin Phosphate®: 150 mg/mL (2 mL, 4 mL, 6 mL, 60 mL)

clindamycin (topical) (klin da MYE sin)

Medication Safety Issues

Sound-alike/look-alike issues:
Cleocin® may be confused with bleomycin, Clinoril®, Cubicin®, Lincocin®
Clindamycin may be confused with clarithromycin, Claritin®, vancomycin

Synonyms clindamycin phosphate

U.S. Brand Names Cleocin T®; Cleocin®; Cleocin® Vaginal Ovule; Clindagel®; ClindaMax®; ClindaReach®; Clindesse®; Evoclin®

Canadian Brand Names Clinda-T; Clindasol™; Clindets; Dalacin® C; Dalacin® T; Dalacin® Vaginal; Taro-Clindamycin

Therapeutic Category Antibiotic, Lincosamide; Topical Skin Product, Acne

Use Treatment of bacterial vaginosis (vaginal cream, vaginal suppository); topically in treatment of severe acne

General Dosage Range

Intravaginal: *Adults:* Insert 1 ovule or applicatorful once daily **or** 1 applicatorful as a single dose (Clindesse®)
Topical: *Children ≥12 years and Adults:* Apply once or twice daily

Dosage Forms

Aerosol, topical: 1% (50 g, 100 g)
  Evoclin®: 1% (50 g, 100 g)
Cream, vaginal: 2% (40 g)
  Cleocin®: 2% (40 g)
  Clindesse®: 2% (5 g)
Gel, topical: 1% (30 g, 60 g)
  Cleocin T®: 1% (30 g, 60 g)
  Clindagel®: 1% (40 mL, 75 mL)
  ClindaMax®: 1% (30 g, 60 g)
Lotion, topical: 1% (60 mL)
  Cleocin T®: 1% (60 mL)
  ClindaMax®: 1% (60 mL)
Pledget, topical: 1% (60s, 69s)
  Cleocin T®: 1% (60s)
  ClindaReach®: 1% (120s)

Solution, topical: 1% (30 mL, 60 mL)
  Cleocin T®: 1% (30 mL, 60 mL)
Suppository, vaginal:
  Cleocin® Vaginal Ovule: 100 mg (3s)

clindamycin and benzoyl peroxide (klin da MYE sin & BEN zoe il peer OKS ide)

Synonyms benzoyl peroxide and clindamycin; clindamycin phosphate and benzoyl peroxide
U.S. Brand Names Acanya®; BenzaClin®; Duac® CS [DSC]
Canadian Brand Names BenzaClin®; Clindoxyl
Therapeutic Category Topical Skin Product; Topical Skin Product, Acne
Use Topical treatment of acne vulgaris
General Dosage Range Topical: *Children ≥12 years and Adults:* Apply once daily (Acanya®, Duac® CS) or twice daily (BenzaClin®) to affected areas
Dosage Forms
  Gel, topical: Clindamycin 1% and benzoyl peroxide 5% (50 g)
  Acanya®: Clindamycin 1.2% and benzoyl peroxide 2.5% (50 g)
  BenzaClin®: Clindamycin 1% and benzoyl peroxide 5% (25 g, 35 g, 50 g)
  Duac®: Clindamycin 1% and benzoyl peroxide 5% (45 g)

clindamycin and tretinoin (klin da MYE sin & TRET i noyn)

Synonyms clindamycin phosphate and tretinoin; tretinoin and clindamycin
U.S. Brand Names Veltin™; Ziana™
Therapeutic Category Acne Products; Retinoic Acid Derivative; Topical Skin Product; Topical Skin Product, Acne
Use Treatment of acne vulgaris
General Dosage Range Topical: *Children ≥12 years and Adults:* Apply pea-size amount to entire face once daily at bedtime
Dosage Forms
  Gel, topical:
  Veltin™: Clindamycin phosphate 1.2% and tretinoin 0.025% (30 g, 60 g)
  Ziana™: Clindamycin phosphate 1.2% and tretinoin 0.025% (30 g, 60 g)

Clindamycine (Can) *see* clindamycin (systemic) *on page 217*
clindamycin hydrochloride *see* clindamycin (systemic) *on page 217*
Clindamycin Injection, USP (Can) *see* clindamycin (systemic) *on page 217*
clindamycin palmitate *see* clindamycin (systemic) *on page 217*
clindamycin phosphate *see* clindamycin (topical) *on page 218*
clindamycin phosphate and benzoyl peroxide *see* clindamycin and benzoyl peroxide *on page 219*
clindamycin phosphate and tretinoin *see* clindamycin and tretinoin *on page 219*
ClindaReach® *see* clindamycin (topical) *on page 218*
Clindasol™ (Can) *see* clindamycin (topical) *on page 218*
Clinda-T (Can) *see* clindamycin (topical) *on page 218*
Clindesse® *see* clindamycin (topical) *on page 218*
Clindets (Can) *see* clindamycin (topical) *on page 218*
Clindoxyl (Can) *see* clindamycin and benzoyl peroxide *on page 219*
Clinisol® *see* amino acid injection *on page 65*
Clinoril® *see* sulindac *on page 839*
Clinpro™ 5000 *see* fluoride *on page 386*

clioquinol and flumethasone *(Canada only)* (klye ok KWIN ole & floo METH a sone)

Synonyms flumethasone and clioquinol; iodochlorhydroxyquin and flumethasone
Canadian Brand Names Locacorten® Vioform®
Therapeutic Category Antibiotic, Topical; Corticosteroid, Topical
Use
  Otic solution: Treatment of otitis externa; otomycosis due to *Aspergillus niger*
  Topical cream: Treatment of corticosteroid-responsive dermatoses complicated by infection with bacterial and/or fungal agents

219

◀ **General Dosage Range**
Otic: *Children >2 years and Adults:* Instill 2-3 drops into affected ear(s) 2 times/day
Topical: *Children >2 years and Adults:* Apply a thin layer to affected area 2-3 times/day
Product Availability Not available in U.S.
Dosage Forms - Canada
Cream, topical:
Locacorten® Vioform®: Clioquinol 3% and flumethasone 0.02% (15 g, 50 g)
Solution, otic:
Locacorten® Vioform®: Clioquinol 1% and flumethasone 0.02% (10 mL)

Clobazam-10 (Can) *see clobazam (Canada only) on page 220*

clobazam *(Canada only)* (KLOE ba zam)

Canadian Brand Names Apo-Clobazam®; Clobazam-10; Dom-Clobazam; Frisium®; Novo-Clobazam; PMS-Clobazam
Therapeutic Category Anticonvulsant; Antidepressant
Use Adjunctive treatment of epilepsy
General Dosage Range Dosage adjustment recommended in patients with hepatic or renal impairment
Oral:
Children <2 years: 0.5-1 mg/kg/day
Children 2-16 years: Initial: 5 mg/day; Maintenance: Up to 40 mg/day
Adults: Initial: 5-15 mg/day; Maintenance: Up to 80 mg/day
Product Availability Not available in U.S.
Dosage Forms - Canada
Tablet:
Alti-Clobazam, Apo-Clobazam®, Clobazam-10, Dom-Clobazam, Frisium®, Novo-Clobazam, PMS-Clobazam, ratio-Clobazam: 10 mg

clobetasol (kloe BAY ta sol)

Medication Safety Issues
International issues:
Clobex [U.S., Canada, and multiple international markets] may be confused with Codex brand name for *Saccharomyces boulardii* [Italy]
Cloderm: Brand name for clobetasol [China, India, Malaysia, Singapore, Thailand], but also brand name for alclometasone [Indonesia]; clocortolone [U.S., Canada]; clotrimazole [Germany]
Synonyms clobetasol propionate
U.S. Brand Names Clobex®; Cormax®; Olux-E™; Olux®; Olux®/Olux-E™ CP [DSC]; Temovate E®; Temovate®
Canadian Brand Names Clobex®; Dermovate®; Gen-Clobetasol; Mylan-Clobetasol Cream; Mylan-Clobetasol Ointment; Mylan-Clobetasol Scalp Application; Novo-Clobetasol; PMS-Clobetasol; ratio-Clobetasol; Taro-Clobetasol
Therapeutic Category Corticosteroid, Topical
Use Short-term relief of inflammation of moderate-to-severe corticosteroid-responsive dermatoses (very high potency topical corticosteroid)
General Dosage Range Topical:
Children ≥12 years: Apply to affected area twice daily (maximum: 50 g/week; 50 mL/week)
Adults: Apply to affected area twice daily **or** apply shampoo to dry scalp once daily (maximum: 50 g/week; 50 mL/week)
Dosage Forms
Aerosol, topical: 0.05% (50 g, 100 g)
Olux-E™: 0.05% (50 g, 100 g)
Olux®: 0.05% (50 g, 100 g)
Cream, topical: 0.05% (15 g, 30 g, 45 g, 60 g)
Temovate E®: 0.05% (60 g)
Gel, topical: 0.05% (15 g, 30 g, 60 g)
Temovate®: 0.05% (60 g)
Lotion, topical:
Clobex®: 0.05% (30 mL, 59 mL, 118 mL)

Ointment, topical: 0.05% (15 g, 30 g, 45 g, 60 g)
  Cormax®: 0.05% (15 g, 45 g)
  Temovate®: 0.05% (15 g, 30 g)
Shampoo, topical:
  Clobex®: 0.05% (118 mL)
Solution, topical: 0.05% (25 mL, 50 mL)
  Clobex®: 0.05% (59 mL, 125 mL)
  Cormax®: 0.05% (25 mL, 50 mL)
  Temovate®: 0.05% (50 mL)

clobetasol propionate *see* clobetasol *on page 220*
Clobex® *see* clobetasol *on page 220*

clocortolone (kloe KOR toe lone)

Medication Safety Issues
  International issues:
    Cloderm: Brand name for clocortolone [U.S., Canada], but also brand name for alclometasone [Indonesia]; clobetasol [China, India, Malaysia, Singapore, Thailand]; clotrimazole [Germany]
Synonyms clocortolone pivalate
U.S. Brand Names Cloderm®
Canadian Brand Names Cloderm®
Therapeutic Category Corticosteroid, Topical
Use Inflammation of corticosteroid-responsive dermatoses (intermediate-potency topical corticosteroid)
General Dosage Range Topical: *Adults:* Apply sparingly to affected area 1-4 times/day
Dosage Forms
  Cream, topical:
    Cloderm®: 0.1% (30 g, 45 g, 90 g)

clocortolone pivalate *see* clocortolone *on page 221*
Cloderm® *see* clocortolone *on page 221*

clodronate *(Canada only)* (KLOE droh nate)

Synonyms clodronate disodium
Canadian Brand Names Bonefos®; Clasteon®
Therapeutic Category Bisphosphonate Derivative
Use Management of hypercalcemia of malignancy; management of osteolysis due to bone metastases of malignancy
General Dosage Range Dosage adjustment recommended in patients with renal impairment
  I.V.: *Adults:* 1500 mg as single dose (Clasteon®) **or** 300 mg/day (Clasteon®, Bonefos®); Maximum therapy: 10 days (Clasteon®); 7 days (Bonefos®)
  Oral: *Adults:* 1600-2400 mg/day in 1-2 divided doses (maximum: 3200 mg/day)
Product Availability Not available in U.S.
Dosage Forms - Canada
  Capsule, oral:
    Bonefos®, Clasteon®: 400 mg
  Injection, solution:
    Bonefos®: 60 mg/mL (5 mL)
    Clasteon®; 30 mg/mL (10 mL)

clodronate disodium *see* clodronate *(Canada only) on page 221*

clofarabine (klo FARE a been)

Medication Safety Issues
  Sound-alike/look-alike issues:
    Clofarabine may be confused with cladribine, clevidipine
  High alert medication:
    This medication is in a class Institute for Safe Medication Practices (ISMP) includes among its list of drug classes which have a heightened risk of causing significant patient harm when used in error.
Synonyms CAFdA; clofarex; NSC606869
U.S. Brand Names Clolar®

◄ **Therapeutic Category** Antineoplastic Agent, Antimetabolite (Purine Antagonist)

Use Treatment of relapsed or refractory acute lymphoblastic leukemia (ALL)

General Dosage Range Dosage adjustment recommended in patients who develop toxicities

  I.V.: *Children >1 year and Adults ≤21 years:* 52 mg/m^2/day days 1 through 5; repeat every 2-6 weeks

Dosage Forms

  Injection, solution [preservative free]:

    Clolar®: 1 mg/mL (20 mL)

clofarex *see clofarabine on page 221*
Clolar® *see clofarabine on page 221*
Clomid® *see clomiphene on page 222*

clomiphene (KLOE mi feen)

Medication Safety Issues

  Sound-alike/look-alike issues:

    ClomiPHENE may be confused with clomiPRAMINE, clonidine

    Clomid® may be confused with clonidine

    Serophene® may be confused with Sarafem®

Synonyms clomiphene citrate

Tall-Man clomiPHENE

U.S. Brand Names Clomid®; Serophene®

Canadian Brand Names Clomid®; Milophene®; Serophene®

Therapeutic Category Ovulation Stimulator

Use Treatment of ovulatory failure in patients desiring pregnancy

General Dosage Range Oral: *Adults (females):* First course: 50 mg/day for 5 days; Second course (if needed): 100 mg/day for 5 days

Dosage Forms

  Tablet, oral: 50 mg

    Clomid®: 50 mg

    Serophene®: 50 mg

clomiphene citrate *see clomiphene on page 222*

clomipramine (kloe MI pra meen)

Medication Safety Issues

  Sound-alike/look-alike issues:

    ClomiPRAMINE may be confused with chlorproMAZINE, clevidipine, clomiPHENE, desipramine, Norpramin®

    Anafranil® may be confused with alfentanil, enalapril, nafarelin

Synonyms clomipramine hydrochloride

Tall-Man clomiPRAMINE

U.S. Brand Names Anafranil®

Canadian Brand Names Anafranil®; Apo-Clomipramine®; CO Clomipramine; Gen-Clomipramine

Therapeutic Category Antidepressant, Tricyclic (Tertiary Amine)

Use Treatment of obsessive-compulsive disorder (OCD)

General Dosage Range Oral:

  Children ≥10 years: Initial: 25 mg/day; Maintenance: Up to 3 mg/kg/day (maximum: 200 mg/day)

  Adults: Initial: 25 mg/day; Maintenance: Up to 250 mg/day

Dosage Forms

  Capsule, oral: 25 mg, 50 mg, 75 mg

    Anafranil®: 25 mg, 50 mg, 75 mg

clomipramine hydrochloride *see clomipramine on page 222*
Clonapam (Can) *see clonazepam on page 222*

clonazepam (kloe NA ze pam)

Medication Safety Issues

  Sound-alike/look-alike issues:

    ClonazePAM may be confused with cloNIDine, clorazepate, cloZAPine, LORazepam

KlonoPIN® may be confused with cloNIDine, clorazepate, cloZAPine, LORazepam

Tall-Man clonazePAM

U.S. Brand Names KlonoPIN®

Canadian Brand Names Alti-Clonazepam; Apo-Clonazepam®; Clonapam; CO Clonazepam; Gen-Clonazepam; Klonopin®; Mylan-Clonazepam; Novo-Clonazepam; Nu-Clonazepam; PMS-Clonazepam; PRO-Clonazepam; Rho®-Clonazepam; Rivotril®; Sandoz-Clonazepam; ZYM-Clonazepam

Therapeutic Category Benzodiazepine

Controlled Substance C-IV

Use Alone or as an adjunct in the treatment of petit mal variant (Lennox-Gastaut), akinetic, and myoclonic seizures; petit mal (absence) seizures unresponsive to succimides; panic disorder with or without agoraphobia

General Dosage Range Oral:

Children <10 years or <30 kg: Initial: 0.01-0.03 mg/kg/day in 2-3 divided doses (maximum: 0.05 mg/kg/day); Maintenance: 0.1-0.2 mg/kg/day in 3 divided doses (maximum: 0.2 mg/kg/day)

Children ≥10 years or ≥30 kg and Adults: Panic disorders: Initial: 0.25 mg twice daily; Maintenance: 1-4 mg/day in 2 divided doses; Seizure disorders: Initial: Up to 1.5 mg/day in 3 divided doses; Maintenance: 0.05-2 mg/kg/day (maximum: 20 mg/day)

Dosage Forms

Tablet, oral: 0.5 mg, 1 mg, 2 mg

KlonoPIN®: 0.5 mg, 1 mg, 2 mg

Tablet, orally disintegrating, oral: 0.125 mg, 0.25 mg, 0.5 mg, 1 mg, 2 mg

clonidine (KLON i deen)

Medication Safety Issues

Sound-alike/look-alike issues:

CloNIDine may be confused with Clomid®, clomiPHENE, clonazePAM, cloZAPine, KlonoPIN®, quiNIDine

Catapres® may be confused with Cataflam®, Combipres

High alert medication:

The Institute for Safe Medication Practices (ISMP) includes this medication (epidural administration) among its list of drug classes which have a heightened risk of causing significant patient harm when used in error.

BEERS Criteria medication:

This drug may be inappropriate for use in geriatric patients (low severity risk).

Administration issues:

Use caution when interpreting dosing information. Pediatric dose for epidural infusion expressed as mcg/kg/**hour**.

Other safety concerns:

Transdermal patch may contain conducting metal (eg, aluminum); remove patch prior to MRI. Errors have occurred when the inactive, optional adhesive cover has been applied instead of the active clonidine-containing patch.

Synonyms clonidine hydrochloride

Tall-Man cloNIDine

U.S. Brand Names Catapres-TTS®-1; Catapres-TTS®-2; Catapres-TTS®-3; Catapres®; Duraclon®; Kapvay™; Nexiclon™ XR

Canadian Brand Names Apo-Clonidine®; Carapres®; Dixarit®; Dom-Clonidine; Novo-Clonidine; Nu-Clonidine

Therapeutic Category Alpha-Adrenergic Agonist

Use

Oral:

Immediate release: Management of hypertension (monotherapy or as adjunctive therapy)

Extended release:

Kapvay™: Treatment of attention-deficit/hyperactivity disorder (ADHD) (monotherapy or as adjunctive therapy)

Nexiclon™ XR: Management of hypertension (monotherapy or as adjunctive therapy)

Epidural (Duraclon®): For continuous epidural administration as adjunctive therapy with opioids for treatment of severe cancer pain in patients tolerant to or unresponsive to opioids alone; epidural clonidine is generally more effective for neuropathic pain and less effective (or possibly ineffective) for somatic or visceral pain

Transdermal patch: Management of hypertension (monotherapy or as adjunctive therapy)

◀ **General Dosage Range Note:** Dosing is expressed as the salt (clonidine hydrochloride) unless otherwise noted.

Epidural:
Children: Initial: 0.5 mcg/kg/**hour**
Adults: Initial: 30 mcg/hour; Maintenance: Up to 40 mcg/hour

Oral, immediate release:
Adults: Initial: 0.1 mg twice daily; Maintenance: 0.1-0.8 mg/day in 2 divided doses (maximum: 2.4 mg/day)
Elderly: Initial: 0.1 mg once daily

Oral, extended release:
Children ≥6 years: (Kapvay™): Initial: 0.1 mg at bedtime; maximum: 0.4 mg/day [ADHD use]
Adults (Nexiclon™ XR): Initial: 0.17 mg clonidine base once daily at bedtime; maintenance: 0.17-0.52 mg/day clonidine base once daily (maximum: 0.52 mg/day clonidine base) [antihypertensive]

Transdermal: *Adults:* Initial: 0.1 mg/24 hour patch applied once every 7 days; Maintenance: 0.1-0.3 mg/24 hour patch applied once every 7 days (maximum: 0.6 mg/24 hours)

Dosage Forms
Injection, solution [preservative free]: 100 mcg/mL (10 mL); 500 mcg/mL (10 mL)
Duraclon®: 100 mcg/mL (10 mL); 500 mcg/mL (10 mL)
Patch, transdermal: 0.1 mg/24 hours (4s); 0.2 mg/24 hours (4s); 0.3 mg/24 hours (4s)
Catapres-TTS®-1: 0.1 mg/24 hours (4s)
Catapres-TTS®-2: 0.2 mg/24 hours (4s)
Catapres-TTS®-3: 0.3 mg/24 hours (4s)
Suspension, extended release, oral:
Nexiclon™ XR: 0.09 mg/mL (118 mL)
Tablet, oral: 0.1 mg, 0.2 mg, 0.3 mg
Catapres®: 0.1 mg, 0.2 mg, 0.3 mg
Tablet, extended release, oral:
Kapvay™: 0.1 mg
Nexiclon™ XR: 0.17 mg

clonidine and chlorthalidone (KLON i deen & klor THAL i done)

Medication Safety Issues
Sound-alike/look-alike issues:
Combipres may be confused with Catapres®
Synonyms chlorthalidone and clonidine; Combipres
U.S. Brand Names Clorpres®
Therapeutic Category Antihypertensive Agent, Combination
Use Management of mild-to-moderate hypertension
General Dosage Range Oral: *Adults:* 1 tablet (clonidine 0.1-0.3 mg/chlorthalidone 15 mg/tablet) 1-2 times/day (maximum: clonidine 0.6 mg; chlorthalidone 30 mg)
Dosage Forms
Tablet:
Clorpres®: 0.1: Clonidine 0.1 mg and chlorthalidone 15 mg; 0.2: Clonidine 0.2 mg and chlorthalidone 15 mg; 0.3: Clonidine 0.3 mg and chlorthalidone 15 mg

clonidine hydrochloride see clonidine on page 223

clopidogrel (kloh PID oh grel)

Medication Safety Issues
Sound-alike/look-alike issues:
Plavix® may be confused with Elavil®, Paxil®
Synonyms clopidogrel bisulfate
U.S. Brand Names Plavix®
Canadian Brand Names Plavix®
Therapeutic Category Antiplatelet Agent

Use Reduces rate of atherothrombotic events (myocardial infarction, stroke, vascular deaths) in patients with recent MI or stroke, or established peripheral arterial disease; reduces rate of atherothrombotic events in patients with unstable angina (UA) or non-ST-segment elevation (NSTEMI) managed medically or with percutaneous coronary intervention (PCI) (with or without stent) or CABG; reduces rate of death and atherothrombotic events in patients with ST-segment elevation MI (STEMI) managed medically

Canadian labeling: Additional use (not in U.S. labeling): Prevention of atherothrombotic and thromboembolic events, including stroke, in patients with atrial fibrillation with at least 1 risk factor for vascular events who are not suitable for treatment with an anticoagulant and are at a low risk for bleeding.

General Dosage Range Oral: *Adults:* Loading dose: 300 mg (maximum: 600 mg); Maintenance: 75 mg once daily

Dosage Forms
Tablet, oral:
Plavix®: 75 mg, 300 mg

clopidogrel bisulfate *see* clopidogrel *on page 224*

Clopixol® (Can) *see* zuclopenthixol *(Canada only) on page 935*

Clopixol-Acuphase® (Can) *see* zuclopenthixol *(Canada only) on page 935*

Clopixol® Depot (Can) *see* zuclopenthixol *(Canada only) on page 935*

clorazepate (klor AZ e pate)

Medication Safety Issues
Sound-alike/look-alike issues:
Clorazepate may be confused with clofibrate, clonazepam, KlonoPIN®
BEERS Criteria medication:
This drug may be inappropriate for use in geriatric patients (high severity risk).

Synonyms clorazepate dipotassium

U.S. Brand Names Tranxene® T-Tab®

Canadian Brand Names Apo-Clorazepate®; Novo-Clopate

Therapeutic Category Anticonvulsant; Benzodiazepine

Controlled Substance C-IV

Use Treatment of generalized anxiety disorder; management of ethanol withdrawal; adjunct anticonvulsant in management of partial seizures

General Dosage Range Oral:
Children 9-12 years: Initial: 3.75-7.5 mg twice daily; Maintenance: Up to 60 mg/day in 2-3 divided doses
Children >12 years: Initial: Up to 7.5 mg 2-3 times/day; Maintenance: Up to 90 mg/day
Adults: Initial: 7.5-15 mg 2-4 times/day; Maintenance: Up to 90 mg/day
Elderly: Anxiety: 7.5 mg 1-2 times/day

Dosage Forms
Tablet, oral: 3.75 mg, 7.5 mg, 15 mg
Tranxene® T-Tab®: 3.75 mg, 7.5 mg, 15 mg

clorazepate dipotassium *see* clorazepate *on page 225*

Clorpactin® WCS-90 [OTC] *see* oxychlorosene *on page 662*

Clorpres® *see* clonidine and chlorthalidone *on page 224*

Clotrimaderm (Can) *see* clotrimazole (topical) *on page 226*

clotrimazole (oral) (kloe TRIM a zole)

Medication Safety Issues
Sound-alike/look-alike issues:
Clotrimazole may be confused with co-trimoxazole
Mycelex may be confused with Myoflex®
International issues:
Cloderm: Brand name for clotrimazole [Germany], but also brand name for alclomethasone [Indonesia]; clobetasol [China, India, Malaysia, Singapore, Thailand]; clocortolone [U.S., Canada]
Canesten: Brand name for clotrimazole [multiple international markets] may be confused with Canesten Bifonazol Comp brand name for bifonazole/urea [Austria]; Canesten Extra brand name for bifonazole [China, Germany]; Canesten Extra Nagelset brand name for bifonazole/urea [Denmark]; Canesten Fluconazole brand name for fluconazole [New Zealand]; Canesten Oasis brand name for sodium citrate [Great Britain]; Canesten Once Daily brand name for bifonazole [Australia]; Canesten Oral ▶

◄ brand name for fluconazole [United Kingdom]; Cenestin® brand name for estrogens (conjugated A/ synthetic) [U.S., Canada]

Mycelex: Brand name for clotrimazole [U.S.] may be confused with Mucolex brand name for bromhexine [Malaysia]; carbocisteine [Thailand]

Synonyms Mycelex

Therapeutic Category Antifungal Agent, Oral Nonabsorbed

Use Treatment of susceptible fungal infections, including oropharyngeal candidiasis; limited data suggest that clotrimazole troches may be effective for prophylaxis against oropharyngeal candidiasis in neutropenic patients

General Dosage Range Oral: *Children >3 years and Adults:* Prophylaxis: 10 mg 3 times/day; Treatment: 10 mg 5 times/day

Dosage Forms
Troche, oral: 10 mg

clotrimazole (topical) (kloe TRIM a zole)

Medication Safety Issues

Sound-alike/look-alike issues:

Clotrimazole may be confused with co-trimoxazole

Lotrimin® may be confused with Lotrisone®

International issues:

Cloderm: Brand name for clotrimazole [Germany], but also brand name for alclomethasone [Indonesia]; clobetasol [China, India, Malaysia, Singapore, Thailand]; clocortolone [U.S., Canada]

Canesten: Brand name for clotrimazole [multiple international markets] may be confused with Canesten Bifonazol Comp brand name for bifonazole/urea [Austria]; Canesten Extra brand name for bifonazole [China, Germany]; Canesten Extra Nagelset brand name for bifonazole/urea [Denmark]; Canesten Fluconazole brand name for fluconazole [New Zealand]; Canesten Oasis brand name for sodium citrate [Great Britain]; Canesten Once Daily brand name for bifonazole [Australia]; Canesten Oral brand name for fluconazole [United Kingdom]; Cenestin® brand name for estrogens (conjugated A/ synthetic) [U.S., Canada]

U.S. Brand Names Anti-Fungal™ [OTC]; Cruex® [OTC]; Gyne-Lotrimin® 3 [OTC]; Gyne-Lotrimin® 7 [OTC]; Lotrimin® AF Athlete's Foot [OTC]; Lotrimin® AF for Her [OTC]; Lotrimin® AF Jock Itch [OTC]

Canadian Brand Names Canesten® Topical; Canesten® Vaginal; Clotrimaderm; Trivagizole-3®

Therapeutic Category Antifungal Agent, Topical; Antifungal Agent, Vaginal

Use Treatment of susceptible fungal infections, including dermatophytoses, superficial mycoses, and cutaneous candidiasis, as well as vulvovaginal candidiasis

General Dosage Range

Intravaginal: *Children >12 years and Adults:* Cream: Insert 1 applicatorful once daily

Topical: *Children >3 years and Adults:* Apply twice daily

Dosage Forms

Cream, topical: 1% (15 g, 30 g, 45 g)
Anti-Fungal™ [OTC]: 1% (113 g)
Cruex® [OTC]: 1% (15 g)
Lotrimin® AF Athlete's Foot [OTC]: 1% (12 g)
Lotrimin® AF for Her [OTC]: 1% (24 g)
Lotrimin® AF Jock Itch [OTC]: 1% (12 g)

Cream, vaginal: 1% (45 g); 2% (21 g)
Gyne-Lotrimin® 7 [OTC]: 1% (45 g)
Gyne-Lotrimin® 3 [OTC]: 2% (21 g)

Solution, topical: 1% (10 mL, 30 mL)

clotrimazole and betamethasone *see* betamethasone and clotrimazole *on page 130*

cloxacillin *(Canada only)* (kloks a SIL in)

Synonyms cloxacillin sodium

Canadian Brand Names Apo-Cloxi®; Novo-Cloxin; Nu-Cloxi

Therapeutic Category Penicillin

Use Treatment of bacterial infections including endocarditis, pneumonia, bone and joint infections, skin and soft-tissue infections, and sepsis that are caused by susceptible strains of penicillinase-producing staphylococci. **Note:** Exhibits good activity against *Staphylococcus aureus*; has activity against many streptococci, but is less active than penicillin and is generally not used in clinical practice to treat streptococcal infections.

General Dosage Range I.M., I.V., oral:
Children ≤20 kg: 25-50 mg/kg/day in divided doses every 6 hours
Children >20 kg and Adults: 250-500 mg every 6 hours

Product Availability Not available in U.S.

Dosage Forms - Canada
Capsule, oral: 250 mg, 500 mg
Injection, powder for reconstitution: 250 mg, 500 mg, 1000 mg, 2000 mg
Powder for suspension, oral: 125 mg/5 mL

cloxacillin sodium *see* cloxacillin *(Canada only) on page 226*

clozapine (KLOE za peen)

Medication Safety Issues
Sound-alike/look-alike issues:
CloZAPine may be confused with clonazePAM, cloNIDine, KlonoPIN®
Clozaril® may be confused with Clinoril®, Colazal®

Tall-Man cloZAPine

U.S. Brand Names Clozaril®; FazaClo®

Canadian Brand Names Apo-Clozapine®; Clozaril®; Gen-Clozapine

Therapeutic Category Antipsychotic Agent, Dibenzodiazepine

Use Treatment-refractory schizophrenia; to reduce risk of recurrent suicidal behavior in schizophrenia or schizoaffective disorder

General Dosage Range Dosage adjustment recommended in patients who develop toxicities
Oral: *Adults:* Initial: 12.5 mg once or twice daily; Maintenance: 12.5-900 mg/day (maximum: 900 mg/day)

Dosage Forms
Tablet, oral: 25 mg, 50 mg, 100 mg, 200 mg
Clozaril®: 25 mg, 100 mg
Tablet, orally disintegrating, oral:
FazaClo®: 12.5 mg, 25 mg, 100 mg, 150 mg, 200 mg

Clozaril® *see* clozapine *on page 227*

CMA-676 *see* gemtuzumab ozogamicin *on page 414*

CMV-IGIV *see* cytomegalovirus immune globulin (intravenous-human) *on page 247*

CNJ-016® *see* vaccinia immune globulin (intravenous) *on page 903*

CNTO-148 *see* golimumab *on page 423*

CNTO 1275 *see* ustekinumab *on page 902*

CoActifed® (Can) *see* triprolidine, pseudoephedrine, and codeine *(Canada only) on page 893*

coagulant complex inhibitor *see* antiinhibitor coagulant complex *on page 83*

coagulation factor I *see* fibrinogen concentrate (human) *on page 376*

coagulation factor VIIa *see* factor VIIa (recombinant) *on page 365*

CO Alendronate (Can) *see* alendronate *on page 49*

coal tar (KOLE tar)

Medication Safety Issues
International issues:
Pentrax [U.S., Canada, Great Britain, Ireland] may be confused with Permax brand name for pergolide [multiple international markets]

Synonyms crude coal tar; LCD; pix carbonis

U.S. Brand Names Balnetar® [OTC]; Betatar Gel® [OTC]; Cutar® [OTC]; Denorex® Therapeutic Protection 2-in-1 Shampoo + Conditioner [OTC]; Denorex® Therapeutic Protection [OTC]; DHS® Tar [OTC]; DHS™ Tar Gel [OTC]; Exorex® Penetrating Emulsion #2 [OTC]; Exorex® Penetrating Emulsion [OTC]; ionil-T® Plus [OTC]; ionil-T® [OTC]; MG217® Medicated Tar Extra Strength [OTC]; MG217® Medicated Tar Intensive Strength [OTC]; MG217® Medicated Tar [OTC]; Neutrogena® T/Gel® Extra

◄ Strength [OTC]; Neutrogena® T/Gel® Stubborn Itch Control [OTC]; Neutrogena® T/Gel® [OTC]; Oxipor® VHC [OTC]; Pentrax® [OTC]; Scytera™ [OTC]; Tera-Gel™ [OTC]; Thera-Gel [OTC]; Zetar® [OTC]

Canadian Brand Names Balnetar®; Estar®; Targel®

Therapeutic Category Antipsoriatic Agent; Antiseborrheic Agent, Topical

Use Topically for controlling dandruff, seborrheic dermatitis, or psoriasis

General Dosage Range Topical: *Adults:*

Bath: Add 60-90 mL (5-20%) or 15-25 mL (30%) to bath water, soak 5-20 minutes, use once daily to every 3 days

Scalp: Apply to lesions 3-12 hours before each shampoo

Shampoo: Rub into wet hair, rinse, repeat leaving on 5 minutes; apply twice weekly for 2 weeks then once weekly

Skin: Apply to affected areas 1-4 times/day, decrease to 2-3 times/week once condition controlled

Soap: Use on affected areas instead of regular soap

Dosage Forms

Aerosol, topical:

Scytera™ [OTC]: Coal tar solution 10% (100 g)

Emulsion, topical:

Cutar® [OTC]: Coal tar solution 7.5% (180 mL, 3840 mL)

Exorex® Penetrating Emulsion [OTC]: Coal tar 1% (100 mL, 250 mL)

Exorex® Penetrating Emulsion #2 [OTC]: Coal tar 2% (100 mL, 250 mL)

Gel, topical:

DHS™ Tar Gel [OTC]: Solubilized coal tar extract 2.9% (240 mL)

Thera-Gel [OTC]: 0.5% (255 mL)

Lotion, topical:

MG217® Medicated Tar [OTC]: Coal tar solution 5% (120 mL)

Oxipor® VHC [OTC]: Coal tar solution 25% (56 mL, 120 mL)

Oil, topical:

Balnetar® [OTC]: Coal tar 2.5% (221 mL)

Ointment, topical:

MG217® Medicated Tar Intensive Strength [OTC]: Coal tar solution 10% (107 g)

Shampoo, topical:

Betatar Gel® [OTC]: Coal tar solution 12.5% (480 mL)

Denorex® Therapeutic Protection [OTC]: Coal tar solution 12.5% (118 mL, 240 mL, 300 mL)

DHS® Tar [OTC]: Solubilized coal tar extract 2.9% (120 mL, 240 mL, 480 mL)

ionil-T® [OTC]: Coal tar 1% (240 mL, 480 mL, 960 mL)

ionil-T® Plus [OTC]: Coal tar 2% (240 mL)

MG217® Medicated Tar Extra Strength [OTC]: Coal tar solution 15% (120 mL, 240 mL)

Neutrogena® T/Gel® [OTC]: Solubilized coal tar extract 2% (130 mL, 255 mL, 480 mL)

Neutrogena® T/Gel® Extra Strength [OTC]: Solubilized coal tar extract 4% (177 mL)

Neutrogena® T/Gel® Stubborn Itch Control [OTC]: Coal tar extract 2% (130 mL)

Pentrax® [OTC]: Coal tar 5% (236 mL)

Tera-Gel™ [OTC]: Solubilized coal tar extract 2% (120 mL, 255 mL)

Zetar® [OTC]: Coal tar 1% (177 mL)

Shampoo/Conditioner, topical:

Denorex® Therapeutic Protection 2-in-1 Shampoo + Conditioner [OTC]: Coal tar solution 12.5% (120 mL, 240 mL, 300 mL)

Solution, topical: 20% (473 mL)

coal tar and salicylic acid (KOLE tar & sal i SIL ik AS id)

Synonyms salicylic acid and coal tar

U.S. Brand Names Tarsum® [OTC]; X-Seb T® Pearl [OTC]; X-Seb T® Plus [OTC]

Canadian Brand Names Sebcur/T®

Therapeutic Category Antipsoriatic Agent; Antiseborrheic Agent, Topical

Use Seborrheal dermatitis, dandruff, psoriasis

General Dosage Range Topical:

Gel: *Adults:* Apply to plaques, leave on up to 1 hour then rinse

Shampoo: *Adults:* Apply to wet hair, massage into scalp then rinse

Dosage Forms

Gel [shampoo]: Coal tar solution 10% [equivalent to coal tar 2%] and salicylic acid (120 mL, 240 mL)

Tarsum® [OTC]: Coal tar solution 10% [equivalent to coal tar 2%] and salicylic acid (120 mL, 240 mL)

Shampoo, topical: Coal tar solution 10% [equivalent to coal tar 2%] and salicylic acid (120 mL, 240 mL)
X-Seb T® Pearl [OTC], X-Seb T® Plus [OTC]: Coal tar solution 10% [equivalent to coal tar 2%] and salicylic acid (120 mL, 240 mL)

CO Amlodipine (Can) see amlodipine on page 69
Coartem® see artemether and lumefantrine on page 94
CO Atenolol (Can) see atenolol on page 101
CO Atorvastatin (Can) see atorvastatin on page 102
CO Azithromycin (Can) see azithromycin (systemic) on page 108
CO Bicalutamide (Can) see bicalutamide on page 133
CO Buspirone (Can) see buspirone on page 151
CO Cabergoline (Can) see cabergoline on page 156

cocaine (koe KANE)
Synonyms cocaine hydrochloride
Therapeutic Category Local Anesthetic
Controlled Substance C-II
Use Topical anesthesia for mucous membranes
General Dosage Range Topical: *Adults:* Do not exceed 1 mg/kg (1% to 10% concentration)
Dosage Forms
Powder, for prescription compounding: USP: 100% (1 g, 5 g, 25 g)
Solution, topical: 4% (4 mL, 10 mL); 10% (4 mL, 10 mL)

cocaine hydrochloride see cocaine on page 229
CO Cilazapril (Can) see cilazapril (Canada only) on page 208
CO Ciprofloxacin (Can) see ciprofloxacin (systemic) on page 210
CO Citalopram (Can) see citalopram on page 213
CO Clomipramine (Can) see clomipramine on page 222
CO Clonazepam (Can) see clonazepam on page 222
Codal-DM [OTC] see phenylephrine, pyrilamine, and dextromethorphan on page 699

codeine (KOE deen)
Medication Safety Issues
Sound-alike/look-alike issues:
Codeine may be confused with Cardene®, Cordran®, iodine, Lodine
High alert medication:
The Institute for Safe Medication Practices (ISMP) includes this medication among its list of drug classes which have a heightened risk of causing significant patient harm when used in error.
Synonyms codeine phosphate; codeine sulfate; methylmorphine
Canadian Brand Names Codeine Contin®
Therapeutic Category Analgesic, Narcotic; Antitussive
Controlled Substance C-II
Use Treatment of mild-to-moderate pain; antitussive in lower doses
General Dosage Range Dosage adjustment recommended in patients with renal impairment
I.M., SubQ:
Children: 0.5-1 mg/kg every 4-6 hours as needed (maximum: 60 mg/dose; 1.5 mg/kg/dose)
Adults: Initial: 30 mg every 4-6 hours; Usual range: 15-120 mg every 4-6 hours as needed (maximum: 1.5 mg/kg/dose)
Oral:
Children: Analgesic: 0.5-1 mg/kg every 4-6 hours as needed (maximum: 60 mg/dose; 1.5 mg/kg/dose); Antitussive: 1-1.5 mg/kg/day divided every 4-6 hours as needed (maximum: 30 mg/day [2-6 years]; 60 mg/day [6-12 years])
Adults: Analgesic: Initial: 30 mg every 4-6 hours as needed; Usual range: 15-120 mg every 4-6 hours as needed (maximum: 1.5 mg/kg/dose); Antitussive: 10-20 mg every 4-6 hours as needed (maximum: 120 mg/day)
Dosage Forms
Powder, for prescription compounding: USP: 100% (10 g, 25 g)
Tablet, oral: 15 mg, 30 mg, 60 mg

◀ **Dosage Forms - Canada**
Tablet, controlled release:
Codeine Contin®: 50 mg, 100 mg, 150 mg, 200 mg

codeine, acetaminophen, butalbital, and caffeine *see* butalbital, acetaminophen, caffeine, and codeine *on page 153*

codeine and acetaminophen *see* acetaminophen and codeine *on page 26*

codeine and butalbital compound *see* butalbital, aspirin, caffeine, and codeine *on page 154*

codeine and guaifenesin *see* guaifenesin and codeine *on page 426*

codeine and promethazine *see* promethazine and codeine *on page 743*

codeine and pseudoephedrine *see* pseudoephedrine and codeine *on page 752*

codeine, aspirin, and carisoprodol *see* carisoprodol, aspirin, and codeine *on page 177*

codeine, butalbital, aspirin, and caffeine *see* butalbital, aspirin, caffeine, and codeine *on page 154*

codeine, chlorpheniramine, and pseudoephedrine *see* chlorpheniramine, pseudoephedrine, and codeine *on page 201*

Codeine Contin® (Can) *see* codeine *on page 229*

codeine, doxylamine, and acetaminophen *see* acetaminophen, codeine, and doxylamine *(Canada only) on page 31*

codeine, guaifenesin, and pseudoephedrine *see* guaifenesin, pseudoephedrine, and codeine *on page 430*

codeine, phenylephrine, and promethazine *see* promethazine, phenylephrine, and codeine *on page 744*

codeine phosphate *see* codeine *on page 229*

codeine phosphate and pseudoephedrine hydrochloride *see* pseudoephedrine and codeine *on page 752*

codeine, pseudoephedrine, and triprolidine *see* triprolidine, pseudoephedrine, and codeine *(Canada only) on page 893*

codeine sulfate *see* codeine *on page 229*

codeine, triprolidine, and pseudoephedrine *see* triprolidine, pseudoephedrine, and codeine *(Canada only) on page 893*

cod liver oil *see* vitamin A and vitamin D *on page 917*

CO Enalapril (Can) *see* enalapril *on page 326*

CO Etidrocal (Can) *see* etidronate and calcium carbonate *(Canada only) on page 360*

Co-Etidronate (Can) *see* etidronate *on page 359*

CO Famciclovir (Can) *see* famciclovir *on page 366*

CO Finasteride (Can) *see* finasteride *on page 378*

CO Fluconazole (Can) *see* fluconazole *on page 381*

CO Fluoxetine (Can) *see* fluoxetine *on page 389*

CO Gabapentin (Can) *see* gabapentin *on page 405*

Cogentin® *see* benztropine *on page 126*

CO Glimepiride (Can) *see* glimepiride *on page 418*

CO Ipra-Sal (Can) *see* ipratropium and albuterol *on page 489*

CO Irbesartan (Can) *see* irbesartan *on page 490*

CO Irbesartan HCT (Can) *see* irbesartan and hydrochlorothiazide *on page 490*

Colace® [OTC] *see* docusate *on page 302*

Colace® (Can) *see* docusate *on page 302*

Colax-C® (Can) *see* docusate *on page 302*

Colazal® *see* balsalazide *on page 113*

ColBenemid *see* colchicine and probenecid *on page 231*

colchicine (KOL chi seen)

Medication Safety Issues
Sound-alike/look-alike issues:
Colchicine may be confused with Cortrosyn®

U.S. Brand Names Colcrys®

Therapeutic Category Antigout Agent

Use Prevention and treatment of acute gout flares; treatment of familial Mediterranean fever (FMF)

General Dosage Range Dosage adjustment recommended in patients with renal impairment or on concomitant therapy

Oral:
  Children 4-6 years: 0.3-1.8 mg/day in 1-2 divided doses
  Children 6-12 years: 0.9-1.8 mg/day in 1-2 divided doses
  Children 12-16 years: 1.2-2.4 mg/day in 1-2 divided doses
  Children >16 years and Adults: 0.6-2.4 mg/day in 1-2 divided doses **or** Initial: 1.2 mg; repeat with 0.6 mg in 1 hour (maximum total therapy: 1.8 mg)

Dosage Forms
  Tablet, oral: 0.6 mg
    Colcrys®: 0.6 mg

Dosage Forms - Canada
  Tablet, oral: 1 mg [scored]

colchicine and probenecid (KOL chi seen & proe BEN e sid)

Synonyms ColBenemid; probenecid and colchicine

Therapeutic Category Antigout Agent

Use Treatment of chronic gouty arthritis when complicated by frequent, recurrent acute attacks of gout

General Dosage Range Dosage adjustment recommended in patients with renal impairment
  Oral: *Adults:* Initial: One tablet daily; Maintenance: 1 tablet twice daily

Dosage Forms
  Tablet: Colchicine 0.5 mg and probenecid 0.5 g

Colcrys® *see* colchicine *on page 230*

Coldamine *see* chlorpheniramine, pseudoephedrine, and methscopolamine *on page 202*

Cold Control PE [OTC] *see* acetaminophen, diphenhydramine, and phenylephrine *on page 33*

Coldcough *see* pseudoephedrine, dihydrocodeine, and chlorpheniramine *on page 754*

Coldcough PD *see* dihydrocodeine, chlorpheniramine, and phenylephrine *on page 285*

colesevelam (koh le SEV a lam)

U.S. Brand Names Welchol®

Canadian Brand Names Welchol®

Therapeutic Category Antihyperlipidemic Agent, Miscellaneous; Bile Acid Sequestrant

Use Management of elevated LDL in primary hypercholesterolemia (Fredrickson type IIa) when used alone or in combination with an HMG-CoA reductase inhibitor; management of heterozygous familial hypercholesterolemia (heFH) in adolescent patients (males and postmenarchal females 10-17 years of age) when used alone or in combination with an HMG-CoA reductase inhibitor, in patients who after an adequate trial of dietary therapy have LDL-C ≥190 mg/dL or LDL-C ≥160 mg/dL with positive family history of premature cardiovascular disease (CVD) or with two or more CVD risk factors; improve glycemic control in type 2 diabetes mellitus (noninsulin-dependent, NIDDM) in conjunction with diet, exercise, and insulin or oral antidiabetic agents

General Dosage Range Oral: *Children 10-17 years (males and postmenarchal females) and Adults:* 3.75 g/day in 1-2 divided doses

Dosage Forms
  Granules for suspension, oral:
    Welchol®: 3.75 g/packet (30s)
  Tablet, oral:
    Welchol®: 625 mg

Colestid® *see* colestipol *on page 231*

Colestid® Flavored *see* colestipol *on page 231*

colestipol (koe LES ti pole)

Medication Safety Issues
  Sound-alike/look-alike issues:
    Colestipol may be confused with calcitriol

Synonyms colestipol hydrochloride

U.S. Brand Names Colestid®; Colestid® Flavored

◀ **Canadian Brand Names** Colestid®

Therapeutic Category Antihyperlipidemic Agent, Miscellaneous

Use Adjunct in management of primary hypercholesterolemia; regression of arteriolosclerosis; relief of pruritus associated with elevated levels of bile acids; possibly used to decrease plasma half-life of digoxin in toxicity

General Dosage Range Oral: *Adults:* Granules: Initial: 5 g 1-2 times/day; Maintenance: 5-30 g/day in 1-4 divided doses; Tablets: Initial: 2 g 1-2 times/day; Maintenance: 2-16 g/day

Dosage Forms

Granules for suspension, oral: 5 g/scoop (500 g); 5 g/packet (30s, 90s)

Colestid®: 5 g/scoop (300 g, 500 g); 5 g/packet (30s, 90s)

Colestid® Flavored: 5 g/scoop (450 g); 5 g/packet (60s)

Tablet, oral: 1 g

Colestid®: 1 g

colestipol hydrochloride *see* colestipol *on page 231*

CO Levetiracetam (Can) *see* levetiracetam *on page 517*

CO Lisinopril (Can) *see* lisinopril *on page 531*

colistimethate (koe lis ti METH ate)

Synonyms colistimethate sodium; colistin methanesulfonate; colistin sulfomethate; pentasodium colistin methanesulfonate

U.S. Brand Names Coly-Mycin® M

Canadian Brand Names Coly-Mycin® M

Therapeutic Category Antibiotic, Miscellaneous

Use Treatment of infections due to sensitive strains of certain gram-negative bacilli which are resistant to other antibacterials or in patients allergic to other antibacterials

General Dosage Range Dosage adjustment recommended in patients with renal impairment

I.M., I.V.: *Children and Adults:* 2.5-5 mg/kg/day in 2-4 divided doses

Dosage Forms

Injection, powder for reconstitution: colistin 150 mg

Coly-Mycin® M: colistin 150 mg

colistimethate sodium *see* colistimethate *on page 232*

colistin, hydrocortisone, neomycin, and thonzonium *see* neomycin, colistin, hydrocortisone, and thonzonium *on page 617*

colistin methanesulfonate *see* colistimethate *on page 232*

colistin sulfomethate *see* colistimethate *on page 232*

collagen *see* collagen hemostat *on page 233*

collagen absorbable hemostat *see* collagen hemostat *on page 233*

collagenase (systemic) (KOL la je nase)

Medication Safety Issues

Sound-alike/look-alike issues:

Collagenase clostridium histolyticum (Xiaflex™) may be confused with topical collagenase formulation (ie, Santyl®)

Xiaflex™ may be confused with Zanaflex®

Synonyms collagenase clostridium histolyticum

U.S. Brand Names Xiaflex™

Therapeutic Category Enzyme

Use Treatment of Dupuytren contracture with a palpable cord

General Dosage Range Intralesional: *Adults:* 0.58 mg per cord

Dosage Forms

Injection, powder for reconstitution:

Xiaflex™: 0.9 mg

collagenase (topical) (KOL la je nase)

Medication Safety Issues
Sound-alike/look-alike issues:
Topical collagenase formulation (Santyl®) may be confused with the injectable collagenase clostridium histolyticum (Xiaflex™)
U.S. Brand Names Santyl®
Canadian Brand Names Santyl®
Therapeutic Category Enzyme
Use Promotes debridement of necrotic tissue in dermal ulcers and severe burns
General Dosage Range Topical: *Children and Adults:* Apply once daily
Dosage Forms
Ointment, topical:
Santyl®: 250 units/g (15 g, 30 g)

collagenase clostridium histolyticum *see* collagenase (systemic) *on page 232*

collagen hemostat (KOL la jen HEE moe stat)

Medication Safety Issues
Sound-alike/look-alike issues:
Avitene® may be confused with Ativan®
Other safety concerns:
Over 100 reports of paralysis or other neural deficits have been received by the FDA, attributable to collagen hemostat-associated neuronal impingement
Synonyms collagen; collagen absorbable hemostat; MCH; microfibrillar collagen hemostat
U.S. Brand Names Avitene®; Avitene® Flour; Avitene® Ultrafoam™; EndoAvitene®; Helistat®; Helitene®; Instat™ MCH; SyringeAvitene™
Therapeutic Category Hemostatic Agent
Use Adjunct to hemostasis when control of bleeding by ligature is ineffective or impractical
General Dosage Range Topical: *Adults:* Apply dry directly to source of bleeding; remove excess material after ~10-15 minutes
Dosage Forms
Powder, topical:
Avitene® Flour: (0.5 g, 1 g, 5 g)
Helitene®: (0.5 g, 1 g)
Instat™ MCH: (0.5 g, 1 g)
SyringeAvitene™: (1 g)
Sheet, topical:
Avitene®: (1s, 6s)
EndoAvitene®: (6s)
Sponge, topical:
Avitene® Ultrafoam™: (6s)
Helistat®: (10s, 18s)

Colocort® *see* hydrocortisone (topical) *on page 450*
CO Lovastatin (Can) *see* lovastatin *on page 540*
Coly-Mycin® M *see* colistimethate *on page 232*
Coly-Mycin® S *see* neomycin, colistin, hydrocortisone, and thonzonium *on page 617*
Colyte® *see* polyethylene glycol-electrolyte solution *on page 718*
Colyte™ (Can) *see* polyethylene glycol-electrolyte solution *on page 718*
Combantrin™ (Can) *see* pyrantel pamoate *on page 756*
Combigan® *see* brimonidine and timolol *on page 141*
CombiPatch® *see* estradiol and norethindrone *on page 345*
Combipres *see* clonidine and chlorthalidone *on page 224*
Combivent® *see* ipratropium and albuterol *on page 489*
Combivent UDV (Can) *see* ipratropium and albuterol *on page 489*
Combivir® *see* lamivudine and zidovudine *on page 509*
CO Meloxicam (Can) *see* meloxicam *on page 556*
CO Memantine (Can) *see* memantine *on page 556*

CONIVAPTAN

CO Metformin (Can) *see* metformin *on page 566*
CO Mirtazapine (Can) *see* mirtazapine *on page 592*
Commit® [OTC] *see* nicotine *on page 625*
Compazine *see* prochlorperazine *on page 740*
Complera™ *see* emtricitabine, rilpivirine, and tenofovir *on page 326*
Compound 347™ *see* enflurane *on page 327*
compound E *see* cortisone *on page 237*
compound F *see* hydrocortisone (systemic) *on page 449*
compound F *see* hydrocortisone (topical) *on page 450*
compound S *see* zidovudine *on page 929*
compound S, abacavir, and lamivudine *see* abacavir, lamivudine, and zidovudine *on page 20*
Compound W® [OTC] *see* salicylic acid *on page 795*
Compound W® One Step Invisible Strip [OTC] *see* salicylic acid *on page 795*
Compound W® One-Step Wart Remover [OTC] *see* salicylic acid *on page 795*
Compound W® One Step Wart Remover for Feet [OTC] *see* salicylic acid *on page 795*
Compound W® One-Step Wart Remover for Kids [OTC] *see* salicylic acid *on page 795*
Compoz® [OTC] *see* diphenhydramine (systemic) *on page 290*
Compro® *see* prochlorperazine *on page 740*
Comtan® *see* entacapone *on page 329*
Comtrex® Maximum Strength, Non-Drowsy Cold & Cough [OTC] *see* acetaminophen, dextromethorphan, and phenylephrine *on page 32*
Comvax® *see Haemophilus* B conjugate and hepatitis B vaccine *on page 432*
Concept DHA™ *see* vitamins (multiple/prenatal) *on page 920*
Concept OB™ *see* vitamins (multiple/prenatal) *on page 920*
Conceptrol® [OTC] *see* nonoxynol 9 *on page 632*
Concerta® *see* methylphenidate *on page 577*
Condyline™ (Can) *see* podofilox *on page 716*
Condylox® *see* podofilox *on page 716*
Congestac® [OTC] *see* guaifenesin and pseudoephedrine *on page 429*

conivaptan (koe NYE vap tan)
Synonyms conivaptan hydrochloride; YM087
U.S. Brand Names Vaprisol®
Therapeutic Category Vasopressin Antagonist
Use Treatment of euvolemic and hypervolemic hyponatremia in hospitalized patients
General Dosage Range Dosage adjustment recommended in patients with hepatic or renal impairment
  I.V.: *Adults:* Loading dose: 20 mg bolus, followed by 20 mg as continuous infusion over 24 hours; Maintenance: 20-40 mg/day as a continuous infusion over 24 hours (maximum therapy: 4 days)
Dosage Forms
  Infusion, premixed in D_5W:
   Vaprisol®: 20 mg (100 mL)

conivaptan hydrochloride *see* conivaptan *on page 234*
conjugated estrogen *see* estrogens (conjugated/equine, systemic) *on page 347*
conjugated estrogen *see* estrogens (conjugated/equine, topical) *on page 348*
CO Norfloxacin (Can) *see* norfloxacin *on page 633*
Conray® *see* iothalamate meglumine *on page 486*
Conray® 30 *see* iothalamate meglumine *on page 486*
Conray® 43 *see* iothalamate meglumine *on page 486*
Constulose *see* lactulose *on page 507*
Contac® Cold 12 Hour Relief Non Drowsy (Can) *see* pseudoephedrine *on page 751*
Contac® Cold and Sore Throat, Non Drowsy, Extra Strength (Can) *see* acetaminophen and pseudoephedrine *on page 29*
Contac® Cold-Chest Congestion, Non Drowsy, Regular Strength (Can) *see* guaifenesin and pseudoephedrine *on page 429*

Contac® Cold + Flu Maximum Strength Non-Drowsy [OTC] *see* acetaminophen and phenylephrine *on page 28*

continuous renal replacement therapy *see* electrolyte solution, renal replacement *on page 323*

ControlRx™ *see* fluoride *on page 386*

ControlRx™ Multi *see* fluoride *on page 386*

ConZip™ *see* tramadol *on page 880*

CO Olanzapine (Can) *see* olanzapine *on page 645*

CO Olanzapine ODT (Can) *see* olanzapine *on page 645*

CO Ondansetron (Can) *see* ondansetron *on page 651*

CO Pantoprazole (Can) *see* pantoprazole *on page 672*

CO Paroxetine (Can) *see* paroxetine *on page 676*

Copaxone® *see* glatiramer acetate *on page 417*

COPD *see* dyphylline and guaifenesin *on page 318*

Copegus® *see* ribavirin *on page 777*

CO Pioglitazone (Can) *see* pioglitazone *on page 706*

copolymer-1 *see* glatiramer acetate *on page 417*

copper (KOP er)

Synonyms cupric chloride; cupric chloride dihydrate

Therapeutic Category Trace Element, Parenteral

Use Supplement to intravenous solutions given for total parenteral nutrition (TPN) to maintain copper serum levels and to prevent depletion of endogenous stores and subsequent deficiency symptoms

General Dosage Range I.V. (as a parenteral nutrition component):
Infants and Children: 20 mcg/kg/day
Adults: 0.3-1.5 mg/day

Dosage Forms
Injection, solution [preservative free]: 0.4 mg/mL (10 mL)

copper *see* trace metals *on page 880*

CO Pramipexole (Can) *see* pramipexole *on page 729*

CO Pravastatin (Can) *see* pravastatin *on page 732*

CO Quetiapine (Can) *see* quetiapine *on page 760*

CO Ramipril (Can) *see* ramipril *on page 766*

CO Ranitidine (Can) *see* ranitidine *on page 767*

Cordarone® *see* amiodarone *on page 67*

Cordran® *see* flurandrenolide *on page 391*

Cordran® SP *see* flurandrenolide *on page 391*

Coreg® *see* carvedilol *on page 178*

Coreg CR® *see* carvedilol *on page 178*

Corfen DM [DSC] *see* chlorpheniramine, phenylephrine, and dextromethorphan *on page 200*

Corgard® *see* nadolol *on page 607*

Coricidin HBP® Chest Congestion and Cough [OTC] *see* guaifenesin and dextromethorphan *on page 427*

Coricidin HBP® Cold and Flu [OTC] *see* chlorpheniramine and acetaminophen *on page 198*

Coricidin® HBP Cough & Cold [OTC] *see* dextromethorphan and chlorpheniramine *on page 271*

Corifact® *see* factor XIII concentrate (human) *on page 366*

CO Risperidone (Can) *see* risperidone *on page 783*

Corlopam® *see* fenoldopam *on page 370*

Cormax® *see* clobetasol *on page 220*

CO Ropinirole (Can) *see* ropinirole *on page 790*

Correctol® [OTC] *see* docusate *on page 302*

Correctol® Tablets [OTC] *see* bisacodyl *on page 134*

Cortaid® Advanced [OTC] *see* hydrocortisone (topical) *on page 450*

Cortaid® Intensive Therapy [OTC] *see* hydrocortisone (topical) *on page 450*

Cortaid® Maximum Strength [OTC] *see* hydrocortisone (topical) *on page 450*

Cortamed® (Can) *see* hydrocortisone (topical) *on page 450*
Cortef® *see* hydrocortisone (systemic) *on page 449*
Cortenema® *see* hydrocortisone (topical) *on page 450*
CortiCool® [OTC] *see* hydrocortisone (topical) *on page 450*

corticorelin (kor ti koe REL in)

Medication Safety Issues
Sound-alike/look-alike issues:
Acthrel® may be confused with Acthar
Corticorelin may be confused with corticotropin
Synonyms corticorelin ovine triflutate; human corticotrophin-releasing hormone, analogue; ovine corticotrophin-releasing hormone
U.S. Brand Names Acthrel®
Therapeutic Category Diagnostic Agent, ACTH-Dependent Hypercortisolism
Use Diagnostic test used in adrenocorticotropic hormone (ACTH)-dependent Cushing syndrome to differentiate between pituitary and ectopic production of ACTH
General Dosage Range I.V.: *Adults:* 1 mcg/kg
Dosage Forms
Injection, powder for reconstitution:
Acthrel®: 100 mcg

corticorelin ovine triflutate *see* corticorelin *on page 236*

corticotropin (kor ti koe TROE pin)

Medication Safety Issues
Sound-alike/look-alike issues:
Corticotropin may be confused with corticorelin, cosyntropin
Synonyms ACTH; Acthar; adrenocorticotropic hormone; corticotropin, repository
U.S. Brand Names H.P. Acthar®
Therapeutic Category Adrenal Corticosteroid
Use Acute exacerbations of multiple sclerosis; infantile spasms; adjunctive therapy for exacerbations/acute episodes of rheumatic disorders (psoriatic arthritis, rheumatoid arthritis, juvenile idiopathic arthritis [JIA], ankylosing spondylitis); exacerbations or maintenance therapy for collagen diseases (systemic lupus erythematosus, systemic dermatomyositis); severe erythema multiforme; Stevens-Johnson syndrome; serum sickness; severe acute/chronic allergic and inflammatory ophthalmic disease (keratitis, iritis, iridocyclitis, diffuse posterior uveitis and choroiditis, optic neuritis, chorioretinitis, anterior segment inflammation); symptomatic sarcoidosis; to induce diuresis for remission of proteinuria in patients with nephrotic syndrome without idiopathic uremia or due to lupus erythematosus
General Dosage Range
I.M.:
Children <2 years: 75 units/m^2/dose twice daily (infantile spasms) followed by gradual downward titration of dose
Children >2 years: 40-80 units every 24-72 hours
Adults: 80-120 units/day for 2-3 weeks (MS) **or** 40-80 units every 24-72 hours (indications other than MS)
SubQ:
Children >2 years: 40-80 units every 24-72 hours
Adults: 80-120 units/day for 2-3 weeks (MS) **or** 40-80 units every 24-72 hours (indications other than MS)
Dosage Forms
Injection, gel:
H.P. Acthar®: 80 units/mL (5 mL)

corticotropin, repository *see* corticotropin *on page 236*
Cortifoam® *see* hydrocortisone (topical) *on page 450*
Cortifoam™ (Can) *see* hydrocortisone (topical) *on page 450*
Cortimyxin® (Can) *see* neomycin, polymyxin B, and hydrocortisone *on page 618*
cortisol *see* hydrocortisone (systemic) *on page 449*
cortisol *see* hydrocortisone (topical) *on page 450*

cortisone (KOR ti sone)

Medication Safety Issues
  Sound-alike/look-alike issues:
    Cortisone may be confused with Cardizem®, Cortizone®
Synonyms compound E; cortisone acetate
Therapeutic Category Adrenal Corticosteroid
Use Management of adrenocortical insufficiency
General Dosage Range Oral:
  Children: 0.5-10 mg/kg/day **or** 20-300 mg/m²/day divided every 6-8 hours
  Adults: 25-300 mg /day divided every 12-24 hours
Dosage Forms
  Tablet, oral: 25 mg

cortisone acetate *see* cortisone *on page 237*
Cortisporin® *see* neomycin, polymyxin B, and hydrocortisone *on page 618*
Cortisporin® Ointment *see* bacitracin, neomycin, polymyxin B, and hydrocortisone *on page 112*
Cortisporin® Otic (Can) *see* neomycin, polymyxin B, and hydrocortisone *on page 618*
Cortisporin®-TC *see* neomycin, colistin, hydrocortisone, and thonzonium *on page 617*
Cortisporin® Topical Ointment (Can) *see* bacitracin, neomycin, polymyxin B, and hydrocortisone *on page 112*
Cortizone-10® Hydratensive Healing [OTC] *see* hydrocortisone (topical) *on page 450*
Cortizone-10® Hydratensive Soothing [OTC] *see* hydrocortisone (topical) *on page 450*
Cortizone-10® Intensive Healing Eczema [OTC] *see* hydrocortisone (topical) *on page 450*
Cortizone-10® Maximum Strength [OTC] *see* hydrocortisone (topical) *on page 450*
Cortizone-10® Maximum Strength Cooling Relief [OTC] *see* hydrocortisone (topical) *on page 450*
Cortizone-10® Maximum Strength Easy Relief [OTC] *see* hydrocortisone (topical) *on page 450*
Cortizone-10® Maximum Strength Intensive Healing Formula [OTC] *see* hydrocortisone (topical) *on page 450*
Cortizone-10® Plus Maximum Strength [OTC] *see* hydrocortisone (topical) *on page 450*
Cortomycin *see* neomycin, polymyxin B, and hydrocortisone *on page 618*
Cortrosyn® *see* cosyntropin *on page 237*
Corvert® *see* ibutilide *on page 462*
Corzall™ Liquid [DSC] *see* carbetapentane and pseudoephedrine *on page 172*
Corzide® *see* nadolol and bendroflumethiazide *on page 608*
CO Sertraline (Can) *see* sertraline *on page 809*
CO Simvastatin (Can) *see* simvastatin *on page 813*
Cosmegen® *see* dactinomycin *on page 249*
Cosopt® *see* dorzolamide and timolol *on page 308*
CO Sotalol (Can) *see* sotalol *on page 828*
CO Sumatriptan (Can) *see* sumatriptan *on page 839*

cosyntropin (koe sin TROE pin)

Medication Safety Issues
  Sound-alike/look-alike issues:
    Cortrosyn® may be confused with colchicine, corticotropin, Cotazym®
    Cosyntropin may be confused with corticotropin
Synonyms synacthen; tetracosactide
U.S. Brand Names Cortrosyn®
Canadian Brand Names Cortrosyn®
Therapeutic Category Diagnostic Agent
Use Diagnostic test to differentiate primary adrenal from secondary (pituitary) adrenocortical insufficiency
General Dosage Range I.M., I.V.:
  Children ≤2 years: 0.125 mg
  Children >2 years and Adults: 0.25 mg

◄ **Dosage Forms**
Injection, powder for reconstitution: 0.25 mg
  Cortrosyn®: 0.25 mg
Injection, solution [preservative free]: 0.25 mg/mL (1 mL)

Cotazym® (Can) *see* pancrelipase *on page 670*
CO Temazepam (Can) *see* temazepam *on page 848*
CO Terbinafine (Can) *see* terbinafine (systemic) *on page 851*
CO Topiramate (Can) *see* topiramate *on page 877*
Cotridin *see* triprolidine, pseudoephedrine, and codeine *(Canada only) on page 893*
co-trimoxazole *see* sulfamethoxazole and trimethoprim *on page 836*
Coumadin® *see* warfarin *on page 922*
CO Valsartan (Can) *see* valsartan *on page 905*
Covan® (Can) *see* triprolidine, pseudoephedrine, and codeine *(Canada only) on page 893*
Covaryx® *see* estrogens (esterified) and methyltestosterone *on page 349*
Covaryx® H.S. *see* estrogens (esterified) and methyltestosterone *on page 349*
CO Venlafaxine XR (Can) *see* venlafaxine *on page 911*
Covera® (Can) *see* verapamil *on page 912*
Covera-HS® *see* verapamil *on page 912*
Coversyl® (Can) *see* perindopril erbumine *on page 690*
Coversyl® Plus (Can) *see* perindopril erbumine and indapamide *(Canada only) on page 691*
Coversyl® Plus HD (Can) *see* perindopril erbumine and indapamide *(Canada only) on page 691*
Coversyl® Plus LD (Can) *see* perindopril erbumine and indapamide *(Canada only) on page 691*
co-vidarabine *see* pentostatin *on page 689*
coviracil *see* emtricitabine *on page 325*
Cozaar® *see* losartan *on page 538*
CO Zopiclone (Can) *see* zopiclone *(Canada only) on page 934*
CP358774 *see* erlotinib *on page 338*
CPC *see* cetylpyridinium *on page 190*
C-Phen [DSC] *see* chlorpheniramine and phenylephrine *on page 198*
CPM *see* cyclophosphamide *on page 242*
CPT-11 *see* irinotecan *on page 491*
CPZ *see* chlorpromazine *on page 203*
Cramp Tabs [OTC] *see* acetaminophen and pamabrom *on page 27*
Crantex® *see* guaifenesin and phenylephrine *on page 428*
Creomulsion® Adult Formula [OTC] *see* dextromethorphan *on page 270*
Creomulsion® for Children [OTC] *see* dextromethorphan *on page 270*
Creon® *see* pancrelipase *on page 670*
Creo-Terpin® [OTC] *see* dextromethorphan *on page 270*
Crestor® *see* rosuvastatin *on page 792*
Cresylate™ *see* m-cresyl acetate *on page 550*
Crinone® *see* progesterone *on page 741*
Critic-Aid® Clear AF [OTC] *see* miconazole (topical) *on page 585*
Critic-Aid Skin Care® [OTC] *see* zinc oxide *on page 930*
Crixivan® *see* indinavir *on page 471*
CroFab® *see* crotalidae polyvalent immune FAB (ovine) *on page 239*
Crolom® [DSC] *see* cromolyn (ophthalmic) *on page 239*
cromoglycic acid *see* cromolyn (nasal) *on page 239*
cromoglycic acid *see* cromolyn (ophthalmic) *on page 239*
cromoglycic acid *see* cromolyn (systemic, oral inhalation) *on page 238*

cromolyn (systemic, oral inhalation) (KROE moe lin)

Synonyms cromoglycic acid; cromolyn sodium; disodium cromoglycate; DSCG
U.S. Brand Names Gastrocrom®
Canadian Brand Names Nalcrom®; Nu-Cromolyn; PMS-Sodium Cromoglycate

Therapeutic Category Mast Cell Stabilizer
Use
Inhalation: May be used as an adjunct in the prophylaxis of allergic disorders, including asthma; prevention of exercise-induced bronchospasm
Oral: Systemic mastocytosis
General Dosage Range
Inhalation: Nebulization: *Children ≥2 years and Adults:* Initial: 20 mg 4 times/day; Maintenance: 20 mg 3-4 times/day **or** 20 mg prior to exercise or allergen exposure
Oral:
Children 2-12 years: 100 mg 4 times/day (maximum: 40 mg/kg/day)
Children >12 years and Adults: 200 mg 4 times/day (maximum: 40 mg/kg/day)
Dosage Forms
Solution, for nebulization: 20 mg/2 mL (60s, 120s)
Solution, oral:
Gastrocrom®: 100 mg/5 mL (96s)

cromolyn (nasal) (KROE moe lin)
Medication Safety Issues
Sound-alike/look-alike issues:
NasalCrom® may be confused with Nasacort®, Nasalide®
Synonyms cromoglycic acid; cromolyn sodium; disodium cromoglycate; DSCG
U.S. Brand Names NasalCrom® [OTC]
Canadian Brand Names Rhinaris-CS Anti-Allergic Nasal Mist
Therapeutic Category Mast Cell Stabilizer
Use Prevention and treatment of seasonal and perennial allergic rhinitis
General Dosage Range Intranasal: *Children ≥2 years and Adults:* Instill 1 spray in each nostril 3-4 times/day
Dosage Forms
Solution, intranasal: 40 mg/mL (13 mL, 26 mL)
NasalCrom® [OTC]: 40 mg/mL (13 mL, 26 mL)

cromolyn (ophthalmic) (KROE moe lin)
Synonyms cromoglycic acid; cromolyn sodium; disodium cromoglycate; DSCG
U.S. Brand Names Crolom® [DSC]
Canadian Brand Names Opticrom®
Therapeutic Category Mast Cell Stabilizer
Use Treatment of vernal keratoconjunctivitis, vernal conjunctivitis, and vernal keratitis
General Dosage Range Ophthalmic: *Adults:* 1-2 drops in each eye 4-6 times/day
Dosage Forms
Solution, ophthalmic: 4% (10 mL)

cromolyn sodium *see* cromolyn (nasal) *on page 239*
cromolyn sodium *see* cromolyn (ophthalmic) *on page 239*
cromolyn sodium *see* cromolyn (systemic, oral inhalation) *on page 238*

crotalidae polyvalent immune FAB (ovine)
(kroe TAL ih die pol i VAY lent i MYUN fab (oh vine))
Synonyms antivenin (crotalidae) polyvalent, FAB (ovine); crotaline antivenin, polyvalent, FAB (ovine); FabAV, FAB (ovine); North American antisnake-bite serum, FAB (ovine); snake antivenin, FAB (ovine)
U.S. Brand Names CroFab®
Therapeutic Category Antivenin
Use Management of patients with North American crotalid envenomations (eg, rattlesnakes [*Crotalus, Sistrurus*], copperheads and cottonmouth/water moccasins [*Agkistrodon*])
General Dosage Range I.V.: *Children and Adults:* Initial dose: 4-6 vials, may repeat with 4-6 vials; Maintenance dose: Administer 2 vials every 6 hours for up to 18 hours

◀ **Dosage Forms**
 Injection, powder for reconstitution:
  CroFab®: Derived from *Crotalus adamanteus, C. atrox, C. scutulatus*, and *Agkistrodon piscivorus* snake venoms

crotaline antivenin, polyvalent, FAB (ovine) *see* crotalidae polyvalent immune FAB (ovine) *on page 239*

crotamiton (kroe TAM i tonn)

Medication Safety Issues
 Sound-alike/look-alike issues:
  Eurax® may be confused with Efudex®, Eulexin, Evoxac®, Serax, Urex
 International issues:
  Eurax [U.S., Canada, and multiple international markets] may be confused with Urex brand name for furosemide [Australia, China,Turkey] and methenamine [U.S., Canada]

U.S. Brand Names Eurax®

Therapeutic Category Scabicides/Pediculicides

Use Treatment of scabies (*Sarcoptes scabiei*) and symptomatic treatment of pruritus

General Dosage Range Topical: *Children and Adults:* Pruritus: Massage into affected areas as needed; Scabies: Apply a thin layer from the neck to the toes, repeat in 24 hours; take a cleansing bath 48 hours after final application, may repeat after 7-10 days

Dosage Forms
 Cream, topical:
  Eurax®: 10% (60 g)
 Lotion, topical:
  Eurax®: 10% (60 mL, 480 mL)

CRRT *see* electrolyte solution, renal replacement *on page 323*

crude coal tar *see* coal tar *on page 227*

Cruex® [OTC] *see* clotrimazole (topical) *on page 226*

Cryselle® 28 *see* ethinyl estradiol and norgestrel *on page 357*

crystalline penicillin *see* penicillin G (parenteral/aqueous) *on page 685*

Crystapen® (Can) *see* penicillin G (parenteral/aqueous) *on page 685*

CS-747 *see* prasugrel *on page 732*

CsA *see* cyclosporine (ophthalmic) *on page 244*

CsA *see* cyclosporine (systemic) *on page 243*

C-Tan D *see* brompheniramine and phenylephrine *on page 143*

C-Tan D Plus *see* brompheniramine and phenylephrine *on page 143*

C-Tanna 12 [DSC] *see* carbetapentane and chlorpheniramine *on page 172*

C-Tanna 12D [DSC] *see* carbetapentane, phenylephrine, and pyrilamine *on page 173*

C-Time [OTC] *see* ascorbic acid *on page 96*

CTLA-4lg *see* abatacept *on page 20*

CTM *see* chlorpheniramine *on page 197*

CTP 30 (Can) *see* citalopram *on page 213*

CTX *see* cyclophosphamide *on page 242*

Cubicin® *see* daptomycin *on page 252*

Culturelle® [OTC] *see* Lactobacillus *on page 506*

cupric chloride *see* copper *on page 235*

cupric chloride dihydrate *see* copper *on page 235*

Cuprimine® *see* penicillamine *on page 683*

Curad® Mediplast® [OTC] *see* salicylic acid *on page 795*

Curasore® [OTC] *see* pramoxine *on page 730*

Curosurf® *see* poractant alfa *on page 722*

Cutar® [OTC] *see* coal tar *on page 227*

Cutivate® *see* fluticasone (topical) *on page 393*

Cutivate™ (Can) *see* fluticasone (topical) *on page 393*

Cuvposa™ *see* glycopyrrolate *on page 422*

CVT-3146 *see* regadenoson *on page 772*
CyA *see* cyclosporine (ophthalmic) *on page 244*
CyA *see* cyclosporine (systemic) *on page 243*
cyanide antidote kit *see* sodium nitrite, sodium thiosulfate, and amyl nitrite *on page 821*
Cyanide Antidote Package *see* sodium nitrite, sodium thiosulfate, and amyl nitrite *on page 821*

cyanocobalamin (sye an oh koe BAL a min)

Synonyms vitamin B_{12}

U.S. Brand Names CaloMist™; Ener-B® [OTC]; Nascobal®; Twelve Resin-K [OTC]

Therapeutic Category Vitamin, Water Soluble

Use Treatment of pernicious anemia; vitamin B_{12} deficiency due to dietary deficiencies or malabsorption diseases, inadequate secretion of intrinsic factor, and inadequate utilization of B_{12} (eg, during neoplastic treatment); increased B_{12} requirements due to pregnancy, thyrotoxicosis, hemorrhage, malignancy, liver or kidney disease

CaloMist™: Maintenance of vitamin B_{12} concentrations after initial correction in patients with B_{12} deficiency without CNS involvement

General Dosage Range
I.M., SubQ: *Children and Adults:* Dosage varies greatly depending on indication
Intranasal: *Adults:* Nascobal®: 500 mcg in one nostril once weekly; CaloMist™: Maintenance therapy (following correction of vitamin B_{12} deficiency): 50-100 mcg/day
Oral: *Adults:* 250-2000 mcg/day

Dosage Forms
Injection, solution: 1000 mcg/mL (1 mL, 10 mL, 30 mL)
Lozenge, oral: 50 mcg (100s); 100 mcg (100s); 250 mcg (100s, 250s); 500 mcg (100s, 250s)
Lozenge, sublingual: 500 mcg (100s)
Solution, intranasal:
CaloMist™: 25 mcg/spray (10.7 mL)
Nascobal®: 500 mcg/spray (2.3 mL)
Tablet, for buccal application/oral/sublingual:
Twelve Resin-K [OTC]: 1000 mcg
Tablet, oral: 50 mcg, 100 mcg, 250 mcg, 500 mcg, 1000 mcg
Ener-B® [OTC]: 100 mcg, 500 mcg, 1000 mcg
Tablet, sublingual: 1000 mcg, 2500 mcg, 5000 mcg
Tablet, timed release, oral: 1000 mcg
Ener-B® [OTC]: 1500 mcg

cyanocobalamin, folic acid, and pyridoxine *see* folic acid, cyanocobalamin, and pyridoxine *on page 396*
Cyclen® (Can) *see* ethinyl estradiol and norgestimate *on page 357*
Cyclessa® *see* ethinyl estradiol and desogestrel *on page 351*

cyclobenzaprine (sye kloe BEN za preen)

Medication Safety Issues
Sound-alike/look-alike issues:
Cyclobenzaprine may be confused with cycloSERINE, cyproheptadine
Flexeril® may be confused with Floxin®
BEERS Criteria medication:
This drug may be inappropriate for use in geriatric patients (high severity risk).
International issues:
Flexin: Brand name for cyclobenzaprine [Chile], but also the brand name for diclofenac [Argentina] and orphenadrine [Israel]
Flexin [Chile] may be confused with Floxin brand name for flunarizine [Thailand], norfloxacin [South Africa], ofloxacin [U.S., Canada], and perfloxacin [Philippines]; Fluoxine brand name for fluoxetine [Thailand]

Synonyms cyclobenzaprine hydrochloride

U.S. Brand Names Amrix®; Fexmid®; Flexeril®

Canadian Brand Names Apo-Cyclobenzaprine®; Dom-Cyclobenzaprine; Flexeril®; Flexitec; Gen-Cyclobenzaprine; Mylan-Cyclobenzaprine; Novo-Cycloprine; Nu-Cyclobenzaprine; PHL-Cyclobenzaprine; PMS-Cyclobenzaprine; ratio-Cyclobenzaprine; Riva-Cycloprine

◄ **Therapeutic Category** Skeletal Muscle Relaxant
Use Treatment of muscle spasm associated with acute, painful musculoskeletal conditions
General Dosage Range Dosage adjustment recommended in patients with hepatic impairment
Oral capsule, extended release: *Adults:* Usual: 15 mg once daily (maximum: 30 mg once daily)
Oral tablet, immediate release:
Children ≥15 years and Adults: Initial: 5 mg 3 times/day; Maintenance: 5-10 mg 3 times/day
Elderly: Initial: 5 mg
Dosage Forms
Capsule, extended release, oral: 15 mg, 30 mg
Amrix®: 15 mg, 30 mg
Tablet, oral: 5 mg, 10 mg
Fexmid®: 7.5 mg
Flexeril®: 5 mg, 10 mg

cyclobenzaprine hydrochloride *see* cyclobenzaprine *on page 241*
Cyclocort® (Can) *see* amcinonide *on page 63*
Cyclogyl® *see* cyclopentolate *on page 242*
Cyclomen® (Can) *see* danazol *on page 251*
Cyclomydril® *see* cyclopentolate and phenylephrine *on page 242*

cyclopentolate (sye kloe PEN toe late)

Synonyms cyclopentolate hydrochloride
U.S. Brand Names AK-Pentolate™; Cyclogyl®; Cylate™
Canadian Brand Names Cyclogyl®; Diopentolate®
Therapeutic Category Anticholinergic Agent
Use Diagnostic procedures requiring mydriasis and cycloplegia
General Dosage Range Ophthalmic:
Children: Instill 1 drop of 0.5%, 1%, or 2% in eye followed by 1 drop of 0.5% or 1% in 5 minutes, if necessary
Adults: Instill 1 drop of 1% followed by another drop in 5 minutes; 2% solution in heavily pigmented iris
Dosage Forms
Solution, ophthalmic: 1% (2 mL, 5 mL, 15 mL)
AK-Pentolate™: 1% (2 mL, 15 mL)
Cyclogyl®: 0.5% (15 mL); 1% (2 mL, 5 mL, 15 mL); 2% (2 mL, 5 mL, 15 mL)
Cylate™: 1% (2 mL, 15 mL)

cyclopentolate and phenylephrine (sye kloe PEN toe late & fen il EF rin)

Synonyms phenylephrine and cyclopentolate
U.S. Brand Names Cyclomydril®
Therapeutic Category Anticholinergic/Adrenergic Agonist
Use Induce mydriasis greater than that produced with cyclopentolate HCl alone
General Dosage Range Ophthalmic: *Children and Adults:* Instill 1 drop into eyes every 5-10 minutes, for up to 3 doses
Dosage Forms
Solution, ophthalmic:
Cyclomydril®: Cyclopentolate 0.2% and phenylephrine 1% (2 mL, 5 mL)

cyclopentolate hydrochloride *see* cyclopentolate *on page 242*

cyclophosphamide (sye kloe FOS fa mide)

Medication Safety Issues
Sound-alike/look-alike issues:
Cyclophosphamide may be confused with cycloSPORINE, ifosfamide
Cytoxan may be confused with cefOXitin, Ciloxan®, cytarabine, CytoGam®, Cytosar®, Cytosar-U, Cytotec®
High alert medication:
This medication is in a class the Institute for Safe Medication Practices (ISMP) includes among its list of drugs which have a heightened risk of causing significant patient harm when used in error.
Synonyms CPM; CTX; CYT; Cytoxan; neosar

Canadian Brand Names Procytox®

Therapeutic Category Antineoplastic Agent

Use

Oncology-related uses: Treatment of Hodgkin lymphoma, non-Hodgkin lymphoma (including Burkitt lymphoma), chronic lymphocytic leukemia (CLL), chronic myelocytic leukemia (CML), acute myelocytic leukemia (AML), acute lymphocytic leukemia (ALL), mycosis fungoides, multiple myeloma, neuroblastoma, retinoblastoma; breast cancer; ovarian adenocarcinoma

Nononcology uses: Treatment of refractory nephrotic syndrome in children

General Dosage Range Dosage adjustment recommended in patients with hepatic or renal impairment

I.V.: *Children and Adults:* Dosage varies greatly depending on indication

Oral: *Children and Adults:* 1-5 mg/kg/day

Dosage Forms

Injection, powder for reconstitution: 500 mg, 1 g, 2 g

Tablet, oral: 25 mg, 50 mg

cycloserine (sye kloe SER een)

Medication Safety Issues

Sound-alike/look-alike issues:

CycloSERINE may be confused with cyclobenzaprine, cycloSPORINE

Tall-Man cyclo**SERINE**

Therapeutic Category Antibiotic, Miscellaneous

Use Adjunctive treatment in pulmonary or extrapulmonary tuberculosis

General Dosage Range Dosage adjustment recommended in patients with renal impairment

Oral:

Children: 10-20 mg/kg/day in 2 divided doses (maximum: 1000 mg/day)

Adults: Initial: 250 mg every 12 hours for 14 days; Maintenance: 500-1000 mg/day in 2 divided doses

Dosage Forms

Capsule, oral:

Seromycin®: 250 mg

Cycloset® *see* bromocriptine *on page 142*

cyclosporin A *see* cyclosporine (ophthalmic) *on page 244*

cyclosporin A *see* cyclosporine (systemic) *on page 243*

cyclosporine (systemic) (SYE kloe spor een)

Medication Safety Issues

Sound-alike/look-alike issues:

CycloSPORINE may be confused with cyclophosphamide, Cyklokapron®, cycloSERINE

CycloSPORINE modified (Neoral®, Gengraf®) may be confused with cycloSPORINE non-modified (SandIMMUNE®)

Gengraf® may be confused with Prograf®

Neoral® may be confused with Neurontin®, Nizoral®

SandIMMUNE® may be confused with SandoSTATIN®

Synonyms CsA; CyA; cyclosporin A

Tall-Man cyclo**SPORINE**

U.S. Brand Names Gengraf®; Neoral®; SandIMMUNE®

Canadian Brand Names Apo-Cyclosporine®; Neoral®; Rhoxal-cyclosporine; Sandimmune® I.V.; Sandoz-Cyclosporine

Therapeutic Category Immunosuppressant Agent

Use Prophylaxis of organ rejection in kidney, liver, and heart transplants, has been used with azathioprine and/or corticosteroids; severe, active rheumatoid arthritis (RA) not responsive to methotrexate alone; severe, recalcitrant plaque psoriasis in nonimmunocompromised adults unresponsive to or unable to tolerate other systemic therapy

General Dosage Range Dosage adjustment recommended in patients with renal impairment

I.V. (non-modified): *Children and Adults:* Initial dose: 5-6 mg/kg/day or one-third of the oral dose as a single dose; Maintenance: 3-7.5 mg/kg/day in 2-3 divided doses or give as continuous infusion over 24 hours ▶

◀ **Oral:**
Modified:
Children and Adults: Transplant: Heart: 7 ± 3 mg/kg/day in 2 divided doses; Liver: 8 ± 4 mg/kg/day in 2 divided doses; Renal: 9 ± 3 mg/kg/day in 2 divided doses
Adults: Initial: 2.5 mg/kg/day in 2 divided doses; Maintenance: Up to 4 mg/kg/day
Non-modified: Children and Adults: Initial: 10-14 mg/kg/day for 1-2 weeks; Maintenance: Taper by 5% per week to 3-10 mg/kg/day

Dosage Forms
Capsule, oral: 25 mg, 100 mg
Gengraf®: 25 mg, 100 mg
Capsule, softgel, oral: 25 mg, 50 mg, 100 mg
Neoral®: 25 mg, 100 mg
SandIMMUNE®: 25 mg, 100 mg
Injection, solution: 50 mg/mL (5 mL)
SandIMMUNE®: 50 mg/mL (5 mL)
Injection, solution [preservative free]: 50 mg/mL (5 mL)
Solution, oral: 100 mg/mL (50 mL)
Gengraf®: 100 mg/mL (50 mL)
Neoral®: 100 mg/mL (50 mL)
SandIMMUNE®: 100 mg/mL (50 mL)

cyclosporine (ophthalmic) (SYE kloe spor een)

Medication Safety Issues
Sound-alike/look-alike issues:
CycloSPORINE may be confused with cyclophosphamide, Cyklokapron®, cycloSERINE
Synonyms CsA; CyA; cyclosporin A
Tall-Man cycloSPORINE
U.S. Brand Names Restasis®
Therapeutic Category Immunosuppressant Agent
Use Increase tear production when suppressed tear production is presumed to be due to keratoconjunctivitis sicca-associated ocular inflammation (in patients not already using topical antiinflammatory drugs or punctal plugs)
General Dosage Range Ophthalmic (Restasis®): Children ≥16 years and Adults: Instill 1 drop in each eye every 12 hours
Dosage Forms
Emulsion, ophthalmic [preservative free]:
Restasis®: 0.05% (0.4 mL)

Cyestra-35 (Can) see cyproterone and ethinyl estradiol (Canada only) on page 245
Cyklokapron® see tranexamic acid on page 881
Cylate™ see cyclopentolate on page 242
Cymbalta® see duloxetine on page 316

cyproheptadine (si proe HEP ta deen)

Medication Safety Issues
Sound-alike/look-alike issues:
Cyproheptadine may be confused with cyclobenzaprine
Periactin may be confused with Percodan®, Persantine®
International issues:
Periactin brand name for cyproheptadine [U.S., multiple international markets] may be confused with Perative brand name for an enteral nutrition preparation [multiple international markets] and brand name for ketoconazole [Argentina]
BEERS Criteria medication:
This drug may be inappropriate for use in geriatric patients (high severity risk).
Synonyms cyproheptadine hydrochloride; Periactin
Therapeutic Category Antihistamine
Use Perennial and seasonal allergic rhinitis and other allergic symptoms including urticaria

General Dosage Range
Oral:
Children 2-6 years: 2 mg every 8-12 hours (not to exceed 12 mg/day)
Children 7-14 years: 4 mg every 8-12 hours (not to exceed 16 mg/day)
Adults: 4-20 mg/day divided every 8 hours (not to exceed 0.5 mg/kg/day)

Dosage Forms
Syrup, oral: 2 mg/5 mL (473 mL, 480 mL)
Tablet, oral: 4 mg

cyproheptadine hydrochloride *see cyproheptadine on page 244*

cyproterone *(Canada only)* (sye PROE ter one)
Synonyms cyproterone acetate
Canadian Brand Names Androcur®; Androcur® Depot; Novo-Cyproterone
Therapeutic Category Antiandrogen; Progestin
Use Palliative treatment of advanced prostate cancer
General Dosage Range
I.M.: *Adults (males):* 300 mg (3 mL) once weekly **or** every 2 weeks
Oral: *Adults (males):* 100-300 mg/day in 2-3 divided doses
Product Availability Not available in U.S.
Dosage Forms - Canada
Injection, solution: 100 mg/mL (3 mL)
Androcur® Depot: 100 mg/mL (3 mL)
Tablet: 50 mg
Androcur®, Apo-Cyproterone®, Gen-Cyproterone: 50 mg

cyproterone and ethinyl estradiol *(Canada only)*
(sye PROE ter one & ETH in il es tra DYE ole)
Synonyms ethinyl estradiol and cyproterone acetate
Canadian Brand Names Cyestra-35; Diane-35®; Novo-Cyproterone/Ethinyl Estradiol
Therapeutic Category Acne Products; Estrogen and Androgen Combination
Use Treatment of females with severe acne, unresponsive to oral antibiotics and other therapies, with associated symptoms of androgenization (including mild hirsutism or seborrhea). **Should not be used solely for contraception;** however, will provide reliable contraception if taken as recommended for approved indications.
General Dosage Range Oral: *Adults (females):* 1 tablet daily
Product Availability Not available in U.S.
Dosage Forms - Canada
Tablet, oral:
Diane-35: Cyproterone 2 mg and ethinyl estradiol 0.035 mg (21s)

cyproterone acetate *see cyproterone (Canada only) on page 245*
Cystadane® *see betaine on page 129*
Cystagon® *see cysteamine on page 245*

cysteamine (sis TEE a meen)
Synonyms cysteamine bitartrate
U.S. Brand Names Cystagon®
Therapeutic Category Urinary Tract Product
Use Treatment of nephropathic cystinosis
General Dosage Range Oral:
Children <12 years: Initial: 1/4 to 1/6 of maintenance dose; Maintenance: 1.3 g/m^2/day **or** 60 mg/kg/day in 4 divided doses (maximum dose: 1.95 g/m^2/day; 90 mg/kg/day)
Children ≥12 years and Adults >110 lbs: Initial: 1/4 to 1/6 of maintenance dose; Maintenance: 2 g/day in 4 divided doses (maximum: 1.95 g/m^2/day; 90 mg/kg/day)
Dosage Forms
Capsule, oral:
Cystagon®: 50 mg, 150 mg

cysteamine bitartrate *see cysteamine on page 245*

cysteine (SIS te een)

Synonyms cysteine hydrochloride
U.S. Brand Names Cysteine-500 [DSC]
Therapeutic Category Nutritional Supplement
Use Supplement to crystalline amino acid solutions, in particular the specialized pediatric formulas (eg, Aminosyn® PF, TrophAmine®) to meet the intravenous amino acid nutritional requirements of infants receiving parenteral nutrition (PN)
General Dosage Range I.V.: *Infants ≤2 years:* Added as a fixed ratio to crystalline amino acid solution: 40 mg cysteine per g of amino acids; dosage will vary with the daily amino acid dosage; individual doses of cysteine of 0.8-1 mmol/kg/day have also been added directly to the daily PN solution
Dosage Forms
Injection, solution: 50 mg/mL (10 mL, 50 mL)

Cysteine-500 [DSC] *see* cysteine *on page 246*
cysteine hydrochloride *see* cysteine *on page 246*
Cystistat® (Can) *see* hyaluronate and derivatives *on page 443*
Cysto-Conray® II *see* iothalamate meglumine *on page 486*
Cystografin® *see* diatrizoate meglumine *on page 274*
Cystografin® Dilute *see* diatrizoate meglumine *on page 274*
Cysview™ *see* hexaminolevulinate *on page 440*
CYT *see* cyclophosphamide *on page 242*

cytarabine (sye TARE a been)

Medication Safety Issues
Sound-alike/look-alike issues:
Cytarabine may be confused with Cytosar®, Cytoxan, vidarabine
Cytarabine (conventional) may be confused with cytarabine liposomal
Cytosar-U may be confused with cytarabine, Cytovene®, Cytoxan, Neosar
High alert medication:
This medication is in a class the Institute for Safe Medication Practices (ISMP) includes among its list of drugs classes which have a heightened risk of causing significant patient harm when used in error.
Administration issues:
Intrathecal medication safety: The American Society of Clinical Oncology (ASCO)/Oncology Nursing Society (ONS) chemotherapy administration safety standards (Jacobson, 2009) encourage the following safety measures for intrathecal chemotherapy:
• Intrathecal medication should not be prepared during the preparation of any other agents
• After preparation, store in an isolated location or container clearly marked with a label identifying as "intrathecal" use only
• Delivery to the patient should only be with other medications also intended for administration into the central nervous system
Synonyms ara-C; arabinosylcytosine; cytarabine (conventional); cytarabine hydrochloride; Cytosar-U; cytosine arabinosine hydrochloride
Canadian Brand Names Cytosar®
Therapeutic Category Antineoplastic Agent
Use Remission induction in acute myeloid leukemia (AML), treatment of acute lymphocytic leukemia (ALL) and chronic myelocytic leukemia (CML; blast phase); prophylaxis and treatment of meningeal leukemia
General Dosage Range Dosage adjustment recommended in patients with hepatic or renal impairment
I.V.: *Children and Adults:* AML Induction: 100-200 mg/m^2/day for 7 days
Dosage Forms
Injection, powder for reconstitution: 100 mg, 500 mg, 1 g
Injection, solution: 20 mg/mL (25 mL); 100 mg/mL (20 mL)
Injection, solution [preservative free]: 20 mg/mL (5 mL, 50 mL); 100 mg/mL (20 mL)

cytarabine (conventional) *see* cytarabine *on page 246*
cytarabine hydrochloride *see* cytarabine *on page 246*
Cytarabine Lipid Complex *see* cytarabine (liposomal) *on page 247*

cytarabine (liposomal) (sye TARE a been lip po SOE mal)

Medication Safety Issues

Sound-alike/look-alike issues:

Cytarabine may be confused with Cytosar®, Cytoxan, vidarabine

Cytarabine liposomal may be confused with conventional cytarabine

High alert medication:

This medication is in a class the Institute for Safe Medication Practices (ISMP) includes among its list of drug classes which have a heightened risk of causing significant patient harm when used in error.

Administration issues:

Intrathecal medication safety: The American Society of Clinical Oncology (ASCO)/Oncology Nursing Society (ONS) chemotherapy administration safety standards (Jacobson, 2009) encourage the following safety measures for intrathecal chemotherapy:

• Intrathecal medication should not be prepared during the preparation of any other agents

• After preparation, store in an isolated location or container clearly marked with a label identifying as "intrathecal" use only

• Delivery to the patient should only be with other medications also intended for administration into the central nervous system

Synonyms Cytarabine Lipid Complex; Cytarabine Liposome; DepoFoam-Encapsulated Cytarabine; DTC 101; Liposomal Cytarabine

U.S. Brand Names DepoCyt®

Canadian Brand Names DepoCyt®

Therapeutic Category Antineoplastic Agent, Antimetabolite (Purine)

Use Treatment of lymphomatous meningitis

General Dosage Range Dosage adjustment recommended in patients who develop toxicities

I.T.: *Adults:* Induction: 50 mg every 14 days for a total of 2 doses (weeks 1 and 3); Consolidation: 50 mg every 14 days for 3 doses (weeks 5, 7, and 9), followed by 50 mg at week 13; Maintenance: 50 mg every 28 days for 4 doses (weeks 17, 21, 25, and 29)

Dosage Forms

Injection, suspension, intrathecal [preservative free]:

DepoCyt®: 10 mg/mL (5 mL)

Cytarabine Liposome *see* cytarabine (liposomal) *on page 247*

CytoGam® *see* cytomegalovirus immune globulin (intravenous-human) *on page 247*

cytomegalovirus immune globulin (intravenous-human)

(sye toe meg a low VYE rus i MYUN GLOB yoo lin in tra VEE nus HYU man)

Medication Safety Issues

Sound-alike/look-alike issues:

CytoGam® may be confused with Cytoxan, Gamimune® N

Synonyms CMV-IGIV

U.S. Brand Names CytoGam®

Canadian Brand Names CytoGam®

Therapeutic Category Immune Globulin

Use Prophylaxis of cytomegalovirus (CMV) disease associated with kidney, lung, liver, pancreas, and heart transplants; concomitant use with ganciclovir should be considered in organ transplants (other than kidney) from CMV seropositive donors to CMV seronegative recipients

General Dosage Range I.V.: *Adults:* Initial: 150 mg/kg with 72 hours of transplant; 2-, 4-, 6- and 8 weeks after transplant: 100 mg/kg (kidney) **or** 150 mg/kg (liver, lung, pancreas, heart); 12 and 16 weeks after transplant: 50 mg/kg (kidney) **or** 100 mg/kg (liver, lung, pancreas, heart)

Dosage Forms

Injection, solution [preservative free]:

CytoGam®: 50 mg ± 10 mg/mL (50 mL)

Cytomel® *see* liothyronine *on page 529*

Cytosar® (Can) *see* cytarabine *on page 246*

Cytosar-U *see* cytarabine *on page 246*

cytosine arabinosine hydrochloride *see* cytarabine *on page 246*

cytostasan *see* bendamustine *on page 119*

Cytotec® *see* misoprostol *on page 592*

Cytovene® (Can) *see* ganciclovir (systemic) *on page 410*

Cytovene®-IV *see* ganciclovir (systemic) *on page 410*

Cytoxan *see* cyclophosphamide *on page 242*

Cytra-3 *see* citric acid, sodium citrate, and potassium citrate *on page 214*

Cytra-K *see* potassium citrate and citric acid *on page 725*

D2 *see* ergocalciferol *on page 336*

D2E7 *see* adalimumab *on page 40*

D₃ *see* cholecalciferol *on page 204*

D-3 [OTC] *see* cholecalciferol *on page 204*

D3-5™ [OTC] *see* cholecalciferol *on page 204*

D3-50™ [OTC] *see* cholecalciferol *on page 204*

D-3-mercaptovaline *see* penicillamine *on page 683*

d4T *see* stavudine *on page 830*

D₅W *see* dextrose *on page 273*

D₁₀W *see* dextrose *on page 273*

D₂₅W *see* dextrose *on page 273*

D₃₀W *see* dextrose *on page 273*

D₄₀W *see* dextrose *on page 273*

D₅₀W *see* dextrose *on page 273*

D₆₀W *see* dextrose *on page 273*

D₇₀W *see* dextrose *on page 273*

D1694 *see* raltitrexed *(Canada only) on page 765*

DAB₃₈₉IL-2 *see* denileukin diftitox *on page 258*

DAB389 interleukin-2 *see* denileukin diftitox *on page 258*

dabigatran etexilate (da BIG a tran ett EX ill ate)

Synonyms dabigatran etexilate mesilate

U.S. Brand Names Pradaxa®

Canadian Brand Names Pradax™

Therapeutic Category Anticoagulant, Thrombin Inhibitor

Use Prevention of stroke and systemic embolism in patients with nonvalvular atrial fibrillation

2011 ACCF/AHA/HRS atrial fibrillation guidelines: Not recommended for patients with coexisting prosthetic heart valve or hemodynamically significant valve disease, severe renal failure (Cl$_{cr}$ <15 mL/minute), or advanced liver disease (impaired baseline clotting function)

Canadian labeling: Additional uses (not in U.S. labeling): Postoperative thromboprophylaxis in patients who have undergone total hip or knee replacement procedures

General Dosage Range Dosage adjustment recommended in patients with renal impairment

Oral: *Adults:* 150 mg twice daily

Dosage Forms

Capsule, oral:

Pradaxa®: 75 mg, 150 mg

Dosage Forms - Canada

Capsule, oral:

Pradax™: 75 mg, 110 mg, 150 mg

dabigatran etexilate mesilate *see* dabigatran etexilate *on page 248*

DABIL2 *see* denileukin diftitox *on page 258*

dacarbazine (da KAR ba zeen)

Medication Safety Issues

Sound-alike/look-alike issues:

Dacarbazine may be confused with procarbazine

High alert medication:

This medication is in a class the Institute for Safe Medication Practices (ISMP) includes among its list of drugs which have a heightened risk of causing significant patient harm when used in error.

Synonyms DIC; dimethyl triazeno imidazole carboxamide; DTIC; DTIC-dome; imidazole carboxamide; imidazole carboxamide dimethyltriazene; WR-139007

Canadian Brand Names Dacarbazine for Injection

Therapeutic Category Antineoplastic Agent

Use Treatment of malignant melanoma, Hodgkin disease

General Dosage Range Dosage adjustment recommended in patients with renal impairment

I.V.:
  Children: 375 mg/m² on days 1 and 15, repeat every 28 days
  Adults: 375 mg/m² days 1 and 15 every 4 weeks **or** 250 mg/m² days 1-5 every 3 weeks

Dosage Forms
  Injection, powder for reconstitution: 100 mg, 200 mg

Dacarbazine for Injection (Can) *see* dacarbazine *on page 248*

dacliximab *see* daclizumab *on page 249*

daclizumab (dac KLYE zue mab)

Synonyms anti-tac monoclonal antibody; dacliximab; MOAB anti-tac

U.S. Brand Names Zenapax® [DSC]

Canadian Brand Names Zenapax®

Therapeutic Category Immunosuppressant Agent

Use Prophylaxis of acute rejection in renal transplantation (in combination with cyclosporine and corticosteroids)

General Dosage Range I.V.: *Children and Adults:* 1 mg/kg within 24 hours before transplantation (day 0), then every 14 days for 4 additional doses

Product Availability Zenapax®: Due to diminishing market demand, the manufacturer of daclizumab has discontinued production; it is anticipated that available supplies will be depleted in January 2010; all remaining lots will expire in 2011.

Dacodyl™ [OTC] *see* bisacodyl *on page 134*

Dacogen® *see* decitabine *on page 256*

DACT *see* dactinomycin *on page 249*

dactinomycin (dak ti noe MYE sin)

Medication Safety Issues
  Sound-alike/look-alike issues:
    DACTINomycin may be confused with DAPTOmycin, DAUNOrubicin
    Actinomycin may be confused with achromycin
  High alert medication:
    This medication is in a class the Institute for Safe Medication Practices (ISMP) includes among its list of drug classes which have a heightened risk of causing significant patient harm when used in error.

Synonyms ACT-D; actinomycin; actinomycin Cl; actinomycin D; DACT

Tall-Man DACTINomycin

U.S. Brand Names Cosmegen®

Canadian Brand Names Cosmegen®

Therapeutic Category Antineoplastic Agent

Use Treatment of Wilms tumor, childhood rhabdomyosarcoma, Ewing sarcoma, metastatic testicular tumors (nonseminomatous), gestational trophoblastic neoplasm; regional perfusion (palliative or adjunctive) of locally recurrent or locoregional solid tumors (sarcomas, carcinomas, and adenocarcinomas)

General Dosage Range
I.V.:
  Children >6 months: 15 mcg/kg/day **or** 400-600 mcg/m²/day for 5 days every 3-6 weeks
  Adults: 12-15 mcg/kg/day **or** 400-600 mcg/m²/day for 5 days every 3-6 weeks **or** 1000 mcg/m² on day 1 **or** 500 mcg/dose days 1 and 2
  Regional perfusion: *Adults:* Lower extremity or pelvis: 50 mcg/kg; Upper extremity: 35 mcg/kg

Dosage Forms
  Injection, powder for reconstitution: 0.5 mg
    Cosmegen®: 0.5 mg

Dairyaid® (Can) *see* lactase *on page 505*

Dakin's Solution *see* sodium hypochlorite solution *on page 820*
Dalacin® C (Can) *see* clindamycin (topical) *on page 218*
Dalacin® T (Can) *see* clindamycin (topical) *on page 218*
Dalacin® Vaginal (Can) *see* clindamycin (topical) *on page 218*

dalfampridine (dal FAM pri deen)

Medication Safety Issues
Sound-alike/look-alike issues:
Ampyra™ may be confused with anakinra
Dalfampridine may be confused with delavirdine, desipramine
Synonyms 4-aminopyridine; 4-AP; EL-970; fampridine-SR
U.S. Brand Names Ampyra™
Therapeutic Category Potassium Channel Blocker
Use Treatment to improve walking in multiple sclerosis (MS) patients
General Dosage Range Oral: Extended release: *Adults:* 10 mg every 12 hours
Dosage Forms
Tablet, extended release, oral:
Ampyra™: 10 mg

dalfopristin and quinupristin *see* quinupristin and dalfopristin *on page 763*
Daliresp™ *see* roflumilast *on page 788*
Dallergy® [DSC] *see* chlorpheniramine, phenylephrine, and methscopolamine *on page 200*
Dallergy Drops [DSC] *see* chlorpheniramine and phenylephrine *on page 198*
Dallergy®-JR [DSC] *see* chlorpheniramine and phenylephrine *on page 198*
Dalmane® (Can) *see* flurazepam *on page 391*
d-Alpha Gems™ [OTC] *see* vitamin E *on page 918*
d-alpha tocopherol *see* vitamin E *on page 918*

dalteparin (dal TE pa rin)

Medication Safety Issues
High alert medication:
The Institute for Safe Medication Practices (ISMP) includes this medication among its list of drugs which have a heightened risk of causing significant patient harm when used in error.
2009 National Patient Safety Goals:
The Joint Commission (TJC) requires healthcare organizations that provide anticoagulant therapy to have a process in place to reduce the risk of anticoagulant-associated patient harm. Patients receiving anticoagulants should receive individualized care through a defined process that includes standardized ordering, dispensing, administration, monitoring and education. This does not apply to routine short-term use of anticoagulants for prevention of venous thromboembolism when the expectation is that the patient's laboratory values will remain within or close to normal values (NPSG.03.05.01).
Synonyms dalteparin sodium; NSC-714371
U.S. Brand Names Fragmin®
Canadian Brand Names Fragmin®
Therapeutic Category Anticoagulant (Other)
Use Prevention of deep vein thrombosis (DVT) which may lead to pulmonary embolism, in patients requiring abdominal surgery who are at risk for thromboembolism complications (eg, patients >40 years of age, obesity, patients with malignancy, history of DVT or pulmonary embolism, and surgical procedures requiring general anesthesia and lasting >30 minutes); prevention of DVT in patients undergoing hip-replacement surgery; patients immobile during an acute illness; prevention of ischemic complications in patients with unstable angina or non-Q-wave myocardial infarction on concurrent aspirin therapy; in patients with cancer, extended treatment (6 months) of acute symptomatic venous thromboembolism (DVT and/or PE) to reduce the recurrence of venous thromboembolism
General Dosage Range SubQ: *Adults:* Prophylaxis: 2500-5000 int. units daily; Treatment: 120 int. units/kg every 12 hours (maximum: 10,000 int. units/dose) **or** ~150-200 int. units/kg (maximum: 18,000 int. units/dose) once daily
Dosage Forms
Injection, solution:
Fragmin®: 25,000 anti-Xa int. units/mL (3.8 mL)

Injection, solution [preservative free]:
Fragmin®: 10,000 anti-Xa int. units/mL (1 mL); 2500 anti-Xa int. units/0.2 mL (0.2 mL); 5000 anti-Xa int. units/0.2 mL (0.2 mL); 7500 anti-Xa int. units/0.3 mL (0.3 mL); 12,500 anti-Xa int. units/0.5 mL (0.5 mL); 15,000 anti-Xa int. units/0.6 mL (0.6 mL); 18,000 anti-Xa int. units/0.72 mL (0.72 mL)

dalteparin sodium see dalteparin on page 250

danaparoid *(Canada only)* (da NAP a roid)

Medication Safety Issues
Sound-alike/look-alike issues:
Orgaran® may be confused with argatroban
Synonyms danaparoid sodium
Canadian Brand Names Orgaran®
Therapeutic Category Anticoagulant (Other)
Use Prevention of postoperative deep vein thrombosis (DVT) following orthopedic or major abdominal and thoracic surgery; prevention of DVT in patients with confirmed diagnosis of non-hemorrhagic stroke; management of heparin-induced thrombocytopenia (HIT)
General Dosage Range Dosage adjustment recommended in patients with renal impairment
SubQ:
Children: 10 units/kg every 12 hours
Adults: Dosage varies greatly depending on indication
I.V.:
Children: Initial bolus: 30 units/kg; maintenance: 1.2-4 units/kg/hour
Adults: Dosage varies greatly depending on indication
Product Availability Not available in U.S.
Dosage Forms - Canada
Injection, solution:
Orgaran®: 750 anti-Xa units/0.6 mL (0.6 mL)

danaparoid sodium see danaparoid (Canada only) on page 251

danazol (DA na zole)

Medication Safety Issues
Sound-alike/look-alike issues:
Danazol may be confused with Dantrium®
Synonyms Danocrine
Canadian Brand Names Cyclomen®
Therapeutic Category Androgen
Use Treatment of endometriosis, fibrocystic breast disease, and hereditary angioedema
General Dosage Range Oral:
Adults (females): 100-800 mg/day in 2 divided doses
Adults (females/males): Hereditary angioedema: Initial: 200 mg 2-3 times/day; after favorable response decrease dosage by 50% or less
Dosage Forms
Capsule, oral: 50 mg, 100 mg, 200 mg

Dandrex see selenium sulfide on page 807
Danocrine see danazol on page 251
Dantrium® see dantrolene on page 251

dantrolene (DAN troe leen)

Medication Safety Issues
Sound-alike/look-alike issues:
Dantrium® may be confused with danazol, Daraprim®
Revonto™ may be confused with Revatio®
Synonyms dantrolene sodium
U.S. Brand Names Dantrium®; Revonto™
Canadian Brand Names Dantrium®
Therapeutic Category Skeletal Muscle Relaxant

◀ **Use** Treatment of spasticity associated with upper motor neuron disorders (eg, spinal cord injury, stroke, cerebral palsy, or multiple sclerosis); management of malignant hyperthermia; prevention of malignant hyperthermia in susceptible individuals (preoperative/postoperative administration)

General Dosage Range
I.V.: *Children and Adults:* 1-2.5 mg/kg; may repeat up to cumulative dose of 10 mg/kg **or** 2.5 mg/kg as a single dose
Oral:
Children: 4-8 mg/kg/day in 4 divided doses **or** 0.5-2 mg/kg/dose 1-3 times/day (maximum: 400 mg/day)
Adults: 4-8 mg/kg/day in 4 divided doses **or** 25-100 mg 1-3 times/day (maximum: 400 mg/day)

Dosage Forms
Capsule, oral: 25 mg, 50 mg, 100 mg
Dantrium®: 25 mg, 50 mg, 100 mg
Injection, powder for reconstitution:
Dantrium®: 20 mg
Revonto™: 20 mg

dantrolene sodium *see* dantrolene *on page* 251

dapcin *see* daptomycin *on page* 252

dapsone (systemic) (DAP sone)

Medication Safety Issues
Sound-alike/look-alike issues:
Dapsone may be confused with Diprosone®
Synonyms diaminodiphenylsulfone
Therapeutic Category Antibiotic, Miscellaneous
Use Treatment of leprosy and dermatitis herpetiformis (infections caused by *Mycobacterium leprae*)
General Dosage Range Oral:
Children: 1-2 mg/kg once daily (maximum: 100 mg/day)
Adults: 50-300 mg once daily
Dosage Forms
Tablet, oral: 25 mg, 100 mg

dapsone (topical) (DAP sone)

Medication Safety Issues
Sound-alike/look-alike issues:
Dapsone may be confused with Diprosone®
Synonyms diaminodiphenylsulfone
U.S. Brand Names Aczone®
Therapeutic Category Topical Skin Product, Acne
Use Topical treatment of acne vulgaris
General Dosage Range Topical: *Children ≥12 years and Adults:* Apply pea-sized amount (approximately) in thin layer to affected areas twice daily
Dosage Forms
Gel, topical:
Aczone®: 5% (30 g, 60 g)

Daptacel® *see* diphtheria, tetanus toxoids, and acellular pertussis vaccine *on page* 296

daptomycin (DAP toe mye sin)

Medication Safety Issues
Sound-alike/look-alike issues:
Cubicin® may be confused with Cleocin®
DAPTOmycin may be confused with DACTINomycin
Synonyms cidecin; dapcin; LY146032
Tall-Man DAPTOmycin
U.S. Brand Names Cubicin®
Canadian Brand Names Cubicin®
Therapeutic Category Antibiotic, Cyclic Lipopeptide

Use Treatment of complicated skin and skin structure infections caused by susceptible aerobic gram-positive organisms; *Staphylococcus aureus* bacteremia, including right-sided native valve infective endocarditis caused by MSSA or MRSA

General Dosage Range Dosage adjustment recommended in patients with renal impairment

I.V.: *Adults:* 4-6 mg/kg once daily

Dosage Forms

Injection, powder for reconstitution:
Cubicin®: 500 mg

Daraprim® *see* pyrimethamine *on page 758*

darbepoetin alfa (dar be POE e tin AL fa)

Medication Safety Issues

Sound-alike/look-alike issues:
Aranesp® may be confused with Aralast, Aricept®
Darbepoetin alfa may be confused with dalteparin, epoetin alfa, epoetin beta

Synonyms erythropoiesis-stimulating agent (ESA); erythropoiesis-stimulating protein; NESP; novel erythropoiesis-stimulating protein

U.S. Brand Names Aranesp®; Aranesp® SingleJect®

Canadian Brand Names Aranesp®

Therapeutic Category Colony-Stimulating Factor; Growth Factor; Recombinant Human Erythropoietin

Use Treatment of anemia due to concurrent myelosuppressive chemotherapy in patients with cancer (nonmyeloid malignancies) receiving chemotherapy (palliative intent) for a planned minimum of 2 additional months of chemotherapy; treatment of anemia due to chronic kidney disease (including patients on dialysis and not on dialysis)

Note: Darbepoetin is **not** indicated for use under the following conditions:
 • Cancer patients receiving hormonal therapy, therapeutic biologic products, or radiation therapy unless also receiving concurrent myelosuppressive chemotherapy
 • Cancer patients receiving myelosuppressive chemotherapy when the expected outcome is curative
 • As a substitute for RBC transfusion in patients requiring immediate correction of anemia

Note: In clinical trials, darbepoetin has not demonstrated improved quality of life, fatigue, or well-being.

General Dosage Range

I.V.:
Children 1-18 years: 6.25-200 mcg/week
Adults: 0.45 mcg/kg once weekly **or** every 4 weeks **or** 0.75 mcg/kg once every 2 weeks **or** 6.25-200 mcg/week

SubQ:
Children 1-18 years: 6.25-200 mcg/week
Adults: 0.45-4.5 mcg/kg/week **or** 0.45 mcg/kg every 4 weeks **or** 0.75 mcg/kg once every 2 weeks **or** 500 mcg once every 3 weeks **or** 6.25-200 mcg/week

Dosage Forms

Injection, solution [preservative free]:
Aranesp®: 25 mcg/mL (1 mL); 40 mcg/mL (1 mL); 60 mcg/mL (1 mL); 100 mcg/mL (1 mL); 150 mcg/0.75 mL (0.75 mL); 200 mcg/mL (1 mL); 300 mcg/mL (1 mL)
Aranesp® SingleJect®: 25 mcg/0.42 mL (0.42 mL); 40 mcg/0.4 mL (0.4 mL); 60 mcg/0.3 mL (0.3 mL); 100 mcg/0.5 mL (0.5 mL); 150 mcg/0.3 mL (0.3 mL); 200 mcg/0.4 mL (0.4 mL); 300 mcg/0.6 mL (0.6 mL); 500 mcg/mL (1 mL)

darifenacin (dar i FEN a sin)

Synonyms darifenacin hydrobromide; UK-88,525

U.S. Brand Names Enablex®

Canadian Brand Names Enablex®

Therapeutic Category Anticholinergic Agent

Use Management of symptoms of bladder overactivity (urge incontinence, urgency, and frequency)

General Dosage Range Dosage adjustment recommended in patients with hepatic impairment or on concomitant therapy

Oral: *Adults:* Initial: 7.5 mg once daily; Maintenance: 7.5-15 mg once daily

◀ **Dosage Forms**
Tablet, extended release, oral:
Enablex®: 7.5 mg, 15 mg

darifenacin hydrobromide *see darifenacin on page 253*

darunavir (dar OO na veer)
Synonyms darunavir ethanolate; TMC-114
U.S. Brand Names Prezista®
Canadian Brand Names Prezista®
Therapeutic Category Antiretroviral Agent, Protease Inhibitor
Use Treatment of HIV-1 infections in combination with ritonavir and other antiretroviral agents
General Dosage Range Dosage adjustment recommended in patients on concomitant therapy or who develop toxicities.
Oral:
Children ≥6 years and ≥20 kg to <30 kg: Darunavir: 375 mg twice daily; Ritonavir: 50 mg twice daily
Children ≥6 years and ≥30 kg to <40 kg: Darunavir: 450 mg twice daily; Ritonavir: 60 mg twice daily
Children ≥6 years and ≥40 kg: Darunavir: 600 mg twice daily; Ritonavir: 100 mg twice daily
Adults: Darunavir: 600 mg twice daily; Ritonavir: 100 mg twice daily **or** Darunavir: 800 mg once daily; Ritonavir: 100 mg once daily
Dosage Forms
Tablet, oral:
Prezista®: 75 mg, 150 mg, 400 mg, 600 mg
Dosage Forms - Canada
Tablet:
Prezista®: 300 mg, 400 mg, 600 mg

darunavir ethanolate *see darunavir on page 254*
Darvocet A500® [DSC] *see propoxyphene and acetaminophen on page 746*
Darvocet-N® 50 [DSC] *see propoxyphene and acetaminophen on page 746*
Darvocet-N® 50 (Can) *see propoxyphene and acetaminophen on page 746*
Darvocet-N® 100 [DSC] *see propoxyphene and acetaminophen on page 746*
Darvocet-N® 100 (Can) *see propoxyphene and acetaminophen on page 746*
Darvon® [DSC] *see propoxyphene on page 746*
Darvon-N® [DSC] *see propoxyphene on page 746*
Darvon-N® (Can) *see propoxyphene on page 746*

dasatinib (da SA ti nib)
Medication Safety Issues
Sound-alike/look-alike issues:
Dasatinib may be confused with imatinib, nilotinib, SUNITinib, vandetanib
High alert medication:
This medication is in a class the Institute for Safe Medication Practices (ISMP) includes among its list of drug classes which have a heightened risk of causing significant patient harm when used in error.
Synonyms BMS-354825
U.S. Brand Names Sprycel®
Canadian Brand Names Sprycel®
Therapeutic Category Antineoplastic Agent, Tyrosine Kinase Inhibitor
Use Treatment of chronic myelogenous leukemia (CML) in chronic, accelerated or blast (myeloid or lymphoid) phase resistant or intolerant to prior therapy (including imatinib); treatment of newly-diagnosed Philadelphia chromosome-positive (Ph+) CML in chronic phase; treatment of Philadelphia chromosome-positive (Ph+) acute lymphoblastic leukemia (ALL) resistant or intolerant to prior therapy
General Dosage Range Dosage adjustment recommended in patients on concomitant therapy or who develop toxicities
Oral: *Adults:* 100-180 mg once daily
Dosage Forms
Tablet, oral:
Sprycel®: 20 mg, 50 mg, 70 mg, 100 mg

daunomycin *see daunorubicin hydrochloride on page 255*

daunorubicin citrate (liposomal) (daw noe ROO bi sin SI trate lip po SOE mal)

Medication Safety Issues

Sound-alike/look-alike issues:
DAUNOrubicin liposomal may be confused with DACTINomycin, DOXOrubicin, DOXOrubicin liposomal, epirubicin, IDArubicin, valrubicin
Liposomal formulation (DaunoXome®) may be confused with the conventional formulation (Cerubidine®, Rubex®)

High alert medication:
The Institute for Safe Medication Practices (ISMP) includes this medication among its list of drug classes which have a heightened risk of causing significant patient harm when used in error.

Synonyms DAUNOrubicin liposomal; liposomal DAUNOrubicin; NSC-697732

Tall-Man DAUNOrubicin citrate (liposomal)

U.S. Brand Names DaunoXome®

Therapeutic Category Antineoplastic Agent

Use First-line treatment of advanced HIV-associated Kaposi sarcoma (KS)

General Dosage Range Dosage adjustment recommended in patients with hepatic or renal impairment
I.V.: *Adults:* 40 mg/m^2 every 2 weeks

Dosage Forms

Injection, solution [preservative free]:
DaunoXome®: 2 mg/mL (25 mL)

daunorubicin hydrochloride (daw noe ROO bi sin hye droe KLOR ide)

Medication Safety Issues

Sound-alike/look-alike issues:
DAUNOrubicin may be confused with DACTINomycin, DOXOrubicin, DOXOrubicin liposomal, epirubicin, IDArubicin, valrubicin
Conventional formulation (Cerubidine®, DAUNOrubicin hydrochloride) may be confused with the liposomal formulation (DaunoXome®)

High alert medication:
The Institute for Safe Medication Practices (ISMP) includes this medication among its list of drug classes which have a heightened risk of causing significant patient harm when used in error.

Synonyms daunomycin; rubidomycin hydrochloride

Tall-Man DAUNOrubicin hydrochloride

U.S. Brand Names Cerubidine®

Canadian Brand Names Cerubidine®

Therapeutic Category Antineoplastic Agent

Use Treatment of acute lymphocytic leukemia (ALL) and acute myeloid leukemia (AML)

General Dosage Range Dosage adjustment recommended in patients with hepatic or renal impairment
I.V.:
Children <2 years or BSA <0.5 m^2: 1 mg/kg/dose per protocol with frequency dependent on regimen employed (maximum cumulative dose: 10 mg/kg)
Children ≥2 years and BSA ≥0.5 m^2: 25 mg/m^2 on day 1 every week for 4 cycles **or** 30-60 mg/m^2/day for 3 days (maximum cumulative dose: 300 mg/m^2)
Adults <60 years: 30-60 mg/m^2/day for 2-3 days (maximum cumulative dose: 550 mg/m^2; 400 mg/m^2 with chest irradiation)
Adults ≥60 years: 30 mg/m^2/day for 2-3 days (maximum cumulative dose: 550 mg/m^2; 400 mg/m^2 with chest irradiation)

Dosage Forms

Injection, powder for reconstitution: 20 mg
Cerubidine®: 20 mg
Injection, solution [preservative free]: 5 mg/mL (4 mL, 10 mL)

DAUNOrubicin liposomal *see* daunorubicin citrate (liposomal) *on page 255*

DaunoXome® *see* daunorubicin citrate (liposomal) *on page 255*

Daxas™ (Can) *see* roflumilast *on page 788*

1-Day™ [OTC] *see* tioconazole *on page 870*

Daypro® *see* oxaprozin *on page 659*

Daytrana® *see* methylphenidate *on page 577*

dCF *see* pentostatin *on page 689*

DDAVP® *see* desmopressin *on page 262*

DDAVP® Melt (Can) *see* desmopressin *on page 262*

ddI *see* didanosine *on page 281*

DDrops® *see* cholecalciferol *on page 204*

DDrops® Baby [OTC] *see* cholecalciferol *on page 204*

DDrops® Kids [OTC] *see* cholecalciferol *on page 204*

1-deamino-8-D-arginine vasopressin *see* desmopressin *on page 262*

Debrox® [OTC] *see* carbamide peroxide *on page 172*

Decadron *see* dexamethasone (systemic) *on page 264*

Decavac® *see* diphtheria and tetanus toxoid *on page 293*

Dec-Chlorphen [DSC] *see* chlorpheniramine and phenylephrine *on page 198*

De-Chlor DM [DSC] *see* chlorpheniramine, phenylephrine, and dextromethorphan *on page 200*

De-Chlor DR [DSC] *see* chlorpheniramine, phenylephrine, and dextromethorphan *on page 200*

decitabine (de SYE ta been)

Medication Safety Issues
High alert medication:
This medication is in a class the Institute for Safe Medication Practices (ISMP) includes among its list of drug classes which have a heightened risk of causing significant patient harm when used in error.

Synonyms 5-Aza-2'-deoxycytidine; 5-Aza-dCyd; deoxyazacytidine; dezocitidine

U.S. Brand Names Dacogen®

Therapeutic Category Antineoplastic Agent, Antimetabolite (Pyrimidine)

Use Treatment of myelodysplastic syndrome (MDS)

General Dosage Range Dosage adjustment recommended in patients who develop toxicities

I.V.: *Adults:* 15 mg/m^2 every 8 hours for 3 days every 6 weeks **or** 20 mg/m^2 daily for 5 days every 28 days

Dosage Forms
Injection, powder for reconstitution:
Dacogen®: 50 mg

Declomycin *see* demeclocycline *on page 258*

Deep Sea [OTC] *see* sodium chloride *on page 818*

deferasirox (de FER a sir ox)

Medication Safety Issues
Sound-alike/look-alike issues:
Deferasirox may be confused with deferoxamine
International issues:
Deferasirox may be confused with deferiprone [Great Britain]

Synonyms ICL670

U.S. Brand Names Exjade®

Canadian Brand Names Exjade®

Therapeutic Category Antidote; Chelating Agent

Use Treatment of chronic iron overload due to blood transfusions (transfusional hemosiderosis)

General Dosage Range Dosage adjustment recommended in patients with renal impairment or on concomitant therapy

Oral: *Children ≥2 years and Adults:* Initial: 20 mg/kg once daily; Maintenance: 20-30 mg/kg once daily (maximum dose: 40 mg/kg/day)

Dosage Forms
Tablet for suspension, oral:
Exjade®: 125 mg, 250 mg, 500 mg

deferoxamine (de fer OKS a meen)

Medication Safety Issues
Sound-alike/look-alike issues:
Deferoxamine may be confused with cefuroxime, deferasirox

Desferal® may be confused with desflurane, Dexferrum®

International issues:

Desferal [U.S., Canada, and multiple international markets] may be confused with Deseril brand name for methysergide [Australia, Belgium, Great Britain, Netherlands]; Disophrol brand name for dexbrompheniramine and pseudoephedrine [Czech Republic, Poland, Turkey]

Synonyms deferoxamine mesylate; desferrioxamine

U.S. Brand Names Desferal®

Canadian Brand Names Desferal®; PMS-Deferoxamine

Therapeutic Category Antidote

Use Adjunct in the treatment of acute iron intoxication; treatment of chronic iron overload secondary to multiple transfusions

Canadian labeling (unlabeled use in the U.S.): Diagnosis of aluminum overload; treatment of chronic aluminum overload in patients with end-stage renal failure undergoing maintenance dialysis

General Dosage Range Dosage adjustment recommended in patients with renal impairment

I.M.:
Children ≥3 years: Maximum: 6 g/24 hours
Adults: Initial: 1000 mg, followed by 500 mg every 4 hours for 2 doses; Maintenance: 500 mg every 4-12 hours **or** 500-1000 mg once daily (maximum: 6 g/day)

I.V.:
Children ≥3 years: 15 mg/kg/hour (maximum: 6 g/24 hours)
Adults: Initial: 1000 mg, followed by 500 mg every 4 hours for 2 doses; Maintenance: 500 mg every 4-12 hours **or** 2000 mg with each unit of blood (maximum: 6 g/day)

SubQ:
Children ≥3 years: 20-40 mg/kg/day (maximum: 1000-2000 mg/day)
Adults: 1-2 g once daily **or** 20-40 mg/kg/day

Dosage Forms
Injection, powder for reconstitution: 500 mg, 2 g
Desferal®: 500 mg, 2 g

deferoxamine mesylate *see deferoxamine on page 256*

Definity® *see perflutren lipid microspheres on page 690*

degarelix (deg a REL ix)

Medication Safety Issues
Sound-alike/look-alike issues:
Degarelix may be confused with cetrorelix, ganirelix

Synonyms degarelix acetate; FE200486

U.S. Brand Names Firmagon®

Canadian Brand Names Firmagon®

Therapeutic Category Antineoplastic Agent, Gonadotropin-Releasing Hormone Antagonist; Gonadotropin Releasing Hormone Antagonist

Use Treatment of advanced prostate cancer

General Dosage Range SubQ: *Adults:* Loading dose: 240 mg; Maintenance dose: 80 mg every 28 days

Dosage Forms
Injection, powder for reconstitution:
Firmagon®: 80 mg, 120 mg

degarelix acetate *see degarelix on page 257*

Dehistine [DSC] *see chlorpheniramine, phenylephrine, and methscopolamine on page 200*

Dehydral® (Can) *see methenamine on page 569*

dehydrobenzperidol *see droperidol on page 314*

Delatestryl® *see testosterone on page 854*

delavirdine (de la VIR deen)

Medication Safety Issues
Sound-alike/look-alike issues:
Delavirdine may be confused with dalfampridine

Synonyms DLV; U-90152S

U.S. Brand Names Rescriptor®

◀ **Canadian Brand Names** Rescriptor®
Therapeutic Category Antiviral Agent
Use Treatment of HIV-1 infection in combination with at least two additional antiretroviral agents
General Dosage Range Oral: *Children ≥16 years and Adults:* 400 mg 3 times/day
Dosage Forms
  Tablet, oral:
    Rescriptor®: 100 mg, 200 mg

Delestrogen® *see* estradiol (systemic) *on page 343*
Delfen® [OTC] *see* nonoxynol 9 *on page 632*
Delsym® [OTC] *see* dextromethorphan *on page 270*
delta-9-tetrahydro-cannabinol *see* dronabinol *on page 314*
delta-9-tetrahydrocannabinol and cannabinol *see* tetrahydrocannabinol and cannabidiol *(Canada only) on page 857*
delta-9 THC *see* dronabinol *on page 314*
deltacortisone *see* prednisone *on page 735*
Delta® D3 [OTC] *see* cholecalciferol *on page 204*
deltadehydrocortisone *see* prednisone *on page 735*
Demadex® *see* torsemide *on page 878*

demeclocycline (dem e kloe SYE kleen)

Synonyms Declomycin; demeclocycline hydrochloride; demethylchlortetracycline
Therapeutic Category Tetracycline Derivative
Use Treatment of susceptible bacterial infections (acne, gonorrhea, pertussis, and urinary tract infections) caused by both gram-negative and gram-positive organisms
General Dosage Range Oral:
  Children ≥8 years: 8-12 mg/kg/day divided every 6-12 hours
  Adults: 600 mg/day in 2 or 4 divided doses
Dosage Forms
  Tablet, oral: 150 mg, 300 mg

demeclocycline hydrochloride *see* demeclocycline *on page 258*
Demerol® *see* meperidine *on page 560*
4-demethoxydaunorubicin *see* idarubicin *on page 463*
demethylchlortetracycline *see* demeclocycline *on page 258*
Demser® *see* metyrosine *on page 584*
Demulen® 30 (Can) *see* ethinyl estradiol and ethynodiol diacetate *on page 353*
Denavir® *see* penciclovir *on page 683*

denileukin diftitox (de ni LOO kin DIF ti toks)

Medication Safety Issues
  High alert medication:
    The Institute for Safe Medication Practices (ISMP) includes this medication among its list of drug classes which have a heightened risk of causing significant patient harm when used in error.
Synonyms DAB389 interleukin-2; $DAB_{389}IL-2$; DABIL2
U.S. Brand Names ONTAK®
Therapeutic Category Antineoplastic Agent, Miscellaneous
Use Treatment of persistent or recurrent cutaneous T-cell lymphoma (CTCL) whose malignant cells express the CD25 component of the IL-2 receptor
General Dosage Range Dosage adjustment recommended in patients who develop toxicities
  I.V.: *Adults:* 9 or 18 mcg/kg/day days 1-5 every 21 days
Dosage Forms
  Injection, solution:
    ONTAK®: 150 mcg/mL (2 mL)

Denorex® Extra Strength Protection [OTC] *see* salicylic acid *on page 795*
Denorex® Extra Strength Protection 2-in-1 [OTC] *see* salicylic acid *on page 795*
Denorex® Therapeutic Protection [OTC] *see* coal tar *on page 227*

Denorex® Therapeutic Protection 2-in-1 Shampoo + Conditioner [OTC] *see* coal tar *on page 227*

denosumab (den OH sue mab)

Medication Safety Issues
Other safety concerns:
Duplicate therapy issues: Prolia® contains denosumab, which is the same ingredient contained in Xgeva™; patients receiving Xgeva™ should not be treated with Prolia®

Synonyms AMG-162

U.S. Brand Names Prolia®; Xgeva™

Canadian Brand Names Prolia®; Xgeva™

Therapeutic Category Monoclonal Antibody

Use Treatment of osteoporosis in postmenopausal women at high risk for fracture; treatment of bone loss in men receiving androgen deprivation therapy (ADT) for nonmetastatic prostate cancer; treatment of bone loss in women receiving aromatase inhibitor (AI) therapy for breast cancer; prevention of skeletal-related events (eg, fracture, spinal cord compression, bone pain requiring surgery/radiation therapy) in patients with bone metastases from solid tumors

General Dosage Range SubQ: *Adults:* Prolia®: 60 mg every 6 months; Xgeva™: 120 mg every 4 weeks

Dosage Forms
Injection, solution [preservative free]:
Prolia®: 60 mg/mL (1 mL)
Xgeva™: 70 mg/mL (1.7 mL)

Denta 5000 Plus™ *see* fluoride *on page 386*

DentaGel™ *see* fluoride *on page 386*

Dentapaine [OTC] *see* benzocaine *on page 121*

Dent's Extra Strength Toothache Gum [OTC] *see* benzocaine *on page 121*

deodorized tincture of opium (error-prone synonym) *see* opium tincture *on page 653*

deoxyazacytidine *see* decitabine *on page 256*

2'-deoxycoformycin *see* pentostatin *on page 689*

deoxycoformycin *see* pentostatin *on page 689*

Depacon® *see* valproic acid *on page 904*

Depakene® *see* valproic acid *on page 904*

Depakote® *see* divalproex *on page 300*

Depakote® ER *see* divalproex *on page 300*

Depakote® Sprinkle *see* divalproex *on page 300*

Depen® *see* penicillamine *on page 683*

Deplin™ *see* methylfolate *on page 576*

DepoCyt® *see* cytarabine (liposomal) *on page 247*

DepoDur® *see* morphine (liposomal) *on page 599*

Depo®-Estradiol *see* estradiol (systemic) *on page 343*

DepoFoam-Encapsulated Cytarabine *see* cytarabine (liposomal) *on page 247*

Depo-Medrol® *see* methylprednisolone *on page 578*

Depo-Prevera® (Can) *see* medroxyprogesterone *on page 554*

Depo-Provera® *see* medroxyprogesterone *on page 554*

Depo-Provera® Contraceptive *see* medroxyprogesterone *on page 554*

depo-subQ provera 104® *see* medroxyprogesterone *on page 554*

Depotest® 100 (Can) *see* testosterone *on page 854*

Depo®-Testosterone *see* testosterone *on page 854*

deprenyl *see* selegiline *on page 806*

depsipeptide *see* romidepsin *on page 789*

DermaFungal [OTC] *see* miconazole (topical) *on page 585*

Dermagran® [OTC] *see* aluminum hydroxide *on page 59*

Dermagran® AF [OTC] *see* miconazole (topical) *on page 585*

Dermamycin® [OTC] *see* diphenhydramine (topical) *on page 291*

Dermarest® Eczema Medicated [OTC] *see* hydrocortisone (topical) *on page 450*

Dermarest® Psoriasis Medicated Moisturizer [OTC] *see* salicylic acid *on page 795*
Dermarest® Psoriasis Medicated Scalp Treatment [OTC] *see* salicylic acid *on page 795*
Dermarest® Psoriasis Medicated Shampoo/Conditioner [OTC] *see* salicylic acid *on page 795*
Dermarest® Psoriasis Medicated Skin Treatment [OTC] *see* salicylic acid *on page 795*
Dermarest® Psoriasis Overnight Treatment [OTC] *see* salicylic acid *on page 795*
Derma-Smoothe/FS® *see* fluocinolone (topical) *on page 384*
Dermatop® *see* prednicarbate *on page 733*
Dermazene® *see* iodoquinol and hydrocortisone *on page 485*
DermaZinc™ [OTC] *see* pyrithione zinc *on page 759*
Dermazole (Can) *see* miconazole (topical) *on page 585*
Dermoplast® Antibacterial [OTC] *see* benzocaine *on page 121*
Dermoplast® Pain Relieving [OTC] *see* benzocaine *on page 121*
DermOtic® *see* fluocinolone (otic) *on page 384*
Dermovate® (Can) *see* clobetasol *on page 220*
Desferal® *see* deferoxamine *on page 256*
desferrioxamine *see* deferoxamine *on page 256*

desflurane (DES flure ane)

Medication Safety Issues
  Sound-alike/look-alike issues:
   Desflurane may be confused with Desferal®
  High alert medication:
   The Institute for Safe Medication Practices (ISMP) includes this medication among its list of drug
   classes which have a heightened risk of causing significant patient harm when used in error.
U.S. Brand Names Suprane®
Canadian Brand Names Suprane®
Therapeutic Category General Anesthetic
Use Induction and/or maintenance of general anesthesia in adults; maintenance of anesthesia in intubated
 children; **Note:** Use of desflurane for induction of general anesthesia is not recommended due to its
 irritant properties and unpleasant odor which causes coughing, breath holding, laryngospasm, oxygen
 desaturation, increased secretions, hypertension, and tachycardia.
General Dosage Range Inhalation:
 Children (intubated): 5.2% to 10% to maintain surgical levels of anesthesia
 Adults: 2.5% to 8.5% to maintain surgical levels of anesthesia
Dosage Forms
 Liquid, for inhalation:
  Suprane®: 100% (240 mL)

desiccated thyroid *see* thyroid, desiccated *on page 865*

desipramine (des IP ra meen)

Medication Safety Issues
  Sound-alike/look-alike issues:
   Desipramine may be confused with clomiPRAMINE, dalfampridine, diphenhydrAMINE, disopyramide,
   imipramine, nortriptyline
   Norpramin® may be confused with clomiPRAMINE, imipramine, Normodyne®, Norpace®, nortriptyline,
   Tenormin®
  International issues:
   Norpramin: Brand name for desipramine [U.S., Canada], but also the brand name for enalapril/
   hydrochlorothiazide [Portugal]; omeprazole [Spain]
Synonyms desipramine hydrochloride; desmethylimipramine hydrochloride
U.S. Brand Names Norpramin®
Canadian Brand Names Alti-Desipramine; Apo-Desipramine®; Norpramin®; Nu-Desipramine; PMS-
 Desipramine
Therapeutic Category Antidepressant, Tricyclic (Secondary Amine)
Use Treatment of depression

General Dosage Range Oral:
Adolescents: 25-100 mg/day in single or divided doses (maximum: 150 mg/day)
Adults: 100-200 mg/day in single or divided doses (maximum: 300 mg/day)
Elderly: 25-100 mg/day in single or divided doses (maximum: 150 mg/day)
Dosage Forms
Tablet, oral: 10 mg, 25 mg, 50 mg, 75 mg, 100 mg, 150 mg
Norpramin®: 10 mg, 25 mg, 50 mg, 75 mg, 100 mg, 150 mg

desipramine hydrochloride *see desipramine on page 260*

desirudin (des i ROO din)
Medication Safety Issues
High alert medication:
The Institute for Safe Medication Practices (ISMP) includes this medication among its list of drugs which have a heightened risk of causing significant patient harm when used in error.
Synonyms CGP-39393; desulfato-hirudin; desulfatohirudin; desulphatohirudin; r-hirudin; recombinant desulfatohirudin; recombinant hirudin
U.S. Brand Names Iprivask®
Therapeutic Category Anticoagulant, Thrombin Inhibitor
Use Prophylaxis of deep vein thrombosis (DVT) in patients undergoing surgery for hip replacement
General Dosage Range Dosage adjustment recommended in patients with renal impairment
SubQ: *Adults:* 15 mg every 12 hours
Dosage Forms
Injection, powder for reconstitution [preservative free]:
Iprivask®: 15 mg

Desitin® [OTC] *see zinc oxide on page 930*
Desitin® Creamy [OTC] *see zinc oxide on page 930*

desloratadine (des lor AT a deen)
Medication Safety Issues
Sound-alike/look-alike issues:
Clarinex® may be confused with Celebrex®
U.S. Brand Names Clarinex®
Canadian Brand Names Aerius®; Aerius® Kids
Therapeutic Category Antihistamine, Nonsedating
Use Relief of nasal and non-nasal symptoms of seasonal allergic rhinitis (SAR) and perennial allergic rhinitis (PAR); treatment of chronic idiopathic urticaria (CIU)
General Dosage Range Dosage adjustment recommended in adult patients with hepatic or renal impairment
Oral:
Children 6-11 months: 1 mg once daily
Children 1-5 years: 1.25 mg once daily
Children 6-11 years: 2.5 mg once daily
Children ≥12 years and Adults: 5 mg once daily
Dosage Forms
Syrup, oral:
Clarinex®: 0.5 mg/mL (480 mL)
Tablet, oral:
Clarinex®: 5 mg
Tablet, orally disintegrating, oral:
Clarinex®: 2.5 mg, 5 mg

desloratadine and pseudoephedrine (des lor AT a deen & soo doe e FED rin)
Synonyms pseudoephedrine and desloratadine
U.S. Brand Names Clarinex-D® 12 Hour; Clarinex-D® 24 Hour
Therapeutic Category Antihistamine/Decongestant Combination, Nonsedating
Use Relief of symptoms of seasonal allergic rhinitis, in children ≥12 years of age and adults
General Dosage Range Dosage adjustment recommended in patients with renal impairment
Oral: *Children ≥12 years and Adults:* 12 hour: 1 tablet twice daily; 24 hour: 1 tablet once daily

◀ **Dosage Forms**
Tablet, variable release:
Clarinex-D® 12 Hour: Desloratadine 2.5 mg [immediate release] and pseudoephedrine 120 mg [extended release]
Clarinex-D® 24 Hour: Desloratadine 5 mg [immediate release] and pseudoephedrine 240 mg [extended release]

desmethylimipramine hydrochloride *see desipramine on page 260*

desmopressin (des moe PRES in)

Synonyms 1-deamino-8-D-arginine vasopressin; desmopressin acetate
U.S. Brand Names DDAVP®; Stimate®
Canadian Brand Names Apo-Desmopressin®; DDAVP®; DDAVP® Melt; Minirin®; Novo-Desmopressin; Octostim®; PMS-Desmopressin
Therapeutic Category Vasopressin Analog, Synthetic
Use
Injection: Treatment of diabetes insipidus; maintenance of hemostasis and control of bleeding in hemophilia A with factor VIII coagulant activity levels >5% and mild-to-moderate classic von Willebrand disease (type 1) with factor VIII coagulant activity levels >5%
Nasal solutions (DDAVP® Nasal Spray and DDAVP® Rhinal Tube): Treatment of central diabetes insipidus
Nasal spray (Stimate®): Maintenance of hemostasis and control of bleeding in hemophilia A with factor VIII coagulant activity levels >5% and mild-to-moderate classic von Willebrand disease (type 1) with factor VIII coagulant activity levels >5%
Tablet: Treatment of central diabetes insipidus, temporary polyuria and polydipsia following pituitary surgery or head trauma, primary nocturnal enuresis
General Dosage Range
I.V.:
Infants and Children ≥3 months: 0.3 mcg/kg as a single dose, may repeat dose if needed
Adults: 2-4 mcg/day in 2 divided doses **or** one-tenth (¹/₁₀) of the intranasal maintenance dose **or** 0.3 mcg/kg as a single dose
Intranasal:
Infants 3-11 months: Initial: 5 mcg/day (0.05 mL/day) in 1-2 divided doses; Maintenance: 5-30 mcg/day (0.05-0.3 mL/day) in 1-2 divided doses
Children 12 months to 12 years: Initial: 5 mcg/day (0.05 mL/day) in 1-2 divided doses; Maintenance: 5-30 mcg/day (0.05-0.3 mL/day) in 1-2 divided doses **or** 150 mcg (1 spray of high concentration) as a single dose
Children >12 years and Adults <50 kg: 10-40 mcg/day (0.1-0.4 mL) in 1-3 divided doses **or** 150 mcg (1 spray of high concentration spray) as a single dose
Children >12 years and Adults ≥50 kg: 10-40 mcg/day in 1-3 divided doses **or** 300 mcg (1 spray each nostril of high concentration spray) as a single dose
Oral:
Children 4-5 years: Initial: 0.05 mg twice daily; Maintenance: 0.1-1.2 mg/day in 2-3 divided doses
Children ≥6 years: Initial: 0.05 mg twice daily **or** 0.2 mg at bedtime; Maintenance: 0.1-1.2 mg/day in 2-3 divided doses **or** 0.2-0.6 mg at bedtime
Adults: 0.2-0.6 mg at bedtime **or** 0.1-1.2 mg/day in 2-3 divided doses
SubQ: *Adults:* 2-4 mcg/day in 2 divided doses **or** one-tenth (¹/₁₀) of the intranasal maintenance dose
Dosage Forms
Injection, solution: 4 mcg/mL (1 mL, 10 mL)
DDAVP®: 4 mcg/mL (1 mL, 10 mL)
Solution, intranasal: 0.1 mg/mL (2.5 mL, 5 mL)
DDAVP®: 0.1 mg/mL (2.5 mL, 5 mL)
Stimate®: 1.5 mg/mL (2.5 mL)
Tablet, oral: 0.1 mg, 0.2 mg
DDAVP®: 0.1 mg, 0.2 mg
Dosage Forms - Canada
Tablet, sublingual:
DDAVP® Melt: 60 mcg, 120 mcg, 240 mcg

desmopressin acetate *see desmopressin on page 262*
Desocort® (Can) *see desonide on page 263*

Desogen® *see ethinyl estradiol and desogestrel on page 351*
desogestrel and ethinyl estradiol *see ethinyl estradiol and desogestrel on page 351*
Desonate® *see desonide on page 263*

desonide (DES oh nide)
U.S. Brand Names Desonate®; DesOwen®; LoKara™; Verdeso®
Canadian Brand Names Desocort®; PMS-Desonide
Therapeutic Category Corticosteroid, Topical
Use Treatment of inflammatory and pruritic manifestations of corticosteroid responsive dermatosis (low-to-medium potency corticosteroid); mild-to-moderate atopic dermatitis
General Dosage Range Topical:
Children ≥3 months: Aerosol, gel: Apply 2 times/day sparingly
Adults: Apply 2-3 times/day sparingly
Dosage Forms
  Aerosol, topical:
   Verdeso®: 0.05% (50 g, 100 g)
  Cream, topical: 0.05% (15 g, 60 g)
   DesOwen®: 0.05% (60 g)
  Gel, topical:
   Desonate®: 0.05% (60 g)
  Lotion, topical: 0.05% (59 mL, 60 mL, 118 mL)
   DesOwen®: 0.05% (60 mL, 120 mL)
   LoKara™: 0.05% (59 mL, 118 mL)
  Ointment, topical: 0.05% (15 g, 60 g)

DesOwen® *see desonide on page 263*

desoximetasone (des oks i MET a sone)
Medication Safety Issues
  Sound-alike/look-alike issues:
   Desoximetasone may be confused with dexamethasone
   Topicort® may be confused with Topic®
U.S. Brand Names Topicort®; Topicort® LP
Canadian Brand Names Taro-Desoximetasone; Topicort®
Therapeutic Category Corticosteroid, Topical
Use Relieves inflammation and pruritic symptoms of corticosteroid-responsive dermatosis (intermediate-to high-potency topical corticosteroid)
General Dosage Range Topical:
  Cream, gel: *Children and Adults:* Apply a thin film to affected area twice daily
  Ointment: *Children ≥10 years and Adults:* Apply a thin film to affected area twice daily
Dosage Forms
  Cream, topical: 0.05% (15 g, 60 g); 0.25% (15 g, 60 g, 100 g)
   Topicort®: 0.25% (15 g, 60 g)
   Topicort® LP: 0.05% (15 g, 60 g)
  Gel, topical: 0.05% (15 g, 60 g)
   Topicort®: 0.05% (15 g, 60 g)
  Ointment, topical: 0.25% (15 g, 60 g)
   Topicort®: 0.25% (15 g, 60 g)

desoxyephedrine hydrochloride *see methamphetamine on page 568*
Desoxyn® *see methamphetamine on page 568*
desoxyphenobarbital *see primidone on page 737*
Desquam-X® (Can) *see benzoyl peroxide on page 124*
Desquam-X® 5 [OTC] *see benzoyl peroxide on page 124*
Desquam-X® 10 [OTC] *see benzoyl peroxide on page 124*
desulfato-hirudin *see desirudin on page 261*
desulphatohirudin *see desirudin on page 261*

desvenlafaxine (des ven la FAX een)

Synonyms O-desmethylvenlafaxine; ODV
U.S. Brand Names Pristiq®
Canadian Brand Names Pristiq®
Therapeutic Category Antidepressant, Serotonin/Norepinephrine Reuptake Inhibitor
Use Treatment of major depressive disorder
General Dosage Range Dosage adjustment recommended in patients with hepatic or renal impairment
  Oral: *Adults:* Initial: 50 mg once daily
Dosage Forms
  Tablet, extended release, oral:
    Pristiq®: 50 mg, 100 mg

Desyrel *see* trazodone *on page 884*
Detane® [OTC] *see* benzocaine *on page 121*
detemir insulin *see* insulin detemir *on page 476*
Detrol® *see* tolterodine *on page 876*
Detrol® LA *see* tolterodine *on page 876*
detryptoreline *see* triptorelin *on page 894*
Dex4® [OTC] *see* dextrose *on page 273*

dexamethasone (systemic) (deks a METH a sone)

Medication Safety Issues
  Sound-alike/look-alike issues:
    Dexamethasone may be confused with desoximetasone, dextroamphetamine
    Decadron® may be confused with Percodan®
Synonyms Decadron; dexamethasone sodium phosphate
U.S. Brand Names Baycadron™; Dexamethasone Intensol™; DexPak® 10 Day TaperPak®; DexPak® 13 Day TaperPak®; DexPak® 6 Day TaperPak®
Canadian Brand Names Apo-Dexamethasone®; Dexasone®
Therapeutic Category Antiemetic; Antiinflammatory Agent; Corticosteroid, Systemic
Use Primarily as an antiinflammatory or immunosuppressant agent in the treatment of a variety of diseases including those of allergic, dermatologic, endocrine, hematologic, inflammatory, neoplastic, nervous system, renal, respiratory, rheumatic, and autoimmune origin; may be used in management of cerebral edema, chronic swelling, as a diagnostic agent, diagnosis of Cushing syndrome, antiemetic
General Dosage Range
  I.M.:
    Children: 0.03-2 mg/kg/day or 0.6-10 mg/m^2/day divided every 6-12 hours
    Adults: 0.75-9 mg/day or 0.03-2 mg/kg/day or 0.6-0.75 mg/m^2/day in divided doses every 6-12 hours **or** 4 mg every 4-6 hours
  I.V.:
    Children: 0.03-2 mg/kg/day or 0.6-10 mg/m^2/day divided every 6-12 hours **or** 10 mg/m^2/dose every 12-24 hours on days of chemotherapy
    Adults: Dosage varies greatly depending on indication
  Intra-articular, intralesional, or soft tissue: *Adults:* 0.4-6 mg/day
  Oral:
    Children: 0.03-2 mg/kg/day or 0.6-10 mg/m^2/day divided every 6-12 hours
    Adults: Dosage varies greatly depending on indication
Dosage Forms
  Elixir, oral: 0.5 mg/5 mL (237 mL)
    Baycadron™: 0.5 mg/5 mL (237 mL)
  Injection, solution: 4 mg/mL (1 mL, 5 mL, 30 mL); 10 mg/mL (1 mL, 10 mL)
  Injection, solution [preservative free]: 10 mg/mL (1 mL)
  Solution, oral: 0.5 mg/5 mL (240 mL, 500 mL)
    Dexamethasone Intensol™: 1 mg/mL (30 mL)
  Tablet, oral: 0.5 mg, 0.75 mg, 1 mg, 1.5 mg, 2 mg, 4 mg, 6 mg
    DexPak® 6 Day TaperPak®: 1.5 mg
    DexPak® 10 Day TaperPak®: 1.5 mg
    DexPak® 13 Day TaperPak®: 1.5 mg

dexamethasone (ophthalmic) (deks a METH a sone)

Medication Safety Issues
Sound-alike/look-alike issues:
Dexamethasone may be confused with desoximetasone, dextroamphetamine
Maxidex® may be confused with Maxzide®
Synonyms dexamethasone sodium phosphate
U.S. Brand Names Maxidex®; Ozurdex®
Canadian Brand Names Diodex®; Maxidex®
Therapeutic Category Antiinflammatory Agent, Ophthalmic; Corticosteroid, Ophthalmic
Use Management of steroid responsive inflammatory conditions such as allergic conjunctivitis, iritis, or cyclitis; symptomatic treatment of corneal injury from chemical, radiation, or thermal burns, or penetration of foreign bodies
Ophthalmic intravitreal implant (Ozurdex®): Treatment of macular edema following branch retinal vein occlusion (BRVO) or central retinal vein occlusion (CRVO); treatment of noninfective uveitis
General Dosage Range
Intravitreal: *Adults:* 0.7 mg implant in affected eye
Ophthalmic:
Children: Instill 1-2 drops into conjunctival sac every hour during the day and every other hour during the night; gradually reduce dose to 2-4 times/day
Adults:
Solution: Instill 1-2 drops into conjunctival sac every hour during the day and every other hour during the night; gradually reduce dose to every 3-4 hours, then to 3-4 times/day
Suspension: Instill 1-2 drops up to 4-6 times/day or hourly in severe cases
Dosage Forms
Implant, intravitreal:
Ozurdex®: 0.7 mg (1s)
Solution, ophthalmic: 0.1% (5 mL)
Suspension, ophthalmic:
Maxidex®: 0.1% (5 mL)

dexamethasone and ciprofloxacin *see* ciprofloxacin and dexamethasone *on page 211*
dexamethasone and tobramycin *see* tobramycin and dexamethasone *on page 874*
Dexamethasone Intensol™ *see* dexamethasone (systemic) *on page 264*
dexamethasone, neomycin, and polymyxin B *see* neomycin, polymyxin B, and dexamethasone *on page 618*
dexamethasone sodium phosphate *see* dexamethasone (ophthalmic) *on page 265*
dexamethasone sodium phosphate *see* dexamethasone (systemic) *on page 264*
Dexasone® (Can) *see* dexamethasone (systemic) *on page 264*

dexbrompheniramine and pseudoephedrine
(deks brom fen EER a meen & soo doe e FED rin)
Synonyms pseudoephedrine and dexbrompheniramine
Canadian Brand Names Drixoral®
Therapeutic Category Antihistamine/Decongestant Combination
Use Relief of symptoms of upper respiratory mucosal congestion in seasonal and perennial nasal allergies, acute rhinitis, rhinosinusitis, and eustachian tube blockage
General Dosage Range Oral: *Children >12 years and Adults:* 1 tablet every 8-12 hours
Dosage Forms
Tablet, sustained action: Dexbrompheniramine 6 mg and pseudoephedrine 120 mg

dexchlorpheniramine (deks klor fen EER a meen)
Medication Safety Issues
BEERS Criteria medication:
This drug may be inappropriate for use in geriatric patients (high severity risk).
Synonyms dexchlorpheniramine maleate
Therapeutic Category Antihistamine
Use Perennial and seasonal allergic rhinitis and other allergic symptoms including urticaria

General Dosage Range Oral:
Regular release:
Children 2-5 years: 0.5 mg every 4-6 hours
Children 6-11 years: 1 mg every 4-6 hours
Adults: 2 mg every 4-6 hours
Timed release:
Children 6-11 years: 4 mg at bedtime
Adults: 4-6 mg at bedtime **or** every 8-10 hours
Dosage Forms
Syrup, oral: 2 mg/5 mL (473 mL)

dexchlorpheniramine maleate *see* dexchlorpheniramine *on page 265*

dexchlorpheniramine tannate, pseudoephedrine tannate, and dextromethorphan tannate
see chlorpheniramine, pseudoephedrine, and dextromethorphan *on page 201*

Dexedrine® (Can) *see* dextroamphetamine *on page 268*

Dexedrine® Spansule® *see* dextroamphetamine *on page 268*

Dexferrum® *see* iron dextran complex *on page 491*

Dexilant™ *see* dexlansoprazole *on page 266*

Dexiron™ (Can) *see* iron dextran complex *on page 491*

dexlansoprazole (deks lan SOE pra zole)

Medication Safety Issues
Sound-alike/look-alike issues:
Dexlansoprazole may be confused with aripiprazole, lansoprazole
Kapidex [DSC] may be confused with Casodex®, Kadian®
International issues:
Kapidex [DSC] may be confused with Capadex which is a brand name for propoxyphene/acetaminophen combination product [Australia, New Zealand]
Synonyms Kapidex; TAK-390MR
U.S. Brand Names Dexilant™
Canadian Brand Names Dexilant™
Therapeutic Category Proton Pump Inhibitor; Substituted Benzimidazole
Use Short-term (4 weeks) treatment of heartburn associated with nonerosive GERD; short-term (up to 8 weeks) treatment of all grades of erosive esophagitis; to maintain healing of erosive esophagitis for up to 6 months
General Dosage Range Dosage adjustment recommended in patients with hepatic impairment
Oral: *Adults:* 30-60 mg once daily
Dosage Forms
Capsule, delayed release, oral:
Dexilant™: 30 mg, 60 mg

dexmedetomidine (deks MED e toe mi deen)

Medication Safety Issues
Sound-alike/look-alike issues:
Precedex® may be confused with Peridex®
Administration issues:
Errors have occurred due to misinterpretation of dosing information; use caution. Maintenance dose expressed as mcg/kg/**hour**.
Synonyms dexmedetomidine hydrochloride
U.S. Brand Names Precedex®
Canadian Brand Names Precedex®
Therapeutic Category Alpha-Adrenergic Agonist - Central-Acting (Alpha$_2$-Agonists); Sedative
Use Sedation of initially intubated and mechanically ventilated patients during treatment in an intensive care setting; sedation prior to and/or during surgical or other procedures of nonintubated patients
General Dosage Range I.V.: *Adults:* Loading infusion: 0.5-1 mcg/kg; Maintenance infusion: 0.2-1 mcg/kg/hour
Dosage Forms
Injection, solution [preservative free]:
Precedex®: 100 mcg/mL (2 mL)

dexmedetomidine hydrochloride *see* dexmedetomidine *on page 266*

dexmethylphenidate (dex meth il FEN i date)

Medication Safety Issues

Sound-alike/look-alike issues:

Dexmethylphenidate may be confused with methadone

Focalin® may be confused with Folotyn®

Synonyms dexmethylphenidate hydrochloride

U.S. Brand Names Focalin XR®; Focalin®

Therapeutic Category Central Nervous System Stimulant, Nonamphetamine

Controlled Substance C-II

Use Treatment of attention-deficit/hyperactivity disorder (ADHD)

General Dosage Range Oral:

Extended release:

Children ≥6 years: Initial: 5 mg once daily; Maintenance: Up to 30 mg/day

Adults: Initial: 10 mg once daily; Maintenance: Up to 40 mg/day

Immediate release: *Children ≥6 years and Adults:* Initial: 2.5 mg twice daily; Maintenance: Up to 20 mg/day in 2 divided doses (at least 4 hours apart)

Dosage Forms

Capsule, extended release, oral:

Focalin XR®: 5 mg, 10 mg, 15 mg, 20 mg, 25 mg, 30 mg, 35 mg, 40 mg

Tablet, oral: 2.5 mg, 5 mg, 10 mg

Focalin®: 2.5 mg, 5 mg, 10 mg

dexmethylphenidate hydrochloride *see* dexmethylphenidate *on page 267*

DexPak® 6 Day TaperPak® *see* dexamethasone (systemic) *on page 264*

DexPak® 10 Day TaperPak® *see* dexamethasone (systemic) *on page 264*

DexPak® 13 Day TaperPak® *see* dexamethasone (systemic) *on page 264*

dexpanthenol (deks PAN the nole)

Synonyms pantothenyl alcohol

Therapeutic Category Gastrointestinal Agent, Stimulant

Use Prophylactic use to minimize paralytic ileus; treatment of postoperative distention; topical to relieve itching and to aid healing of minor dermatoses

General Dosage Range I.M.: *Adults:* Initial: 250-500 mg; repeat in 2 hours, followed by doses every 6 hours if needed

Dosage Forms

Injection, solution [preservative free]: 250 mg/mL (2 mL)

dexrazoxane (deks ray ZOKS ane)

Medication Safety Issues

Sound-alike/look-alike issues:

Zinecard® may be confused with Gemzar®

Synonyms ICRF-187

U.S. Brand Names Totect®; Zinecard®

Canadian Brand Names Zinecard®

Therapeutic Category Cardiovascular Agent, Other

Use

Zinecard®: Reduction of the incidence and severity of cardiomyopathy associated with doxorubicin administration in women with metastatic breast cancer who have received a cumulative doxorubicin dose of 300 mg/m^2 and who would benefit from continuing therapy with doxorubicin. (Not recommended for use with initial doxorubicin therapy.)

Totect®: Treatment of anthracycline-induced extravasation.

General Dosage Range Dosage adjustment recommended in patients with renal impairment

I.V.: *Adults:* A 10:1 ratio of dexrazoxane:doxorubicin (500 mg/m^2 dexrazoxane: 50 mg/m^2 doxorubicin) **or** 1000 mg/m^2 on days 1 and 2 (maximum dose: 2000 mg), followed by 500 mg/m^2 on day 3 (maximum dose: 1000 mg)

◄ Dosage Forms
Injection, powder for reconstitution: 250 mg, 500 mg
Totect®: 500 mg
Zinecard®: 250 mg, 500 mg

dextran (DEKS tran)

Medication Safety Issues
Sound-alike/look-alike issues:
Dextran may be confused with Dexedrine®

Synonyms 10% LMD; dextran 40; dextran, low molecular weight
U.S. Brand Names LMD®
Therapeutic Category Plasma Volume Expander

Use Blood volume expander used in treatment of shock or impending shock when blood or blood products are not available; also used as a priming fluid in pump oxygenators during cardiopulmonary bypass and for prophylaxis of venous thrombosis and pulmonary embolism in surgical procedures associated with a high risk of thromboembolic complications

General Dosage Range I.V.:
Dextran 40:
Children: Infuse 10 mL/kg as rapidly as possible (maximum: 20 mL/kg/day for the first 24 hours; 10 mL/kg/day thereafter); therapy should not be continued beyond 5 days
Adults: Infuse 500-1000 mL (~10 mL/kg) as rapidly as possible (maximum: 20 mL/kg/day for first 24 hours; 10 mL/kg/day thereafter); (5 days total therapy) **or** 50-100 g on the day of surgery, then 50 g (4 mL/minute) every 2-3 days during the period of risk

Dosage Forms
Infusion, premixed in D₅W:
LMD®: 10% Dextran 40 (500 mL)
Infusion, premixed in NS:
LMD®: 10% Dextran 40 (500 mL)

dextran 40 *see dextran on page 268*
dextran, low molecular weight *see dextran on page 268*
dextrin *see wheat dextrin on page 923*

dextroamphetamine (deks troe am FET a meen)

Medication Safety Issues
Sound-alike/look-alike issues:
Dexedrine® may be confused with dextran, Excedrin®
Dextroamphetamine may be confused with dexamethasone
BEERS Criteria medication:
This drug may be inappropriate for use in geriatric patients (high severity risk).

Synonyms dextroamphetamine sulfate
U.S. Brand Names Dexedrine® Spansule®; ProCentra®
Canadian Brand Names Dexedrine®
Therapeutic Category Amphetamine
Controlled Substance C-II
Use Narcolepsy; attention-deficit/hyperactivity disorder (ADHD)

General Dosage Range Oral:
Children 3-5 years: Initial: 2.5 mg once daily; Maintenance: 0.1-0.5 mg/kg once daily (maximum: 40 mg/day)
Children 6-12 years: Initial: 5 mg once or twice daily; Maintenance: 5-20 mg (0.1-0.5 mg/kg) once daily (maximum: 40 mg [ADHD]: 60 mg [narcolepsy])
Children >12 years: Initial: 5-10 mg/day in 1-2 divided doses; Maximum: Up to 40 mg/day [ADHD] or 60 mg/day [narcolepsy]
Adults: Initial: 10 mg once daily; Maximum: Up to 60 mg/day

Dosage Forms
Capsule, extended release, oral: 5 mg, 10 mg, 15 mg
Capsule, sustained release, oral:
Dexedrine® Spansule®: 5 mg, 10 mg, 15 mg

Solution, oral:
  ProCentra®: 5 mg/5 mL (480 mL)
  Tablet, oral: 5 mg, 10 mg

dextroamphetamine and amphetamine (deks troe am FET a meen & am FET a meen)

Medication Safety Issues
  Sound-alike/look-alike issues:
    Adderall® may be confused with Inderal®
  BEERS Criteria medication:
    This drug may be inappropriate for use in geriatric patients (high severity risk).

Synonyms amphetamine and dextroamphetamine

U.S. Brand Names Adderall XR®; Adderall® [DSC]

Canadian Brand Names Adderall XR®

Therapeutic Category Amphetamine

Controlled Substance C-II

Use Attention-deficit/hyperactivity disorder (ADHD); narcolepsy

General Dosage Range Oral:
  Extended release:
    Children 6-12 years: Initial: 5-10 mg once daily; Maintenance: Up to 30 mg/day
    Adolescents 13-17 years: Initial: 10 mg once daily; Maintenance: 10-20 mg once daily (maximum: 60 mg/day)
    Adults: 20 mg once daily (maximum: 60 mg/day)
  Immediate release:
    Children 3-5 years: Initial: 2.5 mg once daily; Maintenance: Up to 40 mg/day in 1-3 divided doses
    Children 6-12 years: Initial: 5 mg once or twice daily; Maintenance: Up to 40 mg/day [ADHD] or 60 mg/day [narcolepsy] in 1-3 divided doses
    Children >12 years and Adults: Initial: 5-10 mg in 1-2 divided doses; Maintenance: Up to 40 mg/day [ADHD] or 60 mg/day [narcolepsy] in 1-3 divided doses

Dosage Forms
  Capsule, extended release:
    5 mg [dextroamphetamine sulfate 1.25 mg, dextroamphetamine saccharate 1.25 mg, amphetamine aspartate monohydrate 1.25 mg, amphetamine sulfate 1.25 mg]
    10 mg [dextroamphetamine sulfate 2.5 mg, dextroamphetamine saccharate 2.5 mg, amphetamine aspartate monohydrate 2.5 mg, amphetamine sulfate 2.5 mg]
    15 mg [dextroamphetamine sulfate 3.75 mg, dextroamphetamine saccharate 3.75 mg, amphetamine aspartate monohydrate 3.75 mg, amphetamine sulfate 3.75 mg]
    20 mg [dextroamphetamine sulfate 5 mg, dextroamphetamine saccharate 5 mg, amphetamine aspartate monohydrate 5 mg, amphetamine sulfate 5 mg]
    25 mg [dextroamphetamine sulfate 6.25 mg, dextroamphetamine saccharate 6.25 mg, amphetamine aspartate monohydrate 6.25 mg, amphetamine sulfate 6.25 mg]
    30 mg [dextroamphetamine sulfate 7.5 mg, dextroamphetamine saccharate 7.5 mg, amphetamine aspartate monohydrate 7.5 mg, amphetamine sulfate 7.5 mg]
    Adderall XR®:
      5 mg [dextroamphetamine 1.25 mg, dextroamphetamine saccharate 1.25 mg, amphetamine aspartate monohydrate 1.25 mg, amphetamine sulfate 1.25 mg]
      10 mg [dextroamphetamine sulfate 2.5 mg, dextroamphetamine saccharate 2.5 mg, amphetamine aspartate monohydrate 2.5 mg, amphetamine sulfate 2.5 mg]
      15 mg [dextroamphetamine sulfate 3.75 mg, dextroamphetamine saccharate 3.75 mg, amphetamine aspartate monohydrate 3.75 mg, amphetamine sulfate 3.75 mg]
      20 mg [dextroamphetamine sulfate 5 mg, dextroamphetamine saccharate 5 mg, amphetamine aspartate monohydrate 5 mg, amphetamine sulfate 5 mg]
      25 mg [dextroamphetamine sulfate 6.25 mg, dextroamphetamine saccharate 6.25 mg, amphetamine aspartate monohydrate 6.25 mg, amphetamine sulfate 6.25 mg]
      30 mg [dextroamphetamine sulfate 7.5 mg, dextroamphetamine saccharate 7.5 mg, amphetamine aspartate monohydrate 7.5 mg, amphetamine sulfate 7.5 mg]

◀ **Tablet:** 5 mg, 7.5 mg, 10 mg, 12.5 mg, 15 mg, 20 mg, 30 mg

5 mg [dextroamphetamine sulfate 1.25 mg, dextroamphetamine saccharate 1.25 mg, amphetamine aspartate monohydrate 1.25 mg, amphetamine sulfate 1.25 mg]

7.5 mg [dextroamphetamine sulfate 1.875 mg, dextroamphetamine saccharate 1.875 mg, amphetamine aspartate monohydrate 1.875 mg, amphetamine sulfate 1.875 mg]

10 mg [dextroamphetamine sulfate 2.5 mg, dextroamphetamine saccharate 2.5 mg, amphetamine aspartate monohydrate 2.5 mg, amphetamine sulfate 2.5 mg]

12.5 mg [dextroamphetamine sulfate 3.125 mg, dextroamphetamine saccharate 3.125 mg, amphetamine aspartate monohydrate 3.125 mg, amphetamine sulfate 3.125 mg]

15 mg [dextroamphetamine sulfate 3.75 mg, dextroamphetamine saccharate 3.75 mg, amphetamine aspartate monohydrate 3.75 mg, amphetamine sulfate 3.75 mg]

20 mg [dextroamphetamine sulfate 5 mg, dextroamphetamine saccharate 5 mg, amphetamine aspartate monohydrate 5 mg, amphetamine sulfate 5 mg]

30 mg [dextroamphetamine sulfate 7.5 mg, dextroamphetamine saccharate 7.5 mg, amphetamine aspartate monohydrate 7.5 mg, amphetamine sulfate 7.5 mg]

dextroamphetamine sulfate *see* dextroamphetamine *on page 268*

dextromethorphan (deks troe meth OR fan)

Medication Safety Issues
Sound-alike/look-alike issues:
Benylin® may be confused with Benadryl®, Ventolin®

Delsym® may be confused with Delfen®, Desyrel

U.S. Brand Names Creo-Terpin® [OTC]; Creomulsion® Adult Formula [OTC]; Creomulsion® for Children [OTC]; Delsym® [OTC]; Father John's® [OTC]; Hold® DM [OTC]; Nycoff [OTC]; PediaCare® Children's Long-Acting Cough [OTC]; Robafen Cough [OTC]; Robitussin® Children's Cough Long-Acting [OTC]; Robitussin® Cough Long Acting [OTC]; Robitussin® CoughGels™ Long-Acting [OTC]; Scot-Tussin® Diabetes [OTC]; Silphen-DM [OTC]; Triaminic Thin Strips® Children's Long Acting Cough [OTC]; Triaminic® Children's Cough Long Acting [OTC]; Trocal® [OTC]; Vicks® 44® Cough Relief [OTC]; Vicks® DayQuil® Cough [OTC]

Therapeutic Category Antitussive

Use Symptomatic relief of coughs caused by the common cold or inhaled irritants

General Dosage Range Oral:
Extended release:

Children 4-6 years: 15 mg twice daily (maximum: 30 mg/day)

Children 6-12 years: 30 mg twice daily (maximum: 60 mg/day)

Children >12 years and Adults: 60 mg twice daily (maximum: 120 mg/day)

Immediate release:

Children 4-6 years: 2.5-7.5 mg every 4-8 hours (maximum: 30 mg/day)

Children 6-12 years: 5-10 mg every 4 hours **or** 15 mg every 6-8 hours (maximum: 60 mg/day)

Children >12 years and Adults: 10-20 mg every 4 hours **or** 30 mg every 6-8 hours (maximum: 120 mg/day)

Dosage Forms
Capsule, liquid filled, oral:

Robafen Cough [OTC]: 15 mg

Robitussin® CoughGels™ Long-Acting [OTC]: 15 mg

Liquid, oral: 15 mg/5 mL (120 mL)

Creo-Terpin® [OTC]: 10 mg/15 mL (120 mL)

Scot-Tussin® Diabetes [OTC]: 10 mg/5 mL (118 mL)

Vicks® 44® Cough Relief [OTC]: 10 mg/5 mL (120 mL)

Lozenge, oral:

Hold® DM [OTC]: 5 mg (10s)

Trocal® [OTC]: 7.5 mg (50s, 300s)

Solution, oral:

PediaCare® Children's Long-Acting Cough [OTC]: 7.5 mg/5 mL (118 mL)

Vicks® DayQuil® Cough [OTC]: 15 mg/15 mL (177 mL, 295 mL)

Strip, orally disintegrating, oral:

Triaminic Thin Strips® Children's Long Acting Cough [OTC]: 7.5 mg (14s, 16s)

Suspension, extended release, oral:

Delsym® [OTC]: Dextromethorphan polistirex [equivalent to dextromethorphan hydrobromide] 30 mg/5 mL (89 mL, 148 mL)

Syrup, oral:
Creomulsion® Adult Formula [OTC]: 20 mg/15 mL (120 mL)
Creomulsion® for Children [OTC]: 5 mg/5 mL (120 mL)
Father John's® [OTC]: 10 mg/5 mL (118 mL, 236 mL)
Robitussin® Children's Cough Long-Acting [OTC]: 7.5 mg/5 mL (118 mL)
Robitussin® Cough Long Acting [OTC]: 15 mg/5 mL (240 mL)
Silphen-DM [OTC]: 10 mg/5 mL (120 mL)
Triaminic® Children's Cough Long Acting [OTC]: 7.5 mg/5 mL (118 mL)
Tablet, oral:
Nycoff [OTC]: 15 mg

dextromethorphan and chlorpheniramine (deks troe meth OR fan & klor fen IR a meen)

Synonyms chlorpheniramine and dextromethorphan; chlorpheniramine maleate and dextromethorphan hydrobromide; dextromethorphan hydrobromide and chlorpheniramine maleate

U.S. Brand Names Coricidin® HBP Cough & Cold [OTC]; Dimetapp® Children's Long Acting Cough Plus Cold [OTC]; Robitussin® Children's Cough & Cold Long-Acting [OTC]; Robitussin® Cough & Cold Long-Acting [OTC]; Scot-Tussin® DM Maximum Strength [OTC]; Triaminic® Children's Softchews® Cough & Runny Nose [OTC]

Therapeutic Category Antitussive; Histamine H_1 Antagonist; Histamine H_1 Antagonist, First Generation

Use Symptomatic relief of runny nose, sneezing, itchy/watery eyes, cough, and other upper respiratory symptoms associated with hay fever, common cold, or upper respiratory allergies

General Dosage Range Oral:
Children 6-11 years: Dextromethorphan 10-15 mg and chlorpheniramine 2 mg every 4-6 hours as needed (maximum: 60 mg dextromethorphan and 10 mg chlorpheniramine/24 hours)
Children ≥12 years and Adults: Dextromethorphan 30 mg and chlorpheniramine 4 mg every 6 hours as needed (maximum: 120 mg dextromethorphan and 16 mg chlorpheniramine/24 hours)

Dosage Forms
Syrup:
Dimetapp® Children's Long Acting Cough Plus Cold [OTC]: Dextromethorphan 7.5 mg and chlorpheniramine 1 mg per 5 mL (118 mL)
Robitussin® Children's Cough and Cold Long-Acting [OTC]: Dextromethorphan 15 mg and chlorpheniramine 2 mg per 5 mL (118 mL)
Robitussin® Cough and Cold Long-Acting [OTC]: Dextromethorphan 15 mg and chlorpheniramine 2 mg per 5 mL (118 mL)
Scot-Tussin® DM Maximum Strength [OTC]: Dextromethorphan 15 mg and chlorpheniramine 2 mg per 5 mL (118 mL)
Tablet:
Coricidin® HBP Cough and Cold [OTC]: Dextromethorphan 30 mg and chlorpheniramine 4 mg
Tablet, softchew:
Triaminic® Children's Softchews® Cough & Runny Nose [OTC]: Dextromethorphan 5 mg and chlorpheniramine 1 mg

dextromethorphan and guaifenesin *see* guaifenesin and dextromethorphan *on page 427*

dextromethorphan and phenylephrine (deks troe meth OR fan & fen il EF rin)

Synonyms dextromethorphan hydrobromide and phenylephrine hydrochloride; phenylephrine and dextromethorphan

U.S. Brand Names PediaCare® Children's Multi-Symptom Cold [OTC]; Safetussin® CD [OTC]; Sudafed PE® Children's Cold & Cough [OTC]; Triaminic Thin Strips® Children's Day Time Cold & Cough [OTC]; Triaminic® Day Time Cold & Cough [OTC]

Therapeutic Category Antitussive; Decongestant

Use Temporary relief of symptoms of hay fever, the common cold, and upper respiratory allergies including sinus/nasal congestion, minor bronchial/throat irritation, and cough

General Dosage Range Oral:
Children ≥4-12 years: Dosage varies greatly depending on product
Children ≥12 years and Adults: Safetussin® CD: 10 mL every 6 hours as needed (maximum: 40 mL/24 hours)

Dosage Forms
Liquid, oral:
Sudafed PE® Children's Cold + Cough [OTC]: Dextromethorphan 5 mg and phenylephrine 2.5 mg per 5 mL (118 mL)

◄ **Strip, orally disintegrating:**
Triaminic Thin Strips® Children's Day Time Cold & Cough [OTC]: Dextromethorphan bromide 5 mg and phenylephrine 2.5 mg (14s, 16s, 48s)
Syrup:
PediaCare® Children's Multi-Symptom Cold [OTC], Triaminic® Day Time Cold & Cough [OTC]: Dextromethorphan 5 mg and phenylephrine 2.5 mg per 5 mL
Safetussin® CD [OTC]: Dextromethorphan 15 mg and phenylephrine 2.5 mg per 5 mL

dextromethorphan and promethazine *see promethazine and dextromethorphan on page 744*
dextromethorphan and pseudoephedrine *see pseudoephedrine and dextromethorphan on page 752*

dextromethorphan and quinidine (deks troe meth OR fan & KWIN i deen)

Synonyms dextromethorphan hydrobromide and quinidine sulfate; quinidine and dextromethorphan
U.S. Brand Names Nuedexta™
Canadian Brand Names Nuedexta™
Therapeutic Category Antiarrhythmic Agent, Class Ia; N-Methyl-D-Aspartate Receptor Antagonist
Use Treatment of pseudobulbar affect (PBA)
General Dosage Range Oral: *Adults:* Initial: Once capsule once daily for 7 days; Maintenance: One capsule twice daily
Dosage Forms
Capsule, oral:
Nuedexta™: Dextromethorphan hydrobromide 20 mg and quinidine sulfate 10 mg

dextromethorphan, chlorpheniramine, and phenylephrine *see chlorpheniramine, phenylephrine, and dextromethorphan on page 200*
dextromethorphan, chlorpheniramine, and pseudoephedrine *see chlorpheniramine, pseudoephedrine, and dextromethorphan on page 201*

dextromethorphan, chlorpheniramine, phenylephrine, and guaifenesin
(deks troe meth OR fan, klor fen IR a meen, fen il EF rin, & gwye FEN e sin)

Synonyms chlorpheniramine, dextromethorphan, phenylephrine, and guaifenesin; guaifenesin, chlorpheniramine, phenylephrine, and dextromethorphan; phenylephrine hydrochloride, chlorpheniramine maleate, dextromethorphan hydrobromide, and guaifenesin
U.S. Brand Names Chlordex GP [DSC]; Donatussin; Quartuss™ [DSC]
Therapeutic Category Antihistamine/Decongestant/Antitussive/Expectorant
Use Symptomatic relief of dry, nonproductive cough and upper respiratory symptoms associated with infections such as the common cold, bronchitis, or sinusitis
General Dosage Range Oral:
Children 2-6 years: 2.5 mL every 6 hours as needed (maximum: 10 mL/24 hours)
Children 6-12 years: 5 mL every 6 hours as needed (maximum: 20 mL/24 hours)
Children ≥12 years and Adults: 10 mL every 6 hours as needed (maximum: 40 mL/24 hours)
Dosage Forms
Syrup:
Donatussin: Dextromethorphan 15 mg, chlorpheniramine 2 mg, phenylephrine 10 mg, and guaifenesin 100 mg per 5 mL (480 mL)

dextromethorphan, guaifenesin, and pseudoephedrine *see guaifenesin, pseudoephedrine, and dextromethorphan on page 430*
dextromethorphan hydrobromide, acetaminophen, and doxylamine succinate *see acetaminophen, dextromethorphan, and doxylamine on page 32*
dextromethorphan hydrobromide, acetaminophen, and phenylephrine hydrochloride *see acetaminophen, dextromethorphan, and phenylephrine on page 32*
dextromethorphan hydrobromide, acetaminophen, doxylamine succinate, and pseudoephedrine hydrochloride *see acetaminophen, dextromethorphan, doxylamine, and pseudoephedrine on page 33*
dextromethorphan hydrobromide and chlorpheniramine maleate *see dextromethorphan and chlorpheniramine on page 271*
dextromethorphan hydrobromide and phenylephrine hydrochloride *see dextromethorphan and phenylephrine on page 271*

dextromethorphan hydrobromide and quinidine sulfate *see* dextromethorphan and quinidine *on page 272*

dextromethorphan hydrobromide, brompheniramine maleate, and pseudoephedrine hydrochloride *see* brompheniramine, pseudoephedrine, and dextromethorphan *on page 144*

dextromethorphan hydrobromide, guaifenesin, and phenylephrine hydrochloride *see* guaifenesin, dextromethorphan, and phenylephrine *on page 429*

dextropropoxyphene *see* propoxyphene *on page 746*

dextrose (DEKS trose)

Medication Safety Issues
Sound-alike/look-alike issues:
Glutose™ may be confused with Glutofac®
High alert medication:
The Institute for Safe Medication Practices (ISMP) includes this medication (hypertonic solutions ≥20%) among its list of drugs which have a heightened risk of causing significant patient harm when used in error.
Other safety concerns:
Inappropriate use of low sodium or sodium-free intravenous fluids (eg D_5W, hypotonic saline) in pediatric patients can lead to significant morbidity and mortality due to hyponatremia (ISMP, 2009).

Synonyms anhydrous glucose; $D_{10}W$; $D_{25}W$; $D_{30}W$; $D_{40}W$; $D_{50}W$; D_5W; $D_{60}W$; $D_{70}W$; dextrose monohydrate; glucose; glucose monohydrate; glycosum

U.S. Brand Names BD™ Glucose [OTC]; Dex4® [OTC]; Enfamil® Glucose [OTC]; GlucoBurst® [OTC]; Glutol™ [OTC]; Glutose 15™ [OTC]; Glutose 45™ [OTC]; Insta-Glucose® [OTC]; Similac® Glucose [OTC]

Therapeutic Category Antidote, Hypoglycemia; Intravenous Nutritional Therapy

Use
Oral: Treatment of hypoglycemia
5% and 10% solutions: Peripheral infusion to provide calories and fluid replacement
25% (hypertonic) solution: Treatment of acute symptomatic episodes of hypoglycemia in infants and children to restore depressed blood glucose levels; adjunctive treatment of hyperkalemia when combined with insulin
50% (hypertonic) solution: Treatment of insulin-induced hypoglycemia (hyperinsulinemia or insulin shock) and adjunctive treatment of hyperkalemia in adolescents and adults
≥10% solutions: Infusion after admixture with amino acids for nutritional support

General Dosage Range
I.V.:
Infants ≤6 months: 0.25-1 g/kg/dose (maximum: 25 g/dose)
Children >6 months to 12 years: 0.5-1 g/kg/dose (maximum: 25 g/dose)
Adolescents and and Adults: 10-50 g/dose
Oral: *Children >2 years and and Adults:* 10-20 g as a single dose, may repeat if needed

Dosage Forms
Gel, oral:
Dex4® [OTC]: 40% (38 g)
GlucoBurst® [OTC]: 40% (37.5 g)
Glutose 15™ [OTC]: 40% (37.5 g)
Glutose 45™ [OTC]: 40% (112.5 g)
Insta-Glucose® [OTC]: 40% (31 g)
Infusion: 5% (25 mL, 50 mL, 100 mL, 150 mL, 250 mL, 500 mL, 1000 mL); 10% (150 mL, 250 mL, 500 mL, 1000 mL); 20% (500 mL, 1000 mL); 30% (500 mL, 1000 mL); 40% (500 mL, 1000 mL); 50% (50 mL, 500 mL, 1000 mL, 2000 mL, 5000 mL); 60% (500 mL, 1000 mL); 70% (250 mL, 500 mL, 1000 mL, 2000 mL)
Injection, solution: 25% (10 mL); 50% (50 mL)
Liquid, oral:
Dex4® [OTC]: 15 g/60 mL (60 mL)
Solution, oral:
Enfamil® Glucose [OTC]: 5% (89 mL); 10% (89 mL)
Glutol™ [OTC]: 55% (180 mL)
Similac® Glucose [OTC]: 5% (59 mL); 10% (59 mL)

◄ **Tablet, chewable, oral**:
BD™ Glucose [OTC]: 5 g
Dex4® [OTC]: 4 g
GlucoBurst® [OTC]: 5 g

dextrose, levulose and phosphoric acid see fructose, dextrose, and phosphoric acid on page 403
dextrose monohydrate see dextrose on page 273
Dex-Tuss see guaifenesin and codeine on page 426
dezocitidine see decitabine on page 256
dFdC see gemcitabine on page 413
dFdCyd see gemcitabine on page 413
DFMO see eflornithine on page 322
DHAD see mitoxantrone on page 593
DHAQ see mitoxantrone on page 593
DHE see dihydroergotamine on page 286
D.H.E. 45® see dihydroergotamine on page 286
DHPG sodium see ganciclovir (systemic) on page 410
DHS™ Sal [OTC] see salicylic acid on page 795
DHS® Tar [OTC] see coal tar on page 227
DHS™ Tar Gel [OTC] see coal tar on page 227
DHS™ Zinc [OTC] see pyrithione zinc on page 759
DiaBeta® see glyburide on page 420
DiabetAid® Antifungal Foot Bath [OTC] see miconazole (topical) on page 585
DiabetAid® Pain and Tingling Relief [OTC] see capsaicin on page 169
DiabetAid Therapeutic Gingivitis Mouth Rinse [OTC] see cetylpyridinium on page 190
Diabetic Siltussin DAS-Na [OTC] see guaifenesin on page 425
Diabetic Siltussin-DM DAS-Na [OTC] see guaifenesin and dextromethorphan on page 427
Diabetic Siltussin-DM DAS-Na Maximum Strength [OTC] see guaifenesin and dextromethorphan on page 427
Diabetic Tussin® DM [OTC] see guaifenesin and dextromethorphan on page 427
Diabetic Tussin® DM Maximum Strength [OTC] see guaifenesin and dextromethorphan on page 427
Diabetic Tussin® EX [OTC] see guaifenesin on page 425
Diabetic Tussin® for Children Allergy Relief [OTC] see chlorpheniramine on page 197
Diaβeta® (Can) see glyburide on page 420
Diamicron® (Can) see gliclazide (Canada only) on page 417
Diamicron® MR (Can) see gliclazide (Canada only) on page 417
diaminocyclohexane oxalatoplatinum see oxaliplatin on page 658
diaminodiphenylsulfone see dapsone (systemic) on page 252
diaminodiphenylsulfone see dapsone (topical) on page 252
Diamode [OTC] see loperamide on page 535
Diamox® (Can) see acetazolamide on page 34
Diamox® Sequels® see acetazolamide on page 34
Diane-35® (Can) see cyproterone and ethinyl estradiol (Canada only) on page 245
Diarr-Eze (Can) see loperamide on page 535
Diastat® see diazepam on page 276
Diastat® AcuDial™ see diazepam on page 276
Diastat® Rectal Delivery System (Can) see diazepam on page 276

diatrizoate meglumine (dye a tri ZOE ate MEG loo meen)

Medication Safety Issues
High alert medication:
The Institute for Safe Medication Practices (ISMP) includes this medication among its list of drugs which have a heightened risk of causing significant patient harm when used in error.
U.S. Brand Names Cystografin®; Cystografin® Dilute
Therapeutic Category Iodinated Contrast Media; Radiological/Contrast Media, Ionic

Use
Solution for instillation: Retrograde cystourethrography; retrograde or ascending pyelography
Solution for injection: Arthrography, cerebral angiography, direct cholangiography, discography, drip infusion pyelography, excretory urography, peripheral arteriography, splenoportography, venography; contrast enhancement of computed tomographic head and body imaging

Dosage Forms
Solution, for instillation:
Cystografin®: 30% (100 mL, 300 mL)
Cystografin® Dilute: 18% (300 mL)

diatrizoate meglumine and diatrizoate sodium
(dye a tri ZOE ate MEG loo meen & dye a tri ZOE ate SOW dee um)

Medication Safety Issues
High alert medication:
The Institute for Safe Medication Practices (ISMP) includes this medication among its list of drug classes which have a heightened risk of causing significant patient harm when used in error.

Synonyms diatrizoate sodium and diatrizoate meglumine; Gastroview

U.S. Brand Names Gastrografin®; MD-76®R; MD-Gastroview®

Therapeutic Category Iodinated Contrast Media; Radiological/Contrast Media, Ionic

Use
Oral/rectal: Examination of GI tract; adjunct to contrast enhancement in computed tomography of the torso
Injection: Angiocardiography, aortography, central venography, cerebral angiography, cholangiography, digital arteriography, excretory urography, nephrotomography, peripheral angiography, peripheral arteriography, renal arteriography, renal venography, splenoportography, visceral arteriography; contrast enhancement of computed tomographic imaging

General Dosage Range
Oral:
Children <5 years: 30 mL, dilute 1:1 (if <10 kg or debilitated, dilute 1:3)
Children 5-10 years: 60 mL, dilute 1:1 (if <10 kg or debilitated, dilute 1:3)
Adults: 30-90 mL **or** 25-77 mL in 1000 mL tap water
Rectal:
Children <5 years: Dilute 1:5 in tap water
Children ≥5 years: Dilute 90 mL in 500 mL tap water
Adults: Dilute 240 mL in 1000 mL tap water

Dosage Forms
Solution, injection:
MD-76®R: Diatrizoate meglumine 660 mg and diatrizoate sodium 100 mg per 1 mL (50 mL, 100 mL, 200 mL)
Solution, oral/rectal:
Gastrografin®: Diatrizoate meglumine 660 mg and diatrizoate sodium 100 mg per 1 mL
MD-Gastroview®: Diatrizoate meglumine 660 mg and diatrizoate sodium 100 mg per 1 mL

diatrizoate meglumine and iodipamide meglumine
(dye a tri ZOE ate MEG loo meen & eye oh DI pa mide MEG loo meen)

Medication Safety Issues
High alert medication:
The Institute for Safe Medication Practices (ISMP) includes this medication among its list of drug classes which have a heightened risk of causing significant patient harm when used in error.

Synonyms iodipamide meglumine and diatrizoate meglumine

U.S. Brand Names Sinografin®

Therapeutic Category Iodinated Contrast Media; Radiological/Contrast Media, Ionic

Use Hysterosalpingography

General Dosage Range Intrauterine: *Adults:* Usual dose: 3-4 mL; Total dosage range: 1.5-10 mL

Dosage Forms
Injection, solution [for intrauterine instillation]:
Sinografin®: Diatrizoate meglumine 524 mg and iodipamide meglumine 268 mg per mL (10 mL)

diatrizoate sodium (dye a tri ZOE ate SOW dee um)
U.S. Brand Names Hypaque™ Sodium

◀ **Therapeutic Category** Iodinated Contrast Media; Radiological/Contrast Media, Ionic

Use Radiographic examination of GI tract

General Dosage Range
Oral:
  Infants and Children: 20% to 40% solution: 30-75 mL
  Adults: 25% to 40% solution: 90-180 mL
Rectal: Enema:
  Infants and Children: 10% to 15% solution: 100-500 mL depending on weight of patient
  Adults: 15% to 25% solution: 500-1000 mL

Dosage Forms
Powder for solution, oral/rectal:
  Hypaque™ Sodium: 100% (250 g)

diatrizoate sodium and diatrizoate meglumine *see diatrizoate meglumine and diatrizoate sodium on page 275*

Diatx®Zn *see vitamins (multiple/oral) on page 919*

Diazemuls® (Can) *see diazepam on page 276*

diazepam (dye AZ e pam)

Medication Safety Issues
Sound-alike/look-alike issues:
  Diazepam may be confused with diazoxide, diltiazem, Ditropan, LORazepam
  Valium® may be confused with Valcyte®
BEERS Criteria medication:
  This drug may be inappropriate for use in geriatric patients (high severity risk).

U.S. Brand Names Diastat®; Diastat® AcuDial™; Diazepam Intensol™; Valium®

Canadian Brand Names Apo-Diazepam®; Diastat®; Diastat® Rectal Delivery System; Diazemuls®; Novo-Dipam; Valium®

Therapeutic Category Benzodiazepine

Controlled Substance C-IV

Use Management of anxiety disorders, ethanol withdrawal symptoms; skeletal muscle relaxant; treatment of convulsive disorders; preoperative or preprocedural sedation and amnesia
  Rectal gel: Management of selected, refractory epilepsy patients on stable regimens of antiepileptic drugs requiring intermittent use of diazepam to control episodes of increased seizure activity

General Dosage Range
I.M.: *Children >30 days and Adults:* Dosage varies greatly depending on indication
I.V.: *Children >30 days and Adults:* Dosage varies greatly depending on indication
Oral:
  Children: 0.12-1 mg/kg/day divided every 6-8 hours **or** 0.2-0.3 mg/kg (maximum: 10 mg) prior to procedures
  Adolescents: 0.12-0.8 mg/kg/day divided every 6-8 hours **or** 10 mg prior to procedures
  Adults: Dosage varies greatly depending on indication
Rectal:
  Gel:
    Children 2-5 years: Initial: 0.5 mg/kg (maximum dose: 20 mg); may repeat in 4-12 hours if needed
    Children 6-11 years: Initial: 0.3 mg/kg (maximum dose: 20 mg); may repeat in 4-12 hours if needed
    Children ≥12 years and Adults: Initial: 0.2 mg/kg (maximum dose: 20 mg); may repeat in 4-12 hours if needed

Dosage Forms
Gel, rectal: 10 mg (2 mL); 20 mg (4 mL); 5 mg/mL (0.5 mL)
  Diastat®: 5 mg/mL (0.5 mL)
  Diastat® AcuDial™: 10 mg (2 mL); 20 mg (4 mL)
Injection, solution: 5 mg/mL (2 mL, 10 mL)
Solution, oral: 5 mg/5 mL (5 mL, 500 mL)
  Diazepam Intensol™: 5 mg/mL (30 mL)
Tablet, oral: 2 mg, 5 mg, 10 mg
  Valium®: 2 mg, 5 mg, 10 mg

Diazepam Intensol™ *see diazepam on page 276*

diazoxide (dye az OKS ide)

Medication Safety Issues
Sound-alike/look-alike issues:
Diazoxide may be confused with diazepam, Dyazide®
U.S. Brand Names Proglycem®
Canadian Brand Names Proglycem®
Therapeutic Category Antihypertensive Agent; Antihypoglycemic Agent
Use Hypoglycemia related to islet cell adenoma, carcinoma, hyperplasia, or adenomatosis; nesidioblastosis; leucine sensitivity; extrapancreatic malignancy
General Dosage Range Oral:
Infants: 8-15 mg/kg/day in divided doses every 8-12 hours
Children and Adults: 3-8 mg/kg/day in divided doses every 8-12 hours
Dosage Forms
Suspension, oral:
Proglycem®: 50 mg/mL (30 mL)
Dosage Forms - Canada
Capsule, oral:
Proglycem®: 50 mg

Dibenzyline® *see* phenoxybenzamine *on page 695*

dibucaine (DYE byoo kane)

U.S. Brand Names Nupercainal® [OTC]
Therapeutic Category Local Anesthetic
Use Fast, temporary relief of pain and itching due to hemorrhoids, minor burns
General Dosage Range Topical:
Children: Apply to affected areas (maximum 7.5 g/24 hour period)
Adults: Apply to affected areas (maximum: 30 g/24 hour period)
Dosage Forms
Ointment, topical: 1% [10 mg/g] (30 g, 454 g)
Nupercainal® [OTC]: 1% [10 mg/g] (30 g, 60 g)

DIC *see* dacarbazine *on page 248*
Dicel® Chewable [OTC] *see* chlorpheniramine and pseudoephedrine *on page 199*
Dicel® DM Chewable [OTC] *see* chlorpheniramine, pseudoephedrine, and dextromethorphan *on page 201*
Dicel® DM Suspension *see* chlorpheniramine, pseudoephedrine, and dextromethorphan *on page 201*
Dicel® Suspension *see* chlorpheniramine and pseudoephedrine *on page 199*
Dicetel® (Can) *see* pinaverium *(Canada only) on page 705*
dichloralphenazone, acetaminophen, and isometheptene *see* acetaminophen, isometheptene, and dichloralphenazone *on page 34*
dichloralphenazone, isometheptene, and acetaminophen *see* acetaminophen, isometheptene, and dichloralphenazone *on page 34*
Dickinson's® Witch Hazel [OTC] *see* witch hazel *on page 923*
Dickinson's® Witch Hazel Astringent Cleanser [OTC] *see* witch hazel *on page 923*
Dickinson's® Witch Hazel Cleansing Astringent [OTC] *see* witch hazel *on page 923*
Diclectin® (Can) *see* doxylamine and pyridoxine *(Canada only) on page 313*

diclofenac (systemic) (dye KLOE fen ak)

Medication Safety Issues
Sound-alike/look-alike issues:
Diclofenac may be confused with Diflucan®
Cataflam® may be confused with Catapres®
Voltaren may be confused with traMADol, Ultram®, Verelan®
International issues:
Diclofenac may be confused with Duphalac brand name for lactulose [multiple international markets]
Flexin: Brand name for diclofenac [Argentina], but also the brand name for cyclobenzaprine [Chile] and orphenadrine [Israel]

◄ Flexin [Argentina] may be confused with Floxin brand name for flunarizine [Thailand], norfloxacin [South Africa], ofloxacin [U.S., Canada], and perfloxacin [Philippines]

Synonyms diclofenac potassium; diclofenac sodium; Voltaren

U.S. Brand Names Cambia™; Cataflam®; Voltaren®-XR; Zipsor™

Canadian Brand Names Apo-Diclo Rapide®; Apo-Diclo®; Apo-Diclo® SR®; Cataflam®; Diclofenac ECT; Diclofenac Sodium; Diclofenac Sodium SR; Diclofenac SR; Dom-Diclofenac; Dom-Diclofenac SR; Novo-Difenac ECT; Novo-Difenac K; Novo-Difenac Suppositories; Novo-Difenac-SR; Nu-Diclo; Nu-Diclo-SR; Pennsaid®; PMS-Diclofenac; PMS-Diclofenac SR; PMS-Diclofenac-K; PRO-Diclo-Rapide; Sandoz-Diclofenac; Sandoz-Diclofenac Rapide; Sandoz-Diclofenac SR; Voltaren Rapide®; Voltaren SR®; Voltaren®

Therapeutic Category Nonsteroidal Antiinflammatory Drug (NSAID)

Use

Capsule: Relief of mild-to-moderate acute pain

Immediate-release tablet: Relief of mild-to-moderate pain; primary dysmenorrhea; acute and chronic treatment of rheumatoid arthritis, osteoarthritis

Delayed-release tablet: Acute and chronic treatment of rheumatoid arthritis, osteoarthritis, ankylosing spondylitis

Extended-release tablet: Chronic treatment of osteoarthritis, rheumatoid arthritis

Oral solution: Treatment of acute migraine with or without aura

Suppository (CAN; not available in U.S.): Symptomatic treatment of rheumatoid arthritis and osteoarthritis (including degenerative joint disease of hip)

General Dosage Range Oral:

Immediate release capsule: *Adults:* 100 mg/day in 4 divided doses

Immediate release tablet: *Adults:* 100-200 mg/day in 2-4 divided doses

Delayed release tablet: *Adults:* 100-200 mg/day in 2-5 divided doses

Extended release tablet: *Adults:* 100-200 mg/day

Oral solution: *Adults:* 50 mg once

Dosage Forms

Capsule, liquid filled, oral:

Zipsor™: 25 mg

Powder for solution, oral:

Cambia™: 50 mg/packet (1s)

Tablet, oral: 50 mg

Cataflam®: 50 mg

Tablet, delayed release, enteric coated, oral: 25 mg, 50 mg, 75 mg

Tablet, extended release, oral: 100 mg

Voltaren®-XR: 100 mg

Dosage Forms - Canada

Suppository:

Voltaren®: 50 mg, 100mg

diclofenac (ophthalmic) (dye KLOE fen ak)

Medication Safety Issues

Sound-alike/look-alike issues:

Diclofenac may be confused with Diflucan®

International Issues:

Diclofenac may be confused with Duphalac brand name for lactulose [multiple international markets]

Flexin: Brand name for diclofenac [Argentina], but also the brand name for cyclobenzaprine [Chile] and orphenadrine [Israel]

Flexin [Argentina] may be confused with Floxin brand name for flunarizine [Thailand], norfloxacin [South Africa], ofloxacin [U.S., Canada], and pefloxacin [Philippines]

Synonyms diclofenac sodium

U.S. Brand Names Voltaren Ophthalmic®

Canadian Brand Names Voltaren Ophtha®

Therapeutic Category Nonsteroidal Antiinflammatory Drug (NSAID), Ophthalmic

Use Treatment of postoperative inflammation following cataract extraction; temporary relief of pain and photophobia in patients undergoing corneal refractive surgery

General Dosage Range Ophthalmic: *Adults:* 1-2 drops into affected eye 4 times/day

Dosage Forms
  Solution, ophthalmic: 0.1% (2.5 mL, 5 mL)
    Voltaren Ophthalmic®: 0.1% (2.5 mL, 5 mL)

diclofenac (topical) (dye KLOE fen ak)

Medication Safety Issues
  Sound-alike/look-alike issues:
    Diclofenac may be confused with Diflucan®
    Voltaren® may be confused with traMADol, Ultram®, Verelan®
  Other safety concerns:
    Transdermal patch (Flector®) contains conducting metal (eg, aluminum); remove patch prior to MRI.
  International issues:
    Diclofenac may be confused with Duphalac brand name for lactulose [multiple international markets]
    Flexin: Brand name for diclofenac [Argentina], but also the brand name for cyclobenzaprine [Chile] and orphenadirine [Israel]
    Flexin [Argentina] may be confused with Floxin brand name for flunarizine [Thailand], norfloxacin [South Africa], ofloxacin [U.S., Canada], and perfloxacin [Philippines]
Synonyms diclofenac diethylamine [CAN]; diclofenac epolamine; diclofenac sodium
U.S. Brand Names Flector®; Pennsaid®; Solaraze®; Voltaren® Gel
Canadian Brand Names Voltaren® Emulgel™
Therapeutic Category Nonsteroidal Antiinflammatory Drug (NSAID), Topical
Use
  Topical gel 1%: Relief of osteoarthritis pain in joints amenable to topical therapy (eg, ankle, elbow, foot, hand, knee, wrist)
    Canadian labeling (not in U.S. labeling): Relief of pain associated with acute, localized joint/muscle injuries (eg, sports injuries, strains) in patients ≥16 years of age
  Topical gel 3%: Actinic keratosis (AK) in conjunction with sun avoidance
  Topical patch: Acute pain due to minor strains, sprains, and contusions
  Topical solution: Relief of osteoarthritis pain of the knee
General Dosage Range Topical: Adults:
  1% gel: Apply 2-4 g to affected joint 4 times/day (maximum: 16 g/day single joint of lower extremity, 8 g/day single joint of upper extremity); Maximum total body dose of 1% gel should not exceed 32 g per day.
  3% gel: Apply to lesion area twice daily
  Patch: Apply 1 patch twice daily
  Solution: Apply 40 drops to each affected knee 4 times/day
Dosage Forms
  Gel, topical:
    Solaraze®: 3% (100 g)
    Voltaren® Gel: 1% (100 g)
  Patch, transdermal:
    Flector®: 1.3% (30s)
  Solution, topical:
    Pennsaid®: 1.5% (150 mL)
Dosage Forms - Canada
  Gel, topical:
    Voltaren® Emulgel™: 1.16% (20 g, 50 g, 100 g)

diclofenac and misoprostol (dye KLOE fen ak & mye soe PROST ole)

Synonyms misoprostol and diclofenac
U.S. Brand Names Arthrotec®
Canadian Brand Names Arthrotec®
Therapeutic Category Analgesic, Nonnarcotic; Prostaglandin
Use Treatment of osteoarthritis and rheumatoid arthritis in patients at high risk for NSAID-induced gastric and duodenal ulceration
General Dosage Range Oral: Adults: Arthrotec® 50: One tablet 2-4 times/day; Arthrotec® 75: One tablet twice daily

◀ **Dosage Forms**
Tablet:
   Arthrotec® 50: Diclofenac 50 mg and misoprostol 200 mcg
   Arthrotec® 75: Diclofenac 75 mg and misoprostol 200 mcg

diclofenac diethylamine [CAN] *see* diclofenac (topical) *on page 279*
Diclofenac ECT (Can) *see* diclofenac (systemic) *on page 277*
diclofenac epolamine *see* diclofenac (topical) *on page 279*
diclofenac potassium *see* diclofenac (systemic) *on page 277*
diclofenac sodium *see* diclofenac (ophthalmic) *on page 278*
diclofenac sodium *see* diclofenac (systemic) *on page 277*
diclofenac sodium *see* diclofenac (topical) *on page 279*
Diclofenac Sodium (Can) *see* diclofenac (systemic) *on page 277*
Diclofenac Sodium SR (Can) *see* diclofenac (systemic) *on page 277*
Diclofenac SR (Can) *see* diclofenac (systemic) *on page 277*

dicloxacillin (dye kloks a SIL in)

Synonyms dicloxacillin sodium
Canadian Brand Names Dycill®; Pathocil®
Therapeutic Category Penicillin
Use Treatment of systemic infections such as pneumonia, skin and soft tissue infections, and osteomyelitis caused by penicillinase-producing staphylococci
General Dosage Range Oral:
   Children <40 kg: 12.5-100 mg/kg/day divided every 6 hours
   Children >40 kg: 125-250 mg every 6 hours
   Adults: 125-1000 mg every 6-8 hours
Dosage Forms
Capsule, oral: 250 mg, 500 mg

dicloxacillin sodium *see* dicloxacillin *on page 280*

dicyclomine (dye SYE kloe meen)

Medication Safety Issues
Sound-alike/look-alike issues:
   Dicyclomine may be confused with diphenhydrAMINE, doxycycline, dyclonine
   Bentyl® may be confused with Aventyl®, Benadryl®, Bontril®, Cantil®, Proventil®, TRENtal®
BEERS Criteria medication:
   This drug may be inappropriate for use in geriatric patients (high severity risk).
Synonyms dicyclomine hydrochloride; dicycloverine hydrochloride
U.S. Brand Names Bentyl®
Canadian Brand Names Bentylol®; Formulex®; Lomine; Riva-Dicyclomine
Therapeutic Category Anticholinergic Agent
Use Treatment of functional bowel/irritable bowel syndrome
General Dosage Range
I.M.: *Adults:* 80 mg/day in 4 divided doses
Oral:
   Adults: Initial: 20 mg 4 times/day; Maintenance: Up to 160 mg/day in 4 divided doses
   Elderly: Initial: 10-20 mg 4 times/day
Dosage Forms
Capsule, oral: 10 mg
   Bentyl®: 10 mg
Injection, solution: 10 mg/mL (2 mL)
   Bentyl®: 10 mg/mL (2 mL)
Syrup, oral:
   Bentyl®: 10 mg/5 mL (480 mL)
Tablet, oral: 20 mg
   Bentyl®: 20 mg

dicyclomine hydrochloride *see* dicyclomine *on page 280*
dicycloverine hydrochloride *see* dicyclomine *on page 280*

Di-Dak-Sol *see* sodium hypochlorite solution *on page 820*

didanosine (dye DAN oh seen)
Medication Safety Issues
 Sound-alike/look-alike issues:
  Videx® may be confused with Lidex®
Synonyms ddI; dideoxyinosine
U.S. Brand Names Videx®; Videx® EC
Canadian Brand Names Videx®; Videx® EC
Therapeutic Category Antiviral Agent
Use Treatment of HIV infection; always to be used in combination with at least two other antiretroviral agents
General Dosage Range Dosage adjustment recommended in patients with renal impairment
 Oral:
  Delayed release:
   Children ≥6 years and 20 kg to <25 kg: 200 mg once daily
   Children ≥6 years and 25 kg to <60 kg and Adults <60 kg: 250 mg once daily
   Children and Adults ≥60 kg: 400 mg once daily
  Pediatric powder for oral solution (Videx®):
   Infants 2 weeks to 8 months: 100 mg/m^2 twice daily
   Children >8 months to 18 years: 120 mg/m^2 twice daily
   Adolescents and Adults <60 kg: 125 mg twice daily **or** 250 mg once daily
   Adolescents and Adults ≥60 kg: 200 mg twice daily **or** 400 mg once daily
Dosage Forms
 Capsule, delayed release, enteric coated beadlets, oral: 125 mg, 200 mg, 250 mg, 400 mg
  Videx® EC: 125 mg, 200 mg, 250 mg, 400 mg
 Capsule, delayed release, enteric coated pellets, oral: 200 mg, 250 mg, 400 mg
 Powder for solution, oral:
  Videx®: 2 g/bottle, 4 g/bottle

dideoxyinosine *see* didanosine *on page 281*
Didrex® *see* benzphetamine *on page 125*
Didrocal® (Can) *see* etidronate and calcium carbonate *(Canada only) on page 360*
Didronel® *see* etidronate *on page 359*
dienogest and estradiol *see* estradiol and dienogest *on page 345*

diethylene triamine penta-acetic acid
(dye ETH i leen TRYE a meen PEN ta a SEE tik AS id)
Synonyms diethylenetriamine pentaacetic acid; DTPA; pentetate calcium trisodium; pentetate zinc trisodium; trisodium calcium diethylenetriaminepentaacetate (Ca-DTPA); zinc diethylenetriaminepentaacetate (Zn-DTPA)
U.S. Brand Names Ca-DTPA; Zn-DTPA
Therapeutic Category Antidote
Use Treatment of known or suspected internal contamination with plutonium, americium, or curium
General Dosage Range I.V.:
 Children <12 years: Initial: Ca-DTPA: 14 mg/kg/day (maximum dose: 1 g/day); Maintenance: Zn-DTPA: 14 mg/kg/day (maximum: 1 g/day)
 Children ≥12 years and Adults: Ca-DTPA: 1 g/day; Zn-DTPA: 1 g/day
Dosage Forms
 Injection, solution:
  Ca-DTPA: 200 mg/mL (5 mL)
  Zn-DTPA: 200 mg/mL (5 mL)

diethylenetriamine pentaacetic acid *see* diethylene triamine penta-acetic acid *on page 281*

diethylpropion (dye eth il PROE pee on)
Medication Safety Issues
 BEERS Criteria medication:
  This drug may be inappropriate for use in geriatric patients (high severity risk).
Synonyms amfepramone; diethylpropion hydrochloride

◀ **Canadian Brand Names** Tenuate®; Tenuate® Dospan®
Therapeutic Category Anorexiant
Controlled Substance C-IV
Use Short-term (few weeks) adjunct in the management of exogenous obesity

Pharmacotherapy for weight loss is recommended only for obese patients with a body mass index ≥30 kg/m^2, or ≥27 kg/m^2 in the presence of other risk factors such as hypertension, diabetes, and/or dyslipidemia or a high waist circumference; therapy should be used in conjunction with a comprehensive weight management program.
General Dosage Range Oral:
Controlled release: *Children >16 years and Adults:* 75 mg at midmorning
Immediate release: *Children >16 years and Adults:* 25 mg 3 times/day
Dosage Forms
Tablet, oral: 25 mg
Tablet, controlled release, oral: 75 mg

diethylpropion hydrochloride *see diethylpropion on page 281*

difenoxin and atropine (dye fen OKS in & A troe peen)
Synonyms atropine and difenoxin
U.S. Brand Names Motofen®
Therapeutic Category Antidiarrheal
Controlled Substance C-IV
Use Treatment of diarrhea
General Dosage Range Oral: *Adults:* 2 tablets (each tablet contains difenoxin hydrochloride 1 mg and atropine sulfate 0.025 mg) initially, then 1 tablet after each loose stool (maximum: 8 tablets/day)
Dosage Forms
Tablet, oral:
Motofen®: Difenoxin 1 mg and atropine 0.025 mg

Differin® *see adapalene on page 40*
Differin® XP (Can) *see adapalene on page 40*
Dificid™ *see fidaxomicin (systemic) on page 377*
Difil-G [DSC] *see dyphylline and guaifenesin on page 318*
Difil-G® 400 *see dyphylline and guaifenesin on page 318*
Difil®-G Forte [DSC] *see dyphylline and guaifenesin on page 318*
difimicin *see fidaxomicin (systemic) on page 377*

diflorasone (dye FLOR a sone)
Medication Safety Issues
International issues:
Florone [Germany, Greece] may be confused with Flogene brand name for piroxicam [Brazil]
Synonyms diflorasone diacetate
U.S. Brand Names ApexiCon® E; ApexiCon™
Therapeutic Category Corticosteroid, Topical
Use Relieves inflammation and pruritic symptoms of corticosteroid-responsive dermatosis (high- to very-high potency topical corticosteroid)
General Dosage Range Topical: *Adults:* Cream: Apply 2-4 times/day; Ointment: Apply 1-3 times/day
Dosage Forms
Cream, topical: 0.05% (15 g, 30 g, 60 g)
ApexiCon® E: 0.05% (30 g, 60 g)
Ointment, topical: 0.05% (15 g, 30 g, 60 g)
ApexiCon™: 0.05% (30 g, 60 g)

diflorasone diacetate *see diflorasone on page 282*
Diflucan® *see fluconazole on page 381*

diflunisal (dye FLOO ni sal)
Synonyms Dolobid
Canadian Brand Names Apo-Diflunisal®; Novo-Diflunisal; Nu-Diflunisal

Therapeutic Category Analgesic, Nonnarcotic; Nonsteroidal Antiinflammatory Drug (NSAID)

Use Management of inflammatory disorders usually including rheumatoid arthritis and osteoarthritis; can be used as an analgesic for treatment of mild-to-moderate pain

General Dosage Range Dosage adjustment recommended in patients with renal impairment

Oral: *Adults:* 250-500 mg every 8-12 hours (maximum: 1.5 g/day)

Dosage Forms

Tablet, oral: 500 mg

difluorodeoxycytidine hydrochlorothiazide *see* gemcitabine *on page 413*

difluprednate (dye floo PRED nate)

Medication Safety Issues

Sound-alike/look-alike issues:

Durezol® may be confused with Durasal™

U.S. Brand Names Durezol®

Therapeutic Category Corticosteroid, Ophthalmic

Use Treatment of inflammation and pain following ocular surgery

General Dosage Range Ophthalmic: *Adults:* Instill 1 drop in affected eye(s) 2-4 times/day

Dosage Forms

Emulsion, ophthalmic:

Durezol®: 0.05% (5 mL)

Digibar™ 190 *see* barium *on page 114*

Digibind® [DSC] *see* digoxin immune Fab *on page 284*

Digibind® (Can) *see* digoxin immune Fab *on page 284*

DigiFab® *see* digoxin immune Fab *on page 284*

digitalis *see* digoxin *on page 283*

digoxin (di JOKS in)

Medication Safety Issues

Sound-alike/look-alike issues:

Digoxin may be confused with Desoxyn®, doxepin

Lanoxin® may be confused with Lasix®, levothyroxine, Levoxyl®, Levsinex®, Lomotil®, Mefoxin®, naloxone, Xanax®

High alert medication:

The Institute for Safe Medication Practices (ISMP) includes this medication among its list of drugs which have a heightened risk of causing significant patient harm when used in error.

BEERS Criteria medication:

This drug may be inappropriate for use in geriatric patients (low severity risk).

International issues:

Lanoxin [U.S., Canada, and multiple international markets] may be confused with Limoxin brand name for ambroxol [Indonesia] and amoxicillin [Mexico]

Synonyms digitalis

U.S. Brand Names Lanoxin®

Canadian Brand Names Apo-Digoxin®; Digoxin CSD; Lanoxin®; Pediatric Digoxin CSD; PMS-Digoxin; Toloxin®

Therapeutic Category Antiarrhythmic Agent, Miscellaneous; Cardiac Glycoside

Use Treatment of mild-to-moderate (or stage C as recommended by the ACCF/AHA) heart failure (HF); atrial fibrillation (rate-control)

Note: In treatment of atrial fibrillation (AF), use is not considered first-line unless AF coexistent with heart failure or in sedentary patients (Fuster, 2006).

General Dosage Range Dosage adjustment recommended in patients with renal impairment

I.M., I.V.:

Preterm infants: Digitalizing dose: 15-25 mcg/kg; Maintenance: 4-6 mcg/kg/day in divided doses every 12 hours

Full-term infants: Digitalizing dose: 20-30 mcg/kg; Maintenance: 5-8 mcg/kg/day in divided doses every 12 hours

Children 1 month to 2 years: Digitalizing dose: 30-50 mcg/kg; Maintenance: 7.5-12 mcg/kg/day in divided doses every 12 hours

◀ *Children 2-5 years:* Digitalizing dose: 25-35 mcg/kg; Maintenance: 6-9 mcg/kg/day in divided doses every 12 hours

Children 5-10 years: Digitalizing dose: 15-30 mcg/kg; Maintenance: 4-8 mcg/kg/day in divided doses every 12 hours

Children >10 years: Digitalizing dose: 8-12 mcg/kg; Maintenance: 2-3 mcg/kg once daily

Adults: Digitalizing dose: 0.5-1 mg; Maintenance: 0.1-0.4 mg once daily

Oral:

Preterm infants: Digitalizing dose: 20-30 mcg/kg; Maintenance: 5-7.5 mcg/kg/day in divided doses every 12 hours

Full-term infants: Digitalizing dose: 25-35 mcg/kg; Maintenance: 6-10 mcg/kg/day in divided doses every 12 hours

Children 1 month to 2 years: Digitalizing dose: 35-60 mcg/kg; Maintenance: 10-15 mcg/kg/day in divided doses every 12 hours

Children 2-5 years: Digitalizing dose: 30-40 mcg/kg; Maintenance: 7.5-10 mcg/kg/day in divided doses every 12 hours

Children 5-10 years: Digitalizing dose: 20-35 mcg/kg; Maintenance: 5-10 mcg/kg/day in divided doses every 12 hours

Children >10 years: Digitalizing dose: 10-15 mcg/kg; Maintenance: 2.5-5 mcg/kg once daily

Adults: Digitalizing dose: 0.75-1.5 mg; Maintenance: 0.125-0.5 mg once daily

Dosage Forms

Injection, solution: 250 mcg/mL (1 mL, 2 mL)

Lanoxin®: 100 mcg/mL (1 mL); 250 mcg/mL (2 mL)

Solution, oral: 50 mcg/mL (2.5 mL, 5 mL, 60 mL)

Tablet, oral: 125 mcg, 250 mcg

Lanoxin®: 125 mcg, 250 mcg

Dosage Forms - Canada

Tablet, oral:

Apo-Digoxin®: 62.5 mcg, 125 mcg, 250 mcg

Digoxin CSD (Can) *see* digoxin *on page 283*

digoxin immune Fab (di JOKS in i MYUN fab)

Synonyms antidigoxin fab fragments, ovine

U.S. Brand Names Digibind® [DSC]; DigiFab®

Canadian Brand Names Digibind®

Therapeutic Category Antidote

Use Treatment of life-threatening or potentially life-threatening digoxin intoxication, including:

• acute digoxin ingestion (ie, >10 mg in adults or >4 mg in children)

• chronic ingestions leading to steady-state digoxin concentrations >6 ng/mL in adults or >4 ng/mL in children

• manifestations of digoxin toxicity due to overdose (life-threatening ventricular arrhythmias, progressive bradycardia, second- or third-degree heart block not responsive to atropine, serum potassium >5 mEq/L in adults or >6 mEq in children)

General Dosage Range I.V.:

Acute ingestion of known amount: *Children and Adults:* Dose (vials) = Total body load (mg) / (0.5 mg digitalis bound/vial)

Based on steady-state digoxin concentration:

Infants and Children ≤20 kg: Dose (mg) = [(serum digoxin concentration [ng/mL] x weight [kg]) / 100] x (mg/vial)

Note: Digibind® 38 mg/vial or DigiFab™ 40 mg/vial

Adults: Dose (vials) = (serum digoxin concentration [ng/mL] x weight [kg]) / 100

Amount ingested and blood level unknown:

Children ≤20 kg: Acute toxicity: 20 vials total in 2 divided doses; Chronic toxicity: 1 vial may be sufficient

Children >20 kg and Adults: Acute toxicity: 20 vials total in 2 divided doses; Chronic toxicity: 6 vials

Dosage Forms

Injection, powder for reconstitution:

DigiFab®: 40 mg

dihematoporphyrin ether *see* porfimer *on page 722*

dihydrocodeine, aspirin, and caffeine (dye hye droe KOE deen, AS pir in, & KAF een)

Medication Safety Issues
Sound-alike/look-alike issues:
Synalgos®-DC may be confused with Synagis®
High alert medication:
The Institute for Safe Medication Practices (ISMP) includes this medication among its list of drug classes which have a heightened risk of causing significant patient harm when used in error.

Synonyms dihydrocodeine compound

U.S. Brand Names Synalgos®-DC

Therapeutic Category Analgesic, Narcotic

Controlled Substance C-III

Use Management of mild-to-moderate pain that requires relaxation

General Dosage Range Oral: *Adults:* 1-2 capsules every 4-6 hours as needed

Dosage Forms
Capsule, oral:
Synalgos®-DC: Dihydrocodeine 16 mg, aspirin 356.4 mg, and caffeine 30 mg

dihydrocodeine bitartrate, acetaminophen, and caffeine *see* acetaminophen, caffeine, and dihydrocodeine *on page 30*

dihydrocodeine bitartrate, pseudoephedrine hydrochloride, and chlorpheniramine maleate *see* pseudoephedrine, dihydrocodeine, and chlorpheniramine *on page 754*

dihydrocodeine, chlorpheniramine, and phenylephrine
(dye hye droe KOE deen, klor fen IR a meen, & fen il EF rin)

Synonyms chlorpheniramine maleate, dihydrocodeine bitartrate, and phenylephrine hydrochloride; phenylephrine, chlorpheniramine, and dihydrocodeine

U.S. Brand Names Coldcough PD; DiHydro-PE [OTC]; Novahistine DH; Tusscough DHC™

Therapeutic Category Antihistamine; Antihistamine/Decongestant/Antitussive; Antitussive; Decongestant

Controlled Substance C-III; C-V

Use Symptomatic relief of cough and congestion associated with the upper respiratory tract

General Dosage Range
Oral:
Children 2-6 years: Novahistine DH: 1.25-2.5 mL every 4-6 hours as needed (maximum: 10 mL/day)
Children 6-12 years: Novahistine DH: 2.5-5 mL every 4-6 hours as needed (maximum: 20 mL/day)
Children >12 years and Adults: Novahistine DH: 5-10 mL every 4-6 hours as needed (maximum: 40 mL/day)

Dosage Forms
Liquid, oral:
Novahistine DH: Dihydrocodeine 7.5 mg, chlorpheniramine 2 mg and phenylephrine 5 mg per 5 mL
Syrup, oral:
Coldcough PD, DiHydro-PE [OTC]: Dihydrocodeine 3 mg, chlorpheniramine 2 mg, and phenylephrine 7.5 mg per 5 mL
Tusscough DHC™: Dihydrocodeine 3 mg, chlorpheniramine 5 mg, and phenylephrine 20 mg per 5 mL

dihydrocodeine compound *see* dihydrocodeine, aspirin, and caffeine *on page 285*

dihydrocodeine, pseudoephedrine, and guaifenesin
(dye hye droe KOE deen, soo doe e FED rin, & gwye FEN e sin)

Synonyms guaifenesin, dihydrocodeine, and pseudoephedrine; pseudoephedrine hydrochloride, guaifenesin, and dihydrocodeine bitartrate

U.S. Brand Names DiHydro-GP; Pancof®-EXP

Therapeutic Category Antitussive/Decongestant/Expectorant

Use Temporary relief of cough and congestion associated with upper respiratory tract infections and allergies

General Dosage Range Oral:
Children 2-6 years: 1.25-2.5 mL every 4-6 hours as needed
Children 6-12 years: 2.5-5 mL every 4-6 hours as needed
Children ≥12 years and Adults: 5-10 mL every 4-6 hours as needed

◄ **Dosage Forms**
Syrup:
DiHydro-GP, Pancof®-EXP: Dihydrocodeine 7.5 mg, pseudoephedrine 15 mg, and guaifenesin 100 mg per 5 mL

DiHydro-CP see pseudoephedrine, dihydrocodeine, and chlorpheniramine on page 754

dihydroergotamine (dye hye droe er GOT a meen)

Synonyms DHE; dihydroergotamine mesylate
U.S. Brand Names D.H.E. 45®; Migranal®
Canadian Brand Names Migranal®
Therapeutic Category Ergot Alkaloid and Derivative
Use Treatment of migraine headache with or without aura; injection also indicated for treatment of cluster headaches
General Dosage Range
I.M., SubQ: *Adults:* 1 mg initially, may repeat hourly up to 3 mg total (maximum: 6 mg/week)
I.V.: *Adults:* 1 mg initially, may repeat hourly up to 2 mg total (maximum: 6 mg/week)
Intranasal: *Adults:* 1 spray (0.5 mg) in each nostril initially, may repeat after 15 minutes up to 4 sprays total (maximum: 6 sprays/24 hours; 8 sprays/week)
Dosage Forms
Injection, solution: 1 mg/mL (1 mL)
D.H.E. 45®: 1 mg/mL (1 mL)
Solution, intranasal:
Migranal®: 4 mg/mL (1 mL)

dihydroergotamine mesylate see dihydroergotamine on page 286
dihydroergotoxine see ergoloid mesylates on page 336
dihydrogenated ergot alkaloids see ergoloid mesylates on page 336
DiHydro-GP see dihydrocodeine, pseudoephedrine, and guaifenesin on page 285
dihydrohydroxycodeinone see oxycodone on page 662
dihydromorphinone see hydromorphone on page 452
DiHydro-PE [OTC] see dihydrocodeine, chlorpheniramine, and phenylephrine on page 285
dihydroxyanthracenedione see mitoxantrone on page 593
dihydroxyanthracenedione dihydrochloride see mitoxantrone on page 593
1,25 dihydroxycholecalciferol see calcitriol on page 159
dihydroxydeoxynorvinkaleukoblastine see vinorelbine on page 916
dihydroxypropyl theophylline see dyphylline on page 318
diiodohydroxyquin see iodoquinol on page 484
Dilacor XR® see diltiazem on page 286
Dilantin® see phenytoin on page 700
Dilantin-125® see phenytoin on page 700
Dilatrate®-SR see isosorbide dinitrate on page 494
Dilaudid® see hydromorphone on page 452
Dilaudid-HP® see hydromorphone on page 452
Dilaudid-HP-Plus® (Can) see hydromorphone on page 452
Dilaudid® Sterile Powder (Can) see hydromorphone on page 452
Dilaudid-XP® (Can) see hydromorphone on page 452
Dilt-CD see diltiazem on page 286
Diltia XT® see diltiazem on page 286

diltiazem (dil TYE a zem)

Medication Safety Issues
Sound-alike/look-alike issues:
Cardizem® may be confused with Cardene®, Cardene SR®, Cardizem CD®, Cardizem SR®, cortisone
Cartia XT® may be confused with Procardia XL®
Diltiazem may be confused with Calan®, diazepam, Dilantin®

Tiazac® may be confused with Tigan®, Tiazac® XC [CAN], Ziac®
High alert medication:
The Institute for Safe Medication Practices (ISMP) includes this medication (I.V. formulation) among its list of drug classes which have a heightened risk of causing significant patient harm when used in error.
Administration issues:
Significant differences exist between oral and I.V. dosing. Use caution when converting from one route of administration to another.
International issues:
Cardizem [U.S., Canada, and multiple international markets] may be confused with Cardem brand name for celiprolol [Spain]
Cartia XT [U.S.] may be confused with Cartia brand name for aspirin [multiple international markets]
Dilacor XR [U.S.] may be confused with Dilacor brand name for verapamil [Brazil]
Dipen [Greece] may be confused with Depen brand name for penicillamine [U.S.]; Depin brand name for nifedipine [India]; Depon brand name for acetaminophen [Greece]
Tiazac: Brand name for diltiazem [U.S, Canada], but also the brand name for pioglitazone [Chile]
Synonyms diltiazem hydrochloride
U.S. Brand Names Cardizem®; Cardizem® CD; Cardizem® LA; Cartia XT®; Dilacor XR®; Dilt-CD; Dilt-XR; Diltia XT®; Diltzac; Matzim™ LA; Taztia XT®; Tiazac®
Canadian Brand Names Apo-Diltiaz CD®; Apo-Diltiaz SR®; Apo-Diltiaz TZ®; Apo-Diltiaz®; Apo-Diltiaz® Injectable; Cardizem® CD; Diltiazem HCl ER®; Diltiazem Hydrochloride Injection; Diltiazem TZ; Diltiazem-CD; Nu-Diltiaz; Nu-Diltiaz-CD; PMS-Diltiazem CD; ratio-Diltiazem CD; Sandoz-Diltiazem CD; Sandoz-Diltiazem T; Teva-Diltiazem; Teva-Diltiazem CD; Teva-Diltiazem HCL ER Capsules; Tiazac®; Tiazac® XC
Therapeutic Category Calcium Channel Blocker
Use
Oral: Essential hypertension; chronic stable angina or angina from coronary artery spasm
Injection: Control of rapid ventricular rate in patients with atrial fibrillation or atrial flutter; conversion of paroxysmal supraventricular tachycardia (PSVT)
General Dosage Range
I.V.: *Adults:* Bolus: 0.25 mg/kg, may repeat 0.35 mg/kg after 15 minutes; Infusion: 5-15 mg/hour
Oral:
Extended release: *Adults:* Initial: 120-240 mg once daily **or** 60-120 mg twice daily; Maintenance: 120-540 mg once daily **or** 240-360 mg/day in 2 divided doses
Immediate release: *Adults:* Initial: 30 mg 4 times/day; Maintenance: 120-320 mg/day in divided doses
Dosage Forms
Capsule, extended release, oral: 60 mg, 90 mg, 120 mg, 180 mg, 240 mg, 300 mg, 360 mg, 420 mg
Cardizem® CD: 120 mg, 180 mg, 240 mg, 300 mg, 360 mg
Cartia XT®: 120 mg, 180 mg, 240 mg, 300 mg
Dilacor XR®: 240 mg
Dilt-CD: 120 mg, 180 mg, 240 mg, 300 mg
Dilt-XR: 120 mg, 180 mg, 240 mg
Diltia XT®: 120 mg, 180 mg, 240 mg
Diltzac: 120 mg, 180 mg, 240 mg, 300 mg, 360 mg
Taztia XT®: 120 mg, 180 mg, 240 mg, 300 mg, 360 mg
Tiazac®: 120 mg, 180 mg, 240 mg, 300 mg, 360 mg, 420 mg
Injection, powder for reconstitution: 100 mg
Injection, solution: 5 mg/mL (5 mL, 10 mL, 25 mL)
Tablet, oral: 30 mg, 60 mg, 90 mg, 120 mg
Cardizem®: 30 mg, 60 mg, 90 mg, 120 mg
Tablet, extended release, oral:
Cardizem® LA: 120 mg, 180 mg, 240 mg, 300 mg, 360 mg, 420 mg
Matzim™ LA: 180 mg, 240 mg, 300 mg, 360 mg, 420 mg
Dosage Forms - Canada
Tablet, extended release:
Tiazac® XC: 120 mg, 180 mg, 240 mg, 300 mg, 360 mg

Diltiazem-CD (Can) *see* diltiazem *on page 286*
Diltiazem HCl ER® (Can) *see* diltiazem *on page 286*
diltiazem hydrochloride *see* diltiazem *on page 286*
Diltiazem Hydrochloride Injection (Can) *see* diltiazem *on page 286*
Diltiazem TZ (Can) *see* diltiazem *on page 286*

Dilt-XR *see* diltiazem *on page* 286
Diltzac *see* diltiazem *on page* 286
Dimaphen Cold & Allergy [OTC] *see* brompheniramine and phenylephrine *on page* 143

dimenhydrinate (dye men HYE dri nate)

Medication Safety Issues
Sound-alike/look-alike issues:
DimenhyDRINATE may be confused with diphenhydrAMINE
Tall-Man dimenhy**DRINATE**
U.S. Brand Names Dramamine® [OTC]; Driminate [OTC]; TripTone® [OTC]
Canadian Brand Names Apo-Dimenhydrinate®; Children's Motion Sickness Liquid; Dimenhydrinate Injection; Dinate®; Gravol®; Nauseatol; Novo-Dimenate; PMS-Dimenhydrinate; Sandoz-Dimenhydrinate
Therapeutic Category Antihistamine
Use Treatment and prevention of nausea, vertigo, and vomiting associated with motion sickness
General Dosage Range
Oral:
Children 2-5 years: 12.5-25 mg every 6-8 hours (maximum: 75 mg/day)
Children 6-12 years: 25-50 mg every 6-8 hours (maximum: 150 mg/day)
I.M.:
Children: 1.25 mg/kg **or** 37.5 mg/m^2 4 times/day (maximum: 300 mg/day)
Adults: 50-100 mg every 4 hours
I.V.: *Adults:* 50-100 mg every 4 hours
Dosage Forms
Injection, solution: 50 mg/mL (1 mL)
Tablet, oral:
Dramamine® [OTC]: 50 mg
Driminate [OTC]: 50 mg
TripTone® [OTC]: 50 mg
Tablet, chewable, oral:
Dramamine® [OTC]: 50 mg

Dimenhydrinate Injection (Can) *see* dimenhydrinate *on page* 288

dimercaprol (dye mer KAP role)

Synonyms BAL; British anti-lewisite; dithioglycerol
U.S. Brand Names BAL in Oil®
Therapeutic Category Chelating Agent
Use Antidote to gold, arsenic (except arsine), or acute mercury poisoning (except nonalkyl mercury); adjunct to edetate CALCIUM disodium in lead poisoning
General Dosage Range I.M.: *Children and Adults:* Dosage varies greatly depending on indication
Dosage Forms
Injection, oil:
BAL in Oil®: 100 mg/mL (3 mL)

Dimetapp® Children's Cold & Allergy [OTC] *see* brompheniramine and phenylephrine *on page* 143
Dimetapp® Children's Long Acting Cough Plus Cold [OTC] *see* dextromethorphan and chlorpheniramine *on page* 271
Dimetapp® Children's Nighttime Cold & Congestion [OTC] *see* diphenhydramine and phenylephrine *on page* 292

dimethyl sulfoxide (dye meth il sul FOKS ide)

Synonyms DMSO
U.S. Brand Names Rimso-50®
Canadian Brand Names Dimethyl Sulfoxide Irrigation, USP; Kemsol®; Rimso-50®
Therapeutic Category Urinary Tract Product
Use Symptomatic relief of interstitial cystitis
General Dosage Range Bladder instillation: *Adults:* Instill 50 mL and allow to remain for 15 minutes, may repeat every 1-2 weeks

Dosage Forms
  Solution, intravesical:
    Rimso-50®: 50% (50 mL)

Dimethyl Sulfoxide Irrigation, USP (Can) *see* dimethyl sulfoxide *on page 288*

dimethyl triazeno imidazole carboxamide *see* dacarbazine *on page 248*

Dinate® (Can) *see* dimenhydrinate *on page 288*

dinoprostone (dye noe PROST one)

Medication Safety Issues
International issues:
  Cervidil brand name for dinoprostone [U.S., Canada, Australia, New Zealand], but also the brand name
    for gemeprost [Italy]

Synonyms PGE_2; prostaglandin E_2

U.S. Brand Names Cervidil®; Prepidil®; Prostin E2®

Canadian Brand Names Cervidil®; Prepidil®; Prostin E_2®

Therapeutic Category Prostaglandin

Use
  Endocervical gel: Promote cervical ripening in patients at or near term in whom there is a medical or
    obstetrical indication for the induction of labor
  Suppositories: Terminate pregnancy from 12th through 20th week of gestation; evacuate uterus in cases
    of missed abortion or intrauterine fetal death up to 28 weeks of gestation; manage benign hydatidiform
    mole (nonmetastatic gestational trophoblastic disease)
  Vaginal insert: Initiation and/or continuation of cervical ripening in patients at or near term in whom there
    is a medical or obstetrical indication for the induction of labor

General Dosage Range
  Endocervical: *Children (females of reproductive age) and Adults (females):* 0.5 mg; may repeat every 6
    hours if needed. Maximum cumulative dose: 1.5 mg/24 hours
  Intravaginal: *Children (females of reproductive age) and Adults (females):* Insert: 10 mg; remove at
    onset of active labor or after 12 hours; Suppository: 20 mg every 3-5 hours until abortion occurs

Dosage Forms
  Gel, endocervical:
    Prepidil®: 0.5 mg/3 g (3 g)
  Insert, vaginal:
    Cervidil®: 10 mg (1s)
  Suppository, vaginal:
    Prostin E2®: 20 mg (5s)

Diocaine® (Can) *see* proparacaine *on page 745*

Diocarpine (Can) *see* pilocarpine (ophthalmic) *on page 704*

Diochloram® (Can) *see* chloramphenicol *on page 193*

Diocto [OTC] *see* docusate *on page 302*

dioctyl calcium sulfosuccinate *see* docusate *on page 302*

dioctyl sodium sulfosuccinate *see* docusate *on page 302*

Diodex® (Can) *see* dexamethasone (ophthalmic) *on page 265*

Diodoquin® (Can) *see* iodoquinol *on page 484*

Diogent® (Can) *see* gentamicin (ophthalmic) *on page 416*

Diomycin® (Can) *see* erythromycin (ophthalmic) *on page 339*

Dionephrine® (Can) *see* phenylephrine (ophthalmic) *on page 697*

Diopentolate® (Can) *see* cyclopentolate *on page 242*

Diopred® (Can) *see* prednisolone (ophthalmic) *on page 734*

Dioptic's Atropine Solution (Can) *see* atropine *on page 103*

Dioptimyd® (Can) *see* sulfacetamide and prednisolone *on page 835*

Dioptrol® (Can) *see* neomycin, polymyxin B, and dexamethasone *on page 618*

Diosulf™ (Can) *see* sulfacetamide (ophthalmic) *on page 835*

Diotame [OTC] *see* bismuth *on page 135*

Diotrope® (Can) *see* tropicamide *on page 895*

Diovan® *see* valsartan *on page 905*

Diovan HCT® *see* valsartan and hydrochlorothiazide *on page 906*
Diovol® (Can) *see* aluminum hydroxide and magnesium hydroxide *on page 60*
Diovol® Ex (Can) *see* aluminum hydroxide and magnesium hydroxide *on page 60*
Diovol Plus® (Can) *see* aluminum hydroxide, magnesium hydroxide, and simethicone *on page 60*
Dipentum® *see* olsalazine *on page 648*
Diphen [OTC] *see* diphenhydramine (systemic) *on page 290*
Diphenhist® [OTC] *see* diphenhydramine (systemic) *on page 290*
Diphenhist® [OTC] [DSC] *see* diphenhydramine (topical) *on page 291*

diphenhydramine (systemic) (dye fen HYE dra meen)

Medication Safety Issues
Sound-alike/look-alike issues:
DiphenhydrAMINE may be confused with desipramine, dicyclomine, dimenhyDRINATE
Benadryl® may be confused with benazepril, Bentyl®, Benylin®, Caladryl®
BEERS Criteria medication:
This drug may be inappropriate for use in geriatric patients (high severity risk).
International issues:
Sominex brand name for diphenhydramine [U.S., Canada], but also the brand name for promethazine [Great Britain]; valerian [Chile]

Synonyms diphenhydramine citrate; diphenhydramine hydrochloride; diphenhydramine tannate

Tall-Man diphenhydrAMINE

U.S. Brand Names Aler-Cap [OTC]; Aler-Dryl [OTC]; Aler-Tab [OTC]; AllerMax® [OTC]; Altaryl [OTC]; Anti-Hist [OTC]; Banophen™ [OTC]; Benadryl® Allergy Quick Dissolve [OTC]; Benadryl® Allergy [OTC]; Benadryl® Children's Allergy FastMelt® [OTC]; Benadryl® Children's Allergy Perfect Measure™ [OTC]; Benadryl® Children's Allergy [OTC]; Benadryl® Children's Dye Free Allergy [OTC]; Benadryl® Dye-Free Allergy [OTC]; Compoz® [OTC]; Diphen [OTC]; Diphenhist® [OTC]; Histaprin [OTC]; Nytol® Quick Caps [OTC]; Nytol® Quick Gels [OTC]; PediaCare® Children's Allergy [OTC]; PediaCare® Children's NightTime Cough [OTC]; Siladryl Allergy [OTC]; Silphen [OTC]; Simply Sleep® [OTC]; Sleep-ettes D [OTC]; Sleep-Tabs [OTC]; Sleepinal® [OTC]; Sominex® Maximum Strength [OTC]; Sominex® [OTC]; Theraflu® Thin Strips® Multi Symptom [OTC]; Triaminic Thin Strips® Children's Cough & Runny Nose [OTC]; Twilite® [OTC]; Unisom® SleepGels® Maximum Strength [OTC]; Unisom® SleepMelts™ [OTC]

Canadian Brand Names Allerdryl®; Allernix; Benadryl®; Nytol®; Nytol® Extra Strength; PMS-Diphenhydramine; Simply Sleep®; Sominex®

Therapeutic Category Histamine H_1 Antagonist; Histamine H_1 Antagonist, First Generation

Use Symptomatic relief of allergic symptoms caused by histamine release including nasal allergies and allergic dermatosis; adjunct to epinephrine in the treatment of anaphylaxis; nighttime sleep aid; prevention or treatment of motion sickness; antitussive; management of parkinsonian syndrome including drug-induced extrapyramidal symptoms

General Dosage Range
I.M., I.V.:
Children: 5 mg/kg/day **or** 150 mg/m²/day in divided every 6-8 hours (maximum: 300 mg/day)
Adults: 10-100 per dose (maximum: 400 mg/day)
Elderly: Initial: 25 mg 2-3 times/day
Oral:
Children 2 to <6 years: 5 mg/kg/day **or** 150 mg/m²/day in divided every 6-8 hours (maximum: 300 mg/day) **or** 6.25 mg every 4-6 hours (maximum: 37.5 mg/day)
Children 6 to <12 years: 5 mg/kg/day **or** 150 mg/m²/day in divided every 6-8 hours (maximum: 300 mg/day) **or** 12.5-25 mg every 4-6 hours (maximum: 150 mg/day)
Children ≥12 years: 5 mg/kg/day **or** 150 mg/m²/day in divided doses every 6-8 hours **or** 25-50 mg every 4-6 hours (maximum: 300 mg/day) **or** 50 mg at bedtime
Adults: 25-50 mg every 4-6 hours (maximum: 400 mg/day) **or** 50 mg at bedtime
Elderly: Initial: 25 mg 2-3 times/day

Dosage Forms
Caplet, oral:
Aler-Dryl [OTC]: 50 mg
AllerMax® [OTC]: 50 mg
Anti-Hist [OTC]: 25 mg
Compoz® [OTC]: 50 mg
Histaprin [OTC]: 25 mg
Nytol® Quick Caps [OTC]: 25 mg

Simply Sleep® [OTC]: 25 mg
Sleep-ettes D [OTC]: 50 mg
Sominex® Maximum Strength [OTC]: 50 mg
Twilite® [OTC]: 50 mg
Capsule, oral: 25 mg, 50 mg
Aler-Cap [OTC]: 25 mg
Banophen™ [OTC]: 25 mg
Benadryl® Allergy [OTC]: 25 mg
Diphen [OTC]: 25 mg
Diphenhist® [OTC]: 25 mg
Sleepinal® [OTC]: 50 mg
Capsule, softgel, oral:
Benadryl® Dye-Free Allergy [OTC]: 25 mg
Compoz® [OTC]: 50 mg
Nytol® Quick Gels [OTC]: 50 mg
Unisom® SleepGels® Maximum Strength [OTC]: 50 mg
Captab, oral:
Diphenhist® [OTC]: 25 mg
Elixir, oral:
Altaryl [OTC]: 12.5 mg/5 mL (120 mL, 480 mL, 3840 mL)
Banophen™ [OTC]: 12.5 mg/5 mL (120 mL, 480 mL)
Injection, solution: 50 mg/mL (1 mL, 10 mL)
Injection, solution [preservative free]: 50 mg/mL (1 mL)
Liquid, oral:
AllerMax® [OTC]: 12.5 mg/5 mL (120 mL)
Benadryl® Children's Allergy [OTC]: 12.5 mg/5 mL (118 mL, 236 mL)
Benadryl® Children's Allergy Perfect Measure™ [OTC]: 12.5 mg/5 mL (5 mL)
Benadryl® Children's Dye Free Allergy [OTC]: 12.5 mg/5 mL (118 mL)
Siladryl Allergy [OTC]: 12.5 mg/5 mL (118 mL, 237 mL, 473 mL)
Solution, oral: 12.5 mg/5 mL (5 mL, 10 mL, 20 mL)
Diphenhist® [OTC]: 12.5 mg/5 mL (120 mL, 480 mL)
Strip, orally disintegrating, oral:
Benadryl® Allergy Quick Dissolve [OTC]: 25 mg (10s)
Theraflu® Thin Strips® Multi Symptom [OTC]: 25 mg (12s, 24s)
Triaminic Thin Strips® Children's Cough & Runny Nose [OTC]: 12.5 mg (14s)
Syrup, oral:
PediaCare® Children's Allergy [OTC]: 12.5 mg/5 mL (118 mL)
PediaCare® Children's NightTime Cough [OTC]: 12.5 mg/5 mL (118 mL)
Silphen [OTC]: 12.5 mg/5 mL (118 mL, 237 mL, 473 mL)
Tablet, oral: 25 mg, 50 mg
Aler-Tab [OTC]: 25 mg
Banophen™ [OTC]: 25 mg
Benadryl® Allergy [OTC]: 25 mg
Sleep-Tabs [OTC]: 25 mg
Sominex® [OTC]: 25 mg
Tablet, orally dissolving, oral:
Benadryl® Children's Allergy FastMelt® [OTC]: 12.5 mg
Unisom® SleepMelts™ [OTC]: 25 mg

diphenhydramine (topical) (dye fen HYE dra meen)
Medication Safety Issues
Sound-alike/look-alike issues:
DiphenhydrAMINE may be confused with desipramine, dicyclomine, dimenhyDRINATE
Benadryl® may be confused with benazepril, Bentyl®, Benylin®, Caladryl®
Administration issues:
Institute for Safe Medication Practices (ISMP) has reported cases of patients mistakenly *swallowing* Benadryl® Itch Stopping [OTC] gel intended for topical application. Unclear labeling and similar packaging of the topical gel in containers resembling an oral liquid are factors believed to be contributing to the administration errors. The topical gel contains camphor which can be toxic if swallowed. ISMP has requested the manufacturer to make the necessary changes to prevent further confusion.
Synonyms diphenhydramine hydrochloride

◄ **Tall-Man** diphenhydrAMINE

U.S. Brand Names Banophen™ Anti-Itch [OTC]; Benadryl® Extra Strength Itch Stopping [OTC]; Benadryl® Itch Relief Extra Strength [OTC]; Benadryl® Itch Stopping Extra Strength [OTC]; Benadryl® Itch Stopping [OTC]; Dermamycin® [OTC]; Diphenhist® [OTC] [DSC]

Canadian Brand Names Benadryl® Cream; Benadryl® Itch Relief Stick; Benadryl® Spray

Therapeutic Category Histamine H$_1$ Antagonist; Histamine H$_1$ Antagonist, First Generation; Topical Skin Product

Use Topically for relief of pain and itching associated with insect bites, minor cuts and burns, or rashes due to poison ivy, poison oak, and poison sumac

General Dosage Range Topical: *Children ≥2 years and Adults:* Apply 1% or 2% up to 3-4 times/day

Dosage Forms
Cream, topical: 2% (30 g)
Banophen™ Anti-Itch [OTC]: 2% (28.4 g)
Benadryl® Itch Stopping [OTC]: 1% (14.2 g, 28.3 g)
Benadryl® Itch Stopping Extra Strength [OTC]: 2% (14.2 g, 28.3 g)
Dermamycin® [OTC]: 2% (28 g)
Gel, topical:
Benadryl® Extra Strength Itch Stopping [OTC]: 2% (120 mL)
Liquid, topical:
Benadryl® Itch Relief Extra Strength [OTC]: 2% (14 mL)
Benadryl® Itch Stopping Extra Strength [OTC]: 2% (59 mL)
Dermamycin® [OTC]: 2% (60 mL)

diphenhydramine and acetaminophen *see* acetaminophen and diphenhydramine *on page 27*
diphenhydramine and ASA *see* aspirin and diphenhydramine *on page 99*
diphenhydramine and aspirin *see* aspirin and diphenhydramine *on page 99*

diphenhydramine and phenylephrine (dye fen HYE dra meen & fen il EF rin)

Synonyms diphenhydramine hydrochloride and phenylephrine hydrochloride; diphenhydramine tannate and phenylephrine tannate; phenylephrine and diphenhydramine; phenylephrine hydrochloride and diphenhydramine hydrochloride; phenylephrine tannate and diphenhydramine tannate

U.S. Brand Names Aldex® CT; Benadryl-D® Allergy & Sinus [OTC]; Benadryl-D® Children's Allergy & Sinus [OTC]; Dimetapp® Children's Nighttime Cold & Congestion [OTC]; Robitussin® Night Time Cough & Cold [OTC]; Triaminic® Children's Night Time Cold & Cough [OTC]; Triaminic® Children's Thin Strips® Night Time Cold & Cough [OTC]

Therapeutic Category Alpha/Beta Agonist; Histamine H$_1$ Antagonist; Histamine H$_1$ Antagonist, First Generation

Use Temporary relief of symptoms of allergic rhinitis, sinusitis, and other upper respiratory conditions, including sinus/nasal congestion, sneezing, stuffy/runny nose, itchy/watery eyes, and cough

General Dosage Range Oral:
Children 6-11 years: Aldex® CT: 1/2 to 1 tablet every 6 hours; OTC labeling: 5-10 mL or 1 strip every 4 hours as needed (maximum: 6 doses/24 hours)
Children ≥12 years and Adults: Aldex® CT: 1-2 tablets every 6 hours; OTC labeling: 10-20 mL every 4 hours as needed or 1 tablet every 4 hours as needed (maximum: 6 doses/24 hours)

Dosage Forms
Liquid, oral:
Benadryl-D® Children's Allergy & Sinus [OTC]: Diphenhydramine 12.5 mg and phenylephrine 5 mg per 5 mL (118 mL)
Strip, orally disintegrating:
Triaminic® Children's Thin Strips® Night Time Cold & Cough [OTC]: Diphenhydramine 12.5 mg and phenylephrine 5 mg
Syrup, oral:
Dimetapp® Children's Nighttime Cold and Congestion [OTC]: Diphenhydramine 6.25 mg and phenylephrine 2.5 mg per 5 mL (120 mL)
Robitussin® Night Time Cough & Cold [OTC]: Diphenhydramine 6.25 mg and phenylephrine 2.5 mg per 5 mL (120 mL)
Triaminic® Children's Night Time Cold & Cough [OTC]: Diphenhydramine 6.25 mg and phenylephrine 2.5 mg per 5 mL (118 mL)

Tablet, oral:
Benadryl-D® Allergy & Sinus [OTC]: Diphenhydramine 25 mg and phenylephrine 10 mg
Tablet, chewable, oral:
Aldex® CT: Diphenhydramine 12.5 mg and phenylephrine 5 mg

diphenhydramine citrate *see* diphenhydramine (systemic) *on page 290*

diphenhydramine citrate and aspirin *see* aspirin and diphenhydramine *on page 99*

diphenhydramine hydrochloride *see* diphenhydramine (systemic) *on page 290*

diphenhydramine hydrochloride *see* diphenhydramine (topical) *on page 291*

diphenhydramine hydrochloride and phenylephrine hydrochloride *see* diphenhydramine and phenylephrine *on page 292*

diphenhydramine, phenylephrine hydrochloride, and acetaminophen *see* acetaminophen, diphenhydramine, and phenylephrine *on page 33*

diphenhydramine tannate *see* diphenhydramine (systemic) *on page 290*

diphenhydramine tannate and phenylephrine tannate *see* diphenhydramine and phenylephrine *on page 292*

diphenoxylate and atropine (dye fen OKS i late & A troe peen)

Medication Safety Issues
Sound-alike/look-alike issues:
Lomotil® may be confused with LaMICtal®, LamISIL®, lamoTRIgine, Lanoxin®, Lasix®
International issues:
Lomotil [U.S., Canada, and multiple international markets] may be confused with Ludiomil brand name for maprotiline [multiple international markets]
Lomotil: Brand name for diphenoxylate [U.S., Canada, and multiple international markets], but also the brand name for loperamide [Mexico, Philippines]

Synonyms atropine and diphenoxylate

U.S. Brand Names Lomotil®

Canadian Brand Names Lomotil®

Therapeutic Category Antidiarrheal

Controlled Substance C-V

Use Treatment of diarrhea

General Dosage Range Oral:
Children 2-12 years: Initial: Diphenoxylate 0.3-0.4 mg/kg/day in 4 divided doses (maximum: 10 mg/day); Maintenance: Reduce as needed, may be as low as 25% of the initial daily dose
Adults: Initial: Diphenoxylate 5 mg 4 times/day (maximum: 20 mg/day); Maintenance: Reduce as needed, may be as low as 5 mg/day

Dosage Forms
Solution, oral: Diphenoxylate 2.5 mg and atropine 0.025 mg per 5 mL
Tablet: Diphenoxylate 2.5 mg and atropine 0.025 mg

diphenylhydantoin *see* phenytoin *on page 700*

diphtheria and tetanus toxoid (dif THEER ee a & TET a nus TOKS oyds)

Medication Safety Issues
Sound-alike/look-alike issues:
Diphtheria and Tetanus Toxoids (Td) may be confused with tuberculin purified protein derivative (PPD)
Pediatric diphtheria and tetanus (DT) may be confused with adult tetanus and diphtheria (Td)

Synonyms DT; Td; tetanus and diphtheria toxoid

U.S. Brand Names Decavac®

Canadian Brand Names Td Adsorbed

Therapeutic Category Toxoid

Use

Diphtheria and tetanus toxoids adsorbed for pediatric use (DT): Infants and children through 6 years of age: Active immunization against diphtheria and tetanus when pertussis vaccine is contraindicated
Tetanus and diphtheria toxoids adsorbed for adult use (Td) (Decavac®): Children ≥7 years of age and Adults: Active immunization against diphtheria and tetanus; tetanus prophylaxis in wound management ▶

293

◀ The Advisory Committee on Immunization Practices (ACIP) recommends routine vaccination for the following:
- Adults and children ≥7 years should receive a booster dose of Td every 10 years; may substitute a single Td booster dose with Tdap
- Children 7-10 years of age, adults, and the elderly (≥65 years) who are wounded in bombings or similar mass casualty events who have penetrating injuries or nonintact skin exposure and who cannot confirm receipt of a tetanus booster within the previous 5 years, may also receive a single dose of Td; children ≥11 years and adults may also receive Td if Tdap is unavailable

General Dosage Range I.M.:
DT: *Children 6 weeks to <7 years:* Primary immunization: 0.5 mL per dose, total of 5 doses
Td: *Children ≥7 years and Adults:* Primary immunization: Two 0.5 mL doses at least 4 weeks apart, followed by third 0.5 mL dose 6 months later, total of 3 doses; Booster immunization: 0.5 mL every 10 years

Dosage Forms
Injection, suspension [Td, adult; preservative free]: Diphtheria 2 Lf units and tetanus 2 Lf units per 0.5 mL (0.5 mL)
Decavac®: Diphtheria 2 Lf units and tetanus 5 Lf units per 0.5 mL (0.5 mL)
Injection, suspension [DT, pediatric; preservative free]: Diphtheria 6.7 Lf units and tetanus 5 Lf units per 0.5 mL (0.5 mL)

diphtheria and tetanus toxoids, acellular pertussis, and poliovirus vaccine

(dif THEER ee a & TET a nus TOKS oyds, ay CEL yoo lar per TUS sis & POE lee oh VYE rus vak SEEN)
Synonyms diphtheria and tetanus toxoids and acellular pertussis adsorbed, and inactivated poliovirus vaccine combined; diphtheria, tetanus toxoids, acellular pertussis (DTaP); DTaP-IPV; poliovirus, inactivated (IPV)

U.S. Brand Names Kinrix®

Therapeutic Category Vaccine, Inactivated

Use Active immunization against diphtheria, tetanus, pertussis, and poliomyelitis, used as the 5th dose in the DTaP series and the 4th dose in the IPV series

The Advisory Committee on Immunization Practices (ACIP) recommends routine vaccination for use as the fifth dose in the DTaP series and the fourth dose in the IPV series in children who received DTaP (Infanrix®) and/or DTaP-Hepatitis B-IPV (Pediarix®) as the first 3 doses and DTaP (Infanrix®) as the fourth dose. Whenever feasible, the same manufacturer should be used to provide the pertussis component; however, vaccination should not be deferred if a specific brand is not known or is not available.

General Dosage Range I.M.: *Children 4-6 years:* 0.5 mL

Dosage Forms
Injection, suspension [preservative free]:
Kinrix®: Diphtheria toxoid 25 Lf, tetanus toxoid 10 Lf, acellular pertussis antigens [inactivated pertussis toxin 25 mcg, filamentous hemagglutinin 25 mcg, pertactin 8 mcg], type 1 poliovirus 40 D-antigen units, type 2 poliovirus 8 D-antigen units, and type 3 poliovirus 32 D-antigen units per 0.5 mL (0.5 mL)

diphtheria and tetanus toxoids, acellular pertussis, hepatitis B (recombinant), poliovirus (inactivated), and *Haemophilus influenzae* B conjugate (adsorbed) vaccine

(dif THEER ee a & TET a nus TOKS oyds, ay CEL yoo lar per TUS sis, hep a TYE tis bee ree KOM be nant, POE lee oh VYE rus in ak ti VAY ted, & hem OF fi lus in floo EN za bee KON joo gate ad SORBED vak SEEN)

Medication Safety Issues
Sound-alike/look-alike issues:
Infanrix Hexa™ may be confused with Infanrix®

Synonyms diphtheria and tetanus toxoids and acellular pertussis, hepatitis B (recombinant), inactivated poliovirus vaccine, and *Haemophilus influenzae* type B combined; DTaP-HepB-IPV-Hib

Canadian Brand Names Infanrix Hexa™

Therapeutic Category Vaccine, Inactivated (Bacterial, Viral)

Use Active primary immunization against diphtheria, tetanus, pertussis, hepatitis B, poliomyelitis and disease caused by *Haemophilus influenzae* type b in infants and children 6 weeks to 2 years of age; booster immunization (at 18 months) in infants who previously received a full primary vaccination course of each component of the vaccine

General Dosage Range I.M.: *Children 6 weeks to 2 years:* Primary immunization: 0.5 mL every 8 weeks for a total of 3 doses; booster dose: 0.5 mL

Product Availability Not available in U.S.

Dosage Forms - Canada
Injection, suspension:
Infanrix Hexa™: Diphtheria toxoid 25 Lf, tetanus toxoid 10 Lf, acellular pertussis antigens [inactivated pertussis toxin 25 mcg, filamentous hemagglutinin 25 mcg, pertactin 8 mcg], HBsAg 10 mcg, type 1 poliovirus 40 D antigen units, type 2 poliovirus 8 D antigen units and type 3 poliovirus 32 D antigen units, *Haemophilus* b capsular polysaccharide 10 mcg [bound to tetanus toxoid 20-40 mcg] per 0.5 mL (0.5 mL) [contains aluminum, neomycin sulfate (trace amounts), polymyxin B (trace amounts), polysorbate 20, polysorbate 80, and yeast protein ≤5%; Pediarix™ vaccine used to reconstitute Hib forms Infanrix Hexa™]

diphtheria and tetanus toxoids, acellular pertussis, poliovirus and *Haemophilus* b conjugate vaccine
(dif THEER ee a & TET a nus TOKS oyds ay CEL yoo lar per TUS sis POE lee oh VYE rus & hem OF fi lus in floo EN za bee KON joo gate vak SEEN)

Medication Safety Issues
Administration issues:
Pentacel® is supplied in two vials, one containing DTaP-IPV liquid and one containing Hib powder, which must be mixed together in order to administer the recommended vaccine components.

Synonyms *Haemophilus* B conjugate (Hib); *Haemophilus* B polysaccharide; diphtheria toxoid; diphtheria, tetanus toxoids, acellular pertussis (DTaP); DTaP-IPV/Hib; pertussis, acellular (adsorbed); poliovirus, inactivated (IPV); tetanus toxoid

U.S. Brand Names Pentacel®

Canadian Brand Names Pediacel®; Pentacel®

Therapeutic Category Vaccine, Inactivated

Use Active immunization against diphtheria, tetanus, pertussis, poliomyelitis, and invasive disease caused by *H. influenzae* type b in children 6 weeks through 4 years of age

Advisory Committee on Immunization Practices (ACIP) recommends that Pentacel® (DTaP-IPV/Hib) may be used to provide the recommended DTaP, IPV, and Hib immunization in children <5 years of age. Whenever feasible, the same manufacturer should be used to provide the pertussis component; however, vaccination should not be deferred if a specific brand is not known or is not available. The Hib component in Pentacel® contains a tetanus toxoid conjugate. A Hib vaccine containing the PRP-OMP conjugate (PedvaxHIB®) may provide a more rapid seroconversion following the first dose and may be preferable to use in certain populations (eg, American Indian or Alaska Native children).

General Dosage Range I.M.: *Children 6 weeks to ≤4 years:* 0.5 mL

Dosage Forms
Injection, suspension:
Pentacel®: Diphtheria toxoid 15 Lf, tetanus toxoid 5 Lf, acellular pertussis antigens, poliovirus, and *Haemophilus* b capsular polysaccharide 10 mcg per 0.5 mL (0.5 mL)

diphtheria and tetanus toxoids and acellular pertussis adsorbed, and inactivated poliovirus vaccine combined *see* diphtheria and tetanus toxoids, acellular pertussis, and poliovirus vaccine *on page 294*

diphtheria and tetanus toxoids and acellular pertussis adsorbed, hepatitis B (recombinant) and inactivated poliovirus vaccine combined *see* diphtheria, tetanus toxoids, acellular pertussis, hepatitis B (recombinant), and poliovirus (inactivated) vaccine *on page 296*

diphtheria and tetanus toxoids and acellular pertussis, hepatitis B (recombinant), inactivated poliovirus vaccine, and *Haemophilus influenzae* type B combined *see* diphtheria and tetanus toxoids, acellular pertussis, hepatitis B (recombinant), poliovirus (inactivated), and *Haemophilus influenzae* B conjugate (adsorbed) vaccine *on page 294*

diphtheria antitoxin (dif THEER ee a an tee TOKS in)
Therapeutic Category Antitoxin

◀ Use Treatment of diphtheria (neutralizes unbound toxin, available from CDC)
General Dosage Range I.M., I.V.: *Children and Adults:* 20,000-120,000 units

diphtheria CRM$_{197}$ protein *see* pneumococcal conjugate vaccine (7-valent) *on page 714*
diphtheria CRM$_{197}$ protein *see* pneumococcal conjugate vaccine (13-valent) *on page 714*
diphtheria, tetanus toxoids, acellular pertussis (DTaP) *see* diphtheria and tetanus toxoids, acellular pertussis, and poliovirus vaccine *on page 294*
diphtheria, tetanus toxoids, acellular pertussis (DTaP) *see* diphtheria and tetanus toxoids, acellular pertussis, poliovirus and *Haemophilus* b conjugate vaccine *on page 295*

diphtheria, tetanus toxoids, acellular pertussis, hepatitis B (recombinant), and poliovirus (inactivated) vaccine
(dif THEER ee a, TET a nus TOKS oyds, ay CEL yoo lar per TUS sis, hep a TYE tis bee ree KOM be nant, & POE lee oh VYE rus vak SEEN)
Synonyms diphtheria and tetanus toxoids and acellular pertussis adsorbed, hepatitis B (recombinant) and inactivated poliovirus vaccine combined; DTap-HepB-IPV
U.S. Brand Names Pediarix®
Canadian Brand Names Pediarix®
Therapeutic Category Vaccine
Use Combination vaccine for the active immunization against diphtheria, tetanus, pertussis, hepatitis B virus (all known subtypes), and poliomyelitis (caused by poliovirus types 1, 2, and 3)

The Advisory Committee on Immunization Practices (ACIP) recommends Pediarix® for the following:
- Primary vaccination for DTaP, Hep B, and IPV in children at 2, 4, and 6 months of age.
- To complete the primary vaccination series in children who have received DTaP (Infanrix®) and who are scheduled to receive the other components of the vaccine. Whenever feasible, the same manufacturer should be used to provide the pertussis component; however, vaccination should not be deferred if a specific brand is not known or is not available. HepB and IPV from different manufacturers are interchangeable.

General Dosage Range I.M.: *Children 6 weeks to <7 years:* 0.5 mL/dose for a total of 3 doses
Dosage Forms
  Injection, suspension [preservative free]:
    Pediarix®: Diphtheria toxoid 25 Lf, tetanus toxoid 10 Lf, acellular pertussis antigens per 0.5 mL (0.5 mL)

diphtheria, tetanus toxoids, and acellular pertussis vaccine
(dif THEER ee a & TET a nus TOKS oyds & ay CEL yoo lar per TUS sis vak SEEN)
Medication Safety Issues
  Sound-alike/look-alike issues:
    Adacel® (Tdap) may be confused with Daptacel® (DTaP)
    Tdap (Adacel®, Boostrix®) may be confused with DTaP (Daptacel®, Infanrix®, Tripedia®)
  Administration issues:
    Carefully review product labeling to prevent inadvertent administration of Tdap when DTaP is indicated. Tdap contains lower amounts of diphtheria toxoid and some pertussis antigens than DTaP.
    Tdap is not indicated for use in children <10 years of age
    DTaP is not indicated for use in persons ≥7 years of age
    Guidelines are available in case of inadvertent administration of these products; refer to ACIP recommendations, February 2006 available at http://www.cdc.gov/mmwr/preview/mmwrhtml/rr55e223a1.htm
  Other safety concerns:
    DTaP: Diphtheria and tetanus toxoids and acellular pertussis vaccine
    DTP: Diphtheria and tetanus toxoids and pertussis vaccine (unspecified pertussis antigens)
    DTwP: Diphtheria and tetanus toxoids and whole-cell pertussis vaccine (no longer available on U.S. market)
    Tdap: Tetanus toxoid, reduced diphtheria toxoid, and acellular pertussis vaccine
Synonyms DTaP; Tdap; tetanus toxoid, reduced diphtheria toxoid, and acellular pertussis, adsorbed
U.S. Brand Names Adacel®; Boostrix®; Daptacel®; Infanrix®; Tripedia® [DSC]
Canadian Brand Names Adacel®; Boostrix®
Therapeutic Category Toxoid

Use

Daptacel®, Infanrix®, Tripedia® (DTaP): Active immunization against diphtheria, tetanus, and pertussis from age 6 weeks through 6 years of age (prior to seventh birthday)

Adacel®, Boostrix® (Tdap): Active booster immunization against diphtheria, tetanus, and pertussis

The Advisory Committee on Immunization Practices (ACIP) recommends routine vaccination for the following:

Children 6 weeks to <7 years (DTaP):
- For primary immunization against diphtheria, tetanus and pertussis
- Pediatric patients who are wounded in bombings or similar mass casualty events and who have penetrating injuries or nonintact skin exposure, and have an uncertain vaccination history should receive a tetanus booster with DTaP (if no contraindications exist) (CDC, 57[RR6], 2008)

Children 7-10 years (Tdap):
- Children not fully vaccinated against pertussis should receive a single dose of Tdap (if no contraindications exist) (CDC, 60[1], 2011)
- Children never vaccinated against diphtheria, tetanus, or pertussis, or whose vaccination status is not known should receive a series of three vaccinations containing tetanus and diphtheria toxoids and the first dose should be with Tdap (CDC, 60[1], 2011)

Adolescents 11-18 years (Tdap):
- A single dose of Tdap as a booster dose in adolescents who have completed the recommended childhood DTaP vaccination series (preferred age of administration is 11-12 years) (CDC, 60[1], 2011)

Adolescents ≥11 years and Adults (Tdap):
- Persons wounded in bombings or similar mass casualty events and who cannot confirm receipt of a tetanus booster within the previous 5 years and who have penetrating injuries or nonintact skin exposure should receive a single dose of Tdap (CDC, 57 [RR6] 2008)

Adults 19-64 years (Tdap): A single dose of Tdap should be given to replace a single dose of the 10-year Td booster in patients who have not previously received Tdap or for whom vaccine status is not known, and as soon as feasible to all:
- Postpartum women (CDC, 57[RR4], 2008; CDC, 60[4], 2011)
- Close contacts of children <12 months of age; Tdap should ideally be administered at least 2 weeks prior to beginning close contact (CDC, 60[4], 2011; CDC, 55[RR17], 2006)
- Healthcare providers with direct patient contact (CDC, 60[4], 2011; CDC, 55[RR17], 2006)

Adults ≥65 years who have not previously received Tdap:
- All adults ≥65 years may receive a single dose of Tdap in place of a dose of Td (CDC, 60[1], 2011)
- Adults ≥65 years who anticipate close contact with children <12 months of age should receive a single dose of Tdap in place a of a dose of Td (CDC, 60[1], 2011)

Note: Tdap is currently recommended for a single dose only (all age groups) (CDC, 60[1], 2011)

General Dosage Range I.M.:

Children 6 weeks to <7 years: Primary immunization: 0.5 mL per dose, total of 5 doses

Children ≥10 years and Adults: Booster immunization: 0.5 mL as a single dose

Dosage Forms

Injection, suspension [Tdap, booster formulation]:

Adacel®: Diphtheria 2 Lf units, tetanus 5 Lf units, and acellular pertussis antigens per 0.5 mL (0.5 mL)

Boostrix®: Diphtheria 2.5 Lf units, tetanus 5 Lf units, and acellular pertussis antigens per 0.5 mL (0.5 mL)

Injection, suspension [DTaP, active immunization formulation]:

Daptacel®: Diphtheria 15 Lf units, tetanus 5 Lf units, and acellular pertussis antigens per 0.5 mL (0.5 mL)

Infanrix®: Diphtheria 25 Lf units, tetanus 10 Lf units, and acellular pertussis antigens per 0.5 mL (0.5 mL) [preservative free]

Tripedia®: Diphtheria 6.7 Lf units, tetanus 5 Lf units, and acellular pertussis antigens per 0.5 mL (0.5 mL)

Note: Tripedia® vaccine is also used to reconstitute ActHIB® to prepare TriHIBit® vaccine (diphtheria, tetanus toxoids, and acellular pertussis and *Haemophilus influenzae* b conjugate vaccine combination)

diphtheria, tetanus toxoids, and acellular pertussis vaccine and *Haemophilus influenzae* b conjugate vaccine

(dif THEER ee a & TET a nus TOKS oyds, ay CEL yoo lar per TUS sis & hem OF fi lus in floo EN za bee KON joo gate vak SEEN)

Synonyms *Haemophilus influenzae* b conjugate vaccine and diphtheria, tetanus toxoids, and acellular pertussis vaccine; DTaP/Hib

◀ **U.S. Brand Names** TriHIBit® [DSC]

Therapeutic Category Toxoid; Vaccine, Inactivated Bacteria

Use Active immunization of children 15-18 months of age for prevention of diphtheria, tetanus, pertussis, and invasive disease caused by *H. influenzae* type b

The Advisory Committee on Immunization Practices (ACIP) recommends the use of TriHIBit® for the fourth dose of the diphtheria, tetanus, pertussis, and *Haemophilus* vaccine series. Whenever feasible, the same manufacturer should be used to provide the pertussis component; however, vaccination should not be deferred if a specific brand is not known or is not available.

General Dosage Range I.M.: *Children 15-18 months:* 0.5 mL

Dosage Forms

Injection, suspension [preservative free]:

TriHIBit®: Diphtheria 6.7 Lf units, tetanus 5 Lf units, acellular pertussis antigens [inactivated pertussis toxin 23.4 mcg, filamentous hemagglutinin 23.4 mcg], and *Haemophilus* b capsular polysaccharide 10 mcg [bound to tetanus toxoid 24 mcg] per 0.5 mL (0.5 mL) [Tripedia® vaccine used to reconstitute ActHIB® forms TriHIBit®]

diphtheria toxoid *see* diphtheria and tetanus toxoids, acellular pertussis, poliovirus and *Haemophilus* b conjugate vaccine *on page 295*

diphtheria toxoid conjugate *see Haemophilus* B conjugate vaccine *on page 432*

dipivalyl epinephrine *see* dipivefrin *on page 298*

dipivefrin (dye PI ve frin)

Synonyms dipivalyl epinephrine; dipivefrin hydrochloride; DPE

Canadian Brand Names Ophtho-Dipivefrin™; PMS-Dipivefrin; Propine®

Therapeutic Category Adrenergic Agonist Agent

Use Reduces elevated intraocular pressure in chronic open-angle glaucoma; also used to treat ocular hypertension, low tension, and secondary glaucomas

General Dosage Range Ophthalmic: *Adults:* Instill 1 drop every 12 hours

dipivefrin hydrochloride *see* dipivefrin *on page 298*

Diprivan® *see* propofol *on page 746*

Diprolene® *see* betamethasone *on page 129*

Diprolene® AF *see* betamethasone *on page 129*

Diprolene® Glycol (Can) *see* betamethasone *on page 129*

dipropylacetic acid *see* valproic acid *on page 904*

Diprosone® (Can) *see* betamethasone *on page 129*

dipyridamole (dye peer ID a mole)

Medication Safety Issues

Sound-alike/look-alike issues:

Dipyridamole may be confused with disopyramide

Persantine® may be confused with Periactin

International issues:

Persantine [U.S., Canada, Belgium, Denmark, France] may be confused with Permitil brand name for sildenafil [Argentina]

BEERS Criteria medication:

This drug may be inappropriate for use in geriatric patients (low severity risk).

U.S. Brand Names Persantine®

Canadian Brand Names Apo-Dipyridamole FC®; Dipyridamole For Injection; Persantine®

Therapeutic Category Antiplatelet Agent; Vasodilator

Use

Oral: Used with warfarin to decrease thrombosis in patients after artificial heart valve replacement

I.V.: Diagnostic agent in CAD

General Dosage Range

I.V.: *Adults:* 0.14 mg/kg/minute for 4 minutes (maximum: 60 mg)

Oral: *Children ≥12 years and Adults:* 75-100 mg 4 times/day

Dosage Forms
   Injection, solution: 5 mg/mL (2 mL, 10 mL)
   Tablet, oral: 25 mg, 50 mg, 75 mg
      Persantine®: 25 mg, 50 mg, 75 mg

dipyridamole and aspirin *see* aspirin and dipyridamole *on page 99*

Dipyridamole For Injection (Can) *see* dipyridamole *on page 298*

disalicylic acid *see* salsalate *on page 799*

DisCoVisc® *see* sodium chondroitin sulfate and sodium hyaluronate *on page 820*

disodium cromoglycate *see* cromolyn (nasal) *on page 239*

disodium cromoglycate *see* cromolyn (ophthalmic) *on page 239*

disodium cromoglycate *see* cromolyn (systemic, oral inhalation) *on page 238*

disodium thiosulfate pentahydrate *see* sodium thiosulfate *on page 824*

d-isoephedrine hydrochloride *see* pseudoephedrine *on page 751*

disopyramide (dye soe PEER a mide)

Medication Safety Issues
   Sound-alike/look-alike issues:
      Disopyramide may be confused with desipramine, dipyridamole
      Norpace® may be confused with Norpramin®
   BEERS Criteria medication:
      This drug may be inappropriate for use in geriatric patients (high severity risk).

Synonyms disopyramide phosphate

U.S. Brand Names Norpace®; Norpace® CR

Canadian Brand Names Norpace®; Rythmodan®; Rythmodan®-LA

Therapeutic Category Antiarrhythmic Agent, Class I-A

Use Suppression and prevention of unifocal and multifocal atrial and premature, ventricular premature complexes, coupled ventricular tachycardia; effective in the conversion of atrial fibrillation, atrial flutter, and paroxysmal atrial tachycardia to normal sinus rhythm and prevention of the recurrence of these arrhythmias after conversion by other methods

General Dosage Range Dosage adjustment recommended in patients with hepatic or renal impairment
   Oral:
      Controlled release:
         Adults <50 kg: 200 mg every 12 hours
         Adults ≥50 kg: 300 mg every 12 hours
      Immediate release:
         Children <1 year: 10-30 mg/kg/day in 4 divided doses
         Children 1-4 years: 10-20 mg/kg/day in 4 divided doses
         Children 4-12 years: 10-15 mg/kg/day in 4 divided doses
         Children 12-18 years: 6-15 mg/kg/day in 4 divided doses
         Adults <50 kg: 100 mg every 6 hours
         Adults ≥50 kg: Initial: 150 mg every 6 hours; Maintenance: 150-400 mg every 6 hours

Dosage Forms
   Capsule, oral: 100 mg, 150 mg
      Norpace®: 100 mg, 150 mg
   Capsule, controlled release, oral:
      Norpace® CR: 100 mg, 150 mg

disopyramide phosphate *see* disopyramide *on page 299*

disulfiram (dye SUL fi ram)

Medication Safety Issues
   Sound-alike/look-alike issues:
      Disulfiram may be confused with Diflucan®

U.S. Brand Names Antabuse®

Therapeutic Category Aldehyde Dehydrogenase Inhibitor Agent

Use Management of chronic alcoholism

General Dosage Range Oral: *Adults:* Initial: 500 mg once daily; Maintenance: 125-500 mg once daily (maximum: 500 mg/day)

◀ **Dosage Forms**
  Tablet, oral: 250 mg, 500 mg
    Antabuse®: 250 mg, 500 mg

dithioglycerol *see* dimercaprol *on page 288*
dithranol *see* anthralin *on page 80*
Ditropan *see* oxybutynin *on page 661*
Ditropan XL® *see* oxybutynin *on page 661*
diurex® [OTC] *see* pamabrom *on page 669*
diurex® Aquagels® [OTC] *see* pamabrom *on page 669*
diurex® Maximum Relief [OTC] *see* pamabrom *on page 669*
Diuril® *see* chlorothiazide *on page 197*

divalproex (dye VAL proe ex)

Medication Safety Issues
  Sound-alike/look-alike issues:
    Depakote® may be confused with Depakene®, Depakote® ER, Senokot®
    Depakote® ER may be confused with Depakote®, divalproex enteric coated
Synonyms divalproex sodium; valproate semisodium; valproic acid derivative
U.S. Brand Names Depakote®; Depakote® ER; Depakote® Sprinkle
Canadian Brand Names Apo-Divalproex®; Dom-Divalproex; Epival®; Mylan-Divalproex; Novo-Divalproex; Nu-Divalproex; PHL-Divalproex; PMS-Divalproex
Therapeutic Category Anticonvulsant, Miscellaneous; Antimanic Agent; Histone Deacetylase Inhibitor
Use Monotherapy and adjunctive therapy in the treatment of patients with complex partial seizures; monotherapy and adjunctive therapy of simple and complex absence seizures; adjunctive therapy in patients with multiple seizure types that include absence seizures
  Depakote®, Depakote® ER: Mania associated with bipolar disorder; migraine prophylaxis
General Dosage Range Dosage adjustment recommended in patients with hepatic impairment
  Oral:
    Children and Adults: Simple and complex absence seizures: Initial: 15 mg/kg/day; Maintenance: Up to 60 mg/kg/day
    Children ≥10 years and Adults: Complex partial seizures: Initial: 10-15 mg/kg/day in 1-3 divided doses; Maintenance: Up to 60 mg/kg/day
    Children ≥16 years and Adults: Migraine prophylaxis: Depakote® ER: 500-1000 mg once daily; Depakote® 250 mg twice daily (maximum: 1000 mg/day)
    Adults: Mania: Depakote®: Initial: 750 mg/day in divided doses; Depakote® ER: Initial: 25 mg/kg/day given once daily; Maintenance: Up to 60 mg/kg/day
Dosage Forms
  Capsule, sprinkle, oral: 125 mg
    Depakote® Sprinkle: 125 mg
  Tablet, delayed release, oral: 125 mg, 250 mg, 500 mg
    Depakote®: 125 mg, 250 mg, 500 mg
  Tablet, extended release, oral: 250 mg, 500 mg
    Depakote® ER: 250 mg, 500 mg

divalproex sodium *see* divalproex *on page 300*
Divigel® *see* estradiol (systemic) *on page 343*
Dixarit® (Can) *see* clonidine *on page 223*
5071-1DL(6) *see* megestrol *on page 555*
dl-alpha tocopherol *see* vitamin E *on page 918*
DLV *see* delavirdine *on page 257*
4-DMDR *see* idarubicin *on page 463*
D-mannitol *see* mannitol *on page 548*
DMSA *see* succimer *on page 832*
DMSO *see* dimethyl sulfoxide *on page 288*
Doan's® Extra Strength [OTC] *see* magnesium salicylate *on page 547*

dobutamine (doe BYOO ta meen)
Medication Safety Issues
  Sound-alike/look-alike issues:
  DOBUTamine may be confused with DOPamine
  High alert medication:
  The Institute for Safe Medication Practices (ISMP) includes this medication among its list of drugs which have a heightened risk of causing significant patient harm when used in error.
Synonyms dobutamine hydrochloride
Tall-Man DOBUTamine
Canadian Brand Names Dobutamine Injection, USP; Dobutrex®
Therapeutic Category Adrenergic Agonist Agent
Use Short-term management of patients with cardiac decompensation
General Dosage Range I.V.: *Children and Adults:* 2.5-20 mcg/kg/minute (maximum: 40 mcg/kg/minute)
Dosage Forms
  Infusion, premixed in D$_5$W: 1 mg/mL (250 mL, 500 mL); 2 mg/mL (250 mL); 4 mg/mL (250 mL)
  Injection, solution: 12.5 mg/mL (20 mL, 40 mL)

dobutamine hydrochloride *see dobutamine on page 301*
Dobutamine Injection, USP (Can) *see dobutamine on page 301*
Dobutrex® (Can) *see dobutamine on page 301*
Docefrez™ *see docetaxel on page 301*

docetaxel (doe se TAKS el)
Medication Safety Issues
  Sound-alike/look-alike issues:
  DOCEtaxel may confused with PACLitaxel
  Taxotere® may be confused with Taxol®
  High alert medication:
  This medication is in a class the Institute for Safe Medication Practices (ISMP) includes among its list of drug classes which have a heightened risk of causing significant patient harm when used in error.
  Administration issues:
  Multiple concentrations: Docetaxel is available as a one-vial formulation at concentrations of 10 mg/mL (generic formulation) and 20 mg/mL (concentrate; Taxotere®), and as a lyophilized powder (Docefrez™) which is reconstituted (with provided diluent) to 20 mg/0.8 mL (20 mg vial) or 24 mg/mL (80 mg vial). Docetaxel was previously available as a two-vial formulation (a concentrated docetaxel solution vial and a diluent vial) resulting in a reconstituted concentration of 10 mg/mL. The two-vial formulation has been discontinued by the manufacturer. Admixture errors have occurred due to the availability of various docetaxel concentrations.
Synonyms RP-6976
Tall-Man DOCEtaxel
U.S. Brand Names Docefrez™; Taxotere®
Canadian Brand Names Docetaxel for Injection; Taxotere®
Therapeutic Category Antineoplastic Agent
Use Treatment of breast cancer (locally advanced/metastatic or adjuvant treatment of operable node-positive); locally-advanced or metastatic nonsmall cell lung cancer (NSCLC); hormone refractory, metastatic prostate cancer; advanced gastric adenocarcinoma; locally-advanced squamous cell head and neck cancer
General Dosage Range Dosage adjustment recommended in patients with hepatic impairment, on concomitant therapy, or who develop toxicities.
I.V.: *Adults:* 60-100 mg/m^2 every 3 weeks
Dosage Forms
  Injection, powder for reconstitution:
  Docefrez™: 20 mg, 80 mg
  Injection, solution: 10 mg/mL (2 mL, 8 mL, 16 mL)
  Taxotere®: 20 mg/mL (1 mL, 4 mL)

Docetaxel for Injection (Can) *see docetaxel on page 301*

docosanol (doe KOE san ole)

Synonyms n-docosanol; behenyl alcohol

U.S. Brand Names Abreva® [OTC]

Therapeutic Category Antiviral Agent, Topical

Use Treatment of herpes simplex of the face or lips

General Dosage Range Topical: *Children ≥12 years and Adults:* Apply 5 times/day to affected area

Dosage Forms

Cream, topical:
Abreva® [OTC]: 10% (2 g)

docusate (DOK yoo sate)

Medication Safety Issues

Sound-alike/look-alike issues:
Colace® may be confused with Calan®, Cozaar®
Dulcolax® (docusate) may be confused with Dulcolax® (bisacodyl)
Surfak® may be confused with Surbex®

International issues:
Docusate may be confused with Doxinate brand name for doxylamine and pyridoxine [India]

Synonyms dioctyl calcium sulfosuccinate; dioctyl sodium sulfosuccinate; docusate calcium; docusate potassium; docusate sodium; DOSS; DSS

U.S. Brand Names Colace® [OTC]; Correctol® [OTC]; Diocto [OTC]; Docu-Soft [OTC]; DocuSoft S™ [OTC]; Dok™ [OTC]; DSS® [OTC]; Dulcolax® Stool Softener [OTC]; Dulcolax® [OTC]; Enemeez® Plus [OTC]; Enemeez® [OTC]; Fleet® Pedia-Lax™ Liquid Stool Softener [OTC]; Fleet® Sof-Lax® [OTC]; Kao-Tin [OTC]; Kaopectate® Stool Softener [OTC]; Phillips'® Liquid-Gels® [OTC]; Phillips'® Stool Softener Laxative [OTC]; Silace [OTC]

Canadian Brand Names Apo-Docusate-Sodium®; Colace®; Colax-C®; Novo-Docusate Calcium; Novo-Docusate Sodium; PMS-Docusate Calcium; PMS-Docusate Sodium; Regulex®; Selax®; Soflax™

Therapeutic Category Stool Softener

Use Stool softener in patients who should avoid straining during defecation and constipation associated with hard, dry stools; prophylaxis for straining (Valsalva) following myocardial infarction. A safe agent to be used in elderly; some evidence that doses <200 mg are ineffective; stool softeners are unnecessary if stool is well hydrated or "mushy" and soft; shown to be ineffective used long-term.

General Dosage Range

Oral:
Children <3 years: 10-40 mg/day in 1-4 divided doses
Children 3-6 years: 20-60 mg/day in 1-4 divided doses
Children 6-12 years: 40-150 mg/day in 1-4 divided doses
Adolescents and Adults: 50-500 mg/day in 1-4 divided doses

Rectal: *Older children and Adults:* Add 50-100 mg to enema fluid

Dosage Forms

Capsule, oral:
Colace® [OTC]: 50 mg, 100 mg

Capsule, liquid, oral:
DocuSoft S™ [OTC]: 100 mg

Capsule, softgel, oral: 100 mg, 240 mg, 250 mg
Correctol® [OTC]: 100 mg
Docu-Soft [OTC]: 100 mg
Dok™ [OTC]: 100 mg, 250 mg
DSS® [OTC]: 100 mg, 250 mg
Dulcolax® [OTC]: 100 mg
Dulcolax® Stool Softener [OTC]: 100 mg
Fleet® Sof-Lax® [OTC]: 100 mg
Kao-Tin [OTC]: 240 mg
Kaopectate® Stool Softener [OTC]: 240 mg
Phillips'® Liquid-Gels® [OTC]: 100 mg
Phillips'® Stool Softener Laxative [OTC]: 100 mg

Liquid, oral: 50 mg/5 mL (10 mL, 25 mL, 473 mL); 150 mg/15 mL (480 mL)
Diocto [OTC]: 150 mg/15 mL (480 mL)
Fleet® Pedia-Lax™ Liquid Stool Softener [OTC]: 50 mg/15 mL (118 mL)
Silace [OTC]: 150 mg/15 mL (473 mL)

Solution, rectal:
Enemeez® [OTC]: 283 mg/5 mL (5 mL)
Enemeez® Plus [OTC]: 283 mg/5 mL (5 mL)
Syrup, oral: 20 mg/5 mL (25 mL, 473 mL)
Colace® [OTC]: 60 mg/15 mL (473 mL)
Diocto [OTC]: 60 mg/15 mL (480 mL)
Silace [OTC]: 60 mg/15 mL (480 mL)
Tablet, oral:
Dok™ [OTC]: 100 mg

docusate and senna (DOK yoo sate & SEN na)

Medication Safety Issues
Sound-alike/look-alike issues:
Senokot® may be confused with Depakote®
Synonyms senna and docusate; senna-S
U.S. Brand Names Dok™ Plus [OTC]; Peri-Colace® [OTC]; Senexon-S [OTC]; Senokot-S® [OTC]; SenoSol™-SS [OTC]
Therapeutic Category Laxative, Stimulant; Stool Softener
Use Short-term treatment of constipation
General Dosage Range Oral:
Children 2-6 years: Initial: 4.3 mg sennosides plus 25 mg docusate (1/2 tablet) once daily (maximum: 1 tablet twice daily)
Children 6-12 years: Initial: 8.6 sennosides plus 50 mg docusate (1 tablet) once daily (maximum: 2 tablets twice daily)
Children ≥12 years and Adults: Initial: 2 tablets (17.2 mg sennosides plus 100 mg docusate) once daily (maximum: 4 tablets twice daily)
Dosage Forms
Tablet: Docusate 50 mg and sennosides 8.6 mg
Dok™ Plus, Peri-Colace® [OTC], Senexon-S [OTC], Senokot-S® [OTC], SenoSol™-SS: Docusate 50 mg and sennosides 8.6 mg

docusate calcium *see* docusate *on page 302*
docusate potassium *see* docusate *on page 302*
docusate sodium *see* docusate *on page 302*
Docu-Soft [OTC] *see* docusate *on page 302*
DocuSoft S™ [OTC] *see* docusate *on page 302*

dofetilide (doe FET il ide)

U.S. Brand Names Tikosyn®
Canadian Brand Names Tikosyn®
Therapeutic Category Antiarrhythmic Agent, Class III
Use Maintenance of normal sinus rhythm in patients with chronic atrial fibrillation/atrial flutter of longer than 1-week duration who have been converted to normal sinus rhythm; conversion of atrial fibrillation and atrial flutter to normal sinus rhythm
General Dosage Range Dosage adjustment recommended in patients with renal impairment
Oral: *Adults:* Initial: 500 mcg twice daily; Maintenance: 125-500 mcg twice daily **or** 125 mcg once daily
Dosage Forms
Capsule, oral:
Tikosyn®: 125 mcg, 250 mcg, 500 mcg

Dofus [OTC] *see* Lactobacillus *on page 506*
Dok™ [OTC] *see* docusate *on page 302*
Dok™ Plus [OTC] *see* docusate and senna *on page 303*

dolasetron (dol A se tron)

Medication Safety Issues
Sound-alike/look-alike issues:
Anzemet® may be confused with Aldomet, Antivert®, Avandamet®
Dolasetron may be confused with granisetron, ondansetron, palonosetron
Synonyms dolasetron mesylate; MDL 73,147EF

▶

◀ **U.S. Brand Names** Anzemet®
Canadian Brand Names Anzemet®
Therapeutic Category Selective 5-HT$_3$ Receptor Antagonist
Use
U.S. labeling:
Injection: Prevention and treatment of postoperative nausea and vomiting
Oral: Prevention of nausea and vomiting associated with emetogenic cancer chemotherapy (initial and repeat courses); prevention of postoperative nausea and vomiting

Canadian labeling: Oral: Prevention of nausea and vomiting associated with emetogenic cancer chemotherapy (initial and repeat courses)
General Dosage Range
I.V.:
Children 2-16 years: 0.35 mg/kg as a single dose (maximum: 12.5 mg)
Adults: 12.5 mg or 100 mg as a single dose
Oral:
Children 2-16 years: 1.2-1.8 mg/kg as a single dose (maximum: 100 mg/dose)
Adults: 100 mg as single dose
Dosage Forms
Injection, solution:
Anzemet®: 20 mg/mL (0.625 mL, 5 mL, 25 mL)
Tablet, oral:
Anzemet®: 50 mg, 100 mg

dolasetron mesylate *see* dolasetron *on page 303*
Dolgic® Plus *see* butalbital, acetaminophen, and caffeine *on page 152*
Dolobid *see* diflunisal *on page 282*
Dolophine® *see* methadone *on page 567*
Doloral (Can) *see* morphine (systemic) *on page 598*
Dom-Alendronate (Can) *see* alendronate *on page 49*
Dom-Amiodarone (Can) *see* amiodarone *on page 67*
Dom-Amitriptyline (Can) *see* amitriptyline *on page 68*
Dom-Amlodipine (Can) *see* amlodipine *on page 69*
Dom-Anagrelide (Can) *see* anagrelide *on page 78*
Dom-Atenolol (Can) *see* atenolol *on page 101*
Dom-Azithromycin (Can) *see* azithromycin (systemic) *on page 108*
Dom-Baclofen (Can) *see* baclofen *on page 112*
Dom-Benzydamine (Can) *see* benzydamine (Canada only) *on page 126*
Dom-Bicalutamide (Can) *see* bicalutamide *on page 133*
Dom-Bromocriptine (Can) *see* bromocriptine *on page 142*
Dom-Buspirone (Can) *see* buspirone *on page 151*
Dom-Captopril (Can) *see* captopril *on page 170*
Dom-Carbamazepine (Can) *see* carbamazepine *on page 171*
Dom-Carvedilol (Can) *see* carvedilol *on page 178*
Dom-Cephalexin (Can) *see* cephalexin *on page 188*
Dom-Cimetidine (Can) *see* cimetidine *on page 209*
Dom-Ciprofloxacin (Can) *see* ciprofloxacin (systemic) *on page 210*
Dom-Citalopram (Can) *see* citalopram *on page 213*
Dom-Clarithromycin (Can) *see* clarithromycin *on page 215*
Dom-Clobazam (Can) *see* clobazam (Canada only) *on page 220*
Dom-Clonidine (Can) *see* clonidine *on page 223*
Dom-Cyclobenzaprine (Can) *see* cyclobenzaprine *on page 241*
Dom-Diclofenac (Can) *see* diclofenac (systemic) *on page 277*
Dom-Diclofenac SR (Can) *see* diclofenac (systemic) *on page 277*
Dom-Divalproex (Can) *see* divalproex *on page 300*
Dom-Domperidone (Can) *see* domperidone (Canada only) *on page 305*
Dom-Doxycycline (Can) *see* doxycycline *on page 312*

Domeboro® [OTC] *see* aluminum sulfate and calcium acetate *on page 61*
dome paste bandage *see* zinc gelatin *on page 930*
Dom-Fenofibrate Micro (Can) *see* fenofibrate *on page 369*
Dom-Fluconazole (Can) *see* fluconazole *on page 381*
Dom-Fluoxetine (Can) *see* fluoxetine *on page 389*
Dom-Furosemide (Can) *see* furosemide *on page 404*
Dom-Gabapentin (Can) *see* gabapentin *on page 405*
Dom-Glyburide (Can) *see* glyburide *on page 420*
Dom-Hydrochlorothiazide (Can) *see* hydrochlorothiazide *on page 445*
Dom-Indapamide (Can) *see* indapamide *on page 470*
Dom-Levetiracetam (Can) *see* levetiracetam *on page 517*
Dom-Levo-Carbidopa (Can) *see* carbidopa and levodopa *on page 174*
Dom-Lisinopril (Can) *see* lisinopril *on page 531*
Dom-Loperamide (Can) *see* loperamide *on page 535*
Dom-Lorazepam (Can) *see* lorazepam *on page 537*
Dom-Lovastatin (Can) *see* lovastatin *on page 540*
Dom-Loxapine (Can) *see* loxapine *on page 541*
Dom-Medroxyprogesterone (Can) *see* medroxyprogesterone *on page 554*
Dom-Mefenamic Acid (Can) *see* mefenamic acid *on page 555*
Dom-Meloxicam (Can) *see* meloxicam *on page 556*
Dom-Metformin (Can) *see* metformin *on page 566*
Dom-Methimazole (Can) *see* methimazole *on page 570*
Dom-Metoprolol (Can) *see* metoprolol *on page 581*
Dom-Minocycline (Can) *see* minocycline *on page 590*
Dom-Mirtazapine (Can) *see* mirtazapine *on page 592*
Dom-Moclobemide (Can) *see* moclobemide *(Canada only) on page 594*
Dom-Ondansetron (Can) *see* ondansetron *on page 651*
Dom-Oxybutynin (Can) *see* oxybutynin *on page 661*
Dom-Paroxetine (Can) *see* paroxetine *on page 676*

domperidone *(Canada only)* (dom PE ri done)

Medication Safety Issues
Sound-alike/look-alike issues:
  Domperidone may be confused with iloperidone
Synonyms domperidone maleate
Canadian Brand Names Apo-Domperidone®; Dom-Domperidone; Mylan-Domperidone; Nu-Domperidone; PHL-Domperidone; PMS-Domperidone; RAN™-Domperidone; ratio-Domperidone; Teva-Domperidone
Therapeutic Category Dopamine Antagonist
Use Symptomatic management of upper GI motility disorders associated with chronic and subacute gastritis and diabetic gastroparesis; prevention of GI symptoms associated with use of dopamine-agonist anti-Parkinson agents
General Dosage Range Dosage adjustment recommended in patients with renal impairment
  Oral: *Adults:* 10-20 mg 3-4 times/day
Product Availability Not available in U.S.
Dosage Forms - Canada
  Tablet: 10 mg
    Apo-Domperidone®, Dom-Domperidone, Novo-Domperidone, Nu-Domperidone, PHL-Domperidone, PMS-Domperidone, ratio-Domperidone: 10 mg

domperidone maleate *see* domperidone *(Canada only) on page 305*
Dom-Pindolol (Can) *see* pindolol *on page 705*
Dom-Pioglitazone (Can) *see* pioglitazone *on page 706*
Dom-Piroxicam (Can) *see* piroxicam *on page 708*
Dom-Pravastatin (Can) *see* pravastatin *on page 732*
Dom-Propranolol (Can) *see* propranolol *on page 747*

Dom-Quetiapine (Can) *see* quetiapine *on page 760*
Dom-Ramipril (Can) *see* ramipril *on page 766*
Dom-Ranitidine (Can) *see* ranitidine *on page 767*
Dom-Risedronate (Can) *see* risedronate *on page 782*
Dom-Risperidone (Can) *see* risperidone *on page 783*
Dom-Salbutamol (Can) *see* albuterol *on page 45*
Dom-Sertraline (Can) *see* sertraline *on page 809*
Dom-Simvastatin (Can) *see* simvastatin *on page 813*
Dom-Sotalol (Can) *see* sotalol *on page 828*
Dom-Sucralfate (Can) *see* sucralfate *on page 833*
Dom-Sumatriptan (Can) *see* sumatriptan *on page 839*
Dom-Temazepam (Can) *see* temazepam *on page 848*
Dom-Terazosin (Can) *see* terazosin *on page 851*
Dom-Terbinafine (Can) *see* terbinafine (systemic) *on page 851*
Dom-Tiaprofenic (Can) *see* tiaprofenic acid *(Canada only) on page 867*
Dom-Ticlopidine (Can) *see* ticlopidine *on page 868*
Dom-Timolol (Can) *see* timolol (ophthalmic) *on page 869*
Dom-Topiramate (Can) *see* topiramate *on page 877*
Dom-Trazodone (Can) *see* trazodone *on page 884*
Dom-Ursodiol C (Can) *see* ursodiol *on page 902*
Dom-Verapamil SR (Can) *see* verapamil *on page 912*
Dom-Zopiclone (Can) *see* zopiclone *(Canada only) on page 934*
Donatussin *see* dextromethorphan, chlorpheniramine, phenylephrine, and guaifenesin *on page 272*
Donatussin DM *see* chlorpheniramine, phenylephrine, and dextromethorphan *on page 200*
Donatussin DM *see* guaifenesin, pseudoephedrine, and dextromethorphan *on page 430*
Donatussin Drops [DSC] *see* guaifenesin and phenylephrine *on page 428*

donepezil (doh NEP e zil)

Medication Safety Issues
  Sound-alike/look-alike issues:
    Aricept® may be confused with AcipHex®, Ascriptin®, and Azilect®
Synonyms E2020
U.S. Brand Names Aricept®; Aricept® ODT
Canadian Brand Names Aricept®; Aricept® RDT
Therapeutic Category Acetylcholinesterase Inhibitor; Cholinergic Agent
Use Treatment of mild, moderate, or severe dementia of the Alzheimer type
General Dosage Range Oral: *Adults:* 5 mg once daily; Maintenance: 5-23 mg once daily
Dosage Forms
  Tablet, oral: 5 mg, 10 mg
    Aricept®: 5 mg, 10 mg, 23 mg
  Tablet, orally disintegrating, oral: 5 mg, 10 mg
    Aricept® ODT: 5 mg, 10 mg

Donnatal® *see* hyoscyamine, atropine, scopolamine, and phenobarbital *on page 459*
Donnatal Extentabs® *see* hyoscyamine, atropine, scopolamine, and phenobarbital *on page 459*

dopamine (DOE pa meen)

Medication Safety Issues
  Sound-alike/look-alike issues:
    DOPamine may be confused with DOBUTamine, Dopram®
  High alert medication:
    The Institute for Safe Medication Practices (ISMP) includes this medication among its list of drugs which have a heightened risk of causing significant patient harm when used in error.
Synonyms dopamine hydrochloride; Intropin
Tall-Man DOPamine
Therapeutic Category Adrenergic Agonist Agent

Use Adjunct in the treatment of shock (eg, MI, open heart surgery, renal failure, cardiac decompensation) which persists after adequate fluid volume replacement

General Dosage Range I.V.:
Children: 1-20 mcg/kg/minute (maximum: 50 mcg/kg/minute)
Adults: 1-50 mcg/kg/minute

Dosage Forms
Infusion, premixed in D₅W: 0.8 mg/mL (250 mL, 500 mL); 1.6 mg/mL (250 mL, 500 mL); 3.2 mg/mL (250 mL)
Injection, solution: 40 mg/mL (5 mL, 10 mL); 80 mg/mL (5 mL, 10 mL); 160 mg/mL (5 mL)

dopamine hydrochloride *see* dopamine *on page 306*
Dopram® *see* doxapram *on page 308*
Doral® *see* quazepam *on page 760*
Doribax® *see* doripenem *on page 307*

doripenem (dore i PEN em)

Medication Safety Issues
Sound-alike/look-alike issues:
Doribax® may be confused with Zovirax®

Synonyms S-4661
U.S. Brand Names Doribax®
Canadian Brand Names Doribax®
Therapeutic Category Antibiotic, Carbapenem

Use Treatment of complicated intraabdominal infections and complicated urinary tract infections (including pyelonephritis) due to susceptible gram-positive, gram-negative (including *Pseudomonas aeruginosa*), and anaerobic bacteria

Canadian labeling: Additional use (not in U.S. labeling): Treatment of nosocomial pneumonia (including ventilator-associated pneumonia)

General Dosage Range Dosage adjustment recommended in patients with renal impairment
I.V.: *Adults:* 500 mg every 8 hours

Dosage Forms
Injection, powder for reconstitution:
Doribax®: 250 mg, 500 mg

dornase alfa (DOOR nase AL fa)

Synonyms recombinant human deoxyribonuclease; rhDNase
U.S. Brand Names Pulmozyme®
Canadian Brand Names Pulmozyme®
Therapeutic Category Enzyme

Use Management of cystic fibrosis patients to reduce the frequency of respiratory infections that require parenteral antibiotics in patients with FVC ≥40% of predicted; in conjunction with standard therapies, to improve pulmonary function in patients with cystic fibrosis

General Dosage Range Inhalation: *Children ≥3 months and Adults:* 2.5 mg once daily

Dosage Forms
Solution, for nebulization [preservative free]:
Pulmozyme®: 2.5 mg/2.5 mL (30s)

Doryx® *see* doxycycline *on page 312*

dorzolamide (dor ZOLE a mide)

Synonyms dorzolamide hydrochloride
U.S. Brand Names Trusopt®
Canadian Brand Names Trusopt®
Therapeutic Category Carbonic Anhydrase Inhibitor

Use Treatment of elevated intraocular pressure in patients with ocular hypertension or open-angle glaucoma

General Dosage Range Ophthalmic: *Children and Adults:* Instill 1 drop into affected eye(s) 3 times/day ▶

◄ **Dosage Forms**
  Solution, ophthalmic: 2% (10 mL)
    Trusopt®: 2% (10 mL)
Dosage Forms - Canada
  Solution, ophthalmic [drops; preservative free]:
    Trusopt®: 2% (0.2 mL)

dorzolamide and timolol (dor ZOLE a mide & TYE moe lole)

Synonyms timolol and dorzolamide
U.S. Brand Names Cosopt®
Canadian Brand Names Apo-Dorzo-Timop; Cosopt®; Sandoz-Dorzolamide/Timolol
Therapeutic Category Beta-Adrenergic Blocker; Carbonic Anhydrase Inhibitor
Use Treatment of elevated intraocular pressure in patients with ocular hypertension or open-angle glaucoma
General Dosage Range Ophthalmic: *Children ≥2 years and Adults:* Instill 1 drop into affected eye(s) twice daily
Dosage Forms
  Solution, ophthalmic [drops]: Dorzolamide 2% and timolol 0.5% (10 mL)
    Cosopt®: Dorzolamide 2% and timolol 0.5% (10 mL)
Dosage Forms - Canada
  Solution, ophthalmic [drops; preservative free]:
    Cosopt®: Dorzolamide hydrochloride 2% and timolol maleate 0.5% (0.2 mL)

dorzolamide hydrochloride *see* dorzolamide *on page 307*
DOSS *see* docusate *on page 302*
Dostinex® (Can) *see* cabergoline *on page 156*
Double Tussin DM [OTC] *see* guaifenesin and dextromethorphan *on page 427*
Dovobet® (Can) *see* calcipotriene and betamethasone *on page 158*
Dovonex® *see* calcipotriene *on page 158*

doxapram (DOKS a pram)

Medication Safety Issues
  Sound-alike/look-alike issues:
    Doxapram may be confused with doxazosin, doxepin, DOXOrubicin
    Dopram® may be confused with DOPamine
  International issues:
    Doxapram may be confused with Doxinate brand name for doxylamine and pyridoxine [Italy]
Synonyms doxapram hydrochloride
U.S. Brand Names Dopram®
Therapeutic Category Respiratory Stimulant
Use Respiratory and CNS stimulant for respiratory depression secondary to anesthesia, drug-induced CNS depression; acute hypercapnia secondary to COPD
General Dosage Range I.V.: *Adults:* 0.5-1 mg/kg every 5 minutes until response (maximum total dose: 2 mg/kg) **or** 1-5 mg/minute until response; should not be continued >2 hours (maximum total dose: 4 mg/kg; 3 g/day)
Dosage Forms
  Injection, solution: 20 mg/mL (20 mL)
    Dopram®: 20 mg/mL (20 mL)

doxapram hydrochloride *see* doxapram *on page 308*

doxazosin (doks AY zoe sin)

Medication Safety Issues
  Sound-alike/look-alike issues:
    Doxazosin may be confused with doxapram, doxepin, DOXOrubicin
    Cardura® may be confused with Cardene®, Cordarone®, Cordran®, Coumadin®, K-Dur®, Ridaura®
  BEERS Criteria medication:
    This drug may be inappropriate for use in geriatric patients (low severity risk).
Synonyms doxazosin mesylate

U.S. Brand Names Cardura®; Cardura® XL

Canadian Brand Names Alti-Doxazosin; Apo-Doxazosin®; Cardura-1™; Cardura-2™; Cardura-4™; Gen-Doxazosin; Mylan-Doxazosin; Novo-Doxazosin

Therapeutic Category Alpha-Adrenergic Blocking Agent

Use

Immediate release formulation: Treatment of hypertension as monotherapy or in conjunction with diuretics, ACE inhibitors, beta-blockers, or calcium antagonists

Immediate release and extended release formulations: Treatment of urinary outflow obstruction and/or obstructive and irritative symptoms associated with benign prostatic hyperplasia (BPH)

General Dosage Range Oral:

Extended release: *Adults:* Initial: 4 mg once daily; Maintenance: 4-8 mg/day (maximum: 8 mg/day)

Immediate release:

Adults: Initial: 1-4 mg once daily; Maintenance: 4-8 mg/day (maximum: 8 mg/day [BPH]; 16 mg/day [Hypertension])

Elderly: Initial: 0.5 mg once daily

Dosage Forms

Tablet, oral: 1 mg, 2 mg, 4 mg, 8 mg

Cardura®: 1 mg, 2 mg, 4 mg, 8 mg

Tablet, extended release, oral:

Cardura® XL: 4 mg, 8 mg

doxazosin mesylate *see* doxazosin *on page 308*

doxepin (systemic) (DOKS e pin)

Medication Safety Issues

Sound-alike/look-alike issues:

Doxepin may be confused with digoxin, doxapram, doxazosin, Doxidan®, doxycycline

SINEquan® may be confused with saquinavir, SEROquel®, Singulair®, Zonegran®

BEERS Criteria medication:

This drug may be inappropriate for use in geriatric patients (high severity risk).

International issues:

Doxal [Finland] may be confused with Doxil brand name for doxorubicin (liposomal) [U.S.. Israel]

Doxal brand name for doxepin [Finland] but also brand name for pyridoxine/thiamine [Brazil]

Synonyms doxepin hydrochloride

U.S. Brand Names Silenor®

Canadian Brand Names Apo-Doxepin®; Doxepine; Novo-Doxepin; Sinequan®

Therapeutic Category Antidepressant, Tricyclic (Tertiary Amine)

Use Depression; treatment of insomnia (with difficulty of sleep maintenance)

General Dosage Range Dosage adjustment recommended for oral route in patients with hepatic impairment

Oral:

Adults: Initial: 25-150 mg/day in 2-3 divided doses; Maintenance: Up to 300 mg/day in single (≤150 mg) or divided doses; 3-6 mg once daily prior to bedtime (insomnia)

Elderly: Initial: 10-25 mg at bedtime; Maintenance: Up to 75 mg at bedtime

Dosage Forms

Capsule, oral: 10 mg, 25 mg, 50 mg, 75 mg, 100 mg, 150 mg

Solution, oral: 10 mg/mL (118 mL, 120 mL)

Tablet, oral:

Silenor®: 3 mg, 6 mg

doxepin (topical) (DOKS e pin)

Medication Safety Issues

Sound-alike/look-alike issues:

Doxepin may be confused with digoxin, doxapram, doxazosin, Doxidan®, doxycycline

Zonalon® may be confused with Zone-A®

International issues:

Doxal [Finland] may be confused with Doxil brand name for doxorubicin (liposomal) [U.S.. Israel]

Doxal brand name for doxepin [Finland] but also brand name for pyridoxine/thiamine [Brazil]

Synonyms doxepin hydrochloride

U.S. Brand Names Prudoxin™; Zonalon®

▶

◀ **Canadian Brand Names** Zonalon®

Therapeutic Category Topical Skin Product

Use Short-term (<8 days) management of moderate pruritus in adults with atopic dermatitis or lichen simplex chronicus

General Dosage Range

Dental: *Adults:* Apply 3-4 times/day

Topical: *Adults:* Apply a thin film 4 times/day (maximum total therapy: 8 days)

Dosage Forms

Cream, topical:
Prudoxin™: 5% (45 g)
Zonalon®: 5% (30 g, 45 g)

Doxepine (Can) *see* doxepin (systemic) *on page 309*

doxepin hydrochloride *see* doxepin (systemic) *on page 309*

doxepin hydrochloride *see* doxepin (topical) *on page 309*

doxercalciferol (doks er kal si fe FEER ole)

Synonyms 1α-hydroxyergocalciferol

U.S. Brand Names Hectorol®

Canadian Brand Names Hectorol®

Therapeutic Category Vitamin D Analog

Use Treatment of secondary hyperparathyroidism in patients with chronic kidney disease

General Dosage Range

I.V.: *Adults:* Initial: 4 mcg 3 times/week after dialysis; Maintenance: Up to 18 mcg/week

Oral:
Adults (dialysis patients): Initial: 10 mcg 3 times/week at dialysis; Maintenance: Up to 60 mcg/week
Adults (predialysis patients): Initial: 1 mcg/day; Maintenance: Up to 3.5 mcg/day

Dosage Forms

Capsule, softgel, oral:
Hectorol®: 0.5 mcg, 1 mcg, 2.5 mcg

Injection, solution:
Hectorol®: 2 mcg/mL (1 mL, 2 mL)

Doxidan® [OTC] *see* bisacodyl *on page 134*

Doxil® *see* doxorubicin (liposomal) *on page 311*

doxorubicin (doks oh ROO bi sin)

Medication Safety Issues

Sound-alike/look-alike issues:
DOXOrubicin may be confused with DACTINomycin, DAUNOrubicin, DAUNOrubicin liposomal, doxapram, doxazosin, DOXOrubicin liposomal, epirubicin, IDArubicin, valrubicin
Adriamycin PFS® may be confused with achromycin, Aredia®, Idamycin®
Conventional formulation (Adriamycin PFS®, Adriamycin RDF®) may be confused with the liposomal formulation (Doxil®)

High alert medication:
The Institute for Safe Medication Practices (ISMP) includes this medication among its list of drug classes which have a heightened risk of causing significant patient harm when used in error.

Administration issues:
Use caution when selecting product for preparation and dispensing; indications, dosages and adverse event profiles differ between conventional DOXOrubicin hydrochloride solution and DOXOrubicin liposomal. Both formulations are the same concentration. As a result, serious errors have occurred.

Other safety concerns:
ADR is an error-prone abbreviation

International issues:
Doxil® may be confused with Doxal® which is a brand name for doxepin in Finland, a brand name for doxycycline in Austria, and a brand name for pyridoxine/thiamine combination in Brazil
Rubex, a discontinued brand name for DOXOrubicin in the U.S, is a brand name for ascorbic acid in Ireland

Synonyms ADR (error-prone abbreviation); adria; doxorubicin hydrochloride; hydroxydaunomycin hydrochloride; hydroxyldaunorubicin hydrochloride

Tall-Man DOXOrubicin
U.S. Brand Names Adriamycin®
Canadian Brand Names Adriamycin®
Therapeutic Category Antineoplastic Agent
Use Treatment of acute lymphocytic leukemia (ALL), acute myeloid leukemia (AML), Hodgkin disease, malignant lymphoma, soft tissue and bone sarcomas, thyroid cancer, small cell lung cancer, breast cancer, gastric cancer, ovarian cancer, bladder cancer, neuroblastoma, and Wilms tumor
General Dosage Range Dosage adjustment recommended in patients with hepatic impairment or who develop toxicities
I.V.: *Children and Adults:* Dosage varies greatly depending on indication
Dosage Forms
Injection, powder for reconstitution:
Adriamycin®: 10 mg, 20 mg, 50 mg
Injection, solution [preservative free]: 2 mg/mL (5 mL, 10 mL, 25 mL, 37.5 mL, 75 mL, 100 mL)
Adriamycin®: 2 mg/mL (5 mL, 10 mL, 25 mL, 100 mL)

doxorubicin hydrochloride *see* doxorubicin *on page 310*
DOXOrubicin hydrochloride (liposomal) *see* doxorubicin (liposomal) *on page 311*
DOXOrubicin hydrochloride liposome *see* doxorubicin (liposomal) *on page 311*

doxorubicin (liposomal) (doks oh ROO bi sin lip pah SOW mal)
Medication Safety Issues
Sound-alike/look-alike issues:
DOXOrubicin liposomal may be confused with DACTINomycin, DAUNOrubicin, DAUNOrubicin liposomal, doxapram, doxazosin, DOXOrubicin, epirubicin, IDArubicin, valrubicin
DOXOrubicin liposomal may be confused with DAUNOrubicin liposomal
Doxil® may be confused with Doxy 100™, Paxil®
Liposomal formulation (Doxil®) may be confused with the conventional formulation (Adriamycin PFS®, Adriamycin RDF®)
High alert medication:
This medication is in a class the Institute for Safe Medication Practices (ISMP) includes among its list of drug classes which have a heightened risk of causing significant patient harm when used in error.
Administration issues:
Use caution when selecting product for preparation and dispensing; indications, dosages and adverse event profiles differ between conventional DOXOrubicin hydrochloride solution and DOXOrubicin liposomal. Both formulations are the same concentration. As a result, serious errors have occurred. Liposomal formulation of doxorubicin should NOT be substituted for doxorubicin hydrochloride on a mg-per-mg basis.
International issues:
Doxil [U.S., Israel] may be confused with Doxal brand name for doxepin [Finland} and pyridoxine/thiamine [Brazil]
Synonyms DOXOrubicin hydrochloride (liposomal); DOXOrubicin hydrochloride liposome; liposomal DOXOrubicin; pegylated DOXOrubicin liposomal; pegylated liposomal DOXOrubicin
Tall-Man DOXOrubicin (liposomal)
U.S. Brand Names Doxil®
Canadian Brand Names Caelyx®; Myocet™
Therapeutic Category Antineoplastic Agent
Use Treatment of ovarian cancer (progressive or recurrent), multiple myeloma (after failure of at least 1 prior therapy), and AIDS-related Kaposi sarcoma (after failure of or intolerance to prior systemic therapy)
General Dosage Range Dosage adjustment recommended in patients with hepatic impairment or who develop toxicities
I.V.: *Adults:* 20-30 mg/m^2 every 3 weeks **or** 50 mg/m^2 every 4 weeks
Dosage Forms
Injection, solution:
Doxil®: 2 mg/mL (10 mL, 25 mL)

Doxy 100™ *see* doxycycline *on page 312*
Doxycin (Can) *see* doxycycline *on page 312*

doxycycline (doks i SYE kleen)

Medication Safety Issues

Sound-alike/look-alike issues:

Doxycycline may be confused with dicyclomine, doxepin, doxylamine

Doxy100™ may be confused with Doxil®

Monodox® may be confused with Maalox®

Oracea® may be confused with Orencia®

Vibramycin® may be confused with vancomycin, Vibativ™

Synonyms doxycycline calcium; doxycycline hyclate; doxycycline monohydrate

U.S. Brand Names Adoxa®; Adoxa® Pak™ 1/150; Adoxa® Pak™ 1/75; Alodox™; Doryx®; Doxy 100™; Monodox®; Ocudox™; Oracea®; Oraxyl™; Periostat®; Vibramycin®

Canadian Brand Names Apo-Doxy Tabs®; Apo-Doxy®; Dom-Doxycycline; Doxycin; Doxytab; Novo-Doxylin; Nu-Doxycycline; Periostat®; PHL-Doxycycline; PMS-Doxycycline; Vibra-Tabs®; Vibramycin®

Therapeutic Category Tetracycline Derivative

Use Principally in the treatment of infections caused by susceptible *Rickettsia*, *Chlamydia*, and *Mycoplasma*; alternative to mefloquine for malaria prophylaxis; treatment for syphilis, uncomplicated *Neisseria gonorrhoeae*, *Listeria*, *Actinomyces israelii*, and *Clostridium* infections in penicillin-allergic patients; used for community-acquired pneumonia and other common infections due to susceptible organisms; anthrax due to *Bacillus anthracis,* including inhalational anthrax (postexposure); treatment of infections caused by uncommon susceptible gram-negative and gram-positive organisms including *Borrelia recurrentis*, *Ureaplasma urealyticum*, *Haemophilus ducreyi*, *Yersinia pestis*, *Francisella tularensis*, *Vibrio cholerae*, *Campylobacter fetus*, *Brucella* spp, *Bartonella bacilliformis*, and *Klebsiella granulomatis*, Q fever, Lyme disease; treatment of inflammatory lesions associated with rosacea; intestinal amebiasis; severe acne

General Dosage Range

I.V.:

Children ≤8 years: 2.2 mg/kg every 12 hours

Children >8 years and ≤45 kg: 2-5 mg/kg/day in 1-2 divided doses (maximum: 200 mg/day)

Children >8 years and >45 kg and Adults: 100-200 mg/day in 1-2 divided doses

Oral:

Children ≤8 years: 2.2 mg/kg every 12 hours

Children >8 years and ≤45 kg: 2-5 mg/kg/day in 1-2 divided doses (maximum: 200 mg/day)

Children >8 years and >45 kg: 100-200 mg/day in 1-2 divided doses

Adults: 100-200 mg/day in 1-2 divided doses **or** 300 mg as a single dose **or** 40 mg/day in 1-2 divided doses

Dosage Forms

Capsule, oral: 50 mg, 100 mg, 150 mg

Adoxa®: 150 mg

Monodox®: 50 mg, 75 mg, 100 mg

Ocudox™: 50 mg

Oraxyl™: 20 mg

Vibramycin®: 100 mg

Capsule, variable release, oral:

Oracea®: 40 mg [30 mg (immediate release) and 10 mg (delayed release)]

Injection, powder for reconstitution: 100 mg

Doxy 100™: 100 mg

Powder for suspension, oral:

Vibramycin®: 25 mg/5 mL (60 mL)

Syrup, oral:

Vibramycin®: 50 mg/5 mL (473 mL)

Tablet, oral: 20 mg, 50 mg, 75 mg, 100 mg, 150 mg

Adoxa®: 50 mg

Adoxa® Pak™ 1/150: 150 mg

Adoxa® Pak™ 1/75: 75 mg

Alodox™: 20 mg

Periostat®: 20 mg

Tablet, delayed release coated beads, oral: 75 mg, 100 mg

Tablet, delayed release coated pellets, oral:

Doryx®: 75 mg, 100 mg, 150 mg

doxycycline calcium *see* doxycycline *on page* 312

doxycycline hyclate *see doxycycline on page 312*
doxycycline monohydrate *see doxycycline on page 312*

doxylamine (dox IL a meen)
Medication Safety Issues
 Sound-alike/look-alike issues:
  Doxylamine may be confused with doxycycline
Synonyms doxylamine succinate
U.S. Brand Names Aldex® AN
Canadian Brand Names Unisom®-2
Therapeutic Category Antihistamine
Use Treatment of short-term insomnia
General Dosage Range Oral: *Adults:* 1 tablet 30 minutes before bedtime
Dosage Forms
 Tablet, chewable, oral:
  Aldex® AN: 5 mg

doxylamine, acetaminophen, and dextromethorphan *see* acetaminophen, dextromethorphan, and doxylamine *on page 32*
doxylamine, acetaminophen, dextromethorphan, and pseudoephedrine *see* acetaminophen, dextromethorphan, doxylamine, and pseudoephedrine *on page 33*

doxylamine and pyridoxine *(Canada only)* (dox IL a meen & peer i DOX een)
Medication Safety Issues
 Sound-alike/look-alike issues:
  Doxylamine may be confused with doxycycline
Synonyms doxylamine succinate and pyridoxine hydrochloride; pyridoxine and doxylamine
Canadian Brand Names Diclectin®
Therapeutic Category Antihistamine; Vitamin
Use Treatment of pregnancy-associated nausea and vomiting
General Dosage Range Oral: *Adults:* 2 tablets (a total of doxylamine 20 mg and pyridoxine 20 mg) at bedtime; may increase by 1 tablet in the morning and/or afternoon in severe cases
Product Availability Not available in U.S.
Dosage Forms - Canada
 Tablet, delayed release:
  Diclectin®: Doxylamine 10 mg and pyridoxine 10 mg

doxylamine succinate *see doxylamine on page 313*
doxylamine succinate and pyridoxine hydrochloride *see doxylamine and pyridoxine (Canada only) on page 313*
doxylamine succinate, codeine phosphate, and acetaminophen *see acetaminophen, codeine, and doxylamine (Canada only) on page 31*
Doxytab (Can) *see doxycycline on page 312*
DPA *see valproic acid on page 904*
DPE *see dipivefrin on page 298*
D-penicillamine *see penicillamine on page 683*
DPH *see phenytoin on page 700*
DPM™ [OTC] *see urea on page 900*
Dramamine® [OTC] *see dimenhydrinate on page 288*
Dramamine® Less Drowsy Formula [OTC] *see meclizine on page 552*
Driminate [OTC] *see dimenhydrinate on page 288*
Drinex [OTC] [DSC] *see acetaminophen, chlorpheniramine, and pseudoephedrine on page 30*
Drinkables® Fruits and Vegetables [OTC] *see vitamins (multiple/oral) on page 919*
Drinkables® MultiVitamins [OTC] *see vitamins (multiple/oral) on page 919*
Drisdol® *see ergocalciferol on page 336*
Dristan® [OTC] *see oxymetazoline (nasal) on page 664*
Dristan® Long Lasting Nasal (Can) *see oxymetazoline (nasal) on page 664*

Dristan® N.D. (Can) *see* acetaminophen and pseudoephedrine *on page 29*
Dristan® N.D., Extra Strength (Can) *see* acetaminophen and pseudoephedrine *on page 29*
Dritho-Creme® *see* anthralin *on page 80*
Dritho-Scalp® *see* anthralin *on page 80*
Drixoral® (Can) *see* dexbrompheniramine and pseudoephedrine *on page 265*
Drixoral® Nasal (Can) *see* oxymetazoline (nasal) *on page 664*
Drixoral® ND (Can) *see* pseudoephedrine *on page 751*

dronabinol (droe NAB i nol)

Medication Safety Issues
Sound-alike/look-alike issues:
Dronabinol may be confused with droperidol

Synonyms delta-9 THC; delta-9-tetrahydro-cannabinol; tetrahydrocannabinol; THC

Canadian Brand Names Marinol®

Therapeutic Category Antiemetic

Controlled Substance C-III

Use Chemotherapy-associated nausea and vomiting refractory to other antiemetic(s); AIDS-related anorexia

General Dosage Range Oral:
Children: Initial: 5 mg/m^2 as a single dose; Maintenance: 5 mg/m^2/dose every 2-4 hours for a total of 4-6 doses/day (maximum: 15 mg/m^2/dose)
Adults: Initial: 5 mg/m^2 as a single dose; Maintenance: 5 mg/m^2/dose every 2-4 hours for a total of 4-6 doses/day (maximum: 15 mg/m^2/dose) **or** Initial: 2.5 mg twice daily; Maintenance: Titrate up to 20 mg/day in 2 divided doses

Dosage Forms
Capsule, soft gelatin, oral: 2.5 mg, 5 mg, 10 mg

dronedarone (droe NE da rone)

Synonyms dronedarone hydrochloride; SR33589

U.S. Brand Names Multaq®

Canadian Brand Names Multaq®

Therapeutic Category Antiarrhythmic Agent, Miscellaneous

Use To reduce the risk of hospitalization related to paroxysmal or persistent atrial fibrillation (AF) or atrial flutter (AFL) in patients with a recent episode of AF/AFL and associated cardiovascular risk factors (eg, age >70 years, hypertension, diabetes, prior cerebrovascular accident, left atrial diameter ≥50 mm or left ventricular ejection fraction <40%), who are in normal sinus rhythm or will be cardioverted

General Dosage Range Oral: *Adults:* 400 mg twice daily

Dosage Forms
Tablet, oral:
Multaq®: 400 mg

dronedarone hydrochloride *see* dronedarone *on page 314*

droperidol (droe PER i dole)

Medication Safety Issues
Sound-alike/look-alike issues:
Droperidol may be confused with dronabinol

Synonyms dehydrobenzperidol

Canadian Brand Names Droperidol Injection, USP

Therapeutic Category Antiemetic; Antipsychotic Agent, Butyrophenone

Use Prevention and/or treatment of nausea and vomiting from surgical and diagnostic procedures

General Dosage Range I.M., I.V.:
Children 2-12 years: Maximum: 0.1 mg/kg; additional doses may be repeated
Adults: Maximum initial dose: 2.5 mg; additional doses of 1.25 mg may be administered

Dosage Forms
Injection, solution: 2.5 mg/mL (2 mL)
Injection, solution [preservative free]: 2.5 mg/mL (2 mL)

Droperidol Injection, USP (Can) *see droperidol on page 314*

drospirenone and estradiol (droh SPYE re none & es tra DYE ole)
Synonyms E2 and DRSP; estradiol and drospirenone
U.S. Brand Names Angeliq®
Canadian Brand Names Angeliq®
Therapeutic Category Estrogen and Progestin Combination
Use Treatment of moderate-to-severe vasomotor symptoms associated with menopause; treatment of vulvar and vaginal atrophy associated with menopause
General Dosage Range Oral: *Adults (females):* 1 tablet daily
Dosage Forms
Tablet:
Angeliq®: Drospirenone 0.5 mg and estradiol 1 mg

drospirenone and ethinyl estradiol *see ethinyl estradiol and drospirenone on page 352*
drospirenone, ethinyl estradiol, and levomefolate calcium *see ethinyl estradiol, drospirenone, and levomefolate on page 358*

drotrecogin alfa (dro TRE coe jin AL fa)
Medication Safety Issues
Administration issues:
Use caution when interpreting dosing information. Maintenance dose expressed as mcg/kg/**hour**.
Synonyms activated protein C, human, recombinant; drotrecogin alfa, activated; protein C (activated), human, recombinant; rhAPC
U.S. Brand Names Xigris®
Canadian Brand Names Xigris®
Therapeutic Category Protein C (Activated)
Use Reduction of mortality from severe sepsis (associated with organ dysfunction) in adults at high risk of death (eg, APACHE II score ≥25)
General Dosage Range I.V.: *Adults:* 24 mcg/kg/**hour** for 96 hours
Dosage Forms
Injection, powder for reconstitution [preservative free]:
Xigris®: 5 mg, 20 mg

drotrecogin alfa, activated *see drotrecogin alfa on page 315*
Droxia® *see hydroxyurea on page 456*
Dr. Scholl's® Callus Removers [OTC] *see salicylic acid on page 795*
Dr. Scholl's® Clear Away® One Step Wart Remover [OTC] *see salicylic acid on page 795*
Dr. Scholl's® Clear Away® Plantar Wart Remover For Feet [OTC] *see salicylic acid on page 795*
Dr. Scholl's® Clear Away® Wart Remover [OTC] *see salicylic acid on page 795*
Dr. Scholl's® Clear Away® Wart Remover Fast-Acting [OTC] *see salicylic acid on page 795*
Dr. Scholl's® Clear Away® Wart Remover Invisible Strips [OTC] *see salicylic acid on page 795*
Dr. Scholl's® Corn/Callus Remover [OTC] *see salicylic acid on page 795*
Dr. Scholl's® Corn Removers [OTC] *see salicylic acid on page 795*
Dr. Scholl's® Extra-Thick Callus Removers [OTC] *see salicylic acid on page 795*
Dr. Scholl's® Extra Thick Corn Removers [OTC] *see salicylic acid on page 795*
Dr. Scholl's® For Her Corn Removers [OTC] *see salicylic acid on page 795*
Dr. Scholl's® OneStep Callus Removers [OTC] *see salicylic acid on page 795*
Dr. Scholl's® OneStep Corn Removers [OTC] *see salicylic acid on page 795*
Dr. Scholl's® Small Corn Removers [OTC] *see salicylic acid on page 795*
Dr. Scholl's® Ultra-Thin Corn Removers [OTC] *see salicylic acid on page 795*
DryMax *see chlorpheniramine, phenylephrine, and methscopolamine on page 200*
Drysol™ *see aluminum chloride hexahydrate on page 59*
DSCG *see cromolyn (nasal) on page 239*
DSCG *see cromolyn (ophthalmic) on page 239*

DSCG see cromolyn (systemic, oral inhalation) on page 238

DSS see docusate on page 302

DSS® [OTC] see docusate on page 302

DT see diphtheria and tetanus toxoid on page 293

DTaP see diphtheria, tetanus toxoids, and acellular pertussis vaccine on page 296

DTap-HepB-IPV see diphtheria, tetanus toxoids, acellular pertussis, hepatitis B (recombinant), and poliovirus (inactivated) vaccine on page 296

DTaP-HepB-IPV-Hib see diphtheria and tetanus toxoids, acellular pertussis, hepatitis B (recombinant), poliovirus (inactivated), and Haemophilus influenzae B conjugate (adsorbed) vaccine on page 294

DTaP/Hib see diphtheria, tetanus toxoids, and acellular pertussis vaccine and Haemophilus influenzae b conjugate vaccine on page 297

DTaP-IPV see diphtheria and tetanus toxoids, acellular pertussis, and poliovirus vaccine on page 294

DTaP-IPV/Hib see diphtheria and tetanus toxoids, acellular pertussis, poliovirus and Haemophilus b conjugate vaccine on page 295

DTC 101 see cytarabine (liposomal) on page 247

DTIC see dacarbazine on page 248

DTIC-dome see dacarbazine on page 248

DTO (error-prone abbreviation) see opium tincture on page 653

DTPA see diethylene triamine penta-acetic acid on page 281

D-Trp(6)-LHRH see triptorelin on page 894

Duac® CS [DSC] see clindamycin and benzoyl peroxide on page 219

Duet® see vitamins (multiple/prenatal) on page 920

Duetact™ see pioglitazone and glimepiride on page 706

Duet® Balanced DHA[ec] see vitamins (multiple/prenatal) on page 920

Duexis® see ibuprofen and famotidine on page 462

Dukoral® (Can) see traveler's diarrhea and cholera vaccine (Canada only) on page 883

Dulcolax® [OTC] see bisacodyl on page 134

Dulcolax® [OTC] see docusate on page 302

Dulcolax® (Can) see bisacodyl on page 134

Dulcolax Balance® [OTC] see polyethylene glycol 3350 on page 718

Dulcolax® Stool Softener [OTC] see docusate on page 302

Dulera® see mometasone and formoterol on page 596

Dull-C® [OTC] see ascorbic acid on page 96

duloxetine (doo LOX e teen)

Medication Safety Issues
Sound-alike/look-alike issues:
  Cymbalta® may be confused with Symbyax®
  DULoxetine may be confused with FLUoxetine

Synonyms (+)-(S)-N-methyl-γ-(1-naphthyloxy)-2-thiophenepropylamine hydrochloride; duloxetine hydrochloride; LY248686

Tall-Man DULoxetine

U.S. Brand Names Cymbalta®

Canadian Brand Names Cymbalta®

Therapeutic Category Antidepressant, Serotonin/Norepinephrine Reuptake Inhibitor

Use Acute and maintenance treatment of major depressive disorder (MDD); treatment of generalized anxiety disorder (GAD); management of diabetic peripheral neuropathic pain (DPNP); management of fibromyalgia (FM); chronic musculoskeletal pain (eg, chronic low back pain, osteoarthritis)

General Dosage Range Oral:
  Adults: 30-60 mg/day in 1-2 divided doses (maximum: 120 mg/day)
  Elderly: Initial: 20 mg 1-2 times/day

Dosage Forms
Capsule, delayed release, enteric coated pellets, oral:
  Cymbalta®: 20 mg, 30 mg, 60 mg

duloxetine hydrochloride see duloxetine on page 316

Duodopa™ (Can) see carbidopa and levodopa on page 174

Duodote™ *see* atropine and pralidoxime *on page 104*
DuoFilm® [OTC] *see* salicylic acid *on page 795*
Duofilm® (Can) *see* salicylic acid *on page 795*
Duoforte® 27 (Can) *see* salicylic acid *on page 795*
DuoNeb® *see* ipratropium and albuterol *on page 489*
DuoTrav™ (Can) *see* travoprost and timolol *(Canada only) on page 883*
Duovent® UDV (Can) *see* ipratropium and fenoterol *(Canada only) on page 490*
DuP 753 *see* losartan *on page 538*
Duraclon® *see* clonidine *on page 223*
Duradryl® *see* chlorpheniramine, phenylephrine, and methscopolamine *on page 200*
Duragesic® *see* fentanyl *on page 371*
Duragesic® MAT (Can) *see* fentanyl *on page 371*
Durahist™ [DSC] *see* chlorpheniramine, pseudoephedrine, and methscopolamine *on page 202*
Duralith® (Can) *see* lithium *on page 532*
Duramist Plus [OTC] *see* oxymetazoline (nasal) *on page 664*
Duramorph *see* morphine (systemic) *on page 598*
Durasal™ *see* salicylic acid *on page 795*
Duratocin™ (Can) *see* carbetocin *(Canada only) on page 173*
Durezol® *see* difluprednate *on page 283*
Duricef *see* cefadroxil *on page 180*
Durolane® (Can) *see* hyaluronate and derivatives *on page 443*

dutasteride (doo TAS teer ide)

U.S. Brand Names Avodart®
Canadian Brand Names Avodart®
Therapeutic Category Antineoplastic Agent, Anthracenedione
Use Treatment of symptomatic benign prostatic hyperplasia (BPH) as monotherapy or combination therapy with tamsulosin
General Dosage Range Oral: *Adults (males):* 0.5 mg once daily
Dosage Forms
  Capsule, softgel, oral:
    Avodart®: 0.5 mg

dutasteride and tamsulosin (doo TAS teer ide & tam SOO loe sin)

Synonyms tamsulosin and dutasteride; tamsulosin hydrochloride and dutasteride
U.S. Brand Names Jalyn™
Therapeutic Category 5 Alpha-Reductase Inhibitor; Alpha$_1$ Blocker
Use Treatment of symptomatic benign prostatic hyperplasia (BPH)
General Dosage Range Oral: *Adults (males):* 1 capsule (0.5 mg dutasteride/0.4 mg tamsulosin) once daily
Dosage Forms
  Capsule, oral:
    Jalyn™: Dutasteride 0.5 mg and tamsulosin hydrochloride 0.4 mg

Duvoid® (Can) *see* bethanechol *on page 131*
D-Vi-Sol® (Can) *see* cholecalciferol *on page 204*
DW286 *see* gemifloxacin *on page 414*
DX-88 *see* ecallantide *on page 318*
Dyazide® *see* hydrochlorothiazide and triamterene *on page 446*
Dycill® (Can) *see* dicloxacillin *on page 280*

dyclonine (DYE kloe neen)

Medication Safety Issues
  Sound-alike/look-alike issues:
    Dyclonine may be confused with dicyclomine
Synonyms dyclonine hydrochloride

◄ **U.S. Brand Names** Sucrets® Children's [OTC]; Sucrets® Maximum Strength [OTC]; Sucrets® Regular Strength [OTC]

Therapeutic Category Local Anesthetic

Use Temporary relief of pain associated with oral mucosa

General Dosage Range Oral: Lozenge: *Children ≥2 years and Adults:* One lozenge every 2 hours as needed (maximum: 10 lozenges/day)

Dosage Forms
Lozenge, oral:
Sucrets® Children's [OTC]: 1.2 mg (18s)
Sucrets® Maximum Strength [OTC]: 3 mg (18s)
Sucrets® Regular Strength [OTC]: 2 mg (18s)

dyclonine hydrochloride *see* dyclonine *on page 317*

DynaCirc CR® *see* isradipine *on page 496*

Dyna-Hex® [OTC] *see* chlorhexidine gluconate *on page 194*

dyphylline (DYE fi lin)

Synonyms dihydroxypropyl theophylline

U.S. Brand Names Lufyllin®

Therapeutic Category Theophylline Derivative

Use Bronchodilator in reversible airway obstruction due to asthma, chronic bronchitis, or emphysema

General Dosage Range Dosage adjustment recommended in patients with renal impairment
Oral: *Adults:* Up to 15 mg/kg 4 times/day

Dosage Forms
Tablet, oral:
Lufyllin®: 200 mg, 400 mg

dyphylline and guaifenesin (DYE fi lin & gwye FEN e sin)

Synonyms guaifenesin and dyphylline

U.S. Brand Names COPD; Difil-G [DSC]; Difil-G® 400; Difil®-G Forte [DSC]; Lufyllin®-GG

Therapeutic Category Expectorant; Theophylline Derivative

Use Treatment of bronchial asthma and reversible bronchospasm associated with chronic bronchitis and emphysema

General Dosage Range Dosage adjustment recommended in patients with renal impairment
Oral: *Children ≥6 years and Adults:* Dosage varies greatly depending on product

Dosage Forms
Elixir: Dyphylline 100 mg and guaifenesin 100 mg per 15 mL
Lufyllin®-GG: Dyphylline 100 mg and guaifenesin 100 mg per 15 mL
Liquid: Dyphylline 100 mg and guaifenesin 100 mg per 5 mL
Tablet: Dyphylline 200 mg and guaifenesin 200 mg
COPD: Dyphylline 200 mg and guaifenesin 200 mg
Difil-G® 400: Dyphylline 200 mg and guaifenesin 400 mg

Dyrenium® *see* triamterene *on page 888*

Dysport™ *see* abobotulinumtoxinA *on page 22*

E2 and DRSP *see* drospirenone and estradiol *on page 315*

7E3 *see* abciximab *on page 21*

E2020 *see* donepezil *on page 306*

E 2080 *see* rufinamide *on page 793*

E7389 *see* eribulin *on page 337*

EACA *see* aminocaproic acid *on page 65*

Ebixa® (Can) *see* memantine *on page 556*

ecallantide (e KAL lan tide)

Synonyms DX-88

U.S. Brand Names Kalbitor®

Therapeutic Category Kallikrein Inhibitor

Use Treatment of acute attacks of hereditary angioedema (HAE)

General Dosage Range SubQ: *Children ≥16 years and Adults:* 30 mg; may repeat once (maximum: 60 mg/24 hours)

Dosage Forms
Injection, solution [preservative free]:
Kalbitor®: 10 mg/mL (1 mL)

echothiophate iodide (ek oh THYE oh fate EYE oh dide)

Synonyms ecostigmine iodide

U.S. Brand Names Phospholine Iodide®

Therapeutic Category Cholinesterase Inhibitor

Use Used as miotic in treatment of chronic, open-angle glaucoma; may be useful in specific cases of angle-closure glaucoma (postiridectomy or where surgery refused/contraindicated); postcataract surgery-related glaucoma; accommodative esotropia

General Dosage Range Ophthalmic:
Children: Diagnosis: Instill 1 drop of (0.125%) into both eyes at bedtime for 2-3 weeks; Treatment: Instill 1 drop of 0.06% once daily **or** 0.125% every other day (maximum: 0.125% daily)
Adults: Initial: 1 drop (0.03%) twice daily; Maintenance: 1 dose daily or every other day

Dosage Forms
Powder for reconstitution, ophthalmic:
Phospholine Iodide®: 6.25 mg (5 mL)

EC-Naprosyn® *see* naproxen *on page* 612
***E. coli* asparaginase** *see* asparaginase *on page* 98

econazole (e KONE a zole)

Synonyms econazole nitrate

Therapeutic Category Antifungal Agent

Use Topical treatment of tinea pedis (athlete's foot), tinea cruris (jock itch), tinea corporis (ringworm), tinea versicolor, and cutaneous candidiasis

General Dosage Range Topical: *Children and Adults:* Apply sufficient quantity once or twice daily

Dosage Forms
Cream, topical: 1% (15 g, 30 g, 85 g)

econazole nitrate *see* econazole *on page* 319
Econopred *see* prednisolone (ophthalmic) *on page* 734
ecostigmine iodide *see* echothiophate iodide *on page* 319
Ecotrin® [OTC] *see* aspirin *on page* 98
Ecotrin® Arthritis Strength [OTC] *see* aspirin *on page* 98
Ecotrin® Low Strength [OTC] *see* aspirin *on page* 98
Ectosone (Can) *see* betamethasone *on page* 129

eculizumab (e kue LIZ oo mab)

Synonyms h5G1.1; Monoclonal Antibody 5G1.1; Monoclonal Antibody Anti-C5

U.S. Brand Names Soliris®

Canadian Brand Names Soliris®

Therapeutic Category Monoclonal Antibody; Monoclonal Antibody, Complement Inhibitor

Use Treatment of paroxysmal nocturnal hemoglobinuria (PNH) to reduce hemolysis; treatment of atypical hemolytic uremic syndrome (aHUS) to inhibit complement-mediated thrombotic microangiopathy

Note: Not indicated for the treatment of hemolytic uremic syndrome related to Shiga toxin *E. coli* (STEC-HUS)

General Dosage Range I.V.:
Children 5 kg to <10 kg: Induction: 300 mg weekly for 1 dose; Maintenance: 300 mg at week 2, then 300 mg every 3 weeks
Children 10 kg to <20 kg: Induction: 600 mg weekly for 1 dose; Maintenance: 300 mg at week 2, then 300 mg every 2 weeks
Children 20 kg to <30 kg: Induction: 600 mg weekly for 2 doses; Maintenance: 600 mg at week 3, then 600 mg every 2 weeks
Children 30 kg to <40 kg: Induction: 600 mg weekly for 2 doses; Maintenance: 900 mg at week 3, then 900 mg every 2 weeks

Children ≥40 kg: Induction: 900 mg weekly for 4 doses; Maintenance: 1200 mg at week 5, then 1200 mg every 2 weeks

Adults: aHUS: Induction: 900 mg weekly for 4 doses; Maintenance: 1200 mg at week 5, then 1200 mg every 2 weeks **or** PNH: Induction: 600 mg weekly for 4 doses; Maintenance: 900 mg at week 5, then 900 mg every 2 weeks

Dosage Forms
Injection, solution [preservative free]:
Soliris®: 10 mg/mL (30 mL)

Ed A-Hist™ [DSC] *see chlorpheniramine and phenylephrine on page 198*
Ed A-Hist DM [DSC] *see chlorpheniramine, phenylephrine, and dextromethorphan on page 200*
Edarbi™ *see azilsartan on page 108*
Ed Chlorped [DSC] *see chlorpheniramine on page 197*
Ed ChlorPed D *see chlorpheniramine and phenylephrine on page 198*
Ed-Chlortan *see chlorpheniramine on page 197*
Edecrin® *see ethacrynic acid on page 350*

edetate CALCIUM disodium (ED e tate KAL see um dye SOW dee um)
Medication Safety Issues
Sound-alike look-alike issues:
To avoid potentially serious errors, the abbreviation "EDTA" should **never** be used.

Edetate CALCIUM disodium (CaEDTA) may be confused with edetate disodium (Na_2EDTA) (not commercially available in the U.S. or Canada). CDC recommends that edetate disodium should **never** be used for chelation therapy in children. Fatal hypocalcemia may result if edetate disodium is used for chelation therapy instead of edetate calcium disodium. ISMP recommends confirming the diagnosis to help distinguish between the two drugs prior to dispensing and/or administering either drug.

Edetate CALCIUM disodium may be confused with etomidate
Synonyms CaEDTA; calcium disodium edetate; edetate disodium CALCIUM; EDTA (CALCIUM disodium) (error-prone abbreviation)
U.S. Brand Names Calcium Disodium Versenate®
Therapeutic Category Chelating Agent
Use Treatment of symptomatic acute and chronic lead poisoning or for symptomatic patients with high blood lead levels
General Dosage Range Dosage adjustment recommended in patients with renal impairment
I.M., I.V.: *Children and Adults:* 1000-1500 mg/m^2/day (25-75 mg/kg/day)
Dosage Forms
Injection, solution:
Calcium Disodium Versenate®: 200 mg/mL (2.5 mL)

edetate disodium CALCIUM *see edetate CALCIUM disodium on page 320*
Edex® *see alprostadil on page 57*
Edluar™ *see zolpidem on page 933*

edrophonium (ed roe FOE nee um)
Synonyms edrophonium chloride
U.S. Brand Names Enlon®
Canadian Brand Names Enlon®; Tensilon®
Therapeutic Category Cholinergic Agent
Use Diagnosis of myasthenia gravis; differentiation of cholinergic crises from myasthenia crises; reversal of nondepolarizing neuromuscular blockers
General Dosage Range
I.M.:
Infants: 0.5-1 mg
Children ≤34 kg: 1 mg
Children >34 kg: 5 mg
Adults: 10 mg, followed by 2 mg if no response

I.V.:
Infants: 0.1 mg, followed by 0.4 mg if no response (maximum total dose: 0.5 mg)
Children ≤34 kg: 0.04 mg/kg as single dose or followed by 0.16 mg/kg if no response **or** 1 mg, followed by 1mg every 30-45 seconds if no response (maximum total dose: 5 mg)
Children >34 kg: 0.04 mg/kg as single dose or followed by 0.16 mg/kg if no response **or** 2 mg, followed by 1 mg every 30-45 seconds if no response (maximum total dose: 10 mg)
Adults: 2 mg test dose, followed by 8 mg if no response **or** 1-10 mg as a single dose **or** 10 mg every 5-10 minutes up to 40 mg **or** 1 mg; may repeat after 1 minute

Dosage Forms
Injection, solution:
Enlon®: 10 mg/mL (15 mL)

edrophonium and atropine (ed roe FOE nee um & A troe peen)

Synonyms atropine sulfate and edrophonium chloride; edrophonium chloride and atropine sulfate
U.S. Brand Names Enlon-Plus®
Therapeutic Category Anticholinergic Agent; Antidote; Cholinergic Agonist
Use Reversal of nondepolarizing neuromuscular blockers; adjunct treatment of respiratory depression caused by curare overdose
General Dosage Range I.V.: *Adults:* 0.05-0.1 mL/kg (0.5-1 mg/kg of edrophonium and 0.007-0.014 mg/kg of atropine)
Dosage Forms
Injection, solution:
Enlon-Plus®: Edrophonium 10 mg/mL and atropine 0.14 mg/mL (5 mL, 15 mL)

edrophonium chloride *see edrophonium on page 320*
edrophonium chloride and atropine sulfate *see edrophonium and atropine on page 321*
EDTA (CALCIUM disodium) (error-prone abbreviation) *see edetate CALCIUM disodium on page 320*
Edurant™ *see rilpivirine on page 781*
EEMT™ *see estrogens (esterified) and methyltestosterone on page 349*
EEMT™ HS *see estrogens (esterified) and methyltestosterone on page 349*
E.E.S.® *see erythromycin (systemic) on page 339*
EES® (Can) *see erythromycin (systemic) on page 339*

efavirenz (e FAV e renz)

U.S. Brand Names Sustiva®
Canadian Brand Names Sustiva®
Therapeutic Category Antiretroviral Agent, Nonnucleoside Reverse Transcriptase Inhibitor (NNRTI)
Use Treatment of HIV-1 infections in combination with at least two other antiretroviral agents
General Dosage Range Dosage adjustment recommended in patients on concomitant therapy
Oral:
Children ≥3 years and 10 kg to <15 kg: 200 mg once daily
Children ≥3 years and 15 kg to <20 kg: 250 mg once daily
Children ≥3 years and 20 kg to <25 kg: 300 mg once daily
Children ≥3 years and 25 kg to <32.5 kg: 350 mg once daily
Children ≥3 years and 32.5 kg to <40 kg: 400 mg once daily
Children ≥3 years and ≥40 kg and Adults: 600 mg once daily
Dosage Forms
Capsule, oral:
Sustiva®: 50 mg, 200 mg
Tablet, oral:
Sustiva®: 600 mg

efavirenz, emtricitabine, and tenofovir
(e FAV e renz, em trye SYE ta been, & te NOE fo veer)

Synonyms emtricitabine, efavirenz, and tenofovir; FTC, TDF, and EFV; tenofovir disoproxil fumarate, efavirenz, and emtricitabine
U.S. Brand Names Atripla®
Canadian Brand Names Atripla®

◀ **Therapeutic Category** Antiretroviral Agent, Nonnucleoside Reverse Transcriptase Inhibitor (NNRTI); Antiretroviral Agent, Nucleoside Reverse Transcriptase Inhibitor (NRTI); Antiretroviral Agent, Reverse Transcriptase Inhibitor (Nucleotide)

Use Treatment of HIV infection

General Dosage Range Oral: *Adults:* 1 tablet (efavirenz 600 mg/emtricitabine 200 mg/tenofovir 300 mg) once daily

Dosage Forms
Tablet:
Atripla®: Efavirenz 600 mg, emtricitabine 200 mg, and tenofovir disoproxil fumarate 300 mg

Effer-K® *see* potassium bicarbonate and potassium citrate *on page 723*

Effexor® *see* venlafaxine *on page 911*

Effexor XR® *see* venlafaxine *on page 911*

Effient® *see* prasugrel *on page 732*

eflornithine (ee FLOR ni theen)

Medication Safety Issues
Sound-alike/look-alike issues:
Vaniqa® may be confused with Viagra®

Synonyms DFMO; eflornithine hydrochloride

U.S. Brand Names Vaniqa®

Canadian Brand Names Vaniqa®

Therapeutic Category Antiprotozoal; Topical Skin Product

Use Cream: Females ≥12 years: Reduce unwanted hair from face and adjacent areas under the chin
Orphan status: Injection: Treatment of meningoencephalitic stage of *Trypanosoma brucei gambiense* infection (sleeping sickness)

General Dosage Range Dosage adjustment recommended in patients with renal impairment
I.V.: *Adults:* 100 mg/kg/dose every 6 hours
Topical: *Children and Adults:* Apply thin layer to affected areas twice daily

Dosage Forms
Cream, topical:
Vaniqa®: 13.9% (30 g)

eflornithine hydrochloride *see* eflornithine *on page 322*

eformoterol and budesonide *see* budesonide and formoterol *on page 146*

Efudex® *see* fluorouracil (topical) *on page 388*

E-Gem® [OTC] *see* vitamin E *on page 918*

E-Gem® Lip Care [OTC] *see* vitamin E *on page 918*

E-Gems® [OTC] *see* vitamin E *on page 918*

E-Gems® Elite [OTC] *see* vitamin E *on page 918*

E-Gems® Plus [OTC] *see* vitamin E *on page 918*

Egrifta™ *see* tesamorelin *on page 853*

EHDP *see* etidronate *on page 359*

EL-970 *see* dalfampridine *on page 250*

Elaprase® *see* idursulfase *on page 464*

Elavil *see* amitriptyline *on page 68*

Eldepryl® *see* selegiline *on page 806*

Eldopaque® [OTC] *see* hydroquinone *on page 453*

Eldopaque® (Can) *see* hydroquinone *on page 453*

Eldopaque Forte® *see* hydroquinone *on page 453*

Eldoquin® [OTC] *see* hydroquinone *on page 453*

Eldoquin® (Can) *see* hydroquinone *on page 453*

Eldoquin Forte® *see* hydroquinone *on page 453*

electrolyte lavage solution *see* polyethylene glycol-electrolyte solution *on page 718*

electrolyte lavage solution *see* polyethylene glycol-electrolyte solution and bisacodyl *on page 719*

electrolyte solution, renal replacement
(ee LEK trow lite soe LOO shun REE nil ree PLASE ment)

Medication Safety Issues
High alert medication:
The Institute for Safe Medication Practices (ISMP) includes this medication among its list of drug classes which have a heightened risk of causing significant patient harm when used in error.

Synonyms continuous renal replacement therapy; CRRT; renal replacement solution

U.S. Brand Names Normocarb HF® 25; Normocarb HF® 35; PrismaSol

Therapeutic Category Alkalinizing Agent; Electrolyte Supplement

Use Used as a replacement solution to replenish water, correct electrolytes, and adjust acid-base balance depleted by hemofiltration or hemodiafiltration (continuous renal replacement therapy [CRRT]); drug poisoning when CRRT is used to remove filterable substances

General Dosage Range Continuous renal replacement circuit: *Children and Adults:*
Pre- or post-filter: Volume of solution administered depends upon the patient's fluid balance, target fluid balance, body weight, and amount of fluid removed during hemofiltration process.
Post-filter replacement: Volume infused/hour should not be greater than 1/3 of blood flow rate (eg, blood flow rate 100 mL/minute [6000 mL/hour]; post-filter replacement rate ≤2000 mL/hour)

Dosage Forms
Injection, solution [concentrate; preservative free]:
Normocarb HF® 25: Bicarbonate 25 mEq/L, chloride 116.5 mEq/L, magnesium 1.5 mEq/L, sodium 140 mEq/L (240 mL) [strength represents final solution after mixing; when diluted as directed, makes 3240 mL of infusate]
Normocarb HF® 35: Bicarbonate 35 mEq/L, chloride 106.5 mEq/L, magnesium 1.5 mEq/L, sodium 140 mEq/L (240 mL) [strength represents final solution after mixing; when diluted as directed, makes 3240 mL of infusate]

Injection, solution [preservative free]:
PrismaSol B22GK 2/0: Bicarbonate 22 mEq/L, chloride 118.5 mEq/L, dextrose 100 mg/dL, lactate 3 mEq/L, magnesium 1.5 mEq/L, potassium 2 mEq/L, sodium 140 mEq/L (5000 mL) [strength represents final solution after mixing]
PrismaSol BGK 2/0: Bicarbonate 32 mEq/L, chloride 108 mEq/L, dextrose 100 mg/dL, lactate 3 mEq/L, magnesium 1 mEq/L, potassium 2 mEq/L, sodium 140 mEq/L (5000 mL) [strength represents final solution after mixing]
PrismaSol BGK 2/3.5: Bicarbonate 32 mEq/L, calcium 3.5 mEq/L, chloride 111.5 mEq/L, dextrose 100 mg/dL, lactate 3 mEq/L, magnesium 1 mEq/L, potassium 2 mEq/L, sodium 140 mEq/L (5000 mL) [strength represents final solution after mixing]
PrismaSol BGK 4/0/1.2: Bicarbonate 32 mEq/L, chloride 110.2 mEq/L, dextrose 100 mg/dL, lactate 3 mEq/L, magnesium 1.2 mEq/L, potassium 4 mEq/L, sodium 140 mEq/L (5000 mL) [strength represents final solution after mixing]
PrismaSol BGK 4/2.5: Bicarbonate 32 mEq/L, calcium 2.5 mEq/L, chloride 113 mEq/L, dextrose 100 mg/dL, lactate 3 mEq/L, magnesium 1.5 mEq/L, potassium 4 mEq/L, sodium 140 mEq/L (5000 mL) [strength represents final solution after mixing]
PrismaSol BK 0/0/1.2: Bicarbonate 32 mEq/L, chloride 106.2 mEq/L, lactate 3 mEq/L, magnesium 1.2 mEq/L, sodium 140 mEq/L (5000 mL) [strength represents final solution after mixing]

Elestat® *see* epinastine *on page 330*
Elestrin® *see* estradiol (systemic) *on page 343*
Eletone® *see* emollients *on page 325*

eletriptan (el e TRIP tan)
Synonyms eletriptan hydrobromide
U.S. Brand Names Relpax®
Canadian Brand Names Relpax®
Therapeutic Category Serotonin 5-HT$_{1B, 1D}$ Receptor Agonist
Use Acute treatment of migraine, with or without aura
General Dosage Range Oral: *Adults:* 20-40 mg as a single dose, may repeat (maximum: 80 mg/day)
Dosage Forms
Tablet, oral:
Relpax®: 20 mg, 40 mg

eletriptan hydrobromide *see* eletriptan *on page 323*

Elidel® *see* pimecrolimus *on page 704*
Eligard® *see* leuprolide *on page 516*
Elimite *see* permethrin *on page 691*
Eliphos™ *see* calcium acetate *on page 160*
Elitek™ *see* rasburicase *on page 769*
Elixophyllin® Elixir *see* theophylline *on page 860*
ella® *see* ulipristal *on page 899*
Ellence® *see* epirubicin *on page 333*
Elmiron® *see* pentosan polysulfate sodium *on page 688*
Elocom® (Can) *see* mometasone (topical) *on page 596*
Elocon® *see* mometasone (topical) *on page 596*
Eloxatin® *see* oxaliplatin *on page 658*
Elspar® *see* asparaginase *on page 98*
Eltor® (Can) *see* pseudoephedrine *on page 751*

eltrombopag (el TROM boe pag)

Synonyms eltrombopag olamine; Revolade®; SB-497115; SB-497115-GR
U.S. Brand Names Promacta®
Canadian Brand Names Revolade™
Therapeutic Category Colony Stimulating Factor; Thrombopoietic Agent
Use Treatment of thrombocytopenia in patients with chronic immune (idiopathic) thrombocytopenic purpura (ITP) at risk for bleeding who have had insufficient response to corticosteroids, immune globulin, or splenectomy
General Dosage Range Dosage adjustment recommended in patients with hepatic impairment, of East-Asian ethnicity, or who develop toxicities
  Oral: Adults: 50 mg once daily (maximum: 75 mg/day)
Dosage Forms
  Tablet, oral:
    Promacta®: 25 mg, 50 mg, 75 mg

eltrombopag olamine *see* eltrombopag *on page 324*
Eltroxin® (Can) *see* levothyroxine *on page 522*
Emadine® *see* emedastine *on page 324*
Embeda™ *see* morphine and naltrexone *on page 599*
Emcyt® *see* estramustine *on page 346*
EMD 68843 *see* vilazodone *on page 914*

emedastine (em e DAS teen)

Synonyms emedastine difumarate
U.S. Brand Names Emadine®
Therapeutic Category Antihistamine, H_1 Blocker, Ophthalmic
Use Treatment of allergic conjunctivitis
General Dosage Range Ophthalmic: *Children ≥3 years and Adults:* Instill 1 drop in affected eye up to 4 times/day
Dosage Forms
  Solution, ophthalmic:
    Emadine®: 0.05% (5 mL)

emedastine difumarate *see* emedastine *on page 324*
Emend® *see* aprepitant *on page 91*
Emend® IV (Can) *see* fosaprepitant *on page 400*
Emend® for Injection *see* fosaprepitant *on page 400*
Emetrol® [OTC] *see* fructose, dextrose, and phosphoric acid *on page 403*
EMLA® *see* lidocaine and prilocaine *on page 526*
Emo-Cort® (Can) *see* hydrocortisone (topical) *on page 450*
emollient cream *see* emollients *on page 325*
emollient foam *see* emollients *on page 325*

emollient lotion *see* emollients *on page 325*

emollients (ee MOL ee ents)

Medication Safety Issues
International issues:
Biafine: Topical emulsion [U.S.], but also a brand name for trolamine [multiple international markets]
Synonyms emollient cream; emollient foam; emollient lotion
U.S. Brand Names Atopiclair®; Biafine®; Eletone®; EpiCeram® Skin Barrier; HylatopicPlus™; HylatopicPlus™- Aurstat; Hylatopic™; Mimyx®; Normlshield®; Promiseb™; PruClair™; PruMyx™; PruTect™; PR™; Tropazone™
Therapeutic Category Skin and Mucous Membrane Agent, Miscellaneous; Topical Skin Product
Use Counteract dryness and itchy skin; lubricate and moisturize skin; aid in protection and healing of superficial wounds, burns, and minor abrasions; relief of itching, burning, and pain experienced with various types of dermatoses (including atopic dermatitis, allergic contact dermatitis, and radiation dermatitis); dermal donor and graft site management
General Dosage Range Topical: *Adults:* Apply to affected area 2-3 times daily
Dosage Forms
Aerosol, topical:
HylatopicPlus™: (100 g, 150 g)
HylatopicPlus™- Aurstat: (100 g)
Hylatopic™: (100 g)
Cream, topical:
Atopiclair®: (100 g)
Eletone®: (100 g)
Normlshield®: (120 g)
Promiseb™: (30 g)
PruClair™: (100 g)
PR™: (56.7 g)
Tropazone™: (120 g)
Cream, topical [preservative free]:
Mimyx®: (140 g)
PruMyx™: (140 g)
Emulsion, topical:
Biafine®: (45 g, 90 g)
EpiCeram® Skin Barrier: (90 g)
PruTect™: (45 g, 90 g)
Lotion, topical:
Tropazone™: (140 g)

Emoquette™ *see* ethinyl estradiol and desogestrel *on page 351*
Emsam® *see* selegiline *on page 806*

emtricitabine (em trye SYE ta been)

Synonyms BW524W91; coviracil; FTC
U.S. Brand Names Emtriva®
Canadian Brand Names Emtriva®
Therapeutic Category Antiretroviral Agent, Nucleoside Reverse Transcriptase Inhibitor (NRTI)
Use Treatment of HIV infection in combination with at least two other antiretroviral agents
General Dosage Range Dosage adjustment recommended in patients with renal impairment
Oral:
Capsule: *Children 3 months to 17 years and >33 kg and Adults:* 200 mg once daily
Solution:
Children <3 months: 3 mg/kg/day
Children 3 months to 17 years: 6 mg/kg once daily (maximum: 240 mg/day)
Adults: 240 mg once daily
Dosage Forms
Capsule, oral:
Emtriva®: 200 mg
Solution, oral:
Emtriva®: 10 mg/mL (170 mL)

emtricitabine and tenofovir (em trye SYE ta been & te NOE fo veer)

Synonyms tenofovir and emtricitabine

U.S. Brand Names Truvada®

Canadian Brand Names Truvada®

Therapeutic Category Antiretroviral Agent, Nucleoside Reverse Transcriptase Inhibitor (NRTI); Antiretroviral Agent, Reverse Transcriptase Inhibitor (Nucleotide)

Use Treatment of HIV infection in combination with other antiretroviral agents

General Dosage Range Dosage adjustment recommended in patients with renal impairment

Oral: *Children ≥12 (and >35 kg) and Adults:* 1 tablet (emtricitabine 200 mg and tenofovir 300 mg) once daily

Dosage Forms

Tablet:

Truvada®: Emtricitabine 200 mg and tenofovir 300 mg

emtricitabine, efavirenz, and tenofovir *see* efavirenz, emtricitabine, and tenofovir *on page* 321

emtricitabine, rilpivirine, and tenofovir
(em trye SYE ta been, ril pi VIR een, & te NOE fo veer)

Synonyms FTC/RPV/TDF; rilpivirine, emtricitabine, and tenofovir; tenofovir, emtricitabine, and rilpivirine

U.S. Brand Names Complera™

Therapeutic Category Antiretroviral Agent, Reverse Transcriptase Inhibitor (Non-nucleoside); Antiretroviral Agent, Reverse Transcriptase Inhibitor (Nucleoside); Antiretroviral Agent, Reverse Transcriptase Inhibitor (Nucleotide)

Use Treatment of human immunodeficiency virus type 1 (HIV 1) infection in antiretroviral treatment-naive adult patients

General Dosage Range Oral: *Adults:* One tablet once daily

Dosage Forms

Tablet, oral:

Complera™: Emtricitabine 200 mg, rilpivirine 25 mg, and tenofovir 300 mg

Emtriva® *see* emtricitabine *on page* 325

ENA 713 *see* rivastigmine *on page* 786

Enablex® *see* darifenacin *on page* 253

enalapril (e NAL a pril)

Medication Safety Issues

Sound-alike/look-alike issues:

Enalapril may be confused with Anafranil®, Elavil®, Eldepryl®, ramipril

Administration issues:

Significant differences exist between oral and I.V. dosing. Use caution when converting from one route of administration to another.

International issues:

Acepril [Hungary, Switzerland] may be confused with Accupril which is a brand name for quinapril [U.S., Canada, multiple international markets]

Acepril: Brand name for enalapril [Hungary, Switzerland], but also brand name for captopril [Great Britain]; lisinopril [Malaysia]

Synonyms enalapril maleate; enalaprilat

U.S. Brand Names Vasotec®

Canadian Brand Names Apo-Enalapril®; CO Enalapril; Mylan-Enalapril; Novo-Enalapril; PMS-Enalapril; PRO-Enalapril; RAN™-Enalapril; ratio-Enalapril; Riva-Enalapril; Sandoz-Enalapril; Sig-Enalapril; Taro-Enalapril; Teva-Enalapril; Vasotec®; Vasotec® I.V.

Therapeutic Category Angiotensin-Converting Enzyme (ACE) Inhibitor

Use Treatment of hypertension; treatment of symptomatic heart failure; treatment of asymptomatic left ventricular dysfunction

General Dosage Range Dosage adjustment recommended in patients with renal impairment

I.V.: *Adults:* 0.625-5 mg every 6 hours

Oral:

Children 1 month to 17 years: Initial: 0.08 mg/kg/day (up to 5 mg) in 1-2 divided doses; Maintenance: Up to 0.58 mg/kg (40 mg)

Adults: Initial: 2.5-5 mg/day in 1-2 divided doses; Maintenance: 2.5-40 mg/day in 1-2 divided doses

Dosage Forms
  Injection, solution: 1.25 mg/mL (1 mL, 2 mL)
  Tablet, oral: 2.5 mg, 5 mg, 10 mg, 20 mg
    Vasotec®: 2.5 mg, 5 mg, 10 mg, 20 mg

enalapril and hydrochlorothiazide (e NAL a pril & hye droe klor oh THYE a zide)

Medication Safety Issues
  International issues:
    Norpramin: Brand name for enalapril/hydrochlorothiazide [Portugal], but also the brand name for desipramine [U.S., Canada]; omeprazole [Spain]

Synonyms enalapril maleate and hydrochlorothiazide; hydrochlorothiazide and enalapril

U.S. Brand Names Vaseretic®

Canadian Brand Names Vaseretic®

Therapeutic Category Antihypertensive Agent, Combination

Use Treatment of hypertension

General Dosage Range Oral: *Adults:* Enalapril 5-10 mg and hydrochlorothiazide 12.5-25 mg once daily (maximum: 40 mg/day [enalapril]; 50 mg/day [hydrochlorothiazide])

Dosage Forms
  Tablet: 5/12.5: Enalapril 5 mg and hydrochlorothiazide 12.5 mg; 10/25: Enalapril 10 mg and hydrochlorothiazide 25 mg
    Vaseretic®: 10/25: enalapril 10 mg and hydrochlorothiazide 25 mg

enalaprilat *see* enalapril *on page 326*

enalapril maleate *see* enalapril *on page 326*

enalapril maleate and hydrochlorothiazide *see* enalapril and hydrochlorothiazide *on page 327*

Enbrel® *see* etanercept *on page 350*

Enbrel® SureClick® *see* etanercept *on page 350*

Encare® [OTC] *see* nonoxynol 9 *on page 632*

Encora® *see* vitamins (multiple/oral) *on page 919*

EndaCof-DC *see* pseudoephedrine and codeine *on page 752*

EndaCof-DM *see* brompheniramine, pseudoephedrine, and dextromethorphan *on page 144*

EndaCof-PD *see* brompheniramine, pseudoephedrine, and dextromethorphan *on page 144*

Endantadine® (Can) *see* amantadine *on page 62*

EndoAvitene® *see* collagen hemostat *on page 233*

Endocet® *see* oxycodone and acetaminophen *on page 662*

Endodan® *see* oxycodone and aspirin *on page 664*

Endo®-Levodopa/Carbidopa (Can) *see* carbidopa and levodopa *on page 174*

Endometrin® *see* progesterone *on page 741*

Enduron *see* methyclothiazide *on page 574*

Enemeez® [OTC] *see* docusate *on page 302*

Enemeez® Plus [OTC] *see* docusate *on page 302*

Ener-B® [OTC] *see* cyanocobalamin *on page 241*

Enerjets [OTC] *see* caffeine *on page 157*

Enfamil® D-Vi-Sol™ [OTC] *see* cholecalciferol *on page 204*

Enfamil® Glucose [OTC] *see* dextrose *on page 273*

enflurane (EN floo rane)

Medication Safety Issues
  Sound-alike/look-alike issues:
    Enflurane may be confused with isoflurane
  High alert medication:
    The Institute for Safe Medication Practices (ISMP) includes this medication among its list of drug classes which have a heightened risk of causing significant patient harm when used in error.

U.S. Brand Names Compound 347™

Therapeutic Category General Anesthetic

Use Maintenance of general anesthesia

Note: Use for induction of general anesthesia is an FDA-labeled indication; however, it is not recommended clinically due to its irritant properties and unpleasant odor which causes breath-holding and coughing. In addition, other labeled indications that are not routinely used and/or recommended clinically include use as analgesia during vaginal delivery and use as an adjunct to other general anesthetic agents during Cesarean section delivery.

General Dosage Range Inhalation: *Adults:* Maintenance: 0.5% to 3% (maximum concentration: 3%)

Dosage Forms
Liquid, for inhalation:
Compound 347™: >99.9% (250 mL)

enfuvirtide (en FYOO vir tide)

Synonyms T-20
U.S. Brand Names Fuzeon®
Canadian Brand Names Fuzeon®
Therapeutic Category Antiretroviral Agent, Fusion Protein Inhibitor
Use Treatment of HIV-1 infection in combination with other antiretroviral agents in treatment-experienced patients with evidence of HIV-1 replication despite ongoing antiretroviral therapy
General Dosage Range Dosage adjustment recommended in patients with renal impairment
SubQ:
Children 6-16 years: 2 mg/kg twice daily (maximum: 90 mg/dose)
Adolescents ≥16 years and Adults: 90 mg twice daily
Dosage Forms
Injection, powder for reconstitution [preservative free]:
Fuzeon®: 108 mg

ENG *see* etonogestrel *on page 361*
Engerix-B® *see* hepatitis B vaccine (recombinant) *on page 438*
Engerix-B® and Havrix® *see* hepatitis A and hepatitis B recombinant vaccine *on page 437*
enhanced-potency inactivated poliovirus vaccine *see* poliovirus vaccine (inactivated) *on page 717*
Enjuva™ *see* estrogens (conjugated B/synthetic) *on page 347*
Enlon® *see* edrophonium *on page 320*
Enlon-Plus® *see* edrophonium and atropine *on page 321*

enoxaparin (ee noks a PA rin)

Medication Safety Issues
Sound-alike/look-alike issues:
Lovenox® may be confused with Lasix®, Levaquin®, Lotronex®, Protonix®
High alert medication:
The Institute for Safe Medication Practices (ISMP) includes this medication among its list of drugs which have a heightened risk of causing significant patient harm when used in error.
2009 National Patient Safety Goals:
The Joint Commission (TJC) requires healthcare organizations that provide anticoagulant therapy to have a process in place to reduce the risk of anticoagulant-associated patient harm. Patients receiving anticoagulants should receive individualized care through a defined process that includes standardized ordering, dispensing, administration, monitoring and education. This does not apply to routine short-term use of anticoagulants for prevention of venous thromboembolism when the expectation is that the patient's laboratory values will remain within or close to normal values (NPSG.03.05.01).
Synonyms enoxaparin sodium
U.S. Brand Names Lovenox®
Canadian Brand Names Enoxaparin Injection; Lovenox®; Lovenox® HP
Therapeutic Category Anticoagulant (Other)
Use
Acute coronary syndromes: Unstable angina (UA), non-ST-elevation (NSTEMI), and ST-elevation myocardial infarction (STEMI)
DVT prophylaxis: Following hip or knee replacement surgery, abdominal surgery, or in medical patients with severely-restricted mobility during acute illness who are at risk for thromboembolic complications
DVT treatment (acute): Inpatient treatment (patients with and without pulmonary embolism) and outpatient treatment (patients without pulmonary embolism)

Note: High-risk patients include those with one or more of the following risk factors: >40 years of age, obesity, general anesthesia lasting >30 minutes, malignancy, history of deep vein thrombosis or pulmonary embolism

General Dosage Range
SubQ:
Adults: Prophylaxis: 30 mg every 12 hours **or** 40 mg once daily; Treatment: 1 mg/kg every 12 hours **or** 1.5 mg/kg once daily
STEMI indication only:
<75 years: 30 mg I.V. bolus plus 1 mg/kg SubQ every 12 hours
≥75 years: 0.75 mg/kg SubQ every 12 hours; **Note:** I.V. bolus is omitted
Elderly: Refer to adult dosing.

Dosage Forms
Injection, solution:
Lovenox®: 100 mg/mL (3 mL)
Injection, solution [preservative free]: 30 mg/0.3 mL (0.3 mL); 40 mg/0.4 mL (0.4 mL); 60 mg/0.6 mL (0.6 mL); 80 mg/0.8 mL (0.8 mL); 100 mg/mL (1 mL); 120 mg/0.8 mL (0.8 mL); 150 mg/mL (1 mL)
Lovenox®: 30 mg/0.3 mL (0.3 mL); 40 mg/0.4 mL (0.4 mL); 60 mg/0.6 mL (0.6 mL); 80 mg/0.8 mL (0.8 mL); 100 mg/mL (1 mL); 120 mg/0.8 mL (0.8 mL); 150 mg/mL (1 mL)

Enoxaparin Injection (Can) *see enoxaparin on page 328*
enoxaparin sodium *see enoxaparin on page 328*
Enpresse® *see ethinyl estradiol and levonorgestrel on page 353*

entacapone (en TA ka pone)
U.S. Brand Names Comtan®
Canadian Brand Names Comtan®
Therapeutic Category Anti-Parkinson Agent; Reverse COMT Inhibitor
Use Adjunct to levodopa/carbidopa therapy in patients with idiopathic Parkinson disease who experience "wearing-off" symptoms at the end of a dosing interval
General Dosage Range Oral: *Adults:* 200 mg with each dose of levodopa/carbidopa (maximum: 1600 mg/day)
Dosage Forms
Tablet, oral:
Comtan®: 200 mg

entacapone, carbidopa, and levodopa *see levodopa, carbidopa, and entacapone on page 519*

entecavir (en TE ka veer)
U.S. Brand Names Baraclude®
Canadian Brand Names Baraclude®
Therapeutic Category Antiretroviral Agent, Reverse Transcriptase Inhibitor (Nucleoside)
Use Treatment of chronic hepatitis B infection, with compensated or decompensated liver disease, in adults with evidence of active viral replication and either evidence of persistent transaminase elevations or histologically-active disease
General Dosage Range
Oral:
Children <16 years: Dosage not established
Adolescents ≥16 years: Nucleoside naive: 0.5 mg once daily; Lamivudine- or telbivudine-resistant: 1 mg once daily
Adults: Nucleoside-naive: 0.5 mg once daily; Lamivudine- or telbivudine-resistant: 1 mg once daily
Dosage Forms
Solution, oral:
Baraclude®: 0.05 mg/mL (210 mL)
Tablet, oral:
Baraclude®: 0.5 mg, 1 mg

Entereg® *see alvimopan on page 61*
Entero-H™ *see barium on page 114*
enterotoxigenic *Escherichia coli* and *Vibrio cholera* vaccine *see traveler's diarrhea and cholera vaccine (Canada only) on page 883*
Entero Vu™ *see barium on page 114*

Entero VU™ 24% *see* barium *on page 114*

Entertainer's Secret® [OTC] *see* saliva substitute *on page 798*

Entex® LA (Can) *see* guaifenesin and pseudoephedrine *on page 429*

Entocort® (Can) *see* budesonide (systemic, oral inhalation) *on page 145*

Entocort® EC *see* budesonide (systemic, oral inhalation) *on page 145*

Entre-S *see* chlorpheniramine, pseudoephedrine, and dextromethorphan *on page 201*

Entrophen® (Can) *see* aspirin *on page 98*

Entsol® [OTC] *see* sodium chloride *on page 818*

Enulose *see* lactulose *on page 507*

Eovist® *see* gadoxetate *on page 409*

EPEG *see* etoposide *on page 361*

ephedrine (systemic) (e FED rin)

Medication Safety Issues
Sound-alike/look-alike issues:
EPHEDrine may be confused with Epifrin®, EPINEPHrine

Synonyms ephedrine sulfate

Tall-Man ePHEDrine

Therapeutic Category Alpha/Beta Agonist

Use Treatment of nasal congestion, anesthesia-induced hypotension

General Dosage Range
I.V.:
  Children: 0.2-0.3 mg/kg/dose every 4-6 hours
  Adults: 5-25 mg/dose; repeat after 5-10 minutes as needed, then every 3-4 hours (maximum: 150 mg/day)
  Oral: *Children ≥12 years and Adults:* 12.5-50 mg every 4 hours as needed (maximum: 150 mg/day)

Dosage Forms
Capsule, oral: 25 mg
Injection, solution [preservative free]: 50 mg/mL (1 mL)

ephedrine, chlorpheniramine, phenylephrine, and carbetapentane *see* chlorpheniramine, ephedrine, phenylephrine, and carbetapentane *on page 199*

ephedrine sulfate *see* ephedrine (systemic) *on page 330*

EpiCeram® Skin Barrier *see* emollients *on page 325*

Epi-Clenz™ [OTC] *see* alcohol (ethyl) *on page 47*

epidoxorubicin *see* epirubicin *on page 333*

Epidrin [DSC] *see* acetaminophen, isometheptene, and dichloralphenazone *on page 34*

Epiduo® *see* adapalene and benzoyl peroxide *on page 40*

Epi E-Z Pen® (Can) *see* epinephrine (systemic, oral inhalation) *on page 331*

Epiflur™ *see* fluoride *on page 386*

Epifoam® *see* pramoxine and hydrocortisone *on page 731*

Epiklor™ *see* potassium chloride *on page 724*

Epiklor™/25 *see* potassium chloride *on page 724*

epinastine (ep i NAS teen)

Synonyms epinastine hydrochloride

U.S. Brand Names Elestat®

Therapeutic Category Antihistamine, H₁ Blocker, Ophthalmic

Use Treatment of allergic conjunctivitis

General Dosage Range Ophthalmic: *Children ≥3 years and Adults:* Instill 1 drop into each eye twice daily

Dosage Forms
Solution, ophthalmic: 0.05% (5 mL)
  Elestat®: 0.05% (5 mL)

epinastine hydrochloride *see* epinastine *on page 330*

epinephrine (systemic, oral inhalation) (ep i NEF rin)

Medication Safety Issues

Sound-alike/look-alike issues:
EPINEPHrine may be confused with ePHEDrine

Epifrin® may be confused with ephedrine, EpiPen®

EpiPen® may be confused with Epifrin®

High alert medication:
The Institute for Safe Medication Practices (ISMP) includes this medication among its list of drugs which have a heightened risk of causing significant patient harm when used in error.

Administration issues:
Medication errors have occurred due to confusion with epinephrine products expressed as ratio strengths (eg, 1:1000 vs 1:10,000).

Epinephrine 1:1000 = 1 mg/mL and is most commonly used I.M.

Epinephrine 1:10,000 = 0.1 mg/mL and is used I.V.

Medication errors have occurred when topical epinephrine 1 mg/mL (1:1000) has been inadvertently injected. Vials of injectable and topical epinephrine look very similar. Epinephrine should always be appropriately labeled with the intended administration.

International issues:
EpiPen [U.S., Canada, and multiple international markets] may be confused with Epigen brand name for glycyrrhizinic acid [Argentina, Mexico, Russia] and Epopen brand name for epoetin alfa [Spain]

Synonyms adrenaline; epinephrine bitartrate; epinephrine hydrochloride; racemic epinephrine; racepinephrine

Tall-Man EPINEPHrine

U.S. Brand Names Adrenaclick™ [DSC]; Adrenalin®; EpiPen 2-Pak®; EpiPen Jr 2-Pak®; EpiPen® Jr. [DSC]; EpiPen® [DSC]; Primatene® Mist [OTC] [DSC]; S2® [OTC]; Twinject®

Canadian Brand Names Adrenalin®; Epi E-Z Pen®; EpiPen®; EpiPen® Jr; Twinject®

Therapeutic Category Alpha/Beta Agonist

Use Treatment of bronchospasms, bronchial asthma, viral croup, anaphylactic reactions, cardiac arrest; added to local anesthetics to decrease systemic absorption of intraspinal and local anesthetics and increase duration of action; decrease superficial hemorrhage

General Dosage Range

I.M.:
Adults: 0.3-0.5 mg (**1:1000** [1 mg/mL] solution) every 15-20 minutes

EpiPen® Jr., Twinject®: *Children 15-29 kg:* 0.15 mg as single dose; may repeat if needed

EpiPen®, Twinject®: *Children ≥30 kg and Adults:* 0.3 mg as single dose; may repeat if needed

Inhalation: *Children ≥4 years and Adults:* 1 inhalation; may repeat once after 1 minute, then do not use again for at least 3 hours

I.V. (**1:10,000** [0.1 mg/mL] solution):
Children: 0.01 mg/kg kg (maximum single dose: 1 mg) every 3-5 minutes as needed **or** 0.1-1 mcg/kg/minute as a continuous infusion **or** 0.01 mg/kg every 20 minutes (hypersensitivity reaction)

Adults: 1 mg every 3-5 minutes (up to 0.2 mg/kg) **or** 1-10 mcg/minute as a continuous infusion

Nebulization (S2® Racepinephrine, OTC):
Children <4 years: Jet nebulizer: 0.05 mL/kg (maximum dose: 0.5 mL) diluted in 3 mL NS up to every 2 hours

Children ≥4 years and Adults:

Hand-bulb nebulizer: Add 0.5 mL (~10 drops) to nebulizer; 1-3 inhalations up to every 3 hours if needed

Jet nebulizer: Add 0.5 mL (~10 drops) to nebulizer and dilute with 3 mL of NS. Administer over ~15 minutes every 3-4 hours as needed.

SubQ:
Children: 0.01 mg/kg (**1:1000** [1 mg/mL] solution) every 20 minutes for 3 doses or as condition requires (maximum: 0.3 mg/dose)

Adults: 0.3-0.5 mg (**1:1000** [1 mg/mL] solution) every 15-20 minutes for 3 doses or as condition requires

EpiPen® Jr, Twinject®: *Children 15-29 kg:* 0.15 mg as single dose; may repeat if needed

EpiPen®, Twinject®: *Children ≥30 kg and Adults:* 0.3 mg as single dose; may repeat if needed

Dosage Forms
Injection, solution: 0.1 mg/mL (10 mL); 0.15 mg/0.15 mL (1.1 mL); 0.3 mg/0.3 mL (1.1 mL); 1 mg/mL (1 mL, 30 mL)
Adrenalin®: 1 mg/mL (1 mL, 30 mL)
EpiPen 2-Pak®: 0.3 mg/0.3 mL (2 mL)
EpiPen Jr 2-Pak®: 0.15 mg/0.3 mL (2 mL)
Twinject®: 0.15 mg/0.15 mL (1.1 mL); 0.3 mg/0.3 mL (1.1 mL)
Injection, solution [preservative free]: 1 mg/mL (1 mL)
Solution, for oral inhalation [preservative free]:
S2® [OTC]: 2.25% (0.5 mL)

epinephrine (nasal) (ep i NEF rin)
Medication Safety Issues
Sound-alike/look-alike issues:
EPINEPHrine may be confused with ePHEDrine
Synonyms adrenaline; epinephrine hydrochloride
Tall-Man EPINEPHrine
U.S. Brand Names Adrenalin®
Canadian Brand Names Adrenalin®
Therapeutic Category Alpha/Beta Agonist
Use Treatment of nasal congestion
General Dosage Range Intranasal: *Children ≥6 years and Adults:* Apply **1:1000** (1 mg/mL) solution locally as drops, spray, or with sterile swab
Dosage Forms
Solution, intranasal:
Adrenalin®: 1 mg/mL (30 mL)

epinephrine and articaine hydrochloride *see* articaine and epinephrine *on page 95*

epinephrine and chlorpheniramine (ep i NEF rin & klor fen IR a meen)
Synonyms insect sting kit
U.S. Brand Names Ana-Kit®
Therapeutic Category Antidote
Use Anaphylaxis emergency treatment of insect bites or stings by the sensitive patient that may occur within minutes of insect sting or exposure to an allergic substance
General Dosage Range
I.M., SubQ: Epinephrine (1:1000):
Children <2 years: 0.05-0.1 mL
Children 2-6 years: 0.15 mL
Children 6-12 years: 0.2 mL
Children >12 years and Adults: 0.3 mL
Oral: Chlorpheniramine (2 mg/tablet):
Children <6 years: 1 tablet
Children 6-12 years: 2 tablets
Children >12 years and Adults: 4 tablets
Dosage Forms
Kit:
Ana-Kit®: Epinephrine 1:1000 (1 mL), chlorpheniramine chewable tablet 2 mg (4), sterile alcohol pads (2), tourniquet (1)

epinephrine and lidocaine *see* lidocaine and epinephrine *on page 525*
epinephrine bitartrate *see* epinephrine (systemic, oral inhalation) *on page 331*
epinephrine bitartrate and bupivacaine hydrochloride *see* bupivacaine and epinephrine *on page 148*
epinephrine hydrochloride *see* epinephrine (nasal) *on page 332*
epinephrine hydrochloride *see* epinephrine (systemic, oral inhalation) *on page 331*
EpiPen® [DSC] *see* epinephrine (systemic, oral inhalation) *on page 331*
EpiPen® (Can) *see* epinephrine (systemic, oral inhalation) *on page 331*
EpiPen 2-Pak® *see* epinephrine (systemic, oral inhalation) *on page 331*

EpiPen® Jr. [DSC] *see* epinephrine (systemic, oral inhalation) *on page 331*
EpiPen® Jr (Can) *see* epinephrine (systemic, oral inhalation) *on page 331*
EpiPen Jr 2-Pak® *see* epinephrine (systemic, oral inhalation) *on page 331*
epipodophyllotoxin *see* etoposide *on page 361*
epipodophyllotoxin *see* etoposide phosphate *on page 361*
EpiQuin® Micro *see* hydroquinone *on page 453*

epirubicin (ep i ROO bi sin)

Medication Safety Issues
Sound-alike/look-alike issues:
Epirubicin may be confused with DOXOrubicin, DAUNOrubicin, eribulin, idarubicin
International issues:
Ellence [U.S.] may be confused with Elase brand name for dornase alfa [Chile, France, Malaysia]
High alert medication:
This drug is in a class the Institute for Safe Medication Practices (ISMP) includes among its list of drug classes which have a heightened risk of causing significant patient harm when used in error.
Synonyms epidoxorubicin; epirubicin hydrochloride; pidorubicin; pidorubicin hydrochloride
U.S. Brand Names Ellence®
Canadian Brand Names Ellence®; Pharmorubicin®
Therapeutic Category Antineoplastic Agent, Anthracycline; Antineoplastic Agent, Antibiotic
Use Adjuvant therapy for primary breast cancer
General Dosage Range Dosage adjustment recommended in patients with hepatic or renal impairment or who develop toxicities
I.V.: *Adults:* 100 mg/m^2 on day 1 every 3 weeks **or** 60 mg/m^2 on days 1 and 8 every 4 weeks
Dosage Forms
Injection, powder for reconstitution: 50 mg
Injection, solution [preservative free]: 2 mg/mL (25 mL, 100 mL)
Ellence®: 2 mg/mL (25 mL, 100 mL)

epirubicin hydrochloride *see* epirubicin *on page 333*
Epitol® *see* carbamazepine *on page 171*
Epival® (Can) *see* divalproex *on page 300*
Epival® I.V. (Can) *see* valproic acid *on page 904*
Epivir® *see* lamivudine *on page 508*
Epivir-HBV® *see* lamivudine *on page 508*

eplerenone (e PLER en one)

Medication Safety Issues
Sound-alike/look-alike issues:
Inspra™ may be confused with Spiriva®
U.S. Brand Names Inspra™
Therapeutic Category Antihypertensive Agent; Selective Aldosterone Blocker
Use Treatment of hypertension (may be used alone or in combination with other antihypertensive agents); treatment of heart failure (HF) following acute MI
General Dosage Range Dosage adjustment recommended in patients on concomitant therapy or based on potassium concentrations
Oral: *Adults:* Initial: 25-50 mg once daily; Maintenance: 50 mg once or twice daily (maximum: 100 mg/day)
Dosage Forms
Tablet, oral: 25 mg, 50 mg
Inspra™: 25 mg, 50 mg

EPO *see* epoetin alfa *on page 333*

epoetin alfa (e POE e tin AL fa)

Medication Safety Issues
Sound-alike/look-alike issues:
Epoetin alfa may be confused with darbepoetin alfa, epoetin beta

▶

◀ Epogen® may be confused with Neupogen®

International issues:

Epopen [Spain] may be confused with EpiPen brand name for epinephrine [U.S., Canada, and multiple international markets]

Synonyms rHuEPO-α; EPO; erythropoiesis-stimulating agent (ESA); erythropoietin

U.S. Brand Names Epogen®; Procrit®

Canadian Brand Names Eprex®

Therapeutic Category Colony-Stimulating Factor

Use Treatment of anemia due to concurrent myelosuppressive chemotherapy in patients with cancer (nonmyeloid malignancies) receiving chemotherapy (palliative intent) for a planned minimum of 2 additional months of chemotherapy; treatment of anemia due to chronic kidney disease (including patients on dialysis and not on dialysis) to decrease the need for RBC transfusion; treatment of anemia associated with HIV (zidovudine) therapy when endogenous erythropoietin levels ≤500 mUnits/mL; reduction of allogeneic RBC transfusion for elective, noncardiac, nonvascular surgery when perioperative hemoglobin is >10 to ≤13 g/dL and there is a high risk for blood loss

Note: Epoetin is **not** indicated for use under the following conditions:

• Cancer patients receiving hormonal therapy, therapeutic biologic products, or radiation therapy unless also receiving concurrent myelosuppressive chemotherapy

• Cancer patients receiving myelosuppressive chemotherapy when the expected outcome is curative

• Surgery patients who are willing to donate autologous blood

• Surgery patients undergoing cardiac or vascular surgery

• As a substitute for RBC transfusion in patients requiring immediate correction of anemia

Note: In clinical trials (and one meta analysis), epoetin has not demonstrated improved quality of life, fatigue, or well-being.

General Dosage Range I.V., SubQ: Children and Adults: Dosage varies greatly depending on indication

Dosage Forms

Injection, solution:

Epogen®: 10,000 units/mL (2 mL); 20,000 units/mL (1 mL)

Procrit®: 10,000 units/mL (2 mL); 20,000 units/mL (1 mL)

Injection, solution [preservative free]:

Epogen®: 2000 units/mL (1 mL); 3000 units/mL (1 mL); 4000 units/mL (1 mL); 10,000 units/mL (1 mL)

Procrit®: 2000 units/mL (1 mL); 3000 units/mL (1 mL); 4000 units/mL (1 mL); 10,000 units/mL (1 mL); 40,000 units/mL (1 mL)

Dosage Forms - Canada

Injection, solution [preservative free]:

Eprex®: 1000 units/0.5 mL (0.5 mL), 2000 units/0.5 mL (0.5 mL), 3000 units/0.3 mL (0.3 mL), 4000 units/ 0.4 mL (0.4 mL), 5000 units/0.5 mL (0.5 mL), 6000 units/0.6 mL (0.6 mL), 8000 units/0.8 mL (0.8 mL), 10,000 units/mL (1 mL), 20,000 units/0.5 mL (0.5 mL), 30,000 units/0.75 mL (0.75 mL), 40,000 units/mL (1 mL) [contains polysorbate 80; prefilled syringe, free of human serum albumin]

Epogen® see epoetin alfa on page 333

epoprostenol (e poe PROST en ole)

Medication Safety Issues

High alert medication:

The Institute for Safe Medication Practices (ISMP) includes this medication among its list of drugs which have a heightened risk of causing significant patient harm when used in error.

Synonyms epoprostenol sodium; PGI$_2$; PGX; prostacyclin

U.S. Brand Names Flolan®; Veletri®

Canadian Brand Names Flolan®

Therapeutic Category Platelet Inhibitor

Use Treatment of pulmonary arterial hypertension (PAH) (WHO Group I) in patients with NYHA Class III or IV symptoms to improve exercise capacity

General Dosage Range

I.V.:

Adults: Initial: 1-2 ng/kg/minute, increase dose in increments of 1-2 ng/kg/minute every 15 minutes or longer until dose-limiting side effects are noted or response to epoprostenol plateaus

Dosage Forms
Injection, powder for reconstitution: 0.5 mg, 1.5 mg
Flolan®: 0.5 mg, 1.5 mg
Veletri®: 1.5 mg

epoprostenol sodium *see* epoprostenol *on page 334*
epothilone B lactam *see* ixabepilone *on page 497*
Eprex® (Can) *see* epoetin alfa *on page 333*

eprosartan (ep roe SAR tan)
U.S. Brand Names Teveten®
Canadian Brand Names Teveten®
Therapeutic Category Angiotensin II Receptor Antagonist
Use Treatment of hypertension; may be used alone or in combination with other antihypertensives
General Dosage Range Oral: *Adults:* Initial: 400-600 mg once daily; Maintenance: 400-800 mg/day in 1-2 divided doses
Dosage Forms
Tablet, oral:
Teveten®: 400 mg, 600 mg

eprosartan and hydrochlorothiazide (ep roe SAR tan & hye droe klor oh THYE a zide)
Synonyms eprosartan mesylate and hydrochlorothiazide; hydrochlorothiazide and eprosartan
U.S. Brand Names Teveten® HCT
Canadian Brand Names Teveten® HCT; Teveten® Plus
Therapeutic Category Angiotensin II Antagonist Combination; Antihypertensive Agent, Combination; Diuretic, Thiazide
Use Treatment of hypertension (not indicated for initial treatment)
General Dosage Range Oral: *Adults:* Eprosartan 600 mg and hydrochlorothiazide 12.5-25 mg once daily
Dosage Forms
Tablet:
Teveten® HCT: 600 mg/12.5 mg: Eprosartan 600 mg and hydrochlorothiazide 12.5 mg; 600 mg/25 mg: Eprosartan 600 mg and hydrochlorothiazide 25 mg

eprosartan mesylate and hydrochlorothiazide *see* eprosartan and hydrochlorothiazide *on page 335*
epsilon aminocaproic acid *see* aminocaproic acid *on page 65*
epsom salts *see* magnesium sulfate *on page 547*
EPT *see* teniposide *on page 850*
eptacog alfa (activated) *see* factor VIIa (recombinant) *on page 365*

eptifibatide (ep TIF i ba tide)
Medication Safety Issues
High alert medication:
The Institute for Safe Medication Practices (ISMP) includes this medication among its list of drugs which have a heightened risk of causing significant patient harm when used in error.
Synonyms intrifiban
U.S. Brand Names Integrilin®
Canadian Brand Names Integrilin®
Therapeutic Category Antiplatelet Agent
Use Treatment of patients with acute coronary syndrome (unstable angina/non-ST-segment elevation myocardial infarction [UA/NSTEMI]), including patients who are to be managed medically and those undergoing percutaneous coronary intervention (PCI including angioplasty, intracoronary stenting)
General Dosage Range Dosage adjustment recommended in patients with renal impairment
I.V.: *Adults:* Bolus: 180 mcg/kg (maximum: 22.6 mg), repeat once for PCI; Infusion: 2 mcg/kg/minute (maximum: 15 mg/hour)
Dosage Forms
Injection, solution:
Integrilin®: 0.75 mg/mL (100 mL); 2 mg/mL (10 mL, 100 mL)

Epzicom® *see* abacavir and lamivudine *on page 20*
Equalactin® [OTC] *see* polycarbophil *on page 717*
Equalizer Gas Relief [OTC] *see* simethicone *on page 812*
Equanil *see* meprobamate *on page 562*
Equetro® *see* carbamazepine *on page 171*
ER-086526 *see* eribulin *on page 337*
Eraxis™ *see* anidulafungin *on page 79*
Erbitux® *see* cetuximab *on page 190*

ergocalciferol (er goe kal SIF e role)

Medication Safety Issues
Sound-alike/look-alike issues:
Calciferol™ may be confused with calcitriol
Drisdol® may be confused with Drysol™
Ergocalciferol may be confused with alfacalcidol, cholecalciferol
Administration issues:
Liquid vitamin D preparations have the potential for dosing errors when administered to infants. Droppers should be clearly marked to easily provide 400 international units. For products intended for infants, the FDA recommends that accompanying droppers deliver no more than 400 international units per dose.

Synonyms activated ergosterol; D2; viosterol; vitamin D2
U.S. Brand Names Calciferol™ [OTC]; Drisdol®; Drisdol® [OTC]
Canadian Brand Names Drisdol®; Ostoforte®
Therapeutic Category Vitamin D Analog
Use Treatment of refractory rickets, hypophosphatemia, hypoparathyroidism; dietary supplement
General Dosage Range Oral:
Children 0-12 months: Adequate intake: 400 int. units/day
Children 1 year to Adults ≤70 years: RDA: 600 int. units/day
Elderly >70 years: RDA: 800 int. units/day
Dosage Forms
Capsule, oral: 50,000 int. units
Drisdol®: 50,000 int. units
Capsule, softgel, oral: 50,000 int. units, 50,000 units
Solution, oral: 8000 int. units/mL (60 mL)
Calciferol™ [OTC]: 8000 int. units/mL (60 mL)
Drisdol® [OTC]: 8000 int. units/mL (60 mL)
Tablet, oral: 400 int. units

ergoloid mesylates (ER goe loid MES i lates)

Medication Safety Issues
BEERS Criteria medication:
This drug may be inappropriate for use in geriatric patients (low severity risk).
Synonyms dihydroergotoxine; dihydrogenated ergot alkaloids; Hydergine [DSC]
Canadian Brand Names Hydergine®
Therapeutic Category Ergot Alkaloid and Derivative
Use Treatment of cerebrovascular insufficiency in primary progressive dementia, Alzheimer dementia, and senile onset
General Dosage Range Oral: *Adults:* Initial: 1 mg 3 times/day; Maintenance: 3-12 mg/day in 3 divided doses
Dosage Forms
Tablet, oral: 1 mg

Ergomar® *see* ergotamine *on page 336*

ergotamine (er GOT a meen)

Synonyms ergotamine tartrate
U.S. Brand Names Ergomar®
Therapeutic Category Ergot Alkaloid and Derivative

Use Abort or prevent vascular headaches, such as migraine, migraine variants, or so-called "histaminic cephalalgia"

General Dosage Range
Sublingual: *Adults:* 1 tablet initially, then 1 tablet every 30 minutes if needed (maximum: 3 tablets/day; 5 tablets/week)

Dosage Forms
Tablet, sublingual:
Ergomar®: 2 mg

ergotamine and caffeine (er GOT a meen & KAF een)

Medication Safety Issues
Sound-alike/look-alike issues:
Cafergot® may be confused with Carafate®

Synonyms caffeine and ergotamine; ergotamine tartrate and caffeine

U.S. Brand Names Cafergot®; Migergot®

Canadian Brand Names Cafergor®

Therapeutic Category Antimigraine Agent; Ergot Derivative; Stimulant

Use Abort or prevent vascular headaches, such as migraine, migraine variants, or so-called "histaminic cephalalgia"

General Dosage Range
Oral: *Adults:* 2 tablets initially, then 1 tablet every 30 minutes as needed (maximum: 6 tablets/attack; 10 tablets/week)
Rectal: *Adults:* 1 suppository initially; may repeat after 1 hour if needed (maximum: 2 doses/attack; 5 doses/week)

Dosage Forms
Suppository, rectal:
Migergot®: Ergotamine tartrate 2 mg and caffeine 100 mg (12s)
Tablet, oral: Ergotamine tartrate 1 mg and caffeine 100 mg
Cafergot®: Ergotamine tartrate 1 mg and caffeine 100 mg

ergotamine tartrate *see* ergotamine *on page* 336

ergotamine tartrate and caffeine *see* ergotamine and caffeine *on page* 337

eribulin (er i BUE lin)

Medication Safety Issues
Sound-alike/look-alike issues:
Eribulin may be confused with epirubicin, erlotinib
High alert medication:
This medication is in a class the Institute for Safe Medication Practices (ISMP) includes among its list of drug classes which have a heightened risk of causing significant patient harm when used in error.

Synonyms B1939; E7389; ER-086526; eribulin mesylate; halichondrin B analog

U.S. Brand Names Halaven™

Therapeutic Category Antineoplastic Agent, Antimicrotubular

Use Treatment of metastatic breast cancer in patients who have received at least 2 prior chemotherapy regimens

General Dosage Range Dosage adjustment recommended in patients with renal or hepatic impairment or who develop toxicities
I.V.: *Adults:* 1.4 mg/m^2/dose days 1 and 8 every 3 weeks

Dosage Forms
Injection, solution:
Halaven™: 0.5 mg/mL (2 mL)

eribulin mesylate *see* eribulin *on page* 337

erlotinib (er LOE tye nib)

Medication Safety Issues
Sound-alike/look-alike issues:
Erlotinib may be confused with crizotinib, eribulin, gefitinib, imatinib, SUNItinib, vandetanib
High alert medication:
This medication is in a class the Institute for Safe Medication Practices (ISMP) includes among its list of drug classes which have a heightened risk of causing significant patient harm when used in error.

Synonyms CP358774; erlotinib hydrochloride; OSI-774

U.S. Brand Names Tarceva®

Canadian Brand Names Tarceva®

Therapeutic Category Antineoplastic Agent, Tyrosine Kinase Inhibitor

Use Treatment of locally advanced or metastatic nonsmall cell lung cancer (NSCLC) refractory to at least 1 prior chemotherapy regimen (as monotherapy); maintenance treatment of locally advanced or metastatic NCSLC which has not progressed after 4-6 cycles of first line platinum-based chemotherapy; locally advanced, unresectable or metastatic pancreatic cancer (first-line therapy in combination with gemcitabine)

General Dosage Range Dosage adjustment recommended in patients with hepatic impairment, on concomitant therapy, who smoke, or who develop toxicities
Oral: *Adults:* 100-150 mg/day

Dosage Forms
Tablet, oral:
Tarceva®: 25 mg, 100 mg, 150 mg

erlotinib hydrochloride *see* erlotinib *on page 338*
E-R-O® [OTC] *see* carbamide peroxide *on page 172*
Errin® *see* norethindrone *on page 633*
Ertaczo® *see* sertaconazole *on page 809*

ertapenem (er ta PEN em)

Medication Safety Issues
Sound-alike/look-alike issues:
Ertapenem may be confused with imipenem, meropenem
INVanz® may be confused with AVINza™, I.V. vancomycin

Synonyms ertapenem sodium; L-749,345; MK0826

U.S. Brand Names INVanz®

Canadian Brand Names Invanz®

Therapeutic Category Antibiotic, Carbapenem

Use Treatment of the following moderate-to-severe infections: Complicated intraabdominal infections, complicated skin and skin structure infections (including diabetic foot infections without osteomyelitis), complicated UTI (including pyelonephritis), acute pelvic infections (including postpartum endomyome-tritis, septic abortion, postsurgical gynecologic infections), and community-acquired pneumonia. Prophylaxis of surgical site infection following elective colorectal surgery. Antibacterial coverage includes aerobic gram-positive organisms, aerobic gram-negative organisms, and anaerobic organisms.

Note: Methicillin-resistant *Staphylococcus aureus, Enterococcus* spp, penicillin-resistant strains of *Streptococcus pneumoniae, Acinetobacter*, and *Pseudomonas aeruginosa*, are **resistant** to ertapenem.

General Dosage Range Dosage adjustment recommended in patients with renal impairment
I.M., I.V.:
Children 3 months to 12 years: 15 mg/kg twice daily (maximum: 1 g/day)
Adolescents ≥13 years and Adults: 1 g once daily or as single dose

Dosage Forms
Injection, powder for reconstitution:
INVanz®: 1 g

ertapenem sodium *see* ertapenem *on page 338*
Erwinia asparaginase *see* asparaginase *on page 98*
Ery *see* erythromycin (topical) *on page 340*
Erybid™ (Can) *see* erythromycin (systemic) *on page 339*
Eryc® (Can) *see* erythromycin (systemic) *on page 339*

Ery-Ped® *see* erythromycin (systemic) *on page 339*
Ery-Tab® *see* erythromycin (systemic) *on page 339*
Erythrocin® *see* erythromycin (systemic) *on page 339*
Erythrocin® Lactobionate-I.V. *see* erythromycin (systemic) *on page 339*

erythromycin (systemic) (er ith roe MYE sin)

Medication Safety Issues
Sound-alike/look-alike issues:
Erythromycin may be confused with azithromycin, clarithromycin, Ethmozine®
Akne-Mycin® may be confused with AK-Mycin®
E.E.S.® may be confused with DES®
Eryc® may be confused with Emcyt®, Ery-Tab®
Ery-Tab® may be confused with Eryc®
Erythrocin® may be confused with Ethmozine®

Synonyms erythromycin base; erythromycin ethylsuccinate; erythromycin lactobionate; erythromycin stearate

U.S. Brand Names E.E.S.®; Ery-Ped®; Ery-Tab®; EryPed®; Erythro-RX; Erythrocin®; Erythrocin® Lactobionate-I.V.; PCE®

Canadian Brand Names Apo-Erythro Base®; Apo-Erythro E-C®; Apo-Erythro-ES®; Apo-Erythro-S®; EES®; Erybid™; Eryc®; Novo-Rythro Estolate; Novo-Rythro Ethylsuccinate; Nu-Erythromycin-S; PCE®

Therapeutic Category Antibiotic, Macrolide

Use Treatment of susceptible bacterial infections including *S. pyogenes*, some *S. pneumoniae,* some *S. aureus*, *M. pneumoniae*, *Legionella pneumophila*, diphtheria, pertussis, *Chlamydia*, erythrasma, *N. gonorrhoeae*, *E. histolytica*, syphilis and nongonococcal urethritis, and *Campylobacter* gastroenteritis; used in conjunction with neomycin for decontaminating the bowel

General Dosage Range
I.V.:
Children: 15-50 mg/kg/day divided every 6 hours (maximum: 4 g/day)
Adults: 15-20 mg/kg/day divided every 6 hours **or** 500 mg to 1 g every 6 hours or as a continuous infusion over 24 hours (maximum: 4 g/day)
Oral:
Children: 30-50 mg/kg/day in 2-4 divided doses (maximum base or stearate: 2 g/day; maximum ethylsuccinate: 3.2 g/day)
Adults: Base: 250-500 mg every 6-12 hours (maximum base or ethylsuccinate: 400-800 mg every 6-12 hours)

Dosage Forms
Capsule, delayed release, enteric coated pellets, oral: 250 mg
Granules for suspension, oral:
E.E.S.®: 200 mg/5 mL (100 mL, 200 mL)
Injection, powder for reconstitution:
Erythrocin® Lactobionate-I.V.: 500 mg
Powder, for prescription compounding:
Erythro-RX: USP: 100% (50 g)
Powder for suspension, oral:
Ery-Ped®: 200 mg/5 mL (100 mL)
EryPed®: 400 mg/5 mL (100 mL)
Tablet, oral: 250 mg, 400 mg, 500 mg
E.E.S.®: 400 mg
Erythrocin®: 250 mg, 500 mg
Tablet, delayed release, enteric coated, oral:
Ery-Tab®: 250 mg, 333 mg, 500 mg
Tablet, polymer coated particles, oral:
PCE®: 333 mg, 500 mg

erythromycin (ophthalmic) (er ith roe MYE sin)

Medication Safety Issues
Sound-alike/look-alike issues:
Erythromycin may be confused with azithromycin
Synonyms erythromycin base
U.S. Brand Names Ilotycin™

◀ **Canadian Brand Names** Diomycin®; PMS-Erythromycin
Therapeutic Category Antibiotic, Macrolide; Antibiotic, Ophthalmic
Use Treatment of superficial eye infections involving the conjunctiva or cornea
General Dosage Range Ophthalmic: *Children and Adults:* Instill ¹/₂" (1.25 cm) 2-6 times/day
Dosage Forms
  Ointment, ophthalmic: 0.5% (1 g, 3.5 g, 3.75 g)
  Ilotycin™: 0.5% (1 g)
  Ointment, ophthalmic [preservative free]: 0.5% (1 g, 3.5 g)

erythromycin (topical) (er ith roe MYE sin)

Medication Safety Issues
  Sound-alike/look-alike issues:
    Erythromycin may be confused with azithromycin, clarithromycin, Ethmozine®
    Akne-Mycin® may be confused with AK-Mycin®
U.S. Brand Names Akne-mycin®; Ery
Canadian Brand Names Sans Acne®
Therapeutic Category Acne Products; Antibiotic, Macrolide; Antibiotic, Topical; Topical Skin Product; Topical Skin Product, Acne
Use Treatment of acne vulgaris
General Dosage Range Topical: *Children and Adults:* Apply over the affected area twice daily
Dosage Forms
  Gel, topical: 2% (30 g, 60 g)
  Ointment, topical:
    Akne-mycin®: 2% (25 g)
  Pledget, topical: 2%
    Ery: 2%
  Solution, topical: 2% (60 mL)
Dosage Forms - Canada
  Solution, topical:
    Sans Acne®: 2% (60 mL)

erythromycin and benzoyl peroxide (er ith roe MYE sin & BEN zoe il per OKS ide)

Synonyms benzoyl peroxide and erythromycin
U.S. Brand Names Benzamycin®; Benzamycin® Pak
Therapeutic Category Acne Products
Use Topical control of acne vulgaris
General Dosage Range Topical: *Adolescents ≥12 years and Adults:* Apply twice daily
Dosage Forms
  Gel, topical: Erythromycin 30 mg and benzoyl peroxide 50 mg per g (23 g, 47g)
  Benzamycin®: Erythromycin 30 mg and benzoyl peroxide 50 mg per g (47 g)
  Benzamycin® Pak: Erythromycin 30 mg and benzoyl peroxide 50 mg per 0.8 g packet (60s)

erythromycin and sulfisoxazole (er ith roe MYE sin & sul fi SOKS a zole)

Medication Safety Issues
  Sound-alike/look-alike issues:
    Pediazole® may be confused with Pediapred®
Synonyms sulfisoxazole and erythromycin
U.S. Brand Names E.S.P.®
Canadian Brand Names Pediazole®
Therapeutic Category Macrolide (Antibiotic); Sulfonamide
Use Treatment of susceptible bacterial infections of the upper and lower respiratory tract, otitis media in children caused by susceptible strains of *Haemophilus influenzae*, and many other infections in patients allergic to penicillin
General Dosage Range Dosage adjustment recommended in patients with renal impaiment
Oral:
  Children ≥2 months: 50 mg/kg/day erythromycin and 150 mg/kg/day sulfisoxazole in divided doses every 6 hours
  Adults: 400 mg erythromycin and 1200 mg sulfisoxazole every 6 hours

Dosage Forms
Powder for oral suspension: Erythromycin 200 mg and sulfisoxazole 600 mg per 5 mL
E.S.P.®: Erythromycin 200 mg and sulfisoxazole 600 mg per 5 mL

erythromycin base *see* erythromycin (ophthalmic) *on page 339*
erythromycin base *see* erythromycin (systemic) *on page 339*
erythromycin ethylsuccinate *see* erythromycin (systemic) *on page 339*
erythromycin lactobionate *see* erythromycin (systemic) *on page 339*
erythromycin stearate *see* erythromycin (systemic) *on page 339*
erythropoiesis-stimulating agent (ESA) *see* darbepoetin alfa *on page 253*
erythropoiesis-stimulating agent (ESA) *see* epoetin alfa *on page 333*
erythropoiesis-stimulating protein *see* darbepoetin alfa *on page 253*
erythropoietin *see* epoetin alfa *on page 333*
Erythro-RX *see* erythromycin (systemic) *on page 339*

escitalopram (es sye TAL oh pram)
Medication Safety Issues
Sound-alike/look-alike issues:
Lexapro® may be confused with Loxitane®
International issues:
Zavesca: Brand name for escitalopram [in multiple international markets; ISMP April 21, 2010], but also brand name for miglustat [Canada, U.S., and multiple international markets]
Synonyms escitalopram oxalate; Lu-26-054; S-citalopram
U.S. Brand Names Lexapro®
Canadian Brand Names Cipralex®
Therapeutic Category Antidepressant, Selective Serotonin Reuptake Inhibitor
Use Treatment of major depressive disorder; generalized anxiety disorders (GAD)
General Dosage Range Dosage adjustment recommended in patients with hepatic impairment
Oral:
Children ≥12 years and Adults: Initial: 10 mg once daily; Maintenance: 10-20 mg once daily
Elderly: 10 mg once daily
Dosage Forms
Solution, oral:
Lexapro®: 1 mg/mL (240 mL)
Tablet, oral:
Lexapro®: 5 mg, 10 mg, 20 mg
Dosage Forms - Canada
Tablet:
Cipralex®: 10 mg, 20 mg

escitalopram oxalate *see* escitalopram *on page 341*
eserine salicylate *see* physostigmine *on page 703*
Esgic® *see* butalbital, acetaminophen, and caffeine *on page 152*
Esgic-Plus™ *see* butalbital, acetaminophen, and caffeine *on page 152*
Eskalith *see* lithium *on page 532*

esmolol (ES moe lol)
Medication Safety Issues
Sound-alike/look-alike issues:
Esmolol may be confused with Osmitrol®
Brevibloc® may be confused with Brevital®, Bumex®, Buprenex®
High alert medication:
The Institute for Safe Medication Practices (ISMP) includes this medication among its list of drugs which have a heightened risk of causing significant patient harm when used in error.
Synonyms esmolol hydrochloride
U.S. Brand Names Brevibloc
Canadian Brand Names Brevibloc®
Therapeutic Category Antiarrhythmic Agent, Class II; Beta-Adrenergic Blocker

◀ **Use** Treatment of supraventricular tachycardia (SVT) and atrial fibrillation/flutter (control ventricular rate); treatment of intraoperative and postoperative tachycardia and/or hypertension; treatment of non-compensatory sinus tachycardia

General Dosage Range I.V.: *Adults:* Bolus: 80 mg **or** 500 mcg/kg; Infusion: 50-200 mcg/kg/minute (maximum: 300 mcg/kg/minute)

Dosage Forms
Infusion, premixed in NS [preservative free]:
Brevibloc: 2000 mg (100 mL); 2500 mg (250 mL)
Injection, solution [preservative free]: 10 mg/mL (10 mL)
Brevibloc: 10 mg/mL (10 mL)

esmolol hydrochloride *see* esmolol *on page 341*

esomeprazole (es oh ME pray zol)

Medication Safety Issues
Sound-alike/look-alike issues:
Esomeprazole may be confused with ARIPiprazole
NexIUM® may be confused with NexAVAR®

Synonyms esomeprazole magnesium; esomeprazole sodium

U.S. Brand Names NexIUM®; NexIUM® I.V.

Canadian Brand Names Apo-Esomeprazole®; Nexium®

Therapeutic Category Proton Pump Inhibitor

Use

Oral: Short-term (4-8 weeks) treatment of erosive esophagitis; maintaining symptom resolution and healing of erosive esophagitis; treatment of symptomatic gastroesophageal reflux disease (GERD); as part of a multidrug regimen for *Helicobacter pylori* eradication in patients with duodenal ulcer disease (active or history of within the past 5 years); prevention of gastric ulcers in patients at risk (age ≥60 years and/or history of gastric ulcer) associated with continuous NSAID therapy; long-term treatment of pathological hypersecretory conditions including Zollinger-Ellison syndrome
Canadian labeling: Additional use (not in U.S. labeling): Oral: Treatment of nonerosive reflux disease (NERD)

I.V.: Short-term (≤10 days) treatment of gastroesophageal reflux disease (GERD) when oral therapy is not possible or appropriate

General Dosage Range Dosage adjustment recommended in patients with hepatic impairment.
I.V.:
Children 1-11 months: 0.5 mg/kg once daily
Children 1-17 years: <55 kg: 10 mg once daily; ≥55 kg: 20 mg once daily
Adults: 20-40 mg once daily
Oral:
Children 1-11 years: <20 kg: 10 mg once daily; ≥20 kg: 10-20 mg once daily
Children 12-17 years: 20-40 mg once daily
Adults: 20-40 mg once daily **or** 80-240 mg/day in divided doses (hypersecretory conditions)

Dosage Forms
Capsule, delayed release, oral:
NexIUM®: 20 mg, 40 mg
Granules for suspension, delayed release, oral:
NexIUM®: 10 mg/packet (30s); 20 mg/packet (30s); 40 mg/packet (30s)
Injection, powder for reconstitution:
NexIUM® I.V.: 20 mg, 40 mg
Dosage Forms - Canada Note: Strength expressed as base.
Granules, for oral suspension, delayed release, as magnesium:
Nexium®: 10 mg/packet (28s)
Tablet, extended release, as magnesium:
Nexium®: 20 mg, 40 mg

esomeprazole and naproxen *see* naproxen and esomeprazole *on page 613*

esomeprazole magnesium *see* esomeprazole *on page 342*

esomeprazole sodium *see* esomeprazole *on page 342*

Esopho-Cat® *see* barium *on page 114*

Esoterica® Daytime [OTC] *see* hydroquinone *on page 453*

Esoterica® Nighttime [OTC] *see* hydroquinone *on page 453*
E.S.P.® *see* erythromycin and sulfisoxazole *on page 340*
Estalis® (Can) *see* estradiol and norethindrone *on page 345*
Estalis-Sequi® (Can) *see* estradiol and norethindrone *on page 345*
Estar® (Can) *see* coal tar *on page 227*

estazolam (es TA zoe lam)
Medication Safety Issues
Sound-alike/look-alike issues:
ProSom® may be confused with PhosLo®, Proscar®, Pro-Sof® Plus, PROzac®, Psorcon®
Synonyms ProSom
Therapeutic Category Benzodiazepine
Controlled Substance C-IV
Use Short-term management of insomnia
General Dosage Range Oral:
Adults: 0.5-2 mg at bedtime
Elderly: Initial: 0.5 mg at bedtime in small or debilitated patients
Dosage Forms
Tablet, oral: 1 mg, 2 mg

Ester-E™ [OTC] *see* vitamin E *on page 918*
esterified estrogen and methyltestosterone *see* estrogens (esterified) and methyltestosterone *on page 349*
esterified estrogens *see* estrogens (esterified) *on page 349*
Estrace® *see* estradiol (systemic) *on page 343*
Estrace® *see* estradiol (topical) *on page 344*
Estraderm® *see* estradiol (systemic) *on page 343*
estradiol *see* estradiol (systemic) *on page 343*
17β-estradiol *see* estradiol (topical) *on page 344*

estradiol (systemic) (es tra DYE ole)
Medication Safety Issues
Sound-alike/look-alike issues:
Alora® may be confused with Aldara®
Elestrin™ may be confused with alosetron
Estraderm® may be confused with Testoderm®
BEERS Criteria medication:
This drug may be inappropriate for use in geriatric patients (low severity risk).
Other safety issues:
Transdermal patch may contain conducting metal (eg, aluminum); remove patch prior to MRI.
International issues:
Vivelle®: Brand name for ethinyl estradiol and norgestimate in Austria
Synonyms estradiol; estradiol acetate; estradiol transdermal; estradiol valerate
U.S. Brand Names Alora®; Climara®; Delestrogen®; Depo®-Estradiol; Divigel®; Elestrin®; Estrace®; Estraderm®; Estrasorb®; EstroGel®; Evamist™; Femring®; Femtrace®; Menostar®; Vivelle-Dot®
Canadian Brand Names Climara®; Depo®-Estradiol; Estraderm®; Estradot®; EstroGel®; Menostar®; Oesclim®; Sandoz-Estradiol Derm 100; Sandoz-Estradiol Derm 50; Sandoz-Estradiol Derm 75
Therapeutic Category Estrogen Derivative
Use Treatment of moderate-to-severe vasomotor symptoms associated with menopause; treatment of moderate-to-severe vulvar and vaginal atrophy associated with menopause; hypoestrogenism (due to hypogonadism, castration, or primary ovarian failure); advanced prostatic cancer (palliation); metastatic breast cancer (palliation) in men and postmenopausal women; postmenopausal osteoporosis (prophylaxis)
General Dosage Range
I.M.:
Cypionate:
Adults (females): Hypoestrogenism: 1.5-2 mg monthly
Adults (females): Menopause: 1-5 mg every 3-4 weeks

◄ Valerate:
  Adults (females): Menopause: 10-20 mg every 4 weeks
  Adults (males): Prostate cancer: 30 mg or more every 1-2 weeks

Oral:
  Adults (females):
    Estrace®: Breast cancer: 10 mg 3 times/day; Hypoestrogenism: 1-2 mg/day; Menopause: 0.5-2 mg/day
    Femtrace®: Menopause: 0.45-1.8 mg/day
  Adults (males): Estrace®: Prostate cancer: 1-2 mg 3 times/day; Breast cancer: 10 mg 3 times/day

Intravaginal: *Adults (females):* (Femring®): 0.05-0.1 mg, leave in place for 3 months

Topical: *Adults (females):*
  Emulsion (Estrasorb®): 3.48 g applied once daily in the morning
  Gel: 1.25 g/day (EstroGel®) or 0.87-1.7 g/day (Elestrin®) or 0.25-1 g/day (Divigel®) applied at the same time each day
  Spray (Evamist™): 1 spray (1.53 mg) per day; dosing range: 1-3 sprays/day

Transdermal: *Adults (females):*
  Alora®, Estraderm®, Vivelle-Dot®: Apply twice weekly continuously or cyclically (3 weeks on, 1 week off)
  Climara®: Apply once weekly continuously or cyclically (3 weeks on, 1 week off)
  Menostar®: Apply once weekly continuously

Dosage Forms

Emulsion, topical:
  Estrasorb®: 2.5 mg/g (56s)

Gel, topical:
  Divigel®: 0.1% (30s)
  Elestrin®: 0.06% (35 g, 70 g)
  EstroGel®: 0.06% (50 g)

Injection, oil: 20 mg/mL (5 mL); 40 mg/mL (5 mL)
  Delestrogen®: 10 mg/mL (5 mL); 20 mg/mL (5 mL); 40 mg/mL (5 mL)
  Depo®-Estradiol: 5 mg/mL (5 mL)

Patch, transdermal: 0.025 mg/24 hours (4s); 0.0375 mg/24 hours (4s); 0.05 mg/24 hours (4s); 0.06 mg/24 hours (4s); 0.075 mg/24 hours (4s); 0.1 mg/24 hours (4s)
  Alora®: 0.025 mg/24 hours (8s); 0.05 mg/24 hours (8s); 0.075 mg/24 hours (8s); 0.1 mg/24 hours (8s)
  Climara®: 0.025 mg/24 hours (4s); 0.0375 mg/24 hours (4s); 0.05 mg/24 hours (4s); 0.06 mg/24 hours (4s); 0.075 mg/24 hours (4s); 0.1 mg/24 hours (4s)
  Estraderm®: 0.05 mg/24 hours (8s); 0.1 mg/24 hours (8s)
  Menostar®: 0.014 mg/24 hours (4s)
  Vivelle-Dot®: 0.025 mg/24 hours (24s); 0.0375 mg/24 hours (24s); 0.05 mg/24 hours (24s); 0.075 mg/24 hours (24s); 0.1 mg/24 hours (24s)

Ring, vaginal:
  Femring®: 0.05 mg/24 hours (1s); 0.1 mg/24 hours (1s)

Solution, topical:
  Evamist™: 1.53 mg/spray (8.1 mL)

Tablet, oral: 0.5 mg, 1 mg, 2 mg
  Estrace®: 0.5 mg, 1 mg, 2 mg
  Femtrace®: 0.45 mg, 0.9 mg, 1.8 mg

estradiol (topical) (es tra DYE ole)

Medication Safety Issues
International issues:
  Estring [U.S., Canada, and multiple international markets] may be confused with Estrena [Finland]

Synonyms 17β-estradiol

U.S. Brand Names Estrace®; Estring®; Vagifem®

Canadian Brand Names Estrace®; Estring®; Vagifem®; Vagifem® 10

Therapeutic Category Estrogen Derivative

Use Treatment of moderate-to-severe vulvar and vaginal atrophy associated with menopause

General Dosage Range Intravaginal: *Adults (females):*
  Cream: Initial: 2-4 g/day for 1-2 weeks, then 1/2 the initial dose for 1-2 weeks; Maintenance: 1 g 1-3 times/week
  Ring: Estring®: Insert 2 mg, leave in place for 3 months
  Tablet: Initial: Insert 1 tablet (10 mcg) once daily for 2 weeks; Maintenance: Insert 1 tablet twice weekly

Dosage Forms
Cream, vaginal:
Estrace®: 0.1 mg/g (42.5 g)
Ring, vaginal:
Estring®: 2 mg (1s)
Tablet, vaginal:
Vagifem®: 10 mcg

estradiol acetate *see* estradiol (systemic) *on page 343*

estradiol and dienogest (es tra DYE ole & dye EN oh jest)

Synonyms dienogest and estradiol; estradiol valerate and dienogest
U.S. Brand Names Natazia™
Therapeutic Category Contraceptive; Estrogen and Progestin Combination
Use Prevention of pregnancy
General Dosage Range Oral: *Children and Adults (females, postmenarche):* 1 tablet daily
Dosage Forms
Tablet, oral [four-phasic formulation]:
Natazia™:
Days 1-2: Estradiol valerate 3 mg [2 dark yellow tablets]
Days 3-7: Estradiol valerate 2 mg and dienogest 2 mg [5 medium red tablets]
Days 8-24: Estradiol valerate 2 mg and dienogest 3 mg [17 light yellow tablets]
Days 25-26: Estradiol valerate 1 mg [2 dark red tablets]
Days 27-28: 2 white inactive tablets (28s)

estradiol and drospirenone *see* drospirenone and estradiol *on page 315*

estradiol and levonorgestrel (es tra DYE ole & LEE voe nor jes trel)

Synonyms levonorgestrel and estradiol
U.S. Brand Names ClimaraPro®
Therapeutic Category Estrogen and Progestin Combination
Use Women with an intact uterus: Treatment of moderate-to-severe vasomotor symptoms associated with menopause; prevention of postmenopausal osteoporosis
General Dosage Range Transdermal: *Adults (females):* Apply 1 patch (estradiol 0.045 mg/ levonorgestrel 0.015 mg) weekly
Dosage Forms
Patch, transdermal:
ClimaraPro®: Estradiol 0.045 mg and levonorgestrel 0.015 mg per 24 hours (4s)

estradiol and NGM *see* estradiol and norgestimate *on page 346*

estradiol and norethindrone (es tra DYE ole & nor eth IN drone)

Synonyms norethindrone and estradiol
U.S. Brand Names Activella®; CombiPatch®; Mimvey™
Canadian Brand Names Estalis-Sequi®; Estalis®
Therapeutic Category Estrogen and Progestin Combination
Use Women with an intact uterus:
Tablet: Treatment of moderate-to-severe vasomotor symptoms associated with menopause; treatment of vulvar and vaginal atrophy; prophylaxis for postmenopausal osteoporosis
Transdermal patch: Treatment of moderate-to-severe vasomotor symptoms associated with menopause; treatment of vulvar and vaginal atrophy; treatment of hypoestrogenism due to hypogonadism, castration, or primary ovarian failure
General Dosage Range
Oral: *Adults (females):* 1 tablet daily
Transdermal: *Adults (females):* Apply 1 patch twice weekly
Dosage Forms
Patch, transdermal:
CombiPatch®:
0.05/0.14: Estradiol 0.05 mg and norethindrone 0.14 mg per day (8s) [9 sq cm]
0.05/0.25: Estradiol 0.05 mg and norethindrone 0.25 mg per day (8s) [16 sq cm]

◀ **Tablet, oral:** Estradiol 1 mg and norethindrone acetate 0.5 mg (28s)
Activella® 0.5/0.1: Estradiol 0.5 mg and norethindrone acetate 0.1 mg (28s)
Activella® 1/0.5, Mimvey™: Estradiol 1 mg and norethindrone acetate 0.5 mg (28s)
Dosage Forms - Canada
Combination pack:
Estalis-Sequi® 140/50:
Patch, transdermal (Vivelle®): Estradiol 50 mcg per day (4s) [14.5 sq cm; total estradiol 4.33 mg]
Patch, transdermal (Estalis®): Norethindrone 140 mcg and estradiol 50 mcg per day (4s) [9 sq cm; total norethindrone 2.7 mg, total estradiol 0.62 mg]
Estalis-Sequi® 250/50:
Patch, transdermal (Vivelle®): Estradiol 50 mcg per day (4s) [14.5 sq cm; total estradiol 4.33 mg]
Patch, transdermal (Estalis®): Norethindrone 250 mcg and estradiol 50 mcg per day (4s) [16 sq cm; total norethindrone 4.8 mg, total estradiol 0.51 mg]
Patch, transdermal:
Estalis®:
140/50: Norethindrone 140 mcg and estradiol 50 mcg per day (8s) [9 sq cm; total norethindrone 2.7 mg, total estradiol 0.62 mg]
250/50 Norethindrone 250 mcg and estradiol 50 mcg per day (8s) [16 sq cm; total norethindrone 4.8 mg, total estradiol 0.51 mg]

estradiol and norgestimate (es tra DYE ole & nor JES ti mate)
Synonyms estradiol and NGM; norgestimate and estradiol; ortho prefest
U.S. Brand Names Prefest™
Therapeutic Category Estrogen and Progestin Combination
Use Women with an intact uterus: Treatment of moderate-to-severe vasomotor symptoms associated with menopause; treatment of atrophic vaginitis; prevention of osteoporosis
General Dosage Range Oral: *Adults (females):* 1 tablet of estradiol 1 mg once daily for 3 days, followed by 1 tablet of estradiol 1 mg and norgestimate 0.09 mg once daily for 3 days; repeat sequence continuously
Dosage Forms
Tablet, oral:
Prefest™: Estradiol 1 mg [15 peach tablets] and estradiol 1 mg and norgestimate 0.09 mg [15 white tablets]

estradiol transdermal *see* estradiol (systemic) *on page 343*
estradiol valerate *see* estradiol (systemic) *on page 343*
estradiol valerate and dienogest *see* estradiol and dienogest *on page 345*
Estradot® (Can) *see* estradiol (systemic) *on page 343*
Estragyn (Can) *see* estrogens (esterified) *on page 349*

estramustine (es tra MUS teen)
Medication Safety Issues
Sound-alike/look-alike issues:
Emcyt® may be confused with Eryc®
Estramustine may be confused with exemestane.
High alert medication:
The Institute for Safe Medication Practices (ISMP) includes this medication among its list of drug classes which have a heightened risk of causing significant patient harm when used in error.
Synonyms estramustine phosphate; estramustine phosphate sodium; NSC-89199
U.S. Brand Names Emcyt®
Canadian Brand Names Emcyt®
Therapeutic Category Antineoplastic Agent
Use Palliative treatment of progressive or metastatic prostate cancer
General Dosage Range Oral: *Adults (males):* 14 mg/kg/day (range: 10-16 mg/kg/day) in 3 or 4 divided doses
Dosage Forms
Capsule, oral:
Emcyt®: 140 mg

estramustine phosphate *see* estramustine *on page 346*

estramustine phosphate sodium *see estramustine on page 346*

Estrasorb® *see estradiol (systemic) on page 343*

Estratab® (Can) *see estrogens (esterified) on page 349*

Estring® *see estradiol (topical) on page 344*

EstroGel® *see estradiol (systemic) on page 343*

estrogenic substances, conjugated *see estrogens (conjugated/equine, systemic) on page 347*

estrogenic substances, conjugated *see estrogens (conjugated/equine, topical) on page 348*

estrogens (conjugated A/synthetic) (ES troe jenz, KON joo gate ed, aye, sin THET ik)

Medication Safety Issues

Sound-alike/look-alike issues:
Cenestin® may be confused with Senexon®

BEERS Criteria medication:
This drug may be inappropriate for use in geriatric patients (low severity risk).

International issues:
Cenestin [U.S., Canada] may be confused with Canesten which is a brand name for clotrimazole [multiple international markets] and a brand name for fluconazole [Great Britain]

U.S. Brand Names Cenestin®

Canadian Brand Names Cenestin

Therapeutic Category Estrogen Derivative

Use Treatment of moderate-to-severe vasomotor symptoms of menopause; treatment of vulvar and vaginal atrophy

General Dosage Range Oral: *Adults (females):* 0.3-1.25 mg once daily

Dosage Forms

Tablet, oral:
Cenestin®: 0.3 mg, 0.45 mg, 0.625 mg, 0.9 mg, 1.25 mg

estrogens (conjugated B/synthetic) (ES troe jenz, KON joo gate ed, bee, sin THET ik)

Medication Safety Issues

Sound-alike/look-alike issues:
Enjuvia™ may be confused with Januvia®

BEERS Criteria medication:
This drug may be inappropriate for use in geriatric patients (low severity risk).

U.S. Brand Names Enjuvia™

Therapeutic Category Estrogen Derivative

Use Treatment of moderate-to-severe vasomotor symptoms of menopause; treatment of vulvar and vaginal atrophy associated with menopause; treatment of moderate-to-severe vaginal dryness and pain with intercourse associated with menopause

General Dosage Range Oral: *Adults (females):* 0.3-1.25 mg once daily

Dosage Forms

Tablet, oral:
Enjuvia™: 0.3 mg, 0.45 mg, 0.625 mg, 0.9 mg, 1.25 mg

estrogens (conjugated/equine, systemic) (ES troe jenz KON joo gate ed, EE kwine)

Medication Safety Issues

Sound-alike/look-alike issues:
Premarin® may be confused with Primaxin®, Provera®, Remeron®

BEERS Criteria medication:
This drug may be inappropriate for use in geriatric patients (low severity risk).

Synonyms C.E.S.; CE; CEE; conjugated estrogen; estrogenic substances, conjugated

U.S. Brand Names Premarin®

Canadian Brand Names C.E.S.®; Premarin®

Therapeutic Category Estrogen Derivative

Use Treatment of moderate-to-severe vasomotor symptoms associated with menopause; treatment of vulvar and vaginal atrophy; hypoestrogenism (due to hypogonadism, castration, or primary ovarian failure); prostatic cancer (palliation); breast cancer (palliation); osteoporosis (prophylaxis, postmenopausal women at significant risk only); abnormal uterine bleeding; moderate-to-severe dyspareunia (pain during intercourse) due to vaginal/vulvar atrophy of menopause

◀ **General Dosage Range** Dosage adjustment recommended in patients with hepatic impairment
I.M., I.V.: *Children (postmenarche) and Adults (females):* Abnormal uterine bleeding: 25 mg, may repeat in 6-12 hours if needed
Oral:
Adolescents and Adult (females): 0.3-1.25 mg daily or cyclically **or** 10 mg 3 times/day [breast cancer]
Adults (males): Breast cancer: 10 mg 3 times/day; Prostate cancer: 1.25-2.5 mg 3 times/day
Dosage Forms
Injection, powder for reconstitution:
Premarin®: 25 mg
Tablet, oral:
Premarin®: 0.3 mg, 0.45 mg, 0.625 mg, 0.9 mg, 1.25 mg

estrogens (conjugated/equine, topical) (ES troe jenz KON joo gate ed, EE kwine)
Medication Safety Issues
Sound-alike/look-alike issues:
Premarin® may be confused with Primaxin®, Provera®, Remeron®
Synonyms C.E.S.; CE; CEE; conjugated estrogen; estrogenic substances, conjugated
U.S. Brand Names Premarin®
Canadian Brand Names Premarin®
Therapeutic Category Estrogen Derivative
Use Treatment of vulvar and vaginal atrophy; moderate-to-severe dyspareunia (pain during intercourse) due to vaginal/vulvar atrophy of menopause
General Dosage Range Intravaginal: *Adults (females):*
Vaginal atrophy: 0.5-2 g/day given cyclically
Moderate-to-severe dyspareunia: 0.5 g twice weekly (eg, Monday and Thursday) or once daily cyclically
Dosage Forms
Cream, vaginal:
Premarin®: 0.625 mg/g (42.5 g)

estrogens (conjugated/equine) and medroxyprogesterone
(ES troe jenz KON joo gate ed/EE kwine & me DROKS ee proe JES te rone)
Medication Safety Issues
Sound-alike/look-alike issues:
Premphase® may be confused with Prempro®
Prempro® may be confused with Premphase®
Synonyms medroxyprogesterone and estrogens (conjugated); MPA and estrogens (conjugated)
U.S. Brand Names Premphase®; Prempro®
Canadian Brand Names Premphase®; Premplus®; Prempro®
Therapeutic Category Estrogen and Progestin Combination
Use Women with an intact uterus: Treatment of moderate-to-severe vasomotor symptoms associated with menopause; treatment of moderate-to-severe vulvar and vaginal atrophy due to menopause; postmenopausal osteoporosis (prophylaxis)
General Dosage Range Oral: *Adults (females):* Prempro®: Conjugated estrogen 0.3-0.625 mg/mPA 1.5-5 mg once daily **or** Premphase®: One 0.625 mg tablet daily on days 1 through 14 and 1 conjugated estrogen 0.625 mg/mPA 5 mg tablet daily on days 15 through 28
Dosage Forms
Tablet:
Premphase® [therapy pack contains two separate tablet formulations]: Conjugated estrogens 0.625 mg [14 maroon tablets] and conjugated estrogen 0.625 mg/medroxyprogesterone 5 mg [14 light blue tablets] (28s)
Prempro®:
0.3/1.5: Conjugated estrogens 0.3 mg and medroxyprogesterone 1.5 mg (28s)
0.45/1.5: Conjugated estrogens 0.45 mg and medroxyprogesterone 1.5 mg (28s)
0.625/2.5: Conjugated estrogens 0.625 mg and medroxyprogesterone 2.5 mg (28s)
0.625/5: Conjugated estrogens 0.625 mg and medroxyprogesterone 5 mg (28s)

estrogens (esterified) (ES troe jenz, es TER i fied)

Medication Safety Issues
Sound-alike/look-alike issues:
Estratab® may be confused with Estratest®, Estratest® H.S.
Beers Criteria medication:
This drug may be inappropriate for use in geriatric patients (low severity risk).
Synonyms esterified estrogens
U.S. Brand Names Menest®
Canadian Brand Names Estragyn; Estratab®; Menest®
Therapeutic Category Estrogen Derivative

Use Treatment of moderate-to-severe vasomotor symptoms associated with menopause; treatment of moderate-to-severe vulvar and vaginal atrophy associated with menopause; hypoestrogenism (due to hypogonadism, castration, or primary ovarian failure); advanced prostatic cancer (palliation), metastatic breast cancer (palliation) in men and postmenopausal women

General Dosage Range
Oral:
Adults (females): Hypogonadism: 2.5-7.5 mg/day for 20 days followed by a 10-day rest, repeat until response; Castration or ovarian failure: 1.25 mg/day, cyclically; Menopause 0.3-1.25 mg/day given cyclically; Breast cancer: 10 mg 3 times/day
Adults (males): Breast cancer: 10 mg 3 times/day; Prostate cancer: 1.25-2.5 mg 3 times/day
Dosage Forms
Tablet, oral:
Menest®: 0.3 mg, 0.625 mg, 1.25 mg, 2.5 mg

estrogens (esterified) and methyltestosterone
(ES troe jenz es TER i fied & meth il tes TOS te rone)

Medication Safety Issues
Sound-alike/look-alike issues:
Estratest® may be confused with Eskalith®, Estratab®, Estratest® H.S.
Estratest® H.S. may be confused with Eskalith®, Estratab®, Estratest®
Synonyms esterified estrogen and methyltestosterone; methyltestosterone and esterified estrogen
U.S. Brand Names Covaryx®; Covaryx® H.S.; EEMT™; EEMT™ HS
Therapeutic Category Estrogen and Androgen Combination
Use Treatment of moderate-to-severe vasomotor symptoms associated with menopause not improved by estrogens alone
General Dosage Range Oral: *Adults (females):* Usual dosage range (based on esterified estrogen component): 0.625-1.25 mg every day for 3 weeks and then discontinued for 1 week off
Dosage Forms
Tablet: Esterified estrogen 0.625 mg and methyltestosterone 1.25 mg; esterified estrogens 1.25 mg and methyltestosterone 2.5 mg
Covaryx® H.S., EEMT™ HS: Esterified estrogen 0.625 mg and methyltestosterone 1.25 mg
Covaryx®, EEMT™: Esterified estrogen 1.25 mg and methyltestosterone 2.5 mg

estropipate (ES troe pih pate)
Medication Safety Issues
BEERS Criteria medication:
This drug may be inappropriate for use in geriatric patients (low severity risk).
Synonyms Ortho Est; piperazine estrone sulfate
Canadian Brand Names Ogen®
Therapeutic Category Estrogen Derivative
Use Treatment of moderate-to-severe vasomotor symptoms associated with menopause; treatment of vulvar and vaginal atrophy; hypoestrogenism (due to hypogonadism, castration, or primary ovarian failure); osteoporosis (prophylaxis, in women at significant risk only)
General Dosage Range Dosage adjustment recommended in patients with hepatic impairment
Oral: *Adults (females):* 0.75-6 mg once daily or cyclically [menopause] **or** 1.5-9 mg for the first 3 weeks, followed by a rest period of 8-10 days [hypoestrogenism] **or** 0.75 mg for 25 days of a 31 day cycle [osteoporosis]

◀ **Dosage Forms**
Tablet, oral: 0.625 mg, 1.25 mg, 2.5 mg

Estrostep® Fe *see ethinyl estradiol and norethindrone on page 355*

eszopiclone (es zoe PIK lone)

Medication Safety Issues
Sound-alike/look-alike issues:
Lunesta® may be confused with Neulasta®
U.S. Brand Names Lunesta®
Therapeutic Category Hypnotic, Nonbenzodiazepine
Controlled Substance C-IV
Use Treatment of insomnia
General Dosage Range Dosage adjustment recommended in patients with hepatic impairment or on concomitant therapy
Oral:
Adults: Initial: 1-2 mg immediately before bedtime (maximum: 3 mg/day)
Elderly: Maximum: 2 mg/day
Dosage Forms
Tablet, oral:
Lunesta®: 1 mg, 2 mg, 3 mg

etanercept (et a NER sept)

Medication Safety Issues
Sound-alike/look-alike issues:
Enbrel® may be confused with Levbid®
U.S. Brand Names Enbrel®; Enbrel® SureClick®
Canadian Brand Names Enbrel®
Therapeutic Category Antirheumatic, Disease Modifying
Use Treatment of moderately- to severely-active rheumatoid arthritis (RA); moderately- to severely-active polyarticular juvenile idiopathic arthritis (JIA); psoriatic arthritis; active ankylosing spondylitis (AS); moderate-to-severe chronic plaque psoriasis
General Dosage Range SubQ:
Children 2-17 years: 0.8 mg/kg (maximum: 50 mg) once weekly **or** 0.4 mg/kg (maximum: 25 mg) twice weekly
Adults: 50 mg once weekly **or** 25-50 mg twice weekly
Dosage Forms
Injection, powder for reconstitution:
Enbrel®: 25 mg
Injection, solution [preservative free]:
Enbrel®: 50 mg/mL (0.51 mL, 0.98 mL)
Enbrel® SureClick®: 50 mg/mL (0.98 mL)

ethacrynate sodium *see ethacrynic acid on page 350*

ethacrynic acid (eth a KRIN ik AS id)

Medication Safety Issues
Sound-alike/look-alike issues:
Edecrin® may be confused with Eulexin, Ecotrin®
BEERS Criteria medication:
This drug may be inappropriate for use in geriatric patients (low severity risk).
Synonyms ethacrynate sodium
U.S. Brand Names Edecrin®; Sodium Edecrin®
Canadian Brand Names Edecrin®
Therapeutic Category Diuretic, Loop
Use Management of edema associated with congestive heart failure; hepatic cirrhosis or renal disease; short-term management of ascites due to malignancy, idiopathic edema, and lymphedema
General Dosage Range
I.V.: *Adults:* 0.5-1 mg/kg/dose (maximum: 100 mg/dose)

Oral:
Children: 1-3 mg/kg/day
Adults: 50-400 mg/day in 1-2 divided doses
Elderly: Initial: 25-50 mg/day

Dosage Forms
Injection, powder for reconstitution:
Sodium Edecrin®: 50 mg
Tablet, oral:
Edecrin®: 25 mg

ethambutol (e THAM byoo tole)

Medication Safety Issues
Sound-alike/look-alike issues:
Myambutol® may be confused with Nembutal®
Synonyms ethambutol hydrochloride
U.S. Brand Names Myambutol®
Canadian Brand Names Etibi®
Therapeutic Category Antimycobacterial Agent
Use Treatment of pulmonary tuberculosis in conjunction with other antituberculosis agents
General Dosage Range Dosage adjustment recommended in patients with renal impairment
Oral:
Children: 15-20 mg/kg/day (maximum: 1 g/day) **or** 50 mg/kg twice weekly (maximum: 2.5 g/dose)
Adults: Daily therapy: 1.5-2.5 g/kg/day (maximum dose: 1.5-2.5 g); 3 times/week DOT: 25-30 mg/kg/dose (maximum dose: 2.4 g/dose); Twice weekly DOT: 50 mg/kg/dose (maximum dose: 4 g/dose)
Dosage Forms
Tablet, oral: 100 mg, 400 mg
Myambutol®: 100 mg, 400 mg

ethambutol hydrochloride *see* ethambutol *on page 351*
Ethamolin® *see* ethanolamine oleate *on page 351*
ethanoic acid *see* acetic acid *on page 35*
ethanol *see* alcohol (ethyl) *on page 47*

ethanolamine oleate (ETH a nol a meen OH lee ate)

Medication Safety Issues
Sound-alike/look-alike issues:
Ethamolin® may be confused with ethanol
Synonyms monoethanolamine
U.S. Brand Names Ethamolin®
Therapeutic Category Sclerosing Agent
Use Orphan drug: Sclerosing agent used for bleeding esophageal varices
General Dosage Range Injection: *Adults:* 1.5-5 mL per varix (maximum: 20 mL total)
Dosage Forms
Injection, solution:
Ethamolin®: 5% (2 mL)

ethinyl estradiol and cyproterone acetate *see* cyproterone and ethinyl estradiol *(Canada only) on page 245*

ethinyl estradiol and desogestrel (ETH in il es tra DYE ole & des oh JES trel)

Medication Safety Issues
Sound-alike/look-alike issues:
Apri® may be confused with Apriso™
Ortho-Cept® may be confused with Ortho-Cyclen®
Synonyms desogestrel and ethinyl estradiol
U.S. Brand Names Apri®; Azurette™; Caziant®; Cesia® [DSC]; Cyclessa®; Desogen®; Emoquette™; Kariva®; Mircette®; Ortho-Cept®; Reclipsen®; Solia® [DSC]; Velivet™
Canadian Brand Names Cyclessa®; Linessa®; Marvelon®; Ortho-Cept®
Therapeutic Category Contraceptive, Oral

◀ **Use** Prevention of pregnancy

General Dosage Range Oral: *Children and Adults (females, postmenarche):* 1 tablet daily

Dosage Forms

Tablet, low-dose formulations:

Azurette™:
Day 1-21: Ethinyl estradiol 0.02 mg and desogestrel 0.15 mg [21 white tablets]
Day 22-23: 2 inactive green tablets
Day 24-28: Ethinyl estradiol 0.01 mg [5 blue tablets] (28s)

Kariva®:
Day 1-21: Ethinyl estradiol 0.02 mg and desogestrel 0.15 mg [21 white tablets]
Day 22-23: 2 inactive light green tablets
Day 24-28: Ethinyl estradiol 0.01 mg [5 light blue tablets] (28s)

Mircette®:
Day 1-21: Ethinyl estradiol 0.02 mg and desogestrel 0.15 mg [21 white tablets]
Day 22-23: 2 inactive green tablets
Day 24-28: Ethinyl estradiol 0.01 mg [5 yellow tablets] (28s)

Tablet, monophasic formulations:

Apri® 28: Ethinyl estradiol 0.03 mg and desogestrel 0.15 mg (28s) [21 rose tablets and 7 white inactive tablets]

Desogen®, Reclipsen®: Ethinyl estradiol 0.03 mg and desogestrel 0.15 mg (28s) [21 white tablets and 7 green inactive tablets]

Emoquette™: Ethinyl estradiol 0.03 mg and desogestrel 0.15 mg (28s) [21 white tablets and 7 light green inactive tablets]

Ortho-Cept® 28: Ethinyl estradiol 0.03 mg and desogestrel 0.15 mg (28s) [21 light orange tablets and 7 green inactive tablets]

Tablet, triphasic formulations:

Caziant®:
Day 1-7: Ethinyl estradiol 0.025 mg and desogestrel 0.1 mg [7 white tablets]
Day 8-14: Ethinyl estradiol 0.025 mg and desogestrel 0.125 mg [7 light blue tablets]
Day 15-21: Ethinyl estradiol 0.025 mg and desogestrel 0.15 mg [7 blue tablets]
Day 22-28: 7 green inactive tablets (28s)

Cyclessa®:
Day 1-7: Ethinyl estradiol 0.025 mg and desogestrel 0.1 mg [7 light yellow tablets]
Day 8-14: Ethinyl estradiol 0.025 mg and desogestrel 0.125 mg [7 orange tablets]
Day 15-21: Ethinyl estradiol 0.025 mg and desogestrel 0.15 mg [7 red tablets]
Day 22-28: 7 green inactive tablets (28s)

Velivet™:
Day 1-7: Ethinyl estradiol 0.025 mg and desogestrel 0.1 mg [7 beige tablets]
Day 8-14: Ethinyl estradiol 0.025 mg and desogestrel 0.125 mg [7 orange tablets]
Day 15-21: Ethinyl estradiol 0.025 mg and desogestrel 0.15 mg [7 pink tablets]
Day 22-28: 7 white inactive tablets (28s)

ethinyl estradiol and drospirenone (ETH in il es tra DYE ole & droh SPYE re none)

Medication Safety Issues

Sound-alike/look-alike issues:

Yasmin® may be confused with Yaz®
Yaz® may be confused with Beyaz™, Yasmin®

Synonyms drospirenone and ethinyl estradiol

U.S. Brand Names Gianvi™; Loryna™; Ocella™; Syeda™; Yasmin®; Yaz®; Zarah®

Canadian Brand Names Yasmin®; Yaz®

Therapeutic Category Contraceptive, Oral

Use Prevention of pregnancy; treatment of premenstrual dysphoric disorder (PMDD); treatment of acne

General Dosage Range Oral: *Children and Adults (females, postmenarche):* 1 tablet daily

Dosage Forms

Tablet, oral:

Gianvi™: Ethinyl estradiol 0.03 mg and drospirenone 3 mg (28s) [24 light pink active tablets and 4 white inactive tablets]

Loryna™: Ethinyl estradiol 0.02 mg and drospirenone 3 mg (28s) [24 peach active tablets and 4 white inactive tablets]

Ocella™, SyedaYasmin®: Ethinyl estradiol 0.03 mg and drospirenone 3 mg (28s) [21 yellow active tablets and 7 white inactive tablets]

Yaz®: Ethinyl estradiol 0.02 mg and drospirenone 3 mg (28s) [24 light pink active tablets and 4 white inactive tablets]

Zarah®: Ethinyl estradiol 0.03 mg and drospirenone 3 mg (28s) [21 blue active tablets and 7 peach inactive tablets]

ethinyl estradiol and ethynodiol diacetate
(ETH in il es tra DYE ole & e thye noe DYE ole dye AS e tate)

Medication Safety Issues
Sound-alike/look-alike issues:
Demulen® may be confused with Dalmane®, Demerol®

Synonyms ethynodiol diacetate and ethinyl estradiol

U.S. Brand Names Kelnor™; Zovia®

Canadian Brand Names Demulen® 30

Therapeutic Category Contraceptive, Oral

Use Prevention of pregnancy

General Dosage Range Oral: *Children and Adults (females, postmenarche):* 1 tablet daily

Dosage Forms
Tablet, monophasic formulations:
Kelnor™ 1/35: Ethinyl estradiol 0.035 mg and ethynodiol diacetate 1 mg [21 light yellow tablets and 7 white inactive tablets] (28s)

Zovia® 1/35-28: Ethinyl estradiol 0.035 mg and ethynodiol diacetate 1 mg [21 light pink tablets and 7 white inactive tablets] (28s)

Zovia® 1/50-28: Ethinyl estradiol 0.05 mg and ethynodiol diacetate 1 mg [21 pink tablets and 7 white inactive tablets] (28s)

ethinyl estradiol and etonogestrel (ETH in il es tra DYE ole & et oh noe JES trel)

Synonyms etonogestrel and ethinyl estradiol

U.S. Brand Names NuvaRing®

Canadian Brand Names NuvaRing®

Therapeutic Category Contraceptive, Oral; Estrogen and Progestin Combination

Use Prevention of pregnancy

General Dosage Range Vaginal: *Children and Adults (females, postmenarche):* Insert one ring and leave in place for 3 consecutive weeks, then remove for 1 week

Dosage Forms
Ring, vaginal:
NuvaRing®: Ethinyl estradiol 0.015 mg/day and etonogestrel 0.12 mg/day (1s) [3-week duration]

ethinyl estradiol and levonorgestrel (ETH in il es tra DYE ole & LEE voe nor jes trel)

Medication Safety Issues
Sound-alike/look-alike issues:
Nordette® may be confused with Nicorette®
Seasonale® may be confused with Seasonique®
Seasonique® may be confused with Seasonale®
Tri-Levlen® may be confused with Trilafon®

Synonyms levonorgestrel and ethinyl estradiol

U.S. Brand Names Amethia™; Amethyst™; Aviane™; Camrese™; Enpresse®; Introvale™; Jolessa™; Lessina®; Levora®; LoSeasonique®; Lutera®; Lybrel®; Nordette® 28; Orsythia™; Portia®; Quasense®; Seasonale®; Seasonique®; Sronyx®; Trivora®

Canadian Brand Names Alesse®; Aviane®; Min-Ovral®; Seasonale®; Triphasil®; Triquilar®

Therapeutic Category Contraceptive, Oral

Use Prevention of pregnancy; postcoital contraception

General Dosage Range Oral: *Children and Adults (females, postmenarche):* 1 tablet daily **or** 2 tablets as soon as possible (but within 72 hours of unprotected intercourse), followed by 2 tablets 12 hours later ▶

◀ **Dosage Forms**
Tablet, oral [low-dose formulation]:
Aviane™: Ethinyl estradiol 0.02 mg and levonorgestrel 0.1 mg (28s) [21 orange tablets and 7 light green inactive tablets]
Lutera®, Sronyx®: Ethinyl estradiol 0.02 mg and levonorgestrel 0.1 mg (28s) [21 white tablets and 7 peach inactive tablets]
Orsythia™: Ethinyl estradiol 0.02 mg and levonorgestrel 0.1 mg (28s) [21 pink tablets and 7 light green inactive tablets]

Tablet, oral [monophasic formulation]:
Levora®: Ethinyl estradiol 0.03 mg and levonorgestrel 0.15 mg (28s) [21 white tablets and 7 peach inactive tablets]
Nordette® 28: Ethinyl estradiol 0.03 mg and levonorgestrel 0.15 mg (28s) [21 light orange tablets and 7 pink inactive tablets]
Portia® 28: Ethinyl estradiol 0.03 mg and levonorgestrel 0.15 mg (28s) [21 pink tablets and 7 white inactive tablets]

Tablet, oral [extended cycle regimen]:
Amethia™: Ethinyl estradiol 0.03 mg and levonorgestrel 0.15 mg (91s) [84 white tablets] and ethinyl estradiol 0.01 mg [7 light blue tablets]
Camrese™: Ethinyl estradiol 0.03 mg and levonorgestrel 0.15 mg (91s) [84 light blue-green tablets] and ethinyl estradiol 0.01 mg [7 yellow tablets]
Introvale™: Ethinyl estradiol 0.03 mg and levonorgestrel 0.15 mg (91s) [84 peach tablets and 7 white inactive tablets]
Jolessa™, Seasonale®: Ethinyl estradiol 0.03 mg and levonorgestrel 0.15 mg (91s) [84 pink tablets and 7 white inactive tablets]
LoSeasonique®: Ethinyl estradiol 0.02 mg and levonorgestrel 0.1 mg (91s) [84 orange tablets] and ethinyl estradiol 0.01 mg [7 yellow tablets]
Quasense®: Ethinyl estradiol 0.03 mg and levonorgestrel 0.15 mg] (91s) [84 white tablets and 7 peach inactive tablets]
Seasonique®: Ethinyl estradiol 0.03 mg and levonorgestrel 0.15 mg (91s) [84 light blue-green tablets] and ethinyl estradiol 0.01 mg [7 yellow tablets]

Tablet, oral [noncyclic regimen]:
Amethyst™: Ethinyl estradiol 0.02 mg and levonorgestrel 0.09 mg (28s) [28 white tablets]
Lybrel®: Ethinyl estradiol 0.02 mg and levonorgestrel 0.09 mg (28s) [28 yellow tablets]

Tablet, oral [triphasic formulation]:
Enpresse®:
Day 1-6: Ethinyl estradiol 0.03 mg and levonorgestrel 0.05 mg [6 pink tablets]
Day 7-11: Ethinyl estradiol 0.04 mg and levonorgestrel 0.075 mg [5 white tablets]
Day 12-21: Ethinyl estradiol 0.03 mg and levonorgestrel 0.125 mg [10 orange tablets]
Day 22-28: 7 light green inactive tablets (28s)
Trivora®:
Day 1-6: Ethinyl estradiol 0.03 mg and levonorgestrel 0.05 mg [6 blue tablets]
Day 7-11: Ethinyl estradiol 0.04 mg and levonorgestrel 0.075 mg [5 white tablets]
Day 12-21: Ethinyl estradiol 0.03 mg and levonorgestrel 0.125 mg [10 pink tablets]
Day 22-28: 7 peach inactive tablets (28s)

ethinyl estradiol and NGM *see* ethinyl estradiol and norgestimate *on page 357*

ethinyl estradiol and norelgestromin (ETH in il es tra DYE ole & nor el JES troe min)

Synonyms norelgestromin and ethinyl estradiol
U.S. Brand Names Ortho Evra®
Canadian Brand Names Evra®
Therapeutic Category Contraceptive, Oral; Estrogen and Progestin Combination
Use Prevention of pregnancy
General Dosage Range Topical: *Children and Adults (females, postmenarche):* Apply one patch weekly for 3 weeks, followed by one week that is patch-free
Dosage Forms
Patch, transdermal:
Ortho Evra®: Ethinyl estradiol 0.75 mg and norelgestromin 6 mg [releases ethinyl estradiol 20 mcg and norelgestromin 150 mcg per day] (1s, 3s)

Dosage Forms - Canada
Patch, transdermal:
Evra®: Ethinyl estradiol 0.6 mg and norelgestromin 6 mg (1s, 3s)

ethinyl estradiol and norethindrone (ETH in il es tra DYE ole & nor eth IN drone)

Medication Safety Issues
Sound-alike/look-alike issues:
femhrt® may be confused with Femara®
Lo Loestrin™ Fe may be confused with Loestrin® Fe
Modicon® may be confused with Mylicon®
Norinyl® may be confused with Nardil®

Synonyms norethindrone acetate and ethinyl estradiol; Ortho Novum

U.S. Brand Names Aranelle®; Balziva™; Brevicon®; Estrostep® Fe; Femcon® Fe; femhrt®; femhrt® Lo; Generess™ Fe; Jevantique™; Jinteli™; Junel® 1.5/30; Junel® 1/20; Junel® Fe 1.5/30; Junel® Fe 1/20; Leena®; Lo Loestrin™ Fe; Loestrin® 21 1.5/30; Loestrin® 21 1/20; Loestrin® 24 Fe; Loestrin® Fe 1.5/30; Loestrin® Fe 1/20; Microgestin® 1.5/30; Microgestin® 1/20; Microgestin® Fe 1.5/30; Microgestin® Fe 1/20; Modicon®; Necon® 0.5/35; Necon® 1/35; Necon® 10/11; Necon® 7/7/7; Norinyl® 1+35; Nortrel® 0.5/35; Nortrel® 1/35; Nortrel® 7/7/7; Ortho-Novum® 1/35; Ortho-Novum® 7/7/7; Ovcon® 35; Ovcon® 50; Tilia™ Fe; Tri-Legest™ Fe; Tri-Norinyl®; Zenchent™; Zeosa™

Canadian Brand Names Brevicon® 0.5/35; Brevicon® 1/35; FemHRT®; Loestrin™ 1.5/30; Minestrin™ 1/20; Ortho® 0.5/35; Ortho® 1/35; Ortho® 7/7/7; Select™ 1/35; Synphasic®

Therapeutic Category Contraceptive, Oral

Use Prevention of pregnancy; treatment of acne; moderate-to-severe vasomotor symptoms associated with menopause; prevention of osteoporosis (in women at significant risk only)

General Dosage Range Oral: *Children and Adults (females, postmenarche):* 1 tablet daily

Dosage Forms
Tablet, oral:
femhrt® 1/5, Jevantique™ 1/5, Jinteli™: Ethinyl estradiol 0.005 mg and norethindrone acetate 1 mg (28s, 90s) [white tablets]
femhrt® Lo 0.5/2.5: Ethinyl estradiol 0.0025 mg and norethindrone acetate 0.5 mg (28s, 90s) [white tablets]

Tablet, oral, monophasic formulations:
Balziva™: Ethinyl estradiol 0.035 mg and norethindrone 0.4 mg (28s) [21 light peach tablets and 7 white inactive tablets]
Brevicon®: Ethinyl estradiol 0.035 mg and norethindrone 0.5 mg (28s) [21 blue tablets and 7 orange inactive tablets]
Junel® 1/20: Ethinyl estradiol 0.02 mg and norethindrone acetate 1 mg (21s) [yellow tablets]
Junel® 1.5/30, Loestrin® 21 1.5/30: Ethinyl estradiol 0.03 mg and norethindrone acetate 1.5 mg (21s) [pink tablets]
Junel® Fe 1/20: Ethinyl estradiol 0.02 mg and norethindrone acetate 1 mg [21 yellow tablets] and ferrous fumarate 75 mg [7 brown tablets] (28s)
Junel® Fe 1.5/30, Loestrin® Fe 21 1.5/30: Ethinyl estradiol 0.03 mg and norethindrone acetate 1.5 mg [21 pink tablets] and ferrous fumarate 75 mg [7 brown tablets] (28s)
Loestrin® 21 1/20: Ethinyl estradiol 0.02 mg and norethindrone acetate 1 mg (21s) [light yellow tablets]
Lo Loestrin™ Fe: Ethinyl estradiol 0.01 mg and norethindrone acetate 1mg [24 blue tablets] and ethinyl estradiol 0.01 mg [2 white tablets] and ferrous fumarate 75 mg [2 brown tablets] (28s)
Loestrin® 24 Fe: Ethinyl estradiol 0.02 mg and norethindrone acetate 1 mg [24 white tablets] and ferrous fumarate 75 mg [4 brown tablets] (28s)
Loestrin® Fe 1/20: Ethinyl estradiol 0.02 mg and norethindrone acetate 1 mg [21 light yellow tablets] and ferrous fumarate 75 mg [7 brown tablets] (28s)
Loestrin® Fe 1.5/30: Ethinyl estradiol 0.03 mg and norethindrone acetate 1.5 mg [21 pink tablets] and ferrous fumarate 75 mg [7 brown tablets] (28s)
Microgestin® 1/20: Ethinyl estradiol 0.02 mg and norethindrone acetate 1 mg (21s) [white tablets]
Microgestin® 1.5/30: Ethinyl estradiol 0.03 mg and norethindrone acetate 1.5 mg (21s) [green tablets]
Microgestin® Fe 1/20: Ethinyl estradiol 0.02 mg and norethindrone acetate 1 mg [21 white tablets] and ferrous fumarate 75 mg [7 brown tablets] (28s)
Microgestin® Fe 1.5/30: Ethinyl estradiol 0.03 mg and norethindrone acetate 1.5 mg [21 green tablets] and ferrous fumarate 75 mg [7 brown tablets] (28s)
Modicon®: Ethinyl estradiol 0.035 mg and norethindrone 0.5 mg (28s) [21 white tablets and 7 green inactive tablets]

ETHINYL ESTRADIOL AND NORETHINDRONE

Necon® 0.5/35, Nortrel® 0.5/35: Ethinyl estradiol 0.035 mg and norethindrone 0.5 mg (28s) [21 light yellow tablets and 7 white inactive tablets]

Necon® 1/35: Ethinyl estradiol 0.035 mg and norethindrone 1 mg (28s) [21 dark yellow tablets and 7 white inactive tablets]

Norinyl® 1+35: Ethinyl estradiol 0.035 mg and norethindrone 1 mg (28s) [21 yellow-green tablets and 7 orange inactive tablets]

Nortrel® 1/35:
Ethinyl estradiol 0.035 mg and norethindrone 1 mg (21s) [yellow tablets]
Ethinyl estradiol 0.035 mg and norethindrone 1 mg (28s) [21 yellow tablets and 7 white inactive tablets]

Ortho-Novum® 1/35: Ethinyl estradiol 0.035 mg and norethindrone 1 mg (28s) [21 peach tablets and 7 green inactive tablets]

Ovcon® 35: Ethinyl estradiol 0.035 mg and norethindrone 0.4 mg (28s) [21 light peach tablets and 7 green inactive tablets]

Ovcon® 50: Ethinyl estradiol 0.05 mg and norethindrone 1 mg (28s) [21 yellow tablets and 7 green inactive tablets]

Zenchent™: Ethinyl estradiol 0.035 mg and norethindrone 0.4 mg (28s) [21 orange tablets and 7 white inactive tablets]

Tablet, chewable, oral, monophasic formulations:

Femcon® Fe: Ethinyl estradiol 0.035 mg and norethindrone 0.4 mg [21 white tablets] and ferrous fumarate 75 mg [7 brown tablets] (28s)

Generess™ Fe: Ethinyl estradiol 0.025 mg and norethindrone 0.8 mg [24 light green tablets] and ferrous fumarate 75 mg [4 brown tablets] (28s)

Zeosa™: Ethinyl estradiol 0.035 mg and norethindrone 0.4 mg [21 light yellow tablets] and ferrous fumarate 75 mg [7 brown tablets] (28s)

Tablet, oral, biphasic formulations:

Necon® 10/11:
Day 1-10: Ethinyl estradiol 0.035 mg and norethindrone 0.5 mg [10 light yellow tablets]
Day 11-21: Ethinyl estradiol 0.035 mg and norethindrone 1 mg [11 dark yellow tablets]
Day 22-28: 7 white inactive tablets (28s)

Tablet, oral, triphasic formulations:

Aranelle®:
Day 1-7: Ethinyl estradiol 0.035 mg and norethindrone 0.5 mg [7 light yellow tablets]
Day 8-16: Ethinyl estradiol 0.035 mg and norethindrone 1 mg [9 white tablets]
Day 17-21: Ethinyl estradiol 0.035 mg and norethindrone 0.5 mg [5 light yellow tablets]
Day 22-28: 7 peach inactive tablets (28s)

Estrostep® Fe, Tilia™ Fe::
Day 1-5: Ethinyl estradiol 0.02 mg and norethindrone acetate 1 mg [5 white triangular tablets]
Day 6-12: Ethinyl estradiol 0.03 mg and norethindrone acetate 1 mg [7 white square tablets]
Day 13-21: Ethinyl estradiol 0.035 mg and norethindrone acetate 1 mg [9 white round tablets]
Day 22-28: Ferrous fumarate 75 mg [7 brown tablets] (28s)

Leena®:
Day 1-7: Ethinyl estradiol 0.035 mg and norethindrone 0.5 mg [7 light blue tablets]
Day 8-16: Ethinyl estradiol 0.035 mg and norethindrone 1 mg [9 light yellow-green tablets]
Day 17-21: Ethinyl estradiol 0.035 mg and norethindrone 0.5 mg [5 light blue tablets]
Day 22-28: 7 orange inactive tablets (28s)

Necon® 7/7/7, Ortho-Novum® 7/7/7:
Day 1-7: Ethinyl estradiol 0.035 mg and norethindrone 0.5 mg [7 white tablets]
Day 8-14: Ethinyl estradiol 0.035 mg and norethindrone 0.75 mg [7 light peach tablets]
Day 15-21: Ethinyl estradiol 0.035 mg and norethindrone 1 mg [7 peach tablets]
Day 22-28: 7 green inactive tablets (28s)

Nortrel® 7/7/7:
Day 1-7: Ethinyl estradiol 0.035 mg and norethindrone 0.5 mg [7 light yellow tablets]
Day 8-14: Ethinyl estradiol 0.035 mg and norethindrone 0.75 mg [7 blue tablets]
Day 15-21: Ethinyl estradiol 0.035 mg and norethindrone 1 mg [7 peach tablets]
Day 22-28: 7 white inactive tablets (28s)

Tri-Legest™ Fe:
Day 1-5: Ethinyl estradiol 0.02 mg and norethindrone acetate 1 mg [5 light pink tablets]
Day 6-12: Ethinyl estradiol 0.03 mg and norethindrone acetate 1 mg [7 light yellow tablets]
Day 13-21: Ethinyl estradiol 0.035 mg and norethindrone acetate 1 mg [9 light blue tablets]
Day 22-28: Ferrous fumarate 75 mg [7 brown tablets] (28s)

Tri-Norinyl®:
Day 1-7: Ethinyl estradiol 0.035 mg and norethindrone 0.5 mg [7 blue tablets]
Day 8-16: Ethinyl estradiol 0.035 mg and norethindrone 1 mg [9 yellow-green tablets]
Day 17-21: Ethinyl estradiol 0.035 mg and norethindrone 0.5 mg [5 blue tablets]
Day 22-28: 7 orange inactive tablets (28s)

ethinyl estradiol and norgestimate (ETH in il es tra DYE ole & nor JES ti mate)

Medication Safety Issues
Sound-alike/look-alike issues:
Ortho-Cyclen® may be confused with Ortho-Cept®
Ortho Tri-Cyclen® may be confused with Ortho Tri-Cyclen® Lo
Ortho Tri-Cyclen® Lo may be confused with Ortho Tri-Cyclen®
International issues:
Vivelle: Brand name for ethinyl estradiol/norgestimate [Austria], but also a brand name for estradiol [U.S. (discontinued), Belgium]

Synonyms ethinyl estradiol and NGM; norgestimate and ethinyl estradiol

U.S. Brand Names MonoNessa®; Ortho Tri-Cyclen®; Ortho Tri-Cyclen® Lo; Ortho-Cyclen®; Sprintec®; Tri-Sprintec®; TriNessa®

Canadian Brand Names Cyclen®; Tri-Cyclen®; Tri-Cyclen® Lo

Therapeutic Category Contraceptive, Oral

Use Prevention of pregnancy; treatment of acne

General Dosage Range Oral: *Children and Adults (females, postmenarche):* 1 tablet daily

Dosage Forms
Tablet, monophasic formulations:
MonoNessa®, Ortho-Cyclen®: Ethinyl estradiol 0.035 mg and norgestimate 0.25 mg (28s) [21 blue tablets and 7 green inactive tablets]
Sprintec®: Ethinyl estradiol 0.035 mg and norgestimate 0.25 mg (28s) [21 blue tablets and 7 white inactive tablets]

Tablet, triphasic formulations:
Ortho Tri-Cyclen®, TriNessa®:
Day 1-7: Ethinyl estradiol 0.035 mg and norgestimate 0.18 mg [7 white tablets]
Day 8-14: Ethinyl estradiol 0.035 mg and norgestimate 0.215 mg [7 light blue tablets]
Day 15-21: Ethinyl estradiol 0.035 mg and norgestimate 0.25 mg [7 blue tablets]
Day 22-28: 7 green inactive tablets (28s)
Tri-Sprintec®:
Day 1-7: Ethinyl estradiol 0.035 mg and norgestimate 0.18 mg [7 gray tablets]
Day 8-14: Ethinyl estradiol 0.035 mg and norgestimate 0.215 mg [7 light blue tablets]
Day 15-21: Ethinyl estradiol 0.035 mg and norgestimate 0.25 mg [7 blue tablets]
Day 22-28: 7 white inactive tablets (28s)
Ortho Tri-Cyclen® Lo:
Day 1-7: Ethinyl estradiol 0.025 mg and norgestimate 0.18 mg [7 white tablets]
Day 8-14: Ethinyl estradiol 0.025 mg and norgestimate 0.215 mg [7 light blue tablets]
Day 15-21: Ethinyl estradiol 0.025 mg and norgestimate 0.25 mg [7 dark blue tablets]
Day 22-28: 7 green inactive tablets (28s)

ethinyl estradiol and norgestrel (ETH in il es tra DYE ole & nor JES trel)

Synonyms Lo Ovral; morning after pill; norgestrel and ethinyl estradiol

U.S. Brand Names Cryselle® 28; Lo/Ovral®-28; Low-Ogestrel®; Ogestrel®

Canadian Brand Names Lo-Femenal 21; Ovral®

Therapeutic Category Contraceptive, Oral

Use Prevention of pregnancy; postcoital contraceptive or "morning after" pill

General Dosage Range Oral: *Children and Adults (females, postmenarche):* 1 tablet daily **or** 2-4 tablets as single dose or in two divided doses (depending on formulation) within 72 hours of unprotected intercourse and 2-4 tablets 12 hours after first dose

Dosage Forms
Tablet, monophasic formulations: Ethinyl estradiol 0.03 mg and norgestrel 0.3 mg [21 white tablets and 7 pink inactive tablets] (28s)
Cryselle® 28: Ethinyl estradiol 0.03 mg and norgestrel 0.3 mg [21 white tablets and 7 light green inactive tablets] (28s)

Low-Ogestrel®: Ethinyl estradiol 0.03 mg and norgestrel 0.3 mg [21 white tablets and 7 peach inactive tablets] (28s)

Lo/Ovral®-28: Ethinyl estradiol 0.03 mg and norgestrel 0.3 mg [21 white tablets and 7 pink inactive tablets] (28s)

Ogestrel®: Ethinyl estradiol 0.05 mg and norgestrel 0.5 mg [21 white tablets and 7 peach inactive tablets] (28s)

ethinyl estradiol, drospirenone, and levomefolate
(ETH in il es tra DYE ole, droh SPYE re none, & lee voe me FOE late)

Medication Safety Issues
Sound-alike/look-alike issues:
Beyaz™ may be confused with Yaz®

Synonyms drospirenone, ethinyl estradiol, and levomefolate calcium; ethinyl estradiol, drospirenone, and levomefolate calcium; levomefolate calcium, drospirenone, and ethinyl estradiol; levomefolate, drospirenone, and ethinyl estradiol

U.S. Brand Names Beyaz™; Safyral™

Therapeutic Category Contraceptive; Estrogen and Progestin Combination

Use Prevention of pregnancy; treatment of premenstrual dysphoric disorder (PMDD); treatment of acne; folate supplementation

General Dosage Range Oral: *Children ≥14 years and Adults:* 1 tablet daily

Dosage Forms
Tablet, oral:
Beyaz™: Ethinyl estradiol 0.02 mg, drospirenone 3 mg, and levomefolate calcium 0.451 mg [24 pink tablets] and levomefolate calcium 0.451 mg [4 light orange tablets] (28s)

Safyral™: Ethinyl estradiol 0.03 mg, drospirenone 3 mg, and levomefolate calcium 0.451 mg [21 orange tablets] and levomefolate calcium 0.451 mg [7 light orange tablets] (28s)

ethinyl estradiol, drospirenone, and levomefolate calcium *see* ethinyl estradiol, drospirenone, and levomefolate *on page 358*

ethiofos *see* amifostine *on page 63*

ethionamide (e thye on AM ide)

U.S. Brand Names Trecator®

Canadian Brand Names Trecator®

Therapeutic Category Antimycobacterial Agent

Use Treatment of tuberculosis and other mycobacterial diseases, in conjunction with other antituberculosis agents, when first-line agents have failed or resistance has been demonstrated

General Dosage Range Dosage adjustment recommended in patients with renal impairment
Oral:
Children: 15-20 mg/kg/day in 2-3 divided doses (maximum: 1 g/day)
Adults: 250-750 mg/day in 1-4 divided doses (maximum: 1 g/day)

Dosage Forms
Tablet, oral:
Trecator®: 250 mg

ethosuximide (eth oh SUKS i mide)

Medication Safety Issues
Sound-alike/look-alike issues:
Ethosuximide may be confused with methsuximide
Zarontin® may be confused with Neurontin®, Xalatan®, Zantac®, Zaroxolyn®

U.S. Brand Names Zarontin®

Canadian Brand Names Zarontin®

Therapeutic Category Anticonvulsant

Use Management of absence (petit mal) seizures

General Dosage Range Oral:
Children 3-6 years: Initial: 250 mg/day; Maintenance: 20 mg/kg/day (maximum: 1.5 g/day in divided doses)
Children ≥6 years: Initial: 500 mg/day; Maintenance: 20 mg/kg/day (maximum: 1.5 g/day in divided doses)
Adults: Initial: 500 mg/day (maximum: 1.5 g/day in divided doses)

Dosage Forms
  Capsule, softgel, oral: 250 mg
    Zarontin®: 250 mg
  Solution, oral: 250 mg/5 mL (473 mL)
    Zarontin®: 250 mg/5 mL (480 mL)
  Syrup, oral: 250 mg/5 mL (473 mL)

ethotoin (ETH oh toyn)

Synonyms ethylphenylhydantoin
U.S. Brand Names Peganone®
Therapeutic Category Hydantoin
Use Generalized tonic-clonic or complex-partial seizures
General Dosage Range Oral:
  Children ≥1 year: Maximum initial dose: 750 mg/day; usual maintenance dose: 0.5-1 g/day; maximum dose: 3 g/day
  Adults: Initial dose: ≤1 g/day; usual maintenance dose: 2-3 g/day
Dosage Forms
  Tablet, oral:
    Peganone®: 250 mg

ethoxynaphthamido penicillin sodium *see* nafcillin *on page 609*
ethyl alcohol *see* alcohol (ethyl) *on page 47*
ethyl aminobenzoate *see* benzocaine *on page 121*

ethyl chloride (ETH il KLOR ide)

Synonyms chloroethane
U.S. Brand Names Gebauer's Ethyl Chloride®
Therapeutic Category Local Anesthetic
Use Local anesthetic in minor operative procedures and to relieve pain caused by insect stings and burns, and irritation caused by myofascial and visceral pain syndromes
General Dosage Range Topical: *Adults:* Dosage varies greatly depending on indication
Dosage Forms
  Aerosol, topical:
    Gebauer's Ethyl Chloride®: 100% (103.5 mL)

ethyl esters of omega-3 fatty acids *see* omega-3-acid ethyl esters *on page 649*
ethylphenylhydantoin *see* ethotoin *on page 359*
ethynodiol diacetate and ethinyl estradiol *see* ethinyl estradiol and ethynodiol diacetate *on page 353*
Ethyol® *see* amifostine *on page 63*
Etibi® (Can) *see* ethambutol *on page 351*

etidronate (e ti DROE nate)

Medication Safety Issues
  Sound-alike/look-alike issues:
    Etidronate may be confused with etidocaine, etomidate, etretinate
Synonyms EHDP; etidronate disodium; sodium etidronate
U.S. Brand Names Didronel®
Canadian Brand Names Co-Etidronate; Mylan-Etidronate
Therapeutic Category Bisphosphonate Derivative
Use Symptomatic treatment of Paget disease; prevention and treatment of heterotopic ossification due to spinal cord injury or after total hip replacement
General Dosage Range Oral: *Adults:* 5-20 mg/kg/day
Dosage Forms
  Tablet, oral: 200 mg, 400 mg
    Didronel®: 400 mg

etidronate and calcium carbonate *(Canada only)*
(e ti DROE nate & KAL see um KAR bun ate)

Synonyms calcium carbonate and etidronate disodium; etidronate disodium and calcium

Canadian Brand Names CO Etidrocal; Didrocal®; Mylan-Eti-Cal Carepac; Novo-Etidronatecal

Therapeutic Category Bisphosphonate Derivative; Calcium Salt

Use Treatment and prevention of postmenopausal osteoporosis; prevention of corticosteroid-induced osteoporosis

General Dosage Range Oral: *Adults:* Etidronate disodium 400 mg once daily for 14 days, followed by calcium carbonate 1250 mg (500 mg elemental calcium) once daily for 76 days

Product Availability Not available in U.S.

Dosage Forms - Canada
  Combination package [each package contains 5 blister cards (90-day supply)]:
  Didrocal®:
    Tablet, etidronate: 400 mg (14s) [first card (white tablets)]
    Tablet, calcium: 1250 mg (76s) [remaining cards (blue tablets)]

etidronate disodium *see* etidronate *on page 359*

etidronate disodium and calcium *see* etidronate and calcium carbonate *(Canada only) on page 360*

etodolac (ee toe DOE lak)

Medication Safety Issues
  Sound-alike/look-alike issues:
    Lodine® may be confused with codeine, iodine, Iopidine®, Lopid®

Synonyms etodolic acid; Lodine

Canadian Brand Names Apo-Etodolac®; Utradol™

Therapeutic Category Analgesic, Nonnarcotic; Nonsteroidal Antiinflammatory Drug (NSAID)

Use Acute and long-term use in the management of signs and symptoms of osteoarthritis; rheumatoid arthritis and juvenile idiopathic arthritis (JIA); management of acute pain

General Dosage Range Oral:
  Extended release:
    Children 6-16 years and 20-30 kg: 400 mg once daily
    Children 6-16 years and 31-45 kg: 600 mg once daily
    Children 6-16 years and 46-60 kg: 800 mg once daily
    Children 6-16 years and >60 kg: 1000 mg once daily
    Adults: 400-1000 mg once daily
  Regular release: *Adults:* 200-400 mg every 6-12 hours as needed **or** 500 mg 2 times/day (maximum: 1 g/day)

Dosage Forms
  Capsule, oral: 200 mg, 300 mg
  Tablet, oral: 400 mg, 500 mg
  Tablet, extended release, oral: 400 mg, 500 mg, 600 mg

etodolic acid *see* etodolac *on page 360*

EtOH *see* alcohol (ethyl) *on page 47*

etomidate (e TOM i date)

Medication Safety Issues
  Sound-alike/look-alike issues:
    Etomidate may be confused with etidronate
  High alert medication:
    The Institute for Safe Medication Practices (ISMP) includes this medication among its list of drugs which have a heightened risk of causing significant patient harm when used in error.

U.S. Brand Names Amidate®

Canadian Brand Names Amidate®

Therapeutic Category General Anesthetic

Use Induction and maintenance of general anesthesia

General Dosage Range I.V.: *Children >10 years and Adults:* Induction: 0.2-0.6 mg/kg; Maintenance: 5-20 mcg/kg/minute

Dosage Forms
 Injection, solution: 2 mg/mL (10 mL, 20 mL)
  Amidate®: 2 mg/mL (10 mL, 20 mL)

etonogestrel (e toe noe JES trel)

Synonyms 3-keto-desogestrel; ENG

U.S. Brand Names Implanon®

Therapeutic Category Contraceptive; Progestin

Use Prevention of pregnancy; for use in women who request long-acting (up to 3 years) contraception

General Dosage Range Subdermal: *Children and Adults (females, postmenarche):* Implant 1 rod for up to 3 years

Product Availability
 Nexplanon®: FDA approved June 2011; availability anticipated October 2011
 Nexplanon® is a radiopaque etonogestrel implant approved for the prevention of pregnancy. Nexplanon® is expected to replace the nonradiopaque etonogestrel implant, Implanon™.

Dosage Forms
 Rod, subdermal:
  Implanon®: 68 mg

etonogestrel and ethinyl estradiol *see* ethinyl estradiol and etonogestrel *on page 353*

ETOP *see* etoposide phosphate *on page 361*

Etopophos® *see* etoposide phosphate *on page 361*

etoposide (e toe POE side)

Medication Safety Issues
 Sound-alike/look-alike issues:
  Etoposide may be confused with teniposide
  Etoposide may be confused with etoposide phosphate (a prodrug of etoposide which is rapidly converted in the plasma to etoposide)
  VePesid® may be confused with Versed
 High alert medication:
  This medication is in a class the Institute for Safe Medication Practices (ISMP) includes among its list of drug classes which have a heightened risk of causing significant patient harm when used in error.

Synonyms EPEG; epipodophyllotoxin; VePesid; VP-16; VP-16-213

U.S. Brand Names Toposar®

Therapeutic Category Antineoplastic Agent

Use Treatment of refractory testicular tumors (injectable formulation); treatment of small cell lung cancer

General Dosage Range Dosage adjustment recommended in patients with hepatic or renal impairment
I.V., oral: *Adults:* Dosage varies greatly depending on indication

Dosage Forms
 Capsule, softgel, oral: 50 mg
 Injection, solution: 20 mg/mL (5 mL, 25 mL, 50 mL, 100 mL)
  Toposar®: 20 mg/mL (5 mL, 25 mL, 50 mL)

etoposide phosphate (e toe POE side FOS fate)

Medication Safety Issues
 Sound-alike/look-alike issues:
  Etoposide phosphate may be confused with etoposide, teniposide
  Etoposide phosphate is a prodrug of etoposide and is rapidly converted in the plasma to etoposide. To avoid confusion or dosing errors, **dosage should be expressed as the desired etoposide dose,** not as the etoposide phosphate dose (eg, etoposide phosphate equivalent to ____ mg etoposide).
 High alert medication:
  This medication is in a class the Institute for Safe Medication Practices (ISMP) includes among its list of drug classes which have a heightened risk of causing significant patient harm when used in error.

Synonyms epipodophyllotoxin; ETOP

U.S. Brand Names Etopophos®

Therapeutic Category Antineoplastic Agent

Use Treatment of refractory testicular tumors; treatment of small cell lung cancer

◀ **General Dosage Range** Dosage adjustment recommended in patients with hepatic or renal impairment
I.V.: *Adults:* Dosage varies greatly depending on indication

Dosage Forms
Injection, powder for reconstitution:
Etopophos®: 100 mg

etravirine (et ra VIR een)

Synonyms TMC125
U.S. Brand Names Intelence®
Canadian Brand Names Intelence®
Therapeutic Category Antiretroviral Agent, Nonnucleoside Reverse Transcriptase Inhibitor (NNRTI)
Use Treatment of HIV-1 infection in combination with at least two additional antiretroviral agents in
treatment-experienced patients exhibiting viral replication with documented nonnucleoside reverse
transcriptase inhibitor (NNRTI) resistance
General Dosage Range Oral: *Adults:* 200 mg twice daily
Dosage Forms
Tablet, oral:
Intelence®: 100 mg, 200 mg

Euflex® (Can) *see* flutamide *on page 392*
Euflexxa® *see* hyaluronate and derivatives *on page 443*
Euglucon® (Can) *see* glyburide *on page 420*
Eulexin *see* flutamide *on page 392*
Eulexin® (Can) *see* flutamide *on page 392*
Eurax® *see* crotamiton *on page 240*
Euro-Lithium (Can) *see* lithium *on page 532*
Euthyrox (Can) *see* levothyroxine *on page 522*
Evac-U-Gen® [OTC] *see* senna *on page 807*
Evamist™ *see* estradiol (systemic) *on page 343*

everolimus (e ver OH li mus)

Medication Safety Issues
Sound-alike/look-alike issues:
Everolimus may be confused with sirolimus, tacrolimus, temsirolimus
High alert medication:
This medication is in a class the Institute for Safe Medication Practices (ISMP) includes among its list of
drug classes which have a heightened risk of causing significant patient harm when used in error.
Synonyms RAD001
U.S. Brand Names Afinitor®; Zortress®
Canadian Brand Names Afinitor®
Therapeutic Category Antineoplastic Agent, mTOR Kinase Inhibitor; mTOR Kinase Inhibitor
Use Treatment of advanced renal cell cancer (RCC), after sunitinib or sorafenib failure (Afinitor®);
treatment of subependymal giant cell astrocytoma (SEGA) associated with tuberous sclerosis, in patients
who are not candidates for curative surgical resection (Afinitor®); treatment of advanced, metastatic or
unresectable pancreatic neuroendocrine tumors (PNET) (Afinitor®); prophylaxis of organ rejection in
patients at low-moderate immunologic risk receiving renal transplants (Zortress®)
General Dosage Range Dosage adjustment recommended in patients with hepatic impairment, on
concomitant therapy, or who develop toxicities
Oral: *Children ≥3 years and Adults:* Dosage varies greatly depending on indication
Dosage Forms
Tablet, oral:
Afinitor®: 2.5 mg, 5 mg, 10 mg
Zortress®: 0.25 mg, 0.5 mg, 0.75 mg

Everone® 200 (Can) *see* testosterone *on page 854*
Evicel™ *see* fibrin sealant *on page 376*
Evista® *see* raloxifene *on page 765*
Evithrom® *see* thrombin (topical) *on page 865*

Evoclin® *see* clindamycin (topical) *on page 218*
Evoxac® *see* cevimeline *on page 191*
Evra® (Can) *see* ethinyl estradiol and norelgestromin *on page 354*
Exactacain® *see* benzocaine, butamben, and tetracaine *on page 123*
Exalgo™ *see* hydromorphone *on page 452*
Excedrin® Extra Strength [OTC] *see* acetaminophen, aspirin, and caffeine *on page 29*
Excedrin® Migraine [OTC] *see* acetaminophen, aspirin, and caffeine *on page 29*
Excedrin® PM® [OTC] *see* acetaminophen and diphenhydramine *on page 27*
Excedrin® Sinus Headache [OTC] *see* acetaminophen and phenylephrine *on page 28*
Excedrin® Tension Headache [OTC] *see* acetaminophen *on page 23*
ExeClear-C *see* guaifenesin and codeine *on page 426*
ExeCof [DSC] *see* guaifenesin, dextromethorphan, and phenylephrine *on page 429*
ExeFen-DMX *see* guaifenesin, pseudoephedrine, and dextromethorphan *on page 430*
ExeFen-IR [DSC] *see* guaifenesin and pseudoephedrine *on page 429*
Exelderm® *see* sulconazole *on page 834*
Exelon® *see* rivastigmine *on page 786*

exemestane (ex e MES tane)

Medication Safety Issues
 Sound-alike/look-alike issues:
  Aromasin® may be confused with Arimidex®
  Exemestane may be confused with estramustine.
U.S. Brand Names Aromasin®
Canadian Brand Names Aromasin®
Therapeutic Category Antineoplastic Agent, Miscellaneous
Use Treatment of advanced breast cancer in postmenopausal women whose disease has progressed following tamoxifen therapy; adjuvant treatment of postmenopausal estrogen receptor-positive early breast cancer following 2-3 years of tamoxifen (for a total of 5 years of adjuvant therapy)
General Dosage Range Dosage adjustment recommended in patients on concomitant therapy
 Oral: *Adults (postmenopausal females):* 25 mg once daily
Dosage Forms
 Tablet, oral: 25 mg
  Aromasin®: 25 mg

exenatide (ex EN a tide)

Synonyms AC 2993; AC002993; exendin-4; LY2148568
U.S. Brand Names Byetta®
Therapeutic Category Antidiabetic Agent, Incretin Mimetic
Use Treatment of type 2 diabetes mellitus (noninsulin-dependent, NIDDM) to improve glycemic control
General Dosage Range SubQ: *Adults:* Initial: 5 mcg twice daily; Maintenance: 5-10 mcg twice daily
Dosage Forms
 Injection, solution:
  Byetta®: 250 mcg/mL (1.2 mL, 2.4 mL)

exendin-4 *see* exenatide *on page 363*
ExeTuss-DM [DSC] *see* guaifenesin, dextromethorphan, and phenylephrine *on page 429*
Exforge® *see* amlodipine and valsartan *on page 71*
Exforge HCT® *see* amlodipine, valsartan, and hydrochlorothiazide *on page 71*
Exjade® *see* deferasirox *on page 256*
ex-lax® [OTC] *see* senna *on page 807*
ex-lax® Maximum Strength [OTC] *see* senna *on page 807*
ex-lax® Ultra [OTC] *see* bisacodyl *on page 134*
Exorex® Penetrating Emulsion [OTC] *see* coal tar *on page 227*
Exorex® Penetrating Emulsion #2 [OTC] *see* coal tar *on page 227*
Extavia® *see* interferon beta-1b *on page 482*
extended release epidural morphine *see* morphine (liposomal) *on page 599*

Extina® *see* ketoconazole (topical) *on page 500*
Extraneal *see* icodextrin *on page 463*
EYE001 *see* pegaptanib *on page 678*
Eyestil (Can) *see* hyaluronate and derivatives *on page 443*
Eye-Stream® (Can) *see* balanced salt solution *on page 113*
E-Z-Cat® *see* barium *on page 114*
E-Z Cat® Dry *see* barium *on page 114*
EZ-Char® [OTC] *see* charcoal *on page 191*
E-Z-Disk™ *see* barium *on page 114*
E-Z-Dose™ with Liquid Polibar Plus® *see* barium *on page 114*

ezetimibe (ez ET i mibe)

Medication Safety Issues
  Sound-alike/look-alike issues:
  Zetia® may be confused with Zebeta®, Zestril®
U.S. Brand Names Zetia®
Canadian Brand Names Ezetrol®
Therapeutic Category Antilipemic Agent, 2-Azetidinone
Use Use in combination with dietary therapy for the treatment of primary hypercholesterolemia (as monotherapy or in combination with HMG-CoA reductase inhibitors); homozygous sitosterolemia; homozygous familial hypercholesterolemia (in combination with atorvastatin or simvastatin); mixed hyperlipidemia (in combination with fenofibrate)
General Dosage Range Oral: *Children ≥10 years and Adults:* 10 mg once daily
Dosage Forms
  Tablet, oral:
  Zetia®: 10 mg

ezetimibe and simvastatin (ez ET i mibe & SIM va stat in)

Medication Safety Issues
  Sound-alike/look-alike issues:
  Vytorin® may be confused with Vyvanse™
Synonyms simvastatin and ezetimibe
U.S. Brand Names Vytorin®
Therapeutic Category Antilipemic Agent, 2-Azetidinone
Use Used in combination with dietary modification for the treatment of primary hypercholesterolemia and homozygous familial hypercholesterolemia
General Dosage Range Dosage adjustment recommended in patients with renal impairment or on concomitant therapy
  Oral: *Adults:* Ezetimibe 10 mg and simvastatin 10-40 mg once daily
Dosage Forms
  Tablet:
  Vytorin®:
    10/10: Ezetimibe 10 mg and simvastatin 10 mg
    10/20: Ezetimibe 10 mg and simvastatin 20 mg
    10/40: Ezetimibe 10 mg and simvastatin 40 mg
    10/80: Ezetimibe 10 mg and simvastatin 80 mg

Ezetrol® (Can) *see* ezetimibe *on page 364*
EZG *see* ezogabine *on page 364*
E-Z-HD™ *see* barium *on page 114*

ezogabine (e ZOG a been)

Synonyms EZG; Potiga™; Retigabine (RTG)
Therapeutic Category Anticonvulsant, Neuronal Potassium Channel Opener
Use Adjuvant treatment of partial seizures
Product Availability Potiga™: FDA approved June 2011; availability expected by the end of 2011

E-Z-Paque® *see* barium *on page 114*

E-Z-Paste® *see* barium *on page 114*
F₃T *see* trifluridine *on page 890*
FabAV, FAB (ovine) *see* crotalidae polyvalent immune FAB (ovine) *on page 239*
FaBB *see* folic acid, cyanocobalamin, and pyridoxine *on page 396*
Fabrazyme® *see* agalsidase beta *on page 43*
Factive® *see* gemifloxacin *on page 414*

factor VIIa (recombinant) (FAK ter SEV en aye ree KOM be nant)
Medication Safety Issues
  Sound-alike/look-alike issues:
    NovoSeven® RT may be confused with Novacet®
Synonyms coagulation factor VIIa; eptacog alfa (activated); rFVIIa
U.S. Brand Names NovoSeven® RT
Canadian Brand Names Niastase®; Niastase® RT
Therapeutic Category Antihemophilic Agent; Blood Product Derivative
Use Treatment of bleeding episodes and prevention of bleeding in surgical interventions in patients with either hemophilia A or B with inhibitors to factor VIII or factor IX, acquired hemophilia, or congenital factor VII deficiency
General Dosage Range I.V.: *Children and Adults:* Dosage varies greatly depending on indication
Dosage Forms
  Injection, powder for reconstitution [preservative free]:
    NovoSeven® RT: 1 mg, 2 mg, 5 mg, 8 mg

factor VIII concentrate *see* antihemophilic factor/von Willebrand factor complex (human) *on page 82*
factor VIII (human) *see* antihemophilic factor (human) *on page 81*
factor VIII (human) *see* antihemophilic factor/von Willebrand factor complex (human) *on page 82*
factor VIII (recombinant) *see* antihemophilic factor (recombinant) *on page 81*

factor IX (FAK ter nyne)
Synonyms factor IX concentrate
U.S. Brand Names AlphaNine® SD; BeneFix®; Mononine®
Canadian Brand Names BeneFix®; Immunine® VH; Mononine®
Therapeutic Category Antihemophilic Agent
Use Prevention and control of bleeding in patients with factor IX deficiency (hemophilia B or Christmas disease)
General Dosage Range I.V.: *Children and Adults:* Dosage varies greatly depending on indication
Dosage Forms
  Injection, powder for reconstitution [recombinant]:
    BeneFix®: ~250 int. units, ~500 int. units, ~1000 int. units, ~2000 int. units [exact potency labeled on each vial]
  Injection, powder for reconstitution [human derived]:
    AlphaNine® SD: ~500 int. units, ~1000 int. units, ~1500 int. units [exact potency labeled on each vial]
    Mononine®: ~500 int. units, ~1000 int. units [exact potency labeled on each vial]

factor IX complex (human) (FAK ter nyne KOM pleks HYU man)
Synonyms PCC; prothrombin complex concentrate
U.S. Brand Names Bebulin® VH; Profilnine® SD
Therapeutic Category Antihemophilic Agent
Use Prevention and control of bleeding in patients with factor IX deficiency (hemophilia B or Christmas disease)
General Dosage Range I.V.: *Children and Adults:* Dosage varies greatly depending on indication
Dosage Forms
  Injection, powder for reconstitution:
    Bebulin® VH: Exact potency labeled on each vial
    Profilnine® SD: ~500 int. units, ~1000 int. units, ~1500 int. units [exact potency labeled on each vial]

factor IX concentrate *see* factor IX *on page 365*
factor 13 *see* factor XIII concentrate (human) *on page 366*

factor XIII concentrate (human) (FAK ter THIR teen KON cen trate HYU man)

Medication Safety Issues

Sound-alike/look-alike issues:

Factor XIII may be confused with Factor VIII

Synonyms activated factor XIII; factor 13; FXIII

U.S. Brand Names Corifact®

Therapeutic Category Antihemophilic Agent; Blood Product Derivative

Use Prophylaxis against bleeding episodes in congenital factor XIII deficiency

General Dosage Range I.V.: *Children and Adults:* Initial: 40 units/kg; Maintenance: Varies depending on desired factor XIII trough levels

Dosage Forms

Injection, powder for reconstitution:

Corifact®: Exact potency labeled on each vial

famciclovir (fam SYE kloe veer)

Medication Safety Issues

Sound-alike/look-alike issues:

Famvir® may be confused with Femara®

U.S. Brand Names Famvir®

Canadian Brand Names Apo-Famciclovir®; CO Famciclovir; Famvir®; PMS-Famciclovir; Sandoz-Famciclovir

Therapeutic Category Antiviral Agent

Use Treatment of acute herpes zoster (shingles); treatment and suppression of recurrent episodes of genital herpes in immunocompetent patients; treatment of herpes labialis (cold sores) in immunocompetent patients; treatment of recurrent mucocutaneous/genital herpes simplex in HIV-infected patients

General Dosage Range Dosage adjustment recommended in patients with renal impairment

Oral: *Adults:* 250-1000 mg twice daily **or** 500 mg every 8 hours **or** 1500 mg once

Dosage Forms

Tablet, oral: 125 mg, 250 mg, 500 mg

Famvir®: 125 mg, 250 mg, 500 mg

famotidine (fa MOE ti deen)

Medication Safety Issues

Sound-alike/look-alike issues:

Famotidine may be confused with FLUoxetine, furosemide

U.S. Brand Names Heartburn Relief Maximum Strength [OTC]; Heartburn Relief [OTC]; Pepcid®; Pepcid® AC Maximum Strength [OTC]; Pepcid® AC [OTC]

Canadian Brand Names Acid Control; Apo-Famotidine®; Apo-Famotidine® Injectable; Famotidine Omega; Mylan-Famotidine; Novo-Famotidine; Nu-Famotidine; Pepcid®; Pepcid® AC; Pepcid® I.V.; Ulcidine

Therapeutic Category Histamine H_2 Antagonist

Use Maintenance therapy and treatment of duodenal ulcer; treatment of gastroesophageal reflux disease (GERD), active benign gastric ulcer; pathological hypersecretory conditions

OTC labeling: Relief of heartburn, acid indigestion, and sour stomach

General Dosage Range Dosage adjustment recommended in patients with renal impairment

I.V.:

Children 1-16 years: 0.25 mg/kg every 12 hours (maximum: 40 mg/day)

Adults: 20 mg every 12 hours

Oral:

Children <3 months: 0.5 mg/kg once daily

Children 3-12 months: 0.5 mg/kg twice daily

Children 1-11 years: 0.5-1 mg/kg/day in 1-2 divided doses (maximum: 80 mg/day)

Children 12-16 years: 0.5-1 mg/kg/day in 1-2 divided doses (maximum: 80 mg/day) **or** 10-20 mg every 12 hours (OTC dosing)

Adults: 20-40 mg/day in 1-2 divided doses **or** 20-160 mg every 6 hours [hypersecretory conditions]

Dosage Forms
 Infusion, premixed in NS [preservative free]: 20 mg (50 mL)
 Injection, solution: 10 mg/mL (4 mL, 20 mL, 50 mL)
 Injection, solution [preservative free]: 10 mg/mL (2 mL)
 Powder for suspension, oral: 40 mg/5 mL (50 mL)
  Pepcid®: 40 mg/5 mL (50 mL)
 Tablet, oral: 10 mg, 20 mg, 40 mg
  Heartburn Relief [OTC]: 10 mg
  Heartburn Relief Maximum Strength [OTC]: 20 mg
  Pepcid®: 20 mg, 40 mg
  Pepcid® AC [OTC]: 10 mg
  Pepcid® AC Maximum Strength [OTC]: 20 mg
 Tablet, chewable, oral:
  Pepcid® AC Maximum Strength [OTC]: 20 mg

famotidine and ibuprofen see ibuprofen and famotidine on page 462

famotidine, calcium carbonate, and magnesium hydroxide
(fa MOE ti deen, KAL see um KAR bun ate, & mag NEE zhum hye DROKS ide)
 Synonyms calcium carbonate, magnesium hydroxide, and famotidine; magnesium hydroxide, famotidine, and calcium carbonate
 U.S. Brand Names Pepcid® Complete® [OTC]; Tums® Dual Action [OTC]
 Canadian Brand Names Pepcid® Complete® [OTC]
 Therapeutic Category Antacid; Histamine H$_2$ Antagonist
 Use Relief of heartburn due to acid indigestion
 General Dosage Range Oral: *Children ≥12 years and Adults:* 1 tablet (famotidine 10 mg/calcium carbonate 800 mg/magnesium hydroxide 165 mg) as needed (maximum: 2 tablets/day)
 Dosage Forms
 Tablet, chewable, oral:
  Pepcid® Complete® [OTC], Tums® Dual Action [OTC]: Famotidine 10 mg, calcium carbonate 800 mg, and magnesium hydroxide 165 mg

Famotidine Omega (Can) see famotidine on page 366
fampridine-SR see dalfampridine on page 250
Famvir® see famciclovir on page 366
Fanapt® see iloperidone on page 465
Fansidar® [DSC] see sulfadoxine and pyrimethamine on page 836
2F-ara-AMP see fludarabine on page 382
Fareston® see toremifene on page 878
Faslodex® see fulvestrant on page 404
Fasturtec® (Can) see rasburicase on page 769

fat emulsion (fat e MUL shun)
 Synonyms intravenous fat emulsion
 U.S. Brand Names Intralipid®; Liposyn® III
 Canadian Brand Names Intralipid®; Liposyn® II
 Therapeutic Category Intravenous Nutritional Therapy
 Use Source of calories and essential fatty acids for patients requiring parenteral nutrition of extended duration; prevention and treatment of essential fatty acid deficiency (EFAD)
 General Dosage Range I.V.:
 Premature infants: Initial: 0.25-0.5 g/kg/day; Maintenance: Up to 3 g/kg/day (≤1 g/kg/day if on phototherapy)
 Infants and Children: Initial: 0.5-1 g/kg/day; Maintenance: Up to 3 g/kg/day
 Adults: Initial: 1 g/kg/day; Maintenance: Up to 2.5-3 g/kg/day **or** 500 mL twice weekly
 Dosage Forms
 Injection, emulsion:
  Intralipid®: 20% (100 mL, 250 mL, 500 mL, 1000 mL); 30% (500 mL)
  Liposyn® III: 10% (250 mL, 500 mL); 20% (250 mL, 500 mL); 30% (500 mL)

Father John's® [OTC] see dextromethorphan on page 270

Father John's® Plus [OTC] *see* chlorpheniramine, phenylephrine, and dextromethorphan *on page* 200

FazaClo® *see* clozapine *on page* 227

5-FC *see* flucytosine *on page* 382

FC1157a *see* toremifene *on page* 878

FE200486 *see* degarelix *on page* 257

febuxostat (feb UX oh stat)

Synonyms TEI-6720; TMX-67

U.S. Brand Names Uloric®

Canadian Brand Names Uloric®

Therapeutic Category Xanthine Oxidase Inhibitor

Use Chronic management of hyperuricemia in patients with gout

General Dosage Range Oral: *Adults:* 40-80 mg once daily

Dosage Forms
Tablet, oral:
Uloric®: 40 mg, 80 mg

Feiba NF *see* antiinhibitor coagulant complex *on page* 83

Feiba VH [DSC] *see* antiinhibitor coagulant complex *on page* 83

felbamate (FEL ba mate)

U.S. Brand Names Felbatol®

Therapeutic Category Anticonvulsant

Use Not as a first-line antiepileptic treatment; only in those patients who respond inadequately to alternative treatments and whose epilepsy is so severe that a substantial risk of aplastic anemia and/or liver failure is deemed acceptable in light of the benefits conferred by its use. Patient must be fully advised of risk and provide signed written informed consent. Felbamate can be used as either monotherapy or adjunctive therapy in the treatment of partial seizures (with and without generalization) and in adults with epilepsy. Used as adjunctive therapy in the treatment of partial and generalized seizures associated with Lennox-Gastaut syndrome in children.

General Dosage Range Dosage adjustment recommended in patients with renal impairment or on concomitant therapy

Oral:
Children 2-14 years: Initial: 15 mg/kg/day in divided doses 3 or 4 times/day; Maintenance: Up to 45 mg/kg/day in divided doses 3 or 4 times/day (maximum: 3600 mg/day)
Children >14 years and Adults: Initial: 1200 mg/day in divided doses 3 or 4 times/day; Maintenance: Up to 3600 mg/day in divided doses 3 or 4 times/day.

Dosage Forms
Suspension, oral:
Felbatol®: 600 mg/5 mL (240 mL, 960 mL)
Tablet, oral: 400 mg, 600 mg
Felbatol®: 400 mg, 600 mg

Felbatol® *see* felbamate *on page* 368

Feldene® *see* piroxicam *on page* 708

felodipine (fe LOE di peen)

Medication Safety Issues
Sound-alike/look-alike issues:
Plendil may be confused with Isordil®, pindolol, Pletal®, PriLOSEC®, Prinivil®

Canadian Brand Names Plendil®; Renedil®; Sandoz-Felodipine

Therapeutic Category Calcium Channel Blocker

Use Treatment of hypertension

General Dosage Range Dosage adjustment recommended in patients with hepatic impairment
Oral:
Adults: Initial: 2.5-10 mg once daily; Maintenance: 2.5-20 mg once daily (maximum: 20 mg/day)
Elderly: Initial: 2.5 mg/day

Dosage Forms
  Tablet, extended release, oral: 2.5 mg, 5 mg, 10 mg

felodipine and ramipril see ramipril and felodipine *(Canada only)* on page 766
Femara® see letrozole on page 515
Femcon® Fe see ethinyl estradiol and norethindrone on page 355
Femecal OB see vitamins (multiple/prenatal) on page 920
femhrt® see ethinyl estradiol and norethindrone on page 355
FemHRT® (Can) see ethinyl estradiol and norethindrone on page 355
femhrt® Lo see ethinyl estradiol and norethindrone on page 355
Femilax™ [OTC] see bisacodyl on page 134
Femiron® [OTC] see ferrous fumarate on page 373
Fem-Prin® [OTC] see acetaminophen, aspirin, and caffeine on page 29
Femring® see estradiol (systemic) on page 343
Femstat® One (Can) see butoconazole on page 155
Femtrace® see estradiol (systemic) on page 343
Fenesin DM IR see guaifenesin and dextromethorphan on page 427
Fenesin IR [OTC] see guaifenesin on page 425
Fenesin PE IR see guaifenesin and phenylephrine on page 428

fenofibrate (fen oh FYE brate)

Medication Safety Issues
  Sound-alike/look-alike issues:
    TriCor® may be confused with Fibricor®, Tracleer®
Synonyms procetofene; proctofene
U.S. Brand Names Antara®; Fenoglide®; Lipofen®; Lofibra®; TriCor®; Triglide®
Canadian Brand Names Apo-Feno-Micro®; Apo-Feno-Super®; Apo-Fenofibrate®; Dom-Fenofibrate Micro; Feno-Micro-200; Fenofibrate Micro; Fenofibrate-S; Fenomax; Lipidil EZ®; Lipidil Micro®; Lipidil Supra®; Mylan-Fenofibrate Micro; Novo-Fenofibrate; Novo-Fenofibrate Micronized; Novo-Fenofibrate-S; Nu-Fenofibrate; PHL-Fenofibrate Micro; PHL-Fenofibrate Supra; PMS-Fenofibrate Micro; PRO-Feno-Super; ratio-Fenofibrate MC; Riva-Fenofibrate Micro; Sandoz-Fenofibrate S
Therapeutic Category Antihyperlipidemic Agent, Miscellaneous
Use Adjunct to dietary therapy for the treatment of adults with elevations of serum triglyceride levels (types IV and V hyperlipidemia); adjunct to dietary therapy for the reduction of low density lipoprotein cholesterol (LDL-C), total cholesterol (total-C), triglycerides, and apolipoprotein B (apo B), and to increase high density lipoprotein cholesterol (HDL-C) in adult patients with primary hypercholesterolemia or mixed dyslipidemia (Fredrickson types IIa and IIb)
General Dosage Range Dosage adjustment recommended in patients with renal impairment
  Oral: *Adults and Elderly:* Dosage varies greatly depending on product
Dosage Forms
  Capsule, oral: 67 mg, 134 mg, 200 mg
    Antara®: 43 mg, 130 mg
    Lipofen®: 50 mg, 150 mg
    Lofibra®: 67 mg, 134 mg, 200 mg
  Tablet, oral: 54 mg, 160 mg
    Fenoglide®: 40 mg, 120 mg
    Lofibra®: 54 mg, 160 mg
    TriCor®: 48 mg, 145 mg
    Triglide®: 50 mg, 160 mg

Fenofibrate Micro (Can) see fenofibrate on page 369
Fenofibrate-S (Can) see fenofibrate on page 369

fenofibric acid (fen oh FYE brik AS id)

Medication Safety Issues
  Sound-alike/look-alike issues:
    Fibricor® may be confused with Tricor®
    TriLipix™ may be confused with Trileptal®, TriLyte®
Synonyms ABT-335; choline fenofibrate

◄ **U.S. Brand Names** Fibricor®; TriLipix®

Therapeutic Category Antilipemic Agent, Fibric Acid

Use Adjunct to dietary therapy for the treatment of severely elevated serum triglyceride levels; adjunct to dietary therapy for the reduction of low density lipoprotein cholesterol (LDL-C), total cholesterol (total-C), triglycerides, and apolipoprotein B (apo B) and to increase high density lipoprotein cholesterol (HDL-C) in patients with primary hypercholesterolemia or mixed dyslipidemia

TriLipix™ is also indicated as adjunct to dietary therapy concomitantly with a statin to reduce triglyceride levels and increase HDL-C levels in patients with mixed dyslipidemia and coronary heart disease (CHD) or at risk for CHD

General Dosage Range Dosage adjustment recommended in patients with renal impairment

Oral: *Adults:* Fibricor®: 35-105 mg once daily (maximum: 105 mg/day); TriLipix™: 45-135 mg once daily (maximum: 135 mg/day)

Dosage Forms
Capsule, delayed release, oral:
TriLipix®: 45 mg, 135 mg
Tablet, oral: 35 mg, 105 mg
Fibricor®: 35 mg, 105 mg

Fenoglide® *see* fenofibrate *on page 369*

fenoldopam (fe NOL doe pam)

Synonyms fenoldopam mesylate

U.S. Brand Names Corlopam®

Canadian Brand Names Corlopam®

Therapeutic Category Antihypertensive Agent

Use Treatment of severe hypertension (up to 48 hours in adults), including in patients with renal compromise; short-term (up to 4 hours) blood pressure reduction in pediatric patients

General Dosage Range I.V.:
Children: Initial: 0.2 mcg/kg/minute, may increase to 0.3-0.5 mcg/kg/minute every 20-30 minutes (maximum: 0.8 mcg/kg/minute)
Adults: Initial: 0.03-0.1 mcg/kg/minute, may increase in increments of 0.05-0.1 mcg/kg/minute every 15 minutes (maximum: 1.6 mcg/kg/minute)

Dosage Forms
Injection, solution: 10 mg/mL (1 mL, 2 mL)
Corlopam®: 10 mg/mL (1 mL, 2 mL)

fenoldopam mesylate *see* fenoldopam *on page 370*
Fenomax (Can) *see* fenofibrate *on page 369*
Feno-Micro-200 (Can) *see* fenofibrate *on page 369*

fenoprofen (fen oh PROE fen)

Medication Safety Issues
Sound-alike/look-alike issues:
Fenoprofen may be confused with flurbiprofen
Nalfon® may be confused with Naldecon®

Synonyms fenoprofen calcium

U.S. Brand Names Nalfon®

Canadian Brand Names Nalfon®

Therapeutic Category Analgesic, Nonnarcotic; Nonsteroidal Antiinflammatory Drug (NSAID)

Use Symptomatic treatment of acute and chronic rheumatoid arthritis and osteoarthritis; relief of mild-to-moderate pain

General Dosage Range Oral: *Adults:* 200 mg every 4-6 hours as needed **or** 300-600 mg 3-4 times/day (maximum: 3.2 g/day)

Dosage Forms
Capsule, oral:
Nalfon®: 200 mg, 400 mg
Tablet, oral: 600 mg

fenoprofen calcium *see* fenoprofen *on page 370*
fenoterol and ipratropium *see* ipratropium and fenoterol *(Canada only) on page 490*

fenoterol hydrobromide and ipratropium bromide *see* ipratropium and fenoterol *(Canada only)* on page 490

fentanyl (FEN ta nil)

Medication Safety Issues

Sound-alike/look-alike issues:

FentaNYL may be confused with alfentanil, SUFentanil

High alert medication:

The Institute for Safe Medication Practices (ISMP) includes this medication among its list of drug classes which have a heightened risk of causing significant patient harm when used in error.

Administration issues:

Fentanyl transdermal system patches: Leakage of fentanyl gel from the patch has been reported; patch may be less effective; do not use. Thoroughly wash any skin surfaces coming into direct contact with gel with water (do not use soap). May contain conducting metal (eg, aluminum); remove patch prior to MRI.

Other safety concerns:

Dosing of transdermal fentanyl patches may be confusing. Transdermal fentanyl patches should always be prescribed in mcg/hour, not size. Patch dosage form of Duragesic®-12 actually delivers 12.5 mcg/hour of fentanyl. Use caution, as orders may be written as "Duragesic 12.5" which can be erroneously interpreted as a 125 mcg dose.

Fentora®, Onsolis™, Abstral®, and Actiq® are not interchangeable; do not substitute doses on a mcg-per-mcg basis.

Synonyms
fentanyl citrate; fentanyl hydrochloride; fentanyl patch; Lazanda®; OTFC (oral transmucosal fentanyl citrate)

Tall-Man fentaNYL

U.S. Brand Names
Abstral®; Actiq®; Duragesic®; Fentora®; Onsolis™

Canadian Brand Names
Abstral™; Actiq®; Duragesic®; Duragesic® MAT; Fentanyl Citrate Injection, USP; Novo-Fentanyl; PMS-Fentanyl MTX; RAN™-Fentanyl Matrix Patch; RAN™-Fentanyl Transdermal System; ratio-Fentanyl

Therapeutic Category
Analgesic, Narcotic; General Anesthetic

Controlled Substance
C-II

Use

Injection: Relief of pain, preoperative medication, adjunct to general or regional anesthesia

Iontophoretic transdermal system (Ionsys™): Short-term, in-hospital management of acute postoperative pain

Transdermal patch (eg, Duragesic®): Management of persistent moderate-to-severe chronic pain

Transmucosal lozenge (eg, Actiq®), buccal tablet (Fentora®), buccal film (Onsolis™), nasal spray (Lazanda®), sublingual tablet (Abstral®): Management of breakthrough cancer pain in opioid-tolerant patients

General Dosage Range

I.M.: *Adults:* 50-100 mcg/dose as a single dose

I.V.:

Children 2-12 years: 2-3 mcg/kg/dose every 1-2 hours

Children >12 years and Adults: 25-100 mcg as a single dose

Transmucosal:

Buccal film (Onsolis™): *Adults:* Initial: 200 mcg; Maintenance dose range: 200-1200 mcg; maximum dose: 1200 mcg film; maximum frequency: 4 applications/day

Buccal tablet (Fentora®): *Adults:* Initial: 100 mcg; may repeat (maximum: 2 doses per breakthrough pain episode every 4 hours)

Lozenge (Actiq®): *Children ≥16 years and Adults:* Initial: 200 mcg; may repeat (maximum: 2 doses per breakthrough pain episode every 4 hours; maximum daily dose: 4 units/day)

Sublingual tablet (Abstral®): *Adults:* Initial: 100 mcg; may repeat (maximum: 2 doses per breakthrough pain episode every 2 hours); usual maximum: 800 mcg/dose

Transdermal: *Children ≥2 years and Adults:* 12.5-300 mcg/hour applied every 72 hours

Product Availability

Lazanda®: FDA approved June 2011; availability expected in the second half of 2011

Lazanda® is a fentanyl nasal spray formulation indicated for the management of breakthrough cancer pain in opioid-tolerant patients.

◀ **Dosage Forms**
Film, for buccal application:
Onsolis™: 200 mcg (30s); 400 mcg (30s); 600 mcg (30s); 800 mcg (30s); 1200 mcg (30s)
Injection, solution [preservative free]: 0.05 mg/mL (2 mL, 5 mL, 10 mL, 20 mL, 30 mL, 50 mL)
Lozenge, oral: 200 mcg (30s); 400 mcg (30s); 600 mcg (30s); 800 mcg (30s); 1200 mcg (30s); 1600 mcg (30s)
Actiq®: 200 mcg (30s); 400 mcg (30s); 600 mcg (30s); 800 mcg (30s); 1200 mcg (30s); 1600 mcg (30s)
Patch, transdermal: 12 [delivers 12.5 mcg/hr] (5s); 25 [delivers 25 mcg/hr] (5s); 50 [delivers 50 mcg/hr] (5s); 75 [delivers 75 mcg/hr] (5s); 100 [delivers 100 mcg/hr] (5s)
Duragesic®: 12 [delivers 12.5 mcg/hr] (5s); 25 [delivers 25 mcg/hr] (5s); 50 [delivers 50 mcg/hr] (5s); 75 [delivers 75 mcg/hr] (5s); 100 [delivers 100 mcg/hr] (5s)
Powder, for prescription compounding: USP: 100% (1 g)
Tablet, for buccal application:
Fentora®: 100 mcg (28s); 200 mcg (28s); 400 mcg (28s); 600 mcg (28s); 800 mcg (28s)
Tablet, sublingual:
Abstral®: 100 mcg (12s, 32s); 200 mcg (12s, 32s); 300 mcg (12s, 32s); 400 mcg (12s, 32s); 600 mcg (32s); 800 mcg (32s)
Dosage Forms - Canada
Patch, transdermal, as base: 12 mcg/hr (5s); 25 mcg/hr (5s); 50 mcg/hr (5s); 75 mcg/hr (5s); 100 mcg/hr (5s)
Duragesic® MAT: 12 mcg/hr (5s); 25 mcg/hr (5s); 50 mcg/hr (5s); 75 mcg/hr (5s); 100 mcg/hr (5s)

fentanyl citrate *see* fentanyl *on page 371*
Fentanyl Citrate Injection, USP (Can) *see* fentanyl *on page 371*
fentanyl hydrochloride *see* fentanyl *on page 371*
fentanyl patch *see* fentanyl *on page 371*
Fentora® *see* fentanyl *on page 371*
Feosol® [OTC] *see* ferrous sulfate *on page 374*
Feraheme® *see* ferumoxytol *on page 374*
Ferate [OTC] *see* ferrous gluconate *on page 373*
Fergon® [OTC] *see* ferrous gluconate *on page 373*
Fer-In-Sol® [OTC] *see* ferrous sulfate *on page 374*
Fer-In-Sol® (Can) *see* ferrous sulfate *on page 374*
Fer-iron [OTC] *see* ferrous sulfate *on page 374*
Fermalac (Can) *see* Lactobacillus *on page 506*
Ferodan™ (Can) *see* ferrous sulfate *on page 374*
Ferretts® [OTC] *see* ferrous fumarate *on page 373*
Ferrex™ 150 [OTC] *see* polysaccharide-iron complex *on page 720*
Ferrex™ 150 Forte *see* polysaccharide-iron complex, vitamin B12, and folic acid *on page 721*
Ferrex™ 150 Forte Plus *see* polysaccharide-iron complex, vitamin B12, and folic acid *on page 721*
Ferrex™ 150 Plus [OTC] *see* polysaccharide-iron complex *on page 720*
ferric (III) hexacyanoferrate (II) *see* ferric hexacyanoferrate *on page 373*

ferric gluconate (FER ik GLOO koe nate)

Medication Safety Issues
Sound-alike/look-alike issues:
Ferric gluconate may be confused with ferumoxytol
Ferrlecit® may be confused with Ferralet®
Synonyms sodium ferric gluconate
U.S. Brand Names Ferrlecit®; Nulecit™
Canadian Brand Names Ferrlecit®
Therapeutic Category Iron Salt
Use Repletion of total body iron content in patients with iron-deficiency anemia who are undergoing hemodialysis in conjunction with erythropoietin therapy
General Dosage Range I.V.:
Children ≥6 years: 1.5 msg/kg of elemental iron at 8 sequential dialysis sessions (maximum: 125 mg/dose)
Adults: 125 mg of elemental iron at ~8 sequential dialysis treatments to make a cumulative dose of 1 g

Dosage Forms
Injection, solution:
Ferrlecit®: Elemental iron 12.5 mg/mL (5 mL)
Nulecit™: Elemental iron 12.5 mg/mL (5 mL)

ferric hexacyanoferrate (FER ik hex a SYE an oh fer ate)

Synonyms ferric (III) hexacyanoferrate (II); insoluble prussian blue; prussian blue
U.S. Brand Names Radiogardase®
Therapeutic Category Antidote
Use Treatment of known or suspected internal contamination with radioactive cesium and/or radioactive or nonradioactive thallium
General Dosage Range Oral:
Children 2-12 years: 1 g 3 times/day
Children >12 years and Adults: 1-3 g 3 times/day
Dosage Forms
Capsule, oral:
Radiogardase®: 0.5 g

Ferrlecit® *see ferric gluconate on page 372*
Ferrocite™ [OTC] *see ferrous fumarate on page 373*
Ferro-Sequels® [OTC] *see ferrous fumarate on page 373*

ferrous fumarate (FER us FYOO ma rate)

Synonyms iron fumarate
U.S. Brand Names Femiron® [OTC]; Ferretts® [OTC]; Ferro-Sequels® [OTC]; Ferrocite™ [OTC]; Hemocyte® [OTC]; Ircon® [OTC]
Canadian Brand Names Palafer®
Therapeutic Category Electrolyte Supplement, Oral
Use Prevention and treatment of iron-deficiency anemias
General Dosage Range Oral:
Children: 1-6 mg elemental iron/kg/day in 1-3 divided doses
Adults: 60 mg elemental iron 2-4 times/day
Dosage Forms
Tablet, oral: 324 mg
Femiron® [OTC]: 63 mg
Ferretts® [OTC]: 325 mg
Ferrocite™ [OTC]: 324 mg
Hemocyte® [OTC]: 324 mg
Ircon® [OTC]: 200 mg
Tablet, timed release, oral:
Ferro-Sequels® [OTC]: 150 mg

ferrous gluconate (FER us GLOO koe nate)

Synonyms iron gluconate
U.S. Brand Names Ferate [OTC]; Fergon® [OTC]
Canadian Brand Names Apo-Ferrous Gluconate®; Novo-Ferrogluc
Therapeutic Category Electrolyte Supplement, Oral
Use Prevention and treatment of iron-deficiency anemias
General Dosage Range Oral:
Children: 1-6 mg Fe/kg/day in 1-3 divided doses
Adults: 60 mg 1-4 times/day
Dosage Forms
Tablet, oral: 246 mg, 324 mg, 325 mg
Ferate [OTC]: 240 mg
Fergon® [OTC]: 240 mg

ferrous sulfate (FER us SUL fate)

Medication Safety Issues
Sound-alike/look-alike issues:
Feosol® may be confused with Fer-In-Sol®
Fer-In-Sol® may be confused with Feosol®
Slow FE® may be confused with Slow-K®
BEERS Criteria medication:
This drug may be inappropriate for use in geriatric patients (dosage-dependent, low-severity risk).
Administration issues:
Fer-In-Sol® (manufactured by Mead Johnson) and a limited number of generic products are available at a concentration of 15 mg/mL. However, many other generics and brand name products of ferrous sulfate oral liquid drops are available at a concentration of 15 mg/0.6 mL. Check concentration closely prior to dispensing. Prescriptions written in milliliters (mL) should be clarified.

Synonyms $FeSO_4$; iron sulfate

U.S. Brand Names Feosol® [OTC]; Fer-In-Sol® [OTC]; Fer-iron [OTC]; MyKidz Iron 10™ [OTC]; Slow FE® [OTC]; Slow Release [OTC]

Canadian Brand Names Apo-Ferrous Sulfate®; Fer-In-Sol®; Ferodan™

Therapeutic Category Electrolyte Supplement, Oral

Use Prevention and treatment of iron-deficiency anemias

General Dosage Range Oral:
Extended release: *Adults:* 250 mg 1-2 times/day
Immediate release:
Children: 1-6 mg Fe/kg/day in 1-3 divided doses (maximum: 15 mg/day [prophylaxis dosing])
Adults: 300 mg 1-4 times/day

Dosage Forms
Elixir, oral: 220 mg/5 mL (473 mL, 480 mL)
Liquid, oral: 300 mg/5 mL (5 mL); 75 mg/mL (50 mL)
Fer-In-Sol® [OTC]: 75 mg/mL (50 mL)
Fer-iron [OTC]: 75 mg/mL (50 mL)
Suspension, oral:
MyKidz Iron 10™ [OTC]: 75 mg/1.5 mL (118 mL)
Tablet, oral: 324 mg, 325 mg
Feosol® [OTC]: 200 mg
Tablet, enteric coated, oral: 324 mg, 325 mg
Tablet, extended release, oral: 140 mg
Tablet, slow release, oral: 160 mg
Slow FE® [OTC]: 142 mg
Slow Release [OTC]: 140 mg

Fertinorm® H.P. (Can) *see* urofollitropin *on page 902*

ferumoxytol (fer ue MOX i tol)

Medication Safety Issues
Sound-alike/look-alike issues:
Ferumoxytol may be confused with ferric gluconate, iron dextran complex, iron sucrose
U.S. Brand Names Feraheme®
Therapeutic Category Iron Salt
Use Treatment of iron-deficiency anemia in chronic kidney disease
General Dosage Range I.V.: *Adults:* 510 mg (17 mL) as a single dose; repeat once 3-8 days later
Dosage Forms
Injection, solution:
Feraheme®: Elemental iron 30 mg/mL (17 mL)

FESO *see* fesoterodine *on page 374*
FeSO$_4$ *see* ferrous sulfate *on page 374*

fesoterodine (fes oh TER oh deen)

Medication Safety Issues
Sound-alike/look-alike issues:
Fesoterodine may be confused with fexofenadine, tolterodine

Synonyms FESO; fesoterodine fumarate

U.S. Brand Names Toviaz™

Therapeutic Category Anticholinergic Agent

Use Treatment of patients with an overactive bladder with symptoms of urinary frequency, urgency, or urge incontinence.

General Dosage Range Dosage adjustment recommended in patients with renal impairment or on concomitant therapy

Oral: *Adults:* 4-8 mg once daily

Dosage Forms

Tablet, extended release, oral:

Toviaz™: 4 mg, 8 mg

fesoterodine fumarate *see* fesoterodine *on page 374*

Feverall® [OTC] *see* acetaminophen *on page 23*

Fexmid® *see* cyclobenzaprine *on page 241*

fexofenadine (feks oh FEN a deen)

Medication Safety Issues

Sound-alike/look-alike issues:

Fexofenadine may be confused with fesoterodine

Allegra® may be confused with Viagra®

International issues:

Allegra [U.S, Canada, and multiple international markets] may be confused with Allegro brand name for fluticasone [Israel] and frovatriptan [Germany]

Synonyms fexofenadine hydrochloride

U.S. Brand Names Allegra®; Allegra® Allergy 12 Hour [OTC]; Allegra® Allergy 24 Hour [OTC]; Allegra® Children's Allergy ODT [OTC]; Allegra® Children's Allergy [OTC]; Allegra® ODT [DSC]

Canadian Brand Names Allegra®

Therapeutic Category Antihistamine

Use Relief of symptoms associated with seasonal allergic rhinitis; treatment of chronic idiopathic urticaria

OTC labeling: Relief of symptoms associated with allergic rhinitis

General Dosage Range Dosage adjustment recommended in patients with renal impairment

Oral:

Children 6 months to <2 years: 15 mg twice daily

Children 2-11 years: 30 mg twice daily

Children ≥12 years and Adults: 60 mg twice daily **or** 180 mg once daily

Dosage Forms

Suspension, oral:

Allegra®: 6 mg/mL (300 mL)

Allegra® Children's Allergy [OTC]: 6 mg/mL (120 mL)

Tablet, oral: 30 mg, 60 mg, 180 mg

Allegra® Allergy 12 Hour [OTC]: 60 mg

Allegra® Allergy 24 Hour [OTC]: 180 mg

Allegra® Children's Allergy [OTC]: 30 mg

Tablet, orally disintegrating, oral:

Allegra® Children's Allergy ODT [OTC]: 30 mg

fexofenadine and pseudoephedrine (feks oh FEN a deen & soo doe e FED rin)

Medication Safety Issues

Sound-alike/look-alike issues:

Allegra-D® may be confused with Viagra®

International issues:

Allegra-D [U.S, Canada, and multiple international markets] may be confused with Allegro brand name for fluticasone [Israel] and frovatriptan [Germany]

Synonyms pseudoephedrine and fexofenadine

U.S. Brand Names Allegra-D® 12 Hour; Allegra-D® 24 Hour

Canadian Brand Names Allegra-D®

Therapeutic Category Antihistamine/Decongestant Combination

◀ **Use** Relief of symptoms associated with seasonal allergic rhinitis in adults and children ≥12 years of age

General Dosage Range Dosage adjustment recommended in patients with renal impairment

Oral: *Children ≥12 years and Adults:* 1 tablet (fexofenadine 60 mg/pseudoephedrine 120 mg) twice daily or 1 tablet (fexofenadine 180 mg/pseudoephedrine 240 mg) once daily

Dosage Forms

Tablet, extended release: Fexofenadine 60 mg [immediate release] and pseudoephedrine 120 mg [extended release]; fexofenadine 180 mg [immediate release] and pseudoephedrine 240 mg [extended release]

Allegra-D® 12 Hour: Fexofenadine 60 mg [immediate release] and pseudoephedrine 120 mg [extended release]

Allegra-D® 24 Hour: Fexofenadine 180 mg [immediate release] and pseudoephedrine 240 mg [extended release]

fexofenadine hydrochloride *see* fexofenadine *on page 375*

Fiberall® [OTC] *see* psyllium *on page 755*

FiberCon® [OTC] *see* polycarbophil *on page 717*

Fiber-Lax [OTC] *see* polycarbophil *on page 717*

Fiber-Tabs™ [OTC] *see* polycarbophil *on page 717*

Fibricor® *see* fenofibric acid *on page 369*

fibrinogen concentrate (human) (fi BRIN o gin KON suhn trate HYU man)

Synonyms coagulation factor I

U.S. Brand Names RiaSTAP®

Therapeutic Category Blood Product Derivative

Use Treatment of acute bleeding episodes in patients with congenital fibrinogen deficiency (afibrinogenemia and hypofibrinogenemia)

General Dosage Range I.V.: *Children and Adults:* When baseline fibrinogen level is known: Dose (mg/kg) = [Target level (mg/dL) - measured level (mg/dL)] **divided by** 1.7 (mg/dL per mg/kg body weight) **or** when baseline fibrinogen level is not known: 70 mg/kg

Dosage Forms

Injection, powder for reconstitution:

RiaSTAP®: 900-1300 mg [contains albumin (human); exact potency labeled on vial]

fibrin sealant (FI brin SEEL ent)

Medication Safety Issues

Administration issues:

Serious and fatal air or gas embolisms have occurred during or after fibrin sealant application using air or gas pressurized spray devices, particularly when used improperly. Manufacturer directions should be followed closely to ensure safe use of spray devices.

Synonyms fibrin sealant (human); FS; FS VH S/D; Tisseel VH S/D

U.S. Brand Names Artiss; Evicel™; TachoSil®; Tisseel

Canadian Brand Names Tisseel

Therapeutic Category Hemostatic Agent

Use

Artiss: Aid in adhering autologous skin grafts in burn patients (not indicated for hemostasis)

Evicel™: Adjunct to hemostasis in surgery when control of bleeding by conventional surgical techniques is ineffective or impractical

TachoSil®: Adjunct to hemostasis in cardiovascular surgery when control of bleeding by conventional surgical technique is ineffective or impractical

Tisseel: Adjunct to hemostasis in cardiopulmonary bypass surgery (including fully heparinized patients) and splenic injury (due to blunt or penetrating trauma to the abdomen) when the control of bleeding by conventional surgical techniques is ineffective or impractical; adjunctive sealant for closure of colostomies

General Dosage Range Topical: *Children >6 months and Adults:* Dosage varies greatly depending on product

Dosage Forms
  Kit:
    Artiss: Solution, topical: Fibrinogen 67-106 mg/mL and thrombin 2.5-6.5 int. units/mL (2 mL, 4 mL, 10 mL)
    Tisseel: Powder for solution, topical: Fibrinogen 67-106 mg/mL and thrombin 400-625 int. units/mL (2 mL, 4 mL, 10 mL)
    Tisseel: Solution, topical: Fibrinogen 67-106 mg/mL and thrombin 400-625 int. units/mL (2 mL, 4 mL, 10 mL)
  Kit [preservative free]:
    Evicel™: Solution, topical: Fibrinogen 55-85 mg/mL and thrombin 800-1200 int. units/mL (2 mL, 4 mL, 10 mL)
  Patch, topical:
    TachoSil®: Fibrinogen 3.6-7.4 mg/cm^2 and thrombin 1.3-2.7 units/cm^2 (1s, 2s)

fibrin sealant (human) *see fibrin sealant on page 376*
Fibro-XL [OTC] *see psyllium on page 755*
Fibro-Lax [OTC] *see psyllium on page 755*
fidaxomicin *see fidaxomicin (systemic) on page 377*

fidaxomicin (systemic) (fye DAX oh mye sin)

Synonyms difimicin; fidaxomicin; lipiarrmycin; OPT-80; PAR-101; tiacumicin B
U.S. Brand Names Dificid™
Therapeutic Category Antibiotic, Macrolide
Use Treatment of *Clostridium difficile*-associated diarrhea (CDAD)
General Dosage Range No dosage adjustment recommended in patients with hepatic or renal impairment.
  Oral: *Adults:* 200 mg twice daily
Dosage Forms
  Tablet, oral:
    Dificid™: 200 mg

filgrastim (fil GRA stim)

Medication Safety Issues
  Sound-alike/look-alike issues:
    Neupogen® may be confused with Epogen®, Neulasta®, Neumega®, Neupro®, Nutramigen®
Synonyms G-CSF; granulocyte colony stimulating factor
U.S. Brand Names Neupogen®
Canadian Brand Names Neupogen®
Therapeutic Category Colony-Stimulating Factor
Use
  Cancer patients (nonmyeloid malignancies) receiving myelosuppressive chemotherapy to decrease the incidence of infection (febrile neutropenia) in regimens associated with a high incidence of neutropenia with fever
  Acute myelogenous leukemia (AML) following induction or consolidation chemotherapy to shorten time to neutrophil recovery and reduce the duration of fever
  Cancer patients (nonmyeloid malignancies) receiving bone marrow transplant to shorten the duration of neutropenia and neutropenia-related events (eg, neutropenic fever)
  Peripheral stem cell transplantation to mobilize hematopoietic progenitor cells for leukapheresis collection
  Severe chronic neutropenia (SCN; chronic administration) to reduce the incidence and duration of neutropenic complications (fever, infections, oropharyngeal ulcers) in symptomatic patients with congenital, cyclic, or idiopathic neutropenia
General Dosage Range
  I.V.: *Children and Adults:* 5-10 mcg/kg/day
  SubQ: *Children and Adults:* 5-10 mcg/kg/day **or** 6 mcg/kg twice daily
Dosage Forms
  Injection, solution [preservative free]:
    Neupogen®: 300 mcg/mL (1 mL, 1.6 mL); 600 mcg/mL (0.5 mL, 0.8 mL)

Finacea® *see azelaic acid on page 107*

Finacea® Plus™ *see azelaic acid on page 107*

finasteride (fi NAS teer ide)

Medication Safety Issues

Sound-alike/look-alike issues:

Finasteride may be confused with furosemide

Proscar® may be confused with ProSom®, Provera®, PROzac®, Psorcon®

U.S. Brand Names Propecia®; Proscar®

Canadian Brand Names CO Finasteride; JAMP-Finasteride; Mylan-Finasteride; Novo-Finasteride; PMS-Finasteride; Propecia®; Proscar®; ratio-Finasteride; Sandoz-Finasteride

Therapeutic Category Antiandrogen

Use

Propecia®: Treatment of male pattern hair loss in **men only**. Safety and efficacy were demonstrated in men between 18-41 years of age.

Proscar®: Treatment of symptomatic benign prostatic hyperplasia (BPH); can be used in combination with an alpha-blocker, doxazosin

General Dosage Range Oral: *Adults:* 1 mg or 5 mg once daily

Dosage Forms

Tablet, oral: 5 mg

Propecia®: 1 mg

Proscar®: 5 mg

fingolimod (fin GOL i mod)

Synonyms FTY720

U.S. Brand Names Gilenya™

Canadian Brand Names Gilenya®

Therapeutic Category Sphingosine 1-Phosphate (S1P) Receptor Modulator

Use Treatment of relapsing forms of multiple sclerosis (MS) to reduce the frequency of clinical exacerbations and delay disability progression

General Dosage Range Oral: *Adults:* 0.5 mg once daily

Dosage Forms

Capsule, oral:

Gilenya™: 0.5 mg

Fioricet® *see butalbital, acetaminophen, and caffeine on page 152*

Fioricet® with Codeine *see butalbital, acetaminophen, caffeine, and codeine on page 153*

Fiorinal® *see butalbital, aspirin, and caffeine on page 154*

Fiorinal®-C 1/2 (Can) *see butalbital, aspirin, caffeine, and codeine on page 154*

Fiorinal®-C 1/4 (Can) *see butalbital, aspirin, caffeine, and codeine on page 154*

Fiorinal® with Codeine *see butalbital, aspirin, caffeine, and codeine on page 154*

Firmagon® *see degarelix on page 257*

First™-Progesterone VGS 25 *see progesterone on page 741*

First™-Progesterone VGS 50 *see progesterone on page 741*

First™-Progesterone VGS 100 *see progesterone on page 741*

First™-Progesterone VGS 200 *see progesterone on page 741*

First™-Progesterone VGS 400 *see progesterone on page 741*

First®-Testosterone *see testosterone on page 854*

First®-Testosterone MC *see testosterone on page 854*

fisalamine *see mesalamine on page 564*

fish oil *see omega-3-acid ethyl esters on page 649*

FK228 *see romidepsin on page 789*

FK506 *see tacrolimus (systemic) on page 842*

Flagyl® *see metronidazole (systemic) on page 582*

Flagyl® 375 *see metronidazole (systemic) on page 582*

Flagyl® ER *see metronidazole (systemic) on page 582*

Flagystatin® (Can) *see metronidazole and nystatin (Canada only) on page 583*

Flamazine® (Can) *see silver sulfadiazine on page 812*

Flarex® see fluorometholone on page 388

flavan see flavocoxid on page 379

flavocoxid (fla vo KOKS id)

Synonyms flavan; flavonoid

U.S. Brand Names Limbrel 250™; Limbrel 500™; Limbrel™ [DSC]

Therapeutic Category Antiinflammatory Agent

Use Clinical dietary management of the metabolic processes of osteoarthritis

General Dosage Range Oral: *Adults:* 250-500 mg every 12 hours

Dosage Forms
  Capsule, oral:
  Limbrel 250™: 250 mg
  Limbrel 500™: 500 mg

flavonoid see flavocoxid on page 379

flavoxate (fla VOKS ate)

Medication Safety Issues
  Sound-alike/look-alike issues:
  FlavoxATE may be confused with fluvoxaMINE
  Urispas may be confused with Urised®

Synonyms flavoxate hydrochloride

Tall-Man flavoxATE

Canadian Brand Names Apo-Flavoxate®; Urispas®

Therapeutic Category Antispasmodic Agent, Urinary

Use Antispasmodic to provide symptomatic relief of dysuria, nocturia, suprapubic pain, urgency, and incontinence due to detrusor instability and hyperreflexia in elderly with cystitis, urethritis, urethrocystitis, urethrotrigonitis, and prostatitis

General Dosage Range Oral: *Children >12 years and Adults:* 100-200 mg 3-4 times/day

Dosage Forms
  Tablet, oral: 100 mg

flavoxate hydrochloride see flavoxate on page 379

Flebogamma® DIF see immune globulin on page 468

flecainide (fle KAY nide)

Medication Safety Issues
  Sound-alike/look-alike issues:
  Flecainide may be confused with fluconazole
  Tambocor™ may be confused with Pamelor®, Temodar®, tamoxifen, Tamiflu®

Synonyms flecainide acetate

U.S. Brand Names Tambocor™

Canadian Brand Names Apo-Flecainide®; Tambocor™

Therapeutic Category Antiarrhythmic Agent, Class I-C

Use Prevention and suppression of documented life-threatening ventricular arrhythmias (eg, sustained ventricular tachycardia); controlling symptomatic, disabling supraventricular tachycardias in patients without structural heart disease in whom other agents fail

General Dosage Range Dosage adjustment recommended in patients with renal impairment
  Oral:
  Children: Initial: 3 mg/kg/day **or** 50-100 mg/m^2/day in 3 divided doses; Maintenance: 3-6 mg/kg/day **or** 100-150 mg/m^2/day in 3 divided doses (maximum: 11 mg/kg/day; 200 mg/m^2/day)
  Adults: Initial: 50-100 mg every 12 hours; Maintenance: 100-400 mg/day in 2 divided doses (maximum: 400 mg/day)

Dosage Forms
  Tablet, oral: 50 mg, 100 mg, 150 mg
  Tambocor™: 50 mg, 100 mg, 150 mg

flecainide acetate see flecainide on page 379

Flector® see diclofenac (topical) on page 279

Fleet® Bisacodyl [OTC] *see* bisacodyl *on page 134*

Fleet® Enema [OTC] *see* sodium phosphates *on page 823*

Fleet Enema® (Can) *see* sodium phosphates *on page. 823*

Fleet® Enema Extra® [OTC] *see* sodium phosphates *on page 823*

Fleet® Glycerin Maximum Strength [OTC] *see* glycerin *on page 421*

Fleet® Glycerin Suppositories [OTC] *see* glycerin *on page 421*

Fleet® Liquid Glycerin [OTC] *see* glycerin *on page 421*

Fleet® Pedia-Lax™ Chewable Tablet [OTC] *see* magnesium hydroxide *on page 545*

Fleet® Pedia-Lax™ Enema [OTC] *see* sodium phosphates *on page 823*

Fleet® Pedia-Lax™ Glycerin Suppositories [OTC] *see* glycerin *on page 421*

Fleet® Pedia-Lax™ Liquid Glycerin Suppositories [OTC] *see* glycerin *on page 421*

Fleet® Pedia-Lax™ Liquid Stool Softener [OTC] *see* docusate *on page 302*

Fleet® Pedia-Lax™ Quick Dissolve [OTC] *see* senna *on page 807*

Fleet® Phospho-soda® [OTC] [DSC] *see* sodium phosphates *on page 823*

Fleet® Phospho-soda® EZ-Prep™ [OTC] [DSC] *see* sodium phosphates *on page 823*

Fleet® Sof-Lax® [OTC] *see* docusate *on page 302*

Fleet® Stimulant Laxative [OTC] *see* bisacodyl *on page 134*

Fletcher's® [OTC] *see* senna *on page 807*

Flexbumin 25% *see* albumin *on page 44*

Flexeril® *see* cyclobenzaprine *on page 241*

Flexitec (Can) *see* cyclobenzaprine *on page 241*

Flex-Power [OTC] *see* trolamine *on page 894*

Flintstones™ Complete [OTC] *see* vitamins (multiple/pediatric) *on page 920*

Flintstones™ Gummies [OTC] *see* vitamins (multiple/pediatric) *on page 920*

Flintstones™ Plus Bone Building Support [OTC] *see* vitamins (multiple/pediatric) *on page 920*

Flintstones™ Plus Bone Building Support Gummies [OTC] *see* vitamins (multiple/pediatric) *on page 920*

Flintstones™ Plus Immunity Support [OTC] *see* vitamins (multiple/pediatric) *on page 920*

Flintstones™ Plus Immunity Support Gummies [OTC] *see* vitamins (multiple/pediatric) *on page 920*

Flintstones™ Plus Iron [OTC] *see* vitamins (multiple/pediatric) *on page 920*

Flintstones™ Sour Gummies [OTC] *see* vitamins (multiple/pediatric) *on page 920*

floctafenina *see* floctafenine *(Canada only) on page 380*

floctafenine *(Canada only)* (flok ta FEN een)

Synonyms floctafenina; floctafeninum

Canadian Brand Names Apo-Floctafenine®

Therapeutic Category Nonsteroidal Antiinflammatory Drug (NSAID), Oral

Use Short-term management of acute, mild-to-moderate pain

General Dosage Range Dosage adjustment recommended in patients with renal impairment
  Oral: *Adults:* 200-400 mg every 6-8 hours as needed (maximum: 1200 mg/day)

Product Availability Not available in U.S.

Dosage Forms - Canada
  Tablet, oral:
    Apo-Floctafenine®: 200 mg, 400 mg

floctafeninum *see* floctafenine *(Canada only) on page 380*

Flolan® *see* epoprostenol *on page 334*

Flomax® *see* tamsulosin *on page 843*

Flomax® CR (Can) *see* tamsulosin *on page 843*

Flonase® *see* fluticasone (nasal) *on page 393*

Flo-Pred™ *see* prednisolone (systemic) *on page 734*

Floranex™ [OTC] *see* Lactobacillus *on page 506*

Flora-Q™ [OTC] *see* Lactobacillus *on page 506*

Florastor® [OTC] *see* Saccharomyces boulardii *on page 794*

Florastor® Kids [OTC] *see Saccharomyces boulardii on page 794*

Florazole® ER (Can) *see metronidazole (systemic) on page 582*

Florical® [OTC] *see calcium carbonate on page 161*

Florinef *see fludrocortisone on page 383*

Florinef® (Can) *see fludrocortisone on page 383*

Flovent *see fluticasone (oral inhalation) on page 392*

Flovent® Diskus® *see fluticasone (oral inhalation) on page 392*

Flovent® HFA *see fluticasone (oral inhalation) on page 392*

floxin otic singles *see ofloxacin (otic) on page 644*

floxuridine (floks YOOR i deen)

Medication Safety Issues
Sound-alike/look-alike issues:
Floxuridine may be confused with Fludara®, fludarabine
FUDR® may be confused with Fludara®

High alert medication:
The Institute for Safe Medication Practices (ISMP) includes this medication among its list of drugs which have a heightened risk of causing significant patient harm when used in error.

Synonyms fluorodeoxyuridine; FUDR

Canadian Brand Names FUDR®

Therapeutic Category Antineoplastic Agent

Use Management of hepatic metastases of colorectal and gastric cancers

General Dosage Range Dosage adjustment recommended in patients with hepatic impairment
Intraarterial: *Adults:* 0.1-0.6 mg/kg/day

Dosage Forms
Injection, powder for reconstitution: 500 mg

Fluanxol® (Can) *see flupenthixol (Canada only) on page 390*

Fluanxol® Depot (Can) *see flupenthixol (Canada only) on page 390*

Fluarix® *see influenza virus vaccine (inactivated) on page 473*

flubenisolone *see betamethasone on page 129*

Flucaine® *see proparacaine and fluorescein on page 745*

fluconazole (floo KOE na zole)

Medication Safety Issues
Sound-alike/look-alike issues:
Fluconazole may be confused with flecainide, FLUoxetine, furosemide, itraconazole
Diflucan® may be confused with diclofenac, Diprivan®, disulfiram

International issues:
Canesten [Great Britain] may be confused with Canesten brand name for clotrimazole [multiple international markets]; Cenestin brand name estrogens (conjugated A/synthetic) [U.S., Canada]

U.S. Brand Names Diflucan®

Canadian Brand Names Apo-Fluconazole®; CanesOral®; CO Fluconazole; Diflucan®; Dom-Fluconazole; Fluconazole Injection; Fluconazole Omega; Mylan-Fluconazole; Novo-Fluconazole; PHL-Fluconazole; PMS-Fluconazole; PRO-Fluconazole; Riva-Fluconazole; Taro-Fluconazole; ZYM-Fluconazole

Therapeutic Category Antifungal Agent

Use Treatment of candidiasis (vaginal, oropharyngeal, esophageal, urinary tract infections, peritonitis, pneumonia, and systemic infections); cryptococcal meningitis; antifungal prophylaxis in allogeneic bone marrow transplant recipients

General Dosage Range Dosage adjustment recommended in patients with renal impairment
I.V., oral:
Children: Loading dose: 6-12 mg/kg; Maintenance: 3-12 mg/kg/day
Adults: 100-800 mg once daily **or** 150 mg as a single dose

◀ **Dosage Forms**
Infusion, premixed iso-osmotic dextrose solution: 200 mg (100 mL); 400 mg (200 mL)
Infusion, premixed iso-osmotic sodium chloride solution: 100 mg (50 mL); 200 mg (100 mL); 400 mg (200 mL)
Diflucan®: 200 mg (100 mL); 400 mg (200 mL)
Infusion, premixed iso-osmotic sodium chloride solution [preservative free]: 200 mg (100 mL); 400 mg (200 mL)
Powder for suspension, oral: 10 mg/mL (35 mL); 40 mg/mL (35 mL)
Diflucan®: 10 mg/mL (35 mL); 40 mg/mL (35 mL)
Tablet, oral: 50 mg, 100 mg, 150 mg, 200 mg
Diflucan®: 50 mg, 100 mg, 150 mg, 200 mg

Fluconazole Injection (Can) *see* fluconazole *on page 381*
Fluconazole Omega (Can) *see* fluconazole *on page 381*

flucytosine (floo SYE toe seen)

Medication Safety Issues
Sound-alike/look-alike issues:
Flucytosine may be confused with fluorouracil
Ancobon® may be confused with Oncovin®
High alert medication:
The Institute for Safe Medication Practices (ISMP) includes this medication among its list of drugs which have a heightened risk of causing significant patient harm when used in error.
Synonyms 5-FC; 5-fluorocytosine; 5-flurocytosine
U.S. Brand Names Ancobon®
Canadian Brand Names Ancobon®
Therapeutic Category Antifungal Agent
Use Adjunctive treatment of systemic fungal infections (eg, septicemia, endocarditis, UTI, meningitis, or pulmonary) caused by susceptible strains of *Candida* or *Cryptococcus*
General Dosage Range Dosage adjustment recommended in patients with renal impairment
Oral: *Adults:* 50-150 mg/kg/day in divided doses every 6 hours
Dosage Forms
Capsule, oral:
Ancobon®: 250 mg, 500 mg

Fludara® *see* fludarabine *on page 382*

fludarabine (floo DARE a been)

Medication Safety Issues
Sound-alike/look-alike issues:
Fludarabine may be confused with cladribine, floxuridine, Flumadine®
Fludara® may be confused with FUDR®
High alert medication:
This medication is in a class the Institute for Safe Medication Practices (ISMP) includes among its list of drug classes which have a heightened risk of causing significant patient harm when used in error.
Synonyms 2F-ara-AMP; fludarabine phosphate
U.S. Brand Names Fludara®; Oforta™
Canadian Brand Names Fludara®
Therapeutic Category Antineoplastic Agent
Use Treatment of progressive or refractory B-cell chronic lymphocytic leukemia (CLL)

Canadian labeling: Second-line treatment of chronic lymphocytic leukemia (CLL); second-line treatment of low-grade, refractory non-Hodgkin lymphoma (NHL)
General Dosage Range Dosage adjustment recommended in patients with renal impairment or who develop toxicities.
Oral: *Adults:* 40 mg/m²/day for 5 days every 28 days
I.V.: *Adults:* 25 mg/m²/day for 5 days every 28 days
Dosage Forms
Injection, powder for reconstitution: 50 mg
Fludara®: 50 mg
Injection, solution [preservative free]: 25 mg/mL (2 mL)

Tablet, oral:
  Oforta™: 10 mg
Dosage Forms - Canada
  Tablet, oral:
  Fludara®: 10 mg

fludarabine phosphate *see* fludarabine *on page 382*

fludrocortisone (floo droe KOR ti sone)

Medication Safety Issues
  Sound-alike/look-alike issues:
  Florinef® may be confused with Fioricet®, Fiorinal®
Synonyms 9α-fluorohydrocortisone acetate; Florinef; fludrocortisone acetate; fluohydrisone acetate; fluohydrocortisone acetate
Canadian Brand Names Florinef®
Therapeutic Category Adrenal Corticosteroid (Mineralocorticoid)
Use Partial replacement therapy for primary and secondary adrenocortical insufficiency in Addison disease; treatment of salt-losing adrenogenital syndrome
General Dosage Range Oral:
  Children: 0.05-0.1 mg/day
  Adults: 0.05-0.2 mg/day (range: 0.1 mg 3 times/week to 0.2 mg/day)
Dosage Forms
  Tablet, oral: 0.1 mg

fludrocortisone acetate *see* fludrocortisone *on page 383*
FluLaval® *see* influenza virus vaccine (inactivated) *on page 473*
Flumadine® *see* rimantadine *on page 782*

flumazenil (FLOO may ze nil)

Medication Safety Issues
  Sound-alike/look-alike issues:
  Flumazenil may be confused with influenza virus vaccine
U.S. Brand Names Romazicon®
Canadian Brand Names Anexate®; Flumazenil Injection; Flumazenil Injection, USP; Romazicon®
Therapeutic Category Antidote
Use Benzodiazepine antagonist; reverses sedative effects of benzodiazepines used in conscious sedation and general anesthesia; treatment of benzodiazepine overdose
General Dosage Range I.V.:
  Children: Initial: 0.01 mg/kg (maximum dose: 0.2 mg), may repeat 0.01 mg/kg (maximum dose: 0.2 mg) as needed (maximum cumulative total: 1 mg or 0.05 mg/kg, whichever is lower)
  Adults: Benzodiazepine overdose: Initial: 0.2 mg, may repeat with 0.3 mg, then 0.5 mg (maximum cumulative total dose: 5 mg); Reversal of conscious sedation/general anesthesia: Initial: 0.2 mg, may repeat (maximum total dose: 1 mg)
Dosage Forms
  Injection, solution: 0.1 mg/mL (5 mL, 10 mL)
  Romazicon®: 0.1 mg/mL (5 mL, 10 mL)

Flumazenil Injection (Can) *see* flumazenil *on page 383*
Flumazenil Injection, USP (Can) *see* flumazenil *on page 383*
flumethasone and clioquinol *see* clioquinol and flumethasone *(Canada only) on page 219*
FluMist® *see* influenza virus vaccine (live/attenuated) *on page 474*

flunarizine *(Canada only)* (floo NAR i zeen)

Synonyms flunarizine hydrochloride
Canadian Brand Names Apo-Flunarizine®; Novo-Flunarizine; Sibelium®
Therapeutic Category Calcium-Entry Blocker (Selective)
Use Prophylaxis of classic (with aura) or common (without aura) migraine; symptomatic treatment of vestibular vertigo (due to a diagnosed functional disorder of the vestibular system)

◀ **General Dosage Range Oral:**
Adults <65 years: 5-10 mg once daily
Elderly ≥65 years: 2.5-5 mg once daily
Product Availability Not available in U.S.
Dosage Forms - Canada
Capsule, oral:
Apo-Flunarizine®, Novo-Flunarizine, Sibelium®: 5 mg

flunarizine hydrochloride *see* flunarizine *(Canada only) on page 383*

flunisolide (nasal) (floo NISS oh lide)

Medication Safety Issues
Sound-alike/look-alike issues:
Flunisolide may be confused with Flumadine®, fluocinonide
Nasarel may be confused with Nizoral®
Canadian Brand Names Apo-Flunisolide®; Nasalide®; Rhinalar®
Therapeutic Category Corticosteroid, Nasal
Use Seasonal or perennial rhinitis
General Dosage Range Intranasal:
Children 6-14 years: 1-2 sprays 2-3 times/day (maximum: 4 sprays/day in each nostril)
Children ≥15 years and Adults: 2 sprays twice daily (maximum: 8 sprays/day in each nostril)
Dosage Forms
Solution, intranasal: 25 mcg/actuation (25 mL); 29 mcg/actuation (25 mL)

fluocinolone (ophthalmic) (floo oh SIN oh lone)

Medication Safety Issues
Sound-alike/look-alike issues:
Fluocinolone may be confused with fluocinonide
Synonyms fluocinolone acetonide
U.S. Brand Names Retisert®
Therapeutic Category Corticosteroid, Ophthalmic
Use Treatment of chronic, noninfectious uveitis affecting the posterior segment of the eye
General Dosage Range Ocular implant: *Children ≥12 years and Adults:* One silicone-encased tablet (0.59 mg) is designed to release 0.6 mcg/day, decreasing over 30 days to a steady-state release rate of 0.3-0.4 mcg/day for 30 months
Dosage Forms
Implant, intravitreal:
Retisert®: 0.59 mg (1s)

fluocinolone (otic) (floo oh SIN oh lone)

Medication Safety Issues
Sound-alike/look-alike issues:
Fluocinolone may be confused with fluocinonide
Synonyms fluocinolone acetonide
U.S. Brand Names DermOtic®
Therapeutic Category Corticosteroid, Otic
Use Relief of chronic eczematous external otitis
General Dosage Range Otic: *Children ≥2 years and Adults:* 5 drops into affected ear twice daily
Dosage Forms
Oil, otic:
DermOtic®: 0.01% (20 mL)

fluocinolone (topical) (floo oh SIN oh lone)

Medication Safety Issues
Sound-alike/look-alike issues:
Fluocinolone may be confused with fluocinonide
Synonyms fluocinolone acetonide
U.S. Brand Names Capex®; Derma-Smoothe/FS®

Canadian Brand Names Capex®; Derma-Smoothe/FS®; Synalar®
Therapeutic Category Corticosteroid, Topical
Use Relief of susceptible inflammatory dermatosis [low, medium corticosteroid]; dermatitis or psoriasis of the scalp; atopic dermatitis in adults and children ≥3 months of age
General Dosage Range Topical:
Children ≥3 months: Apply a thin layer to affected area 2-4 times/day
Adults: Body: Apply thin layer to affected area 2-4 times/day; Scalp: 1 ounce daily (Capex®) **or** massage into wet hair and leave on for at least 4 hours (Derma-Smoothe/FS®)
Dosage Forms
Cream, topical: 0.01% (15 g, 60 g); 0.025% (15 g, 60 g)
Oil, topical:
Derma-Smoothe/FS®: 0.01% (120 mL)
Ointment, topical: 0.025% (15 g, 60 g)
Shampoo, topical:
Capex®: 0.01% (120 mL)
Solution, topical: 0.01% (60 mL)

fluocinolone acetonide *see* fluocinolone (ophthalmic) *on page 384*
fluocinolone acetonide *see* fluocinolone (otic) *on page 384*
fluocinolone acetonide *see* fluocinolone (topical) *on page 384*

fluocinolone, hydroquinone, and tretinoin
(floo oh SIN oh lone, HYE droe kwin one, & TRET i noyn)
Synonyms hydroquinone, fluocinolone acetonide, and tretinoin; tretinoin, fluocinolone acetonide, and hydroquinone
U.S. Brand Names Tri-Luma®
Therapeutic Category Corticosteroid, Topical; Depigmenting Agent; Retinoic Acid Derivative
Use Short-term treatment of moderate-to-severe melasma of the face
General Dosage Range Topical: *Adults:* Apply a thin film once daily to affected areas.
Dosage Forms
Cream, topical:
Tri-Luma®: Fluocinolone acetonide 0.01%, hydroquinone 4%, and tretinoin 0.05% (30 g)

fluocinonide (floo oh SIN oh nide)
Medication Safety Issues
Sound-alike/look-alike issues:
Fluocinonide may be confused with flunisolide, fluocinolone
Lidex® may be confused with Lasix®, Videx®, Wydase®
Synonyms Lidex
U.S. Brand Names Vanos®
Canadian Brand Names Lidemol®; Lidex®; Lyderm®; Tiamol®; Topactin; Topsyn®
Therapeutic Category Corticosteroid, Topical
Use Antiinflammatory, antipruritic; treatment of plaque-type psoriasis (up to 10% of body surface area) [high-potency topical corticosteroid]
General Dosage Range Topical:
Children <12 years: Apply thin layer of 0.05% cream to affected area 2-4 times/day
Children ≥12 years and Adults: Apply thin layer of 0.05% cream to affected area 2-4 times/day **or** apply a thin layer of 0.1% cream once or twice daily to affected area
Dosage Forms
Cream, topical:
Vanos®: 0.1% (30 g, 60 g, 120 g)
Cream, anhydrous, emollient, topical: 0.05% (15 g, 30 g, 60 g, 120 g)
Cream, aqueous, emollient, topical: 0.05% (15 g, 30 g, 60 g)
Gel, topical: 0.05% (15 g, 30 g, 60 g)
Ointment, topical: 0.05% (15 g, 30 g, 60 g)
Solution, topical: 0.05% (20 mL, 60 mL)

fluohydrisone acetate *see* fludrocortisone *on page 383*
fluohydrocortisone acetate *see* fludrocortisone *on page 383*
Fluorabon™ *see* fluoride *on page 386*

Fluor-A-Day® *see* fluoride *on page 386*
Fluor-A-Day (Can) *see* fluoride *on page 386*

fluorescein (FLURE e seen)
Synonyms fluorescein sodium; sodium fluorescein; soluble fluorescein
U.S. Brand Names AK-Fluor®; Angiofluor™ Lite [DSC]; Angiofluor™ [DSC]; BioGlo™; Fluorescite®; Fluorets®; Ful-Glo®
Canadian Brand Names Fluorescite®
Therapeutic Category Diagnostic Agent
Use
  Injection: Diagnostic aid in ophthalmic angiography and angioscopy
  Topical: To stain the anterior segment of the eye for procedures (such as fitting contact lenses), disclosing corneal injury, and in applanation tonometry
General Dosage Range Dosage adjustment recommended in patients with renal impairment
I.V.:
  Children: 3.5 mg/lb (7.7 mg/kg) as a single dose
  Adults: 500-750 mg as a single dose
  Ophthalmic: *Children and Adults:* Apply moistened strip until desired amount of staining obtained
Dosage Forms
  Injection, solution: 10% (5 mL); 25% (2 mL)
  AK-Fluor®: 10% (5 mL)
  Injection, solution [preservative free]:
  Fluorescite®: 10% (5 mL)
  Strip, ophthalmic:
  BioGlo™: 1 mg (100s, 300s)
  Fluorets®: 1 mg (100s)
  Ful-Glo®: 0.6 mg (300s); 1 mg (100s)

fluorescein and proparacaine *see* proparacaine and fluorescein *on page 745*
fluorescein sodium *see* fluorescein *on page 386*
Fluorescite® *see* fluorescein *on page 386*
Fluorets® *see* fluorescein *on page 386*

fluoride (FLOR ide)
Medication Safety Issues
  Sound-alike/look-alike issues:
  Phos-Flur® may be confused with PhosLo®
  International issues:
  Fluorex [France] may be confused with Flarex brand name for fluorometholone [U.S., Canada, and multiple international markets] and Fluarix brand name for influenza virus vaccine (inactivated) [U.S., and multiple international markets]
Synonyms acidulated phosphate fluoride; sodium fluoride; stannous fluoride
U.S. Brand Names Act® Kids [OTC]; Act® Restoring™ [OTC]; Act® Total Care™ [OTC]; Act® [OTC]; CaviRinse™; Clinpro™ 5000; ControlRx™; ControlRx™ Multi; Denta 5000 Plus™; DentaGel™; Epiflur™; Fluor-A-Day®; Fluorabon™; Fluorinse®; Fluoritab; Flura-Drops®; Gel-Kam® Rinse; Gel-Kam® [OTC]; Just For Kids™ [OTC]; Lozi-Flur™; NeutraCare®; NeutraGard® Advanced; Omni Gel™ [OTC]; OrthoWash™; PerioMed™; Phos-Flur®; Phos-Flur® Rinse [OTC]; PreviDent®; PreviDent® 5000 Booster; PreviDent® 5000 Dry Mouth; PreviDent® 5000 Plus®; PreviDent® 5000 Sensitive; StanGard® Perio; Stop®
Canadian Brand Names Fluor-A-Day
Therapeutic Category Mineral, Oral
Use Prevention of dental caries
General Dosage Range Oral:
  Cream: *Children ≥6 years and Adults:* Brush on teeth once daily
  Fluorinse®, PreviDent® rinse: *Children >6 years and Adults:* Once weekly, vigorously swish 5-10 mL (Fluorinse®) or 10 mL (PreviDent®) in mouth for 1 minute, then spit
  Gel or Rinse:
    Children 6-12 years: 5-10 mL rinse or apply to teeth and spit daily after brushing
    Adults: 10 mL rinse or apply to teeth and spit daily after brushing
  Lozenge: *Adults:* 1 daily

Lozenge/oral drops/tablets:
  Fluoride content of drinking water <0.3 ppm:
    Children 6 months to 3 years: 0.25 mg/day
    Children 3-6 years: 0.5 mg/day
    Children 6-16 years: 1 mg/day
  Fluoride content of drinking water 0.3-0.6 ppm:
    Children 3-6 years: 0.25 mg/day
    Children 6-16 years: 0.5 mg/day

Dosage Forms
  Cream, oral: 1.1% (51 g)
    Denta 5000 Plus™: 1.1% (51 g)
    PreviDent® 5000 Plus®: 1.1% (51 g)
  Gel, oral:
    PreviDent® 5000 Booster: 1.1% (100 mL, 106 mL)
    PreviDent® 5000 Dry Mouth: 1.1% (100 mL)
    PreviDent® 5000 Sensitive: 1.1% (100 mL)
  Gel, topical: 1.1% (56 g)
    DentaGel™: 1.1% (56 g)
    Gel-Kam® [OTC]: 0.4% (129 g)
    Just For Kids™ [OTC]: 0.4% (122 g)
    NeutraCare®: 1.1% (60 g)
    NeutraGard® Advanced: 1.1% (60 g)
    Omni Gel™ [OTC]: 0.4% (122 g); 0.4% (122 g)
    Phos-Flur®: 1.1% (51 g)
    PreviDent®: 1.1% (56 g)
    Stop®: 0.4% (120 g)
  Liquid, oral:
    Fluoritab: 0.125 mg/drop
  Lozenge, oral:
    Lozi-Flur™: 2.21 mg (90s)
  Paste, oral:
    Clinpro™ 5000: 1.1% (113 g)
    ControlRx™: 1.1% (57 g)
    ControlRx™ Multi: 1.1% (57 g)
  Solution, oral: 1.1 mg/mL (50 mL); 0.2% (473 mL); 0.63% (300 mL)
    Act® [OTC]: 0.05% (532 mL)
    Act® Kids [OTC]: 0.05% (500 mL, 532 mL)
    Act® Restoring™ [OTC]: 0.02% (1000 mL); 0.05% (532 mL)
    Act® Total Care™ [OTC]: 0.02% (1000 mL); 0.05% (88 mL, 532 mL)
    CaviRinse™: 0.2% (240 mL)
    Fluor-A-Day®: 0.278 mg/drop (30 mL)
    Fluorabon®: 0.55 mg/0.6 mL (60 mL)
    Fluorinse®: 0.2% (480 mL)
    Flura-Drops®: 0.55 mg/drop (24 mL)
    Gel-Kam® Rinse: 0.63% (300 mL)
    OrthoWash™: 0.044% (480 mL)
    PerioMed™: 0.63% (284 mL)
    Phos-Flur® Rinse [OTC]: 0.044% (473 mL, 500 mL)
    PreviDent®: 0.2% (473 mL)
    StanGard® Perio: 0.63% (284 mL)
  Tablet, chewable, oral: 0.55 mg, 1.1 mg, 2.2 mg
    Epiflur™: 0.55 mg, 1.1 mg, 2.2 mg
    Fluor-A-Day®: 1.1 mg, 2.2 mg
    Fluoritab: 1.1 mg, 2.2 mg

Fluorinse® *see* fluoride *on page 386*

Fluoritab *see* fluoride *on page 386*

5-fluorocytosine *see* flucytosine *on page 382*

fluorodeoxyuridine *see* floxuridine *on page 381*

9α-fluorohydrocortisone acetate *see* fludrocortisone *on page 383*

fluorometholone (flure oh METH oh lone)

Medication Safety Issues
International issues:
Flarex [U.S., Canada, and multiple international markets] may be confused with Fluarix brand name for influenza virus vaccine (inactivated) [U.S. and multiple international markets] and Fluorex brand name for fluoride [France]

U.S. Brand Names Flarex®; FML Forte®; FML®

Canadian Brand Names Flarex®; FML Forte®; FML®; PMS-Fluorometholone

Therapeutic Category Adrenal Corticosteroid

Use Treatment of steroid-responsive inflammatory conditions of the eye

General Dosage Range Ophthalmic:
Ointment: *Children >2 years and Adults:* Apply small amount (~1/2" ribbon) every 4 hours (initial: 24-48 hours) **or** 1-3 times/day
Suspension:
Children >2 years: Instill 1 drop every 4 hours (initial: 24-48 hours) **or** 1 drop 2-4 times/day
Adults: Instill 2 drops (initial: 24-48 hours) **or** 1-2 drops 2-4 times/day

Dosage Forms
Ointment, ophthalmic:
FML®: 0.1% (3.5 g)
Suspension, ophthalmic: 0.1% (5 mL, 10 mL, 15 mL)
Flarex®: 0.1% (5 mL)
FML Forte®: 0.25% (5 mL, 10 mL)
FML®: 0.1% (5 mL, 10 mL, 15 mL)

Fluoroplex® *see* fluorouracil (topical) *on page 388*

5-fluorouracil *see* fluorouracil (systemic) *on page 388*

5-fluorouracil *see* fluorouracil (topical) *on page 388*

fluorouracil (systemic) (flure oh YOOR a sil)

Medication Safety Issues
Sound-alike/look-alike issues:
Fluorouracil may be confused with flucytosine
High alert medication:
This medication is in a class the Institute for Safe Medication Practices (ISMP) includes among its list of drugs which have a heightened risk of causing significant patient harm when used in error.

Synonyms 5-fluorouracil; 5-FU; FU

U.S. Brand Names Adrucil®

Therapeutic Category Antineoplastic Agent, Antimetabolite (Pyrimidine Analog)

Use Treatment of carcinomas of the breast, colon, rectum, pancreas, or stomach

General Dosage Range Dosage adjustment recommended in patients with hepatic or renal impairment
I.V.: *Adults:* Dosage varies greatly depending on indication

Dosage Forms
Injection, solution: 50 mg/mL (10 mL, 20 mL, 50 mL, 100 mL)
Adrucil®: 50 mg/mL (10 mL, 50 mL, 100 mL)

fluorouracil (topical) (flure oh YOOR a sil)

Medication Safety Issues
Sound-alike/look-alike issues:
Fluorouracil may be confused with flucytosine
Efudex® may be confused with Efidac (Efidac 24®), Eurax®
High alert medication:
The Institute for Safe Medication Practices (ISMP) includes this medication among its list of drugs which have a heightened risk of causing significant patient harm when used in error.
International issues:
Carac® [U.S.] may be confused with Carace brand name for lisinopril [Ireland]

Synonyms 5-fluorouracil; 5-FU; FU

U.S. Brand Names Carac®; Efudex®; Fluoroplex®

Canadian Brand Names Efudex®; Fluoroplex®

Therapeutic Category Antineoplastic Agent, Antimetabolite (Pyrimidine Analog)

Use Management of actinic or solar keratoses and superficial basal cell carcinomas

General Dosage Range Topical: *Adults:* Apply to lesions once (Carac™) or twice daily (Efudex®; Fluoroplex®)

Dosage Forms
Cream, topical: 5% (40 g)
Carac®: 0.5% (30 g)
Efudex®: 5% (40 g)
Fluoroplex®: 1% (30 g)
Solution, topical: 2% (10 mL); 5% (10 mL)
Efudex®: 5% (10 mL)

fluoxetine (floo OKS e teen)

Medication Safety Issues
Sound-alike/look-alike issues:
FLUoxetine may be confused with DULoxetine, famotidine, Feldene®, fluconazole, fluvastatin, fluvoxaMINE, fosinopril, furosemide, PARoxetine, thiothixene
PROzac® may be confused with Paxil®, Prelone®, PriLOSEC®, Prograf®, Proscar®, ProSom®, ProStep®, Provera®
Sarafem® may be confused with Serophene®
BEERS Criteria medication:
This drug may be inappropriate for use in geriatric patients (high severity risk).
International issues:
Reneuron [Spain] may be confused with Remeron brand name for mirtazapine [U.S., Canada, and multiple international markets]
Synonyms fluoxetine hydrochloride
Tall-Man FLUoxetine
U.S. Brand Names PROzac®; PROzac® Weekly™; Sarafem®; Selfemra® [DSC]
Canadian Brand Names Apo-Fluoxetine®; CO Fluoxetine; Dom-Fluoxetine; Fluoxetine; FXT 40; Gen-Fluoxetine; Mylan-Fluoxetine; Novo-Fluoxetine; Nu-Fluoxetine; PHL-Fluoxetine; PMS-Fluoxetine; PRO-Fluoxetine; Prozac®; ratio-Fluoxetine; Riva-Fluoxetine; Sandoz-Fluoxetine; Teva-Fluoxetine; ZYM-Fluoxetine
Therapeutic Category Antidepressant, Selective Serotonin Reuptake Inhibitor
Use Treatment of major depressive disorder (MDD); treatment of binge-eating and vomiting in patients with moderate-to-severe bulimia nervosa; obsessive-compulsive disorder (OCD); premenstrual dysphoric disorder (PMDD); panic disorder with or without agoraphobia; in combination with olanzapine for treatment-resistant or bipolar I depression
General Dosage Range Dosage adjustment recommended in patients with hepatic impairment
Oral:
Children 7-18 years: Initial: 10-20 mg once daily; Maintenance: 10-60 mg once daily
Adults: 10-80 mg once daily **or** 90 mg once weekly
Elderly: 10 mg/day
Dosage Forms
Capsule, oral: 10 mg, 20 mg, 40 mg
PROzac®: 10 mg, 20 mg, 40 mg
Capsule, delayed release, enteric coated pellets, oral: 90 mg
PROzac® Weekly™: 90 mg
Solution, oral: 20 mg/5 mL (5 mL, 120 mL)
Tablet, oral: 10 mg, 20 mg
Sarafem®: 10 mg, 15 mg, 20 mg

Fluoxetine (Can) *see* fluoxetine *on page 389*
fluoxetine and olanzapine *see* olanzapine and fluoxetine *on page 645*
fluoxetine hydrochloride *see* fluoxetine *on page 389*

fluoxymesterone (floo oks i MES te rone)

Medication Safety Issues
Sound-alike/look-alike issues:
Halotestin® may be confused with Haldol®, haloperidol
U.S. Brand Names Androxy™
Therapeutic Category Androgen

◄ **Controlled Substance** C-III
Use Replacement of endogenous testicular hormone; in females, palliative treatment of breast cancer
General Dosage Range Oral:
Adults (females): 10-40 mg/day in divided doses
Adults (males): 2.5-20 mg/day
Dosage Forms
Tablet, oral:
Androxy™: 10 mg

flupenthixol *(Canada only)* (floo pen THIKS ol)

Synonyms flupenthixol decanoate; flupenthixol dihydrochloride
Canadian Brand Names Fluanxol®; Fluanxol® Depot
Therapeutic Category Antipsychotic Agent; Thioxanthene Derivative
Use Maintenance therapy of chronic schizophrenic patients whose main manifestations do **not** include excitement, agitation, or hyperactivity
General Dosage Range
I.M. (Depot): *Adults:* Initial test dose: 5-20 mg; Maintenance: 2- to 3-week intervals
Oral: *Adults:* Initial: 1 mg 3 times/day; Maintenance: 3-6 mg/day in divided doses
Product Availability Not available in U.S.
Dosage Forms - Canada
Injection, solution [depot]:
Fluanxol®: 20 mg/mL (10 mL); 100 mg/mL (2 mL)
Tablet, oral:
Fluanxol®: 0.5 mg, 3 mg

flupenthixol decanoate *see* flupenthixol *(Canada only) on page 390*
flupenthixol dihydrochloride *see* flupenthixol *(Canada only) on page 390*

fluphenazine (floo FEN a zeen)

Medication Safety Issues
Sound-alike/look-alike issues:
FluPHENAZine may be confused with fluvoxaMINE
International issues:
Prolixin [Turkey] may be confused with Prolixan brand name for azapropazone [Greece]
Synonyms fluphenazine decanoate; fluphenazine hydrochloride
Tall-Man fluPHENAZine
Canadian Brand Names Apo-Fluphenazine Decanoate®; Apo-Fluphenazine®; Modecate®; Modecate® Concentrate; PMS-Fluphenazine Decanoate
Therapeutic Category Phenothiazine Derivative
Use Management of manifestations of psychotic disorders and schizophrenia; depot formulation may offer improved outcome in individuals with psychosis who are nonadherent with oral antipsychotics
General Dosage Range
I.M. (hydrochloride): *Adults:* Initial: 1.25 mg as a single dose; Maintenance: 2.5-10 mg/day in divided doses every 6-8 hours
I.M., SubQ (Depot): *Adults:* Initial: 6.25-25 mg every 2-4 weeks (maximum: 100 mg)
Oral: *Adults:* 1-20 mg/day in divided doses every 6-8 hours (maximum: 40 mg/day)
Dosage Forms
Elixir, oral: 2.5 mg/5 mL (60 mL, 473 mL)
Injection, oil: 25 mg/mL (5 mL)
Injection, solution: 2.5 mg/mL (10 mL)
Solution, oral: 5 mg/mL (118 mL)
Tablet, oral: 1 mg, 2.5 mg, 5 mg, 10 mg

fluphenazine decanoate *see* fluphenazine *on page 390*
fluphenazine hydrochloride *see* fluphenazine *on page 390*
Flura-Drops® *see* fluoride *on page 386*

flurandrenolide (flure an DREN oh lide)

Medication Safety Issues
Sound-alike/look-alike issues:
Cordran® may be confused with Cardura®, codeine, Cordarone®

Synonyms flurandrenolone

U.S. Brand Names Cordran®; Cordran® SP

Canadian Brand Names Cordran®

Therapeutic Category Corticosteroid, Topical

Use Inflammation of corticosteroid-responsive dermatoses [medium potency topical corticosteroid]

General Dosage Range Topical:
Children: Apply 1-2 times/day
Adults: Apply 2-3 times/day

Dosage Forms
Cream, topical:
Cordran® SP: 0.05% (15 g, 30 g, 60 g)
Lotion, topical:
Cordran®: 0.05% (15 mL, 60 mL)
Tape, topical:
Cordran®: 4 mcg/cm^2 (24 inch, 80 inch)

flurandrenolone *see* flurandrenolide *on page 391*

flurazepam (flure AZ e pam)

Medication Safety Issues
Sound-alike/look-alike issues:
Flurazepam may be confused with temazepam
Dalmane® may be confused with Demulen®, Dialume®
BEERS Criteria medication:
This drug may be inappropriate for use in geriatric patients (high severity risk).

Synonyms flurazepam hydrochloride

Canadian Brand Names Apo-Flurazepam®; Dalmane®; Som Pam

Therapeutic Category Benzodiazepine

Controlled Substance C-IV

Use Short-term treatment of insomnia

General Dosage Range Oral:
Children ≥15 years and Elderly: 15 mg at bedtime
Adults: 15-30 mg at bedtime

Dosage Forms
Capsule, oral: 15 mg, 30 mg

flurazepam hydrochloride *see* flurazepam *on page 391*

flurbiprofen (systemic) (flure BI proe fen)

Medication Safety Issues
Sound-alike/look-alike issues:
Flurbiprofen may be confused with fenoprofen
Ansaid® may be confused with Asacol®, Axid®

Synonyms flurbiprofen sodium

Canadian Brand Names Alti-Flurbiprofen; Ansaid®; Apo-Flurbiprofen®; Froben-SR®; Froben®; Novo-Flurprofen; Nu-Flurprofen

Therapeutic Category Nonsteroidal Antiinflammatory Drug (NSAID)

Use Treatment of rheumatoid arthritis and osteoarthritis

General Dosage Range Oral: *Adults:* 200-300 mg/day in 2-4 divided doses (maximum: 100 mg/dose; 300 mg/day)

Dosage Forms
Tablet, oral: 50 mg, 100 mg

flurbiprofen (ophthalmic) (flure BI proe fen)

Medication Safety Issues
Sound-alike/look-alike issues:
Flurbiprofen may be confused with fenoprofen
Ocufen® may be confused with Ocuflox®, Ocupress®
Synonyms flurbiprofen sodium
U.S. Brand Names Ocufen®
Canadian Brand Names Ocufen®
Therapeutic Category Nonsteroidal Antiinflammatory Drug (NSAID), Ophthalmic
Use Inhibition of intraoperative miosis
General Dosage Range Ophthalmic: *Adults:* Instill 1 drop to each eye every 30 minutes (maximum: 4 doses)
Dosage Forms
Solution, ophthalmic: 0.03% (2.5 mL)
Ocufen®: 0.03% (2.5 mL)

flurbiprofen sodium *see* flurbiprofen (ophthalmic) *on page 392*
flurbiprofen sodium *see* flurbiprofen (systemic) *on page 391*
5-flurocytosine *see* flucytosine *on page 382*

flutamide (FLOO ta mide)

Medication Safety Issues
Sound-alike/look-alike issues:
Flutamide may be confused with Flumadine®, thalidomide
Eulexin may be confused with Edecrin®, Eurax®
Synonyms 4'-nitro-3'-trifluoromethylisobutyrantide; Eulexin; Niftolid; NSC-147834; SCH 13521
Canadian Brand Names Apo-Flutamide®; Euflex®; Eulexin®; Novo-Flutamide; PMS-Flutamide; Teva-Flutamide
Therapeutic Category Antiandrogen
Use Treatment of metastatic prostatic carcinoma in combination therapy with LHRH agonist analogues
General Dosage Range Oral: *Adults:* 250 mg 3 times/day
Dosage Forms
Capsule, oral: 125 mg

fluticasone (oral inhalation) (floo TIK a sone)

Medication Safety Issues
Sound-alike/look-alike issues:
Flovent® may be confused with Flonase®
International issues:
Allegro: Brand name for fluticasone [Israel], but also the brand name for frovatriptan [Germany]
Allegro [Israel] may be confused with Allegra and Allegra-D brand names for fexofenadine and fexofenadine/pseudoephedrine, respectively, [U.S., Canada, and multiple international markets]
Flovent® [U.S., Canada] may be confused with Flogen brand name for naproxen [Mexico]
Synonyms Flovent; fluticasone propionate
U.S. Brand Names Flovent® Diskus®; Flovent® HFA
Canadian Brand Names Flovent® Diskus®; Flovent® HFA
Therapeutic Category Corticosteroid, Inhalant (Oral)
Use Maintenance treatment of asthma as prophylactic therapy; also indicated for patients requiring oral corticosteroid therapy for asthma to assist in total discontinuation or reduction of total oral dose
General Dosage Range Inhalation:
Flovent® HFA:
Children 4-11 years: 88 mcg twice daily (maximum: >352 mcg/day in 2 divided doses)
Children ≥12 years and Adults: 88-880 mcg twice daily
Flovent® Diskus®:
Children 4-11 years: 50-100 mcg twice daily
Children >11 years and Adults: 100-1000 mcg twice daily

Dosage Forms
  Aerosol, for oral inhalation:
    Flovent® HFA: 44 mcg/inhalation (10.6 g); 110 mcg/inhalation (12 g); 220 mcg/inhalation (12 g)
  Powder, for oral inhalation:
    Flovent® Diskus®: 50 mcg (60s); 100 mcg (60s); 250 mcg (60s)
Dosage Forms - Canada
  Powder, for oral inhalation [prefilled blister pack]:
    Flovent® Diskus®: 50 mcg (28s, 60s); 100 mcg (28s, 60s); 250 mcg (28s, 60s); 500 mcg (28s, 60s)

fluticasone (nasal) (floo TIK a sone)

Medication Safety Issues
  Sound-alike/look-alike issues:
    Flonase® may be confused with Flovent®
  International issues:
    Allegro: Brand name for fluticasone [Israel], but also the brand name for frovatriptan [Germany]
    Allegro [Israel] may be confused with Allegra and Allegra-D brand names for fexofenadine and fexofenadine/pseudoephedrine, respectively, [U.S., Canada, and multiple international markets]
Synonyms fluticasone furoate; fluticasone propionate
U.S. Brand Names Flonase®; Veramyst®
Canadian Brand Names Apo-Fluticasone®; Avamys®; Flonase®; ratio-Fluticasone
Therapeutic Category Corticosteroid, Nasal
Use
  Flonase®: Management of seasonal and perennial allergic rhinitis and nonallergic rhinitis
  Veramyst®, Avamys® [CAN]: Management of seasonal and perennial allergic rhinitis
General Dosage Range Intranasal:
  Propionate (Flonase®):
    Children ≥4 years: Initial: 1 spray (50 mcg/spray) per nostril once daily; Maintenance: 1-2 sprays (100 mcg) per nostril once daily (maximum: 2 sprays in each nostril [200 mcg]/day)
    Adults: Initial: 2 sprays (50 mcg/spray) per nostril once daily; Maintenance: 1-2 sprays per nostril once daily
  Furoate (Veramyst®):
    Children 2-11 years: Initial: 1 spray (27.5 mcg/spray) per nostril once daily; Maintenance 1-2 sprays per nostril once daily (55-110 mcg/day) (maximum: 2 sprays in each nostril [110 mcg]/day)
    Children ≥12 years and Adults: Initial: 2 sprays (27.5 mcg/spray) per nostril once daily; Maintenance 1-2 sprays per nostril once daily (55-110 mcg/day) (maximum: 2 sprays in each nostril [110 mcg]/day)
Dosage Forms
  Suspension, intranasal: 50 mcg/inhalation (16 g)
    Flonase®: 50 mcg/inhalation (16 g)
    Veramyst®: 27.5 mcg/inhalation (10 g)
Dosage Forms - Canada
  Suspension, intranasal, as furoate [spray]:
    Avamys®: 27.5 mcg/inhalation (4.5 g, 10 g)

fluticasone (topical) (floo TIK a sone)

Medication Safety Issues
  Sound-alike/look-alike issues:
    Cutivate® may be confused with Ultravate®
  International issues:
    Allegro: Brand name for fluticasone [Israel], but also the brand name for frovatriptan [Germany]
    Allegro [Israel] may be confused with Allegra and Allegra-D brand names for fexofenadine and fexofenadine/pseudoephedrine, respectively, [U.S., Canada, and multiple international markets]
Synonyms fluticasone propionate
U.S. Brand Names Cutivate®
Canadian Brand Names Cutivate™
Therapeutic Category Corticosteroid, Topical
Use Relief of inflammation and pruritus associated with corticosteroid-responsive dermatoses; atopic dermatitis
General Dosage Range Topical:
  Cream: *Children ≥3 months and Adults:* Apply sparingly to affected area once or twice daily

◄ Lotion:
Children ≥1 year: Apply sparingly to affected area once daily
Adults: Apply sparingly to affected area once or twice daily
Dosage Forms
Cream, topical: 0.05% (15 g, 30 g, 60 g)
Cutivate®: 0.05% (30 g, 60 g)
Lotion, topical:
Cutivate®: 0.05% (120 mL)
Ointment, topical: 0.005% (15 g, 30 g, 60 g)
Cutivate®: 0.005% (30 g, 60 g)

fluticasone and salmeterol (floo TIK a sone & sal ME te role)

Medication Safety Issues
Sound-alike/look-alike issues:
Advair® may be confused with Adcirca®, Advicor®
Synonyms fluticasone propionate and salmeterol xinafoate; salmeterol and fluticasone
U.S. Brand Names Advair Diskus®; Advair® HFA
Canadian Brand Names Advair Diskus®; Advair®
Therapeutic Category Beta$_2$-Adrenergic Agonist Agent; Corticosteroid, Inhalant
Use Maintenance treatment of asthma; maintenance treatment of COPD
General Dosage Range Oral inhalation:
Children 4-11 years: Advair Diskus®: Fluticasone 100 mcg/salmeterol 50 mcg/inhalation: One inhalation twice daily (maximum dose)
Children ≥12 years:
Advair Diskus®: Fluticasone 100-500 mcg/salmeterol 50 mcg/inhalation: One inhalation twice daily. Maximum: Fluticasone 500 mcg/salmeterol 50 mcg/inhalation twice daily
Advair® HFA: Fluticasone 45-230 mcg/salmeterol 21 mcg/inhalation: Two inhalations twice daily
Adults:
Advair Diskus®: Initial, maximum: Fluticasone 250 mcg/salmeterol 50 mcg twice daily [COPD]; Maximum dose: Fluticasone 500 mcg/salmeterol 50 mcg/inhalation: One inhalation twice daily [Asthma]
Advair® HFA: Fluticasone 45-230 mcg/salmeterol 50 mcg/inhalation: Two inhalations twice daily
Dosage Forms
Aerosol, for oral inhalation:
Advair® HFA:
45/21: Fluticasone propionate 45 mcg and salmeterol 21 mcg (8 g, 12 g) [chlorofluorocarbon free]
115/21: Fluticasone propionate 115 mcg and salmeterol 21 mcg (8 g, 12 g) [chlorofluorocarbon free]
230/21: Fluticasone propionate 230 mcg and salmeterol 21 mcg (8 g, 12 g) [chlorofluorocarbon free]
Powder, for oral inhalation:
Advair Diskus®:
100/50: Fluticasone propionate 100 mcg and salmeterol 50 mcg (14s, 60s)
250/50: Fluticasone propionate 250 mcg and salmeterol 50 mcg (60s)
500/50: Fluticasone propionate 500 mcg and salmeterol 50 mcg (60s)
Dosage Forms - Canada
Aerosol, for oral inhalation:
Advair®: 125/25: Fluticasone propionate 125 mcg and salmeterol 25 mcg (12 g); 250/25: Fluticasone propionate 250 mcg and salmeterol 25 mcg (12 g)

fluticasone furoate *see* fluticasone (nasal) *on page 393*
fluticasone propionate *see* fluticasone (nasal) *on page 393*
fluticasone propionate *see* fluticasone (oral inhalation) *on page 392*
fluticasone propionate *see* fluticasone (topical) *on page 393*
fluticasone propionate and salmeterol xinafoate *see* fluticasone and salmeterol *on page 394*

fluvastatin (FLOO va sta tin)

Medication Safety Issues
Sound-alike/look-alike issues:
Fluvastatin may be confused with fluoxetine, nystatin, pitavastatin
U.S. Brand Names Lescol®; Lescol® XL
Canadian Brand Names Lescol®; Lescol® XL

Therapeutic Category HMG-CoA Reductase Inhibitor

Use To be used as a component of multiple risk factor intervention in patients at risk for atherosclerosis vascular disease due to hypercholesterolemia

Adjunct to dietary therapy to reduce elevated total cholesterol (total-C), LDL-C, triglyceride, and apolipoprotein B (apo-B) levels and to increase HDL-C in primary hypercholesterolemia and mixed dyslipidemia (Fredrickson types IIa and IIb); to slow the progression of coronary atherosclerosis in patients with coronary heart disease; reduce risk of coronary revascularization procedures in patients with coronary heart disease

General Dosage Range Oral:
Extended release: *Children 10-16 years (females 1 year postmenarche) and Adults:* 80 mg once daily
Immediate release:
  Adolescents 10-16 years (females 1 year postmenarche): Initial: 20 mg once daily; Maintenance: Up to 80 mg/day in 2 divided doses
  Adults: Initial: 20-40 mg once daily; Maintenance: Up to 80 mg/day in 2 divided doses

Dosage Forms
Capsule, oral:
  Lescol®: 20 mg, 40 mg
Tablet, extended release, oral:
  Lescol® XL: 80 mg

Fluviral S/F® (Can) *see* influenza virus vaccine (inactivated) *on page 473*
Fluvirin® *see* influenza virus vaccine (inactivated) *on page 473*

fluvoxamine (floo VOKS a meen)

Medication Safety Issues
Sound-alike/look-alike issues:
  FluvoxaMINE may be confused with flavoxATE, FLUoxetine, fluPHENAZine
  Luvox may be confused with Lasix®, Levoxyl®, Lovenox®

Synonyms Luvox

Tall-Man fluvoxaMINE

U.S. Brand Names Luvox® CR

Canadian Brand Names Alti-Fluvoxamine; Apo-Fluvoxamine®; Luvox®; Novo-Fluvoxamine; Nu-Fluvoxamine; PMS-Fluvoxamine; Rhoxal-fluvoxamine; Riva-Fluvox; Sandoz-Fluvoxamine

Therapeutic Category Antidepressant, Selective Serotonin Reuptake Inhibitor

Use Treatment of obsessive-compulsive disorder (OCD)

General Dosage Range Dosage adjustment recommended in patients with hepatic impairment
Oral:
  Children 8-11 years: Initial: 25 mg at bedtime; Maintenance: 50-200 mg/day (maximum: 200 mg/day)
  Children 12-17 years: Initial: 25 mg at bedtime; Maintenance: 50-200 mg/day (maximum: 300 mg/day)
  Adults: Initial: 50-100 mg at bedtime; Maintenance: 100-300 mg/day in 1-2 divided doses

Dosage Forms
Capsule, extended release, oral:
  Luvox® CR: 100 mg, 150 mg
Tablet, oral: 25 mg, 50 mg, 100 mg

Fluzone® *see* influenza virus vaccine (inactivated) *on page 473*
Fluzone® High-Dose *see* influenza virus vaccine (inactivated) *on page 473*
Fluzone® Intradermal *see* influenza virus vaccine (inactivated) *on page 473*
FML® *see* fluorometholone *on page 388*
FML Forte® *see* fluorometholone *on page 388*
Focalin® *see* dexmethylphenidate *on page 267*
Focalin XR® *see* dexmethylphenidate *on page 267*
Foille® [OTC] *see* benzocaine *on page 121*
folacin *see* folic acid *on page 396*
Folacin-800 [OTC] *see* folic acid *on page 396*
folacin, vitamin B$_{12}$, and vitamin B$_6$ *see* folic acid, cyanocobalamin, and pyridoxine *on page 396*
folate *see* folic acid *on page 396*
Folbee *see* folic acid, cyanocobalamin, and pyridoxine *on page 396*

Folbic *see* folic acid, cyanocobalamin, and pyridoxine *on page 396*
Folcaps™ *see* folic acid, cyanocobalamin, and pyridoxine *on page 396*
Folcaps™ Care One *see* vitamins (multiple/prenatal) *on page 920*
Folgard® [OTC] *see* folic acid, cyanocobalamin, and pyridoxine *on page 396*
Folgard RX® *see* folic acid, cyanocobalamin, and pyridoxine *on page 396*

folic acid (FOE lik AS id)

Medication Safety Issues
Sound-alike/look-alike issues:
Folic acid may be confused with folinic acid
Synonyms folacin; folate; pteroylglutamic acid
U.S. Brand Names Folacin-800 [OTC]
Canadian Brand Names Apo-Folic®
Therapeutic Category Vitamin, Water Soluble
Use Treatment of megaloblastic and macrocytic anemias due to folate deficiency; dietary supplement to prevent neural tube defects
General Dosage Range
I.M., I.V., SubQ:
Infants: 0.1 mg/day
Children <4 years: Up to 0.3 mg/day
Children ≥4 years and Adults: 0.4 mg/day
Pregnant and lactating women: 0.8 mg/day
Oral:
Infants: 0.1 mg/day
Children <4 years: Up to 0.3 mg/day
Children ≥4 years and Adults: 0.4 mg/day
Pregnant and lactating women: 0.8 mg/day (anemia) **or** 4 mg/day (prevention of neural tube defects)
Females of childbearing potential: Prevention of neural tube defects: 0.4-0.8 mg/day
Dosage Forms
Injection, solution: 5 mg/mL (10 mL)
Tablet, oral: 0.4 mg, 0.8 mg, 1 mg
Folacin-800 [OTC]: 0.8 mg

folic acid and polysaccharide-iron complex *see* polysaccharide-iron complex and folic acid *on page 721*

folic acid, cyanocobalamin, and pyridoxine

(FOE lik AS id, sye an oh koe BAL a min, & peer i DOKS een)
Synonyms cyanocobalamin, folic acid, and pyridoxine; folacin, vitamin B_{12}, and vitamin B_6; pyridoxine, folic acid, and cyanocobalamin
U.S. Brand Names FaBB; Folbee; Folbic; Folcaps™; Folgard RX®; Folgard® [OTC]; Foltabs™ 800 [OTC]; Foltx®; Homocysteine Guard [OTC]; Lev-Tov [OTC]; Tri-B® [OTC]; Tricardio B; Vita-Respa®
Therapeutic Category Vitamin
Use Nutritional supplement in end-stage renal failure, dialysis, hyperhomocysteinemia, homocystinuria, malabsorption syndromes, dietary deficiencies
General Dosage Range Oral: *Adults:* 1 tablet (folic acid 0.4-2.5 mg/cyanocobalamin 115-2000 mcg/pyridoxine 10-25 mg) daily
Dosage Forms
Tablet: Folic acid 0.8 mg, cyanocobalamin 1000 mcg, and pyridoxine 50 mg
FaBB, Folgard RX®: Folic acid 2.2 mg, cyanocobalamin 1000 mcg, and pyridoxine 25 mg
Folbee: Folic acid 2.5 mg, cyanocobalamin 1000 mcg, and pyridoxine 25 mg
Folbic, Foltx®: Folic acid 2.5 mg, cyanocobalamin 2000 mcg, and pyridoxine 25 mg
Folcaps™: Folic acid 2.2 mg, cyanocobalamin 500 mcg, and pyridoxine 25 mg
Folgard® [OTC], Foltabs™ 800 [OTC]: Folic acid 0.8 mg, cyanocobalamin 115 mcg, and pyridoxine 10 mg
Homocysteine Guard [OTC], Tri-B® [OTC]: Folic acid 0.8 mg, cyanocobalamin 400 mcg, and pyridoxine 25 mg
Lev-Tov [OTC]: Folic acid 0.8 mg, cyanocobalamin 250 mcg, and pyridoxine 25 mg
Tricardio B: Folic acid 0.4 mg, cyanocobalamin 250 mcg, and pyridoxine 25 mg
Vita-Respa®: Folic acid 2.2 mg, cyanocobalamin 1300 mcg, and pyridoxine 25 mg

folic acid, magnesium carbonate, and calcium carbonate *see* magnesium carbonate, calcium carbonate, and folic acid *on page 544*

folinate calcium *see* leucovorin calcium *on page 515*

folinic acid (error prone synonym) *see* leucovorin calcium *on page 515*

follicle-stimulating hormone, human *see* urofollitropin *on page 902*

follicle stimulating hormone, recombinant *see* follitropin alfa *on page 397*

follicle stimulating hormone, recombinant *see* follitropin beta *on page 397*

Follistim® AQ *see* follitropin beta *on page 397*

Follistim® AQ Cartridge *see* follitropin beta *on page 397*

follitropin alfa (foe li TRO pin AL fa)

Synonyms follicle stimulating hormone, recombinant; FSH; rFSH-alpha; rhFSH-alpha

U.S. Brand Names Gonal-f®; Gonal-f® RFF; Gonal-f® RFF Pen

Canadian Brand Names Gonal-f®; Gonal-f® Pen

Therapeutic Category Ovulation Stimulator

Use

Gonal-f®: Ovulation induction in patients in whom the cause of infertility is functional and not caused by primary ovarian failure; development of multiple follicles with Assisted Reproductive Technology (ART); spermatogenesis induction

Gonal-f® RFF: Ovulation induction in patients in whom the cause of infertility is functional and not caused by primary ovarian failure; development of multiple follicles with ART

General Dosage Range SubQ:

Adults (females): Initial: 75-225 int. units once daily for 5-7 days; Maintenance: Up to 300-450 int. units/ day

Adults (males): Gonal-f®: Initial: 150 int. units 3 times/week; Maintenance: Up to 300 int. units 3 times/ week (maximum: 18 months of therapy)

Dosage Forms

Injection, powder for reconstitution:

Gonal-f®: 450 int. units, 1050 int. units

Gonal-f® RFF: 75 int. units

Injection, solution:

Gonal-f® RFF Pen: 300 int. units/0.5 mL (0.5 mL); 450 int. units/0.75 mL (0.75 mL); 900 int. units/1.5 mL (1.5 mL)

follitropin beta (foe li TRO pin BAY ta)

Synonyms follicle stimulating hormone, recombinant; FSH; rFSH-beta; rhFSH-beta

U.S. Brand Names Follistim® AQ; Follistim® AQ Cartridge

Canadian Brand Names Puregon®

Therapeutic Category Ovulation Stimulator

Use

Females: Induction of ovulation and pregnancy in anovulatory infertile patients in whom the cause of infertility is functional and not caused by primary ovarian failure; development of multiple follicles with Assisted Reproductive Technology (ART)

Males: Induction of spermatogenesis in men with primary and secondary hypogonadotropic hypogonadism in whom the cause of infertility is not due to primary testicular failure.

General Dosage Range

I.M., SubQ: *Adults (females):* Initial: 75-225 int. units/day; Maintenance: Up to 175-600 int. units/day

SubQ: *Adults (males):* 450 int. units/week

Dosage Forms

Injection, solution:

Follistim® AQ: 75 int. units/0.5 mL (0.5 mL); 150 int. units/0.5 mL (0.5 mL)

Follistim® AQ Cartridge: 350 int. units/0.42 mL (0.42 mL); 650 int. units/0.78 mL (0.78 mL); 975 int. units/1.17 mL (1.17 mL)

Folotyn® *see* pralatrexate *on page 728*

Foltabs™ 800 [OTC] *see* folic acid, cyanocobalamin, and pyridoxine *on page 396*

Foltabs™ Prenatal *see* vitamins (multiple/prenatal) *on page 920*

Foltabs™ Prenatal Plus DHA *see* vitamins (multiple/prenatal) *on page 920*

Foltrin® *see* vitamins (multiple/oral) *on page 919*

Foltx® *see* folic acid, cyanocobalamin, and pyridoxine *on page 396*

fomepizole (foe ME pi zole)

Medication Safety Issues
Sound-alike/look-alike issues:
Fomepizole may be confused with omeprazole

Synonyms 4-methylpyrazole; 4-MP

U.S. Brand Names Antizol®

Therapeutic Category Antidote

Use Treatment of methanol or ethylene glycol poisoning alone or in combination with hemodialysis

General Dosage Range Dosage adjustment recommended in patients with renal impairment

I.V.: *Adults:* Loading dose of 15 mg/kg, followed by 10 mg/kg every 12 hours for 4 doses, then 15 mg/kg every 12 hours

Dosage Forms
Injection, solution [preservative free]: 1 g/mL (1.5 mL)
Antizol®: 1 g/mL (1.5 mL)

fondaparinux (fon da PARE i nuks)

Medication Safety Issues
High alert medication:
The Institute for Safe Medication Practices (ISMP) includes this medication among its list of drugs which have a heightened risk of causing significant patient harm when used in error.

Synonyms fondaparinux sodium

U.S. Brand Names Arixtra®

Canadian Brand Names Arixtra®

Therapeutic Category Factor Xa Inhibitor

Use Prophylaxis of deep vein thrombosis (DVT) in patients undergoing surgery for hip replacement, knee replacement, hip fracture (including extended prophylaxis following hip fracture surgery), or abdominal surgery (in patients at risk for thromboembolic complications); treatment of acute pulmonary embolism (PE); treatment of acute DVT without PE

Canadian labeling: Additional uses (not approved in U.S.): Unstable angina or non-ST segment elevation myocardial infarction (UA/NSTEMI) for the prevention of death and subsequent MI; ST segment elevation MI (STEMI) for the prevention of death and myocardial reinfarction

General Dosage Range SubQ:
Adults <50 kg: Treatment: 5 mg once daily
Adults 50-100 kg: Prophylaxis: 2.5 mg once daily; Treatment: 7.5 mg once daily
Adults >100 kg: Prophylaxis: 2.5 mg once daily; Treatment: 10 mg once daily

Dosage Forms
Injection, solution [preservative free]: 2.5 mg/0.5 mL (0.5 mL); 5 mg/0.4 mL (0.4 mL); 7.5 mg/0.6 mL (0.6 mL); 10 mg/0.8 mL (0.8 mL)
Arixtra®: 2.5 mg/0.5 mL (0.5 mL); 5 mg/0.4 mL (0.4 mL); 7.5 mg/0.6 mL (0.6 mL); 10 mg/0.8 mL (0.8 mL)

fondaparinux sodium *see* fondaparinux *on page 398*

Foradil® (Can) *see* formoterol *on page 398*

Foradil® Aerolizer® *see* formoterol *on page 398*

Forane® *see* isoflurane *on page 493*

formoterol (for MOH te rol)

Medication Safety Issues
Sound-alike/look-alike issues:
Foradil® may be confused with Toradol®
Administration issues:
Foradil® capsules for inhalation are for administration via Aerolizer™ inhaler and are **not** for oral use.
International issues:
Foradil [U.S., Canada, and multiple international markets] may be confused with Theradol brand name for tramadol [Netherlands]

Synonyms formoterol fumarate; formoterol fumarate dihydrate

U.S. Brand Names Foradil® Aerolizer®; Perforomist®

Canadian Brand Names Foradil®; Oxeze® Turbuhaler®

Therapeutic Category Beta$_2$-Adrenergic Agonist Agent

Use Maintenance treatment of asthma and prevention of bronchospasm (as concomitant therapy) in patients ≥5 years of age with reversible obstructive airway disease, including patients with symptoms of nocturnal asthma; maintenance treatment of bronchoconstriction in patients with COPD; prevention of exercise-induced bronchospasm in patients ≥5 years of age (monotherapy may be indicated in patients without persistent asthma)

Canadian labeling: Oxeze®: Also approved for acute relief of symptoms ("on demand" treatment) in patients ≥6 years of age

General Dosage Range Inhalation:

Foradil®: *Children ≥5 years and Adults:* 12 mcg capsule inhaled every 12 hours (maximum: 24 mcg/day) **or** 12 mcg capsule inhaled prior to exercise

Perforomist™: *Adults:* 20 mcg twice daily (maximum dose: 40 mcg/day)

Dosage Forms

Powder, for oral inhalation:

Foradil® Aerolizer®: 12 mcg/capsule (12s, 60s)

Solution, for nebulization:

Perforomist®: 20 mcg/2 mL (60s)

Dosage Forms - Canada

Powder for oral inhalation:

Oxeze® Turbuhaler®: 6 mcg/inhalation, 12 mcg/inhalation

formoterol and budesonide *see* budesonide and formoterol *on page 146*

formoterol and mometasone *see* mometasone and formoterol *on page 596*

formoterol and mometasone furoate *see* mometasone and formoterol *on page 596*

formoterol fumarate *see* formoterol *on page 398*

formoterol fumarate dihydrate *see* formoterol *on page 398*

formoterol fumarate dihydrate and budesonide *see* budesonide and formoterol *on page 146*

formoterol fumarate dihydrate and mometasone *see* mometasone and formoterol *on page 596*

Formula EM [OTC] *see* fructose, dextrose, and phosphoric acid *on page 403*

Formulation R™ [OTC] *see* phenylephrine (topical) *on page 698*

Formulex® (Can) *see* dicyclomine *on page 280*

5-formyl tetrahydrofolate *see* leucovorin calcium *on page 515*

Fortamet® *see* metformin *on page 566*

Fortaz® *see* ceftazidime *on page 184*

Forteo® *see* teriparatide *on page 853*

Fortesta™ *see* testosterone *on page 854*

Fortical® *see* calcitonin *on page 159*

Fosamax® *see* alendronate *on page 49*

Fosamax Plus D® *see* alendronate and cholecalciferol *on page 49*

fosamprenavir (FOS am pren a veer)

Medication Safety Issues

Sound-alike/look-alike issues:

Lexiva® may be confused with Levitra®

Synonyms fosamprenavir calcium; GW433908G

U.S. Brand Names Lexiva®

Canadian Brand Names Telzir®

Therapeutic Category Antiretroviral Agent, Protease Inhibitor

Use Treatment of HIV infections in combination with at least two other antiretroviral agents

General Dosage Range Dosage adjustment recommended in patients with hepatic impairment or on concomitant therapy

Oral:

Children 2-5 years: 30 mg/kg/dose twice daily (maximum: 1400 mg twice daily)

◀ *Children ≥6 years:*
Unboosted regimen: 30 mg/kg/dose twice daily (maximum: 1400 mg twice daily)
Ritonavir-boosted regimen: 18 mg/kg/dose twice daily (maximum: 700 mg twice daily)
Adults:
Unboosted regimen: 1400 mg twice daily
Ritonavir-boosted regimen: 700 mg twice daily **or** 1400 mg once daily
Dosage Forms
Suspension, oral:
Lexiva®: 50 mg/mL (225 mL)
Tablet, oral:
Lexiva®: 700 mg
Dosage Forms - Canada
Tablet:
Telzir®: 700 mg
Suspension, oral:
Telzir®: 50 mg/mL

fosamprenavir calcium *see fosamprenavir on page 399*

fosaprepitant (fos a PRE pi tant)
Medication Safety Issues
Sound-alike/look-alike issues:
Fosaprepitant may be confused with aprepitant, fosamprenavir, fospropofol
Emend® for Injection (fosaprepitant) may be confused with Emend® (aprepitant) which is an oral capsule formulation.
Synonyms aprepitant injection; fosaprepitant dimeglumine; L-758,298; MK 0517
U.S. Brand Names Emend® for Injection
Canadian Brand Names Emend® IV
Therapeutic Category Antiemetic; Substance P/Neurokinin 1 Receptor Antagonist
Use Prevention of acute and delayed nausea and vomiting associated with moderately- and highly-emetogenic chemotherapy (in combination with other antiemetics)
General Dosage Range I.V.: *Adults:* 115 or 150 mg as a single dose
Dosage Forms
Injection, powder for reconstitution:
Emend® for Injection: 150 mg

fosaprepitant dimeglumine *see fosaprepitant on page 400*
Fosavance (Can) *see alendronate and cholecalciferol on page 49*

foscarnet (fos KAR net)
Synonyms PFA; phosphonoformate; phosphonoformic acid
Canadian Brand Names Foscavir®
Therapeutic Category Antiviral Agent
Use Treatment of acyclovir-resistant mucocutaneous herpes simplex virus (HSV) infections in immunocompromised persons (eg, with advanced AIDS); treatment of CMV retinitis in persons with HIV
General Dosage Range Dosage adjustment recommended in patients with renal impairment
I.V.: *Children >12 years and Adults:* Induction: CMV: 180 mg/kg/day in 2-3 evenly divided doses; HSV: 40 mg/kg/dose every 8-12 hours; Maintenance: CMV: 90-120 mg/kg once daily
Dosage Forms
Injection, solution [preservative free]: 24 mg/mL (250 mL, 500 mL)

Foscavir® (Can) *see foscarnet on page 400*

fosfomycin (fos foe MYE sin)
Medication Safety Issues
Sound-alike/look-alike issues:
Monurol® may be confused with Monopril®
Synonyms fosfomycin tromethamine
U.S. Brand Names Monurol®
Canadian Brand Names Monurol®

Therapeutic Category Antibiotic, Miscellaneous

Use Single oral dose in the treatment of uncomplicated urinary tract infections in women due to susceptible strains of *E. coli* and *Enterococcus faecalis*

General Dosage Range Oral: *Adults (females):* 3 g once

Dosage Forms
Powder for solution, oral:
Monurol®: 3 g/sachet (3s)

fosfomycin tromethamine *see* fosfomycin *on page 400*

fosinopril (foe SIN oh pril)

Medication Safety Issues
Sound-alike/look-alike issues:
Fosinopril may be confused with FLUoxetine, Fosamax®, furosemide, lisinopril
Monopril may be confused with Accupril®, minoxidil, moexipril, Monoket®, Monurol®, ramipril

Synonyms fosinopril sodium; Monopril

Canadian Brand Names Apo-Fosinopril®; Jamp-Fosinopril; Monopril®; Mylan-Fosinopril; PMS-Fosinopril; RAN™-Fosinopril; Riva-Fosinopril; Teva-Fosinopril

Therapeutic Category Angiotensin-Converting Enzyme (ACE) Inhibitor

Use Treatment of hypertension, either alone or in combination with other antihypertensive agents; treatment of heart failure (HF)

General Dosage Range Oral:
Children ≥6 years and >50 kg: Initial: 5-10 mg once daily (maximum: 40 mg/day)
Adults: Initial: 10 mg once daily; Maintenance: 10-40 mg/day in 1-2 divided doses (maximum: 80 mg/day)

Dosage Forms
Tablet, oral: 10 mg, 20 mg, 40 mg

fosinopril and hydrochlorothiazide (foe SIN oh pril & hye droe klor oh THYE a zide)

Medication Safety Issues
Sound-alike/look-alike issues:
Monopril® may be confused with Accupril®, minoxidil, moexipril, Monoket®, Monurol®, ramipril

Synonyms hydrochlorothiazide and fosinopril

U.S. Brand Names Monopril-HCT® [DSC]

Canadian Brand Names Monopril-HCT®

Therapeutic Category Angiotensin-Converting Enzyme (ACE) Inhibitor

Use Treatment of hypertension; not indicated for first-line treatment

General Dosage Range Oral: *Adults:* Fosinopril 10-80 mg and hydrochlorothiazide 12.5-50 mg once daily

Dosage Forms
Tablet: 10/12.5: Fosinopril 10 mg and hydrochlorothiazide 12.5 mg; 20/12.5: Fosinopril 20 mg and hydrochlorothiazide 12.5 mg

fosinopril sodium *see* fosinopril *on page 401*

fosphenytoin (FOS fen i toyn)

Medication Safety Issues
Sound-alike/look-alike issues:
Cerebyx® may be confused with Celebrex®, Celexa™, Cerezyme®, Cervarix®
Fosphenytoin may be confused with fospropofol
Administration issues:
Overdoses have occurred due to confusion between the **mg per mL concentration** of fosphenytoin (50 mg PE/mL) and **total drug content per vial** (either 100 mg PE/2 mL vial or 500 mg PE/10 mL vial). ISMP recommends that the total drug content per container is identified instead of the concentration in mg per mL to avoid confusion and potential overdosages. Additionally, since most errors have occurred with overdoses in children, they recommend that pediatric hospitals should consider stocking only the 2 mL vial.

Synonyms fosphenytoin sodium

U.S. Brand Names Cerebyx®

Canadian Brand Names Cerebyx®

◀ **Therapeutic Category** Hydantoin

Use Used for the control of generalized convulsive status epilepticus and prevention and treatment of seizures occurring during neurosurgery; indicated for short-term parenteral administration when other means of phenytoin administration are unavailable, inappropriate, or deemed less advantageous (the safety and effectiveness of fosphenytoin use for more than 5 days has not been systematically evaluated)

General Dosage Range

I.M.: *Adults:* Loading: 15-20 mg PE/kg; Maintenance: 4-6 mg PE/kg/day

I.V.: *Adults:* Loading: 10-20 mg PE/kg; Maintenance: 4-6 mg PE/kg/day

Dosage Forms

Injection, **solution**: 75 mg/mL (2 mL, 10 mL)
  Cerebyx®: 75 mg/mL (2 mL)
Injection, **solution** [preservative free]: 75 mg/mL (2 mL)

fosphenytoin sodium *see* fosphenytoin *on page 401*

fospropofol (fos PROE po fole)

Medication Safety Issues

Sound-alike/look-alike issues:
  Fospropofol may be confused with fosaprepitant, fosphenytoin, propofol

High alert medication:
  The Institute for Safe Medication Practices (ISMP) includes this medication among its list of drugs which have a heightened risk of causing significant patient harm when used in error.

Administration issues:
  Onset of action: The onset of action will be delayed due to need for conversion to the active metabolite, propofol. If supplemental doses are administered before full effect occurs, the risk of dose-stacking may be elevated resulting in deeper sedation than intended.

Synonyms aquavan; fospropofol disodium; GPI 15715

U.S. Brand Names Lusedra™

Therapeutic Category Sedative

Controlled Substance C-IV

Use Monitored anesthesia care (MAC) sedation in patients undergoing diagnostic or therapeutic procedures

General Dosage Range I.V.:

Adults <65 years or with mild systemic disease (ASA-PS1 or -PS2): Initial: 6.5 mg/kg (maximum initial dose: 577.5 mg or 16.5 mL); Supplemental: 1.6 mg/kg (maximum supplemental dose: 140 mg or 4 mL) no more frequently than every 4 minutes as needed

Elderly ≥65 years or patients with severe systemic disease (ASA-PS3 or -PS4): Initial: 4.9 mg/kg (maximum initial dose: 437.5 mg or 12.5 mL); Supplemental 1.2 mg/kg (maximum supplemental dose: 105 mg or 3 mL) no more frequently than every 4 minutes as needed

Dosage Forms

Injection, **solution** [preservative free]:
  Lusedra™: 35 mg/mL (30 mL)

fospropofol disodium *see* fospropofol *on page 402*

Fosrenol® *see* lanthanum *on page 512*

FR901228 *see* romidepsin *on page 789*

Fragmin® *see* dalteparin *on page 250*

Fraxiparine™ (Can) *see* nadroparin *(Canada only) on page 608*

Fraxiparine™ Forte (Can) *see* nadroparin *(Canada only) on page 608*

FreAmine® III *see* amino acid injection *on page 65*

FreAmine® HBC *see* amino acid injection *on page 65*

Freedavite [OTC] *see* vitamins (multiple/oral) *on page 919*

Freezone® [OTC] *see* salicylic acid *on page 795*

Frisium® (Can) *see* clobazam *(Canada only) on page 220*

Froben® (Can) *see* flurbiprofen (systemic) *on page 391*

Froben-SR® (Can) *see* flurbiprofen (systemic) *on page 391*

Frova® *see* frovatriptan *on page 403*

frovatriptan (froe va TRIP tan)

Medication Safety Issues

International issues:

Allegro: Brand name for frovatriptan [Germany], but also the brand name for fluticasone [Israel]

Allegro [Germany] may be confused with Allegra and Allegra-D brand names for fexofenadine and fexofenadine/pseudoehedrine, respectively, in the [U.S., Canada, and multiple international markets]

Synonyms frovatriptan succinate

U.S. Brand Names Frova®

Canadian Brand Names Frova®

Therapeutic Category Antimigraine Agent; Serotonin 5-HT$_{1B, 1D}$ Receptor Agonist

Use Acute treatment of migraine with or without aura

General Dosage Range Oral: *Adults:* 2.5 mg as a single dose, may repeat after 2 hours (maximum: 7.5 mg/day)

Dosage Forms

Tablet, oral:

Frova®: 2.5 mg

frovatriptan succinate *see* frovatriptan *on page* 403

fructose, dextrose, and phosphoric acid (FRUK tose, DEKS trose, & foss FOR ik AS id)

Medication Safety Issues

Sound-alike/look-alike issues:

Emetrol® may be confused with emetine

Synonyms dextrose, levulose and phosphoric acid; levulose, dextrose and phosphoric acid; phosphorated carbohydrate solution; phosphoric acid, levulose and dextrose

U.S. Brand Names Emetrol® [OTC]; Formula EM [OTC]; Kalmz [OTC]; Nausea Relief [OTC]; Nausetrol® [OTC]

Therapeutic Category Antiemetic

Use Relief of nausea associated with upset stomach that occurs with intestinal or stomach flu, and food indiscretions

General Dosage Range Oral:

Children ≥2-12 years: 5-10 mL every 15 minutes as needed; do not take for more than 1 hour (5 doses)

Children ≥12 years and Adults: 15-30 mL every 15 minutes as needed; do not take for more than 1 hour (5 doses)

Dosage Forms

Liquid, oral: Fructose 1.87 g, dextrose 1.87 g, and phosphoric acid 21.5 mg per 5 mL

Formula EM [OTC], Kalmz [OTC], Nausea Relief [OTC], Nausetrol® [OTC]: Fructose 1.87 g, dextrose 1.87 g, and phosphoric acid 21.5 mg per 5 mL

frusemide *see* furosemide *on page* 404

FS *see* fibrin sealant *on page* 376

FSH *see* follitropin alfa *on page* 397

FSH *see* follitropin beta *on page* 397

FSH *see* urofollitropin *on page* 902

FS VH S/D *see* fibrin sealant *on page* 376

FTC *see* emtricitabine *on page* 325

FTC/RPV/TDF *see* emtricitabine, rilpivirine, and tenofovir *on page* 326

FTC, TDF, and EFV *see* efavirenz, emtricitabine, and tenofovir *on page* 321

FTY720 *see* fingolimod *on page* 378

FU *see* fluorouracil (systemic) *on page* 388

FU *see* fluorouracil (topical) *on page* 388

5-FU *see* fluorouracil (systemic) *on page* 388

5-FU *see* fluorouracil (topical) *on page* 388

Fucidin® (Can) *see* fusidic acid *(Canada only) on page* 405

Fucidin H (Can) *see* fusidic acid and hydrocortisone *(Canada only) on page* 405

Fucithalmic® (Can) *see* fusidic acid *(Canada only) on page* 405

FUDR *see* floxuridine *on page* 381

FUDR® (Can) *see floxuridine on page 381*
Ful-Glo® *see fluorescein on page 386*

fulvestrant (fool VES trant)

Synonyms ICI-182,780; ZD9238

U.S. Brand Names Faslodex®

Canadian Brand Names Faslodex®

Therapeutic Category Antineoplastic Agent, Estrogen Receptor Antagonist

Use Treatment of hormone receptor-positive metastatic breast cancer in postmenopausal women with disease progression following antiestrogen therapy

General Dosage Range Dosage adjustment recommended in patients with hepatic impairment
    I.M.: *Adults (postmenopausal women):* Initial: 500 mg on days 1, 15, and 29; Maintenance: 500 mg once monthly

Dosage Forms
    Injection, solution:
      Faslodex®: 50 mg/mL (5 mL)

Fungi-Nail® [OTC] *see undecylenic acid and derivatives on page 899*
Fungizone® (Can) *see amphotericin B (conventional) on page 75*
Fung-O® [OTC] *see salicylic acid on page 795*
Fungoid® [OTC] *see miconazole (topical) on page 585*
Furadantin® *see nitrofurantoin on page 629*
furazosin *see prazosin on page 733*

furosemide (fyoor OH se mide)

Medication Safety Issues
    Sound-alike/look-alike issues:
      Furosemide may be confused with famotidine, finasteride, fluconazole, FLUoxetine, fosinopril, loperamide, torsemide
      Lasix® may be confused with Esidrix®, Lanoxin®, Lidex®, Lomotil®, Lovenox®, Luvox®, Luxiq®
    International issues:
      Diuril: Brand name for furosemide [Philippines], but also the brand name for chlorothiazide [U.S., Canada]
      Urex: Brand name for furosemide [Australia], but is also brand name for methenamine [multiple international markets]
      Urex [Australia] may be confused with Eurax brand name for crotamiton [U.S., Canada, and multiple international markets]

Synonyms frusemide

U.S. Brand Names Lasix®

Canadian Brand Names Apo-Furosemide®; Bio-Furosemide; Dom-Furosemide; Furosemide Injection, USP; Furosemide Special; Lasix®; Lasix® Special; Novo-Semide; Nu-Furosemide; PMS-Furosemide

Therapeutic Category Diuretic, Loop

Use Management of edema associated with heart failure and hepatic or renal disease; acute pulmonary edema; treatment of hypertension (alone or in combination with other antihypertensives)

General Dosage Range
    I.M.:
      Children: Initial: 1 mg/kg/dose; Maintenance: Up to 6 mg/kg/dose every 6-12 hours
      Adults: Initial: 20-40 mg/dose; Usual maintenance dose interval: 6-12 hours (maximum: 200 mg/dose)
      Elderly: Initial: 20 mg/day
    I.V.:
      Children: Initial: 1 mg/kg/dose; Maintenance: Up to 6 mg/kg/dose every 6-12 hours
      Adults: Initial: 20-40 mg/dose; Usual maintenance dose interval: 6-12 hours (maximum: 200 mg/dose) **or** 40 mg, followed by 80 mg within 1 hour if inadequate response **or** 20-40 mg bolus, followed by continuous I.V. infusion doses of 10-40 mg/hour, doubled as needed up to a maximum 160 mg/hour
      Elderly: Initial: 20 mg/day

Oral:
  Children: Initial: 2 mg/kg/dose every 6-8 hours (maximum: 6 mg/kg/dose)
  Adults: Initial: 20-80 mg/dose every 6-8 hours; Usual maintenance dose interval: Once or twice daily
    (maximum: 600 mg/day)
  Elderly: Initial: 20 mg/day
Dosage Forms
  Injection, solution [preservative free]: 10 mg/mL (2 mL, 4 mL, 10 mL)
  Solution, oral: 40 mg/5 mL (5 mL, 500 mL); 10 mg/mL (4 mL, 60 mL, 120 mL)
  Tablet, oral: 20 mg, 40 mg, 80 mg
    Lasix®: 20 mg, 40 mg, 80 mg

Furosemide Injection, USP (Can) *see furosemide on page 404*

Furosemide Special (Can) *see furosemide on page 404*

fusidic acid *(Canada only)* (fyoo SI dik AS id)

Synonyms sodium fusidate
Canadian Brand Names Fucidin®; Fucithalmic®
Therapeutic Category Antifungal Agent, Systemic
Use
  Topical: Treatment of primary and secondary skin infections caused by susceptible organisms
  Ophthalmic: Treatment of superficial infections of the eye and conjunctiva caused by susceptible
    organisms
General Dosage Range
  Ophthalmic: *Children ≥2 years and Adults:* Instill 1 drop in each eye every 12 hours
  Topical: *Children and Adults:* Apply to affected area 3-4 times/day or 1-2 times/day if gauze dressing
    used
Product Availability Not available in U.S.
Dosage Forms - Canada
  Cream, topical:
    Fucidin®: 2% (15 g, 30 g)
  Ointment, topical:
    Fucidin®: 2% (15 g, 30 g)
  Suspension, ophthalmic:
    Fucithalmic®: 10 mg/g [1%] (0.2 g) [unit-dose, without preservative]; (3 g, 5 g) [multidose, contains
      benzalkonium chloride]

fusidic acid and hydrocortisone *(Canada only)*
(fyoo SI dik AS id & hye droe KOR ti sone)
Synonyms hydrocortisone and fusidic acid
Canadian Brand Names Fucidin H
Therapeutic Category Antibiotic, Topical; Corticosteroid, Topical
Use Treatment of mild- to moderately-severe atopic dermatitis caused by susceptible organisms
General Dosage Range Topical: *Children ≥3 years and Adults:* Apply 3 times/day
Product Availability Not available in U.S.
Dosage Forms - Canada
  Cream, topical:
    Fusidin H: Fusidic acid 2% and hydrocortisone 1% (5 g, 15 g, 30 g)

Fusilev™ *see LEVOleucovorin on page 521*

Fuzeon® *see enfuvirtide on page 328*

FVIII/vWF *see antihemophilic factor/von Willebrand factor complex (human) on page 82*

FXIII *see factor XIII concentrate (human) on page 366*

FXT 40 (Can) *see fluoxetine on page 389*

GAA *see alglucosidase alfa on page 51*

gabapentin (GA ba pen tin)

Medication Safety Issues
  Sound-alike/look-alike issues:
    Neurontin® may be confused with Motrin®, Neoral®, nitrofurantoin, Noroxin®, Zarontin®
U.S. Brand Names Neurontin®

▶

Canadian Brand Names Apo-Gabapentin®; CO Gabapentin; Dom-Gabapentin; Mylan-Gabapentin; Neurontin®; PHL-Gabapentin; PMS-Gabapentin; PRO-Gabapentin; RAN™-Gabapentin; ratio-Gabapentin; Riva-Gabapentin; Teva-Gabapentin

Therapeutic Category Anticonvulsant

Use Adjunct for treatment of partial seizures with and without secondary generalized seizures in patients >12 years of age with epilepsy; adjunct for treatment of partial seizures in pediatric patients 3-12 years of age; management of postherpetic neuralgia (PHN) in adults

General Dosage Range Dosage adjustment recommended in patients with renal impairment
Oral:
Children 3-4 years: Initial: 10-15 mg/kg/day in 3 divided doses; Maintenance: 40 mg/kg/day in 3 divided doses (maximum: 50 mg/kg/day)
Children 5-12 years: Initial: 10-15 mg/kg/day in 3 divided doses; Maintenance: 25-35 mg/kg/day in 3 divided doses (maximum: 50 mg/kg/day)
Children >12 years: Initial: 300 mg 3 times/day; Maintenance: 900-1800 mg/day in 3 divided doses (maximum: 3600 mg/day [short-term])
Adults: Initial: 300 mg 1-3 times/day; Maintenance: 900-3600 mg/day in 3 divided doses (maximum: 3600 mg/day [short-term])

Product Availability
Gralise™: FDA approved January 2011; availability expected in late 2011
Gralise™ is a once-daily formulation of gabapentin approved for the treatment of postherpetic neuralgia.

Dosage Forms
Capsule, oral: 100 mg, 300 mg, 400 mg
Neurontin®: 100 mg, 300 mg, 400 mg
Solution, oral: 250 mg/5 mL (470 mL)
Neurontin®: 250 mg/5 mL (470 mL)
Tablet, oral: 600 mg, 800 mg
Neurontin®: 600 mg, 800 mg

gabapentin enacarbil (gab a PEN tin en a KAR bil)

Synonyms GSK 1838262; Solzira; XP13512
U.S. Brand Names Horizant™
Therapeutic Category Anticonvulsant, Miscellaneous
Use Treatment of moderate-to-severe restless leg syndrome (RLS)
General Dosage Range Dosage adjustment recommended in patients with renal impairment.
Oral: *Adults:* 600 mg once daily
Dosage Forms
Tablet, extended release, oral:
Horizant™: 600 mg

Gabitril® *see* tiagabine *on page 866*
Gablofen® *see* baclofen *on page 112*

gadobenate dimeglumine (gad oh BEN ate dye MEG loo meen)

Medication Safety Issues
High alert medication:
The Institute for Safe Medication Practices (ISMP) includes this medication among its list of drugs which have a heightened risk of causing significant patient harm when used in error.
Synonyms gadolinum-BOPTA; Gd-BOPTA
U.S. Brand Names Multihance®; Multihance® Multipack™
Therapeutic Category Diagnostic Agent; Radiological/Contrast Media, Nonionic
Use Contrast medium for magnetic resonance imaging (MRI) to visualize CNS lesions with abnormal vascularity in the brain, spine, and associated tissues
General Dosage Range I.V.: *Children ≥3 years and Adults:* 0.1 mmol/kg (0.2 mL/kg)
Dosage Forms
Injection, solution [preservative free]:
Multihance®: 529 mg/mL (5 mL, 10 mL, 15 mL, 20 mL)
Multihance® Multipack™: 529 mg/mL (50 mL, 100 mL)

gadobutrol *(Canada only)* (gad oh BYOO trol)

Medication Safety Issues
Sound-alike/look-alike issues:
Gadovist® may be confused with Magnevist®, Vasovist™
High alert medication:
The Institute for Safe Medication Practices (ISMP) includes this medication among its list of drug classes which have a heightened risk of causing significant patient harm when used in error.

Synonyms gadovist 1.0

Canadian Brand Names Gadovist®

Therapeutic Category Gadolinium-Containing Contrast Agent; Radiological/Contrast Media, Nonionic

Use Contrast medium for magnetic resonance imaging (MRI) of CNS lesions (brain, spine, and associated tissues); perfusion studies to diagnose stroke, or to detect focal cerebral ischemia or tumor perfusion; contrast-enhanced magnetic resonance angiography (CE-MRA)

General Dosage Range Dosage adjustment recommended in patients with renal impairment
I.V.: *Adults:* 0.1-0.3 mL/kg **or** 7.5-20 mL

Product Availability
Gadavist™: FDA approved March 2011; expected availability undetermined
Gadavist™ is a gadolinium-based contrast agent approved for use in diagnostic magnetic resonance imaging (MRI) for the enhancement and detection of disruptions in the blood brain barrier and/or CNS vasculature abnormalities in patients >2 years or age.

Dosage Forms - Canada
Injection, solution [preservative free]:
Gadovist®: 604.72 mg/mL (15 mL)

gadodiamide (gad oh DYE a mide)

Medication Safety Issues
High alert medication:
The Institute for Safe Medication Practices (ISMP) includes this medication among its list of drugs which have a heightened risk of causing significant patient harm when used in error.

Synonyms gadolinium-DTPA-BMA; Gd-DTPA-BMA

U.S. Brand Names Omniscan®

Therapeutic Category Radiological/Contrast Media, Nonionic

Use Contrast medium for magnetic resonance imaging (MRI) to visualize CNS lesions with abnormal vascularity in the brain, spine, and associated tissues, and to visualize body lesions with abnormal vascularity within the thoracic (noncardiac), abdominal, pelvic cavities, and retroperitoneal space

General Dosage Range I.V.:
Children ≥2 years: 0.05-0.1 mmol/kg (0.1-0.2 mL/kg)
Adults: 0.05-0.1 mmol/kg (0.1-0.2 mL/kg); may repeat 0.2 mmol/kg (0.4 mL/kg) once if needed [CNS imaging]

Dosage Forms
Injection, solution [preservative free]:
Omniscan®: 287 mg/mL (5 mL, 10 mL, 15 mL, 20 mL, 50 mL)

gadofosveset (gad oh FOS ve set)

Medication Safety Issues
Sound-alike/look-alike issues:
Vasovist® may be confused with Magnevist®, Gadovist®
High alert medication:
The Institute for Safe Medication Practices (ISMP) includes this medication among its list of drug classes which have a heightened risk of causing significant patient harm when used in error.

Synonyms gadofosveset trisodium

U.S. Brand Names Ablavar®

Therapeutic Category Gadolinium-Containing Contrast Agent; Radiological/Contrast Media, Paramagnetic Agent

Use Contrast medium used in magnetic resonance angiography (MRA) to evaluate or better define aortoiliac occlusive disease

General Dosage Range I.V.: *Adults:* 0.03 mmol/kg (0.12 mL/kg)

◀ **Dosage Forms**
  Injection, solution [preservative free]:
    Ablavar®: 0.25 mmol/mL (10 mL, 15 mL)
Dosage Forms - Canada
  Injection, solution [preservative free]:
    Vasovist®: 0.25 mmoL/mL (10 mL, 15 mL, 20 mL)

gadofosveset trisodium *see gadofosveset on page 407*
gadolinium-DTPA *see gadopentetate dimeglumine on page 408*
gadolinium-DTPA-BMA *see gadodiamide on page 407*
gadolinium-DTPA-BMEA *see gadoversetamide on page 408*
gadolinium-HP-DO3A *see gadoteridol on page 408*
gadolinum-BOPTA *see gadobenate dimeglumine on page 406*

gadopentetate dimeglumine (gad oh PEN te tate dye MEG loo meen)

Medication Safety Issues
  High alert medication:
    The Institute for Safe Medication Practices (ISMP) includes this medication among its list of drugs which have a heightened risk of causing significant patient harm when used in error.
Synonyms gadolinium-DTPA; Gd-DTPA
U.S. Brand Names Magnevist®
Canadian Brand Names Magnevist®
Therapeutic Category Radiological/Contrast Media, Paramagnetic Agent
Use Contrast medium for magnetic resonance imaging (MRI) to visualize CNS lesions with abnormal vascularity in the brain, spine and associated tissues, extracranial/extraspinal lesions with abnormal vascularity in the head and neck, and body lesions with abnormal vascularity (excluding the heart)
General Dosage Range I.V.: *Children ≥2 years and Adults:* 0.1 mmol/kg (0.2 mL/kg)
Dosage Forms
  Injection, solution [preservative free]:
    Magnevist®: 469.01 mg/mL (5 mL, 10 mL, 15 mL, 20 mL, 50 mL, 100 mL)

gadoteridol (gad oh TER i dol)

Medication Safety Issues
  High alert medication:
    The Institute for Safe Medication Practices (ISMP) includes this medication among its list of drugs which have a heightened risk of causing significant patient harm when used in error.
Synonyms gadolinium-HP-DO3A; Gd-HP-DO3A
U.S. Brand Names ProHance®; ProHance® Multipack™
Therapeutic Category Radiological/Contrast Media, Nonionic
Use Contrast medium for magnetic resonance imaging (MRI) to visualize CNS lesions with abnormal vascularity in the brain, spine, and associated tissues and to visualize extracranial/extraspinal tissues in the head and neck
General Dosage Range I.V.:
  Children ≥2 years: 0.1 mmol/kg (0.2 mL/kg)
  Adults: 0.1 mmol/kg (0.2 mL/kg); may repeat 0.2 mmol/kg (0.4 mL/kg) once if needed [CNS imaging]
Dosage Forms
  Injection, solution [preservative free]:
    ProHance®: 279.3 mg/mL (5 mL, 10 mL, 15 mL, 17 mL, 20 mL)
    ProHance® Multipack™: 279.3 mg/mL (50 mL)

gadoversetamide (gad oh ver SET a mide)

Medication Safety Issues
  High alert medication:
    The Institute for Safe Medication Practices (ISMP) includes this medication among its list of drugs which have a heightened risk of causing significant patient harm when used in error.
Synonyms gadolinium-DTPA-BMEA; Gd-DTPA-BMEA
U.S. Brand Names OptiMARK®
Therapeutic Category Radiological/Contrast Media, Nonionic

Use Contrast medium for magnetic resonance imaging (MRI) to visualize CNS lesions with abnormal vascularity in the brain, spine, and associated tissues and to visualize liver lesions with abnormal vascularity in patients highly suspect for liver structural abnormalities

General Dosage Range I.V.: *Adults:* 0.1 mmol/kg (0.2 mL/kg)

Dosage Forms
Injection, solution [preservative free]:
OptiMARK®: 330.9 mg/mL (5 mL, 10 mL, 15 mL, 20 mL, 30 mL, 50 mL)

Gadovist® (Can) *see gadobutrol (Canada only) on page 407*

gadovist 1.0 *see gadobutrol (Canada only) on page 407*

gadoxetate (gad OX e tate)

Medication Safety Issues
Sound-alike/look-alike issues:
Eovist® may be confused with Evista®
High alert medication:
The Institute for Safe Medication Practices (ISMP) includes this medication among its list of drugs which have a heightened risk of causing significant patient harm when used in error.

Synonyms gadoxetate disodium; Gd-EOB-DTPA

U.S. Brand Names Eovist®

Canadian Brand Names Primovist

Therapeutic Category Gadolinium-Containing Contrast Agent; Radiological/Contrast Media, Ionic (Low Osmolality); Radiological/Contrast Media, Paramagnetic Agent

Use Contrast medium for magnetic resonance imaging (MRI) to detect and characterize lesions within focal liver disease

General Dosage Range I.V.: *Adults:* 0.025 mmol/kg (0.1 mL/kg)

Dosage Forms
Injection, solution [preservative free]:
Eovist®: 181.43 mg/mL (10 mL)

gadoxetate disodium *see gadoxetate on page 409*

galantamine (ga LAN ta meen)

Medication Safety Issues
Sound-alike/look-alike issues:
Razadyne® may be confused with Rozerem™
Reminyl® may be confused with Amaryl®, Robinul®
Due to patient safety concerns regarding prescribing and dispensing errors between Reminyl® and Amaryl®, Reminyl® (galantamine) is being renamed to Razadyne® (immediate-release) and Razadyne® ER (extended-release). The brand name Reminyl® was discontinued with the July, 2005 distribution of Razadyne®.
International issues:
Reminyl [multiple international markets] may be confused with Amarel [France] and Amaryl [U.S., Canada, and multiple international markets], brand names for glimepiride

Synonyms galantamine hydrobromide

U.S. Brand Names Razadyne®; Razadyne® ER

Canadian Brand Names Mylan-Galantamine ER; PAT-Galantamine ER; Reminyl®; Reminyl® ER

Therapeutic Category Acetylcholinesterase Inhibitor (Central)

Use Treatment of mild-to-moderate dementia of Alzheimer disease

General Dosage Range Dosage adjustment recommended in patients with hepatic or renal impairment
Oral:
Extended-release: *Adults:* Initial: 8 mg once daily; Maintenance: 16-24 mg once daily
Immediate release: *Adults:* Initial: 4 mg twice daily; Maintenance: 16-24 mg/day in 2 divided doses

Dosage Forms
Capsule, extended release, oral: 8 mg, 16 mg, 24 mg
Razadyne® ER: 8 mg, 16 mg, 24 mg
Solution, oral: 4 mg/mL (100 mL)
Razadyne®: 4 mg/mL (100 mL)
Tablet, oral: 4 mg, 8 mg, 12 mg
Razadyne®: 4 mg, 8 mg, 12 mg

galantamine hydrobromide *see galantamine on page 409*

galsulfase (gal SUL fase)

Synonyms recombinant N-acetylgalactosamine 4-sulfatase; rhASB

U.S. Brand Names Naglazyme®

Therapeutic Category Enzyme

Use Replacement therapy in mucopolysaccharidosis VI (MPS VI; Maroteaux-Lamy Syndrome) for improvement of walking and stair-climbing capacity

General Dosage Range I.V.: *Children >5 years and Adults:* 1 mg/kg once weekly

Dosage Forms

Injection, solution [preservative free]:
Naglazyme®: 5 mg/5 mL (5 mL)

Galzin® *see zinc acetate on page 930*

GamaSTAN™ S/D *see immune globulin on page 468*

Gamimune® N (Can) *see immune globulin on page 468*

gamma benzene hexachloride *see lindane on page 528*

Gamma E-Gems® [OTC] *see vitamin E on page 918*

Gamma-E PLUS [OTC] *see vitamin E on page 918*

Gammagard® Liquid *see immune globulin on page 468*

Gammagard Liquid (Can) *see immune globulin on page 468*

Gammagard S/D® *see immune globulin on page 468*

Gammagard S/D (Can) *see immune globulin on page 468*

gamma globulin *see immune globulin on page 468*

gamma hydroxybutyric acid *see sodium oxybate on page 822*

gammaphos *see amifostine on page 63*

Gammaplex® *see immune globulin on page 468*

Gamunex® [DSC] *see immune globulin on page 468*

Gamunex® (Can) *see immune globulin on page 468*

Gamunex®-C *see immune globulin on page 468*

ganciclovir (systemic) (gan SYE kloe veer)

Medication Safety Issues

Sound-alike/look-alike issues:
Cytovene® may be confused with Cytosar®, Cytosar-U®
Ganciclovir may be confused with acyclovir

Synonyms DHPG sodium; GCV sodium; nordeoxyguanosine

U.S. Brand Names Cytovene®-IV

Canadian Brand Names Cytovene®

Therapeutic Category Antiviral Agent

Use Treatment of CMV retinitis in immunocompromised individuals, including patients with acquired immunodeficiency syndrome; prophylaxis of CMV infection in transplant patients

General Dosage Range Dosage adjustment recommended in patients with renal impairment

I.V.: *Children and Adults:* Induction: 5 mg/kg every 12 hours; Maintenance: 30-35 mg/kg/week, given as once-daily dose for 5-7 days per week

Dosage Forms

Injection, powder for reconstitution: 500 mg
Cytovene®-IV: 500 mg

ganciclovir (ophthalmic) (gan SYE kloe veer)

Medication Safety Issues

Sound-alike/look-alike issues:
Ganciclovir may be confused with acyclovir

Synonyms nordeoxyguanosine

U.S. Brand Names Vitrasert®; Zirgan®

Canadian Brand Names Vitrasert®

Therapeutic Category Antiviral Agent

Use
Intravitreal implant: Treatment of CMV retinitis in patients with acquired immunodeficiency syndrome
Ophthalmic gel: Treatment of acute herpetic keratitis (dendritic ulcers)

General Dosage Range
Ocular implant: *Children ≥9 years and Adults:* 1 implant for 5-8 month period
Ophthalmic gel: *Children ≥2 months and Adults:* 1 drop in affected eye 3-5 times/day

Dosage Forms
Gel, ophthalmic:
Zirgan®: 0.15% (5 g)
Implant, intravitreal:
Vitrasert®: 4.5 mg (1s)

Ganidin® NR [OTC] [DSC] *see* guaifenesin *on page* 425

ganirelix (ga ni REL ix)

Medication Safety Issues
International issues:
Antagon® (former U.S. brand name for ganirelix): Brand name for astemizole in Mexico; brand name for ranitidine in Brazil

Synonyms antagon; ganirelix acetate

Canadian Brand Names Orgalutran®

Therapeutic Category Antigonadotropic Agent

Use Inhibits premature luteinizing hormone (LH) surges in women undergoing controlled ovarian hyperstimulation

General Dosage Range SubQ: *Adults:* 250 mcg/day

Dosage Forms
Injection, solution: 250 mcg/0.5 mL (0.5 mL)

ganirelix acetate *see* ganirelix *on page* 411

Gani-Tuss DM NR [DSC] *see* guaifenesin and dextromethorphan *on page* 427

Gani-Tuss® NR *see* guaifenesin and codeine *on page* 426

GAR-936 *see* tigecycline *on page* 868

Garamycin® *see* gentamicin (ophthalmic) *on page* 416

Garasone (Can) *see* gentamicin (ophthalmic) *on page* 416

Gardasil® *see* papillomavirus (types 6, 11, 16, 18) vaccine (human, recombinant) *on page* 674

Gas-X® [OTC] *see* simethicone *on page* 812

Gas-X® Children's Tongue Twisters™ [OTC] *see* simethicone *on page* 812

Gas-X® Extra Strength [OTC] *see* simethicone *on page* 812

Gas-X® Maximum Strength [OTC] *see* simethicone *on page* 812

Gas-X® Thin Strips™ [OTC] *see* simethicone *on page* 812

Gas Ban™ [OTC] *see* calcium carbonate and simethicone *on page* 162

Gas Free Extra Strength [OTC] *see* simethicone *on page* 812

Gas Relief Ultra Strength [OTC] *see* simethicone *on page* 812

Gastrocrom® *see* cromolyn (systemic, oral inhalation) *on page* 238

Gastrografin® *see* diatrizoate meglumine and diatrizoate sodium *on page* 275

Gastroview *see* diatrizoate meglumine and diatrizoate sodium *on page* 275

gatifloxacin (gat i FLOKS a sin)

U.S. Brand Names Zymar® [DSC]; Zymaxid™

Canadian Brand Names Zymar®

Therapeutic Category Antibiotic, Quinolone

Use Treatment of bacterial conjunctivitis

General Dosage Range Ophthalmic: *Children ≥1 year and Adults:* 1 drop into affected eye(s) every 2 hours while awake (maximum: 8 times/day) for 1-2 days; followed by 1 drop into affected eye(s) 2-4 times/day

Dosage Forms
Solution, ophthalmic:
Zymaxid™: 0.5% (2.5 mL)

GaviLyte™-C *see* polyethylene glycol-electrolyte solution *on page 718*

GaviLyte™-G *see* polyethylene glycol-electrolyte solution *on page 718*

GaviLyte™-N *see* polyethylene glycol-electrolyte solution *on page 718*

Gaviscon® Extra Strength [OTC] *see* aluminum hydroxide and magnesium carbonate *on page 59*

Gaviscon® Liquid [OTC] *see* aluminum hydroxide and magnesium carbonate *on page 59*

Gaviscon® Tablet [OTC] *see* aluminum hydroxide and magnesium trisilicate *on page 60*

Gax-X® Infant [OTC] *see* simethicone *on page 812*

G-CSF *see* filgrastim *on page 377*

G-CSF (PEG conjugate) *see* pegfilgrastim *on page 679*

GCV sodium *see* ganciclovir (systemic) *on page 410*

GD-Amlodipine (Can) *see* amlodipine *on page 69*

GD-Atorvastatin (Can) *see* atorvastatin *on page 102*

Gd-BOPTA *see* gadobenate dimeglumine *on page 406*

Gd-DTPA *see* gadopentetate dimeglumine *on page 408*

Gd-DTPA-BMA *see* gadodiamide *on page 407*

Gd-DTPA-BMEA *see* gadoversetamide *on page 408*

Gd-EOB-DTPA *see* gadoxetate *on page 409*

Gd-HP-DO3A *see* gadoteridol *on page 408*

GD-Sertraline (Can) *see* sertraline *on page 809*

Gebauer's Ethyl Chloride® *see* ethyl chloride *on page 359*

gefitinib (ge FI tye nib)

Medication Safety Issues

Sound-alike/look-alike issues:

Gefitinib may be confused with crizotinib, erlotinib, imatinib, SORAfenib, SUNItinib, vandetanib

High alert medication:

This medication is in a class the Institute for Safe Medication Practices (ISMP) includes among its list of drug classes which have a heightened risk of causing significant patient harm when used in error.

Synonyms ZD1839

U.S. Brand Names Iressa®

Canadian Brand Names IRESSA®

Therapeutic Category Antineoplastic Agent, Tyrosine Kinase Inhibitor

Use Treatment of locally advanced or metastatic nonsmall cell lung cancer (NSCLC) after failure of platinum-based and docetaxel therapies. Treatment is limited to patients who are benefiting or have benefited from treatment with gefitinib.

Note: Due to the lack of improved survival data from clinical trials of gefitinib, and in response to positive survival data with another EGFR inhibitor, according to the U.S. labeling, physicians are advised to use treatment options other than gefitinib in patients with advanced nonsmall cell lung cancer following one or two prior chemotherapy regimens when they are refractory/intolerant to their most recent regimen.

Canada labeling: First-line treatment of locally advanced or metastatic NSCLC with activating mutations of EGFR-TK

General Dosage Range Dosage adjustment recommended in patients on concomitant therapy or who develop toxicities.

Oral: *Adults:* 250 mg once daily

Dosage Forms

Tablet, oral:

Iressa®: 250 mg

gelatin (absorbable) (JEL a tin, ab SORB a ble)

Synonyms absorbable gelatin sponge

U.S. Brand Names Gelfilm®; Gelfoam®

Therapeutic Category Hemostatic Agent

Use Adjunct to provide hemostasis in surgery; open prostatic surgery

General Dosage Range Topical: *Children and Adults:* Apply packs or sponges dry or saturated with sodium chloride

Dosage Forms
  Film, ophthalmic:
    Gelfilm®: (6s)
  Film, topical:
    Gelfilm®: (1s)
  Powder, topical:
    Gelfoam®: (1 g)
  Sponge, oral topical:
    Gelfoam®: (12s)
  Sponge, topical:
    Gelfoam®: (4s, 6s, 12s)

gelatin, pectin, and methylcellulose (JEL a tin, PEK tin, & meth il SEL yoo lose)
  Synonyms methylcellulose, gelatin, and pectin; pectin, gelatin, and methylcellulose
  Therapeutic Category Protectant, Topical
  Use Temporary relief from minor oral irritations
  General Dosage Range Topical: *Children and Adults:* Press small dabs into place until the involved area is coated with a thin film as needed

Gelclair® *see* mucosal barrier gel, oral *on page 602*
Gelfilm® *see* gelatin (absorbable) *on page 412*
Gelfoam® *see* gelatin (absorbable) *on page 412*
Gel-Kam® [OTC] *see* fluoride *on page 386*
Gel-Kam® Rinse *see* fluoride *on page 386*
Gelnique® *see* oxybutynin *on page 661*
GelRite™ [OTC] *see* alcohol (ethyl) *on page 47*
Gel-Stat™ [OTC] *see* alcohol (ethyl) *on page 47*
Gelucast® *see* zinc gelatin *on page 930*
Gelusil® [OTC] *see* aluminum hydroxide, magnesium hydroxide, and simethicone *on page 60*
Gelusil® (Can) *see* aluminum hydroxide, magnesium hydroxide, and simethicone *on page 60*
Gelusil® Extra Strength (Can) *see* aluminum hydroxide and magnesium hydroxide *on page 60*

gemcitabine (jem SITE a been)
  Medication Safety Issues
    Sound-alike/look-alike issues:
      Gemcitabine may be confused with gemtuzumab
      Gemzar® may be confused with Zinecard®
    High alert medication:
      This medication is in a class the Institute for Safe Medication Practices (ISMP) includes among its list of drug classes which have a heightened risk of causing significant patient harm when used in error.
  Synonyms dFdC; dFdCyd; difluorodeoxycytidine hydrochlorothiazide; gemcitabine hydrochloride; LY-188011
  U.S. Brand Names Gemzar®
  Canadian Brand Names Gemcitabine For Injection, USP; Gemzar®
  Therapeutic Category Antineoplastic Agent
  Use Treatment of metastatic breast cancer; inoperable locally-advanced or metastatic nonsmall cell lung cancer (NSCLC); locally advanced or metastatic pancreatic cancer; advanced, relapsed ovarian cancer
  General Dosage Range Dosage adjustment recommended in patients with hepatic impairment or who develop toxicities
    I.V.: *Adults:* Dosage varies greatly depending on indication
  Dosage Forms
    Injection, powder for reconstitution: 200 mg, 1 g, 2 g
      Gemzar®: 200 mg, 1 g

Gemcitabine For Injection, USP (Can) *see* gemcitabine *on page 413*
gemcitabine hydrochloride *see* gemcitabine *on page 413*

gemfibrozil (jem FI broe zil)

Medication Safety Issues
Sound-alike/look-alike issues:
Lopid® may be confused with Levbid®, Lipitor®, Lodine®, Lorabid®, Slo-bid™

Synonyms CI-719

U.S. Brand Names Lopid®

Canadian Brand Names Apo-Gemfibrozil®; Gen-Gemfibrozil; GMD-Gemfibrozil; Lopid®; Mylan-Gemfibrozil; Novo-Gemfibrozil; Nu-Gemfibrozil; PMS-Gemfibrozil

Therapeutic Category Antihyperlipidemic Agent, Miscellaneous

Use Treatment of hypertriglyceridemia in Fredrickson types IV and V hyperlipidemia for patients who are at greater risk for pancreatitis and who have not responded to dietary intervention; to reduce the risk of CHD development in Fredrickson type IIb patients without a history or symptoms of existing CHD who have not responded to dietary and other interventions (including pharmacologic treatment) and who have decreased HDL, increased LDL, and increased triglycerides

General Dosage Range Oral: *Adults:* 600 mg twice daily

Dosage Forms
Tablet, oral: 600 mg
Lopid®: 600 mg

gemifloxacin (je mi FLOKS a sin)

Synonyms DW286; gemifloxacin mesylate; LA 20304a; SB-265805

U.S. Brand Names Factive®

Canadian Brand Names Factive®

Therapeutic Category Antibiotic, Quinolone

Use Treatment of acute exacerbation of chronic bronchitis; treatment of community-acquired pneumonia (CAP), including pneumonia caused by multidrug-resistant strains of *S. pneumoniae* (MDRSP)

General Dosage Range Dosage adjustment recommended in patients with renal impairment
Oral: *Adults:* 320 mg once daily

Dosage Forms
Tablet, oral:
Factive®: 320 mg

gemifloxacin mesylate *see* gemifloxacin *on page 414*

gemtuzumab ozogamicin (gem TOO zoo mab oh zog a MY sin)

Medication Safety Issues
Sound-alike/look-alike issues:
Gemtuzumab may be confused with gemcitabine
High alert medication:
This medication is in a class the Institute for Safe Medication Practices (ISMP) includes among its list of drug classes which have a heightened risk of causing significant patient harm when used in error.

Synonyms CMA-676; Mylotarg

Therapeutic Category Antineoplastic Agent, Natural Source (Plant) Derivative

Use Due to safety concerns, as well as lack of clinical benefit demonstrated in a post-approval clinical trial, gemtuzumab was withdrawn from the U.S. commercial market in 2010.

Product Availability No longer commercially available in the U.S. market for new patients. Available in Canada through a special access program.

Gemzar® *see* gemcitabine *on page 413*
Genac™ [OTC] [DSC] *see* triprolidine and pseudoephedrine *on page 893*
Gen-Acyclovir (Can) *see* acyclovir (systemic) *on page 39*
Gen-Amilazide (Can) *see* amiloride and hydrochlorothiazide *on page 64*
Gen-Amoxicillin (Can) *see* amoxicillin *on page 73*
Genaphed™ [OTC] [DSC] *see* pseudoephedrine *on page 751*
Genaton™ [OTC] *see* aluminum hydroxide and magnesium carbonate *on page 59*
Gen-Beclo (Can) *see* beclomethasone (nasal) *on page 117*
Gen-Budesonide AQ (Can) *see* budesonide (nasal) *on page 146*
Gen-Buspirone (Can) *see* buspirone *on page 151*

Gen-Clindamycin (Can) *see* clindamycin (systemic) *on page 217*
Gen-Clobetasol (Can) *see* clobetasol *on page 220*
Gen-Clomipramine (Can) *see* clomipramine *on page 222*
Gen-Clonazepam (Can) *see* clonazepam *on page 222*
Gen-Clozapine (Can) *see* clozapine *on page 227*
Gen-Combo Sterinebs (Can) *see* ipratropium and albuterol *on page 489*
Gen-Cyclobenzaprine (Can) *see* cyclobenzaprine *on page 241*
Gen-Doxazosin (Can) *see* doxazosin *on page 308*
gene-activated human acid-beta-glucosidase *see* velaglucerase alfa *on page 910*
Generess™ Fe *see* ethinyl estradiol and norethindrone *on page 355*
Generlac *see* lactulose *on page 507*
Genfiber™ [OTC] [DSC] *see* psyllium *on page 755*
Gen-Fluoxetine (Can) *see* fluoxetine *on page 389*
Gen-Gemfibrozil (Can) *see* gemfibrozil *on page 414*
Gengraf® *see* cyclosporine (systemic) *on page 243*
Gen-Hydroxychloroquine (Can) *see* hydroxychloroquine *on page 454*
Gen-Hydroxyurea (Can) *see* hydroxyurea *on page 456*
Gen-Ipratropium (Can) *see* ipratropium (oral inhalation) *on page 489*
Gen-Lovastatin (Can) *see* lovastatin *on page 540*
Gen-Medroxy (Can) *see* medroxyprogesterone *on page 554*
Gen-Nabumetone (Can) *see* nabumetone *on page 607*
Gen-Nizatidine (Can) *see* nizatidine *on page 631*
Gen-Nortriptyline (Can) *see* nortriptyline *on page 634*
Genotropin® *see* somatropin *on page 826*
Genotropin Miniquick® *see* somatropin *on page 826*
Gen-Piroxicam (Can) *see* piroxicam *on page 708*
Gen-Selegiline (Can) *see* selegiline *on page 806*
Gen-Sumatriptan (Can) *see* sumatriptan *on page 839*
Gentak® *see* gentamicin (ophthalmic) *on page 416*

gentamicin (systemic) (jen ta MYE sin)

Medication Safety Issues
Sound-alike/look-alike issues:
Gentamicin may be confused with gentian violet, kanamycin, vancomycin
High alert medication:
The Institute for Safe Medication Practices (ISMP) includes this medication (intrathecal administration) among its list of drug classes which have a heightened risk of causing significant patient harm when used in error.

Synonyms gentamicin sulfate

Canadian Brand Names Gentamicin Injection, USP

Therapeutic Category Antibiotic, Aminoglycoside

Use Treatment of susceptible bacterial infections, normally gram-negative organisms, including *Pseudomonas, Proteus, Serratia,* and gram-positive *Staphylococcus*; treatment of bone infections, respiratory tract infections, skin and soft tissue infections, as well as abdominal and urinary tract infections, and septicemia; treatment of infective endocarditis

General Dosage Range Dosage adjustment recommended for the I.M. and I.V. routes in patients with renal impairment
I.M., I.V.:
Children <5 years: 2.5 mg/kg/dose every 8 hours
Children ≥5 years: 2-2.5 mg/kg/dose every 8 hours
Adults: 1-2.5 mg/kg/dose every 8-12 hours **or** 4-7 mg/kg once daily
Intrathecal: *Adults:* 4-8 mg/day

Dosage Forms
Infusion, premixed in NS: 60 mg (50 mL, 100 mL); 80 mg (50 mL, 100 mL); 100 mg (50 mL, 100 mL); 120 mg (50 mL, 100 mL)
Injection, solution: 40 mg/mL (2 mL, 20 mL, 50 mL)
Injection, solution [preservative free]: 10 mg/mL (2 mL)

gentamicin (ophthalmic) (jen ta MYE sin)

Medication Safety Issues
Sound-alike/look-alike issues:
Gentamicin may be confused with gentian violet, kanamycin, vancomycin
Synonyms gentamicin sulfate
U.S. Brand Names Garamycin®; Gentak®
Canadian Brand Names Diogent®; Garamycin®; Garasone; Gentak®; Gentocin; PMS-Gentamicin
Therapeutic Category Antibiotic, Aminoglycoside; Antibiotic, Ophthalmic
Use Treatment of ophthalmic infections caused by susceptible bacteria
General Dosage Range Ophthalmic: *Children and Adults:* Ointment: Instill 1/2" (1.25 cm) 2-3 times/day to every 3-4 hours; Solution: Instill 1-2 drops every 4 hours, up to 2 drops every hour for severe infections
Dosage Forms
Ointment, ophthalmic:
Gentak®: 0.3% (3.5 g)
Ointment, ophthalmic [preservative free]:
Garamycin®: 0.3% (3.5 g)
Solution, ophthalmic: 0.3% (5 mL, 15 mL)
Garamycin®: 0.3% (5 mL)
Gentak®: 0.3% (5 mL)

gentamicin (topical) (jen ta MYE sin)

Medication Safety Issues
Sound-alike/look-alike issues:
Gentamicin may be confused with gentian violet, kanamycin, vancomycin
Canadian Brand Names PMS-Gentamicin; ratio-Gentamicin
Therapeutic Category Antibiotic, Aminoglycoside; Antibiotic, Topical
Use Used topically to treat superficial infections of the skin
General Dosage Range Topical: *Children and Adults:* Apply 3-4 times/day to affected area
Dosage Forms
Cream, topical: 0.1% (15 g, 30 g)
Ointment, topical: 0.1% (15 g, 30 g)

Geritol Extend® [OTC] *see* vitamins (multiple/oral) *on page 919*
Geritol® Tonic [OTC] *see* vitamins (multiple/oral) *on page 919*
Geri-Tussin [OTC] *see* guaifenesin *on page 425*
Gesticare® *see* vitamins (multiple/prenatal) *on page 920*
Gesticare® DHA *see* vitamins (multiple/prenatal) *on page 920*
Gets-It® [OTC] *see* salicylic acid *on page 795*
GF196960 *see* tadalafil *on page 842*
GG *see* guaifenesin *on page 425*
GHB *see* sodium oxybate *on page 822*
GI87084B *see* remifentanil *on page 773*
Gianvi™ *see* ethinyl estradiol and drospirenone *on page 352*
Gilenya™ *see* fingolimod *on page 378*
Gilenya® (Can) *see* fingolimod *on page 378*
Giltuss® [DSC] *see* guaifenesin, dextromethorphan, and phenylephrine *on page 429*
Giltuss Pediatric® [DSC] *see* guaifenesin, dextromethorphan, and phenylephrine *on page 429*
Giltuss TR® [DSC] *see* guaifenesin, dextromethorphan, and phenylephrine *on page 429*
glargine insulin *see* insulin glargine *on page 476*
Glassia™ *see* alpha$_1$-proteinase inhibitor *on page 55*

glatiramer acetate (gla TIR a mer AS e tate)

Medication Safety Issues
Sound-alike/look-alike issues:
Copaxone® may be confused with Compazine®
Synonyms copolymer-1
U.S. Brand Names Copaxone®
Canadian Brand Names Copaxone®
Therapeutic Category Biological, Miscellaneous
Use Management of relapsing-remitting type multiple sclerosis, including patients with a first clinical episode with MRI features consistent with multiple sclerosis
General Dosage Range SubQ: *Adults:* 20 mg daily
Dosage Forms
Injection, solution [preservative free]:
Copaxone®: 20 mg/mL (1 mL)

glcCerase *see* velaglucerase alfa *on page 910*
Gleevec® *see* imatinib *on page 465*
Gliadel® *see* carmustine *on page 177*
Gliadel Wafer® (Can) *see* carmustine *on page 177*
glibenclamide *see* glyburide *on page 420*
Gliclazide-80 (Can) *see* gliclazide *(Canada only) on page 417*

gliclazide *(Canada only)* (GLYE kla zide)

Medication Safety Issues
High alert medication:
This medication is in a class the Institute for Safe Medication Practices (ISMP) includes among its list of drugs which have a heightened risk of causing significant patient harm when used in error.
Canadian Brand Names Apo-Gliclazide®; Apo-Gliclazide® MR; Diamicron®; Diamicron® MR; Gliclazide MR; Gliclazide-80; Mylan-Gliclazide; Novo-Gliclazide; PMS-Gliclazide
Therapeutic Category Antidiabetic Agent, Oral; Hypoglycemic Agent, Oral; Sulfonylurea Agent
Use Management of type 2 diabetes mellitus (noninsulin-dependent, NIDDM)
General Dosage Range Oral:
Immediate release: *Adults:* Initial: 80 mg twice daily; Maintenance: 80-320 mg/day (maximum: 320 mg/day)
Modified release: *Adults:* 30-120 mg once daily (maximum: 120 mg/day)
Product Availability Not available in U.S.

▶

◀ **Dosage Forms - Canada**
Tablet, oral:
Diamicron®: 80 mg
Tablet, modified release, oral:
Diamicron® MR: 30 mg, 60 mg

Gliclazide MR (Can) *see gliclazide (Canada only) on page 417*

glimepiride (GLYE me pye ride)

Medication Safety Issues
Sound-alike/look-alike issues:
Glimepiride may be confused with glipiZIDE
Amaryl® may be confused with Altace®, Amerge®, Reminyl®
High alert medication:
The Institute for Safe Medication Practices (ISMP) includes this medication among its list of drugs which
have a heightened risk of causing significant patient harm when used in error.
International issues:
Amarel [France], Amaryl [U.S., Canada, and multiple international markets] may be confused with
Reminyl brand name for galantamine [multiple international markets]
Amaryl [U.S., Canada, and multiple international markets] may be confused with Almarl brand name for
arotinolol [Japan]
U.S. Brand Names Amaryl®

Canadian Brand Names Amaryl®; Apo-Glimepiride®; CO Glimepiride; Novo-Glimepiride; PMS-
Glimepiride; ratio-Glimepiride; Rhoxal-glimepiride; Sandoz-Glimepiride

Therapeutic Category Antidiabetic Agent, Oral

Use Management of type 2 diabetes mellitus (noninsulin-dependent, NIDDM) as an adjunct to diet and
exercise to lower blood glucose; may be used in combination with metformin or insulin in patients whose
hyperglycemia cannot be controlled by diet and exercise in conjunction with a single oral hypoglycemic
agent

General Dosage Range Dosage adjustment recommended in patients with renal impairment
Oral:
Adults: Initial: 1-2 mg once daily; Maintenance: 1-4 mg once daily (maximum: 8 mg/day)
Elderly: Initial: 1 mg/day
Dosage Forms
Tablet, oral: 1 mg, 2 mg, 4 mg
Amaryl®: 1 mg, 2 mg, 4 mg

glimepiride and pioglitazone *see pioglitazone and glimepiride on page 706*
glimepiride and pioglitazone hydrochloride *see pioglitazone and glimepiride on page 706*
glimepiride and rosiglitazone maleate *see rosiglitazone and glimepiride on page 791*

glipizide (GLIP i zide)

Medication Safety Issues
Sound-alike/look-alike issues:
GlipiZIDE may be confused with glimepiride, glyBURIDE
Glucotrol® may be confused with Glucophage®, Glucotrol® XL, glyBURIDE
Glucotrol XL® may be confused with Glucotrol®
High alert medication:
The Institute for Safe Medication Practices (ISMP) includes this medication among its list of drugs which
have a heightened risk of causing significant patient harm when used in error.

Synonyms glydiazinamide

Tall-Man glipiZIDE

U.S. Brand Names Glucotrol XL®; Glucotrol®

Therapeutic Category Antidiabetic Agent, Oral

Use Management of type 2 diabetes mellitus (noninsulin-dependent, NIDDM)

General Dosage Range Dosage adjustment recommended in patients with hepatic impairment
Oral:
Immediate release:
Adults: Initial: 5 mg/day; Maintenance: Up to 40 mg/day
Elderly: Initial: 2.5 mg/day

Extended release: *Adults:* Initial: 5 mg/day; Maintenance: Up to 20 mg/day

Dosage Forms
Tablet, oral: 5 mg, 10 mg
  Glucotrol®: 5 mg, 10 mg
Tablet, extended release, oral: 2.5 mg, 5 mg, 10 mg
  Glucotrol XL®: 2.5 mg, 5 mg, 10 mg

glipizide and metformin (GLIP i zide & met FOR min)

Medication Safety Issues
High alert medication:
  The Institute for Safe Medication Practices (ISMP) includes this medication among its list of drugs which have a heightened risk of causing significant patient harm when used in error.
Synonyms glipizide and metformin hydrochloride; metformin and glipizide
U.S. Brand Names Metaglip™
Therapeutic Category Antidiabetic Agent (Biguanide); Antidiabetic Agent (Sulfonylurea)
Use Indicated as an adjunct to diet and exercise to improve glycemic control in adults with type 2 diabetes mellitus (noninsulin-dependent, NIDDM)
General Dosage Range Oral: *Adults:* Initial: Glipizide 2.5 mg and metformin 250 mg once daily; Maintenance: Up to glipizide 20 mg/day and metformin 2000 mg/day in divided doses
Dosage Forms
Tablet, oral: 2.5/250: Glipizide 2.5 mg and metformin 250 mg; 2.5/500: Glipizide 2.5 mg and metformin 500 mg; 5/500: Glipizide 5 mg and metformin 500 mg
  Metaglip™: 2.5/500: Glipizide 2.5 mg and metformin 500 mg; 5/500: Glipizide 5 mg and metformin 500 mg

glipizide and metformin hydrochloride *see* glipizide and metformin *on page 419*
glivec *see* imatinib *on page 465*
GlucaGen® *see* glucagon *on page 419*
GlucaGen® Diagnostic Kit *see* glucagon *on page 419*
GlucaGen® HypoKit® *see* glucagon *on page 419*

glucagon (GLOO ka gon)

Medication Safety Issues
Sound-alike/look-alike issues:
  Glucagon may be confused with Glaucon®
Synonyms glucagon hydrochloride
U.S. Brand Names GlucaGen®; GlucaGen® Diagnostic Kit; GlucaGen® HypoKit®; Glucagon Emergency Kit
Therapeutic Category Antihypoglycemic Agent
Use Management of hypoglycemia; diagnostic aid in radiologic examinations to temporarily inhibit GI tract movement
General Dosage Range
I.M.:
  Children <20 kg: 0.5 mg **or** 20-30 mcg/kg/dose, may repeat
  Children ≥20 kg: 1 mg, may repeat
  Adults: 1 mg, may repeat **or** 1-2 mg prior to gastrointestinal procedure
I.V.:
  Children <20 kg: 0.5 mg or 20-30 mcg/kg/dose, may repeat
  Children ≥20 kg: 1 mg, may repeat
  Adults: 1 mg, may repeat in 20 minutes **or** 0.25-2 mg 10 minutes prior to gastrointestinal procedure
SubQ:
  Children <20 kg: 0.5 mg **or** 20-30 mcg/kg/dose, may repeat
  Children ≥20 kg and Adults: 1 mg, may repeat
Dosage Forms
Injection, powder for reconstitution:
  GlucaGen®: 1 mg
  GlucaGen® Diagnostic Kit: 1 mg
  GlucaGen® HypoKit®: 1 mg
  Glucagon Emergency Kit: 1 mg

Glucagon Emergency Kit *see* glucagon *on page 419*
glucagon hydrochloride *see* glucagon *on page 419*
Glucobay™ (Can) *see* acarbose *on page 23*
GlucoBurst® [OTC] *see* dextrose *on page 273*
glucocerebrosidase *see* alglucerase *on page 51*
GlucoNorm® (Can) *see* repaglinide *on page 773*
Glucophage® *see* metformin *on page 566*
Glucophage® XR *see* metformin *on page 566*
glucose *see* dextrose *on page 273*
glucose monohydrate *see* dextrose *on page 273*

glucose polymers (GLOO kose POL i merz)
U.S. Brand Names Moducal® [OTC]; Polycose® [OTC]
Therapeutic Category Nutritional Supplement
Use Supplies calories for those persons not able to meet the caloric requirement with usual food intake
General Dosage Range Oral: *Children and Adults:* Add to foods, beverages, or water as needed
Dosage Forms
  Powder for suspension, oral:
    Moducal® [OTC]: 368 g
    Polycose® [OTC]: 350 g

Glucotrol® *see* glipizide *on page 418*
Glucotrol XL® *see* glipizide *on page 418*
Glucovance® *see* glyburide and metformin *on page 421*
glulisine insulin *see* insulin glulisine *on page 477*
Glumetza® *see* metformin *on page 566*

glutamic acid (gloo TAM ik AS id)
Synonyms glutamic acid hydrochloride
Therapeutic Category Gastrointestinal Agent, Miscellaneous
Use Treatment of hypochlorhydria and achlorhydria
General Dosage Range Oral: *Adults:* 500-1000 mg/day in 3 divided doses
Dosage Forms
  Tablet, oral: 500 mg

glutamic acid hydrochloride *see* glutamic acid *on page 420*
Glutofac®-MX *see* vitamins (multiple/oral) *on page 919*
Glutofac®-ZX *see* vitamins (multiple/oral) *on page 919*
Glutol™ [OTC] *see* dextrose *on page 273*
Glutose 15™ [OTC] *see* dextrose *on page 273*
Glutose 45™ [OTC] *see* dextrose *on page 273*
glybenclamide *see* glyburide *on page 420*
glybenzcyclamide *see* glyburide *on page 420*

glyburide (GLYE byoor ide)
Medication Safety Issues
  Sound-alike/look-alike issues:
    GlyBURIDE may be confused with glipiZIDE, Glucotrol®
    DiaβBeta® may be confused with Diabinese®, Zebeta®
    Micronase may be confused with microK®, miconazole, Micronor®, Microzide™
  High alert medication:
    The Institute for Safe Medication Practices (ISMP) includes this medication among its list of drugs which have a heightened risk of causing significant patient harm when used in error.
Synonyms glibenclamide; glybenclamide; glybenzcyclamide; Micronase
Tall-Man glyBURIDE
U.S. Brand Names DiaBeta®; Glynase® PresTab®

Canadian Brand Names Apo-Glyburide®; Diaβeta®; Dom-Glyburide; Euglucon®; Med-Glybe; Mylan-Glybe; Novo-Glyburide; Nu-Glyburide; PMS-Glyburide; PRO-Glyburide; ratio-Glyburide; Riva-Glyburide; Sandoz-Glyburide; Teva-Glyburide

Therapeutic Category Antidiabetic Agent, Oral

Use Adjunct to diet and exercise for the management of type 2 diabetes mellitus (noninsulin-dependent, NIDDM)

General Dosage Range Oral:
Regular tablets: *Adults:* Initial: 1.25-5 mg once daily; Maintenance: 1.25-20 mg/day as single or divided doses (maximum: 20 mg/day)
Micronized tablets: *Adults:* Initial: 0.75-3 mg once daily; Maintenance: 0.75-12 mg/day as single or divided doses (maximum: 12 mg/day)

Dosage Forms
Tablet, oral: 1.25 mg, 1.5 mg, 2.5 mg, 3 mg, 5 mg, 6 mg
DiaBeta®: 1.25 mg, 2.5 mg, 5 mg
Glynase® PresTab®: 1.5 mg, 3 mg, 6 mg

glyburide and metformin (GLYE byoor ide & met FOR min)

Medication Safety Issues
Sound-alike/look-alike issues:
Glucovance® may be confused with Vyvanse™
High alert medication:
The Institute for Safe Medication Practices (ISMP) includes this medication among its list of drugs which have a heightened risk of causing significant patient harm when used in error.

Synonyms glyburide and metformin hydrochloride; metformin and glyburide

U.S. Brand Names Glucovance®

Therapeutic Category Antidiabetic Agent (Sulfonylurea); Antidiabetic Agent, Oral

Use Adjunct to diet and exercise for the management of type 2 diabetes mellitus (noninsulin-dependent, NIDDM)

General Dosage Range Oral: *Adults:* Initial: Glyburide 1.25-5 mg and metformin 250-500 mg once or twice daily; Maintenance: Up to glyburide 20 mg/day and metformin 2000 mg/day

Dosage Forms
Tablet: Glyburide 1.25 mg and metformin 250 mg; glyburide 2.5 mg and metformin 500 mg; glyburide 5 mg and metformin 500 mg
Glucovance®: 2.5 mg/500 mg: Glyburide 2.5 mg and metformin 500 mg; 5 mg/500 mg: Glyburide 5 mg and metformin 500 mg

glyburide and metformin hydrochloride *see* glyburide and metformin *on page 421*

glycerin (GLIS er in)

Synonyms glycerol

U.S. Brand Names Fleet® Glycerin Maximum Strength [OTC]; Fleet® Glycerin Suppositories [OTC]; Fleet® Liquid Glycerin [OTC]; Fleet® Pedia-Lax™ Glycerin Suppositories [OTC]; Fleet® Pedia-Lax™ Liquid Glycerin Suppositories [OTC]; Orajel® Dry Mouth [OTC]; Sani-Supp® [OTC]

Therapeutic Category Laxative; Ophthalmic Agent, Miscellaneous

Use Constipation; reduction of intraocular pressure; reduction of corneal edema; glycerin has been administered orally to reduce intracranial pressure

General Dosage Range
Ophthalmic: *Children and Adults:* Instill 1-2 drops in eye(s) once or every 3-4 hours
Oral: *Children and Adults:* 1.5 g/kg/day divided every 4 hours **or** 1 g/kg/dose every 6 hours **or** 1-1.8 g/kg once
Rectal:
Children <6 years: 1 infant suppository 1-2 times/day as needed **or** 2-5 mL as an enema
Children ≥6 years and Adults: 1 adult suppository 1-2 times/day as needed **or** 5-15 mL as an enema

Dosage Forms
Gel, oral:
Orajel® Dry Mouth [OTC]: 18% (42 g)
Liquid, for prescription compounding: USP: 100% (3840 mL)
Liquid, topical: USP: 100% (120 mL, 180 mL, 480 mL, 3840 mL)

Solution, rectal:
Fleet® Liquid Glycerin [OTC]: 5.6 g/5.5 mL (7.5 mL)
Fleet® Pedia-Lax™ Liquid Glycerin Suppositories [OTC]: 2.3 g/2.3 mL (4 mL)
Suppository, rectal: 1.5 g (12s, 25s); 80.7% (25s, 50s, 100s); 82.5% (12s, 25s, 50s, 100s)
Fleet® Glycerin Maximum Strength [OTC]: 3 g (18s)
Fleet® Glycerin Suppositories [OTC]: 2 g (12s, 50s)
Fleet® Pedia-Lax™ Glycerin Suppositories [OTC]: 1 g (12s)
Sani-Supp® [OTC]: 82.5% (10s, 25s)

glycerol see glycerin on page 421
glycerol guaiacolate see guaifenesin on page 425
glyceryl trinitrate see nitroglycerin on page 629
Glycon (Can) see metformin on page 566

glycopyrrolate (glye koe PYE roe late)
Medication Safety Issues
Sound-alike/look-alike issues:
Robinul® may be confused with Reminyl®
Synonyms glycopyrronium bromide
U.S. Brand Names Cuvposa™; Robinul®; Robinul® Forte
Canadian Brand Names Glycopyrrolate Injection, USP
Therapeutic Category Anticholinergic Agent
Use Inhibit salivation and excessive secretions of the respiratory tract preoperatively; control of upper airway secretions; intraoperatively to counteract drug-induced or vagal mediated bradyarrhythmias; adjunct in treatment of peptic ulcer (indication listed in product labeling but currently has no place in management of peptic ulcer disease)

Cuvposa™: Reduce chronic, severe drooling in those with neurologic conditions (eg, cerebral palsy) associated with drooling
General Dosage Range
I.M.:
Children <2 years: 4-9 mcg/kg once **or** 4-10 mcg/kg every 3-4 hours (maximum: 0.2 mg/dose; 0.8 mg/day)
Children ≥2 years: 4 mcg/kg once **or** 4-10 mcg/kg every 3-4 hours (maximum: 0.2 mg/dose; 0.8 mg/day)
Adults: 4 mcg/kg once **or** 0.1-0.2 mg 3-4 times/day
I.V.:
Children: 4-10 mcg/kg every 3-4 hours (maximum: 0.2 mg/dose; 0.8 mg/day) **or** 4 mcg/kg (maximum: 0.1 mg); repeat as needed
Adults: 0.1-0.2 mg 3-4 times/day **or** 0.1 mg repeated as needed
Oral: Children 3-16 years: 0.02-0.1 mg/kg/dose 3 times/day (maximum 3 mg/dose)
Dosage Forms
Injection, solution: 0.2 mg/mL (1 mL, 2 mL, 5 mL, 20 mL)
Robinul®: 0.2 mg/mL (1 mL, 2 mL, 5 mL, 20 mL)
Solution, oral:
Cuvposa™: 1 mg/5 mL (473 mL)
Tablet, oral: 1 mg, 2 mg
Robinul®: 1 mg
Robinul® Forte: 2 mg

Glycopyrrolate Injection, USP (Can) see glycopyrrolate on page 422
glycopyrronium bromide see glycopyrrolate on page 422
glycosum see dextrose on page 273
glydiazinamide see glipizide on page 418
Glynase® PresTab® see glyburide on page 420
Gly-Oxide® [OTC] see carbamide peroxide on page 172
Glyquin® XM (Can) see hydroquinone on page 453
Glyset® see miglitol on page 588
GM-CSF see sargramostim on page 802
GMD-Gemfibrozil (Can) see gemfibrozil on page 414
GnRH see gonadorelin (Canada only) on page 423

gold sodium thiomalate (gold SOW dee um thye oh MAL ate)

Synonyms sodium aurothiomalate

U.S. Brand Names Myochrysine®

Canadian Brand Names Myochrysine®

Therapeutic Category Gold Compound

Use Adjunctive treatment of active rheumatoid arthritis

General Dosage Range Dosage adjustment recommended in patients with renal impairment or who develop toxicities

I.M.:

Children: Test dose (recommended): 10 mg first week; Initial dosing: 1 mg/kg/week (maximum: 50 mg/injection); Maintenance: 1 mg/kg/dose (maximum: 50 mg/injection)

Adults: Test dose: 10 mg first week; Initial dosing: 25 mg second week, then 25-50 mg/week until 1 g cumulative dose has been given; Maintenance: 25-50 mg every other week for 2-20 weeks, then every 3-4 weeks

Dosage Forms

Injection, solution:

Myochrysine®: 50 mg/mL (1 mL)

golimumab (goe LIM ue mab)

Synonyms CNTO-148

U.S. Brand Names Simponi®

Canadian Brand Names Simponi®

Therapeutic Category Antipsoriatic Agent; Antirheumatic, Disease Modifying; Monoclonal Antibody; Tumor Necrosis Factor (TNF) Blocking Agent

Use Treatment of active rheumatoid arthritis (moderate-to-severe), active psoriatic arthritis, and active ankylosing spondylitis

General Dosage Range SubQ: *Adults:* 50 mg once per month

Dosage Forms

Injection, solution [preservative free]:

Simponi®: 50 mg/0.5 mL (0.5 mL)

GoLYTELY® *see* polyethylene glycol-electrolyte solution *on page 718*

gonadorelin acetate *see* gonadorelin *(Canada only) on page 423*

gonadorelin *(Canada only)* (goe nad oh RELL in)

Medication Safety Issues

Sound-alike/look-alike issues:

Gonadorelin may be confused with gonadotropin, guanadrel

Synonyms GnRH; gonadorelin acetate; gonadotropin releasing hormone; LHRH; LRH; luteinizing hormone releasing hormone

Canadian Brand Names Lutrepulse™

Therapeutic Category Gonadotropin

Use Induction of ovulation in females with hypothalamic amenorrhea

General Dosage Range I.V., SubQ: *Adults:* 1-20 mcg every 90 minutes

Product Availability Not available in U.S.

Dosage Forms - Canada

Injection, powder for reconstitution:

Lutrepulse®: 0.8 mg, 3.2 mg

gonadotropin releasing hormone *see* gonadorelin *(Canada only) on page 423*

Gonak™ *see* hydroxypropyl methylcellulose *on page 455*

Gonal-f® *see* follitropin alfa *on page 397*

Gonal-f® Pen (Can) *see* follitropin alfa *on page 397*

Gonal-f® RFF *see* follitropin alfa *on page 397*

Gonal-f® RFF Pen *see* follitropin alfa *on page 397*

gonioscopic ophthalmic solution *see* hydroxypropyl methylcellulose *on page 455*

Goniosoft™ [OTC] *see* hydroxypropyl methylcellulose *on page 455*

Goody's® Extra Strength Headache Powder [OTC] *see* acetaminophen, aspirin, and caffeine *on page 29*

Goody's® Extra Strength Pain Relief [OTC] *see* acetaminophen, aspirin, and caffeine *on page 29*

Goody's PM® [OTC] *see* acetaminophen and diphenhydramine *on page 27*

Gordofilm [OTC] *see* salicylic acid *on page 795*

Gordon Boro-Packs [OTC] *see* aluminum sulfate and calcium acetate *on page 61*

Gordon's® Urea [OTC] *see* urea *on page 900*

Gormel® [OTC] *see* urea *on page 900*

Gormel® Ten [OTC] *see* urea *on page 900*

goserelin (GOE se rel in)

Synonyms goserelin acetate; ICI-118630; ZDX

U.S. Brand Names Zoladex®

Canadian Brand Names Zoladex®; Zoladex® LA

Therapeutic Category Gonadotropin-Releasing Hormone Analog

Use Treatment of locally confined prostate cancer; palliative treatment of advanced prostate cancer; palliative treatment of advanced breast cancer in pre- and perimenopausal women; treatment of endometriosis, including pain relief and reduction of endometriotic lesions; endometrial thinning agent as part of treatment for dysfunctional uterine bleeding

General Dosage Range SubQ: *Adults:* 3.6 mg every 28 days **or** 10.8 mg every 12 weeks

Dosage Forms
Implant, subcutaneous:
Zoladex®: 3.6 mg (1s); 10.8 mg (1s)

goserelin acetate *see* goserelin *on page 424*

GP 47680 *see* oxcarbazepine *on page 660*

GPI 15715 *see* fospropofol *on page 402*

GR38032R *see* ondansetron *on page 651*

gramicidin, neomycin, and polymyxin B *see* neomycin, polymyxin B, and gramicidin *on page 618*

granisetron (gra NI se tron)

Medication Safety Issues
Sound-alike/look-alike issues:
Granisetron may be confused with dolasetron, ondansetron, palonosetron

Synonyms BRL 43694

U.S. Brand Names Granisol™; Kytril®; Sancuso®

Canadian Brand Names Granisetron Hydrochloride Injection; Kytril®

Therapeutic Category Selective 5-HT$_3$ Receptor Antagonist

Use Prophylaxis of nausea and vomiting associated with emetogenic chemotherapy and radiation therapy; prophylaxis and treatment of postoperative nausea and vomiting (PONV)

General Dosage Range
I.V.:
Children ≥2 years: 10 mcg/kg/dose (maximum: 1 mg/dose) as a single dose or every 12 hours
Adults: 10 mcg/kg/dose (maximum: 1 mg/dose) as a single dose or every 12 hours **or** 1 mg as a single dose
Oral: *Adults:* 2 mg/day in 1-2 divided dose
Transdermal: *Adults:* 1 patch prior to chemotherapy; Maximum duration: Patch may be worn up to 7 days

Dosage Forms
Injection, solution: 1 mg/mL (1 mL, 4 mL)
Injection, solution [preservative free]: 0.1 mg/mL (1 mL); 1 mg/mL (1 mL)
Patch, transdermal:
Sancuso®: 3.1 mg/24 hours (1s)
Solution, oral:
Granisol™: 2 mg/10 mL (30 mL)
Tablet, oral: 1 mg
Kytril®: 1 mg

Granisetron Hydrochloride Injection (Can) *see* granisetron *on page 424*

Granisol™ *see* granisetron *on page 424*
Granulex® *see* trypsin, balsam Peru, and castor oil *on page 896*
granulocyte colony stimulating factor *see* filgrastim *on page 377*
granulocyte colony stimulating factor (PEG conjugate) *see* pegfilgrastim *on page 679*
granulocyte-macrophage colony-stimulating factor *see* sargramostim *on page 802*
Gravol® (Can) *see* dimenhydrinate *on page 288*
green tea extract *see* sinecatechins *on page 814*
Grifulvin V® *see* griseofulvin *on page 425*

griseofulvin (gri see oh FUL vin)

Medication Safety Issues
  International issues:
    Fulvicin® (brand name used in international markets) may be confused with Furacin®
Synonyms griseofulvin microsize; griseofulvin ultramicrosize
U.S. Brand Names Grifulvin V®; Gris-PEG®
Therapeutic Category Antifungal Agent
Use Treatment of susceptible tinea infections of the skin, hair, and nails
General Dosage Range Oral:
  Microsize:
    Children >2 years: 10-20 mg/kg/day in single or divided doses
    Adults: 500-1000 mg/day in single or divided doses
  Ultramicrosize:
    Children >2 years: 5-15 mg/kg/day in single dose or 2 divided doses (maximum: 750 mg/day)
    Adults: 375-750 mg/day in single or divided doses
Dosage Forms
  Suspension, oral: 125 mg/5 mL (120 mL)
  Tablet, oral:
    Grifulvin V®: 500 mg
    Gris-PEG®: 125 mg, 250 mg

griseofulvin microsize *see* griseofulvin *on page 425*
griseofulvin ultramicrosize *see* griseofulvin *on page 425*
Gris-PEG® *see* griseofulvin *on page 425*
growth hormone, human *see* somatropin *on page 826*
GSK-580299 *see* papillomavirus (types 16, 18) vaccine (human, recombinant) *on page 673*
GSK 1838262 *see* gabapentin enacarbil *on page 406*
Guaiatussin AC *see* guaifenesin and codeine *on page 426*
Guaicon DM [OTC] [DSC] *see* guaifenesin and dextromethorphan *on page 427*
Guaicon DMS [OTC] *see* guaifenesin and dextromethorphan *on page 427*
Guaifen™ DM [DSC] *see* guaifenesin, dextromethorphan, and phenylephrine *on page 429*

guaifenesin (gwye FEN e sin)

Medication Safety Issues
  Sound-alike/look-alike issues:
    GuaiFENesin may be confused with guanFACINE
    Mucinex® may be confused with Mucomyst®
    Naldecon® may be confused with Nalfon®
  International issues:
    Mucolex® [Hong Kong] may be confused with Mycelex® which is a brand name for clotrimazole in the U.S.
Synonyms cheratussin; GG; glycerol guaiacolate
Tall-Man guaiFENesin
U.S. Brand Names Allfen [OTC]; Bidex®-400 [OTC]; Diabetic Siltussin DAS-Na [OTC]; Diabetic Tussin® EX [OTC]; Fenesin IR [OTC]; Ganidin® NR [OTC] [DSC]; Geri-Tussin [OTC]; Humibid® Maximum Strength [OTC]; Mucinex® Kid's Mini-Melts™ [OTC]; Mucinex® Kid's [OTC]; Mucinex® Maximum Strength [OTC]; Mucinex® [OTC]; Mucus Relief [OTC]; Organidin® NR [OTC] [DSC]; Refenesen™ 400 [OTC]; Refenesen™ [OTC]; Robafen [OTC]; Scot-Tussin® Expectorant [OTC]; Siltussin DAS [OTC]

[DSC]; Siltussin SA [OTC]; Vicks® Casero™ Chest Congestion Relief [OTC]; Vicks® DayQuil® Mucus Control [OTC]; Xpect™ [OTC]

Canadian Brand Names Balminil Expectorant; Benylin® E Extra Strength; Koffex Expectorant; Robitussin®

Therapeutic Category Expectorant

Use Help loosen phlegm and thin bronchial secretions to make coughs more productive

General Dosage Range Oral:
Extended release: *Children ≥12 years and Adults:* 600-1200 mg every 12 hours (maximum: 2.4 g/day)
Immediate release:
  Children 6 months to 2 years: 25-50 mg every 4 hours (maximum: 300 mg/day)
  Children 2-5 years: 50-100 mg every 4 hours (maximum: 600 mg/day)
  Children 6-11 years: 100-200 mg every 4 hours (maximum: 1.2 g/day)
  Children ≥12 years and Adults: 200-400 mg every 4 hours (maximum: 2.4 g/day)

Dosage Forms
  Caplet, oral:
  Fenesin IR [OTC]: 400 mg
  Refenesen™ 400 [OTC]: 400 mg
  Granules, oral:
  Mucinex® Kid's Mini-Melts™ [OTC]: 50 mg/packet (12s); 100 mg/packet (12s)
  Liquid, oral:
  Diabetic Tussin® EX [OTC]: 100 mg/5 mL (118 mL)
  Mucinex® Kid's [OTC]: 100 mg/5 mL (118 mL)
  Scot-Tussin® Expectorant [OTC]: 100 mg/5 mL (120 mL)
  Vicks® Casero™ Chest Congestion Relief [OTC]: 100 mg/6.25 mL (120 mL, 240 mL)
  Vicks® DayQuil® Mucus Control [OTC]: 200 mg/15 mL (295 mL)
  Syrup, oral: 100 mg/5 mL (5 mL, 10 mL, 15 mL, 118 mL, 120 mL, 240 mL, 473 mL, 480 mL)
  Diabetic Siltussin DAS-Na [OTC]: 100 mg/5 mL (118 mL)
  Geri-Tussin [OTC]: 100 mg/5 mL (120 mL, 240 mL, 480 mL)
  Robafen [OTC]: 100 mg/5 mL (120 mL, 240 mL, 480 mL)
  Siltussin SA [OTC]: 100 mg/5 mL (120 mL, 240 mL, 480 mL)
  Tablet, oral: 400 mg
  Allfen [OTC]: 400 mg
  Bidex®-400 [OTC]: 400 mg
  Mucus Relief [OTC]: 400 mg
  Refenesen™ [OTC]: 200 mg
  Xpect™ [OTC]: 400 mg
  Tablet, extended release, oral:
  Humibid® Maximum Strength [OTC]: 1200 mg
  Mucinex® [OTC]: 600 mg
  Mucinex® Maximum Strength [OTC]: 1200 mg

guaifenesin and codeine (gwye FEN e sin & KOE deen)

Synonyms codeine and guaifenesin; Robitussin AC

U.S. Brand Names Allfen CD; Allfen CDX; Dex-Tuss; ExeClear-C; Gani-Tuss® NR; Guaiatussin AC; Mar-Cof® CG; Robafen AC; Tusso-C™

Therapeutic Category Antitussive/Expectorant

Controlled Substance C-V

Use Temporary control of cough due to minor throat and bronchial irritation

General Dosage Range Oral: *Children ≥6 years and Adults:* Dosage varies greatly depending on product

Dosage Forms
  Liquid, oral:
  Dex-Tuss: Guaifenesin 300 mg and codeine 10 mg per 5 mL
  Gani-Tuss® NR: Guaifenesin 100 mg and codeine 10 mg per 5 mL
  Solution, oral: Guaifenesin 100 mg and codeine 10 mg per 5 mL
  Mar-Cof® CG: Guaifenesin 225 mg and codeine 7.5 mg per 5 mL
  Syrup, oral: Guaifenesin 100 mg and codeine 10 mg per 5 mL (473 mL)
  ExeClear-C, Tusso-C™: Guaifenesin 200 mg and codeine 10 mg per 5 mL
  Guaiatussin AC, Robafen AC: Guaifenesin 100 mg and codeine 10 mg per 5 mL

Tablet, oral:
Allfen CD: Guaifenesin 400 mg and codeine 10 mg
Allfen CDX: Guaifenesin 400 mg and codeine 20 mg

guaifenesin and dextromethorphan (gwye FEN e sin & deks troe meth OR fan)

Medication Safety Issues

Sound-alike/look-alike issues:
Benylin® may be confused with Benadryl®, Ventolin®

Synonyms dextromethorphan and guaifenesin

U.S. Brand Names Allfen DM [OTC] [DSC]; Cheracol® D [OTC]; Cheracol® Plus [OTC]; Coricidin HBP® Chest Congestion and Cough [OTC]; Diabetic Siltussin-DM DAS-Na Maximum Strength [OTC]; Diabetic Siltussin-DM DAS-Na [OTC]; Diabetic Tussin® DM Maximum Strength [OTC]; Diabetic Tussin® DM [OTC]; Double Tussin DM [OTC]; Fenesin DM IR; Gani-Tuss DM NR [DSC]; Guaicon DM [OTC] [DSC]; Guaicon DMS [OTC]; Guia-D [DSC]; Guiadrine™ DX [DSC]; Kolephrin® GG/DM [OTC]; Mintab DM [DSC]; Mucinex® DM Maximum Strength [OTC]; Mucinex® DM [OTC]; Mucinex® Kid's Cough Mini-Melts™ [OTC]; Mucinex® Kid's Cough [OTC]; Refenesen™ DM [OTC]; Robafen DM Clear [OTC]; Robafen DM [OTC]; Robitussin® Cough & Chest Congestion DM Max [OTC]; Robitussin® Cough & Chest Congestion DM [OTC]; Robitussin® Cough & Chest Congestion Sugar-Free DM [OTC]; Safe Tussin® DM [OTC]; Scot-Tussin® Senior [OTC]; Silexin [OTC]; Siltussin DM DAS [OTC]; Siltussin DM [OTC]; Simuc-DM [DSC]; Su-Tuss DM [DSC]; Tussi-Bid®; Vicks® 44E [OTC]; Vicks® DayQuil® Mucus Control DM [OTC]; Vicks® Pediatric Formula 44E [OTC]

Canadian Brand Names Balminil DM E; Benylin® DM-E; Koffex DM-Expectorant; Robitussin® DM

Therapeutic Category Antitussive/Expectorant

Use Temporary control of cough due to minor throat and bronchial irritation

General Dosage Range Oral:

Children 2-6 years: Guaifenesin 50-100 mg and dextromethorphan 2.5-5 mg every 4 hours (maximum: Guaifenesin 600 mg/day; Dextromethorphan 30 mg/day)

Children 6-12 years: Guaifenesin 100-200 mg and dextromethorphan 5-10 mg every 4 hours (maximum: Guaifenesin 1200 mg/day; Dextromethorphan 60 mg/day)

Children ≥12 years and Adults: Guaifenesin 200-400 mg and dextromethorphan 10-20 mg every 4 hours (maximum: Guaifenesin 2400 mg/day; Dextromethorphan 120 mg/day)

Dosage Forms

Caplet, oral:
Fenesin DM IR: Guaifenesin 400 mg and dextromethorphan 15 mg
Refenesen™ DM [OTC]: Guaifenesin 400 mg and dextromethorphan 20 mg

Capsule, softgel, oral:
Coricidin HBP® Chest Congestion and Cough [OTC]: Guaifenesin 200 mg and dextromethorphan 10 mg

Granules, oral:
Mucinex® Kid's Cough Mini-Melts™: Guaifenesin 100 mg and dextromethorphan hydrobromide 5 mg per packet (12s)

Liquid, oral: Guaifenesin 100 mg and dextromethorphan 10 mg per 5 mL; guaifenesin 300 mg and dextromethorphan 10 mg per 5 mL
Diabetic Tussin® DM [OTC]: Guaifenesin 100 mg and dextromethorphan 10 mg per 5 mL
Diabetic Tussin® DM Maximum Strength [OTC]: Guaifenesin 200 mg and dextromethorphan 10 mg per 5 mL
Double Tussin DM [OTC]: Guaifenesin 300 mg and dextromethorphan 20 mg per 5 mL
Kolephrin® GG/DM [OTC]: Guaifenesin 150 mg and dextromethorphan 10 mg per 5 mL
Mucinex® Kid's Cough: Guaifenesin 100 mg and dextromethorphan 5 mg per 5 mL
Safe Tussin® DM [OTC]: Guaifenesin 100 mg and dextromethorphan 15 mg per 5 mL
Scot-Tussin® Senior [OTC]: Guaifenesin 200 mg and dextromethorphan 15 mg per 5 mL
Vicks® 44E [OTC]: Guaifenesin 200 mg and dextromethorphan hydrobromide 20 mg per 15 mL
Vicks® DayQuil® Mucus Control DM [OTC]: Guaifenesin 200 mg and dextromethorphan hydrobromide 10 mg per 15 mL
Vicks® Pediatric Formula 44E [OTC]: Guaifenesin 100 mg and dextromethorphan hydrobromide 10 mg per 15 mL

◄ **Syrup, oral:** Guaifenesin 100 mg and dextromethorphan 10 mg per 5 mL
Cheracol® D [OTC], Cheracol® Plus [OTC], Diabetic Siltussin-DM DAS-Na [OTC], Diabetic Siltussin-DM DAS-Na Maximum Strength [OTC], Guaicon DMS [OTC], Robafen DM [OTC], Robafen DM Clear [OTC], Robitussin® Cough & Chest Congestion DM [OTC], Robitussin® Cough & Chest Congestion Sugar-Free DM [OTC], Silexin [OTC], Siltussin DM [OTC], Siltussin DM DAS [OTC]: Guaifenesin 100 mg and dextromethorphan 10 mg per 5 mL
Robitussin® Cough & Chest Congestion DM Max [OTC]: Guaifenesin 200 mg and dextromethorphan hydrobromide 10 mg per 5 mL
Tablet, oral: Guaifenesin 1000 mg and dextromethorphan hydrobromide 60 mg; guaifenesin 1200 mg and dextromethorphan hydrobromide 60 mg
Silexin [OTC]: Guaifenesin 100 mg and dextromethorphan hydrobromide 10 mg
Tablet, extended release, oral: Guaifenesin 800 mg and dextromethorphan 30 mg; Guaifenesin 1200 mg and dextromethorphan 20 mg
Mucinex® DM [OTC]: Guaifenesin 600 mg and dextromethorphan 30 mg
Mucinex® DM Maximum Strength [OTC]: Guaifenesin 1200 mg and dextromethorphan 60 mg
Tablet, long-acting, oral: Guaifenesin 1000 mg and dextromethorphan 60 mg
Tablet, sustained release, oral:
Tussi-Bid®: Guaifenesin 1200 mg and dextromethorphan 60 mg
Tablet, timed release, oral [scored]: Guaifenesin 1200 mg and dextromethorphan 60 mg

guaifenesin and dyphylline see dyphylline and guaifenesin on page 318

guaifenesin and phenylephrine (gwye FEN e sin & fen il EF rin)

Medication Safety Issues
Sound-alike/look-alike issues:
Entex® may be confused with Tenex®
Entex® LA brand name represents a different product in the U.S. than it does in Canada. Formerly available in the U.S., Entex® LA contains guaifenesin and phenylephrine, while in Canada the product bearing this brand name contains guaifenesin and pseudoephedrine.

Synonyms guaifenesin and phenylephrine tannate; phenylephrine hydrochloride and guaifenesin

U.S. Brand Names Ambi 10PEH/400GFN [OTC]; Crantex®; Donatussin Drops [DSC]; Fenesin PE IR; Guiatex PE™ [DSC]; Liquibid® D-R [OTC]; Liquibid® PD-R [OTC]; Maxiphen [OTC] [DSC]; Medent®-PEI [OTC]; Mucinex® Cold [OTC]; Mucus Relief Sinus [OTC]; OneTab™ Congestion & Cold [OTC]; Refenesen™ PE [OTC]; Rescon GG [OTC]; Sina-12X® [DSC]; Sudafed PE® Non-Drying Sinus [OTC]; Triaminic® Children's Chest & Nasal Congestion [OTC]

Therapeutic Category Cold Preparation

Use Temporary relief of nasal congestion, sinusitis, rhinitis, and hay fever; temporary relief of cough associated with upper respiratory tract conditions, especially when associated with dry, nonproductive cough

General Dosage Range Oral: *Children >2 years and Adults:* Dosage varies greatly depending on product

Dosage Forms
Caplet, oral:
Fenesin PE IR, OneTab™ Congestion & Cold [OTC], Refenesen™ PE [OTC]: Guaifenesin 400 mg and phenylephrine 10 mg
Sudafed PE® Non-Drying Sinus [OTC]: Guaifenesin 200 mg and phenylephrine 5 mg
Liquid, oral:
Crantex®: Guaifenesin 100 mg and phenylephrine 7.5 mg per 5 mL (473 mL)
Mucinex® Cold [OTC]: Guaifenesin 100 mg and phenylephrine 2.5 mg per 5 mL (480 mL)
Rescon GG [OTC]: Guaifenesin 100 mg and phenylephrine 5 mg per 5 mL (120 mL, 480 mL)
Syrup, oral:
Triaminic® Children's Chest & Nasal Congestion [OTC]: Guaifenesin 50 mg and phenylephrine 2.5 mg per 5 mL (118 mL)
Tablet, oral:
Ambi 10PEH/400GFN [OTC], Liquibid® D-R [OTC], Medent®-PEI [OTC], Mucus Relief Sinus [OTC]: Guaifenesin 400 mg and phenylephrine 10 mg
Liquibid® PD-R [OTC]: Guaifenesin 200 mg and phenylephrine 5 mg
Tablet, long acting: Guaifenesin 900 mg and phenylephrine 25 mg; guaifenesin 1200 mg and phenylephrine 25 mg
Tablet, prolonged release: Guaifenesin 600 mg and phenylephrine 15 mg

guaifenesin and phenylephrine tannate see guaifenesin and phenylephrine on page 428

guaifenesin and pseudoephedrine (gwye FEN e sin & soo doe e FED rin)

Medication Safety Issues

Sound-alike/look-alike issues:

Entex® may be confused with Tenex®

Entex® LA brand name represents a different product in the U.S. than it does in Canada. In the U.S., Entex® LA contains guaifenesin and phenylephrine, while in Canada the product bearing this brand name contains guaifenesin and pseudoephedrine.

Synonyms pseudoephedrine and guaifenesin

U.S. Brand Names Ambifed [OTC] [DSC]; Ambifed-G [OTC]; Congestac® [OTC]; ExeFen-IR [DSC]; Maxifed [OTC]; Maxifed-G [OTC]; Mucinex® D Maximum Strength [OTC]; Mucinex® D [OTC]; Refenesen Plus [OTC]; Respaire®-30 [DSC]; SudaTex-G [OTC]; Tenar™ PSE [DSC]

Canadian Brand Names Contac® Cold-Chest Congestion, Non Drowsy, Regular Strength; Entex® LA; Novahistex® Expectorant with Decongestant

Therapeutic Category Expectorant/Decongestant

Use Temporary relief of nasal congestion and to help loosen phlegm and thin bronchial secretions in the treatment of cough

General Dosage Range Oral: *Children >2 years and Adults:* Dosage varies greatly depending on product

Dosage Forms

Caplet, oral:

Congestac® [OTC], Refenesen Plus [OTC]: Guaifenesin 400 mg and pseudoephedrine 60 mg

Tablet, oral:

Ambifed-G [OTC]: Guaifenesin 400 mg and pseudoephedrine 20 mg

Maxifed [OTC]: Guaifenesin 400 mg and pseudoephedrine 60 mg

Maxifed-G [OTC], SudaTex-G [OTC]: Guaifenesin 400 mg and pseudoephedrine 40 mg

Tablet, extended release, oral:

Mucinex® D [OTC]: Guaifenesin 600 mg and pseudoephedrine 60 mg

Mucinex® D Maximum Strength [OTC]: Guaifenesin 1200 mg and pseudoephedrine 120 mg

guaifenesin, chlorpheniramine, phenylephrine, and dextromethorphan see dextromethorphan, chlorpheniramine, phenylephrine, and guaifenesin on page 272

guaifenesin, dextromethorphan, and phenylephrine
(gwye FEN e sin, deks troe meth OR fan, & fen il EF rin)

Synonyms dextromethorphan hydrobromide, guaifenesin, and phenylephrine hydrochloride; guaifenesin, dextromethorphan hydrobromide, and phenylephrine hydrochloride; phenylephrine hydrochloride, guaifenesin, and dextromethorphan hydrobromide

U.S. Brand Names Certuss-D® [DSC]; ExeCof [DSC]; ExeTuss-DM [DSC]; Giltuss Pediatric® [DSC]; Giltuss TR® [DSC]; Giltuss® [DSC]; Guaifen™ DM [DSC]; Maxiphen DM; Maxiphen DMX; Mucinex® Children's Multi-Symptom Cold [OTC]; Robafen CF Cough & Cold [OTC]; Robitussin® Children's Cough & Cold CF [OTC]; Robitussin® Cough & Cold CF Max [OTC]; Robitussin® Cough & Cold CF [OTC]; SINUtuss® DM [DSC]; Tusso™-DMR [DSC]

Therapeutic Category Antitussive; Decongestant

Use Symptomatic relief of dry nonproductive coughs and upper respiratory symptoms associated with hay fever, colds, or the flu

General Dosage Range Oral: *Children >4 years and Adults:* Dosage varies greatly depending on product

Dosage Forms

Liquid, oral:

Maxiphen DMX: Guaifenesin 200 mg, dextromethorphan 20 mg, and phenylephrine 10 mg per 5 mL

Mucinex® Children's Multi-Symptom Cold [OTC]: Guaifenesin 100 mg, dextromethorphan 5 mg, and phenylephrine 2.5 mg per 5 mL

Robitussin® Children's Cough & Cold CF [OTC]: Guaifenesin 50 mg, dextromethorphan 5 mg, and phenylephrine 2.5 mg per 5 mL

Robitussin® Cough & Cold CF [OTC]: Guaifenesin 100 mg, dextromethorphan 10 mg, and phenylephrine 5 mg per 5 mL

Robitussin® Cough & Cold CF Max [OTC]: Guaifenesin 200 mg, dextromethorphan 10 mg, and phenylephrine 5 mg per 5 mL

Syrup, oral:
Robafen CF Cough & Cold [OTC]: Guaifenesin 100 mg, dextromethorphan 10 mg, and phenylephrine 5 mg per 5 mL
Tablet, oral [scored]:
Maxiphen DM: Guaifenesin 400 mg, dextromethorphan 20 mg, and phenylephrine 10 mg

guaifenesin, dextromethorphan hydrobromide, and phenylephrine hydrochloride *see* guaifenesin, dextromethorphan, and phenylephrine *on page 429*

guaifenesin, dihydrocodeine, and pseudoephedrine *see* dihydrocodeine, pseudoephedrine, and guaifenesin *on page 285*

guaifenesin, phenylephrine, and chlorpheniramine *see* chlorpheniramine, phenylephrine, and guaifenesin *on page 200*

guaifenesin, phenylephrine tannate, and pyrilamine tannate *see* phenylephrine, pyrilamine, and guaifenesin *on page 700*

guaifenesin, pseudoephedrine, and codeine
(gwye FEN e sin, soo doe e FED rin, & KOE deen)

Synonyms codeine, guaifenesin, and pseudoephedrine; pseudoephedrine, guaifenesin, and codeine

U.S. Brand Names Mytussin® DAC

Canadian Brand Names Benylin® 3.3 mg-D-E; Calmylin with Codeine

Therapeutic Category Antitussive/Decongestant/Expectorant

Controlled Substance C-V

Use Temporarily relieves nasal congestion and controls cough associated with upper respiratory infections and related conditions (common cold, sinusitis, bronchitis, influenza)

General Dosage Range Oral:
Children 6-12 years: 5 mL every 4 hours (maximum: 20 mL/24 hours)
Children >12 years and Adults: 10 mL every 4 hours (maximum: 40 mL/24 hours)

Dosage Forms
Syrup, oral: Guaifenesin 100 mg, pseudoephedrine 30 mg, and codeine 10 mg per 5 mL (473 mL)
Mytussin® DAC: Guaifenesin 100 mg, pseudoephedrine 30 mg, and codeine 10 mg per 5 mL (118 mL, 473 mL)

guaifenesin, pseudoephedrine, and dextromethorphan
(gwye FEN e sin, soo doe e FED rin, & deks troe meth OR fan)

Synonyms dextromethorphan, guaifenesin, and pseudoephedrine; pseudoephedrine, dextromethorphan, and guaifenesin

U.S. Brand Names Ambifed DM; Ambifed-G DM; Donatussin DM; ExeFen-DMX; Maxifed DM; Maxifed DMX

Canadian Brand Names Balminil DM + Decongestant + Expectorant; Benylin® DM-D-E

Therapeutic Category Cold Preparation

Use Temporarily relieves nasal congestion and controls cough due to minor throat and bronchial irritation; helps loosen phlegm and thin bronchial secretions to make coughs more productive

General Dosage Range Oral: *Children ≥6 years and Adults:* Dosage varies greatly depending on product

Dosage Forms
Liquid, oral:
Maxifed DM: Guaifenesin 200 mg, pseudoephedrine 20 mg, and dextromethorphan 10 mg per 5 mL
Syrup, oral:
Donatussin DM: Guaifenesin 150 mg, pseudoephedrine 30 mg, and dextromethorphan 15 mg per 5 mL
Tablet, oral:
Ambifed DM: Guaifenesin 400 mg, pseudoephedrine 30 mg, and dextromethorphan 20 mg
Ambifed-G DM: Guaifenesin 400 mg, pseudoephedrine 20 mg, and dextromethorphan 20 mg
ExeFen-DMX, Maxifed DMX: Guaifenesin 400 mg, pseudoephedrine 60 mg, and dextromethorphan 20 mg
Maxifed DM: Guaifenesin 400 mg, pseudoephedrine 40 mg, and dextromethorphan 20 mg

guanabenz (GWAHN a benz)

Medication Safety Issues
Sound-alike/look-alike issues:
Guanabenz may be confused with guanadrel, guanfacine

Synonyms guanabenz acetate

Canadian Brand Names Wytensin®
Therapeutic Category Alpha-Adrenergic Agonist
Use Management of hypertension
General Dosage Range Oral:
  Adults: Initial: 4 mg twice daily; Maintenance: 4-32 mg twice daily
  Elderly: Initial: 4 mg once daily
Dosage Forms
  Tablet, oral: 4 mg

guanabenz acetate *see* guanabenz *on page 430*

guanfacine (GWAHN fa seen)
Medication Safety Issues
  Sound-alike/look-alike issues:
    GuanFACINE may be confused with guaiFENesin, guanabenz, guanidine
    Tenex® may be confused with Entex®, Ten-K®, Xanax®
  International issues:
    Tenex [U.S., Canada] may be confused with Kinex brand name for biperiden [Mexico]
Synonyms guanfacine hydrochloride
Tall-Man guanFACINE
U.S. Brand Names Intuniv™; Tenex®
Therapeutic Category Alpha-Adrenergic Agonist
Use
  Tablet, immediate release: Management of hypertension
  Tablet, extended release: Treatment of attention-deficit/hyperactivity disorder (ADHD) as monotherapy or adjunctive therapy to stimulants
General Dosage Range Oral:
  Immediate release: *Children ≥12 years and Adults:* 0.5-2 mg once daily
  Extended release: *Children ≥6 years and Adolescents:* 1-4 mg once daily
Dosage Forms
  Tablet, oral: 1 mg, 2 mg
    Tenex®: 1 mg, 2 mg
  Tablet, extended release, oral:
    Intuniv™: 1 mg, 2 mg, 3 mg, 4 mg

guanfacine hydrochloride *see* guanfacine *on page 431*

guanidine (GWAHN i deen)
Medication Safety Issues
  Sound-alike/look-alike issues:
    Guanidine may be confused with guanfacine, guanethidine
Synonyms guanidine hydrochloride
Therapeutic Category Cholinergic Agent
Use Reduction of the symptoms of muscle weakness associated with the myasthenic syndrome of Eaton-Lambert, not for myasthenia gravis
General Dosage Range Oral: *Adults:* Initial: 10-15 mg/kg/day in 3-4 divided doses; Maintenance: Up to 35 mg/kg/day
Dosage Forms
  Tablet, oral: 125 mg

guanidine hydrochloride *see* guanidine *on page 431*
Guia-D [DSC] *see* guaifenesin and dextromethorphan *on page 427*
Guiadrine™ DX [DSC] *see* guaifenesin and dextromethorphan *on page 427*
Guiatex PE™ [DSC] *see* guaifenesin and phenylephrine *on page 428*
gum benjamin *see* benzoin *on page 123*
GW506U78 *see* nelarabine *on page 616*
GW-1000-02 *see* tetrahydrocannabinol and cannabidiol *(Canada only) on page 857*
GW433908G *see* fosamprenavir *on page 399*
GW572016 *see* lapatinib *on page 512*

GW786034 *see* pazopanib *on page 676*
Gynazole-1® *see* butoconazole *on page 155*
Gyne-Lotrimin® 3 [OTC] *see* clotrimazole (topical) *on page 226*
Gyne-Lotrimin® 7 [OTC] *see* clotrimazole (topical) *on page 226*
Gynol II® [OTC] *see* nonoxynol 9 *on page 632*
Gynol II® Extra Strength [OTC] *see* nonoxynol 9 *on page 632*
Gynovite® Plus [OTC] *see* vitamins (multiple/oral) *on page 919*
H1N1 influenza vaccine *see* influenza virus vaccine (inactivated) *on page 473*
H1N1 influenza vaccine *see* influenza virus vaccine (live/attenuated) *on page 474*
h5G1.1 *see* eculizumab *on page 319*
H5N1 influenza vaccine *see* influenza virus vaccine (H5N1) *on page 473*
Habitrol *see* nicotine *on page 625*
Habitrol® (Can) *see* nicotine *on page 625*

Haemophilus B conjugate and hepatitis B vaccine
(he MOF i lus bee KON joo gate & hep a TYE tis bee vak SEEN)

Medication Safety Issues
Sound-alike/look-alike issues:
Comvax® may be confused with Recombivax [Recombivax HB®]

Synonyms *Haemophilus* b (meningococcal protein conjugate) conjugate vaccine; hepatitis B vaccine (recombinant); hib conjugate vaccine; hib-hepB

U.S. Brand Names Comvax®

Therapeutic Category Vaccine, Inactivated Virus

Use
Immunization against invasive disease caused by *H. influenzae* type b and against infection caused by all known subtypes of hepatitis B virus in infants 6 weeks to 15 months of age born of hepatitis B surface antigen (HB$_s$Ag)-negative mothers
Infants born of HB$_s$Ag-positive mothers or mothers of unknown HB$_s$Ag status should receive hepatitis B vaccine (recombinant) at birth and should complete the hepatitis B vaccination series given according to a particular schedule (refer to current ACIP recommendations).

General Dosage Range I.M.: *Infants ≥6 weeks:* 0.5 mL (series includes 3 doses)

Dosage Forms
Injection, suspension [preservative free]:
Comvax®: *Haemophilus* b capsular polysaccharide 7.5 mcg and hepatitis B surface antigen 5 mcg per 0.5 mL (0.5 mL)

Haemophilus B conjugate (Hib) *see* diphtheria and tetanus toxoids, acellular pertussis, poliovirus and *Haemophilus* b conjugate vaccine *on page 295*

Haemophilus B conjugate vaccine (he MOF fi lus bee KON joo gate vak SEEN)

Medication Safety Issues
International issues:
Hiberix is also a brand name for influenza virus vaccine in multiple international markets

Synonyms *Haemophilus* b oligosaccharide conjugate vaccine; *Haemophilus* b polysaccharide vaccine; diphtheria toxoid conjugate; HbCV; hib; hib conjugate vaccine; hib polysaccharide conjugate; PRP-OMP; PRP-T

U.S. Brand Names ActHIB®; Hiberix®; PedvaxHIB®

Canadian Brand Names ActHIB®; PedvaxHIB®

Therapeutic Category Vaccine, Inactivated Bacteria

Use Routine immunization of children against invasive disease caused by *H. influenzae* type b

The Advisory Committee on Immunization Practices (ACIP) recommends routine vaccination of all children through age 59 months. Efficacy data are not available for use in older children and adults with chronic conditions associated with an increased risk of Hib disease. However, a single dose may also be considered for older children, adolescents, and adults who did not receive the childhood series and who have had splenectomies or who have sickle cell disease, leukemia, or HIV infection.

General Dosage Range I.M.: *Children:* 0.5 mL (number of doses determined by age at first dose)

Dosage Forms
Injection, powder for reconstitution [preservative free]:
ActHIB® *Haemophilus* b capsular polysaccharide 10 mcg per 0.5 mL
Hiberix®: *Haemophilus* b capsular polysaccharide 10 mcg per 0.5 mL
Injection, suspension:
PedvaxHIB®: *Haemophilus* b capsular polysaccharide 7.5 mcg

Haemophilus b (meningococcal protein conjugate) conjugate vaccine *see Haemophilus* B conjugate and hepatitis B vaccine *on page 432*

Haemophilus b oligosaccharide conjugate vaccine *see Haemophilus* B conjugate vaccine *on page 432*

Haemophilus B polysaccharide *see* diphtheria and tetanus toxoids, acellular pertussis, poliovirus and *Haemophilus* b conjugate vaccine *on page 295*

Haemophilus b polysaccharide vaccine *see Haemophilus* B conjugate vaccine *on page 432*

Haemophilus influenzae b conjugate vaccine and diphtheria, tetanus toxoids, and acellular pertussis vaccine *see* diphtheria, tetanus toxoids, and acellular pertussis vaccine and *Haemophilus influenzae* b conjugate vaccine *on page 297*

HAL *see* hexaminolevulinate *on page 440*

Halaven™ *see* eribulin *on page 337*

halcinonide (hal SIN oh nide)

Medication Safety Issues
Sound-alike/look-alike issues:
Halcinonide may be confused with Halcion®
Halog® may be confused with Haldol®, Mycolog®
U.S. Brand Names Halog®
Canadian Brand Names Halog®
Therapeutic Category Corticosteroid, Topical
Use Inflammation of corticosteroid-responsive dermatoses [high potency topical corticosteroid]
General Dosage Range Topical: *Children and Adults:* Apply sparingly 1-3 times/day
Dosage Forms
Cream, topical:
Halog®: 0.1% (30 g, 60 g)
Ointment, topical:
Halog®: 0.1% (30 g, 60 g)

Halcion® *see* triazolam *on page 888*

Haldol® *see* haloperidol *on page 434*

Haldol® Decanoate *see* haloperidol *on page 434*

Haley's M-O *see* magnesium hydroxide and mineral oil *on page 546*

HalfLytely® and Bisacodyl *see* polyethylene glycol-electrolyte solution and bisacodyl *on page 719*

Halfprin® [OTC] *see* aspirin *on page 98*

halichondrin B analog *see* eribulin *on page 337*

halobetasol (hal oh BAY ta sol)

Medication Safety Issues
Sound-alike/look-alike issues:
Ultravate® may be confused with Cutivate®
Synonyms halobetasol propionate
U.S. Brand Names Ultravate®
Canadian Brand Names Ultravate®
Therapeutic Category Corticosteroid, Topical
Use Relief of inflammatory and pruritic manifestations of corticosteroid-response dermatoses [super high potency topical corticosteroid]
General Dosage Range Topical: *Children ≥12 years and Adults:* Apply sparingly to lesion/skin twice daily (maximum: 50 g/week; 2 consecutive weeks)
Dosage Forms
Cream, topical: 0.05% (15 g, 50 g)
Ultravate®: 0.05% (15 g, 50 g)

◄ **Ointment, topical**: 0.05% (15 g, 50 g)
 Ultravate®: 0.05% (15 g, 50 g)

halobetasol propionate *see halobetasol on page 433*
Halog® *see halcinonide on page 433*

haloperidol (ha loe PER i dole)
Medication Safety Issues
 Sound-alike/look-alike issues:
  Haloperidol may be confused Halotestin®
  Haldol® may be confused with Halcion®, Halenol®, Halog®, Halotestin®, Stadol®
Synonyms haloperidol decanoate; haloperidol lactate
U.S. Brand Names Haldol®; Haldol® Decanoate
Canadian Brand Names Apo-Haloperidol LA®; Apo-Haloperidol®; Haloperidol Injection, USP; Haloperidol Long Acting; Haloperidol-LA; Haloperidol-LA Omega; Novo-Peridol; PMS-Haloperidol; PMS-Haloperidol LA
Therapeutic Category Antipsychotic Agent, Butyrophenone
Use Management of schizophrenia; control of tics and vocal utterances of Tourette disorder in children and adults; severe behavioral problems in children
General Dosage Range
 I.M.:
  Decanoate: *Adults:* Initial: 10-20 times daily oral dose at 4-week intervals; Maintenance: 10-15 times initial oral dose
  Lactate:
   Children 6-12 years: 1-3 mg/dose every 4-8 hours (maximum: 0.15 mg/kg/day)
   Adults: 2-5 mg every 4-8 hours as needed
 Oral:
  Children 3-12 years (15-40 kg): Initial: 0.5 mg/day in 2-3 divided doses; Maintenance: 0.05-0.15 mg/kg/day in 2-3 divided doses
  Adults: Initial: 0.5-5 mg 2-3 times/day; Maintenance: Up to 30 mg/day in 2-3 divided doses
Dosage Forms
 Injection, oil: 50 mg/mL (1 mL, 5 mL); 100 mg/mL (1 mL, 5 mL)
  Haldol® Decanoate: 50 mg/mL (1 mL); 100 mg/mL (1 mL)
 Injection, solution: 5 mg/mL (1 mL, 10 mL)
  Haldol®: 5 mg/mL (1 mL)
 Solution, oral: 2 mg/mL (5 mL, 15 mL, 120 mL)
 Tablet, oral: 0.5 mg, 1 mg, 2 mg, 5 mg, 10 mg, 20 mg

haloperidol decanoate *see haloperidol on page 434*
Haloperidol Injection, USP (Can) *see haloperidol on page 434*
Haloperidol-LA (Can) *see haloperidol on page 434*
haloperidol lactate *see haloperidol on page 434*
Haloperidol-LA Omega (Can) *see haloperidol on page 434*
Haloperidol Long Acting (Can) *see haloperidol on page 434*
hamamelis water *see witch hazel on page 923*
harkoseride *see lacosamide on page 505*
Havrix® *see hepatitis A vaccine on page 437*
HAVRIX® (Can) *see hepatitis A vaccine on page 437*
Havrix® and Engerix-B® *see hepatitis A and hepatitis B recombinant vaccine on page 437*
HbCV *see Haemophilus B conjugate vaccine on page 432*
HBIG *see hepatitis B immune globulin (human) on page 438*
hBNP *see nesiritide on page 620*
hCG *see chorionic gonadotropin (human) on page 206*
HCTZ (error-prone abbreviation) *see hydrochlorothiazide on page 445*
HDA® Toothache [OTC] *see benzocaine on page 121*
HDCV *see rabies vaccine on page 764*
Head & Shoulders® Citrus Breeze [OTC] *see pyrithione zinc on page 759*
Head & Shoulders® Citrus Breeze 2-in-1 [OTC] *see pyrithione zinc on page 759*
Head & Shoulders® Classic Clean [OTC] *see pyrithione zinc on page 759*

Head & Shoulders® Classic Clean 2-in-1 [OTC] *see* pyrithione zinc *on page 759*
Head & Shoulders® Dry Scalp [OTC] *see* pyrithione zinc *on page 759*
Head & Shoulders® Dry Scalp 2-in-1 [OTC] *see* pyrithione zinc *on page 759*
Head & Shoulders® Dry Scalp Care [OTC] *see* pyrithione zinc *on page 759*
Head & Shoulders® Dry Scalp Care 2-in-1 [OTC] *see* pyrithione zinc *on page 759*
Head & Shoulders® Extra Volume [OTC] *see* pyrithione zinc *on page 759*
Head & Shoulders® intensive solutions 2 in 1 [OTC] *see* pyrithione zinc *on page 759*
Head & Shoulders® intensive solutions for dry/damaged hair [OTC] *see* pyrithione zinc *on page 759*
Head & Shoulders® intensive solutions for fine/oily hair [OTC] *see* pyrithione zinc *on page 759*
Head & Shoulders® intensive solutions for normal hair [OTC] *see* pyrithione zinc *on page 759*
Head & Shoulders® Intensive Treatment [OTC] *see* selenium sulfide *on page 807*
Head & Shoulders® Ocean Lift [OTC] *see* pyrithione zinc *on page 759*
Head & Shoulders® Ocean Lift 2-in-1 [OTC] *see* pyrithione zinc *on page 759*
Head & Shoulders® Refresh [OTC] *see* pyrithione zinc *on page 759*
Head & Shoulders® Refresh 2-in-1 [OTC] *see* pyrithione zinc *on page 759*
Head & Shoulders® Restoring Shine [OTC] *see* pyrithione zinc *on page 759*
Head & Shoulders® Restoring Shine 2 in 1 [OTC] *see* pyrithione zinc *on page 759*
Head & Shoulders® Sensitive Care [OTC] *see* pyrithione zinc *on page 759*
Head & Shoulders® Sensitive Care 2 in 1 [OTC] *see* pyrithione zinc *on page 759*
Head & Shoulders® Smooth & Silky [OTC] *see* pyrithione zinc *on page 759*
Head & Shoulders® Smooth & Silky 2-in-1 [OTC] *see* pyrithione zinc *on page 759*
Healon® (Can) *see* hyaluronate and derivatives *on page 443*
Healon GV® (Can) *see* hyaluronate and derivatives *on page 443*
Heartburn Relief [OTC] *see* famotidine *on page 366*
Heartburn Relief Maximum Strength [OTC] *see* famotidine *on page 366*
Heather *see* norethindrone *on page 633*
Hectorol® *see* doxercalciferol *on page 310*
Helidac® *see* bismuth, metronidazole, and tetracycline *on page 136*
Helistat® *see* collagen hemostat *on page 233*
Helitene® *see* collagen hemostat *on page 233*
Helixate® FS *see* antihemophilic factor (recombinant) *on page 81*
Hemabate® *see* carboprost tromethamine *on page 175*
hematin *see* hemin *on page 435*
hemiacidrin *see* citric acid, magnesium carbonate, and glucono-delta-lactone *on page 214*

hemin (HEE min)

Synonyms hematin
U.S. Brand Names Panhematin®
Therapeutic Category Blood Modifiers
Use Treatment of recurrent attacks of acute intermittent porphyria (AIP)
General Dosage Range I.V.: *Children ≥16 years and Adults:* 1-4 mg/kg/day divided every 12 hours (maximum: 6 mg/kg/24 hours)
Dosage Forms
Injection, powder for reconstitution:
Panhematin®: 313 mg

Hemocyte® [OTC] *see* ferrous fumarate *on page 373*
Hemocyte Plus® *see* vitamins (multiple/oral) *on page 919*
Hemofil M *see* antihemophilic factor (human) *on page 81*
hemorrhoidal HC *see* hydrocortisone (topical) *on page 450*
Hemril® -30 *see* hydrocortisone (topical) *on page 450*
HepA *see* hepatitis A vaccine *on page 437*
HepaGam B® *see* hepatitis B immune globulin (human) *on page 438*

HepaGam B™ (Can) *see* hepatitis B immune globulin (human) *on page 438*

HepA-HepB *see* hepatitis A and hepatitis B recombinant vaccine *on page 437*

Hepalean® (Can) *see* heparin *on page 436*

Hepalean® Leo (Can) *see* heparin *on page 436*

Hepalean®-LOK (Can) *see* heparin *on page 436*

heparin (HEP a rin)

Medication Safety Issues

Sound-alike/look-alike issues:
Heparin may be confused with Hespan®

High alert medication:
The Institute for Safe Medication Practices (ISMP) includes this medication among its list of drugs which have a heightened risk of causing significant patient harm when used in error.

2009 National Patient Safety Goals:
The Joint Commission (TJC) requires healthcare organizations that provide anticoagulant therapy to have a process in place to reduce the risk of anticoagulant-associated patient harm. Patients receiving anticoagulants should receive individualized care through a defined process that includes standardized ordering, dispensing, administration, monitoring, and education. This does not apply to routine short-term use of anticoagulants for prevention of venous thromboembolism when the expectation is that the patient's laboratory values will remain within or close to normal values (NPSG.03.05.01).

Administration issues:
The 100 unit/mL concentration should not be used to flush heparin locks, I.V. lines, or intra-arterial lines in neonates or infants <10 kg (systemic anticoagulation may occur). The 10 unit/mL flush concentration may inadvertently cause systemic anticoagulation in infants <1 kg who receive frequent flushes.

Other safety concerns:
Heparin sodium injection 10,000 units/mL and Hep-Lock U/P 10 units/mL have been confused with each other. Fatal medication errors have occurred between the two whose labels are both blue. **Never rely on color as a sole indicator to differentiate product identity.**

Heparin lock flush solution is intended only to maintain patency of I.V. devices and is **not** to be used for anticoagulant therapy.

Synonyms heparin calcium; heparin lock flush; heparin sodium

U.S. Brand Names Hep-Lock; Hep-Lock U/P; HepFlush®-10

Canadian Brand Names Hepalean®; Hepalean® Leo; Hepalean®-LOK

Therapeutic Category Anticoagulant (Other)

Use Prophylaxis and treatment of thromboembolic disorders; as an anticoagulant for extracorporeal and dialysis procedures

Note: Heparin lock flush solution is intended only to maintain patency of I.V. devices and is **not** to be used for systemic anticoagulant therapy.

General Dosage Range

I.V.:
Children: Bolus: 50-100 units/kg; Initial infusion: 15-25 units/kg/hour; Maintenance: Increase dose by 2-4 units/kg/hour every 6-8 hours as needed **or** 50-100 units/kg every 4 hours intermittently

Adults: Bolus: 60-80 units/kg; Infusion: 10-30 units/kg/hour **or** 10,000 units (initially), then 50-70 units/kg (5000-10,000 units) every 4-6 hours intermittently

SubQ: *Adults:* Thromboprophylaxis: 5000 units every 8-12 hours; Treatment: 17,500 units every 12 hours

Dosage Forms

Infusion, premixed in 1/2 NS: 25,000 units (250 mL, 500 mL)

Infusion, premixed in D₅W: 10,000 units (100 mL, 250 mL); 12,500 units (250 mL); 20,000 units (500 mL); 25,000 units (250 mL, 500 mL)

Infusion, premixed in NS: 1000 units (500 mL); 2000 units (1000 mL)

Infusion, premixed in NS [preservative free]: 1000 units (500 mL); 2000 units (1000 mL)

Injection, solution: 10 units/mL (1 mL, 2 mL, 3 mL, 5 mL, 10 mL, 30 mL); 100 units/mL (1 mL, 2 mL, 3 mL, 5 mL, 10 mL, 30 mL); 1000 units/mL (1 mL, 10 mL, 30 mL); 5000 units/mL (1 mL, 10 mL); 10,000 units/mL (1 mL, 4 mL, 5 mL); 20,000 units/mL (1 mL)

Hep-Lock: 10 units/mL (1 mL, 2 mL, 10 mL, 30 mL); 100 units/mL (1 mL, 2 mL, 10 mL, 30 mL)

Injection, solution [preservative free]: 1 units/mL (2 mL, 3 mL, 5 mL); 2 units/mL (3 mL); 10 units/mL (1 mL, 2 mL, 2.5 mL, 3 mL, 5 mL, 6 mL, 10 mL); 100 units/mL (1 mL, 2 mL, 2.5 mL, 3 mL, 5 mL, 10 mL); 1000 units/mL (2 mL); 5000 units/mL (0.5 mL); 10,000 units/mL (0.5 mL)
Hep-Lock U/P: 10 units/mL (1 mL); 100 units/mL (1 mL)
HepFlush®-10: 10 units/mL (10 mL)
Injection, solution, oral: 10,000 units/mL (1 mL)

heparin calcium *see* heparin *on page* 436
heparin lock flush *see* heparin *on page* 436
heparin sodium *see* heparin *on page* 436
HepatAmine® *see* amino acid injection *on page* 65
Hepatasol® *see* amino acid injection *on page* 65

hepatitis A and hepatitis B recombinant vaccine
(hep a TYE tis aye & hep a TYE tis bee ree KOM be nant vak SEEN)

Synonyms Engerix-B® and Havrix®; Havrix® and Engerix-B®; HepA-HepB; hepatitis B and hepatitis A vaccine

U.S. Brand Names Twinrix®

Canadian Brand Names Twinrix®; Twinrix® Junior

Therapeutic Category Vaccine

Use Active immunization against disease caused by hepatitis A virus and hepatitis B virus (all known subtypes) in populations desiring protection against or at high risk of exposure to these viruses.

Populations include travelers or people living in or relocating to areas of intermediate/high endemicity for **both** HAV and HBV and are at increased risk of HBV infection due to behavioral or occupational factors; patients with chronic liver disease; laboratory workers who handle live HAV and HBV; healthcare workers, police, and other personnel who render first-aid or medical assistance; workers who come in contact with sewage; employees of day care centers and correctional facilities; patients/staff of hemodialysis units; men who have sex with men; patients frequently receiving blood products; military personnel; users of injectable illicit drugs; close household contacts of patients with hepatitis A and hepatitis B infection; residents of drug and alcohol treatment centers

General Dosage Range I.M.: *Adults:* 3 doses (1 mL each) given on a 0-, 1-, and 6-month schedule

Dosage Forms

Injection, suspension [preservative free]:
Twinrix®: Hepatitis A virus antigen 720 ELISA units and hepatitis B surface antigen 20 mcg per mL (1 mL)

Dosage Forms - Canada

Injection, suspension [preservative free]:
Twinrix® Junior: Hepatitis A virus antigen 360 ELISA units and hepatitis B surface antigen 10 mcg per 0.5 mL (0.5 mL)

hepatitis A vaccine (hep a TYE tis aye vak SEEN)

Medication Safety Issues

International issues:
Avaxim [Canada and multiple international markets] may be confused with Avastin brand name for bevacizumab [U.S., Canada, and multiple international markets]

Synonyms HepA

U.S. Brand Names Havrix®; VAQTA®

Canadian Brand Names Avaxim®; Avaxim®-Pediatric; HAVRIX®; VAQTA®

Therapeutic Category Vaccine, Inactivated Virus

Use

Active immunization against disease caused by hepatitis A virus (HAV)

The Advisory Committee on Immunization Practices (ACIP) recommends routine vaccination for:
- All children ≥12 months of age
- All unvaccinated adults requesting protection from HAV infection
- All unvaccinated adults at risk for HAV infection, such as:
  Behavioral risks: Men who have sex with men; injection drug users
  Occupational risks: Persons who work with HAV-infected primates or with HAV in a research laboratory setting

◄ Medical risks: Persons with chronic liver disease; patients who receive clotting-factor concentrates
- Other risks: International travelers to regions with high or intermediate levels of endemic HAV infection (a list of countries is available at http://wwwn.cdc.gov/travel/contentdiseases.aspx)
- Unvaccinated persons who anticipate close personal contact with international adoptee from a country of intermediate to high endemicity of HAV, during their first 60 days of arrival into the United States (eg, household contacts, babysitters)

General Dosage Range I.M.:
Children 12 months to 18 years: 0.5 mL
Adults: 1 mL

Dosage Forms
Injection, suspension [preservative free]:
Havrix®: Hepatitis A virus antigen 720 ELISA units/0.5 mL (0.5 mL); Hepatitis A virus antigen 1440 ELISA units/mL (1 mL)
VAQTA®: Hepatitis A virus antigen 25 units/0.5 mL (0.5 mL); Hepatitis A virus antigen 50 units/mL (1 mL)

hepatitis B and hepatitis A vaccine *see* hepatitis A and hepatitis B recombinant vaccine
on page 437

hepatitis B immune globulin (human) (hep a TYE tis bee i MYUN GLOB yoo lin YU man)

Medication Safety Issues
Sound-alike/look-alike issues:
HBIG may be confused with BabyBIG

Synonyms HBIG

U.S. Brand Names HepaGam B®; HyperHEP B™ S/D; Nabi-HB®

Canadian Brand Names HepaGam B™; HyperHep B®

Therapeutic Category Immune Globulin

Use
Passive prophylactic immunity to hepatitis B following: Acute exposure to blood containing hepatitis B surface antigen (HBsAg); perinatal exposure of infants born to HBsAg-positive mothers; sexual exposure to HBsAg-positive persons; household exposure to persons with acute HBV infection
Prevention of hepatitis B virus recurrence after liver transplantation in HBsAg-positive transplant patients
Note: Hepatitis B immune globulin is not indicated for treatment of active hepatitis B infection and is ineffective in the treatment of chronic active hepatitis B infection.

General Dosage Range
I.M.:
Newborns and Infants <12 months: 0.5 mL as a single dose
Children ≥12 months and Adults: 0.06 mL/kg as a single dose; may repeat in 28-30 days
I.V.: *Adults:* 20,000 int. units/dose daily for 8 days, then every 2 weeks, then once monthly

Dosage Forms
Injection, solution [preservative free]:
HepaGam B®: Anti-HBs > 312 int. units/mL (1 mL, 5 mL)
HyperHEP B™ S/D: Anti-HBs ≥ 220 int. units/mL (0.5 mL, 1 mL, 5 mL)
Nabi-HB®: Anti-HBs > 312 int. units/mL (1 mL, 5 mL)

hepatitis B inactivated virus vaccine (recombinant DNA) *see* hepatitis B vaccine (recombinant) on page 438

hepatitis B vaccine (recombinant) (hep a TYE tis bee vak SEEN ree KOM be nant)

Medication Safety Issues
Sound-alike/look-alike issues:
Engerix-B® adult may be confused with Engerix-B® pediatric/adolescent
Recombivax HB® may be confused with Comvax®

Synonyms hepatitis B inactivated virus vaccine (recombinant DNA); HepB

U.S. Brand Names Engerix-B®; Recombivax HB®

Canadian Brand Names Engerix-B®; Recombivax HB®

Therapeutic Category Vaccine, Inactivated Virus

Use Immunization against infection caused by all known subtypes of hepatitis B virus (HBV)

The Advisory Committee on Immunization Practices (ACIP) recommends routine vaccination for the following (CDC 2006; CDC 2005):
- All infants at birth
- All infants and children (post-birth dose; refer to recommended vaccination schedule)
- All unvaccinated adults requesting protection from HBV infection
- All unvaccinated adults at risk for HBV infection such as those with:
  Behavioral risks: Sexually-active persons with >1 partner in a 6-month period; persons seeking evaluation or treatment for a sexually-transmitted disease; men who have sex with men; injection drug users
  Occupational risks: Healthcare and public safety workers with reasonably anticipated risk for exposure to blood or blood contaminated body fluids
  Medical risks: Persons with end-stage renal disease (including predialysis, hemodialysis, peritoneal dialysis, and home dialysis); persons with HIV infection; persons with chronic liver disease
  Other risks: Household contacts and sex partners of persons with chronic HBV infection; residents and staff of facilities for developmentally disabled persons; international travelers to regions with high or intermediate levels of endemic HBV infection

In addition, the ACIP recommends vaccination for any persons who are wounded in bombings or similar mass casualty events who have penetrating injuries or nonintact skin exposure, or who have contact with mucous membranes (exception - superficial contact with intact skin), and who cannot confirm receipt of a hepatitis B vaccination (CDC, 2008).

General Dosage Range Dosage adjustment recommended in patients with renal impairment.
I.M.:
Birth to 19 years: 0.5 mL
Adults ≥20 years: 1 mL

Dosage Forms
Injection, suspension [preservative free]:
  Engerix-B®: Hepatitis B surface antigen 10 mcg/0.5 mL (0.5 mL); Hepatitis B surface antigen 20 mcg/mL (1 mL)
  Recombivax HB®: Hepatitis B surface antigen 5 mcg/0.5 mL (0.5 mL); Hepatitis B surface antigen 10 mcg/mL (1 mL); Hepatitis B surface antigen 40 mcg/mL (1 mL)

hepatitis B vaccine (recombinant) *see Haemophilus* B conjugate and hepatitis B vaccine *on page 432*

HepB *see hepatitis B vaccine (recombinant) on page 438*

HepFlush®-10 *see heparin on page 436*

Hep-Lock *see heparin on page 436*

Hep-Lock U/P *see heparin on page 436*

Hepsera® *see adefovir on page 41*

Hepsera™ (Can) *see adefovir on page 41*

Heptovir® (Can) *see lamivudine on page 508*

Herceptin® *see trastuzumab on page 882*

HES *see hetastarch on page 439*

HES *see pentastarch on page 686*

HES *see tetrastarch on page 858*

HES 130/0.4 *see tetrastarch on page 858*

Hespan® *see hetastarch on page 439*

hetastarch (HET a starch)

Medication Safety Issues
  Sound-alike/look-alike issues:
    Hespan® may be confused with heparin
Synonyms HES; hydroxyethyl starch
U.S. Brand Names Hespan®; Hextend®
Canadian Brand Names Hextend®
Therapeutic Category Plasma Volume Expander
Use Blood volume expander used in treatment of hypovolemia; adjunct in leukapheresis to improve harvesting and increase the yield of granulocytes by centrifugation (Hespan®)

◀ **General Dosage Range** Dosage adjustment recommended in patients with renal impairment
I.V.: *Adults:* 500-1500 mL/day **or** 20 mL/kg/day (up to 1500 mL/day)
Leukapheresis: *Adults:* 250-700 mL
Dosage Forms
Infusion:
Hextend®: 6% (500 mL)
Infusion, premixed in NS: 6% (500 mL)
Hespan®: 6% (500 mL)

Hexabrix™ *see* ioxaglate meglumine and ioxaglate sodium *on page 487*
hexachlorocyclohexane *see* lindane *on page 528*

hexachlorophene (heks a KLOR oh feen)

Medication Safety Issues
Sound-alike/look-alike issues:
pHisoHex® may be confused with Fostex®, pHisoDerm®
U.S. Brand Names pHisoHex®
Canadian Brand Names pHisoHex®
Therapeutic Category Antibacterial, Topical
Use Surgical scrub and as a bacteriostatic skin cleanser; control an outbreak of gram-positive infection when other procedures have been unsuccessful
General Dosage Range Topical: *Children and Adults:* Apply 5 mL cleanser and water to area to be cleansed
Dosage Forms
Liquid, topical:
pHisoHex®: 3% (150 mL, 480 mL)

Hexalen® *see* altretamine *on page 59*
hexamethylenetetramine *see* methenamine *on page 569*
hexamethylmelamine *see* altretamine *on page 59*

hexaminolevulinate (hex a mee noe LEV ue lin ate)

Synonyms HAL; hexaminolevulinate hydrochloride
U.S. Brand Names Cysview™
Therapeutic Category Contrast Agent
Use Detection of non-muscle invasive papillary cancer of the bladder; used in conjunction with the Karl Storz D-Light C Photodynamic Diagnostic (PDD) system
General Dosage Range Intravesical instillation: *Adults:* 50 mL instilled into empty bladder via urinary catheter
Dosage Forms
Powder for solution, intravesical:
Cysview™: 100 mg

hexaminolevulinate hydrochloride *see* hexaminolevulinate *on page 440*
Hexit™ (Can) *see* lindane *on page 528*
HEXM *see* altretamine *on page 59*
Hextend® *see* hetastarch *on page 439*

hexylresorcinol (heks il re ZOR si nole)

U.S. Brand Names Sucrets® Original [OTC]
Therapeutic Category Local Anesthetic
Use Minor antiseptic and local anesthetic for sore throat; topical antiseptic for minor cuts or abrasions
General Dosage Range Oral: *Children ≥6 years and Adults:* Up to 10 lozenges/day
Dosage Forms
Lozenge, oral:
Sucrets® Original [OTC]: 2.4 mg (18s)

hFSH *see* urofollitropin *on page 902*
hGH *see* somatropin *on page 826*
hib *see* Haemophilus B conjugate vaccine *on page 432*

hib conjugate vaccine *see Haemophilus* B conjugate and hepatitis B vaccine *on page 432*
hib conjugate vaccine *see Haemophilus* B conjugate vaccine *on page 432*
Hiberix® *see Haemophilus* B conjugate vaccine *on page 432*
hib-hepB *see Haemophilus* B conjugate and hepatitis B vaccine *on page 432*
Hibiclens® [OTC] *see* chlorhexidine gluconate *on page 194*
Hibidil® 1:2000 (Can) *see* chlorhexidine gluconate *on page 194*
Hibistat® [OTC] *see* chlorhexidine gluconate *on page 194*
hib polysaccharide conjugate *see Haemophilus* B conjugate vaccine *on page 432*
High Gamma Vitamin E Complete™ [OTC] *see* vitamin E *on page 918*
high-molecular-weight iron dextran (DexFerrum®) *see* iron dextran complex *on page 491*
Hi-Kovite [OTC] *see* vitamins (multiple/oral) *on page 919*
Hiprex® *see* methenamine *on page 569*
hirulog *see* bivalirudin *on page 137*
Histacol™ BD [DSC] *see* brompheniramine, pseudoephedrine, and dextromethorphan *on page 144*
Histantil (Can) *see* promethazine *on page 742*
Histaprin [OTC] *see* diphenhydramine (systemic) *on page 290*
Histatab PH [DSC] *see* chlorpheniramine, phenylephrine, and methscopolamine *on page 200*
Hista-Vent® PSE [DSC] *see* chlorpheniramine, pseudoephedrine, and methscopolamine *on page 202*
Hizentra® *see* immune globulin *on page 468*
hMG *see* menotropins *on page 559*
HMM *see* altretamine *on page 59*
HMR 3647 *see* telithromycin *on page 847*
HN$_2$ *see* mechlorethamine *on page 552*
Hold® DM [OTC] *see* dextromethorphan *on page 270*

homatropine (hoe MA troe peen)

Medication Safety Issues
Sound-alike/look-alike issues:
Homatropine may be confused with Humatrope®, somatropin
Synonyms homatropine hydrobromide
U.S. Brand Names Isopto® Homatropine
Therapeutic Category Anticholinergic Agent
Use Producing cycloplegia and mydriasis for refraction; treatment of acute inflammatory conditions of the uveal tract; optical aid in axial lens opacities
General Dosage Range Ophthalmic:
Children: Instill 1 drop (2% solution) 2-3 times/day **or** immediately prior to procedure, repeat every 10 minutes as needed
Adults: Instill 1-2 drops (2% or 5% solution) 2-3 times/day, up to every 3-4 hours as needed **or** 1-2 drops (2% solution) or 1 drop (5% solution) prior to procedure, repeat every 5-10 minutes as needed up to 3 doses
Dosage Forms
Solution, ophthalmic:
Isopto® Homatropine: 2% (5 mL); 5% (5 mL)

homatropine and hydrocodone *see* hydrocodone and homatropine *on page 448*
homatropine hydrobromide *see* homatropine *on page 441*
Homocysteine Guard [OTC] *see* folic acid, cyanocobalamin, and pyridoxine *on page 396*
Horizant™ *see* gabapentin enacarbil *on page 406*
horse antihuman thymocyte gamma globulin *see* antithymocyte globulin (equine) *on page 83*
12 Hour Nasal Relief [OTC] *see* oxymetazoline (nasal) *on page 664*
H.P. Acthar® *see* corticotropin *on page 236*
hpAT *see* antithrombin III *on page 83*
Hp-PAC® (Can) *see* lansoprazole, amoxicillin, and clarithromycin *on page 511*
HPV2 *see* papillomavirus (types 16, 18) vaccine (human, recombinant) *on page 673*
HPV4 *see* papillomavirus (types 6, 11, 16, 18) vaccine (human, recombinant) *on page 674*

HPV 16/18 L1 VLP/AS04 VAC *see* papillomavirus (types 16, 18) vaccine (human, recombinant) *on page 673*

HPV vaccine *see* papillomavirus (types 6, 11, 16, 18) vaccine (human, recombinant) *on page 674*

HPV vaccine *see* papillomavirus (types 16, 18) vaccine (human, recombinant) *on page 673*

HRIG *see* rabies immune globulin (human) *on page 764*

HTF919 *see* tegaserod *on page 846*

HumaLOG® *see* insulin lispro *on page 478*

Humalog® (Can) *see* insulin lispro *on page 478*

HumaLOG® KwikPen™ *see* insulin lispro *on page 478*

Humalog® Mix 25 (Can) *see* insulin lispro protamine and insulin lispro *on page 478*

HumaLOG® Mix 50/50™ *see* insulin lispro protamine and insulin lispro *on page 478*

HumaLOG® Mix 50/50™ KwikPen™ *see* insulin lispro protamine and insulin lispro *on page 478*

HumaLOG® Mix 75/25™ *see* insulin lispro protamine and insulin lispro *on page 478*

HumaLOG® Mix 75/25™ KwikPen™ *see* insulin lispro protamine and insulin lispro *on page 478*

Human Albumin Grifols® 25% *see* albumin *on page 44*

human antitumor necrosis factor alpha *see* adalimumab *on page 40*

human C1 inhibitor *see* C1 inhibitor (human) *on page 156*

human corticotrophin-releasing hormone, analogue *see* corticorelin *on page 236*

human diploid cell cultures rabies vaccine *see* rabies vaccine *on page 764*

human growth hormone *see* somatropin *on page 826*

humanized IgG1 anti-CD52 monoclonal antibody *see* alemtuzumab *on page 48*

human LFA-3/IgG(1) fusion protein *see* alefacept *on page 48*

human menopausal gonadotropin *see* menotropins *on page 559*

human papillomavirus vaccine *see* papillomavirus (types 6, 11, 16, 18) vaccine (human, recombinant) *on page 674*

human papillomavirus vaccine *see* papillomavirus (types 16, 18) vaccine (human, recombinant) *on page 673*

human rotavirus vaccine, attenuated (HRV) *see* rotavirus vaccine *on page 792*

human thyroid stimulating hormone *see* thyrotropin alpha *on page 866*

Humate-P® *see* antihemophilic factor/von Willebrand factor complex (human) *on page 82*

Humatin® (Can) *see* paromomycin *on page 675*

Humatrope® *see* somatropin *on page 826*

huMax-CD20 *see* ofatumumab *on page 643*

Humibid® Maximum Strength [OTC] *see* guaifenesin *on page 425*

Humira® *see* adalimumab *on page 40*

Humira® Pen *see* adalimumab *on page 40*

HuMist® [OTC] *see* sodium chloride *on page 818*

HuMist® for Kids [OTC] *see* sodium chloride *on page 818*

Humulin® 20/80 (Can) *see* insulin NPH and insulin regular *on page 479*

HumuLIN® 70/30 *see* insulin NPH and insulin regular *on page 479*

Humulin® 70/30 (Can) *see* insulin NPH and insulin regular *on page 479*

HumuLIN® N *see* insulin NPH *on page 479*

Humulin® N (Can) *see* insulin NPH *on page 479*

HumuLIN® R *see* insulin regular *on page 480*

Humulin® R (Can) *see* insulin regular *on page 480*

HumuLIN® R U-500 *see* insulin regular *on page 480*

Hurricaine® [OTC] *see* benzocaine *on page 121*

HXM *see* altretamine *on page 59*

Hyalgan® *see* hyaluronate and derivatives *on page 443*

hyaluronan *see* hyaluronate and derivatives *on page 443*

hyaluronate and derivatives (hye al yoor ON ate & dah RIV ah tives)

Medication Safety Issues

Sound-alike/look-alike issues:

Synvisc® may be confused with Synagis®

Synonyms hyaluronan; hyaluronic acid; hylan G-F 20; hylan polymers; sodium hyaluronate

U.S. Brand Names Amvisc®; Amvisc® Plus; Bionect®; Euflexxa®; Hyalgan®; Juvéderm® Ultra; Juvéderm® Ultra Plus; Juvéderm® Ultra Plus XC; Juvéderm® Ultra XC; Orthovisc®; Perlane®; Provisc®; Restylane®; Supartz®; Synvisc-One®; Synvisc®

Canadian Brand Names Cystistat®; Durolane®; Eyestil; Healon GV®; Healon®; OrthoVisc®; Suplasyn®

Therapeutic Category Antirheumatic Miscellaneous; Ophthalmic Agent, Viscoelastic; Skin and Mucous Membrane Agent

Use

Intraarticular injection: Treatment of pain in osteoarthritis in knee in patients who have failed nonpharmacologic treatment and simple analgesics

Intradermal: Correction of moderate-to-severe facial wrinkles or folds

Ophthalmic: Surgical aid in cataract extraction, intraocular implantation, corneal transplant, glaucoma filtration, and retinal attachment surgery

Topical cream, gel: Management of skin ulcers and wounds

General Dosage Range

Intraarticular: *Adults:* 16-30 mg once weekly for 3-5 doses (total injections: 3-5) **or** 48 mg once

Intradermal: *Adults:* Inject as required for cosmetic effect (maximum: 20 mL/60 kg/year [Juvederm® all formulations] or maximum: 6 mL/treatment [Perlane®, Restylane®])

Ophthalmic: *Adults:* Depends upon procedure (slowly introduce a sufficient quantity into eye)

Topical: *Adults:* Apply to affected area 2-3 times daily

Dosage Forms

Cream, topical:

Bionect®: 0.2% (25 g)

Gel, topical:

Bionect®: 0.2% (30 g, 60 g)

Injection, gel, intradermal [hyaluronate acid]:

Juvéderm® Ultra: 24 mg/mL (0.4 mL, 0.8 mL)

Juvéderm® Ultra Plus: 24 mg/mL (0.4 mL, 0.8 mL)

Juvéderm® Ultra Plus XC: Hyaluronic acid 24 mg/mL and lidocaine 0.3% (0.4 mL, 0.8 mL)

Juvéderm® Ultra XC: Hyaluronic acid 24 mg/mL and lidocaine 0.3% (0.4 mL, 0.8 mL)

Injection, gel, intradermal [sodium hyaluronate]:

Perlane®: 20 mg/mL (1 mL)

Restylane®: 20 mg/mL (0.4 mL, 1 mL, 2 mL)

Injection, solution, intra-articular:

Euflexxa®: 10 mg/mL (2 mL)

Hyalgan®: 10 mg/mL (2 mL)

Orthovisc®: 15 mg/mL (2 mL)

Supartz®: 10 mg/mL (2.5 mL)

Synvisc-One®: 8 mg/mL (6 mL)

Synvisc®: 8 mg/mL (2 mL)

Injection, solution, intraocular:

Amvisc®: 12 mg/mL (0.5 mL, 0.8 mL)

Amvisc® Plus: 16 mg/mL (0.5 mL, 0.8 mL)

Provisc®: 10 mg/mL (0.4 mL, 0.55 mL, 0.85 mL)

hyaluronic acid *see* hyaluronate and derivatives *on page 443*

hyaluronidase (hye al yoor ON i dase)

Medication Safety Issues

Sound-alike/look-alike issues:

Wydase may be confused with Lidex®, Wyamine®

U.S. Brand Names Amphadase™; Hylenex; Vitrase®

Therapeutic Category Enzyme

Use Increase the dispersion and absorption of other injected drugs; increase rate of absorption of parenteral fluids given by subcutaneous administration (hypodermoclysis)

◀ **General Dosage Range**
Intradermal: *Children and Adults:* 0.02 mL (3 units) of a 150 units/mL solution
SubQ:
Premature Infants: Volume of a single clysis/day should not exceed 25 mL/kg; rate of administration should not exceed 2 mL/minute
Children <3 years: Volume of a single clysis should not exceed 200 mL **or** 75 units over each scapula followed by injection of contrast medium at the same site
Children ≥3 years and Adults: Rate and volume of a single clysis should not exceed those used for infusion of I.V. fluids **or** 75 units over each scapula followed by injection of contrast medium at the same site

Dosage Forms
Injection, solution:
Amphadase™: 150 units/mL (1 mL)
Injection, solution [preservative free]:
Hylenex: 150 units/mL (1 mL)
Vitrase®: 200 units/mL (2 mL)

hycamptamine *see* topotecan *on page 878*
Hycamtin® *see* topotecan *on page 878*
hycet® *see* hydrocodone and acetaminophen *on page 446*
Hycodan® [DSC] *see* hydrocodone and homatropine *on page 448*
Hycort™ (Can) *see* hydrocortisone (topical) *on page 450*
Hydeltra T.B.A.® (Can) *see* prednisolone (systemic) *on page 734*
Hydergine [DSC] *see* ergoloid mesylates *on page 336*
Hydergine® (Can) *see* ergoloid mesylates *on page 336*
Hyderm (Can) *see* hydrocortisone (topical) *on page 450*

hydralazine (hye DRAL a zeen)

Medication Safety Issues
Sound-alike/look-alike issues:
HydrALAZINE may be confused with hydrOXYzine
Synonyms Apresoline [DSC]; hydralazine hydrochloride
Tall-Man hydrALAZINE
Canadian Brand Names Apo-Hydralazine®; Apresoline®; Novo-Hylazin; Nu-Hydral
Therapeutic Category Vasodilator
Use Management of moderate-to-severe hypertension
General Dosage Range Dosage adjustment recommended in patients with renal impairment
I.M., I.V.:
Children: 0.1-0.2 mg/kg/dose (not to exceed 20 mg) every 4-6 hours as needed (maximum: 3.5 mg/kg/day in 4-6 divided doses)
Adults: Initial: 10-20 mg/dose every 4-6 hours as needed; Maintenance: Up to 40 mg/dose every 4-6 hours **or** Eclampsia/pre-eclampsia: 5 mg/dose then 5-10 mg every 20-30 minutes as needed
Oral:
Children: Initial: 0.75-1 mg/kg/day in 2-4 divided doses; Maintenance: Up to 7.5 mg/kg/day in 2-4 divided doses (maximum: 200 mg/day)
Adults: Initial: 10-25 mg 3-4 times/day; Maintenance: 25-300 mg/day (target dose: 225-300 mg/day for CHF) in 2-4 divided doses (maximum: 300 mg/day)
Elderly: Initial: 10 mg 2-3 times/day, increase by 10-25 mg/day every 2-5 days; Target dose: 225-300 mg/day for CHF

Dosage Forms
Injection, solution: 20 mg/mL (1 mL)
Tablet, oral: 10 mg, 25 mg, 50 mg, 100 mg

hydralazine and isosorbide dinitrate *see* isosorbide dinitrate and hydralazine *on page 494*
hydralazine hydrochloride *see* hydralazine *on page 444*
hydrated chloral *see* chloral hydrate *on page 193*
Hydrea® *see* hydroxyurea *on page 456*
Hydrisalic® [OTC] *see* salicylic acid *on page 795*
Hydro 35™ *see* urea *on page 900*

Hydro 40™ *see* urea *on page 900*

hydrochlorothiazide (hye droe klor oh THYE a zide)
Medication Safety Issues
  Sound-alike/look-alike issues:
   Esidrix may be confused with Lasix®
   HCTZ is an error-prone abbreviation (mistaken as hydrocortisone)
   Hydrochlorothiazide may be confused with hydrocortisone, hydroflumethiazide, Viskazide®
   Microzide™ may be confused with Maxzide®, Micronase®
Synonyms HCTZ (error-prone abbreviation); Hydrodiuril
U.S. Brand Names Microzide®
Canadian Brand Names Apo-Hydro®; Bio-Hydrochlorothiazide; Dom-Hydrochlorothiazide; Novo-Hydrazide; Nu-Hydro; PMS-Hydrochlorothiazide
Therapeutic Category Diuretic, Thiazide
Use Management of mild-to-moderate hypertension; treatment of edema in heart failure and nephrotic syndrome
General Dosage Range Oral:
  Children <6 months: 1-3 mg/kg/day in 2 divided doses
  Children >6 months to 2 years: 1-3 mg/kg/day in 2 divided doses (maximum: 37.5 mg/day)
  Children >2-17 years: Initial: 1 mg/kg/day (maximum: 3 mg/kg/day [50 mg/day])
  Adults: 12.5-100 mg/day in 1-2 divided doses (maximum: 200 mg/day)
  Elderly: 12.5-25 once daily
Dosage Forms
  Capsule, oral: 12.5 mg
   Microzide®: 12.5 mg
  Tablet, oral: 12.5 mg, 25 mg, 50 mg

hydrochlorothiazide, aliskiren, and amlodipine *see* aliskiren, amlodipine, and hydrochlorothiazide *on page 52*
hydrochlorothiazide, amlodipine, and aliskiren *see* aliskiren, amlodipine, and hydrochlorothiazide *on page 52*
hydrochlorothiazide, amlodipine, and valsartan *see* amlodipine, valsartan, and hydrochlorothiazide *on page 71*
hydrochlorothiazide and aliskiren *see* aliskiren and hydrochlorothiazide *on page 52*
hydrochlorothiazide and amiloride *see* amiloride and hydrochlorothiazide *on page 64*
hydrochlorothiazide and benazepril *see* benazepril and hydrochlorothiazide *on page 119*
hydrochlorothiazide and bisoprolol *see* bisoprolol and hydrochlorothiazide *on page 136*
hydrochlorothiazide and candesartan *see* candesartan and hydrochlorothiazide *on page 167*
hydrochlorothiazide and captopril *see* captopril and hydrochlorothiazide *on page 170*
hydrochlorothiazide and cilazapril *see* cilazapril and hydrochlorothiazide *(Canada only) on page 208*
hydrochlorothiazide and enalapril *see* enalapril and hydrochlorothiazide *on page 327*
hydrochlorothiazide and eprosartan *see* eprosartan and hydrochlorothiazide *on page 335*
hydrochlorothiazide and fosinopril *see* fosinopril and hydrochlorothiazide *on page 401*
hydrochlorothiazide and irbesartan *see* irbesartan and hydrochlorothiazide *on page 490*
hydrochlorothiazide and lisinopril *see* lisinopril and hydrochlorothiazide *on page 532*
hydrochlorothiazide and losartan *see* losartan and hydrochlorothiazide *on page 538*
hydrochlorothiazide and methyldopa *see* methyldopa and hydrochlorothiazide *on page 575*
hydrochlorothiazide and metoprolol *see* metoprolol and hydrochlorothiazide *on page 582*
hydrochlorothiazide and metoprolol tartrate *see* metoprolol and hydrochlorothiazide *on page 582*
hydrochlorothiazide and moexipril *see* moexipril and hydrochlorothiazide *on page 595*
hydrochlorothiazide and olmesartan medoxomil *see* olmesartan and hydrochlorothiazide *on page 647*
hydrochlorothiazide and pindolol *see* pindolol and hydrochlorothiazide *(Canada only) on page 705*
hydrochlorothiazide and propranolol *see* propranolol and hydrochlorothiazide *on page 748*
hydrochlorothiazide and quinapril *see* quinapril and hydrochlorothiazide *on page 761*
hydrochlorothiazide and ramipril *see* ramipril and hydrochlorothiazide *(Canada only) on page 766*

hydrochlorothiazide and spironolactone
(hye droe klor oh THYE a zide & speer on oh LAK tone)

Medication Safety Issues

Sound-alike/look-alike issues:
Aldactazide® may be confused with Aldactone®

Synonyms spironolactone and hydrochlorothiazide

U.S. Brand Names Aldactazide®

Canadian Brand Names Aldactazide 25®; Aldactazide 50®; Novo-Spirozine

Therapeutic Category Antihypertensive Agent, Combination

Use Management of mild-to-moderate hypertension; treatment of edema in congestive heart failure and nephrotic syndrome, and cirrhosis of the liver accompanied by edema and/or ascites

General Dosage Range Oral: *Adults:* 12.5-50 mg hydrochlorothiazide and 12.5-50 mg spironolactone/day in 1-2 divided doses

Dosage Forms

Tablet: Hydrochlorothiazide 25 mg and spironolactone 25 mg
Aldactazide®: 25/25: Hydrochlorothiazide 25 mg and spironolactone 25 mg; 50/50: Hydrochlorothiazide 50 mg and spironolactone 50 mg

hydrochlorothiazide and telmisartan *see* telmisartan and hydrochlorothiazide *on page 848*

hydrochlorothiazide and triamterene (hye droe klor oh THYE a zide & trye AM ter een)

Medication Safety Issues

Sound-alike/look-alike issues:
Dyazide® may be confused with diazoxide, Dynacin®
Maxzide® may be confused with Maxidex®, Microzide®

Synonyms triamterene and hydrochlorothiazide

U.S. Brand Names Dyazide®; Maxzide®; Maxzide®-25

Canadian Brand Names Apo-Triazide®; Nu-Triazide; Pro-Triazide; Riva-Zide; Teva-Triamterene HCTZ

Therapeutic Category Antihypertensive Agent, Combination

Use Treatment of hypertension or edema (not recommended for initial treatment) when hypokalemia has developed on hydrochlorothiazide alone or when the development of hypokalemia must be avoided

General Dosage Range Oral: *Adults:* 25-50 mg hydrochlorothiazide and 37.5-75 mg triamterene once daily

Dosage Forms

Capsule: Hydrochlorothiazide 25 mg and triamterene 37.5 mg; hydrochlorothiazide 25 mg and triamterene 50 mg
Dyazide®: Hydrochlorothiazide 25 mg and triamterene 37.5 mg

Tablet: Hydrochlorothiazide 25 mg and triamterene 37.5 mg; hydrochlorothiazide 50 mg and triamterene 75 mg
Maxzide®: Hydrochlorothiazide 50 mg and triamterene 75 mg [scored]
Maxzide®-25: Hydrochlorothiazide 25 mg and triamterene 37.5 mg [scored]

hydrochlorothiazide and valsartan *see* valsartan and hydrochlorothiazide *on page 906*
hydrochlorothiazide, olmesartan, and amlodipine *see* olmesartan, amlodipine, and hydrochlorothiazide *on page 646*
Hydrocil® Instant [OTC] *see* psyllium *on page 755*

hydrocodone and acetaminophen (hye droe KOE done & a seet a MIN oh fen)

Medication Safety Issues

Sound-alike/look-alike issues:
Lorcet® may be confused with Fioricet®
Lortab® may be confused with Cortef®, Lorabid®
Vicodin® may be confused with Hycodan®, Hycomine®, Indocin®, Uridon®
Zydone® may be confused with Vytone®

High alert medication:
The Institute for Safe Medication Practices (ISMP) includes this medication among its list of drug classes which have a heightened risk of causing significant patient harm when used in error.

Other safety concerns:
Duplicate therapy issues: This product contains acetaminophen, which may be a component of other combination products. Do not exceed the maximum recommended daily dose of acetaminophen.

Synonyms acetaminophen and hydrocodone

U.S. Brand Names hycet®; Lorcet® 10/650; Lorcet® Plus; Lortab®; Margesic® H; Maxidone®; Norco®; Stagesic™; Vicodin®; Vicodin® ES; Vicodin® HP; Xodol® 10/300; Xodol® 5/300; Xodol® 7.5/300; Zamicet™; Zolvit™; Zydone®

Therapeutic Category Analgesic, Narcotic

Controlled Substance C-III

Use Relief of moderate-to-severe pain

General Dosage Range Oral:

Children 2-13 years or <50 kg: Hydrocodone 0.1-0.2 mg/kg/dose every 4-6 hours (maximum: 6 doses/day or maximum recommended dose of acetaminophen for age/weight)

Children ≥50 kg and Adults: Hydrocodone 2.5-10 mg every 4-6 hours (maximum: 4 g/day [acetaminophen])

Elderly: Hydrocodone 2.5-5 mg every 4-6 hours

Dosage Forms

Capsule, oral: Hydrocodone 5 mg and acetaminophen 500 mg

Margesic® H, Stagesic™: Hydrocodone 5 mg and acetaminophen 500 mg

Elixir, oral:

Lortab®: Hydrocodone 7.5 mg and acetaminophen 500 mg per 15 mL

Solution, oral: Hydrocodone 7.5 mg and acetaminophen 325 mg per 15 mL; hydrocodone 7.5 mg and acetaminophen 500 mg per 15 mL; hydrocodone 10 mg and acetaminophen 325 mg per 15 mL

hycet®: Hydrocodone 7.5 mg and acetaminophen 325 mg per 15 mL

Zamicet™: Hydrocodone 10 mg and acetaminophen 325 mg per 15 mL

Zolvit™: Hydrocodone 10 mg and acetaminophen 300 mg per 15 mL (480 mL)

Tablet, oral:

Generics:

Hydrocodone 2.5 mg and acetaminophen 500 mg

Hydrocodone 5 mg and acetaminophen 300 mg

Hydrocodone 5 mg and acetaminophen 325 mg

Hydrocodone 5 mg and acetaminophen 500 mg

Hydrocodone 7.5 mg and acetaminophen 300 mg

Hydrocodone 7.5 mg and acetaminophen 325 mg

Hydrocodone 7.5 mg and acetaminophen 500 mg

Hydrocodone 7.5 mg and acetaminophen 650 mg

Hydrocodone 7.5 mg and acetaminophen 750 mg

Hydrocodone 10 mg and acetaminophen 300 mg

Hydrocodone 10 mg and acetaminophen 325 mg

Hydrocodone 10 mg and acetaminophen 500 mg

Hydrocodone 10 mg and acetaminophen 650 mg

Hydrocodone 10 mg and acetaminophen 660 mg

Hydrocodone 10 mg and acetaminophen 750 mg

Brands:

Lorcet® 10/650: Hydrocodone 10 mg and acetaminophen 650 mg

Lorcet® Plus: Hydrocodone 7.5 mg and acetaminophen 650 mg

Lortab®: 5/500: Hydrocodone 5 mg and acetaminophen 500 mg; 7.5/500: Hydrocodone 7.5 mg and acetaminophen 500 mg; 10/500: Hydrocodone 10 mg and acetaminophen 500 mg

Maxidone®: Hydrocodone 10 mg and acetaminophen 750 mg

Norco®: Hydrocodone 5 mg and acetaminophen 325 mg; hydrocodone 7.5 mg and acetaminophen 325 mg; hydrocodone 10 mg and acetaminophen 325 mg

Vicodin®: Hydrocodone 5 mg and acetaminophen 500 mg

Vicodin® ES: Hydrocodone 7.5 mg and acetaminophen 750 mg

Vicodin® HP: Hydrocodone 10 mg and acetaminophen 660 mg

Xodol®: 5/300: Hydrocodone 5 mg and acetaminophen 300 mg; 7.5/300: Hydrocodone 7.5 mg and acetaminophen 300 mg; 10/300: Hydrocodone 10 mg and acetaminophen 300 mg

Zydone®: Hydrocodone 5 mg and acetaminophen 400 mg; hydrocodone 7.5 mg and acetaminophen 400 mg; hydrocodone 10 mg and acetaminophen 400 mg

hydrocodone and chlorpheniramine (hye droe KOE done & klor fen IR a meen)

Medication Safety Issues

Sound-alike/look-alike issues:

Tussionex® represents a different product in the U.S. than it does in Canada. In the U.S., Tussionex® contains hydrocodone and chlorpheniramine, while in Canada the product bearing this name contains hydrocodone and phenyltoloxamine.

Synonyms chlorpheniramine maleate and hydrocodone bitartrate; hydrocodone polistirex and chlorpheniramine polistirex

U.S. Brand Names TussiCaps®; Tussionex®

Therapeutic Category Antihistamine/Antitussive

Controlled Substance C-III

Use Symptomatic relief of cough and upper respiratory symptoms associated with cold and allergy

General Dosage Range Oral:

Children 6-12 years: TussiCaps® 5 mg/4 mg: 1 capsule every 12 hours (maximum: 2 capsules/24 hours); Tussionex®: 2.5 mL every 12 hours (maximum: 5 mL/24 hours)

Children >12 years and Adults: TussiCaps® 10 mg/8 mg: 1 capsule every 12 hours (maximum: 2 capsules/24 hours); Tussionex®: 5 mL every 12 hours (maximum: 10 mL/24 hours)

Dosage Forms

Capsule, extended release:

TussiCaps® 5/4: Hydrocodone bitartrate 5 mg and chlorpheniramine maleate 4 mg

TussiCaps® 10/8: Hydrocodone bitartrate 10 mg and chlorpheniramine maleate 8 mg

Suspension, extended release: Hydrocodone bitartrate 10 mg and chlorpheniramine maleate 8 mg per 5 mL

Tussionex®: Hydrocodone bitartrate 10 mg and chlorpheniramine maleate 8 mg per 5 mL

hydrocodone and homatropine (hye droe KOE done & hoe MA troe peen)

Medication Safety Issues

Sound-alike/look-alike issues:

Hycodan® may be confused with Hycomine®, Vicodin®

Synonyms homatropine and hydrocodone; hydrocodone bitartrate and homatropine methylbromide

U.S. Brand Names Hycodan® [DSC]; Hydromet®; Tussigon®

Therapeutic Category Antitussive

Controlled Substance C-III

Use Symptomatic relief of cough

General Dosage Range Oral:

Children 6-11 years: 1/2 tablet or 2.5 mL every 4-6 hours as needed (maximum: 3 tablets or 15 mL/24 hours)

Children ≥12 years and Adults: 1 tablet or 5 mL every 4-6 hours as needed (maximum: 6 tablets/24 hours or 30 mL/24 hours)

Dosage Forms

Syrup: Hydrocodone 5 mg and homatropine 1.5 mg per 5 mL

Hydromet®: Hydrocodone 5 mg and homatropine 1.5 mg per 5 mL

Tablet:

Tussigon®: Hydrocodone 5 mg and homatropine 1.5 mg

hydrocodone and ibuprofen (hye droe KOE done & eye byoo PROE fen)

Medication Safety Issues

Sound-alike/look-alike issues:

Reprexain™ may be confused with ZyPREXA®

High alert medication:

The Institute for Safe Medication Practices (ISMP) includes this medication among its list of drug classes which have a heightened risk of causing significant patient harm when used in error.

Synonyms hydrocodone bitartrate and ibuprofen; ibuprofen and hydrocodone

U.S. Brand Names Ibudone™; Reprexain™; Vicoprofen®

Canadian Brand Names Vicoprofen®

Therapeutic Category Analgesic, Narcotic

Controlled Substance C-III

Use Short-term (generally <10 days) management of moderate-to-severe acute pain; is not indicated for treatment of such conditions as osteoarthritis or rheumatoid arthritis

General Dosage Range Oral: *Adults:* 1 tablet every 4-6 hours (maximum: 5 tablets/day; <10 days total therapy)

Dosage Forms
Tablet: Hydrocodone 5 mg and ibuprofen 200 mg; hydrocodone 7.5 mg and ibuprofen 200 mg
   Ibudone™: 5/200: Hydrocodone 5 mg and ibuprofen 200 mg; 10/200: Hydrocodone 10 mg and ibuprofen 200 mg
   Reprexain™: 2.5/200: Hydrocodone 2.5 mg and ibuprofen 200 mg; 5/200: Hydrocodone 5 mg and ibuprofen 200 mg; 10/200: Hydrocodone 10 mg and ibuprofen 200 mg
   Vicoprofen®: 7.5/200: Hydrocodone 7.5 mg and ibuprofen 200 mg

hydrocodone and pseudoephedrine (hye droe KOE done & soo doe e FED rin)

Synonyms pseudoephedrine and hydrocodone; pseudoephedrine hydrochloride and hydrocodone bitartrate

U.S. Brand Names Rezira™

Therapeutic Category Antitussive/Decongestant

Controlled Substance C-III

Use Symptomatic relief of cough and nasal congestion associated with common cold

General Dosage Range Oral: *Adults:* 5 mL every 4-6 hours as needed (maximum: 20 mL/24 hours)

Dosage Forms
Solution, oral:
   Rezira™: Hydrocodone 5 mg and pseudoephedrine 60 mg per 5 mL (480 mL)

hydrocodone bitartrate and homatropine methylbromide *see* hydrocodone and homatropine *on page 448*

hydrocodone bitartrate and ibuprofen *see* hydrocodone and ibuprofen *on page 448*

hydrocodone, chlorpheniramine, and pseudoephedrine
(hye droe KOE done, klor fen IR a meen, & soo doe e FED rin)

Synonyms chlorpheniramine, pseudoephedrine, and hydrocodone; pseudoephedrine hydrochloride, hydrocodone bitartrate, and chlorpheniramine maleate; pseudoephedrine, hydrocodone, and chlorpheniramine

U.S. Brand Names Zutripro™

Therapeutic Category Alpha/Beta Agonist; Analgesic, Opioid; Antitussive; Decongestant; Histamine H$_1$ Antagonist; Histamine H$_1$ Antagonist, First Generation

Controlled Substance C-III

Use Temporary relief of cough and nasal congestion due to colds or upper respiratory allergies

General Dosage Range
Oral: *Adults:* 5 mL every 4-6 hours as needed (maximum: 4 doses/24 hours)

Dosage Forms
Solution, oral:
   Zutripro™: Hydrocodone bitartrate 5 mg, chlorpheniramine maleate 4 mg, and pseudoephedrine hydrochloride 60 mg per 5 mL (480 mL) [contains propylene glycol; grape flavor]

hydrocodone polistirex and chlorpheniramine polistirex *see* hydrocodone and chlorpheniramine *on page 448*

hydrocortisone (systemic) (hye droe KOR ti sone)

Medication Safety Issues
Sound-alike/look-alike issues:
   Hydrocortisone may be confused with hydrocodone, hydroxychloroquine, hydrochlorothiazide
   Cortef® may be confused with Coreg®, Lortab®
   HCT (occasional abbreviation for hydrocortisone) is an error-prone abbreviation (mistaken as hydrochlorothiazide)
   Solu-CORTEF® may be confused with Solu-MEDROL®

Synonyms A-hydroCort; compound F; cortisol; hydrocortisone sodium succinate

U.S. Brand Names A-Hydrocort®; Cortef®; Solu-CORTEF®

Canadian Brand Names Cortef®; Solu-Cortef®

Therapeutic Category Corticosteroid, Systemic

◀ **Use** Management of adrenocortical insufficiency; antiinflammatory or immunosuppressive

General Dosage Range

I.M., I.V. (succinate): *Children and Adults:* Dosage varies greatly depending on indication

Oral:

Children: 0.5-10 mg/kg/day **or** 10-300 mg/m^2/day divided every 6-8 hours

Adolescents: 0.5-10 mg/kg/day **or** 10-300 mg/m^2/day divided every 6-8 hours **or** 15-240 mg every 12 hours

Adults: 20-480 mg/day in divided doses every 8-12 hours **or** 10-20 mg/m^2/day in 3 divided doses

Dosage Forms

Injection, powder for reconstitution:

A-Hydrocort®: 100 mg

Solu-CORTEF®: 100 mg

Injection, powder for reconstitution [preservative free]:

Solu-CORTEF®: 100 mg, 250 mg, 500 mg, 1000 mg

Tablet, oral: 5 mg, 10 mg, 20 mg

Cortef®: 5 mg, 10 mg, 20 mg

hydrocortisone (topical) (hye droe KOR ti sone)

Medication Safety Issues

Sound-alike/look-alike issues:

Hydrocortisone may be confused with hydrocodone, hydroxychloroquine, hydrochlorothiazide

Anusol® may be confused with Anusol-HC®, Aplisol®, Aquasol®

Anusol-HC® may be confused with Anusol®

Cortizone® may be confused with cortisone

HCT (occasional abbreviation for hydrocortisone) is an error-prone abbreviation (mistaken as hydrochlorothiazide)

Hytone® may be confused with Vytone®

Proctocort® may be confused with ProctoCream®

ProctoCream® may be confused with Proctocort®

International issues:

Nutracort [U.S. and multiple international markets] may be confused with Nitrocor brand name of nitroglycerin [Italy, Russia, and Venezuela]

Synonyms A-hydroCort; compound F; cortisol; hemorrhoidal HC; hydrocortisone acetate; hydrocortisone butyrate; hydrocortisone probutate; hydrocortisone valerate

U.S. Brand Names Ala-Cort; Ala-Scalp; Anu-med HC; Anucort-HC™; Anusol-HC®; Aquanil HC® [OTC]; Beta-HC® [OTC]; Caldecort® [OTC]; Colocort®; Cortaid® Advanced [OTC]; Cortaid® Intensive Therapy [OTC]; Cortaid® Maximum Strength [OTC]; Cortenema®; CortiCool® [OTC]; Cortifoam®; Cortizone-10® Hydratensive Healing [OTC]; Cortizone-10® Hydratensive Soothing [OTC]; Cortizone-10® Intensive Healing Eczema [OTC]; Cortizone-10® Maximum Strength Cooling Relief [OTC]; Cortizone-10® Maximum Strength Easy Relief [OTC]; Cortizone-10® Maximum Strength Intensive Healing Formula [OTC]; Cortizone-10® Maximum Strength [OTC]; Cortizone-10® Plus Maximum Strength [OTC]; Dermarest® Eczema Medicated [OTC]; Hemril® -30; Hydrocortisone Plus [OTC]; Hydroskin® [OTC]; Locoid Lipocream®; Locoid®; Pandel®; Pediaderm™ HC; Preparation H® Hydrocortisone [OTC]; Procto-Pak™; Proctocort®; ProctoCream®-HC; Proctosol-HC®; Proctozone-HC 2.5%™; Recort [OTC]; Scalpana [OTC]; Texacort®; U-Cort®; Westcort®

Canadian Brand Names Aquacort®; Cortamed®; Cortenema®; Cortifoam™; Emo-Cort®; Hycort™; Hyderm; HydroVal®; Locoid®; Prevex® HC; Sarna® HC; Westcort®

Therapeutic Category Corticosteroid, Rectal; Corticosteroid, Topical

Use Relief of inflammation of corticosteroid-responsive dermatoses (low and medium potency topical corticosteroid); adjunctive treatment of ulcerative colitis

General Dosage Range

Rectal: *Adults:* 10-100 mg 1-2 times/day

Topical: *Children >2 years and Adults:* Apply to affected area 2-4 times/day

Dosage Forms

Aerosol, rectal:

Cortifoam®: 10% (15 g)

Cream, topical: 0.1% (15 g, 45 g); 0.2% (15 g, 45 g, 60 g); 0.5% (0.9 g, 15 g, 28.4 g, 30 g, 60 g); 1% (0.9 g, 1 g, 1.5 g, 15 g, 20 g, 28.35 g, 28.4 g, 30 g, 114 g, 120 g, 454 g); 2% (43 g); 2.5% (20 g, 28 g, 28.35 g, 30 g, 454 g)

Ala-Cort: 1% (28.4 g, 85.2 g)

Anusol-HC®: 2.5% (30 g)

Caldecort® [OTC]: 1% (28.4 g)
Cortaid® Advanced [OTC]: 1% (42 g)
Cortaid® Intensive Therapy [OTC]: 1% (37 g, 56 g)
Cortaid® Maximum Strength [OTC]: 1% (14 g, 28 g, 37 g, 56 g)
Cortizone-10® Maximum Strength [OTC]: 1% (15 g, 28 g, 56 g)
Cortizone-10® Maximum Strength Intensive Healing Formula [OTC]: 1% (28 g, 56 g)
Cortizone-10® Plus Maximum Strength [OTC]: 1% (28 g, 56 g)
Hydrocortisone Plus [OTC]: 1% (28.4 g)
Hydroskin® [OTC]: 1% (28 g)
Locoid Lipocream®: 0.1% (15 g, 45 g, 60 g)
Locoid®: 0.1% (15 g, 45 g)
Pandel®: 0.1% (15 g, 45 g, 80 g)
Preparation H® Hydrocortisone [OTC]: 1% (26 g)
Procto-Pak™: 1% (28.4 g)
Proctocort®: 1% (28.35 g)
ProctoCream®-HC: 2.5% (30 g)
Proctosol-HC®: 2.5% (28.35 g)
Proctozone-HC 2.5%™: 2.5% (30 g)
Recort [OTC]: 1% (30 g)
U-Cort®: 1% (28 g)
Gel, topical:
CortiCool® [OTC]: 1% (0.9 g, 42.5 g)
Cortizone-10® Maximum Strength Cooling Relief [OTC]: 1% (28 g)
Liquid, topical:
Cortizone-10® Maximum Strength Easy Relief [OTC]: 1% (36 mL)
Scalpana [OTC]: 1% (85.5 mL)
Lotion, topical: 1% (114 g, 118 mL, 120 mL); 2.5% (59 mL, 60 mL, 118 mL)
Ala-Scalp: 2% (29.6 mL)
Aquanil HC® [OTC]: 1% (120 mL)
Beta-HC® [OTC]: 1% (60 mL)
Cortaid® Intensive Therapy [OTC]: 1% (98 g)
Cortizone-10® Hydratensive Healing [OTC]: 1% (113 g)
Cortizone-10® Hydratensive Soothing [OTC]: 1% (113 g)
Cortizone-10® Intensive Healing Eczema [OTC]: 1% (99 g)
Dermarest® Eczema Medicated [OTC]: 1% (118 mL)
Hydroskin® [OTC]: 1% (118 mL)
Locoid®: 0.1% (60 mL)
Pediaderm™ HC: 2% (29.6 mL)
Ointment, topical: 0.1% (15 g, 45 g); 0.2% (15 g, 45 g, 60 g); 0.5% (30 g); 1% (25 g, 28.4 g, 30 g, 110 g, 430 g, 454 g); 2.5% (20 g, 28.35 g, 30 g, 454 g)
Cortaid® Maximum Strength [OTC]: 1% (28 g, 37 g)
Cortizone-10® Maximum Strength [OTC]: 1% (28 g, 56 g)
Locoid®: 0.1% (15 g, 45 g)
Westcort®: 0.2% (15 g, 45 g, 60 g)
Powder, for prescription compounding: USP: 100% (10 g, 25 g, 50 g, 100 g, 1000 g)
Solution, topical: 0.1% (20 mL, 60 mL)
Cortaid® Intensive Therapy [OTC]: 1% (59 mL)
Locoid®: 0.1% (20 mL, 60 mL)
Texacort®: 2.5% (30 mL)
Suppository, rectal: 25 mg (12s, 24s, 1000s); 30 mg (12s)
Anu-med HC: 25 mg (12s)
Anucort-HC™: 25 mg (12s, 24s, 100s)
Anusol-HC®: 25 mg (12s, 24s)
Hemril® -30: 30 mg (12s, 24s)
Proctocort®: 30 mg (12s, 24s)
Suspension, rectal: 100 mg/60 mL (60 mL)
Colocort®: 100 mg/60 mL (60 mL)
Cortenema®: 100 mg/60 mL (60 mL)

hydrocortisone acetate *see* hydrocortisone (topical) *on page 450*
hydrocortisone, acetic acid, and propylene glycol diacetate *see* acetic acid, propylene glycol diacetate, and hydrocortisone *on page 35*
hydrocortisone and acyclovir *see* acyclovir and hydrocortisone *on page 39*

hydrocortisone and benzoyl peroxide *see* benzoyl peroxide and hydrocortisone *on page 125*

hydrocortisone and ciprofloxacin *see* ciprofloxacin and hydrocortisone *on page 211*

hydrocortisone and fusidic acid *see* fusidic acid and hydrocortisone *(Canada only) on page 405*

hydrocortisone and iodoquinol *see* iodoquinol and hydrocortisone *on page 485*

hydrocortisone and lidocaine *see* lidocaine and hydrocortisone *on page 526*

hydrocortisone and pramoxine *see* pramoxine and hydrocortisone *on page 731*

hydrocortisone and urea *see* urea and hydrocortisone *on page 901*

hydrocortisone, bacitracin, neomycin, and polymyxin B *see* bacitracin, neomycin, polymyxin B, and hydrocortisone *on page 112*

hydrocortisone butyrate *see* hydrocortisone (topical) *on page 450*

hydrocortisone, neomycin, and polymyxin B *see* neomycin, polymyxin B, and hydrocortisone *on page 618*

hydrocortisone, neomycin, colistin, and thonzonium *see* neomycin, colistin, hydrocortisone, and thonzonium *on page 617*

Hydrocortisone Plus [OTC] *see* hydrocortisone (topical) *on page 450*

hydrocortisone probutate *see* hydrocortisone (topical) *on page 450*

hydrocortisone sodium succinate *see* hydrocortisone (systemic) *on page 449*

hydrocortisone valerate *see* hydrocortisone (topical) *on page 450*

Hydrodiuril *see* hydrochlorothiazide *on page 445*

Hydromet® *see* hydrocodone and homatropine *on page 448*

Hydromorph Contin® (Can) *see* hydromorphone *on page 452*

Hydromorph-IR® (Can) *see* hydromorphone *on page 452*

hydromorphone (hye droe MOR fone)

Medication Safety Issues

Sound-alike/look-alike issues:

Dilaudid® may be confused with Demerol®, Dilantin®

HYDROmorphone may be confused with morphine; significant overdoses have occurred when hydromorphone products have been inadvertently administered instead of morphine sulfate. Commercially available prefilled syringes of both products looks similar and are often stored in close proximity to each other. **Note:** Hydromorphone 1 mg oral is approximately equal to morphine 4 mg oral; hydromorphone 1 mg I.V. is approximately equal to morphine 5 mg I.V.

High alert medication:

The Institute for Safe Medication Practices (ISMP) includes this medication among its list of drug classes which have a heightened risk of causing significant patient harm when used in error.

Administration issues:

Dilaudid®, Dilaudid-HP®: Extreme caution should be taken to avoid confusing the highly-concentrated (Dilaudid-HP®) injection with the less-concentrated (Dilaudid®) injectable product.

Exalgo™: Extreme caution should be taken to avoid confusing the extended release Exalgo™ 8 mg tablets with immediate release hydromorphone 8 mg tablets

Significant differences exist between oral and I.V. dosing. Use caution when converting from one route of administration to another.

Synonyms dihydromorphinone; hydromorphone hydrochloride

Tall-Man HYDROmorphone

U.S. Brand Names Dilaudid-HP®; Dilaudid®; Exalgo™

Canadian Brand Names Dilaudid-HP-Plus®; Dilaudid-HP®; Dilaudid-XP®; Dilaudid®; Dilaudid® Sterile Powder; Hydromorph Contin®; Hydromorph-IR®; Hydromorphone HP; Hydromorphone HP® 10; Hydromorphone HP® 20; Hydromorphone HP® 50; Hydromorphone HP® Forte; Hydromorphone Hydrochloride Injection, USP; Jurnista™; PMS-Hydromorphone

Therapeutic Category Analgesic, Narcotic

Controlled Substance C-II

Use Management of moderate-to-severe pain

Exalgo™: Management of moderate-to-severe pain in opioid-tolerant patients (requiring around-the-clock analgesia for an extended period of time)

General Dosage Range Dosage adjustment recommended in patients with hepatic or renal impairment

I.M., SubQ: *Children >50 kg and Adults:* 0.8-2 mg every 4-6 hours

I.V.:
Children ≥6 months and <50 kg: 0.015 mg/kg/dose every 3-6 hours as needed
Children >50 kg and Adults: 0.2-0.6 mg every 2-3 hours as needed
Adults (mechanically ventilated): Infusion: 0.5-1 mg/**hour** (based on 70 kg patient) **or** 7-15 mcg/kg/**hour**
Epidural PCA: *Children >50 kg and Adults:* Bolus: 0.4-1 mg; Infusion: 0.03-0.3 mg/**hour**; Demand dose: 0.02-0.5 mg; Lockout interval: 10-15 minutes
Oral:
Children ≥6 months and <50 kg: 0.03-0.08 mg/kg/dose every 3-4 hours as needed
Children >50 kg: 2-8 mg every 3-4 hours as needed
Adults: 2-8 mg every 3-4 hours as needed; Extended release: 8-64 mg every 24 hours
Elderly: 1-2 mg every 3-6 hours
PCA:
Children <50 kg: Usual concentration: 0.2 mg/mL; Demand dose: 0.003-0.005 mg/kg/dose; Lockout interval: 6-10 minutes; Usual basal rate: 0-0.004 mg/kg/hour
Children >50 kg and Adults: Usual concentration: 0.2 mg/mL; Demand dose: 0.05-0.4 mg; Lockout interval: 5-10 minutes
Rectal: *Children >50 kg and Adults:* 3 mg every 6-8 hours as needed

Dosage Forms
Injection, powder for reconstitution:
Dilaudid-HP®: 250 mg
Injection, solution: 1 mg/mL (1 mL); 2 mg/mL (1 mL, 20 mL); 4 mg/mL (1 mL); 10 mg/mL (1 mL, 5 mL, 50 mL)
Dilaudid-HP®: 10 mg/mL (1 mL, 5 mL, 50 mL)
Dilaudid®: 1 mg/mL (1 mL); 2 mg/mL (1 mL); 4 mg/mL (1 mL)
Injection, solution [preservative free]: 10 mg/mL (1 mL, 5 mL, 50 mL)
Liquid, oral:
Dilaudid®: 1 mg/mL (473 mL)
Powder, for prescription compounding: USP: 100% (972 mg)
Suppository, rectal: 3 mg (6s)
Tablet, oral: 2 mg, 4 mg, 8 mg
Dilaudid®: 2 mg, 4 mg, 8 mg
Tablet, extended release, oral:
Exalgo™: 8 mg, 12 mg, 16 mg

Dosage Forms - Canada
Capsule, controlled release:
Hydromorph Contin®: 3 mg, 6 mg, 12 mg, 18 mg, 24 mg, 30 mg [not available in U.S.]

Hydromorphone HP (Can) *see* hydromorphone *on page 452*
Hydromorphone HP® 10 (Can) *see* hydromorphone *on page 452*
Hydromorphone HP® 20 (Can) *see* hydromorphone *on page 452*
Hydromorphone HP® 50 (Can) *see* hydromorphone *on page 452*
Hydromorphone HP® Forte (Can) *see* hydromorphone *on page 452*
hydromorphone hydrochloride *see* hydromorphone *on page 452*
Hydromorphone Hydrochloride Injection, USP (Can) *see* hydromorphone *on page 452*
hydroquinol *see* hydroquinone *on page 453*

hydroquinone (HYE droe kwin one)

Medication Safety Issues
Sound-alike/look-alike issues:
Eldopaque® may be confused with Eldoquin®
Eldoquin® may be confused with Eldopaque®
Eldopaque Forte® may be confused with Eldoquin Forte®
Eldoquin Forte® may be confused with Eldopaque Forte®

Synonyms hydroquinol; quinol

U.S. Brand Names Aclaro PD®; Aclaro®; Alphaquin HP®; Eldopaque Forte®; Eldopaque® [OTC]; Eldoquin Forte®; Eldoquin® [OTC]; EpiQuin® Micro; Esoterica® Daytime [OTC]; Esoterica® Nighttime [OTC]; Lustra-AF®; Lustra-Ultra™; Lustra®; Melanex® [DSC]; Melpaque HP®; Melquin HP®; Melquin-3®; NeoStrata® HQ Skin Lightening [OTC]; Nuquin HP®; Palmer's® Skin Success® Eventone® Fade Cream [OTC]; Palmer's® Skin Success® Eventone® Fade Milk [OTC]; Palmer's® Skin Success® Eventone® Ultra Fade Serum [OTC]

◄ **Canadian Brand Names** Eldopaque®; Eldoquin®; Glyquin® XM; Lustra®; NeoStrata® HQ; Solaquin Forte®; Solaquin®; Ultraquin™

Therapeutic Category Topical Skin Product

Use Gradual bleaching of hyperpigmented skin conditions

General Dosage Range Topical: *Children >12 years and Adults:* Apply thin layer and rub in twice daily

Dosage Forms

 Cream, topical: 4% (28.35 g, 28.4 g, 30 g)
  Alphaquin HP®: 4% (28.4 g, 56.7 g)
  Eldopaque Forte®: 4% (28.35 g)
  Eldopaque® [OTC]: 2% (28.35 g)
  Eldoquin Forte®: 4% (28.4 g)
  Eldoquin® [OTC]: 2% (28.35 g)
  EpiQuin® Micro: 4% (40 g)
  Esoterica® Daytime [OTC]: 2% (70 g, 85 g)
  Esoterica® Nighttime [OTC]: 2% (85 g)
  Lustra-AF®: 4% (56.8 g)
  Lustra-Ultra™: 4% (56.8 g)
  Lustra®: 4% (56.8 g)
  Melpaque HP®: 4% (14.2 g, 28.4 g)
  Melquin HP®: 4% (14.2 g, 28.4 g)
  Nuquin HP®: 4% (14.2 g, 28.4 g, 56.7 g)
  Palmer's® Skin Success® Eventone® Fade Cream [OTC]: 2% (75 g, 125 g)
 Emulsion, topical:
  Aclaro PD®: 4% (42.5 g)
  Aclaro®: 4% (48.2 g)
 Gel, topical: 4% (28.35 g, 30 g)
  NeoStrata® HQ Skin Lightening [OTC]: 2% (30 g)
  Nuquin HP®: 4% (14.2 g, 28.4 g)
 Lotion, topical:
  Palmer's® Skin Success® Eventone® Fade Milk [OTC]: 2% (250 mL)
 Solution, topical:
  Melquin-3®: 3% (29.57 mL)
  Palmer's® Skin Success® Eventone® Ultra Fade Serum [OTC]: 2% (30 mL)

hydroquinone, fluocinolone acetonide, and tretinoin *see* fluocinolone, hydroquinone, and tretinoin *on page 385*

Hydroskin® [OTC] *see* hydrocortisone (topical) *on page 450*

HydroVal® (Can) *see* hydrocortisone (topical) *on page 450*

hydroxyamphetamine and tropicamide (hye droks ee am FET a meen & troe PIK a mide)

Synonyms hydroxyamphetamine hydrobromide and tropicamide; tropicamide and hydroxyamphetamine

U.S. Brand Names Paremyd®

Therapeutic Category Adrenergic Agonist Agent, Ophthalmic

Use Short-term pupil dilation for diagnostic procedures and exams

General Dosage Range Ophthalmic: *Adults:* Instill 1-2 drops into conjunctival sac(s)

Dosage Forms
 Solution, ophthalmic:
  Paremyd®: Hydroxyamphetamine 1% and tropicamide 0.25% (15 mL)

hydroxyamphetamine hydrobromide and tropicamide *see* hydroxyamphetamine and tropicamide *on page 454*

4-hydroxybutyrate *see* sodium oxybate *on page 822*

hydroxycarbamide *see* hydroxyurea *on page 456*

hydroxychloroquine (hye droks ee KLOR oh kwin)

Medication Safety Issues
 Sound-alike/look-alike issues:
  Hydroxychloroquine may be confused with hydrocortisone
  Plaquenil® may be confused with Platinol®

Synonyms hydroxychloroquine sulfate

U.S. Brand Names Plaquenil®

Canadian Brand Names Apo-Hydroxyquine®; Gen-Hydroxychloroquine; Mylan-Hydroxychloroquine; Plaquenil®; PRO-Hydroxyquine

Therapeutic Category Aminoquinoline (Antimalarial)

Use Suppression and treatment of acute attacks of malaria; treatment of systemic lupus erythematosus (SLE) and rheumatoid arthritis

General Dosage Range Oral:
Children: 13 mg/kg for 1-2 doses, followed by 6.5 mg/kg for 3 doses or once weekly
Adults: Initial: 400-800 mg/day divided 1-2 times/day; Maintenance: 200-400 mg/day **or** 800 mg for 1-2 doses, followed by 400 mg for 3 doses or once weekly

Dosage Forms
Tablet, oral: 200 mg
Plaquenil®: 200 mg

hydroxychloroquine sulfate *see hydroxychloroquine on page 454*
1-α-hydroxycholecalciferol *see alfacalcidol (Canada only) on page 50*
hydroxydaunomycin hydrochloride *see doxorubicin on page 310*
hydroxyethylcellulose *see artificial tears on page 96*
hydroxyethyl starch *see hetastarch on page 439*
hydroxyethyl starch *see pentastarch on page 686*
hydroxyethyl starch *see tetrastarch on page 858*
hydroxyldaunorubicin hydrochloride *see doxorubicin on page 310*

hydroxyprogesterone caproate (hye droks ee proe JES te rone CAP ro ate)

Medication Safety Issues
Sound-alike/look-alike issues:
Hydroxyprogesterone caproate may be confused with medroxyPROGESTERone

Synonyms 17OHPC

U.S. Brand Names Makena™

Therapeutic Category Progestin

Use To reduce the risk of preterm birth in women with singleton pregnancies who have a history of spontaneous preterm birth (delivery <37 weeks gestation) with previous singleton pregnancies

General Dosage Range I.M.: *Pregnant females:* 250 mg every 7 days

Dosage Forms
Injection, solution:
Makena™: 250 mg/mL (5 mL)

hydroxypropyl cellulose (hye droks ee PROE pil SEL yoo lose)

U.S. Brand Names Lacrisert®

Canadian Brand Names Lacrisert®

Therapeutic Category Ophthalmic Agent, Miscellaneous

Use Dry eyes (moderate-to-severe)

General Dosage Range Ophthalmic: *Adults:* Apply once daily

Dosage Forms
Insert, ophthalmic [preservative free]:
Lacrisert®: 5 mg (60s)

hydroxypropyl methylcellulose (hye droks ee PROE pil meth il SEL yoo lose)

Medication Safety Issues
Sound-alike/look-alike issues:
Isopto® Tears may be confused with Isoptin®

Synonyms gonioscopic ophthalmic solution; hypromellose

U.S. Brand Names Cellugel®; GenTeal® Mild [OTC]; GenTeal® [OTC]; Gonak™; Goniosoft™ [OTC]; Isopto® Tears [OTC]; Natural Balance Tears [OTC]; Nature's Tears [OTC]; Tears Again® MC Gel Drops™ [OTC]

Canadian Brand Names Genteal®; Isopto® Tears

Therapeutic Category Ophthalmic Agent, Miscellaneous

Use Relief of burning and minor irritation due to dry eyes; diagnostic agent in gonioscopic examination

◀ **General Dosage Range Ophthalmic:** *Adults:* Instill 1-2 drops in affected eye(s) as needed
Dosage Forms
  Gel, ophthalmic [preservative free]:
    GenTeal® [OTC]: 0.3% (10 mL)
  Injection, solution, ophthalmic:
    Cellugel®: 2% (1 mL)
  Solution, ophthalmic:
    Gonak™: 2.5% (15 mL)
    Goniosoft™ [OTC]: 2.5% (15 mL)
    Isopto® Tears [OTC]: 0.5% (15 mL)
    Natural Balance Tears [OTC]: 0.4% (15 mL)
    Nature's Tears [OTC]: 0.4% (15 mL)
    Tears Again® MC Gel Drops™ [OTC]: 0.3% (15 mL)
  Solution, ophthalmic [preservative free]:
    GenTeal® [OTC]: 0.3% (15 mL, 25 mL)
    GenTeal® Mild [OTC]: 0.2% (15 mL, 25 mL)

9-hydroxy-risperidone *see* paliperidone *on page* 668

hydroxyurea (hye droks ee yoor EE a)
Medication Safety Issues
  Sound-alike/look-alike issues:
    Hydroxyurea may be confused with hydrOXYzine
  High alert medication:
    This medication is in a class the Institute for Safe Medication Practices (ISMP) includes among its list of drugs which have a heightened risk of causing significant patient harm when used in error.
  International issues:
    Hydrea [U.S., Canada, and multiple international markets] may be confused with Hydra brand name for isoniazid [Japan]
Synonyms hydroxycarbamide; hydurea
U.S. Brand Names Droxia®; Hydrea®
Canadian Brand Names Apo-Hydroxyurea®; Gen-Hydroxyurea; Hydrea®; Mylan-Hydroxyurea
Therapeutic Category Antineoplastic Agent
Use Treatment of melanoma, refractory chronic myelocytic leukemia (CML); recurrent, metastatic, or inoperable ovarian cancer; radiosensitizing agent in the treatment of squamous cell head and neck cancer (excluding lip cancer); adjunct in the management of sickle cell patients who have had at least three painful crises in the previous 12 months (to reduce frequency of these crises and the need for blood transfusions)
General Dosage Range Dosage adjustment recommended in patients with renal impairment
  Oral: *Adults:* 15-35 mg/kg/day **or** 500-3000 mg/day as single or divided dose **or** 80 mg/kg as a single dose every third day
Dosage Forms
  Capsule, oral: 500 mg
    Droxia®: 200 mg, 300 mg, 400 mg
    Hydrea®: 500 mg

1-α-hydroxyvitamin D₃ *see* alfacalcidol *(Canada only) on page* 50

hydroxyzine (hye DROKS i zeen)
Medication Safety Issues
  Sound-alike/look-alike issues:
    HydrOXYzine may be confused with hydrALAZINE, hydroxyurea
    Atarax® may be confused with Ativan®
    Vistaril® may be confused with Restoril™, Versed, Zestril®
  BEERS Criteria medication:
    This drug may be inappropriate for use in geriatric patients (high severity risk).
  International issues:
    Vistaril [U.S. and Turkey] may be confused with Vastarel brand name for trimetazidine [multiple international markets]
Synonyms hydroxyzine hydrochloride; hydroxyzine pamoate
Tall-Man hydrOXYzine

456

U.S. Brand Names Vistaril®

Canadian Brand Names Apo-Hydroxyzine®; Atarax®; Hydroxyzine Hydrochloride Injection, USP; Novo-Hydroxyzin; Nu-Hydroxyzine; PMS-Hydroxyzine; Riva-Hydroxyzine

Therapeutic Category Antiemetic; Antihistamine

Use Treatment of anxiety/agitation (including adjunctive therapy in alcoholism); adjunct to pre- and postoperative analgesia and anesthesia; antipruritic; antiemetic

General Dosage Range Dosage adjustment recommended in patients with hepatic impairment

I.M.:
Children: 1.1 mg/kg/dose
Adults: 25-100 mg/dose

Oral:
Children: 0.6 mg/kg/dose (sedation)
Children <6 years: 50 mg/day in divided doses
Children ≥6 years: 50-100 mg/day in divided doses
Adults: 25-100 mg/dose

Dosage Forms
Capsule, oral: 25 mg, 50 mg, 100 mg
Vistaril®: 25 mg, 50 mg
Injection, solution: 25 mg/mL (1 mL); 50 mg/mL (1 mL, 2 mL, 10 mL)
Solution, oral: 10 mg/5 mL (473 mL)
Syrup, oral: 10 mg/5 mL (118 mL, 473 mL, 480 mL)
Tablet, oral: 10 mg, 25 mg, 50 mg

hydroxyzine hydrochloride *see* hydroxyzine *on page 456*
Hydroxyzine Hydrochloride Injection, USP (Can) *see* hydroxyzine *on page 456*
hydroxyzine pamoate *see* hydroxyzine *on page 456*
hydurea *see* hydroxyurea *on page 456*
Hygroton *see* chlorthalidone *on page 204*
hylan G-F 20 *see* hyaluronate and derivatives *on page 443*
hylan polymers *see* hyaluronate and derivatives *on page 443*
Hylatopic™ *see* emollients *on page 325*
HylatopicPlus™ *see* emollients *on page 325*
HylatopicPlus™- Aurstat *see* emollients *on page 325*
Hylenex *see* hyaluronidase *on page 443*
HyoMax™-DT *see* hyoscyamine *on page 457*
HyoMax™-FT *see* hyoscyamine *on page 457*
HyoMax®-SL *see* hyoscyamine *on page 457*
HyoMax® -SR *see* hyoscyamine *on page 457*
Hyonatol *see* hyoscyamine, atropine, scopolamine, and phenobarbital *on page 459*
hyoscine butylbromide *see* scopolamine (systemic) *on page 804*
hyoscine hydrobromide *see* scopolamine (ophthalmic) *on page 805*

hyoscyamine (hye oh SYE a meen)

Medication Safety Issues
Sound-alike/look-alike issues:
Anaspaz® may be confused with Anaprox®, Antispas®
Levbid® may be confused with Enbrel®, Lithobid®, Lopid®, Lorabid®
Levsinex® may be confused with Lanoxin®
Levsin/SL® maybe confused with Levaquin®
BEERS Criteria medication:
This drug may be inappropriate for use in geriatric patients (high severity risk).

Synonyms *l*-hyoscyamine sulfate; hyoscyamine sulfate

U.S. Brand Names Anaspaz®; HyoMax® -SR; HyoMax®-SL; HyoMax™-DT; HyoMax™-FT; Hyosyne; Levbid®; Levsin®; Levsin®/SL; Symax® DuoTab; Symax® FasTab; Symax® SL; Symax® SR

Canadian Brand Names Levsin®

Therapeutic Category Anticholinergic Agent

◀ **Use**

Oral: Adjunctive therapy for peptic ulcers, irritable bowel, neurogenic bladder/bowel; treatment of infant colic, GI tract disorders caused by spasm; to reduce rigidity, tremors, sialorrhea, and hyperhidrosis associated with parkinsonism; as a drying agent in acute rhinitis

Injection: Preoperative antimuscarinic to reduce secretions and block cardiac vagal inhibitory reflexes; to improve radiologic visibility of the kidneys; symptomatic relief of biliary and renal colic; reduce GI motility to facilitate diagnostic procedures (ie, endoscopy, hypotonic duodenography); reduce pain and hypersecretion in pancreatitis, certain cases of partial heart block associated with vagal activity; reversal of neuromuscular blockade

General Dosage Range

I.M., SubQ: *Adults:* 0.25-0.5 mg 4 times/day as needed

I.V.:

Children ≥2 years: 5 mcg/kg given 30-60 minutes prior to induction of anesthesia

Adults: 0.125-0.5 mg 4 times/day as needed **or** 0.25-0.5 mg or 5 mcg/kg as a single dose **or** 0.2 mg for every 1 mg neostigmine

Oral:

Regular release:

Children <2 years and 3.4 kg: 4 drops every 4 hours as needed (maximum: 24 drops/day)

Children <2 years and 5 kg: 5 drops every 4 hours as needed (maximum: 30 drops/day)

Children <2 years and 7 kg: 6 drops every 4 hours as needed (maximum: 36 drops/day)

Children <2 years and 10 kg: 8 drops every 4 hours as needed (maximum: 48 drops/day)

Children ≥2 years and 10 kg: 0.031-0.033 mg every 4 hours as needed (maximum: 0.75 mg/day)

Children ≥2 years and 20 kg: 0.0625 mg every 4 hours as needed (maximum: 0.75 mg/day)

Children ≥2 years and 40 kg: 0.0938 mg every 4 hours as needed (maximum: 0.75 mg/day)

Children ≥2 years and 50 kg: 0.125 mg every 4 hours as needed (maximum: 0.75 mg/day)

Adults: 0.125-0.25 mg every 4 hours or as needed (maximum: 1.5 mg/day)

Timed release: *Adults:* 0.375-0.75 mg every 12 hours (maximum: 1.5 mg/day)

S.L.:

Children ≥2 years and 10 kg: 0.031-0.033 mg every 4 hours as needed (maximum: 0.75 mg/day)

Children ≥2 years and 20 kg: 0.0625 mg every 4 hours as needed (maximum: 0.75 mg/day)

Children ≥2 years and 40 kg: 0.0938 mg every 4 hours as needed (maximum: 0.75 mg/day)

Children ≥2 years and 50 kg: 0.125 mg every 4 hours as needed (maximum: 0.75 mg/day)

Adults: 0.125-0.25 mg every 4 hours or as needed (maximum: 1.5 mg/day)

Dosage Forms

Elixir, oral: 0.125 mg/5 mL (473 mL, 480 mL)

Hyosyne: 0.125 mg/5 mL (473 mL)

Injection, solution:

Levsin®: 0.5 mg/mL (1 mL)

Solution, oral: 0.125 mg/mL (15 mL)

Hyosyne: 0.125 mg/mL (15 mL)

Tablet, oral: 0.125 mg

Levsin®: 0.125 mg

Tablet, sublingual: 0.125 mg

HyoMax®-SL: 0.125 mg

Levsin®/SL: 0.125 mg

Symax® SL: 0.125 mg

Tablet, chewable/disintegrating, oral:

HyoMax™-FT: 0.125 mg

Symax® FasTab: 0.125 mg

Tablet, extended release, oral: 0.375 mg

Levbid®: 0.375 mg

Tablet, orally disintegrating, oral: 0.125 mg

Anaspaz®: 0.125 mg

Tablet, sustained release, oral: 0.375 mg

HyoMax® -SR: 0.375 mg

Symax® SR: 0.375 mg

Tablet, variable release, oral:

HyoMax™-DT: Hyoscyamine sulfate 0.125 mg [immediate release] and hyoscyamine sulfate 0.25 mg [sustained release]

Symax® DuoTab: Hyoscyamine sulfate 0.125 mg [immediate release] and hyoscyamine sulfate 0.25 mg [sustained release]

hyoscyamine, atropine, scopolamine, and phenobarbital
(hye oh SYE a meen, A troe peen, skoe POL a meen, & fee noe BAR bi tal)

Medication Safety Issues
Sound-alike/look-alike issues:
Donnatal® may be confused with Donnagel®, Donnatal Extentabs®
BEERS Criteria medication:
This drug may be inappropriate for use in geriatric patients (high severity risk).

Synonyms atropine, hyoscyamine, phenobarbital, and scopolamine; belladonna alkaloids with phenobarbital; phenobarbital, hyoscyamine, atropine, and scopolamine; scopolamine, hyoscyamine, atropine, and phenobarbital

U.S. Brand Names Donnatal Extentabs®; Donnatal®; Hyonatol

Therapeutic Category Anticholinergic Agent

Use Adjunct in treatment of irritable bowel syndrome, acute enterocolitis, duodenal ulcer

General Dosage Range Oral:
Extended release: *Adults:* 1 tablet every 8-12 hours
Regular release:
  Children 4.5 kg: 0.5 mL every 4 hours **or** 0.75 mL every 6 hours
  Children 10 kg: 1 mL every 4 hours **or** 1.5 mL every 6 hours
  Children 14 kg: 1.5 mL every 4 hours **or** 2 mL every 6 hours
  Children 23 kg: 2.5 mL every 4 hours **or** 3.8 mL every 6 hours
  Children 34 kg: 3.8 mL every 4 hours **or** 5 mL every 6 hours
  Children ≥45 kg: 5 mL every 4 hours **or** 7.5 mL every 6 hours
  Adults: 1-2 tablets **or** 5-10 mL of elixir 3-4 times/day

Dosage Forms
Elixir: Hyoscyamine sulfate 0.1037 mg, atropine sulfate 0.0194 mg, scopolamine hydrobromide 0.0065 mg, and phenobarbital 16.2 mg per 5 mL
  Donnatal®: Hyoscyamine 0.1037 mg, atropine 0.0194 mg, scopolamine 0.0065 mg, and phenobarbital 16.2 mg per 5 mL
Tablet: Hyoscyamine 0.1037 mg, atropine 0.0194 mg, scopolamine 0.0065 mg, and phenobarbital 16.2 mg
  Donnatal®: Hyoscyamine 0.1037 mg, atropine 0.0194 mg, scopolamine 0.0065 mg, and phenobarbital 16.2 mg
  Hyonatol: Hyoscyamine 0.1037 mg, atropine 0.0194 mg, scopolamine 0.0065 mg, and phenobarbital 16.2 mg
Tablet, extended release:
  Donnatal Extentabs®: Hyoscyamine 0.3111 mg, atropine 0.0582 mg, scopolamine 0.0195 mg, and phenobarbital 48.6 mg

Hytrin® (Can) *see* terazosin *on page 851*
Hyzaar® *see* losartan and hydrochlorothiazide *on page 538*
Hyzaar® DS (Can) *see* losartan and hydrochlorothiazide *on page 538*
HZT-501 *see* ibuprofen and famotidine *on page 462*
I^{123} iobenguane *see* iobenguane I 123 *on page 483*
I-123 MIBG *see* iobenguane I 123 *on page 483*

ibandronate (eye BAN droh nate)
Synonyms ibandronate sodium; ibandronic acid
U.S. Brand Names Boniva®
Therapeutic Category Bisphosphonate Derivative
Use Treatment and prevention of osteoporosis in postmenopausal females
General Dosage Range
I.V.: *Adults:* 3 mg every 3 months
Oral: *Adults:* 2.5 mg once daily **or** 150 mg once a month
Dosage Forms
Injection, solution:
Boniva®: 1 mg/mL (3 mL)
Tablet, oral:
Boniva®: 150 mg

ibandronate sodium *see* ibandronate *on page 460*
ibandronic acid *see* ibandronate *on page 460*
Iberet®-500 [OTC] [DSC] *see* vitamins (multiple/oral) *on page 919*
ibidomide hydrochloride *see* labetalol *on page 504*

ibritumomab (ib ri TYOO mo mab)
Medication Safety Issues
High alert medication:
The Institute for Safe Medication Practices (ISMP) includes this medication among its list of drug classes which have a heightened risk of causing significant patient harm when used in error.
Administration issues:
Dosage maximum: Do not exceed the Y-90 Ibritumomab maximum allowable dose of 32 mCi, regardless of the patient's body weight.
Synonyms ibritumomab tiuxetan; IDEC-Y2B8; In-111 ibritumomab; In-111 zevalin; Y-90 ibritumomab; Y-90 zevalin
U.S. Brand Names Zevalin®
Canadian Brand Names Zevalin®
Therapeutic Category Antineoplastic Agent, Monoclonal Antibody; Radiopharmaceutical
Use Treatment of relapsed or refractory low-grade or follicular B-cell non-Hodgkin lymphoma (NHL); treatment of follicular NHL in patients who achieve a response (partial or complete) to first-line chemotherapy
General Dosage Range I.V.: *Adults:*
Day 1: In-111: 5 mCi (1.6 mg total antibody dose)
Day 7, 8, or 9: Y-90: 0.3-0.4 mCi/kg (11.1-14.8 MBq/kg actual body weight) (maximum: 32 mCi [1184 MBq])
Dosage Forms
Injection, solution [preservative free]:
Zevalin®: 1.6 mg/mL (2 mL)

ibritumomab tiuxetan *see* ibritumomab *on page 460*
Ibu® *see* ibuprofen *on page 460*
Ibu-200 [OTC] *see* ibuprofen *on page 460*
Ibudone™ *see* hydrocodone and ibuprofen *on page 448*

ibuprofen (eye byoo PROE fen)
Medication Safety Issues
Sound-alike/look-alike issues:
Haltran® may be confused with Halfprin®

Motrin® may be confused with Neurontin®

Administration issues:

Injectable formulations: Both ibuprofen and ibuprofen lysine are available for parenteral use. Ibuprofen lysine is **only** indicated for closure of a clinically-significant patent ductus arteriosus.

Synonyms *p*-isobutylhydratropic acid; ibuprofen lysine

U.S. Brand Names Addaprin [OTC]; Advil® Children's [OTC]; Advil® Infants' [OTC]; Advil® Migraine [OTC]; Advil® [OTC]; Caldolor™; I-Prin [OTC]; Ibu-200 [OTC]; Ibu®; Midol® Cramps & Body Aches [OTC]; Motrin® Children's [OTC]; Motrin® IB [OTC]; Motrin® Infants' [OTC]; Motrin® Junior [OTC]; NeoProfen®; Proprinal® [OTC]; TopCare® Junior Strength [OTC]; Ultraprin [OTC]

Canadian Brand Names Advil®; Apo-Ibuprofen®; Motrin® (Children's); Motrin® IB; Novo-Profen; Nu-Ibuprofen

Therapeutic Category Analgesic, Nonnarcotic; Antipyretic; Nonsteroidal Antiinflammatory Drug (NSAID)

Use

Oral: Inflammatory diseases and rheumatoid disorders including juvenile idiopathic arthritis (JIA), mild-to-moderate pain, fever, dysmenorrhea, osteoarthritis

Ibuprofen injection (Caldolor™): Management of mild-to-moderate pain; management moderate-to-severe pain when used concurrently with an opioid analgesic; reduction of fever

Ibuprofen lysine injection (NeoProfen®): To induce closure of a clinically-significant patent ductus arteriosus (PDA) in premature infants weighing between 500-1500 g and who are ≤32 weeks gestational age (GA) when usual treatments are ineffective

General Dosage Range

I.V. (ibuprofen [Caldolor™]): *Adults:* 100-400 mg every 4-6 hours or 400-800 mg every 6 hours (maximum: 3.2 g/day)

I.V. (ibuprofen lysine [NeoProfen®]): *Infants between 500-1500 g and ≤32 weeks GA:* Initial: 10 mg/kg, followed by two doses of 5 mg/kg at 24 and 48 hours; **Note:** Dose should be based on birth weight.

Oral:

Analgesic/antipyretic:

Children 6-11 months and 12-17 lbs: 50 mg every 6-8 hours (maximum: 4 doses/day) **or** 4-10 mg/kg every 6-8 hours (maximum: 40 mg/kg/day)

Children 12-23 months and 18-23 lbs: 75 mg every 6-8 hours (maximum: 4 doses/day) **or** 4-10 mg/kg every 6-8 hours (maximum: 40 mg/kg/day)

Children 2-3 years and 24-35 lbs: 100 mg every 6-8 hours (maximum: 4 doses/day) **or** 4-10 mg/kg every 6-8 hours (maximum: 40 mg/kg/day)

Children 4-5 years and 36-47 lbs: 150 mg every 6-8 hours (maximum: 4 doses/day) **or** 4-10 mg/kg every 6-8 hours (maximum: 40 mg/kg/day)

Children 6-8 years and 48-59 lbs: 200 mg every 6-8 hours (maximum: 4 doses/day) **or** 4-10 mg/kg every 6-8 hours (maximum: 40 mg/kg/day)

Children 9-10 years and 60-71 lbs: 250 mg every 6-8 hours (maximum: 4 doses/day) **or** 4-10 mg/kg every 6-8 hours (maximum: 40 mg/kg/day)

Children 11-12 years and 72-95 lbs: 300 mg every 6-8 hours (maximum: 4 doses/day) **or** 4-10 mg/kg every 6-8 hours (maximum: 40 mg/kg/day)

Children >12 years: 200 mg every 4-6 hours as needed (maximum: 1200 mg/day) **or** 4-10 mg/kg every 6-8 hours (maximum: 40 mg/kg/day)

Adults: 200-400 mg every 4-6 hours

Inflammatory disease: *Adults:* 400-800 mg 3-4 times/day (maximum: 3200 mg/day)

JIA: *Children >6 months:* 30-50 mg/kg/day divided every 8 hours (maximum: 2.4 g/day)

Dosage Forms

Caplet, oral: 200 mg

Advil® [OTC]: 200 mg

Motrin® IB [OTC]: 200 mg

Motrin® Junior [OTC]: 100 mg

Capsule, liquid filled, oral: 200 mg

Advil® [OTC]: 200 mg

Advil® Migraine [OTC]: 200 mg

Capsule, softgel, oral: 200 mg

Gelcap, oral:

Advil® [OTC]: 200 mg

Injection, solution:

Caldolor™: 100 mg/mL (4 mL, 8 mL)

Injection, solution [preservative free]:

NeoProfen®: 17.1 mg/mL (2 mL)

◄ **Suspension, oral**: 100 mg/5 mL (5 mL, 10 mL, 120 mL, 240 mL, 480 mL); 40 mg/mL (15 mL)
  Advil® Children's [OTC]: 100 mg/5 mL (120 mL)
  Advil® Infants' [OTC]: 40 mg/mL (15 mL)
  Motrin® Children's [OTC]: 100 mg/5 mL (60 mL, 120 mL)
  Motrin® Infants' [OTC]: 40 mg/mL (15 mL)
Tablet, oral: 200 mg, 400 mg, 600 mg, 800 mg
  Addaprin [OTC]: 200 mg
  Advil® [OTC]: 200 mg
  I-Prin [OTC]: 200 mg
  Ibu-200 [OTC]: 200 mg
  Ibu®: 400 mg, 600 mg, 800 mg
  Midol® Cramps & Body Aches [OTC]: 200 mg
  Motrin® IB [OTC]: 200 mg
  Proprinal® [OTC]: 200 mg
  Ultraprin [OTC]: 200 mg
Tablet, chewable, oral:
  Motrin® Junior [OTC]: 100 mg
  TopCare® Junior Strength [OTC]: 100 mg

ibuprofen and famotidine (eye byoo PROE fen & fa MOE ti deen)
Synonyms Duexis®; famotidine and ibuprofen; HZT-501
Therapeutic Category Histamine H$_2$ Antagonist; Nonsteroidal Anti-inflammatory Drug (NSAID), Oral
Use Reduction of the risk of NSAID-associated gastric ulcers in patients who require an NSAID for the treatment of rheumatoid arthritis or osteoarthritis
General Dosage Range Oral: *Adults:* One tablet (800 mg ibuprofen/26.6 mg famotidine) 3 times daily
Product Availability Duexis®: FDA approved April 2011; availability currently undetermined; consult prescribing information for additional information

ibuprofen and hydrocodone see hydrocodone and ibuprofen on page 448
ibuprofen and oxycodone see oxycodone and ibuprofen on page 664
ibuprofen and pseudoephedrine see pseudoephedrine and ibuprofen on page 753
ibuprofen lysine see ibuprofen on page 460

ibuprofen, pseudoephedrine, and chlorpheniramine
(eye byoo PROE fen, soo doe e FED rin, & klor fen IR a meen)
Synonyms chlorpheniramine maleate, ibuprofen, and pseudoephedrine; ibuprofen, pseudoephedrine, and chlorpheniramine maleate; pseudoephedrine, chlorpheniramine, and ibuprofen
U.S. Brand Names Advil® Allergy Sinus; Advil® Multi-Symptom Cold
Canadian Brand Names Advil® Cold and Sinus Nighttime; Advil® Cold and Sinus Plus; Children's Advil® Cold and Flu Multi-Symptom
Therapeutic Category Antihistamine/Decongestant/Analgesic
Use Temporary relief of symptoms associated with the common cold, hay fever, or other respiratory allergies
General Dosage Range Oral: *Children ≥12 years and Adults:* 1 caplet every 4-6 hours (maximum: 6 caplets/day)
Dosage Forms
Caplet:
  Advil® Allergy Sinus, Advil® Multi-Symptom Cold: Ibuprofen 200 mg, pseudoephedrine 30 mg, and chlorpheniramine 2 mg

ibuprofen, pseudoephedrine, and chlorpheniramine maleate see ibuprofen, pseudoephedrine, and chlorpheniramine on page 462

ibutilide (i BYOO ti lide)
Medication Safety Issues
High alert medication:
  The Institute for Safe Medication Practices (ISMP) includes this medication among its list of drugs which have a heightened risk of causing significant patient harm when used in error.
Synonyms ibutilide fumarate
U.S. Brand Names Corvert®
Therapeutic Category Antiarrhythmic Agent, Class III

Use Acute termination of atrial fibrillation or flutter of recent onset; the effectiveness of ibutilide has not been determined in patients with arrhythmias >90 days in duration

General Dosage Range I.V.:
Adults <60 kg: 0.01 mg/kg; may repeat once
Adults ≥60 kg: 1 mg; may repeat once

Dosage Forms
Injection, solution: 0.1 mg/mL (10 mL)
Corvert®: 0.1 mg/mL (10 mL)

ibutilide fumarate *see* ibutilide *on page 462*
IC51 *see* Japanese encephalitis virus vaccine (inactivated) *on page 498*
IC-Green™ *see* indocyanine green *on page 471*
ICI-182,780 *see* fulvestrant *on page 404*
ICI-204,219 *see* zafirlukast *on page 926*
ICI-46474 *see* tamoxifen *on page 843*
ICI-118630 *see* goserelin *on page 424*
ICI-176334 *see* bicalutamide *on page 133*
ICI-D1033 *see* anastrozole *on page 79*
ICI-D1694 *see* raltitrexed *(Canada only) on page 765*
ICL670 *see* deferasirox *on page 256*

icodextrin (eye KOE dex trin)

Medication Safety Issues
Other safety concerns:
Special care is warranted in patients with diabetes: Due to potential interference by maltose, careful attention must be given to glucose monitoring; only glucose monitors and test strips which employ the glucose-specific method should be used. Inaccurate methods (glucose dehydrogenase pyrroloquinolinequinone [GDH-PQQ] or glucose-dye-oxidoreductase methods [GDO]) can result in falsely-elevated readings. Inaccurate readings may mask recognition of true hypoglycemia, or may prompt the administration of insulin, potentially leading to life-threatening consequences.

U.S. Brand Names Extraneal
Therapeutic Category Adhesiolytic; Peritoneal Dialysate, Osmotic
Use
Adept®: Reduction of postsurgical adhesions in gynecologic laparoscopic procedures
Extraneal®: Daily exchange for the long dwell (8- to 16-hour) during continuous ambulatory peritoneal dialysis (CAPD) or automated peritoneal dialysis (APD) for the management of end-stage renal disease (ESRD); improvement of long-dwell ultrafiltration and clearance of creatinine and urea nitrogen (compared to 4.25% dextrose) in patients with high/average or greater transport characteristics as measured by peritoneal equilibration test (PET)

General Dosage Range Intraperitoneal: *Adults:*
CAPD or APD (Extraneal®): Given as a single daily exchange in CAPD or APD; dwell time of 8-16 hours is suggested
Laparoscopic gynecologic surgery (Adept®): Irrigate with at least 100 mL every 30 minutes during surgery; aspirate remaining fluid after surgery is completed, then instill 1 L into the cavity

Dosage Forms
Solution, intraperitoneal [preservative free]:
Extraneal: 7.5% (1.5 L, 2 L, 2.5 L)

ICRF-187 *see* dexrazoxane *on page 267*
Icy Hot® [OTC] *see* methyl salicylate and menthol *on page 579*
Idamycin® (Can) *see* idarubicin *on page 463*
Idamycin PFS® *see* idarubicin *on page 463*

idarubicin (eye da ROO bi sin)

Medication Safety Issues
Sound-alike/look-alike issues:
IDArubicin may be confused with DOXOrubicin, DAUNOrubicin, epirubicin

463

◀ Idamycin PFS® may be confused with Adriamycin

High alert medication:
The Institute for Safe Medication Practices (ISMP) includes this medication among its list of drugs which have a heightened risk of causing significant patient harm when used in error.

Synonyms 4-demethoxydaunorubicin; 4-DMDR; idarubicin hydrochloride; IDR; IMI 30; SC 33428

Tall-Man IDArubicin

U.S. Brand Names Idamycin PFS®

Canadian Brand Names Idamycin®

Therapeutic Category Antineoplastic Agent

Use Treatment of acute myeloid leukemia (AML)

General Dosage Range Dosage adjustment recommended in patients with hepatic or renal impairment
I.V.: *Adults:* Induction: 12 mg/m^2/day for 3 days; Consolidation: 10-12 mg/m^2/day for 2 days

Dosage Forms
Injection, solution [preservative free]: 1 mg/mL (5 mL, 10 mL, 20 mL)
Idamycin PFS®: 1 mg/mL (5 mL, 10 mL, 20 mL)

idarubicin hydrochloride *see* idarubicin *on page 463*

IDEC-C2B8 *see* rituximab *on page 784*

IDEC-Y2B8 *see* ibritumomab *on page 460*

IDR *see* idarubicin *on page 463*

idursulfase (eye dur SUL fase)

Medication Safety Issues
Sound-alike/look-alike issues:
Elaprase® may be confused with Elspar®

U.S. Brand Names Elaprase®

Canadian Brand Names Elaprase®

Therapeutic Category Enzyme

Use Replacement therapy in mucopolysaccharidosis II (MPS II, Hunter syndrome) for improvement of walking capacity

General Dosage Range I.V.: *Children ≥5 years and Adults:* 0.5 mg/kg once weekly

Dosage Forms
Injection, solution [preservative free]:
Elaprase®: 2 mg/mL (5 mL)

Ifex *see* ifosfamide *on page 464*

ifosfamide (eye FOSS fa mide)

Medication Safety Issues
Sound-alike/look-alike issues:
Ifosfamide may be confused with cyclophosphamide
High alert medication:
The Institute for Safe Medication Practices (ISMP) includes this medication among its list of drugs which have a heightened risk of causing significant patient harm when used in error.

Synonyms isophosphamide; Z4942

U.S. Brand Names Ifex

Canadian Brand Names Ifex

Therapeutic Category Antineoplastic Agent

Use Treatment of testicular cancer

General Dosage Range Dosage adjustment recommended in patients with hepatic or renal impairment
I.V.: *Adults:* 4000-5000 mg/m^2/day for 1 day every 14-28 days **or** 1000-3000 mg/m^2/day for 2-5 days every 21-28 days

Dosage Forms
Injection, powder for reconstitution: 1 g, 3 g
Ifex: 1 g, 3 g
Injection, solution: 50 mg/mL (20 mL, 60 mL)

IG *see* immune globulin *on page 468*

IgG4-kappa monoclonal antibody *see* natalizumab *on page 614*

IGIM *see* immune globulin *on page 468*
IGIV *see* immune globulin *on page 468*
IGIVnex® (Can) *see* immune globulin *on page 468*
IL-1Ra *see* anakinra *on page 78*
IL-2 *see* aldesleukin *on page 47*
IL-11 *see* oprelvekin *on page 653*
Ilaris® *see* canakinumab *on page 167*

iloperidone (eye loe PER i done)

Medication Safety Issues
Sound-alike/look-alike issues:
Fanapt® may be confused with Xanax®
Iloperidone may be confused with domperidone
U.S. Brand Names Fanapt®
Therapeutic Category Antipsychotic Agent, Atypical
Use Acute treatment of schizophrenia
General Dosage Range Oral: *Adults:* Initial: 1 mg twice daily; Dosage range: 6-12 mg twice daily (maximum: 24 mg/day)
Dosage Forms
Tablet, oral:
Fanapt®: 1 mg, 2 mg, 4 mg, 6 mg, 8 mg, 10 mg, 12 mg, 1 mg (2s), 2 mg (2s), 4 mg (2s), and 6 mg (2s)

iloprost (EYE loe prost)

Synonyms iloprost tromethamine; prostacyclin PGI$_2$
U.S. Brand Names Ventavis®
Therapeutic Category Prostaglandin
Use Treatment of pulmonary arterial hypertension (PAH) (WHO Group I) in patients with NYHA Class III or IV symptoms to improve exercise tolerance, symptoms, and diminish clinical deterioration
General Dosage Range Dosage adjustment recommended in patients with hepatic impairment.
Inhalation: *Adults:* Initial: 2.5 mcg/dose; Maintenance: 2.5-5 mcg/dose 6-9 times/day (maximum: 45 mcg/day)
Dosage Forms
Solution, for oral inhalation [preservative free]:
Ventavis®: 10 mcg/mL (1 mL); 20 mcg/mL (1 mL)

iloprost tromethamine *see* iloprost *on page 465*
Ilotycin™ *see* erythromycin (ophthalmic) *on page 339*

imatinib (eye MAT eh nib)

Medication Safety Issues
Sound-alike/look-alike issues:
Imatinib may be confused with dasatinib, erlotinib, gefitinib, nilotinib, SORAfenib, SUNItinib, vandetanib
High alert medication:
The Institute for Safe Medication Practices (ISMP) includes this medication among its list of drug classes which have a heightened risk of causing significant patient harm when used in error.
Synonyms CGP-57148B; glivec; imatinib mesylate; STI-571
U.S. Brand Names Gleevec®
Canadian Brand Names Gleevec®
Therapeutic Category Antineoplastic Agent, Tyrosine Kinase Inhibitor
Use Treatment of:
Gastrointestinal stromal tumors (GIST) kit-positive (CD117), including unresectable and/or metastatic malignant and adjuvant treatment following complete resection
Philadelphia chromosome-positive (Ph+) chronic myeloid leukemia (CML) in chronic phase (newly-diagnosed)
Ph+ CML in chronic phase in pediatric patients recurring following stem cell transplant or who are resistant to interferon-alpha therapy (**not** an approved use in Canada)
Ph+ CML in blast crisis, accelerated phase, or chronic phase after failure of interferon therapy
Ph+ acute lymphoblastic leukemia (ALL) (relapsed or refractory)

◄ Aggressive systemic mastocytosis (ASM) without D816V c-Kit mutation (or c-Kit mutation status unknown)

Dermatofibrosarcoma protuberans (DFSP) (unresectable, recurrent and/or metastatic)

Hypereosinophilic syndrome (HES) and/or chronic eosinophilic leukemia (CEL)

Myelodysplastic/myeloproliferative disease (MDS/MPD) associated with platelet-derived growth factor receptor (PDGFR) gene rearrangements

Canada labeling (not an approved indication in the U.S.): Ph+ ALL induction therapy (newly diagnosed)

General Dosage Range Dosage adjustment recommended in patients with hepatic or renal impairment, on concomitant therapy, and/or who develop toxicities

Oral:
Children ≥2 years: 260-340 mg/m^2/day in 1-2 divided doses (maximum: 600 mg/day)
Adults: 100-800 mg/day in 1-2 divided doses

Dosage Forms
Tablet, oral:
Gleevec®: 100 mg, 400 mg

imatinib mesylate *see* imatinib *on page 465*

IMC-C225 *see* cetuximab *on page 190*

Imdur® *see* isosorbide mononitrate *on page 495*

123I-metaiodobenzylguanidine (MIBG) *see* iobenguane I 123 *on page 483*

imferon *see* iron dextran complex *on page 491*

IMI 30 *see* idarubicin *on page 463*

IMid-1 *see* lenalidomide *on page 514*

imidazole carboxamide *see* dacarbazine *on page 248*

imidazole carboxamide dimethyltriazene *see* dacarbazine *on page 248*

imiglucerase (i mi GLOO ser ace)

Medication Safety Issues
Sound-alike/look-alike issues:
Cerezyme® may be confused with Cerebyx®, Ceredase®

U.S. Brand Names Cerezyme®

Canadian Brand Names Cerezyme®

Therapeutic Category Enzyme

Use Long-term enzyme replacement therapy for patients with Type 1 Gaucher disease

General Dosage Range I.V.: *Children ≥2 years and Adults:* Initial: 30-60 units/kg every 2 weeks; Range: 2.5 units/kg 3 times/week to 60 units/kg once weekly; Average dose: 60 units/kg every 2 weeks

Dosage Forms
Injection, powder for reconstitution:
Cerezyme®: 200 units, 400 units

imipemide *see* imipenem and cilastatin *on page 466*

imipenem and cilastatin (i mi PEN em & sye la STAT in)

Medication Safety Issues
Sound-alike/look-alike issues:
Imipenem may be confused with ertapenem, meropenem
Primaxin® may be confused with Premarin®, Primacor®

Synonyms imipemide; Primaxin® I.M. [DSC]

U.S. Brand Names Primaxin® I.V.

Canadian Brand Names Imipenem and Cilastatin for Injection; Primaxin® I.V. Infusion; RAN™-Imipenem-Cilastatin

Therapeutic Category Carbapenem (Antibiotic)

Use Treatment of lower respiratory tract, urinary tract, intraabdominal, gynecologic, bone and joint, skin and skin structure, endocarditis (caused by *Staphylococcus aureus*) and polymicrobic infections as well as bacterial septicemia. Antibacterial activity includes gram-positive bacteria (methicillin-sensitive *S. aureus* and *Streptococcus* spp), resistant gram-negative bacilli (including extended spectrum beta-lactamase-producing *Escherichia coli* and *Klebsiella* spp, *Enterobacter* spp, and *Pseudomonas aeruginosa*), and anaerobes.

General Dosage Range Dosage adjustment recommended in patients with renal impairment

I.V.:
Children >3 months: 15-25 mg/kg every 6 hours (maximum: 4 g/day)
Adults 30 to <70 kg: 125 mg every 12 hours up to 1000 mg every 8 hours
Adults ≥70 kg: 250-1000 mg every 6-8 hours (maximum: 50 mg/kg/day; 4 g/day)

Dosage Forms

Injection, powder for reconstitution:
Primaxin® I.V.: Imipenem 250 mg and cilastatin 250 mg; imipenem 500 mg and cilastatin 500 mg

Imipenem and Cilastatin for Injection (Can) *see* imipenem and cilastatin *on page 466*

imipramine (im IP ra meen)

Medication Safety Issues

Sound-alike/look-alike issues:
Imipramine may be confused with amitriptyline, desipramine, Norpramin®

Synonyms imipramine hydrochloride; imipramine pamoate

U.S. Brand Names Tofranil-PM®; Tofranil®

Canadian Brand Names Apo-Imipramine®; Novo-Pramine; Tofranil®

Therapeutic Category Antidepressant, Tricyclic (Tertiary Amine)

Use Treatment of depression; treatment of nocturnal enuresis in children

General Dosage Range Oral:
Children ≥6-12 years: Initial: 25 mg at bedtime, may increase to 50 mg at bedtime if no response (maximum: 2.5 mg/kg/day; 50 mg/day)
Children >12 years: Initial: 25 mg at bedtime, may increase to 75 mg at bedtime if not response (maximum: 75 mg/day) **or** 30-40 mg/day, increase gradually, to a maximum of 100 mg/day in single or divided doses
Adults: Initial: 75-150 mg/day, increase gradually to a maximum of 200 mg/day (outpatients) or 300 mg/day (inpatients) in divided doses or a single dose at bedtime
Elderly: Initial: 25-50 mg at bedtime (maximum: 100 mg/day)

Dosage Forms

Capsule, oral: 75 mg, 100 mg, 125 mg, 150 mg
Tofranil-PM®: 75 mg, 100 mg, 125 mg, 150 mg
Tablet, oral: 10 mg, 25 mg, 50 mg
Tofranil®: 10 mg, 25 mg, 50 mg

imipramine hydrochloride *see* imipramine *on page 467*

imipramine pamoate *see* imipramine *on page 467*

imiquimod (i mi KWI mod)

Medication Safety Issues

Sound-alike/look-alike issues:
Aldara® may be confused with Alora®, Lialda®

U.S. Brand Names Aldara®; Zyclara®

Canadian Brand Names Aldara®; Vyloma™; Zyclara®

Therapeutic Category Immune Response Modifier

Use Treatment of external genital and perianal warts/condyloma acuminata; nonhyperkeratotic actinic keratosis on face or scalp; superficial basal cell carcinoma (sBCC) with a maximum tumor diameter of 2 cm located on the trunk, neck, or extremities (excluding hands or feet)

General Dosage Range Topical:
Children ≥12 years: Apply a thin layer 3 times/week on alternate days, leave on for 6-10 hours
Adults:
Actinic keratosis: Apply twice weekly or once daily at bedtime for 2 treatment cycles (14 days each) separated by a 14-day rest period with no treatment; leave on for 8 hours
External genital and/or perianal warts/condyloma acuminata: Apply a thin layer 3 times/week on alternate days; leave on for 6-10 hours
Superficial basal cell carcinoma: Apply once daily at bedtime 5 days/week; leave on for 8 hours before washing

Product Availability
Zyclara® 2.5% cream: FDA approved July 2011; availability currently undetermined
Zyclara® 2.5% cream is a topical immunomodulator approved for the treatment of actinic keratoses. ▶

◀ **Dosage Forms**
Cream, topical: 5% (24s)
Aldara®: 5% (24s)
Zyclara®: 3.75% (28s)

Imitrex® see sumatriptan on page 839
Imitrex® DF (Can) see sumatriptan on page 839
Imitrex® Injection (Can) see sumatriptan on page 839
Imitrex® Nasal Spray (Can) see sumatriptan on page 839
ImmuCyst® (Can) see BCG on page 115

immune globulin (i MYUN GLOB yoo lin)

Medication Safety Issues

Sound-alike/look-alike issues:
Gamimune® N may be confused with CytoGam®
Immune globulin (intravenous) may be confused with hepatitis B immune globulin

Synonyms gamma globulin; IG; IGIM; IGIV; immune globulin subcutaneous (human); immune serum globulin; ISG; IV immune globulin; IVIG; panglobulin; SCIG

U.S. Brand Names Carimune® NF; Flebogamma® DIF; GamaSTAN™ S/D; Gammagard S/D®; Gammagard® Liquid; Gammaplex®; Gamunex® [DSC]; Gamunex®-C; Hizentra®; Octagam®; Privigen®; Vivaglobin® [DSC]

Canadian Brand Names BayGam®; Gamimune® N; Gammagard Liquid; Gammagard S/D; Gamunex®; IGIVnex®; Privigen®; Vivaglobin®

Therapeutic Category Blood Product Derivative; Immune Globulin

Use

Treatment of primary humoral immunodeficiency syndromes (congenital agammaglobulinemia, severe combined immunodeficiency syndromes [SCIDS], common variable immunodeficiency, X-linked immunodeficiency, Wiskott-Aldrich syndrome) (Carimune® NF, Flebogamma® DIF, Gammagard® Liquid, Gammagard S/D®, Gammaplex®, Gamunex®, Gamunex®-C, Hizentra®, Octagam®, Privigen®, Vivaglobin®)

Treatment of acute and chronic immune (idiopathic) thrombocytopenic purpura (ITP) (Carimune® NF, Gammagard S/D®, Gamunex®, Gamunex®-C, Privigen® [chronic only])

Treatment of chronic inflammatory demyelinating polyneuropathy (CIDP) (Gamunex®, Gamunex®-C)

Prevention of coronary artery aneurysms associated with Kawasaki syndrome (in combination with aspirin) (Gammagard S/D®)

Prevention of bacterial infection in patients with hypogammaglobulinemia and/or recurrent bacterial infections with B-cell chronic lymphocytic leukemia (CLL) (Gammagard S/D®)

Prevention of serious infection in immunoglobulin deficiency (select agammaglobulinemias) (GamaSTAN™ S/D)

Provision of passive immunity in the following susceptible individuals (GamaSTAN™ S/D):
Hepatitis A: Pre-exposure prophylaxis; postexposure: within 14 days and/or prior to manifestation of disease

Measles: For use within 6 days of exposure in an unvaccinated person, who has not previously had measles

Rubella: Postexposure prophylaxis (within 72 hours) to reduce the risk of infection and fetal damage in exposed pregnant women who will not consider therapeutic abortion

Varicella: For immunosuppressed patients when varicella zoster immune globulin is not available

General Dosage Range

I.M.: *Children and Adults:*
Hepatitis A:
Preexposure prophylaxis upon travel into endemic areas:
0.02 mL/kg for anticipated risk of exposure <3 months
0.06 mL/kg for anticipated risk of exposure ≥3 months
Postexposure prophylaxis: 0.02 mL/kg
Measles:
Postexposure, immunocompetent: 0.25 mL/kg
Postexposure, immunocompromised: 0.5 mL/kg (maximum dose: 15 mL)
Rubella: Prophylaxis during pregnancy: 0.55 mL/kg
Varicella: Prophylaxis: 0.6-1.2 mL/kg
Immune globulin deficiency: 0.66 mL/kg; administer a double dose at onset of therapy

I.V.: *Children and Adults:*
B-cell chronic lymphocytic leukemia (CLL): 400 mg/kg
Chronic inflammatory demyelinating polyneuropathy (CIDP): Loading dose: 2000 mg/kg; Maintenance: 500-1000 mg/kg
Immune (idiopathic) thrombocytopenic purpura (ITP): Dosage varies greatly depending on product
Kawasaki syndrome: 400-2000 mg/kg
Measles: >400 mg/kg
Primary humoral immunodeficiency disorders: 200-800 mg/kg
SubQ: *Children and Adults:*
Measles: ≥200 mg/kg
Primary humoral immunodeficiency disorders: Dosage varies greatly depending on product

Dosage Forms
Injection, powder for reconstitution [preservative free]:
Carimune® NF: 3 g, 6 g, 12 g
Gammagard S/D®: 2.5 g, 5 g, 10 g
Injection, solution [preservative free]:
Flebogamma® DIF: 5% [50 mg/mL] (10 mL, 50 mL, 100 mL, 200 mL, 400 mL); 10% [100 mg/mL] (100 mL, 200 mL)
GamaSTAN™ S/D: 15% to 18% [150 to 180 mg/mL] (2 mL, 10 mL)
Gammagard® Liquid: 10% [100 mg/mL] (10 mL, 25 mL, 50 mL, 100 mL, 200 mL)
Gammaplex®: 5% [50 mg/mL] (50 mL, 100 mL, 200 mL)
Gamunex®-C: 10% [100 mg/mL] (10 mL, 25 mL, 50 mL, 100 mL, 200 mL)
Hizentra®: 200 mg/mL (5 mL, 10 mL, 20 mL)
Octagam®: 5% [50 mg/mL] (20 mL, 50 mL, 100 mL, 200 mL)
Privigen®: 10% [100 mg/mL] (50 mL, 100 mL, 200 mL)

immune globulin subcutaneous (human) *see* immune globulin *on page 468*
immune serum globulin *see* immune globulin *on page 468*
Immunine® VH (Can) *see* factor IX *on page 365*
Imodium® (Can) *see* loperamide *on page 535*
Imodium® A-D [OTC] *see* loperamide *on page 535*
Imodium® A-D for children [OTC] *see* loperamide *on page 535*
Imodium® Advanced Multi-Symptom (Can) *see* loperamide and simethicone *on page 535*
Imodium® Multi-Symptom Relief [OTC] *see* loperamide and simethicone *on page 535*
Imogam® Rabies-HT *see* rabies immune globulin (human) *on page 764*
Imogam® Rabies Pasteurized (Can) *see* rabies immune globulin (human) *on page 764*
Imovane® (Can) *see* zopiclone *(Canada only) on page 934*
Imovax® Polio (Can) *see* poliovirus vaccine (inactivated) *on page 717*
Imovax® Rabies *see* rabies vaccine *on page 764*
Implanon® *see* etonogestrel *on page 361*
Imuran® *see* azathioprine *on page 107*
In-111 ibritumomab *see* ibritumomab *on page 460*
In-111 zevalin *see* ibritumomab *on page 460*

inamrinone *(eye NAM ri none)*

Medication Safety Issues
Sound-alike/look-alike issues:
Amrinone (former name for inamrinone) may be confused with aMILoride, amiodarone
High alert medication:
The Institute for Safe Medication Practices (ISMP) includes this medication among its list of drug classes which have a heightened risk of causing significant patient harm when used in error.
Synonyms amrinone lactate
Therapeutic Category Adrenergic Agonist Agent
Use Short-term therapy in patients with intractable heart failure
General Dosage Range Dosage adjustment recommended in patients with renal impairment
I.V.: *Adults:* Bolus: 0.75 mg/kg; may repeat; Infusion: 5-10 mcg/kg/minute

Incivek™ *see* telaprevir *on page 846*

incobotulinumtoxinA (in kuh BOT yoo lin num TOKS in aye)

Medication Safety Issues
Other safety concerns:
Botulinum products are not interchangeable; potency differences may exist between the products.
Synonyms botulinum toxin type A
U.S. Brand Names Xeomin®
Canadian Brand Names Xeomin®
Therapeutic Category Neuromuscular Blocker Agent, Toxin; Ophthalmic Agent, Toxin
Use Treatment of blepharospasm in patients previously treated with onabotulinumtoxinA (Botox®); treatment of cervical dystonia in botulinum toxin-naïve and previously treated patients; temporary improvement in the appearance of moderate-to-severe glabellar lines associated with corrugator and/or procerus muscle activity

Canadian labeling: Treatment of hypertonicity disorders of the seventh nerve (eg, blepharospasm, hemifacial spasm); treatment of poststroke spasticity of upper limb(s); treatment of cervical dystonia (spasmodic torticollis)
General Dosage Range I.M.: *Adults:*
Blepharospasm: Initial: Total dose should be the same as previously administered onabotulinumtoxinA dose or 1.25-2.5 units/injection site (maximum dose: 35 units/eye or 70 units/both eyes/every 3 months)
Cervical dystonia: Initial total dose: 120 units
Reduction of glabellar lines: 4 units/injection site into each of the 5 sites (maximum dose: 20 units/ treatment session every 3 months)
Dosage Forms
Injection, powder for reconstitution:
Xeomin®: 50 units, 100 units

Increlex® *see* mecasermin *on page 552*

indacaterol (in da KA ter ol)

Synonyms Arcapta™ Neohaler™; indacaterol maleate; OnBrez Breezehaler; QAB149
Therapeutic Category Beta$_2$-Adrenergic Agonist; Beta$_2$-Adrenergic Agonist, Long-Acting
Use Long-term maintenance treatment of bronchoconstriction in chronic obstructive pulmonary disease (COPD), including chronic bronchitis and emphysema
Product Availability Arcapta™ Neohaler™: FDA approved July 2011; expected availability first quarter 2012; consult prescribing information for additional information

indacaterol maleate *see* indacaterol *on page 470*

indapamide (in DAP a mide)

Medication Safety Issues
Sound-alike/look-alike issues:
Indapamide may be confused with Iopidine®
International issues:
Pretanix [Hungary] may be confused with Protonix brand name for pantoprazole [U.S., Canada]
Canadian Brand Names Apo-Indapamide®; Dom-Indapamide; Lozide®; Lozol®; Mylan-Indapamide; Novo-Indapamide; Nu-Indapamide; PHL-Indapamide; PMS-Indapamide; PRO-Indapamide; Riva-Indapamide
Therapeutic Category Diuretic, Miscellaneous
Use Management of mild-to-moderate hypertension; treatment of edema in heart failure and nephrotic syndrome
General Dosage Range Oral: *Adults:* 1.25-5 mg once daily
Dosage Forms
Tablet, oral: 1.25 mg, 2.5 mg

indapamide and perindopril erbumine *see* perindopril erbumine and indapamide *(Canada only) on page 691*
Inderal® (Can) *see* propranolol *on page 747*
Inderal® LA *see* propranolol *on page 747*
Inderide *see* propranolol and hydrochlorothiazide *on page 748*
indigo carmine *see* indigotindisulfonate sodium *on page 471*

indigotindisulfonate sodium (in di goe tin dye SUL foe nate SOW dee um)

Synonyms indigo carmine
Therapeutic Category Diagnostic Agent, Kidney Function
Use Localizing ureteral orifices during cystoscopy and ureteral catheterization
General Dosage Range I.M., I.V.:
Infants and Children: <5 mL
Adults: 5 mL
Dosage Forms
Injection, solution: 8 mg/mL (5 mL)

indinavir (in DIN a veer)

Medication Safety Issues
Sound-alike/look-alike issues:
Indinavir may be confused with Denavir™
Synonyms indinavir sulfate
U.S. Brand Names Crixivan®
Canadian Brand Names Crixivan®
Therapeutic Category Antiviral Agent
Use Treatment of HIV infection; should always be used as part of a multidrug regimen (at least three antiretroviral agents)
General Dosage Range Dosage adjustment recommended in patients with hepatic impairment or on concomitant therapy
Oral: *Adults:* 800 mg every 8 hours; Boosted regimen: 800 mg every 12 hours
Dosage Forms
Capsule, oral:
Crixivan®: 100 mg, 200 mg, 400 mg

indinavir sulfate *see* indinavir *on page 471*
Indocid® P.D.A. (Can) *see* indomethacin *on page 471*
Indocin® *see* indomethacin *on page 471*
Indocin® I.V. *see* indomethacin *on page 471*

indocyanine green (in doe SYE a neen green)

U.S. Brand Names IC-Green™
Therapeutic Category Diagnostic Agent
Use Determining hepatic function, cardiac output, and liver blood flow; ophthalmic angiography
General Dosage Range
Cardiac catheter:
Infants: 1.25 mg (maximum total dose: 2 mg/kg)
Children: 2.5 mg (maximum total dose: 2 mg/kg)
Adults: 5 mg (maximum total dose: 2 mg/kg)
I.V.: *Adults:* Hepatic function: 0.5 mg/kg; Ophthalmic angiography: ≤40 mg bolus
Dosage Forms
Injection, powder for reconstitution: 25 mg
IC-Green™: 25 mg

indometacin *see* indomethacin *on page 471*

indomethacin (in doe METH a sin)

Medication Safety Issues
Sound-alike/look-alike issues:
Indocin® may be confused with Imodium®, Lincocin®, Minocin®, Vicodin®
BEERS Criteria medication:
This drug may be inappropriate for use in geriatric patients (high severity risk).
International issues:
Flexin® [Great Britain] may be confused with Floxin® which is a brand name for ofloxacin in the U.S.
Flexin® [Great Britain]: Brand name for orphenadrine in Israel
Synonyms indometacin; indomethacin sodium trihydrate
U.S. Brand Names Indocin®; Indocin® I.V.

◄ **Canadian Brand Names** Apo-Indomethacin®; Indocid® P.D.A.; Novo-Methacin; Nu-Indo; Pro-Indo; ratio-Indomethacin; Sandoz-Indomethacin

Therapeutic Category Analgesic, Nonnarcotic; Nonsteroidal Antiinflammatory Drug (NSAID)

Use Acute gouty arthritis, acute bursitis/tendonitis, moderate-to-severe osteoarthritis, rheumatoid arthritis, ankylosing spondylitis; I.V. form used as alternative to surgery for closure of patent ductus arteriosus in neonates

General Dosage Range
I.V.:
Neonates <48 hours old at time of first dose: Initial: 0.2 mg/kg, followed by 2 doses of 0.1 mg/kg at 12- to 24-hour intervals
Neonates 2-7 days old at time of first dose: Initial: 0.2 mg/kg, followed by 2 doses of 0.2 mg/kg at 12- to 24-hour intervals
Neonates >7 days old at time of first dose: Initial: 0.2 mg/kg, followed by 2 doses of 0.25 mg/kg at 12- to 24-hour intervals
Oral:
Extended release: Children >14 years and Adults: 75-150 mg/day in 1-2 divided doses (maximum: 150 mg/day)
Immediate release:
Children ≥2 years: 1-2 mg/kg/day in 2-4 divided doses (maximum: 4 mg/kg/day; 200 mg/day)
Adults: 50-150 mg/day in 2-4 divided doses (maximum: 200 mg/day)

Dosage Forms
Capsule, oral: 25 mg, 50 mg
Capsule, extended release, oral: 75 mg
Injection, powder for reconstitution: 1 mg
Indocin® I.V.: 1 mg
Suppository, rectal: 50 mg (30s)
Suspension, oral:
Indocin®: 25 mg/5 mL (237 mL)

indomethacin sodium trihydrate see indomethacin on page 471

INF-alpha 2 see interferon alfa-2b on page 481

Infanrix® see diphtheria, tetanus toxoids, and acellular pertussis vaccine on page 296

Infanrix Hexa™ (Can) see diphtheria and tetanus toxoids, acellular pertussis, hepatitis B (recombinant), poliovirus (inactivated), and Haemophilus influenzae B conjugate (adsorbed) vaccine on page 294

Infantaire [OTC] see acetaminophen on page 23

Infantaire Gas [OTC] see simethicone on page 812

Infants Gas Relief Drops [OTC] see simethicone on page 812

Infasurf® see calfactant on page 166

INFeD® see iron dextran complex on page 491

Infergen® see interferon alfacon-1 on page 481

infliximab (in FLIKS e mab)

Medication Safety Issues
Sound-alike/look-alike issues:
InFLIXimab may be confused with riTUXimab
Remicade® may be confused with Renacidin®, Rituxan®

Synonyms avakine; infliximab, recombinant

Tall-Man inFLIXimab

U.S. Brand Names Remicade®

Canadian Brand Names Remicade®

Therapeutic Category Monoclonal Antibody

Use
Treatment of moderately- to severely-active rheumatoid arthritis (with methotrexate)
Treatment of moderately- to severely-active Crohn disease with inadequate response to conventional therapy (to reduce signs/symptoms and induce and maintain clinical remission) or to reduce the number of draining enterocutaneous and rectovaginal fistulas and maintain fistula closure
Treatment of psoriatic arthritis (to reduce signs/symptoms of active arthritis and inhibit progression of structural damage and improve physical function)
Treatment of chronic severe plaque psoriasis

Treatment of active ankylosing spondylitis (reduce signs/symptoms)
Treatment of moderately- to severely-active ulcerative colitis with inadequate response to conventional therapy (reduce signs/symptoms and induce and maintain clinical remission, mucosal healing and eliminate corticosteroid use)

General Dosage Range Dosage adjustment is required in heart failure patients.
I.V.:
Children ≥6 years: Initial: 5 mg/kg at 0, 2, and 6 weeks; Maintenance: 5 mg/kg every 8 weeks
Adults: Initial: 3-10 mg/kg at 0, 2, and 6 weeks; Maintenance: 3-10 mg/kg every 8 weeks **or** 5 mg/kg every 6 weeks

Dosage Forms
Injection, powder for reconstitution:
Remicade®: 100 mg

infliximab, recombinant *see* infliximab *on page 472*

influenza vaccine *see* influenza virus vaccine (inactivated) *on page 473*

influenza vaccine *see* influenza virus vaccine (live/attenuated) *on page 474*

influenza virus vaccine (H5N1) (in floo EN za VYE rus vak SEEN H5N1)

Medication Safety Issues
Sound-alike/look-alike issues:
Influenza virus vaccine (H5N1) may be confused with the nonavian strain of influenza virus vaccine

Synonyms avian influenza virus vaccine; bird flu vaccine; H5N1 influenza vaccine; influenza virus vaccine (monovalent)

Therapeutic Category Vaccine

Use Active immunization of adults at increased risk of exposure to the H5N1 viral subtype of influenza

General Dosage Range I.M.: *Adults 18-64 years:* 1 mL, followed by second 1 mL dose given 28 days later

Dosage Forms
Injection, suspension: Hemagglutinin (H5N1strain) 90 mcg/mL (5 mL)

influenza virus vaccine (inactivated) (in floo EN za VYE rus vak SEEN, in ak ti VAY ted)

Medication Safety Issues
Sound-alike/look-alike issues:
Fluarix® may be confused with Flarex®
Influenza virus vaccine may be confused with flumazenil
Influenza virus vaccine may be confused with tetanus toxoid and tuberculin products. Medication errors have occurred when tuberculin skin tests (PPD) have been inadvertently administered instead of tetanus toxoid products and influenza virus vaccine. These products are refrigerated and often stored in close proximity to each other.

International issues:
Fluarix [U.S., Canada, and multiple international markets] may be confused with Flarex brand name for fluorometholone [U.S. and multiple international markets] and Fluorex brand name for fluoride [France]

Synonyms H1N1 influenza vaccine; influenza vaccine; influenza virus vaccine (purified surface antigen); influenza virus vaccine (split-virus); trivalent inactivated influenza vaccine (TIV)

U.S. Brand Names Afluria®; Fluarix®; FluLaval®; Fluvirin®; Fluzone®; Fluzone® High-Dose; Fluzone® Intradermal

Canadian Brand Names Fluviral S/F®; Vaxigrip®

Therapeutic Category Vaccine, Inactivated (Viral)

Use Provide active immunity to influenza virus strains contained in the vaccine

The Advisory Committee on Immunization Practices (ACIP) recommends annual vaccination with the seasonal trivalent inactivated influenza vaccine (TIV) (injection) for all persons ≥6 months of age.
When vaccine supply is limited, target groups for vaccination (those at higher risk of complications from influenza infection and their close contacts) include the following:
• Persons ≥50 years of age
• Residents of nursing homes and other chronic-care facilities that house persons of any age with chronic medical conditions
• Adults and children with chronic disorders of the pulmonary or cardiovascular systems (except hypertension), including asthma

- Adults and children who have chronic metabolic diseases (including diabetes mellitus), hepatic disease, renal dysfunction, hematologic disorders, or immunosuppression (including immunosuppression caused by medications or HIV)
- Adults and children with cognitive or neurologic/neuromuscular conditions (including conditions such as spinal cord injuries or seizure disorders) which may compromise respiratory function, the handling of respiratory secretions, or that can increase the risk of aspiration
- Children and adolescents (6 months to 18 years of age) who are receiving long-term aspirin therapy, and therefore, may be at risk for developing Reye syndrome after influenza
- Women who are or will be pregnant during the influenza season
- Children 6-59 months of age
- Healthcare personnel
- Household contacts and caregivers of children <5 years (particularly children <6 months) and adults ≥50 years
- Household contacts and caregivers of persons with medical conditions which put them at high risk of complications from influenza infection
- American Indians/Alaska Natives
- Morbidly obese (BMI ≥40)

The Advisory Committee on Immunization Practices (ACIP) states that healthy, nonpregnant persons aged 2-49 years may receive vaccination with either the seasonal live, attenuated influenza vaccine (LAIV) (nasal spray) or the seasonal trivalent inactivated influenza vaccine (TIV) (injection).

General Dosage Range
I.M.:
  Children 6-35 months: 0.25 mL/dose (1 or 2 doses per season)
  Children 3-9 years: 0.5 mL/dose (1 or 2 doses per season)
  Children ≥9 years and Adults: 0.5 mL/dose (1 dose per season)
Intradermal: *Adults:* 18-64 years: 0.1 mL/dose (1 dose per season)

Dosage Forms
Injection, suspension:
  Afluria®: Hemagglutinin 45 mcg/0.5 mL (5 mL)
  FluLaval®: Hemagglutinin 45 mcg/0.5 mL (5 mL)
  Fluvirin®: Hemagglutinin 45 mcg/0.5 mL (5 mL)
  Fluzone®: Hemagglutinin 45 mcg/0.5 mL (5 mL)
Injection, suspension [preservative free]:
  Afluria®: Hemagglutinin 45 mcg/0.5 mL (0.5 mL)
  Fluarix®: Hemagglutinin 45 mcg/0.5 mL (0.5 mL)
  Fluvirin®: Hemagglutinin 45 mcg/0.5 mL (0.5 mL)
  Fluzone®: Hemagglutinin 22.5 mcg/0.25 mL (0.25 mL); Hemagglutinin 45 mcg/0.5 mL (0.5 mL)
  Fluzone® High-Dose: Hemagglutinin 180 mcg/0.5 mL (0.5 mL)
  Fluzone® Intradermal: Hemagglutinin 27 mcg/0.1 mL (0.1 mL)

influenza virus vaccine (live/attenuated) (in floo EN za VYE rus vak SEEN)

Medication Safety Issues
Sound-alike/look-alike issues:
  Influenza virus vaccine may be confused with flumazenil
Synonyms H1N1 influenza vaccine; influenza vaccine; influenza virus vaccine (trivalent, live); live attenuated influenza vaccine (LAIV)
U.S. Brand Names FluMist®
Canadian Brand Names FluMist®
Therapeutic Category Vaccine, Live (Viral)
Use Provide active immunity to influenza virus strains contained in the vaccine

The Advisory Committee on Immunization Practices (ACIP) states that healthy, nonpregnant persons aged 2-49 years may receive vaccination with either the seasonal live, attenuated influenza vaccine (LAIV) (nasal spray) or the seasonal trivalent inactivated influenza vaccine (TIV) (injection).

General Dosage Range Intranasal:
  Children 2-8 years: 0.2 mL/dose (1 or 2 doses per season)
  Children ≥9 years and Adults ≤49 years: 0.2 mL/dose (1 dose per season)

Dosage Forms
Solution, intranasal [preservative free]:
  FluMist®: (0.2 mL)

influenza virus vaccine (monovalent) *see* influenza virus vaccine (H5N1) *on page 473*

influenza virus vaccine (purified surface antigen) *see* influenza virus vaccine (inactivated) *on page 473*

influenza virus vaccine (split-virus) *see* influenza virus vaccine (inactivated) *on page 473*

influenza virus vaccine (trivalent, live) *see* influenza virus vaccine (live/attenuated) *on page 474*

Infufer® (Can) *see* iron dextran complex *on page 491*

Infumorph 200 *see* morphine (systemic) *on page 598*

Infumorph 500 *see* morphine (systemic) *on page 598*

Infuvite® Adult *see* vitamins (multiple/injectable) *on page 919*

Infuvite® Pediatric *see* vitamins (multiple/injectable) *on page 919*

INH *see* isoniazid *on page 493*

Inhibace® (Can) *see* cilazapril (Canada only) *on page 208*

Inhibace® Plus (Can) *see* cilazapril and hydrochlorothiazide (Canada only) *on page 208*

Innohep® [DSC] *see* tinzaparin *on page 870*

Innohep® (Can) *see* tinzaparin *on page 870*

InnoPran XL® *see* propranolol *on page 747*

INOmax® *see* nitric oxide *on page 628*

Inova™ *see* benzoyl peroxide *on page 124*

insect sting kit *see* epinephrine and chlorpheniramine *on page 332*

insoluble prussian blue *see* ferric hexacyanoferrate *on page 373*

Inspra™ *see* eplerenone *on page 333*

Insta-Glucose® [OTC] *see* dextrose *on page 273*

Instat™ MCH *see* collagen hemostat *on page 233*

insulin aspart (IN soo lin AS part)

Medication Safety Issues
Sound-alike/look-alike issues:
NovoLOG® may be confused with HumaLOG®, HumuLIN® R, NovoLIN® N, NovoLIN® R, NovoLOG® Mix 70/30
High alert medication:
The Institute for Safe Medication Practices (ISMP) includes this medication among its list of drugs which have a heightened risk of causing significant patient harm when used in error. *Due to the number of insulin preparations, it is essential to identify/clarify the type of insulin to be used.*
Other safety concerns:
Cross-contamination may occur if insulin pens are shared among multiple patients. Steps should be taken to prohibit sharing of insulin pens.

Synonyms aspart insulin

U.S. Brand Names NovoLOG®; NovoLOG® FlexPen®; NovoLOG® Penfill®

Canadian Brand Names NovoRapid®

Therapeutic Category Antidiabetic Agent, Insulin

Use Treatment of type 1 diabetes mellitus (insulin-dependent, IDDM) and type 2 diabetes mellitus (noninsulin-dependent, NIDDM) to improve glycemic control

General Dosage Range Dosage adjustment recommended in patients with renal impairment
I.V.: *Adults:* Refer to Insulin Regular on page 480
SubQ: *Children ≥2 years and Adults:* Refer to Insulin Regular on page 480

Dosage Forms
Injection, solution:
NovoLOG®: 100 units/mL (10 mL)
NovoLOG® FlexPen®: 100 units/mL (3 mL)
NovoLOG® Penfill®: 100 units/mL (3 mL)

insulin aspart and insulin aspart protamine *see* insulin aspart protamine and insulin aspart *on page 476*

insulin aspart protamine and insulin aspart
(IN soo lin AS part PROE ta meen & IN soo lin AS part)

Medication Safety Issues

Sound-alike/look-alike issues:
NovoLOG® Mix 70/30 may be confused with HumaLOG® Mix 75/25™, HumuLIN® 70/30, NovoLIN® 70/30, NovoLOG®

High alert medication:
The Institute for Safe Medication Practices (ISMP) includes this medication among its list of drugs which have a heightened risk of causing significant patient harm when used in error. ***Due to the number of insulin preparations, it is essential to identify/clarify the type of insulin to be used.***

Other safety concerns:
Cross-contamination may occur if insulin pens are shared among multiple patients. Steps should be taken to prohibit sharing of insulin pens.

Synonyms insulin aspart and insulin aspart protamine; NovoLog 70/30

U.S. Brand Names NovoLOG® Mix 70/30; NovoLOG® Mix 70/30 FlexPen®

Canadian Brand Names NovoMix® 30

Therapeutic Category Antidiabetic Agent, Insulin

Use Treatment of type 1 diabetes mellitus (insulin-dependent, IDDM) and type 2 diabetes mellitus (noninsulin-dependent, NIDDM) to improve glycemic control

General Dosage Range Dosage adjustment recommended in patients with renal impairment
SubQ: *Adults:* Refer to Insulin Regular on page 480

Dosage Forms

Injection, suspension:
NovoLOG® Mix 70/30: Insulin aspart protamine suspension 70% [intermediate acting] and insulin aspart solution 30% [rapid acting]: 100 units/mL (10 mL)
NovoLOG® Mix 70/30 FlexPen®: Insulin aspart protamine suspension 70% [intermediate acting] and insulin aspart solution 30% [rapid acting]: 100 units/mL (3 mL)

insulin detemir (IN soo lin DE te mir)

Medication Safety Issues

High alert medication:
The Institute for Safe Medication Practices (ISMP) includes this medication among its list of drugs which have a heightened risk of causing significant patient harm when used in error. ***Due to the number of insulin preparations, it is essential to identify/clarify the type of insulin to be used.***

Administration issues:
Insulin detemir is a clear solution, but it is NOT intended for I.V. or I.M. administration.

Other safety concerns:
Cross-contamination may occur if insulin pens are shared among multiple patients. Steps should be taken to prohibit sharing of insulin pens.

Synonyms detemir insulin

U.S. Brand Names Levemir®; Levemir® FlexPen®

Canadian Brand Names Levemir®

Therapeutic Category Antidiabetic Agent, Insulin

Use Treatment of type 1 diabetes mellitus (insulin-dependent, IDDM) and type 2 diabetes mellitus (noninsulin-dependent, NIDDM) to improve glycemic control

General Dosage Range Dosage adjustment recommended in patients with renal impairment
SubQ:
Children ≥6 years: Refer to Insulin Regular on page 480
Adults: Refer to Insulin Regular on page 480; 0.1-0.2 units/kg once daily **or** 10 units once- or twice daily (manufacturer recommendations)

Dosage Forms

Injection, solution:
Levemir®: 100 units/mL (10 mL)
Levemir® FlexPen®: 100 units/mL (3 mL)

insulin glargine (IN soo lin GLAR jeen)

Medication Safety Issues

Sound-alike/look-alike issues:
Insulin glargine may be confused with insulin glulisine

Lantus® may be confused with latanoprost, Latuda®, Xalatan®

High alert medication:

The Institute for Safe Medication Practices (ISMP) includes this medication among its list of drugs which have a heightened risk of causing significant patient harm when used in error. *Due to the number of insulin preparations, it is essential to identify/clarify the type of insulin to be used.*

Administration issues:

Insulin glargine is a clear solution, but it is NOT intended for I.V. or I.M. administration.

Other safety concerns:

Cross-contamination may occur if insulin pens are shared among multiple patients. Steps should be taken to prohibit sharing of insulin pens.

International issues:

Lantus [U.S., Canada, and multiple international markets] may be confused with Lanvis brand name for thioguanine [Canada and multiple international markets]

Synonyms glargine insulin

U.S. Brand Names Lantus®; Lantus® Solostar®

Canadian Brand Names Lantus®; Lantus® OptiSet®

Therapeutic Category Antidiabetic Agent, Insulin

Use Treatment of type 1 diabetes mellitus (insulin-dependent, IDDM) and type 2 diabetes mellitus (noninsulin-dependent, NIDDM) to improve glycemic control

General Dosage Range Dosage adjustment recommended in patients with renal impairment

SubQ: *Children ≥6 years and Adults:* Refer to Insulin Regular on page 480

Dosage Forms

Injection, solution:

Lantus®: 100 units/mL (3 mL, 10 mL)

Lantus® Solostar®: 100 units/mL (3 mL)

insulin glulisine (IN soo lin gloo LIS een)

Medication Safety Issues

Sound-alike/look-alike issues:

Insulin glulisine may be confused with insulin glargine

High alert medication:

The Institute for Safe Medication Practices (ISMP) includes this medication among its list of drugs which have a heightened risk of causing significant patient harm when used in error. *Due to the number of insulin preparations, it is essential to identify/clarify the type of insulin to be used.*

Other safety concerns:

Cross-contamination may occur if insulin pens are shared among multiple patients. Steps should be taken to prohibit sharing of insulin pens.

Synonyms glulisine insulin

U.S. Brand Names Apidra®; Apidra® SoloStar®

Canadian Brand Names Apidra®

Therapeutic Category Antidiabetic Agent, Insulin

Use Treatment of type 1 diabetes mellitus (insulin-dependent, IDDM) and type 2 diabetes mellitus (noninsulin-dependent, NIDDM) to improve glycemic control

General Dosage Range Dosage adjustment recommended in patients with renal impairment

I.V.: *Adults:* Refer to Insulin Regular on page 480

SubQ: *Children ≥4 years and Adults:* Refer to Insulin Regular on page 480

Dosage Forms

Injection, solution:

Apidra®: 100 units/mL (3 mL, 10 mL)

Apidra® SoloStar®: 100 units/mL (3 mL)

insulin lispro (IN soo lin LYE sproe)

Medication Safety Issues

Sound-alike/look-alike issues:

HumaLOG® may be confused with HumaLOG® Mix 50/50, Humira®, HumuLIN® N, HumuLIN® R, NovoLOG®

High alert medication:

The Institute for Safe Medication Practices (ISMP) includes this medication among its list of drugs which have a heightened risk of causing significant patient harm when used in error. *Due to the number of insulin preparations, it is essential to identify/clarify the type of insulin to be used.*

Other safety concerns:

Cross-contamination may occur if insulin pens are shared among multiple patients. Steps should be taken to prohibit sharing of insulin pens.

Synonyms lispro insulin

U.S. Brand Names HumaLOG®; HumaLOG® KwikPen™

Canadian Brand Names Humalog®

Therapeutic Category Antidiabetic Agent, Insulin

Use Treatment of type 1 diabetes mellitus (insulin-dependent, IDDM) and type 2 diabetes mellitus (noninsulin-dependent, NIDDM) to improve glycemic control

General Dosage Range Dosage adjustment recommended in patients with renal impairment

SubQ: *Children and Adults:* Refer to Insulin Regular on page 480

Dosage Forms

Injection, solution:

HumaLOG®: 100 units/mL (3 mL, 10 mL)

HumaLOG® KwikPen™: 100 units/mL (3 mL)

insulin lispro and insulin lispro protamine *see* insulin lispro protamine and insulin lispro on page 478

insulin lispro protamine and insulin lispro

(IN soo lin LYE sproe PROE ta meen & IN soo lin LYE sproe)

Medication Safety Issues

Sound-alike/look-alike issues:

HumaLOG® Mix 50/50™ may be confused with HumaLOG®

HumaLOG® Mix 75/25™ may be confused with HumuLIN® 70/30, NovoLIN® 70/30, and NovoLOG® Mix 70/30

High alert medication:

The Institute for Safe Medication Practices (ISMP) includes this medication among its list of drugs which have a heightened risk of causing significant patient harm when used in error. *Due to the number of insulin preparations, it is essential to identify/clarify the type of insulin to be used.*

Other safety concerns:

Cross-contamination may occur if insulin pens are shared among multiple patients. Steps should be taken to prohibit sharing of insulin pens.

Synonyms insulin lispro and insulin lispro protamine

U.S. Brand Names HumaLOG® Mix 50/50™; HumaLOG® Mix 50/50™ KwikPen™; HumaLOG® Mix 75/25™; HumaLOG® Mix 75/25™ KwikPen™

Canadian Brand Names Humalog® Mix 25

Therapeutic Category Antidiabetic Agent, Insulin

Use Treatment of type 1 diabetes mellitus (insulin-dependent, IDDM) and type 2 diabetes mellitus (noninsulin-dependent, NIDDM) to improve glycemic control

General Dosage Range Dosage adjustment recommended in patients with renal impairment

SubQ: *Adults:* Refer to Insulin Regular on page 480

Dosage Forms

Injection, suspension:

HumaLOG® Mix 50/50™: Insulin lispro protamine suspension 50% [intermediate acting] and insulin lispro solution 50% [rapid acting]: 100 units/mL (10 mL)

HumaLOG® Mix 50/50™ KwikPen™: Insulin lispro protamine suspension 50% [intermediate acting] and insulin lispro solution 50% [rapid acting]: 100 units/mL (3 mL)

HumaLOG® Mix 75/25™: Insulin lispro protamine suspension 75% [intermediate acting] and insulin lispro solution 25% [rapid acting]: 100 units/mL (10 mL)

HumaLOG® Mix 75/25™ KwikPen™: Insulin lispro protamine suspension 75% [intermediate acting] and insulin lispro solution 25% [rapid acting]: 100 units/mL (3 mL)

insulin NPH (IN soo lin N P H)

Medication Safety Issues

Sound-alike/look-alike issues:
HumuLIN® N may be confused with HumuLIN® R, HumaLOG®, Humira®
NovoLIN® N may be confused with NovoLIN® R, NovoLOG®

High alert medication:
The Institute for Safe Medication Practices (ISMP) includes this medication among its list of drugs which have a heightened risk of causing significant patient harm when used in error. *Due to the number of insulin preparations, it is essential to identify/clarify the type of insulin to be used.*

Other safety concerns:
Cross-contamination may occur if insulin pens are shared among multiple patients. Steps should be taken to prohibit sharing of insulin pens.

Synonyms isophane insulin; NPH insulin

U.S. Brand Names HumuLIN® N; NovoLIN® N

Canadian Brand Names Humulin® N; Novolin® ge NPH

Therapeutic Category Antidiabetic Agent, Insulin

Use Treatment of type 1 diabetes mellitus (insulin-dependent, IDDM) and type 2 diabetes mellitus (noninsulin-dependent, NIDDM) to improve glycemic control

General Dosage Range Dosage adjustment recommended in patients with renal impairment
SubQ: *Children and Adults:* Refer to Insulin Regular on page 480

Dosage Forms
Injection, suspension:
HumuLIN® N: 100 units/mL (3 mL, 10 mL)
NovoLIN® N: 100 units/mL (10 mL)

Dosage Forms - Canada
Injection, suspension:
Novolin® ge NPH: 100 units/mL (3 mL, 10 mL)

insulin NPH and insulin regular (IN soo lin N P H & IN soo lin REG yoo ler)

Medication Safety Issues

Sound-alike/look-alike issues:
HumuLIN® 70/30 may be confused with HumaLOG® Mix 75/25, HumuLIN® R, NovoLIN® 70/30, NovoLOG® Mix 70/30
NovoLIN® 70/30 may be confused with HumaLOG® Mix 75/25, HumuLIN® 70/30, HumuLIN® R, NovoLIN® R, and NovoLOG® Mix 70/30

High alert medication:
The Institute for Safe Medication Practices (ISMP) includes this medication among its list of drugs which have a heightened risk of causing significant patient harm when used in error. *Due to the number of insulin preparations, it is essential to identify/clarify the type of insulin to be used.*

Other safety concerns:
Cross-contamination may occur if insulin pens are shared among multiple patients. Steps should be taken to prohibit sharing of insulin pens.

Synonyms insulin regular and insulin NPH; isophane insulin and regular insulin; NPH insulin and regular insulin

U.S. Brand Names HumuLIN® 70/30; NovoLIN® 70/30

Canadian Brand Names Humulin® 20/80; Humulin® 70/30; Novolin® ge 30/70; Novolin® ge 40/60; Novolin® ge 50/50

Therapeutic Category Antidiabetic Agent, Insulin

Use Treatment of type 1 diabetes mellitus (insulin-dependent, IDDM) and type 2 diabetes mellitus (noninsulin-dependent, NIDDM) to improve glycemic control

General Dosage Range Dosage adjustment recommended in patients with renal impairment
SubQ: *Children and Adults:* Refer to Insulin Regular on page 480

◄ **Dosage Forms**
Injection, suspension:
HumuLIN® 70/30: Insulin NPH suspension 70% [intermediate acting] and insulin regular solution 30% [short acting]: 100 units/mL (3 mL, 10 mL)
NovoLIN® 70/30: Insulin NPH suspension 70% [intermediate acting] and insulin regular solution 30% [short acting]: 100 units/mL (10 mL)

Dosage Forms - Canada
Injection, suspension:
Humulin® 20/80: Insulin regular solution 20% [short acting] and insulin NPH suspension 80% [intermediate acting]: 100 units/mL (3 mL)
Novolin® ge 30/70: Insulin regular solution 30% [short acting] and insulin NPH suspension 70% [intermediate acting]: 100 units/mL (3 mL)
Novolin® ge 40/60: Insulin regular solution 40% [short acting] and insulin NPH suspension 60% [intermediate acting]: 100 units/mL (3 mL)
Novolin® ge 50/50: Insulin regular solution 50% [short acting] and insulin NPH suspension 50% [intermediate acting]: 100 units/mL (3 mL)

insulin regular (IN soo lin REG yoo ler)

Medication Safety Issues
Sound-alike/look-alike issues:
HumuLIN® R may be confused with HumaLOG®, Humira®, HumuLIN® 70/30, HumuLIN® N, NovoLIN® 70/30, NovoLIN® R, NovoLOG®
NovoLIN® R may be confused with HumuLIN® R, NovoLIN® 70/30, NovoLIN® N, NovoLOG®
High alert medication:
The Institute for Safe Medication Practices (ISMP) includes this medication among its list of drugs which have a heightened risk of causing significant patient harm when used in error. *Due to the number of insulin preparations, it is essential to identify/clarify the type of insulin to be used.*
Administration issues:
Concentrated solutions (eg, U-500) should not be available in patient care areas. U-500 regular insulin should be stored, dispensed, and administered separately from U-100 regular insulin. For patients who receive U-500 insulin in the hospital setting, highlighting the strength prominently on the patient's medical chart and medication record may help to reduce dispensing errors.
Other safety concerns:
Cross-contamination may occur if insulin pens are shared among multiple patients. Steps should be taken to prohibit sharing of insulin pens.

Synonyms regular insulin

U.S. Brand Names HumuLIN® R; HumuLIN® R U-500; NovoLIN® R

Canadian Brand Names Humulin® R; Novolin® ge Toronto

Therapeutic Category Antidiabetic Agent, Insulin; Antidote

Use Treatment of type 1 diabetes mellitus (insulin-dependent, IDDM) and type 2 diabetes mellitus (noninsulin-dependent, NIDDM) to improve glycemic control

General Dosage Range Dosage adjustment recommended in patients with renal impairment
I.V., SubQ: *Children and Adults:*
Diabetes mellitus, type 1: Initial: 0.5-1 unit/kg/day in divided doses; Usual maintenance: 0.5-1.2 units/kg/day in divided doses. **Note:** Generally, 50% to 75% of the total daily dose (TDD) is given as an intermediate- or long-acting form of insulin (1-2 daily injections) and the remaining portion is then divided and administered before or at mealtime (depending on the formulation) as a rapid-acting or short-acting form of insulin.
Diabetes mellitus, type 2: Initial basal insulin dose: 0.2 units/kg or 10 units/day given as an intermediate- or long-acting insulin at bedtime or long-acting insulin given in the morning

Dosage Forms
Injection, solution:
HumuLIN® R: 100 units/mL (3 mL, 10 mL)
HumuLIN® R U-500: 500 units/mL (20 mL)
NovoLIN® R: 100 units/mL (10 mL)

insulin regular and insulin NPH *see* insulin NPH and insulin regular *on page 479*
Integrilin® *see* eptifibatide *on page 335*
Intelence® *see* etravirine *on page 362*
α-2-interferon *see* interferon alfa-2b *on page 481*

interferon alfa-2a (PEG conjugate) *see* peginterferon alfa-2a *on page* 679
interferon alfa-2b (PEG conjugate) *see* peginterferon alfa-2b *on page* 680

interferon alfa-2b (in ter FEER on AL fa too bee)

Medication Safety Issues
Sound-alike/look-alike issues:
Interferon alfa-2b may be confused with interferon alfa-2a, interferon alfa-n3, pegylated interferon alfa-2b
Intron® A may be confused with PEG-Intron®
International issues:
Interferon alfa-2b may be confused with interferon alpha multi-subtype which is available in international markets
Synonyms INF-alpha 2; interferon alpha-2b; rLFN-α2; α-2-interferon
U.S. Brand Names Intron® A
Canadian Brand Names Intron® A
Therapeutic Category Biological Response Modulator
Use
Patients ≥1 year of age: Chronic hepatitis B
Patients ≥3 years of age: Chronic hepatitis C (in combination with ribavirin)
Patients ≥18 years of age: Condyloma acuminata, chronic hepatitis B, chronic hepatitis C, hairy cell leukemia, malignant melanoma, AIDS-related Kaposi sarcoma, follicular non-Hodgkin lymphoma
General Dosage Range Dosage adjustment is recommended in patients who develop toxicities
I.M.:
Children 1-17 years: 3-5 million units/m^2 3 times/week (maximum: 3 million units/dose)
Adults: Dosage varies greatly depending on indication
I.V.: *Adults:* 20 million units/m^2 for 5 consecutive days per week
Intralesional: *Adults:* 1 million units/lesion 3 times/week, on alternate days (maximum: 5 lesions/treatment)
SubQ:
Children 1-17 years: Initial: 3 million units/m^2 3 times/week for 1 week; Maintenance: 6 million units/m^2 3 times/week (maximum: 10 million units 3 times/week)
Adults: Dosage varies greatly depending on indication
Dosage Forms
Injection, powder for reconstitution [preservative free]:
Intron® A: 10 million int. units, 18 million int. units, 50 million int. units
Injection, solution:
Intron® A: 6 million int. units/mL (3 mL); 10 million int. units/mL (2.5 mL); 3 million int. units/0.2 mL (1.2 mL); 5 million int. units/0.2 mL (1.2 mL); 10 million int. units/0.2 mL (1.2 mL)

interferon alfacon-1 (in ter FEER on AL fa con one)

Medication Safety Issues
Sound-alike/look-alike issues:
Interferon alfacon-1 may be confused with interferon alfa-2a, interferon alfa-2b, interferon alfa-n3, peginterferon alfa-2b
International issues:
Interferon alfacon-1 may be confused with interferon alpha multi-subtype which is available in international markets
U.S. Brand Names Infergen®
Therapeutic Category Interferon
Use Treatment of chronic hepatitis C virus (HCV) infection in patients ≥18 years of age with compensated liver disease and anti-HCV serum antibodies or HCV RNA; concurrent use with ribavirin in HCV-infected patients who have failed treatment with pegylated interferon/ribavirin (Bacon, 2009)
General Dosage Range Dosage adjustment recommended in patients who develop toxicities
SubQ: *Adults:* 9-15 mcg 3 times/week; may increase to 15 mcg 3 times/week
Dosage Forms
Injection, solution [preservative free]:
Infergen®: 30 mcg/mL (0.3 mL, 0.5 mL)

interferon alfa-n3 (in ter FEER on AL fa en three)

Medication Safety Issues
Sound-alike/look-alike issues:
Alferon® may be confused with Alkeran®

U.S. Brand Names Alferon® N

Canadian Brand Names Alferon® N

Therapeutic Category Biological Response Modulator

Use Patients ≥18 years of age: Intralesional treatment of refractory or recurring genital or venereal warts (condylomata acuminata)

General Dosage Range Intralesional: *Adults:* Inject 250,000 units (0.05 mL) in each wart twice weekly (maximum: 8 weeks)

Dosage Forms
Injection, solution:
Alferon® N: 5 million int. units (1 mL)

interferon alpha-2b *see* interferon alfa-2b *on page 481*

interferon beta-1a (in ter FEER on BAY ta won aye)

Medication Safety Issues
Sound-alike/look-alike issues:
Avonex® may be confused with Avelox®

Synonyms rIFN beta-1a

U.S. Brand Names Avonex®; Rebif®

Canadian Brand Names Avonex®; Rebif®

Therapeutic Category Biological Response Modulator

Use Treatment of relapsing forms of multiple sclerosis (MS)

General Dosage Range Dosage adjustment recommended in patients who develop toxicities
I.M.: *Adults:* 30 mcg once weekly
SubQ: *Adults:* Initial: 4.4 or 8.8 mcg 3 times/week for 2 weeks; Titration: 11 or 22 mcg 3 times/week for 2 weeks; Maintenance: 22 or 44 mcg 3 times/week

Dosage Forms
Injection, powder for reconstitution [preservative free]:
Avonex®: 33 mcg [contains albumin (human); 6.6 million units; provides 30 mcg/mL following reconstitution; supplied with diluent]
Injection, solution:
Avonex®: 30 mcg/0.5 mL (0.5 mL)
Injection, solution [preservative free]:
Rebif®: 22 mcg/0.5 mL (0.5 mL), 44 mcg/0.5 mL (0.5 mL)
Injection, solution [preservative free, combination package]:
Rebif®: Titration Pack: 22 mcg/0.5 mL (6s) and 8.8 mcg/0.2 mL (6s)

interferon beta-1b (in ter FEER on BAY ta won bee)

Synonyms rIFN beta-1b

U.S. Brand Names Betaseron®; Extavia®

Canadian Brand Names Betaseron®; Extavia®

Therapeutic Category Biological Response Modulator

Use Treatment of relapsing forms of multiple sclerosis (MS); treatment of first clinical episode with MRI features consistent with MS

Canadian labeling: Additional use (not in U.S. labeling): Treatment of secondary-progressive MS

General Dosage Range SubQ: *Adults:* 0.0625-0.25 mg (2-8 million units) every other day

Dosage Forms
Injection, powder for reconstitution:
Betaseron®: 0.3 mg [~9.6 million int. units]
Injection, powder for reconstitution [preservative free]:
Extavia®: 0.3 mg [~9.6 million int. units]

interferon gamma-1b (in ter FEER on GAM ah won bee)

U.S. Brand Names Actimmune®

Canadian Brand Names Actimmune®

Therapeutic Category Biological Response Modulator

Use Reduce frequency and severity of serious infections associated with chronic granulomatous disease; delay time to disease progression in patients with severe, malignant osteopetrosis

General Dosage Range Dosage adjustment recommended in patients who develop toxicities

  SubQ: *Children and Adults:*
    BSA ≤0.5 m^2: 1.5 mcg/kg/dose 3 times/week
    BSA >0.5 m^2: 50 mcg/m^2 (1 million int. units/m^2) 3 times/week

Dosage Forms

  Injection, solution [preservative free]:
    Actimmune®: 100 mcg (0.5 mL)

interleukin-1 receptor antagonist *see* anakinra *on page 78*

interleukin 2 *see* aldesleukin *on page 47*

interleukin-11 *see* oprelvekin *on page 653*

Intralipid® *see* fat emulsion *on page 367*

intrapleural talc *see* talc (sterile) *on page 843*

intravenous fat emulsion *see* fat emulsion *on page 367*

intrifiban *see* eptifibatide *on page 335*

Intron® A *see* interferon alfa-2b *on page 481*

Intropin *see* dopamine *on page 306*

Introvale™ *see* ethinyl estradiol and levonorgestrel *on page 353*

Intuniv™ *see* guanfacine *on page 431*

INVanz® *see* ertapenem *on page 338*

Invanz® (Can) *see* ertapenem *on page 338*

Invega® *see* paliperidone *on page 668*

Invega® Sustenna® *see* paliperidone *on page 668*

Invirase® *see* saquinavir *on page 802*

iobenguane I 123 (eye oh BEN gwane eye one TWEN tee three)

Synonyms 123 meta-iodobenzlyguanidine sulfate; 123I-metaiodobenzylguanidine (MIBG); I-123 MIBG; I^{123} iobenguane; iobenguane sulfate I 123

U.S. Brand Names AdreView™

Therapeutic Category Radiopharmaceutical

Use As an adjunct to other diagnostic tests, in the detection of primary or metastatic pheochromocytoma or neuroblastoma

Dosage Forms

  Injection, solution:
    AdreView™: Iobenguane sulfate 0.08 mg and I 123 74 MBq (2 mCi) per mL (5 mL)

iobenguane sulfate I 123 *see* iobenguane I 123 *on page 483*

Iodex® [OTC] *see* iodine *on page 483*

iodine (EYE oh dyne)

Medication Safety Issues

  Sound-alike/look-alike issues:
    Iodine may be confused with codeine, Iopidine®, Lodine®

U.S. Brand Names Iodex® [OTC]; Iodoflex™ [OTC]; Iodosorb® [OTC]

Therapeutic Category Topical Skin Product

Use Used topically as an antiseptic in the management of minor, superficial skin wounds and has been used to disinfect the skin preoperatively

General Dosage Range Topical: *Adults:* Antiseptic: Apply to affected area 1-3 times/day; Ulcer/wound cleansing: Apply to clean wound 3 times/week (maximum: 50 g/application; 150 g/week)

Dosage Forms

  Dressing, topical:
    Iodoflex™ [OTC]: 0.9% (3s, 5s)
  Gel, topical:
    Iodosorb® [OTC]: 0.9% (40 g)

◀ **Ointment, topical**:
Iodex® [OTC]: 4.7% (30 g, 720 g)
Tincture, topical: 2% (30 mL, 59 mL, 473 mL); 7% (30 mL, 473 mL)

iodine *see* trace metals *on page 880*

iodine I 131 tositumomab and tositumomab *see* tositumomab and iodine I 131 tositumomab
on page 879

iodipamide meglumine (eye oh DI pa mide MEG loo meen)

Medication Safety Issues
High alert medication:
The Institute for Safe Medication Practices (ISMP) includes this medication among its list of drugs which have a heightened risk of causing significant patient harm when used in error.

U.S. Brand Names Cholografin® Meglumine

Therapeutic Category Iodinated Contrast Media; Radiological/Contrast Media, Ionic

Use Contrast medium for intravenous cholangiography and cholecystography

General Dosage Range I.V.:
Infants and Children: 0.3-0.6 mL/kg (maximum: 20 mL)
Adults: 20 mL

Dosage Forms
Injection, solution:
Cholografin® Meglumine: 520 mg/mL (20 mL)

iodipamide meglumine and diatrizoate meglumine *see* diatrizoate meglumine and iodipamide meglumine *on page 275*

iodixanol (EYE oh dix an ole)

Medication Safety Issues
High alert medication:
The Institute for Safe Medication Practices (ISMP) includes this medication among its list of drugs which have a heightened risk of causing significant patient harm when used in error.
Administration issues:
Not for intrathecal use.

U.S. Brand Names Visipaque™

Canadian Brand Names Visipaque™

Therapeutic Category Iodinated Contrast Media; Radiological/Contrast Media, Nonionic

Use
Intraarterial: Digital subtraction angiography, angiocardiography, peripheral arteriography, visceral arteriography, cerebral arteriography
Intravenous: Contrast enhanced computed tomography imaging, excretory urography, and peripheral venography

General Dosage Range
I.V.:
Children >1-12 years: Iodixanol 270 mg iodine/mL: 1-2 mL/kg (maximum: 2 mL/kg)
Children >12 years and Adults: Iodixanol 270 mg and 320 mg iodine/mL: Concentration and dose vary based on study type; refer to product labeling (maximum total dose: 80 g iodine)
Intraarterial:
Children >1-12 years: Iodixanol 320 mg iodine/mL: 1-2 mL/kg (maximum: 4 mL/kg)
Children >12 years and Adults: Iodixanol 320 mg iodine/mL: Dose individualized based on injection site and study type; refer to product labeling (maximum total dose: 80 g iodine)

Dosage Forms
Injection, solution [preservative free]:
Visipaque™: 270: 550 mg/mL (50 mL, 100 mL, 125 mL, 150 mL, 200 mL, 500 mL); 320: 652 mg/mL (50 mL, 100 mL, 125 mL, 150 mL, 200 mL, 500 mL)

iodochlorhydroxyquin and flumethasone *see* clioquinol and flumethasone *(Canada only)* *on page 219*

Iodoflex™ [OTC] *see* iodine *on page 483*

iodoquinol (eye oh doe KWIN ole)

Synonyms diiodohydroxyquin

U.S. Brand Names Yodoxin®
Canadian Brand Names Diodoquin®
Therapeutic Category Amebicide
Use Treatment of acute and chronic intestinal amebiasis; asymptomatic cyst passers; *Blastocystis hominis* infections; ineffective for amebic hepatitis or hepatic abscess
General Dosage Range Oral:
   Children: 30-40 mg/kg/day in 3 divided doses (maximum: 1.95 g/day)
   Adults: 650 mg 3 times/day (maximum: 2 g/day)
Dosage Forms
   Tablet, oral:
      Yodoxin®: 210 mg, 650 mg

iodoquinol and hydrocortisone (eye oh doe KWIN ole & hye droe KOR ti sone)
Medication Safety Issues
   Sound-alike/look-alike issues:
      Vytone may be confused with Hytone®, Zydone®
Synonyms hydrocortisone and iodoquinol
U.S. Brand Names Alcortin® A; Dermazene®
Therapeutic Category Antifungal/Corticosteroid
Use Treatment of eczema (including impetiginized, nuchal, and nummular); acne urticaria; anogenital pruritus, atopic dermatitis, chronic infectious dermatitis; chronic eczematoid otitis externa; folliculitis; intertrigo; lichen simplex chronicus; moniliasis; mycotic dermatoses; neurodermatitis (localized or systemic); pyoderma, stasis dermatitis
General Dosage Range Topical: *Children ≥12 years and Adults:* Apply 3-4 times/day
Dosage Forms
   Cream, topical: Iodoquinol 1% and hydrocortisone 1% (30 g)
      Dermazene®: Iodoquinol 1% and hydrocortisone 1% (30 g)
   Gel, topical:
      Alcortin® A: Iodoquinol 1% and hydrocortisone 2% (2 g)

Iodosorb® [OTC] see iodine on page 483

iohexol (eye oh HEX ole)
Medication Safety Issues
   High alert medication:
      The Institute for Safe Medication Practices (ISMP) includes this medication among its list of drugs which have a heightened risk of causing significant patient harm when used in error.
U.S. Brand Names Omnipaque™ 140; Omnipaque™ 180; Omnipaque™ 240; Omnipaque™ 300; Omnipaque™ 350
Canadian Brand Names Omnipaque™
Therapeutic Category Polypeptide Hormone; Radiological/Contrast Media, Nonionic
Use
   Intrathecal: Myelography; contrast enhancement for computerized tomography
   Intravascular: Angiocardiography, aortography, digital subtraction angiography, peripheral arteriography, excretory urography; contrast enhancement for computed tomographic imaging
   Oral/body cavity: Arthrography, GI tract examination, hysterosalpingography, pancreatography, cholangiopancreatography, herniography, cystourethrography; enhanced computed tomography of the abdomen
Dosage Forms
   Injection, solution [preservative free]:
      Omnipaque™ 140: 302 mg/mL (50 mL)
      Omnipaque™ 180: 388 mg/mL (10 mL, 20 mL)
      Omnipaque™ 240: 518 mg/mL (10 mL, 20 mL, 50 mL, 75 mL, 100 mL, 150 mL, 200 mL)
      Omnipaque™ 300: 647 mg/mL (10 mL, 30 mL, 50 mL, 75 mL, 100 mL, 125 mL, 150 mL, 200 mL, 500 mL)
      Omnipaque™ 350: 755 mg/mL (50 mL, 75 mL, 100 mL, 125 mL, 150 mL, 200 mL, 250 mL, 500 mL)
   Injection, solution, oral [preservative free]:
      Omnipaque™ 240: 518 mg/mL (50 mL)
      Omnipaque™ 300: 647 mg/mL (50 mL)
      Omnipaque™ 350: 755 mg/mL (50 mL)

Ionil® [OTC] *see* salicylic acid *on page 795*

Ionil Plus® [OTC] *see* salicylic acid *on page 795*

ionil-T® [OTC] *see* coal tar *on page 227*

ionil-T® Plus [OTC] *see* coal tar *on page 227*

iopamidol (eye oh PA mi dole)

Medication Safety Issues
High alert medication:
The Institute for Safe Medication Practices (ISMP) includes this medication among its list of drugs which have a heightened risk of causing significant patient harm when used in error.
U.S. Brand Names Isovue Multipack®; Isovue-M®; Isovue®; Isovue® 200; Isovue® 300; Isovue® 370
Therapeutic Category Iodinated Contrast Media; Radiological/Contrast Media, Nonionic
Use
Intrathecal (Isovue-M®): Myelography contrast enhancement of computed tomographic cisternography and ventriculography; thoracolumbar myelography
Intravascular (Isovue®, Isovue Multipack®): Angiography (eg, coronary, cerebral, peripheral arteriogram), pediatric angiocardiography, excretory urography; contrast enhancement of computed tomographic imaging (in adults and children); evaluation of certain malignancies; image enhancement of non-neoplastic lesions
Dosage Forms
Injection, solution:
Isovue Multipack®: 51% (200 mL); 61% (200 mL, 500 mL); 76% (200 mL, 500 mL)
Isovue® 200: 41% (50 mL, 200 mL)
Isovue®: 51% (50 mL, 100 mL, 150 mL, 200 mL)
Isovue® 300: 61% (30 mL, 50 mL, 75 mL, 100 mL, 125 mL, 150 mL)
Isovue® 370: 76% (50 mL, 75 mL, 100 mL, 125 mL, 150 mL)
Injection, solution, intrathecal:
Isovue-M®: 41% (10 mL, 20 mL); 61% (15 mL)

Iopidine® *see* apraclonidine *on page 91*

iopromide (eye oh PROE mide)

Medication Safety Issues
High alert medication:
The Institute for Safe Medication Practices (ISMP) includes this medication among its list of drugs which have a heightened risk of causing significant patient harm when used in error.
U.S. Brand Names Ultravist®
Therapeutic Category Radiological/Contrast Media, Nonionic
Use Enhance imaging in cerebral arteriography and peripheral arteriography; coronary arteriography and left ventriculography, visceral angiography and aortography; contrast-enhanced computed tomographic imaging of the head and body, excretory urography, intraarterial digital subtraction angiography, peripheral venography
Dosage Forms
Injection, solution:
Ultravist®: Iodine 240 mg/mL (100 mL, 200 mL); Iodine 300 mg/mL (50 mL, 100 mL, 125 mL, 150 mL, 200 mL, 500 mL); Iodine 370 mg/mL (50 mL, 100 mL, 150 mL, 200 mL, 250 mL, 500 mL)

iOSAT™ [OTC] *see* potassium iodide *on page 726*

iothalamate meglumine (eye oh thal A mate MEG loo meen)

Medication Safety Issues
High alert medication:
The Institute for Safe Medication Practices (ISMP) includes this medication among its list of drugs which have a heightened risk of causing significant patient harm when used in error.
U.S. Brand Names Conray®; Conray® 30; Conray® 43; Cysto-Conray® II
Therapeutic Category Iodinated Contrast Media; Radiological/Contrast Media, Ionic

Use
Solution for injection: Arthrography, cerebral angiography, cranial computerized angiotomography, digital subtraction angiography, direct cholangiography, endoscopic retrograde cholangiopancreatography, excretory urography, peripheral arteriography, urography, venography; contrast enhancement of computed tomographic images
Solution for instillation: Retrograde cystography and cystourethrography

Dosage Forms
Injection, solution:
Conray® 30: 30% (50 mL, 150 mL)
Conray® 43: 43% (50 mL, 100 mL, 200 mL, 250 mL)
Conray®: 60% (30 mL, 50 mL, 100 mL, 150 mL)
Injection, solution for instillation:
Cysto-Conray® II: 17.2% (250 mL)

iotrolan *(Canada only)* (eye OH troe lan)

Medication Safety Issues
Sound-alike/look-alike issues:
Osmovist® may be confused with Gadovist®, Magnevist®, Vasovist®
Canadian Brand Names Osmovist®
Therapeutic Category Iodinated Contrast Media; Radiological/Contrast Media, Nonionic (Iso-Osmolality)
Use Myelography (lumbar, cervical, total columnar); computerized tomography (CT) of spinal and subarachnoid spaces
Product Availability Not available in U.S.
Dosage Forms - Canada
Injection, solution, intrathecal [preservative free]:
Osmovist®:
240 [contains iotrolan 513 mg equivalent to iodine 240 mg/mL] (10 mL)
300 [contains iotrolan 641 mg equivalent to iodine 300 mg /mL] (10 mL)

ioversol (EYE oh ver sole)

Medication Safety Issues
High alert medication:
The Institute for Safe Medication Practices (ISMP) includes this medication among its list of drugs which have a heightened risk of causing significant patient harm when used in error.
U.S. Brand Names Optiray® 160; Optiray® 240; Optiray® 300; Optiray® 320; Optiray® 350
Therapeutic Category Iodinated Contrast Media; Radiological/Contrast Media, Nonionic
Use Arteriography, angiography, angiocardiography, ventriculography, excretory urography, and venography procedures; contrast enhanced tomographic imaging; intraarterial digital substraction angiography (Optiray® 160)
Dosage Forms
Injection, solution [preservative free]:
Optiray® 160: 34% (50 mL, 100 mL)
Optiray® 240: 51% (50 mL, 100 mL, 125 mL, 150 mL, 200 mL)
Optiray® 300: 64% (50 mL, 100 mL, 125 mL, 150 mL, 200 mL)
Optiray® 320: 68% (20 mL, 30 mL, 50 mL, 75 mL, 100 mL, 125 mL, 150 mL, 200s)
Optiray® 350: 74% (30 mL, 50 mL, 75 mL, 100 mL, 125 mL, 150 mL, 200 mL)

ioxaglate meglumine and ioxaglate sodium
(eye ox AG late MEG loo meen & eye ox AG late SOW dee um)

Medication Safety Issues
High alert medication:
The Institute for Safe Medication Practices (ISMP) includes this medication among its list of drugs which have a heightened risk of causing significant patient harm when used in error.
Synonyms ioxaglate sodium and ioxaglate meglumine
U.S. Brand Names Hexabrix™
Therapeutic Category Iodinated Contrast Media; Radiological/Contrast Media, Ionic
Use Angiocardiography, arteriography, aortography, arthrography, angiography, hysterosalpingography, venography, and urography procedures; contrast enhancement of computed tomographic imaging ▶

◀ **Dosage Forms**
Injection, solution:
Hexabrix™: Ioxaglate meglumine 39.3% and ioxaglate sodium 19.6% (20 mL, 50 mL, 100 mL, 150 mL, 200 mL)

ioxaglate sodium and ioxaglate meglumine *see* ioxaglate meglumine and ioxaglate sodium
on page 487

ioxilan (eye OKS ee lan)

Medication Safety Issues
High alert medication:
The Institute for Safe Medication Practices (ISMP) includes this medication among its list of drugs which have a heightened risk of causing significant patient harm when used in error.

U.S. Brand Names Oxilan® 300; Oxilan® 350

Canadian Brand Names Oxilan® 300; Oxilan® 350

Therapeutic Category Iodinated Contrast Media; Radiological/Contrast Media, Nonionic

Use
Intraarterial: Ioxilan 300 mgI/mL is indicated for cerebral arteriography. Ioxilan 350 mgI/mL is indicated for coronary arteriography and left ventriculography, visceral angiography, aortography, and peripheral arteriography
Intravenous: Both products are indicated for excretory urography and contrast-enhanced computed tomographic (CECT) imaging of the head and body

Dosage Forms
Injection, solution [preservative free]:
Oxilan® 300: 62% (50 mL, 100 mL, 150 mL, 200 mL, 500 mL)
Oxilan® 350: 73% (50 mL, 100 mL, 150 mL, 200 mL, 500 mL)

ipecac syrup (IP e kak SIR up)

Synonyms syrup of ipecac

Therapeutic Category Antidote

Use Treatment of acute oral drug overdosage and in certain poisonings

General Dosage Range Oral:
Children 6-12 months: 5-10 mL followed by 10-20 mL/kg of water, may repeat if vomiting does not occur within 20 minutes
Children 1-12 years: 15 mL followed by 10-20 mL/kg of water, may repeat if vomiting does not occur within 20 minutes
Adults: 15-30 mL followed by 200-300 mL of water, may repeat if vomiting does not occur within 20 minutes

ipilimumab (ip i LIM u mab)

Medication Safety Issues
High alert medication:
This medication is in a class the Institute for Safe Medication Practices (ISMP) includes among its list of drug classes which have a heightened risk of causing significant patient harm when used in error.

Synonyms MDX-010; MDX-CTLA-4; MOAB-CTLA-4

U.S. Brand Names Yervoy™

Therapeutic Category Antineoplastic Agent, Monoclonal Antibody; Monoclonal Antibody

Use Treatment of unresectable or metastatic melanoma

General Dosage Range Dosage adjustment recommended in patients who develop toxicities.
I.V.: *Adults:* 3 mg/kg every 3 weeks

Dosage Forms
Injection, solution [preservative free]:
Yervoy™: 5 mg/mL (10 mL, 40 mL)

Iplex *see* mecasermin *on page 552*
IPOL® *see* poliovirus vaccine (inactivated) *on page 717*

ipratropium (oral inhalation) (i pra TROE pee um)

Medication Safety Issues
  Sound-alike/look-alike issues:
    Atrovent® may be confused with Alupent®, Serevent®
    Ipratropium may be confused with tiotropium

Synonyms ipratropium bromide

U.S. Brand Names Atrovent® HFA

Canadian Brand Names Atrovent® HFA; Gen-Ipratropium; Mylan-Ipratropium Sterinebs; Novo-Ipramide; Nu-Ipratropium; PMS-Ipratropium

Therapeutic Category Anticholinergic Agent

Use Anticholinergic bronchodilator used in bronchospasm associated with COPD, bronchitis, and emphysema

General Dosage Range
  Inhalation: *Children >12 years and Adults:* 2 inhalations 4 times/day (maximum: 12 inhalations/day)
  Nebulization: *Children >12 years and Adults:* 500 mcg every 6-8 hours

Dosage Forms
  Aerosol, for oral inhalation:
    Atrovent® HFA: 17 mcg/actuation (12.9 g)
  Solution, for nebulization: 0.02% [500 mcg/2.5 mL] (25s, 30s, 60s)
  Solution, for nebulization [preservative free]: 0.02% [500 mcg/2.5 mL] (25s, 30s, 60s)

ipratropium (nasal) (i pra TROE pee um)

Medication Safety Issues
  Sound-alike/look-alike issues:
    Ipratropium may be confused with tiotropium
    Atrovent® may be confused with Alupent®, Serevent®

Synonyms ipratropium bromide

U.S. Brand Names Atrovent®

Canadian Brand Names Alti-Ipratropium; Apo-Ipravent®; Atrovent®; Mylan-Ipratropium Solution

Therapeutic Category Anticholinergic Agent

Use Symptomatic relief of rhinorrhea associated with the common cold and allergic and nonallergic rhinitis

General Dosage Range Intranasal:
  0.03% solution: *Children ≥6 years and Adults:* 2 sprays in each nostril 2-3 times/day
  0.06% solution: *Children ≥5 years and Adults:* 2 sprays in each nostril 3-4 times/day

Dosage Forms
  Solution, intranasal: 0.03% (30 mL); 0.06% (15 mL)
  Atrovent®: 0.03% (30 mL); 0.06% (15 mL)

ipratropium and albuterol (i pra TROE pee um & al BYOO ter ole)

Medication Safety Issues
  Sound-alike/look-alike issues:
    Combivent® may be confused with Combivir®, Serevent®
  International issues:
    DuoNeb® may be confused with DuoTrav™ which is a brand name for travoprost/timolol combination product in Canada or may be confused with Duovent® UDV which is a brand name for ipratropium/fenoterol combination product in Canada

Synonyms albuterol and ipratropium; salbutamol and ipratropium

U.S. Brand Names Combivent®; DuoNeb®

Canadian Brand Names CO Ipra-Sal; Combivent UDV; Gen-Combo Sterinebs; ratio-Ipra Sal UDV

Therapeutic Category Bronchodilator

Use Treatment of COPD in those patients who are currently on a regular bronchodilator who continue to have bronchospasms and require a second bronchodilator

General Dosage Range
  Inhalation: *Adults:* 2 inhalations 4 times/day (maximum: 12 inhalations/day)
  Nebulization: *Adults:* 3 mL every 4-6 hours

Dosage Forms
Aerosol for oral inhalation:
Combivent®: Ipratropium bromide 18 mcg and albuterol (base) 90 mcg per inhalation (14.7 g) [200 metered actuations]
Solution for nebulization: Ipratropium 0.5 mg and albuterol (base) 2.5 mg per 3 mL (30s, 60s)
DuoNeb®: Ipratropium 0.5 mg and albuterol (base) 2.5 mg per 3 mL (30s, 60s)

ipratropium and fenoterol *(Canada only)* (i pra TROE pee um & fen oh TER ole)
Medication Safety Issues
Sound-alike/look-alike issues:
Duovent® UDV may be confused with Combivent® UDV
International issues:
Duovent® UDV may be confused with DuoNeb® which is a brand name for ipratropium/albuterol combination product in the U.S.
Synonyms fenoterol and ipratropium; fenoterol hydrobromide and ipratropium bromide; ipratropium bromide and fenoterol hydrobromide
Canadian Brand Names Duovent® UDV
Therapeutic Category Anticholinergic Agent; Beta$_2$-Adrenergic Agonist
Use Treatment of bronchospasm associated with acute severe exacerbation of COPD or bronchial asthma
General Dosage Range Nebulization: *Children ≥12 years and Adults:* Usual dose: 4 mL; may repeat every 6 hours as needed
Product Availability Not available in U.S.
Dosage Forms - Canada
Solution for nebulization:
Duovent® UDV: Ipratropium bromide 0.5 mg and fenoterol 1.25 mg per 4 mL (20s)

ipratropium bromide *see* ipratropium (nasal) *on page 489*
ipratropium bromide *see* ipratropium (oral inhalation) *on page 489*
ipratropium bromide and fenoterol hydrobromide *see* ipratropium and fenoterol *(Canada only) on page 490*
I-Prin [OTC] *see* ibuprofen *on page 460*
Iprivask® *see* desirudin *on page 261*
iproveratril hydrochloride *see* verapamil *on page 912*
IPV *see* poliovirus vaccine (inactivated) *on page 717*
Iquix® *see* levofloxacin (ophthalmic) *on page 520*

irbesartan (ir be SAR tan)
Medication Safety Issues
Sound-alike/look-alike issues:
Avapro® may be confused with Anaprox®
U.S. Brand Names Avapro®
Canadian Brand Names Avapro®; CO Irbesartan; PMS-Irbesartan; ratio-Irbesartan; Sandoz-Irbesartan; Teva-Irbesartan
Therapeutic Category Angiotensin II Receptor Antagonist
Use Treatment of hypertension alone or in combination with other antihypertensives; treatment of diabetic nephropathy in patients with type 2 diabetes mellitus (noninsulin-dependent, NIDDM) and hypertension
General Dosage Range Oral:
Children 6-12 years: Initial: 75 mg once daily; Maintenance: 75-150 mg once daily
Children ≥13 years and Adults: Initial: 75-150 mg once daily; Maintenance: 75 to 300 mg once daily
Dosage Forms
Tablet, oral:
Avapro®: 75 mg, 150 mg, 300 mg

irbesartan and hydrochlorothiazide (ir be SAR tan & hye droe klor oh THYE a zide)
Medication Safety Issues
Sound-alike/look-alike issues:
Avalide® may be confused with Avandia®
Synonyms Avapro® HCT; hydrochlorothiazide and irbesartan
U.S. Brand Names Avalide®

Canadian Brand Names Avalide®; CO Irbesartan HCT; Irbesartan-HCTZ; PMS-Irbesartan HCTZ; Ran™-Irbesartan HCTZ; ratio-Irbesartan HCTZ; Sandoz-Irbesartan HCT; Teva-Irbesartan HCTZ

Therapeutic Category Antihypertensive Agent, Combination

Use Combination therapy for the management of hypertension; may be used as initial therapy in patients likely to need multiple drugs to achieve blood pressure goals

General Dosage Range Oral: *Adults:* Irbesartan 150-300 mg and hydrochlorothiazide 12.5-25 mg once daily

Dosage Forms

Tablet:

Avalide®: Irbesartan 150 mg and hydrochlorothiazide 12.5 mg; irbesartan 300 mg and hydrochlorothiazide 12.5 mg; irbesartan 300 mg and hydrochlorothiazide 25 mg

Irbesartan-HCTZ (Can) *see* irbesartan and hydrochlorothiazide *on page 490*

Ircon® [OTC] *see* ferrous fumarate *on page 373*

Iressa® *see* gefitinib *on page 412*

IRESSA® (Can) *see* gefitinib *on page 412*

irinotecan (eye rye no TEE kan)

Medication Safety Issues

Sound-alike/look-alike issues:

Irinotecan may be confused with topotecan

High alert medication:

This medication is in a class the Institute for Safe Medication Practices (ISMP) includes among its list of drug classes which have a heightened risk of causing significant patient harm when used in error.

Synonyms camptothecin-11; CPT-11; irinotecan HCl; irinotecan hydrochloride

U.S. Brand Names Camptosar®

Canadian Brand Names Camptosar®; Irinotecan Hydrochloride Trihydrate

Therapeutic Category Antineoplastic Agent

Use Treatment of metastatic carcinoma of the colon or rectum

General Dosage Range Dosage adjustment recommended in patients with hepatic impairment or who develop toxicities

I.V.: *Adults:* Dosage varies greatly depending on indication

Dosage Forms

Injection, solution: 20 mg/mL (2 mL, 5 mL, 25 mL)

Camptosar®: 20 mg/mL (2 mL, 5 mL, 15 mL)

irinotecan HCl *see* irinotecan *on page 491*

irinotecan hydrochloride *see* irinotecan *on page 491*

Irinotecan Hydrochloride Trihydrate (Can) *see* irinotecan *on page 491*

iron dextran *see* iron dextran complex *on page 491*

iron dextran complex (EYE ern DEKS tran KOM pleks)

Medication Safety Issues

Sound-alike/look-alike issues:

Dexferrum® may be confused with Desferal®

Iron dextran complex may be confused with ferumoxytol

Synonyms high-molecular-weight iron dextran (DexFerrum®); imferon; iron dextran; low-Molecular-weight iron dextran (INFeD®)

U.S. Brand Names Dexferrum®; INFeD®

Canadian Brand Names Dexiron™; Infufer®

Therapeutic Category Electrolyte Supplement, Oral

Use Treatment of iron deficiency in patients in whom oral administration is infeasible or ineffective

General Dosage Range Note: A 0.5 mL test dose (0.25 mL in infants) should be given prior to starting iron dextran therapy.

I.M., I.V.:

Children <5 kg and >4 months: Replacement iron (mg) = blood loss (mL) x Hct; **Note:** Total dose should be divided daily at not more than 25 mg/day

Children 5-15 kg and >4 months: Total Dose (mL) = 0.0442 (desired Hgb [usually 12 g/dL] - observed Hgb) x W (in kg) + (0.26 x W [in kg]) **or** replacement iron (mg) = blood loss (mL) x hematocrit; **Note:** Total dose should be divided daily at not more than 50 mg/day (5-10 kg) or 100 mg/day (10-15 kg)

Children >15 kg: Total Dose (mL) = 0.0442 (desired Hgb [usually 14.8 g/dL] - observed Hgb) x LBW + (0.26 x LBW) **or** replacement iron (mg) = blood loss (mL) x Hct; **Note:** Total dose should be divided daily at not more than 100 mg/day

Adults: Total Dose (mL) = 0.0442 (desired Hgb [usually 14.8 g/dL] - observed Hgb) x LBW + (0.26 x LBW) **or** replacement iron (mg) = blood loss (mL) x Hct; **Note:** Total dose should be divided daily at not more than 100 mg/day

Dosage Forms

Injection, solution:
Dexferrum®: Elemental iron 50 mg/mL (1 mL, 2 mL)
INFeD®: Elemental iron 50 mg/mL (2 mL)

iron fumarate *see* ferrous fumarate *on page 373*

iron gluconate *see* ferrous gluconate *on page 373*

iron-polysaccharide complex *see* polysaccharide-iron complex *on page 720*

iron-polysaccharide complex and folic acid *see* polysaccharide-iron complex and folic acid *on page 721*

iron-polysaccharide complex, vitamin B12, and folic acid *see* polysaccharide-iron complex, vitamin B12, and folic acid *on page 721*

iron sucrose (EYE ern SOO krose)

Medication Safety Issues

Sound-alike/look-alike issues:
Iron sucrose may be confused with ferumoxytol

U.S. Brand Names Venofer®

Canadian Brand Names Venofer®

Therapeutic Category Iron Salt

Use Treatment of iron-deficiency anemia in chronic renal failure, including nondialysis-dependent patients (with or without erythropoietin therapy) and dialysis-dependent patients receiving erythropoietin therapy

General Dosage Range I.V.: *Adults:* 100 mg (5 mL) 1-3 times/week during dialysis **or** 200 mg on 5 different occasions within a 14-day period **or** two 300 mg infusion 14 days apart, followed by a single 400 mg infusion 14 days later (maximum: 1000 mg cumulative total)

Dosage Forms

Injection, solution [preservative free]:
Venofer®: Elemental iron 20 mg/mL (5 mL, 10 mL)

iron sulfate *see* ferrous sulfate *on page 374*

Isagel® [OTC] *see* alcohol (ethyl) *on page 47*

ISD *see* isosorbide dinitrate *on page 494*

ISDN *see* isosorbide dinitrate *on page 494*

Isentress® *see* raltegravir *on page 765*

ISG *see* immune globulin *on page 468*

ISMN *see* isosorbide mononitrate *on page 495*

Ismo® *see* isosorbide mononitrate *on page 495*

isoamyl nitrite *see* amyl nitrite *on page 77*

isobamate *see* carisoprodol *on page 176*

isocarboxazid (eye soe kar BOKS a zid)

U.S. Brand Names Marplan®

Therapeutic Category Antidepressant, Monoamine Oxidase Inhibitor

Use Treatment of depression

General Dosage Range Oral: *Adults:* Initial: 10 mg 2-4 times/day; may increase to a maximum of 60 mg/day divided in 2-4 doses

Dosage Forms

Tablet, oral:
Marplan®: 10 mg

isoflurane (eye soe FLURE ane)

Medication Safety Issues
Sound-alike/look-alike issues:
Isoflurane may be confused with enflurane, isoflurophate
High alert medication:
The Institute for Safe Medication Practices (ISMP) includes this medication among its list of drug classes which have a heightened risk of causing significant patient harm when used in error.
U.S. Brand Names Forane®; Terrell™
Canadian Brand Names Forane®
Therapeutic Category General Anesthetic
Use Maintenance of general anesthesia
Note: Use of isoflurane for induction of general anesthesia is an FDA-labeled indication; however, it is not recommended clinically due to its irritant properties and unpleasant odor, which causes breath-holding or coughing.
General Dosage Range Inhalation: *Adults:* Maintenance: With nitrous oxide: 1% to 2.5%; without nitrous oxide: 1.5% to 3.5%
Dosage Forms
Liquid, for inhalation: USP: ≥ 99.9 mL/100 mL (100 mL, 250 mL)
Forane®: USP: ≥ 99.9 mL/100 mL (100 mL, 250 mL)
Terrell™: USP: ≥ 99.9 mL/100 mL (100 mL, 250 mL)

isometheptene, acetaminophen, and dichloralphenazone *see* acetaminophen, isometheptene, and dichloralphenazone *on page 34*
isometheptene, dichloralphenazone, and acetaminophen *see* acetaminophen, isometheptene, and dichloralphenazone *on page 34*
IsonaRif™ *see* rifampin and isoniazid *on page 779*

isoniazid (eye soe NYE a zid)

Medication Safety Issues
International issues:
Hydra [Japan] may be confused with Hydrea brand name for hydroxyurea [U.S., Canada, and multiple international markets]
Synonyms INH; isonicotinic acid hydrazide
Canadian Brand Names Isotamine®; PMS-Isoniazid
Therapeutic Category Antitubercular Agent
Use Treatment of susceptible tuberculosis infections; treatment of latent tuberculosis infection (LTBI)
General Dosage Range Oral, I.M.:
Children: 10-20 mg/kg/day once daily (maximum: 300 mg/day) **or** 20-40 mg/kg 2-3 times/week (maximum: 900 mg/dose)
Adults: 300 mg (5 mg/kg) once daily **or** 900 mg (15 mg/kg) 2-3 times/week
Dosage Forms
Injection, solution: 100 mg/mL (10 mL)
Solution, oral: 50 mg/5 mL (473 mL)
Tablet, oral: 100 mg, 300 mg

isoniazid and rifampin *see* rifampin and isoniazid *on page 779*
isoniazid, pyrazinamide, and rifampin *see* rifampin, isoniazid, and pyrazinamide *on page 780*
isonicotinic acid hydrazide *see* isoniazid *on page 493*
isonipecaine hydrochloride *see* meperidine *on page 560*
isophane insulin *see* insulin NPH *on page 479*
isophane insulin and regular insulin *see* insulin NPH and insulin regular *on page 479*
isophosphamide *see* ifosfamide *on page 464*

isoproterenol (eye soe proe TER e nole)

Medication Safety Issues
Sound-alike/look-alike issues:
Isuprel® may be confused with Disophrol®, Ismelin®, Isordil®
Synonyms isoproterenol hydrochloride
U.S. Brand Names Isuprel®

▶

Therapeutic Category Adrenergic Agonist Agent

Use Manufacturer's labeled indications (see **"Note"**): Mild or transient episodes of heart block that do not require electric shock or pacemaker therapy; serious episodes of heart block and Adams-Stokes attacks (except when caused by ventricular tachycardia or fibrillation); cardiac arrest until electric shock or pacemaker therapy is available; bronchospasm during anesthesia; adjunct to fluid and electrolyte replacement therapy and other drugs and procedures in the treatment of hypovolemic or septic shock and low cardiac output states (eg, decompensated heart failure, cardiogenic shock)

Note: The use of isoproterenol in advanced cardiac life support (ACLS) has largely been supplanted by the use of other adrenergic agents (eg, epinephrine and dopamine). The use of isoproterenol for bronchospasm during anesthesia and cardiogenic, hypovolemic, or septic shock is no longer recommended.

General Dosage Range Continuous I.V. infusion:
Children: 0.05-2 mcg/**kg**/minute; titrate to patient response
Adults: 2-10 mcg/minute; titrate to patient response

Dosage Forms
Injection, solution:
Isuprel®: 0.2 mg/mL (1 mL, 5 mL)

isoproterenol hydrochloride *see* isoproterenol *on page 493*

Isoptin® SR *see* verapamil *on page 912*

Isopto® Atropine *see* atropine *on page 103*

Isopto® Carbachol *see* carbachol *on page 170*

Isopto® Carpine *see* pilocarpine (ophthalmic) *on page 704*

Isopto® Homatropine *see* homatropine *on page 441*

Isopto® Hyoscine *see* scopolamine (ophthalmic) *on page 805*

Isopto® Tears [OTC] *see* hydroxypropyl methylcellulose *on page 455*

Isopto® Tears (Can) *see* hydroxypropyl methylcellulose *on page 455*

Isordil® Titradose™ *see* isosorbide dinitrate *on page 494*

Isosorbide (Can) *see* isosorbide dinitrate *on page 494*

isosorbide dinitrate (eye soe SOR bide dye NYE trate)

Medication Safety Issues
Sound-alike/look-alike issues:
Isordil® may be confused with Inderal®, Isuprel®, Plendil®

Synonyms ISD; ISDN

U.S. Brand Names Dilatrate®-SR; Isordil® Titradose™

Canadian Brand Names ISDN; Isosorbide; Novo-Sorbide; PMS-Isosorbide

Therapeutic Category Vasodilator

Use Prevention and treatment of angina pectoris

Note: Due to slower onset of action, not the drug of choice to abort an acute anginal episode.

General Dosage Range
Oral:
Immediate release: *Adults:* 5-40 mg 2-3 times/day
Sustained release: *Adults:* 40-160 mg/day in divided doses
Sublingual: *Adults:* 2.5-5 mg every 5-10 minutes for maximum of 3 doses in 15-30 minutes **or** 2.5-5 mg 15 minutes prior to activities which may provoke an anginal episode.

Dosage Forms
Capsule, sustained release, oral:
Dilatrate®-SR: 40 mg
Tablet, oral: 5 mg, 10 mg, 20 mg, 30 mg
Isordil® Titradose™: 5 mg, 40 mg
Tablet, sublingual: 2.5 mg, 5 mg
Tablet, extended release, oral: 40 mg

isosorbide dinitrate and hydralazine
(eye soe SOR bide dye NYE trate & hye DRAL a zeen)

Synonyms hydralazine and isosorbide dinitrate

U.S. Brand Names BiDil®

Therapeutic Category Vasodilator

Use Treatment of heart failure, adjunct to standard therapy, in self-identified African-Americans

General Dosage Range Dosage adjustment recommended in patients who develop toxicities.
Oral: *Adults:* 1-2 tablets 3 times/day

Dosage Forms
Tablet:
BiDil®: Isosorbide dinitrate 20 mg and hydralazine 37.5 mg

isosorbide mononitrate (eye soe SOR bide mon oh NYE trate)

Medication Safety Issues
Sound-alike/look-alike issues:
Imdur® may be confused with Imuran®, Inderal LA®, K-Dur®
Monoket® may be confused with Monopril®

Synonyms ISMN

U.S. Brand Names Imdur®; Ismo®; Monoket®

Canadian Brand Names Apo-ISMN®; Imdur®; PMS-ISMN; PRO-ISMN

Therapeutic Category Vasodilator

Use Prevention of angina pectoris

General Dosage Range Oral:
Extended release: *Adults:* Initial: 30-60 mg once daily; Maintenance: 30-240 mg once daily (maximum: 240 mg/day)
Regular release: *Adults:* 5-20 mg twice daily

Dosage Forms
Tablet, oral: 10 mg, 20 mg
Ismo®: 20 mg
Monoket®: 10 mg, 20 mg
Tablet, extended release, oral: 30 mg, 60 mg, 120 mg
Imdur®: 30 mg, 60 mg, 120 mg

isosulfan blue (eye soe SUL fan bloo)

U.S. Brand Names Lymphazurin™

Therapeutic Category Contrast Agent

Use Adjunct to lymphography for visualization of the lymphatic system; sentinel node identification

General Dosage Range SubQ: *Adults:* Inject 0.5 mL into 3 interdigital spaces of each extremity per study (maximum: 3 mL [30 mg])

Dosage Forms
Injection, solution [preservative free]:
Lymphazurin™: 1% (5 mL)

Isotamine® (Can) *see* isoniazid *on page 493*

isotretinoin (eye soe TRET i noyn)

Medication Safety Issues
Sound-alike/look-alike issues:
Accutane® may be confused with Accolate®, Accupril®
Claravis™ may be confused with Cleviprex™
ISOtretinoin may be confused with tretinoin

Synonyms 13-*cis*-retinoic acid

Tall-Man ISOtretinoin

U.S. Brand Names Amnesteem®; Claravis™; Sotret®

Canadian Brand Names Accutane®; Clarus™; Isotrex®

Therapeutic Category Retinoic Acid Derivative

Use Treatment of severe recalcitrant nodular acne unresponsive to conventional therapy

General Dosage Range Dosage adjustments recommended in patients with hepatic impairment
Oral:
Children 12-17 years: 0.05-1 mg/kg/day in 2 divided doses
Adults: 0.05-2 mg/kg/day in 2 divided doses

◀ **Dosage Forms**
  Capsule, oral:
    Claravis™: 10 mg, 20 mg, 30 mg, 40 mg
  Capsule, softgel, oral:
    Amnesteem®: 10 mg, 20 mg, 40 mg
    Sotret®: 10 mg, 20 mg, 30 mg, 40 mg

Isotrex® (Can) see isotretinoin on page 495
Isovue® see iopamidol on page 486
Isovue® 200 see iopamidol on page 486
Isovue® 300 see iopamidol on page 486
Isovue® 370 see iopamidol on page 486
Isovue-M® see iopamidol on page 486
Isovue Multipack® see iopamidol on page 486

isoxsuprine (eye SOKS syoo preen)

Medication Safety Issues
  Sound-alike/look-alike issues:
    Vasodilan® may be confused with Vasocidin®
  BEERS Criteria medication:
    This drug may be inappropriate for use in geriatric patients (low severity risk).
Synonyms isoxsuprine hydrochloride; Vasodilan
Therapeutic Category Vasodilator
Use Treatment of peripheral vascular diseases, such as arteriosclerosis obliterans and Raynaud disease
General Dosage Range Oral: *Adults:* 10-20 mg 3-4 times/day
Dosage Forms
  Tablet, oral: 10 mg, 20 mg

isoxsuprine hydrochloride see isoxsuprine on page 496

isradipine (iz RA di peen)

Medication Safety Issues
  Sound-alike/look-alike issues:
    DynaCirc® may be confused with Dynabac®, Dynacin®
U.S. Brand Names DynaCirc CR®
Therapeutic Category Calcium Channel Blocker
Use Treatment of hypertension
General Dosage Range Dosage adjustment recommended in patients with hepatic or renal impairment
  Oral: *Adults:*
    Capsule: Initial: 2.5 mg twice daily; Usual range: 2.5-10 mg/day
    Controlled release tablet: Initial: 5 mg once daily; Maintenance: 5-20 mg once daily (maximum: 20 mg/day)
Dosage Forms
  Capsule, oral: 2.5 mg, 5 mg
  Tablet, controlled release, oral:
    DynaCirc CR®: 5 mg, 10 mg

Istalol® see timolol (ophthalmic) on page 869
Istodax® see romidepsin on page 789
Isuprel® see isoproterenol on page 493
Itch-X® [OTC] see pramoxine on page 730

itraconazole (i tra KOE na zole)

Medication Safety Issues
  Sound-alike/look-alike issues:
    Itraconazole may be confused with fluconazole
    Sporanox® may be confused with Suprax®, Topamax®
U.S. Brand Names Sporanox®
Canadian Brand Names Sporanox®

Therapeutic Category Antifungal Agent
Use
  Oral capsules: Treatment of susceptible fungal infections in immunocompromised and immunocompetent patients including blastomycosis and histoplasmosis; indicated for aspergillosis (in patients intolerant/refractory to amphotericin B), and onychomycosis of the toenail and fingernail (in nonimmunocompromised patients)
  Oral solution: Treatment of oral and esophageal candidiasis
General Dosage Range Dosage adjustment recommended in patients with renal impairment
  Oral: *Adults:* 100-800 mg/day; doses >200 mg/day are given in 2-3 divided doses
Dosage Forms
  Capsule, oral: 100 mg
    Sporanox®: 100 mg
  Solution, oral:
    Sporanox®: 10 mg/mL (150 mL)

ivermectin (eye ver MEK tin)
U.S. Brand Names Stromectol®
Therapeutic Category Antibiotic, Miscellaneous
Use Treatment of the following infections: Strongyloidiasis of the intestinal tract due to the nematode parasite *Strongyloides stercoralis*. Onchocerciasis due to the immature form of the nematode parasite *Onchocerca volvulus*
General Dosage Range Oral: *Children ≥15 kg and Adults:* 150-200 mcg/kg as a single dose
Dosage Forms
  Tablet, oral:
    Stromectol®: 3 mg

IVIG *see* immune globulin *on page 468*
IV immune globulin *see* immune globulin *on page 468*
Ivy Block® [OTC] *see* bentoquatam *on page 120*
Ivy-Rid® [OTC] *see* benzocaine *on page 121*

ixabepilone (ix ab EP i lone)
Medication Safety Issues
  High alert medication:
    This medication is in a class the Institute for Safe Medication Practices (ISMP) includes among its list of drug classes which have a heightened risk of causing significant patient harm when used in error.
Synonyms azaepothilone B; BMS-247550; epothilone B lactam
U.S. Brand Names Ixempra®
Therapeutic Category Antineoplastic Agent, Antimicrotubular; Antineoplastic Agent, Epothilone B Analog
Use Treatment of metastatic or locally-advanced breast cancer (refractory or resistant)
General Dosage Range Dosage adjustment recommended in patients with hepatic impairment or who develop toxicities
  I.V.: *Adults:* 40 mg/m^2 every 3 weeks (maximum dose: 88 mg)
Dosage Forms
  Injection, powder for reconstitution:
    Ixempra®: 15 mg, 45 mg

Ixempra® *see* ixabepilone *on page 497*
Ixiaro® *see* Japanese encephalitis virus vaccine (inactivated) *on page 498*
Jalyn™ *see* dutasteride and tamsulosin *on page 317*
JAMP-Amlodipine (Can) *see* amlodipine *on page 69*
JAMP-Atenolol (Can) *see* atenolol *on page 101*
JAMP-Bicalutamide (Can) *see* bicalutamide *on page 133*
JAMP-Carvedilol (Can) *see* carvedilol *on page 178*
JAMP-Citalopram (Can) *see* citalopram *on page 213*
JAMP-Finasteride (Can) *see* finasteride *on page 378*
Jamp-Fosinopril (Can) *see* fosinopril *on page 401*
JAMP-Lisinopril (Can) *see* lisinopril *on page 531*

JAMP-Metoprolol-L (Can) *see* metoprolol *on page 581*

JAMP-Ondansetron (Can) *see* ondansetron *on page 651*

JAMP-Pioglitazone (Can) *see* pioglitazone *on page 706*

JAMP-Quetiapine (Can) *see* quetiapine *on page 760*

JAMP-Ramipril (Can) *see* ramipril *on page 766*

JAMP-Risperidone (Can) *see* risperidone *on page 783*

JAMP-Ropinirole (Can) *see* ropinirole *on page 790*

JAMP-Simvastatin (Can) *see* simvastatin *on page 813*

JAMP-Tamsulosin (Can) *see* tamsulosin *on page 843*

JAMP-Terbinafine (Can) *see* terbinafine (systemic) *on page 851*

Jantoven® *see* warfarin *on page 922*

Janumet® *see* sitagliptin and metformin *on page 816*

Januvia® *see* sitagliptin *on page 815*

Japanese encephalitis virus vaccine (inactivated)

(jap a NEESE en sef a LYE tis VYE rus vak SEEN, in ak ti VAY ted)

Synonyms IC51; JE-VC (Ixiaro®)

U.S. Brand Names Ixiaro®

Therapeutic Category Vaccine, Inactivated Virus

Use Active immunization against Japanese encephalitis

Japanese encephalitis vaccine is not recommended for all persons traveling to or residing in Asia. The Advisory Committee on Immunization Practices (ACIP) recommends vaccination for:
- Persons spending ≥1 month in endemic areas during transmission season
- Research laboratory workers who may be exposed to the Japanese encephalitis virus

Vaccination may also be considered for the following:
- Travelers to areas with an ongoing outbreak
- Travelers spending <30 days in endemic areas during the transmission season and planning to go outside of urban areas and have an increased risk of exposure. For example, high-risk activities include extensive outdoor activity in rural areas especially at night; extensive outdoor activities such as camping, hiking, etc; staying in accommodations without air conditioning, screens or bed nets.
- Travelers to endemic areas who are unsure of specific destination, activities, or duration of travel

General Dosage Range I.M.: *Adults ≥17 years:* 0.5 mL/dose on days 0 and 28

Dosage Forms

Injection, suspension:

Ixiaro®: Inactivated JEV proteins 6 mcg/0.5 mL (0.5 mL)

Jevantique™ *see* ethinyl estradiol and norethindrone *on page 355*

JE-VC (Ixiaro®) *see* Japanese encephalitis virus vaccine (inactivated) *on page 498*

Jevtana® *see* cabazitaxel *on page 156*

Jinteli™ *see* ethinyl estradiol and norethindrone *on page 355*

Jolessa™ *see* ethinyl estradiol and levonorgestrel *on page 353*

Jolivette® *see* norethindrone *on page 633*

Junel® 1.5/30 *see* ethinyl estradiol and norethindrone *on page 355*

Junel® 1/20 *see* ethinyl estradiol and norethindrone *on page 355*

Junel® Fe 1.5/30 *see* ethinyl estradiol and norethindrone *on page 355*

Junel® Fe 1/20 *see* ethinyl estradiol and norethindrone *on page 355*

Jurnista™ (Can) *see* hydromorphone *on page 452*

Just For Kids™ [OTC] *see* fluoride *on page 386*

Juvéderm® Ultra *see* hyaluronate and derivatives *on page 443*

Juvéderm® Ultra XC *see* hyaluronate and derivatives *on page 443*

Juvéderm® Ultra Plus *see* hyaluronate and derivatives *on page 443*

Juvéderm® Ultra Plus XC *see* hyaluronate and derivatives *on page 443*

K-10® (Can) *see* potassium chloride *on page 724*

Kadian® *see* morphine (systemic) *on page 598*

Kala® [OTC] *see* Lactobacillus *on page 506*

Kalbitor® *see* ecallantide *on page 318*

Kaletra® *see* lopinavir and ritonavir *on page 536*
Kalexate *see* sodium polystyrene sulfonate *on page 823*
Kalmz [OTC] *see* fructose, dextrose, and phosphoric acid *on page 403*

kanamycin (kan a MYE sin)

Medication Safety Issues
Sound-alike/look-alike issues:
Kanamycin may be confused with Garamycin®, gentamicin
Synonyms kanamycin sulfate
Therapeutic Category Aminoglycoside (Antibiotic)
Use Treatment of serious infections caused by susceptible strains of *E. coli, Proteus* species, *Enterobacter aerogenes, Klebsiella pneumoniae, Serratia marcescens,* and *Acinetobacter* species; second-line treatment of *Mycobacterium tuberculosis*
General Dosage Range Dosage adjustment of I.M. and I.V. route recommended in patients with renal impairment
I.M., I.V.:
Children: 15 mg/kg/day divided every 8-12 hours
Adults: 5-7.5 mg/kg every 8-12 hours
Elderly: 5-7.5 mg/kg every 12-24 hours
Inhalation, aerosol: *Adults:* 250 mg 2-4 times/day
Intraperitoneal: *Adults:* 500 mg
Irrigation: *Adults:* 0.25% (maximum: 1.5 g/day)
Dosage Forms
Injection, solution: 1 g/3 mL (3 mL)

kanamycin sulfate *see* kanamycin *on page 499*
Kank-A® Soft Brush [OTC] *see* benzocaine *on page 121*
Kaon-CL® 10 *see* potassium chloride *on page 724*
Kaopectate® [OTC] *see* bismuth *on page 135*
Kaopectate® Extra Strength [OTC] *see* bismuth *on page 135*
Kaopectate® Stool Softener [OTC] *see* docusate *on page 302*
Kao-Tin [OTC] *see* bismuth *on page 135*
Kao-Tin [OTC] *see* docusate *on page 302*
Kapidex *see* dexlansoprazole *on page 266*
Kapvay™ *see* clonidine *on page 223*
Kariva® *see* ethinyl estradiol and desogestrel *on page 351*
Kayexalate® *see* sodium polystyrene sulfonate *on page 823*
KCl *see* potassium chloride *on page 724*
kdur *see* potassium chloride *on page 724*
K-Dur® (Can) *see* potassium chloride *on page 724*
Keflex® *see* cephalexin *on page 188*
Keftab® (Can) *see* cephalexin *on page 188*
Kelnor™ *see* ethinyl estradiol and ethynodiol diacetate *on page 353*
Kemsol® (Can) *see* dimethyl sulfoxide *on page 288*
Kenalog® *see* triamcinolone (topical) *on page 887*
Kenalog®-10 *see* triamcinolone (systemic) *on page 886*
Kenalog®-40 *see* triamcinolone (systemic) *on page 886*
keoxifene hydrochloride *see* raloxifene *on page 765*
Kepivance® *see* palifermin *on page 668*
Keppra® *see* levetiracetam *on page 517*
Keppra XR™ *see* levetiracetam *on page 517*
Kerafoam® *see* urea *on page 900*
Kerafoam® 42 *see* urea *on page 900*
Keralac™ *see* urea *on page 900*
Keralac™ Nailstik *see* urea *on page 900*
Keralyt® *see* salicylic acid *on page 795*

Keratol 40™ [DSC] *see* urea *on page 900*
Kerlone® *see* betaxolol (systemic) *on page 130*
Kerol™ *see* urea *on page 900*
Kerol™ AD *see* urea *on page 900*
Kerol™ Redi-Cloths *see* urea *on page 900*
Kerol™ ZX *see* urea *on page 900*
Kerr Insta-Char® [OTC] *see* charcoal *on page 191*
Ketalar® *see* ketamine *on page 500*

ketamine (KEET a meen)

Medication Safety Issues
 Sound-alike/look-alike issues:
  Ketalar® may be confused with Kenalog®, ketorolac
 High alert medication:
  The Institute for Safe Medication Practices (ISMP) includes this medication among its list of drugs which have a heightened risk of causing significant patient harm when used in error.
Synonyms ketamine hydrochloride
U.S. Brand Names Ketalar®
Canadian Brand Names Ketalar®; Ketamine Hydrochloride Injection, USP
Therapeutic Category General Anesthetic
Controlled Substance C-III
Use Induction and maintenance of general anesthesia
General Dosage Range
 I.M.: *Children ≥16 years and Adults:* 2-6 mg/kg
 I.V.: *Children ≥16 years and Adults:* 0.2-2 mg/kg **or** 0.1-0.5 mg/minute as a continuous infusion
Dosage Forms
 Injection, solution: 10 mg/mL (20 mL); 50 mg/mL (10 mL); 100 mg/mL (5 mL, 10 mL)
  Ketalar®: 10 mg/mL (20 mL); 50 mg/mL (10 mL); 100 mg/mL (5 mL)

ketamine hydrochloride *see* ketamine *on page 500*
Ketamine Hydrochloride Injection, USP (Can) *see* ketamine *on page 500*
Ketek® *see* telithromycin *on page 847*

ketoconazole (systemic) (kee toe KOE na zole)

Medication Safety Issues
 Sound-alike/look-alike issues:
  Nizoral® may be confused with Nasarel, Neoral®, Nitrol®
Canadian Brand Names Apo-Ketoconazole®; Novo-Ketoconazole
Therapeutic Category Antifungal Agent, Oral
Use Treatment of susceptible fungal infections, including candidiasis, oral thrush, blastomycosis, histoplasmosis, paracoccidioidomycosis, coccidioidomycosis, chromomycosis, candiduria, chronic mucocutaneous candidiasis, as well as certain recalcitrant cutaneous dermatophytoses
General Dosage Range Oral:
 Children ≥2 years: 3.3-6.6 mg/kg once daily
 Adults: 200-400 mg once daily
Dosage Forms
 Tablet, oral: 200 mg

ketoconazole (topical) (kee toe KOE na zole)

Medication Safety Issues
 Sound-alike/look-alike issues:
  Nizoral® may be confused with Nasarel, Neoral®, Nitrol®
U.S. Brand Names Extina®; Nizoral®; Nizoral® A-D [OTC]; Xolegel®
Canadian Brand Names Ketoderm®; Xolegel®
Therapeutic Category Antifungal Agent, Topical

Use
  Cream: Treatment of tinea corporis, tinea cruris, tinea versicolor, cutaneous candidiasis, seborrheic dermatitis
  Foam, gel: Treatment of seborrheic dermatitis
  Shampoo: Treatment of dandruff, seborrheic dermatitis, tinea versicolor

General Dosage Range Topical:
  Cream: *Children ≥12 years and Adults:* Rub gently into the affected area 1-2 times daily
  Foam: *Children ≥12 years and Adults:* Apply to affected area twice daily
  Gel: *Children ≥12 years and Adults:* Apply gently to affected area once daily
  Shampoo: *Children ≥12 years and Adults:* Apply up to twice weekly

Dosage Forms
  Aerosol, topical:
    Extina®: 2% (50 g, 100 g)
  Cream, topical: 2% (15 g, 30 g, 60 g)
  Gel, topical:
    Xolegel®: 2% (45 g)
  Shampoo, topical: 2% (120 mL)
    Nizoral®: 2% (120 mL)
    Nizoral® A-D [OTC]: 1% (120 mL, 210 mL)

Ketoderm® (Can) see ketoconazole (topical) *on page 500*
3-keto-desogestrel see etonogestrel *on page 361*

ketoprofen (kee toe PROE fen)

Medication Safety Issues
  Sound-alike/look-alike issues:
    Ketoprofen may be confused with ketotifen

Canadian Brand Names Apo-Keto SR®; Apo-Keto-E®; Apo-Keto®; Ketoprofen SR; Ketoprofen-E; Nu-Ketoprofen; Nu-Ketoprofen-E; PMS-Ketoprofen; PMS-Ketoprofen-E

Therapeutic Category Analgesic, Nonnarcotic; Nonsteroidal Antiinflammatory Drug (NSAID)

Use Acute and long-term treatment of rheumatoid arthritis and osteoarthritis; primary dysmenorrhea; mild-to-moderate pain

General Dosage Range Dosage adjustment recommended in patients with hepatic and renal impairment
  Oral:
    Extended release: *Adults:* 200 mg once daily
    Regular release: *Adults:* 25-50 mg 4 times/day or 75 mg 3 times/day (maximum: 300 mg/day)

Dosage Forms
  Capsule, oral: 50 mg, 75 mg
  Capsule, extended release, oral: 200 mg

Ketoprofen-E (Can) see ketoprofen *on page 501*
Ketoprofen SR (Can) see ketoprofen *on page 501*

ketorolac (systemic) (KEE toe role ak)

Medication Safety Issues
  Sound-alike/look-alike issues:
    Ketorolac may be confused with Ketalar®
    Toradol® may be confused with Foradil®, Inderal®, TEGretol®, Torecan®, traMADol, tromethamine
  Beers Criteria medication:
    This drug may be inappropriate for use in geriatric patients (high severity risk).
  International issues:
    Toradol [Canada and multiple international markets] may be confused with Theradol brand name for tramadol [Netherlands]

Synonyms ketorolac tromethamine; Toradol

Canadian Brand Names Apo-Ketorolac Injectable®; Apo-Ketorolac®; Ketorolac Tromethamine Injection, USP; Novo-Ketorolac; Nu-Ketorolac; Toradol®; Toradol® IM

Therapeutic Category Nonsteroidal Antiinflammatory Drug (NSAID), Oral; Nonsteroidal Antiinflammatory Drug (NSAID), Parenteral

Use Short-term (≤5 days) management of moderate-to-severe acute pain requiring analgesia at the opioid level ▶

◄ **General Dosage Range** Dosage adjustment recommended in patients with renal impairment

I.M.:

Children ≥16 years and Adults <50 kg and Elderly ≥65 years: 30 mg as a single dose **or** 15 mg every 6 hours (maximum: 60 mg/day)

Children ≥16 years and Adults ≥50 kg: 60 mg as a single dose **or** 30 mg every 6 hours (maximum: 120 mg/day)

I.V.:

Children ≥16 years and Adults <50 kg and Elderly ≥65 years: 15 mg as a single dose **or** 15 mg every 6 hours (maximum: 60 mg/day)

Children ≥16 years and Adults ≥50 kg: 30 mg as a single dose **or** 30 mg every 6 hours (maximum: 120 mg/day)

Oral:

Children ≥17 years and Adults <50 kg and Elderly ≥65 years: 10 mg every 4-6 hours (maximum: 40 mg/day)

Children ≥17 years and Adults ≥50 kg: 20 mg, followed by 10 mg every 4-6 hours (maximum: 40 mg/day)

Dosage Forms

Injection, solution: 15 mg/mL (1 mL, 2 mL); 30 mg/mL (1 mL, 2 mL, 10 mL)

Tablet, oral: 10 mg

ketorolac (nasal) (KEE toe role ak)

Medication Safety Issues

Sound-alike/look-alike issues:

Ketorolac may be confused with Ketalar®

BEERS Criteria medication:

This drug may be inappropriate for use in geriatric patients (high severity risk).

Synonyms ketorolac tromethamine

U.S. Brand Names Sprix®

Therapeutic Category Nonsteroidal Antiinflammatory Drug (NSAID), Nasal

Use Short-term (≤5 days) management of moderate-to-moderately-severe acute pain requiring analgesia at the opioid level

General Dosage Range Dosage adjustment recommended in patients with renal impairment.

Intranasal:

Adults <65 years and ≥50 kg: one spray (15.75 mg) in each nostril (total dose: 31.5 mg) every 6-8 hours; maximum dose: 4 doses (126 mg)/day

Adults <50 kg and/or Elderly ≥65 years: One spray (15.75 mg) in 1 nostril (total dose: 15.75 mg) every 6-8 hours; maximum dose: 4 doses (63 mg)/day

Dosage Forms

Solution, intranasal [preservative free]:

Sprix®: 15.75 mg/spray (1.7 g)

ketorolac (ophthalmic) (KEE toe role ak)

Medication Safety Issues

Sound-alike/look-alike issues:

Acular® may be confused with Acthar®, Ocular®

Ketorolac may be confused with Ketalar®

Synonyms ketorolac tromethamine

U.S. Brand Names Acular LS®; Acular®; Acuvail®

Canadian Brand Names Acular LS®; Acular®; ratio-Ketorolac

Therapeutic Category Nonsteroidal Antiinflammatory Drug (NSAID), Ophthalmic

Use Temporary relief of ocular itching due to seasonal allergic conjunctivitis; postoperative inflammation following cataract extraction; reduction of ocular pain and photophobia following incisional refractive surgery; reduction of ocular pain, burning, and stinging following corneal refractive surgery

General Dosage Range Ophthalmic: *Children ≥3 years and Adults:* Instill 1 drop (0.25 mg) 4 times/day to eye(s)

Dosage Forms
Solution, ophthalmic: 0.4% (5 mL); 0.5% (3 mL, 5 mL, 10 mL)
Acular LS®: 0.4% (5 mL)
Acular®: 0.5% (5 mL)
Solution, ophthalmic [preservative free]:
Acuvail®: 0.45% (0.4 mL)

ketorolac tromethamine *see* ketorolac (nasal) *on page 502*
ketorolac tromethamine *see* ketorolac (ophthalmic) *on page 502*
ketorolac tromethamine *see* ketorolac (systemic) *on page 501*
Ketorolac Tromethamine Injection, USP (Can) *see* ketorolac (systemic) *on page 501*

ketotifen (ophthalmic) (kee toe TYE fen)

Medication Safety Issues
Sound-alike/look-alike issues:
Claritin™ Eye (ketotifen) may be confused with Claritin® (loratadine)
Ketotifen may be confused with ketoprofen
ZyrTEC® Itchy Eye (ketotifen) may be confused with ZyrTEC® (cetirizine)
Synonyms ketotifen fumarate
U.S. Brand Names Alaway™ [OTC]; Claritin™ Eye [OTC]; Zaditor® [OTC]; ZyrTEC® Itchy Eye [OTC]
Canadian Brand Names Zaditor®
Therapeutic Category Antihistamine, H_1 Blocker, Ophthalmic
Use Temporary relief of eye itching due to allergic conjunctivitis
General Dosage Range Ophthalmic: *Children ≥3 years and Adults:* Instill 1 drop into the affected eye(s) twice daily, every 8-12 hours
Dosage Forms
Solution, ophthalmic: 0.025% (5 mL)
Alaway™ [OTC]: 0.025% (10 mL)
Claritin™ Eye [OTC]: 0.025% (5 mL)
Zaditor® [OTC]: 0.025% (5 mL)
ZyrTEC® Itchy Eye [OTC]: 0.025% (5 mL)
Dosage Forms - Canada
Solution, ophthalmic [drops]:
Zaditor®: 0.025% (5 mL)
Solution, ophthalmic [drops], preservative free:
Zaditor®: 0.025% (0.4 mL) (30s)

ketotifen fumarate *see* ketotifen (ophthalmic) *on page 503*
Key-E® [OTC] *see* vitamin E *on page 918*
Key-E® Kaps [OTC] *see* vitamin E *on page 918*
Key-E® Powder [OTC] *see* vitamin E *on page 918*
Keygesic [OTC] *see* magnesium salicylate *on page 547*
khloditan *see* mitotane *on page 593*
KI *see* potassium iodide *on page 726*
Kidkare Children's Cough/Cold [OTC] *see* chlorpheniramine, pseudoephedrine, and dextromethorphan *on page 201*
Kidrolase® (Can) *see* asparaginase *on page 98*
Kineret® *see* anakinra *on page 78*
Kinevac® *see* sincalide *on page 814*
Kinrix® *see* diphtheria and tetanus toxoids, acellular pertussis, and poliovirus vaccine *on page 294*
Kionex® *see* sodium polystyrene sulfonate *on page 823*
Kivexa™ (Can) *see* abacavir and lamivudine *on page 20*
Klaron® *see* sulfacetamide (topical) *on page 835*
Klean-Prep® (Can) *see* polyethylene glycol-electrolyte solution *on page 718*
KlonoPIN® *see* clonazepam *on page 222*
Klonopin® (Can) *see* clonazepam *on page 222*
Klor-Con® *see* potassium chloride *on page 724*
Klor-Con® 8 *see* potassium chloride *on page 724*

Klor-Con® 10 *see* potassium chloride *on page 724*
Klor-Con®/25 *see* potassium chloride *on page 724*
Klor-Con®/EF *see* potassium bicarbonate and potassium citrate *on page 723*
Klor-Con® M10 *see* potassium chloride *on page 724*
Klor-Con® M15 *see* potassium chloride *on page 724*
Klor-Con® M20 *see* potassium chloride *on page 724*
K-Lyte/Cl *see* potassium bicarbonate and potassium chloride *on page 723*
KMD 3213 *see* silodosin *on page 811*
Koffex DM-D (Can) *see* pseudoephedrine and dextromethorphan *on page 752*
Koffex DM-Expectorant (Can) *see* guaifenesin and dextromethorphan *on page 427*
Koffex Expectorant (Can) *see* guaifenesin *on page 425*
Kogenate® FS *see* antihemophilic factor (recombinant) *on page 81*
Kolephrin® GG/DM [OTC] *see* guaifenesin and dextromethorphan *on page 427*
Kombiglyze™ XR *see* saxagliptin and metformin *on page 803*
Konakion (Can) *see* phytonadione *on page 703*
Konsyl® [OTC] *see* psyllium *on page 755*
Konsyl-D™ [OTC] *see* psyllium *on page 755*
Konsyl® Easy Mix™ [OTC] *see* psyllium *on page 755*
Konsyl® Fiber [OTC] *see* polycarbophil *on page 717*
Konsyl® Orange [OTC] *see* psyllium *on page 755*
Konsyl® Original [OTC] *see* psyllium *on page 755*
Koāte®-DVI *see* antihemophilic factor (human) *on page 81*
K-Phos® MF *see* potassium phosphate and sodium phosphate *on page 727*
K-Phos® Neutral *see* potassium phosphate and sodium phosphate *on page 727*
K-Phos® No. 2 *see* potassium phosphate and sodium phosphate *on page 727*
K-Phos® Original *see* potassium acid phosphate *on page 723*
KPN Prenatal [OTC] *see* vitamins (multiple/prenatal) *on page 920*
Kristalose® *see* lactulose *on page 507*
Krystexxa™ *see* pegloticase *on page 682*
K-Tab® *see* potassium chloride *on page 724*
kunecatechins *see* sinecatechins *on page 814*
Kuvan™ *see* sapropterin *on page 802*
Kwellada-P™ (Can) *see* permethrin *on page 691*
Kytril® *see* granisetron *on page 424*
L-749,345 *see* ertapenem *on page 338*
L-758,298 *see* fosaprepitant *on page 400*
L-M-X® 4 [OTC] *see* lidocaine (topical) *on page 524*
L-M-X® 5 [OTC] *see* lidocaine (topical) *on page 524*
L 754030 *see* aprepitant *on page 91*
LA 20304a *see* gemifloxacin *on page 414*

labetalol (la BET a lole)

Medication Safety Issues
Sound-alike/look-alike issues:
Labetalol may be confused with betaxolol, Hexadrol®, lamoTRIgine, Lipitor®
Normodyne® may be confused with Norpramin®
Trandate® may be confused with traMADol, Trendar®, Trental®, Tridrate®
High alert medication:
The Institute for Safe Medication Practices (ISMP) includes this medication among its list of drugs which have a heightened risk of causing significant patient harm when used in error.
Administration issues:
Significant differences exist between oral and I.V. dosing. Use caution when converting from one route of administration to another.
Synonyms ibidomide hydrochloride; labetalol hydrochloride
U.S. Brand Names Trandate®

Canadian Brand Names Apo-Labetalol®; Labetalol Hydrochloride Injection, USP; Normodyne®; Trandate®

Therapeutic Category Alpha-/Beta- Adrenergic Blocker

Use Treatment of mild-to-severe hypertension; I.V. for severe hypertension (eg, hypertensive emergencies)

General Dosage Range
I.V.:
Children: 0.3-1 mg/kg/dose intermittently **or** 0.4-1 mg/kg/hour infusion (maximum: 3 mg/kg/hour)
Adults: Bolus: 20 mg, may give 40-80 mg at 10-minute intervals; Infusion: 2 mg/minute (maximum: 300 mg total cumulative dose)
Oral: *Adults:* Initial: 100 mg twice daily; Maintenance: 200-800 mg/day in 2 divided doses (maximum: 2.4 g/day)

Dosage Forms
Injection, solution: 5 mg/mL (4 mL, 8 mL, 20 mL, 40 mL)
Trandate®: 5 mg/mL (20 mL, 40 mL)
Tablet, oral: 100 mg, 200 mg, 300 mg
Trandate®: 100 mg, 200 mg, 300 mg

labetalol hydrochloride *see* labetalol *on page 504*

Labetalol Hydrochloride Injection, USP (Can) *see* labetalol *on page 504*

Lac-Dose® [OTC] *see* lactase *on page 505*

Lac-Hydrin® *see* lactic acid and ammonium hydroxide *on page 506*

Lac-Hydrin® Five [OTC] *see* lactic acid and ammonium hydroxide *on page 506*

LAClotion™ *see* lactic acid and ammonium hydroxide *on page 506*

lactosamide (la KOE sa mide)

Medication Safety Issues
Sound-alike/look-alike issues:
Lacosamide may be confused with zonisamide
Vimpat® may be confused with Vimovo™

Synonyms ADD 234037; harkoseride; LCM; SPM 927

U.S. Brand Names Vimpat®

Canadian Brand Names Vimpat®

Therapeutic Category Anticonvulsant, Miscellaneous

Controlled Substance C-V

Use Adjunctive therapy in the treatment of partial-onset seizures

General Dosage Range Dosage adjustment recommended in patients with hepatic or renal impairment
Oral: *Adolescents ≥17 years and Adults:* Initial: 50 mg twice daily; Maintenance dose: 200-400 mg/day

Dosage Forms
Injection, solution:
Vimpat®: 10 mg/mL (20 mL)
Solution, oral:
Vimpat®: 10 mg/mL (20 mL)
Tablet, oral:
Vimpat®: 50 mg, 100 mg, 150 mg, 200 mg

Lacrisert® *see* hydroxypropyl cellulose *on page 455*

LaCrosse Complete [OTC] *see* sodium phosphates *on page 823*

Lactaid® Fast Act [OTC] *see* lactase *on page 505*

Lactaid® Original [OTC] *see* lactase *on page 505*

lactase (LAK tase)

U.S. Brand Names Lac-Dose® [OTC]; Lactaid® Fast Act [OTC]; Lactaid® Original [OTC]; Lactose Intolerance [OTC]; Lactrase® [OTC]

Canadian Brand Names Dairyaid®

Therapeutic Category Nutritional Supplement

Use Help digest lactose in milk for patients with lactose intolerance

General Dosage Range Oral: *Adults:* 1-2 capsules with meals **or** 5-15 drops or 1-2 capsules/quart of milk **or** 1-3 tablets with meals

▶

◀ **Dosage Forms**
Caplet, oral: 3000 FCC lactase units
  Lactaid® Fast Act [OTC]: 9000 FCC lactase units
  Lactaid® Original [OTC]: 3000 FCC lactase units
Capsule, oral:
  Lactrase® [OTC]: 250 mg standardized enzyme lactase
Capsule, softgel, oral:
  Lactose Intolerance [OTC]: 250 mg standardized enzyme lactase
Tablet, oral:
  Lac-Dose® [OTC]: 3000 FCC lactase units
Tablet, chewable, oral:
  Lactaid® Fast Act [OTC]: 9000 FCC lactase units

lactic acid (LAK tik AS id)

Synonyms sodium-PCA and lactic acid
Therapeutic Category Topical Skin Product
Use Lubricate and moisturize the skin counteracting dryness and itching
General Dosage Range Topical: *Adults:* Apply twice daily
Dosage Forms
Cream, topical: 10% (113 g, 113.4 g, 227 g)
Lotion, topical: 10% (355 mL, 360 mL, 473 mL)

lactic acid and ammonium hydroxide (LAK tik AS id & a MOE nee um hye DROKS ide)

Synonyms ammonium hydroxide and lactic acid; ammonium lactate
U.S. Brand Names AmLactin® [OTC]; Geri-Hydrolac™ [OTC]; Geri-Hydrolac™-12 [OTC]; Lac-Hydrin®; Lac-Hydrin® Five [OTC]; LAClotion™
Therapeutic Category Topical Skin Product
Use Treatment of moderate-to-severe xerosis and ichthyosis vulgaris
General Dosage Range Topical:
Cream: *Children ≥2 years and Adults:* Apply twice daily to affected area
Lotion: *Children and Adults:* Apply twice daily to affected area
Dosage Forms
Cream, topical: Lactic acid 12% with ammonium hydroxide (140 g, 280 g, 385 g)
  AmLactin® [OTC]: Lactic acid 12% with ammonium hydroxide (140 g)
  Lac-Hydrin®: Lactic acid 12% with ammonium hydroxide (280 g, 385 g)
Lotion, topical: Lactic acid 12% with ammonium hydroxide (225 g, 400 g)
  AmLactin® [OTC], Lac-Hydrin®, LAClotion™: Lactic acid 12% with ammonium hydroxide (225 g, 400 g)
  Geri-Hydrolac™ [OTC], Lac-Hydrin® Five: Lactic acid 5% with ammonium hydroxide (120 mL, 240 mL)
  Geri-Hydrolac™-12 [OTC]: Lactic acid 12% with ammonium hydroxide (120 mL, 240 mL)

Lactinex™ [OTC] *see Lactobacillus on page 506*

Lactobacillus (lak toe ba SIL us)

Synonyms *Lactobacillus acidophilus*; *Lactobacillus bifidus*; *Lactobacillus bulgaricus*; *Lactobacillus casei*; *Lactobacillus paracasei*; *Lactobacillus plantarum*; *Lactobacillus reuteri*; *Lactobacillus rhamnosus* GG
U.S. Brand Names Bacid® [OTC]; Culturelle® [OTC]; Dofus [OTC]; Flora-Q™ [OTC]; Floranex™ [OTC]; Kala® [OTC]; Lactinex™ [OTC]; Lacto-Bifidus [OTC]; Lacto-Key [OTC]; Lacto-Pectin [OTC]; Lacto-TriBlend [OTC]; Megadophilus® [OTC]; MoreDophilus® [OTC]; RisaQuad®-2 [OTC]; RisaQuad™ [OTC]; Superdophilus® [OTC]; VSL #3® [OTC]; VSL #3®-DS
Canadian Brand Names Bacid®; Fermalac
Therapeutic Category Gastrointestinal Agent, Miscellaneous
Use Promote normal bacterial flora of the intestinal tract
General Dosage Range Oral: *Children and Adults:* Dosage varies greatly depending on product
Dosage Forms
Capsule:
  Culturelle® [OTC]: *L. rhamnosus* GG 10 billion colony-forming units
  Dofus [OTC]: *L. acidophilus* and *L. bifidus* 10:1 ratio
  Flora-Q™ [OTC]: *L. acidophilus* and *L. paracasei* ≥8 billion colony-forming units
  Lacto-Key [OTC]:
    100: *L. acidophilus* 1 billion colony-forming units
    600: *L. acidophilus* 6 billion colony-forming units

Lacto-Bifidus [OTC]:
  100: *L. bifidus* 1 billion colony-forming units
  600: *L. bifidus* 6 billion colony-forming units
Lacto-Pectin [OTC]: *L. acidophilus* and *L. casei* ≥5 billion colony-forming units
Lacto-TriBlend [OTC]:
  100: *L. acidophilus, L. bifidus,* and *L. bulgaricus* 1 billion colony-forming units
  600: *L. acidophilus, L. bifidus,* and *L. bulgaricus* 6 billion colony-forming units
Megadophilus® [OTC], Superdophilus® [OTC]: *L. acidophilus* 2 billion units
RisaQuad™ [OTC]: *L. acidophilus* and *L. paracasei* 8 billion colony-forming units
VSL #3® [OTC]: *L. acidophilus, L. plantarum, L. paracasei, L. bulgaricus* 112 billion live cells
Capsule, double strength:
RisaQuad®-2 [OTC]: *L. acidophilus* and *L. paracasei* 16 billion colony-forming units
Capsule, softgel: *L. acidophilus* 100 active units
Caplet:
Bacid® [OTC]: *L. acidophilus* 80% and *L. bulgaricus* 10%
Granules:
Floranex™ [OTC], Lactinex™ [OTC]: *L. acidophilus* and *L. bulgaricus* 100 million live cells per 1 g packet (12s)
Powder:
Lacto-TriBlend [OTC]: *L. acidophilus, L. bifidus,* and *L. bulgaricus* 10 billion colony-forming units per ¼ teaspoon
Megadophilus® [OTC], Superdophilus® [OTC]: *L. acidophilus* 2 billion units per half-teaspoon
MoreDophilus® [OTC]: *L. acidophilus* 12.4 billion units per teaspoon
VSL #3® [OTC]: *L. acidophilus, L. plantarum, L. paracasei, L. bulgaricus* 450 billion live cells
VSL #3®-DS: *L. acidophilus, L. plantarum, L. paracasei, L. bulgaricus* 900 billion live cells
Tablet:
Kala® [OTC]: *L. acidophilus* 200 million units
Tablet, chewable: *L. reuteri* 100 million organisms
Floranex™ [OTC]: *L. acidophilus* and *L. bulgaricus* 1 million colony-forming units
Lactinex™ [OTC]: *L. acidophilus* and *L. bulgaricus* 1 million live cells
Wafer: *L. acidophilus* 90 mg and *L. bifidus* 25 mg (100s)

Lactobacillus acidophilus see Lactobacillus *on page 506*
Lactobacillus bifidus see Lactobacillus *on page 506*
Lactobacillus bulgaricus see Lactobacillus *on page 506*
Lactobacillus casei see Lactobacillus *on page 506*
Lactobacillus paracasei see Lactobacillus *on page 506*
Lactobacillus plantarum see Lactobacillus *on page 506*
Lactobacillus reuteri see Lactobacillus *on page 506*
Lactobacillus rhamnosus GG see Lactobacillus *on page 506*
Lacto-Bifidus [OTC] see Lactobacillus *on page 506*
lactoflavin see riboflavin *on page 778*
Lacto-Key [OTC] see Lactobacillus *on page 506*
Lacto-Pectin [OTC] see Lactobacillus *on page 506*
Lactose Intolerance [OTC] see lactase *on page 505*
Lacto-TriBlend [OTC] see Lactobacillus *on page 506*
Lactrase® [OTC] see lactase *on page 505*

lactulose (LAK tyoo lose)

Medication Safety Issues
 Sound-alike/look-alike issues:
  Lactulose may be confused with lactose
U.S. Brand Names Constulose; Enulose; Generlac; Kristalose®
Canadian Brand Names Acilac; Apo-Lactulose®; Laxilose; PMS-Lactulose
Therapeutic Category Ammonium Detoxicant; Laxative
Use Prevention and treatment of portal-systemic encephalopathy (including hepatic precoma and coma); treatment of constipation

◄ **General Dosage Range**
Oral:
Infants: 1.7-6.7 g/day (2.5-10 mL/day) in divided doses
Older Children and Adolescents: 26.7-60 g/day (40-90 mL/day) in divided doses
Adults: PSE: 20-30 g (30-45 mL) every hour initially, then 3-4 times/day; Constipation: 10-40 g (15-60 mL) daily
Rectal: *Adults:* Constipation: 200 g (300 mL); may repeat every 4-6 hours

Dosage Forms
Crystals for solution, oral:
Kristalose®: 10 g/packet (30s); 20 g/packet (30s)
Solution, oral: 10 g/15 mL (15 mL, 30 mL, 237 mL, 240 mL, 473 mL, 480 mL, 500 mL, 946 mL, 960 mL, 1000 mL, 1890 mL, 1892 mL, 1920 mL)
Constulose: 10 g/15 mL (946 mL)
Enulose: 10 g/15 mL (473 mL)
Solution, oral/rectal: 10 g/15 mL (237 mL, 473 mL, 946 mL, 1920 mL)
Generlac: 10 g/15 mL (473 mL, 1892 mL)

ladakamycin *see* azacitidine *on page 106*
Lagesic™ [DSC] *see* acetaminophen and phenyltoloxamine *on page 28*
L-AmB *see* amphotericin B liposomal *on page 76*
LaMICtal® *see* lamotrigine *on page 509*
Lamictal® (Can) *see* lamotrigine *on page 509*
LaMICtal® ODT™ *see* lamotrigine *on page 509*
LaMICtal® XR™ *see* lamotrigine *on page 509*
LamISIL® *see* terbinafine (systemic) *on page 851*
Lamisil® (Can) *see* terbinafine (systemic) *on page 851*
Lamisil® (Can) *see* terbinafine (topical) *on page 852*
LamISIL AT® [OTC] *see* terbinafine (topical) *on page 852*

lamivudine (la MI vyoo deen)

Medication Safety Issues
Sound-alike/look-alike issues:
LamiVUDine may be confused with lamoTRIgine
Epivir® may be confused with Combivir®
Synonyms 3TC
Tall-Man lamiVUDine
U.S. Brand Names Epivir-HBV®; Epivir®
Canadian Brand Names 3TC®; Heptovir®
Therapeutic Category Antiviral Agent
Use
Epivir®: Treatment of HIV infection when antiretroviral therapy is warranted; should always be used as part of a multidrug regimen (at least three antiretroviral agents)
Epivir-HBV®: Treatment of chronic hepatitis B associated with evidence of hepatitis B viral replication and active liver inflammation. Resistance develops rapidly in hepatitis B; consider use only if other anti-HBV antiviral agents with more favorable resistance patterns cannot be used.
General Dosage Range Dosage adjustment recommended in patients with renal impairment
Oral:
Infants 1-3 months: HIV (DHHS [pediatric], 2010): 4 mg/kg/dose twice daily
Children 3 months to 2 years: HIV: 4 mg/kg/dose twice daily (maximum: 150 mg/dose twice daily)
Children 2-16 years and >16 years and <50 kg: Hepatitis B: 3 mg/kg/dose once daily (maximum: 100 mg/day); HIV: 4 mg/kg/dose twice daily (maximum: 150 mg/dose twice daily)
Children >16 years and ≥50 kg: Hepatitis B: 3 mg/kg/dose once daily (maximum: 100 mg/day); HIV: 150 mg twice daily **or** 300 mg once daily
Adults <50 kg: Hepatitis B: 100 mg/day; HIV (DHHS [pediatric], 2010): 4 mg/kg/dose twice daily (maximum: 150 mg/dose twice daily)
Adults ≥50 kg: Hepatitis B: 100 mg/day; HIV: 150 mg twice daily **or** 300 mg once daily

Dosage Forms
  Solution, oral:
    Epivir-HBV®: 5 mg/mL
    Epivir®: 10 mg/mL
  Tablet, oral:
    Epivir-HBV®: 100 mg
    Epivir®: 150 mg, 300 mg

lamivudine, abacavir, and zidovudine *see* abacavir, lamivudine, and zidovudine *on page 20*
lamivudine and abacavir *see* abacavir and lamivudine *on page 20*

lamivudine and zidovudine (la MI vyoo deen & zye DOE vyoo deen)
Medication Safety Issues
  Sound-alike/look-alike issues:
    Combivir® may be confused with Combivent®, Epivir®
  Other safety concerns:
    AZT is an error-prone abbreviation (mistaken as azaTHIOprine, aztreonam)
Synonyms AZT + 3TC (error-prone abbreviation); zidovudine and lamivudine
U.S. Brand Names Combivir®
Canadian Brand Names Combivir®
Therapeutic Category Antiviral Agent
Use Treatment of HIV infection when therapy is warranted based on clinical and/or immunological evidence of disease progression
General Dosage Range Oral: *Adolescents ≥30 kg and Adults:* 1 tablet (lamivudine 150 mg/zidovudine 300 mg) twice daily
Dosage Forms
  Tablet:
    Combivir®: Lamivudine 150 mg and zidovudine 300 mg [scored]

lamotrigine (la MOE tri jeen)
Medication Safety Issues
  Sound-alike/look-alike issues:
    LamoTRIgine may be confused with labetalol, Lamisil®, lamiVUDine, levothyroxine, Lomotil®
    LaMICtal® may be confused with LamISIL®, Lomotil®
  Administration issues:
    Potential exists for medication errors to occur among different formulations of Lamictal® (tablets, extended release tablets, orally disintegrating tablets, and chewable/dispersible tablets). Patients should be instructed to visually inspect tablets dispensed to verify receiving the correct medication and formulation. The medication guide includes illustrations to aid in tablet verification.
  International issues:
    Lamictal [U.S., Canada, and multiple international markets] may be confused with Ludiomil brand name for maprotiline [multiple international markets]
    Lamotrigine [U.S., Canada, and multiple international markets] may be confused with Ludiomil brand name for maprotiline [multiple international markets]
Synonyms BW-430C; LTG
Tall-Man lamoTRIgine
U.S. Brand Names LaMICtal®; LaMICtal® ODT™; LaMICtal® XR™
Canadian Brand Names Apo-Lamotrigine®; Lamictal®; Mylan-Lamotrigine; Novo-Lamotrigine; PMS-Lamotrigine; ratio-Lamotrigine; Teva-Lamotrigine
Therapeutic Category Anticonvulsant
Use Adjunctive therapy in the treatment of generalized seizures of Lennox-Gastaut syndrome, primary generalized tonic-clonic seizures, and partial seizures; conversion to monotherapy in patients with partial seizures who are receiving treatment with valproic acid or a single enzyme-inducing antiepileptic drug (specifically carbamazepine, phenytoin, phenobarbital or primidone); maintenance treatment of bipolar I disorder

◀ **General Dosage Range** Dosage adjustment recommended in patients with hepatic or renal impairment or on concomitant therapy

Oral:

Immediate release formulation:

Children 2-12 years: Dosage varies greatly depending on indication

Children ≥13 years and Adults: Dosage varies greatly depending on indication

Extended release formulation: *Children ≥13 years and Adults:* Dosage varies greatly depending on indication

Dosage Forms

Tablet, oral: 25 mg, 100 mg, 150 mg, 200 mg

LaMICtal®: 25 mg, 100 mg, 150 mg, 200 mg, 25 mg (42s) [white tablets] and 100 mg (7s) [peach tablets], 25 mg (84s) [white tablets] and 100 mg (14s) [peach tablets]

Tablet, chewable/dispersible, oral: 5 mg, 25 mg

LaMICtal®: 2 mg, 5 mg, 25 mg

Tablet, extended release, oral:

LaMICtal® XR™: 25 mg, 50 mg, 100 mg, 200 mg, 300 mg, 25 mg (21s) [yellow/white tablets] and 50 mg (7s) [green/white tablets], 50 mg (14s) [green/white tablets], 100 mg (14s) [orange/white tablets], and 200 mg (7s) [blue/white tablets], 25 mg (14s) [yellow/white tablets], 50 mg (14s) [green/white tablets], and 100 mg (7s) [orange/white tablets]

Tablet, orally disintegrating, oral:

LaMICtal® ODT™: 25 mg, 50 mg, 100 mg, 200 mg, 25 mg (21s) and 50 mg (7s), 50 mg (42s) and 100 mg (14s), 25 mg (14s), 50 mg (14s), and 100 mg (7s)

Lanacane® [OTC] *see* benzocaine *on page 121*

Lanacane® Maximum Strength [OTC] *see* benzocaine *on page 121*

Lanaphilic® with Urea [OTC] *see* urea *on page 900*

lanolin, cetyl alcohol, glycerin, petrolatum, and mineral oil
(LAN oh lin, SEE til AL koe hol, GLIS er in, pe troe LAY tum, & MIN er al oyl)

Synonyms cetyl alcohol, glycerin, lanolin, mineral oil, and petrolatum; mineral oil, petrolatum, lanolin, cetyl alcohol, and glycerin

U.S. Brand Names Lubriderm® Fragrance Free [OTC]; Lubriderm® [OTC]

Therapeutic Category Topical Skin Product

Use Treatment of dry skin

General Dosage Range Topical: *Adults:* Apply to skin as necessary

Dosage Forms

Lotion, topical [bottle]: 180 mL, 300 mL, 480 mL

Lubriderm® Fragrance Free [OTC], Lubriderm® [OTC]: 180 mL, 300 mL, 480 mL

Lotion, topical [tube]: 100 mL

Lubriderm® Fragrance Free [OTC], Lubriderm® [OTC]: 100 mL

Lanoxin® *see* digoxin *on page 283*

lanreotide (lan REE oh tide)

Medication Safety Issues

Sound-alike/look-alike issues:

Somatuline® may be confused with somatropin, SUMAtriptan

International issues:

Somatuline® may be confused with Soma® which is a brand name for carisoprodol in the U.S.

Synonyms lanreotide acetate

U.S. Brand Names Somatuline® Depot

Canadian Brand Names Somatuline® Autogel®

Therapeutic Category Somatostatin Analog

Use Long-term treatment of acromegaly in patients who are not candidates for or are unresponsive to surgery and/or radiotherapy

Canadian labeling: Also approved in Canada for relief of symptoms of acromegaly

General Dosage Range Dosage adjustment recommended in patients with hepatic or renal impairment

SubQ: *Adults:* Initial: 90 mg once every 4 weeks for 3 months; Maintenance: 60-120 mg every 4 weeks **or** 120 mg every 6-8 weeks

Dosage Forms
Injection, solution:
   Somatuline® Depot: 60 mg/0.4 mL (0.4 mL); 90 mg/0.4 mL (0.4 mL); 120 mg/0.5 mL (0.5 mL)
Dosage Forms - Canada
Injection, solution:
   Somatuline® Autogel®: 60 mg/~0.3 mL (~0.3 mL); 90 mg/~0.4 mL (~0.4 mL); 120 mg/~0.5 mL (~0.5 mL)

lanreotide acetate *see* lanreotide *on page 510*

lansoprazole (lan SOE pra zole)

Medication Safety Issues
   Sound-alike/look-alike issues:
   Lansoprazole may be confused with aripiprazole, dexlansoprazole
   Prevacid® may be confused with Pravachol®, Prevpac®, PriLOSEC®, Prinivil®
U.S. Brand Names Prevacid®; Prevacid® 24 HR [OTC]; Prevacid® SoluTab™

Canadian Brand Names Apo-Lansoprazole®; Mylan-Lansoprazole; Prevacid®; Prevacid® FasTab; Teva-Lansoprazole

Therapeutic Category Gastric Acid Secretion Inhibitor

Use Short-term treatment of active duodenal ulcers; maintenance treatment of healed duodenal ulcers; as part of a multidrug regimen for *H. pylori* eradication to reduce the risk of duodenal ulcer recurrence; short-term treatment of active benign gastric ulcer; treatment of NSAID-associated gastric ulcer; to reduce the risk of NSAID-associated gastric ulcer in patients with a history of gastric ulcer who require an NSAID; short-term treatment of symptomatic GERD; short-term treatment for all grades of erosive esophagitis; to maintain healing of erosive esophagitis; long-term treatment of pathological hypersecretory conditions, including Zollinger-Ellison syndrome

OTC labeling: Relief of frequent heartburn (≥2 days/week)

General Dosage Range Oral:
   Children 1-11 years and ≤30 kg: 15 mg once daily (maximum: 30 mg twice daily)
   Children 1-11 years and >30 kg: 30 mg once daily (maximum: 30 mg twice daily)
   Children 12-17 years: 15-30 mg once daily
   Adults: 15-180 mg/day in 1-2 divided doses
Dosage Forms
   Capsule, delayed release, oral: 15 mg, 30 mg
      Prevacid®: 15 mg, 30 mg
      Prevacid® 24 HR [OTC]: 15 mg
   Tablet, delayed release, orally disintegrating, oral: 15 mg, 30 mg
      Prevacid® SoluTab™: 15 mg, 30 mg

lansoprazole, amoxicillin, and clarithromycin
(lan SOE pra zole, a moks i SIL in, & kla RITH roe mye sin)
Medication Safety Issues
   Sound-alike/look-alike issues:
   Prevpac® may be confused with Prevacid®
Synonyms amoxicillin, clarithromycin, and lansoprazole; clarithromycin, lansoprazole, and amoxicillin; lansoprazole, amoxicillin, and clarithromycin
U.S. Brand Names Prevpac®
Canadian Brand Names Hp-PAC®
Therapeutic Category Antibiotic, Macrolide Combination; Antibiotic, Penicillin; Gastrointestinal Agent, Miscellaneous
Use Eradication of *H. pylori* to reduce the risk of recurrent duodenal ulcer
General Dosage Range Oral: *Adults:* Lansoprazole 30 mg, amoxicillin 1 g, and clarithromycin 500 mg taken together twice daily
Dosage Forms
   Combination package [each administration card contains]:
      Prevpac®:
         Capsule: Amoxicillin 500 mg (4 capsules/day)
         Capsule, delayed release (Prevacid®): Lansoprazole 30 mg (2 capsules/day)
         Tablet (Biaxin®): Clarithromycin 500 mg (2 tablets/day)

lansoprazole, amoxicillin, and clarithromycin *see* lansoprazole, amoxicillin, and clarithromycin *on page 511*

lanthanum (LAN tha num)

Medication Safety Issues
Sound-alike/look-alike issues:
Lanthanum may be confused with lithium
Synonyms lanthanum carbonate
U.S. Brand Names Fosrenol®
Canadian Brand Names Fosrenol®
Therapeutic Category Phosphate Binder
Use Reduction of serum phosphate in patients with stage 5 chronic kidney disease (end-stage renal disease [ESRD]; kidney failure: GFR <15 mL/minute/1.73 m² or dialysis)
General Dosage Range Oral: *Adults:* Initial: 1500 mg/day in divided doses; Usual range: 1500-3000 mg/day
Dosage Forms
Tablet, chewable, oral:
Fosrenol®: 500 mg, 750 mg, 1000 mg

lanthanum carbonate *see* lanthanum *on page 512*
Lantus® *see* insulin glargine *on page 476*
Lantus® OptiSet® (Can) *see* insulin glargine *on page 476*
Lantus® Solostar® *see* insulin glargine *on page 476*
Lanvis® (Can) *see* thioguanine *on page 862*

lapatinib (la PA ti nib)

Medication Safety Issues
Sound-alike/look-alike issues:
Lapatinib may be confused with dasatinib, erlotinib, imatinib, SUNItinib, vandetanib
High alert medication:
This medication is in a class of medications the Institute for Safe Medication Practices (ISMP) includes among its list of drug classes which have a heightened risk of causing significant patient harm when used in error.
Synonyms GW572016; lapatinib ditosylate
U.S. Brand Names Tykerb®
Canadian Brand Names Tykerb®
Therapeutic Category Antineoplastic Agent, Tyrosine Kinase Inhibitor; Epidermal Growth Factor Receptor (EGFR) Inhibitor
Use Treatment of HER2 overexpressing advanced or metastatic breast cancer (in combination with capecitabine) in patients who have received prior therapy (with an anthracycline, a taxane, and trastuzumab) and HER2 overexpressing hormone receptor positive metastatic breast cancer in postmenopausal women (in combination with letrozole)
General Dosage Range Dosage adjustment recommended in patients with hepatic impairment, on concomitant therapy, or who develop toxicities
Oral: *Adults:* 1250-1500 mg once daily
Dosage Forms
Tablet, oral:
Tykerb®: 250 mg

lapatinib ditosylate *see* lapatinib *on page 512*
Largactil® (Can) *see* chlorpromazine *on page 203*
L-arginine *see* arginine *on page 93*
L-arginine hydrochloride *see* arginine *on page 93*
Lariam® (Can) *see* mefloquine *on page 555*

laronidase (lair OH ni days)

Synonyms recombinant α-L-iduronidase (glycosaminoglycan α-L-iduronohydrolase)
U.S. Brand Names Aldurazyme®
Canadian Brand Names Aldurazyme®

Therapeutic Category Enzyme

Use Treatment of Hurler and Hurler-Scheie forms of mucopolysaccharidosis I (MPS I); treatment of Scheie form of MPS I in patients with moderate-to-severe symptoms

General Dosage Range I.V.: *Children ≥5 years and Adults:* 0.58 mg/kg once weekly

Dosage Forms
Injection, solution [preservative free]:
Aldurazyme®: 2.9 mg/5 mL (5 mL)

Lasix® *see furosemide on page 404*

Lasix® Special (Can) *see furosemide on page 404*

L-asparaginase *see asparaginase on page 98*

L-asparaginase with polyethylene glycol *see pegaspargase on page 678*

lassar's zinc paste *see zinc oxide on page 930*

Lastacaft™ *see alcaftadine on page 46*

latanoprost (la TA noe prost)

Medication Safety Issues
Sound-alike/look-alike issues:
Latanoprost may be confused with Lantus®
Xalatan® may be confused with Lantus®, Travatan®, Xalacom™, Zarontin®

U.S. Brand Names Xalatan®

Canadian Brand Names Xalatan®

Therapeutic Category Prostaglandin

Use Reduction of elevated intraocular pressure in patients with open-angle glaucoma or ocular hypertension

General Dosage Range Ophthalmic: *Adults:* 1 drop (1.5 mcg) in the affected eye(s) once daily

Dosage Forms
Solution, ophthalmic: 0.005% (2.5 mL)
Xalatan®: 0.005% (2.5 mL)

latanoprost and timolol *(Canada only)* (la TA noe prost & TIM oh lol)

Medication Safety Issues
Sound-alike/look-alike issues:
Xalacom™ may be confused with Xalatan®

Synonyms timolol maleate and latanoprost

Canadian Brand Names Xalacom™

Therapeutic Category Beta Blocker, Nonselective; Ophthalmic Agent, Antiglaucoma; Prostaglandin, Ophthalmic

Use Reduction of intraocular pressure (IOP) in patients with open-angle glaucoma or ocular hypertension who are insufficiently responsive to topical beta-blockers, prostaglandin analogues, or other IOP-reducing agents and in whom combination therapy is appropriate

General Dosage Range Ophthalmic: *Adults:* Instill 1 drop once daily

Product Availability Not available in U.S.

Dosage Forms - Canada
Solution, ophthalmic:
Xalacom™: Latanoprost (0.005%) and timolol 0.5% (as base) (2.5 mL)

Latisse® *see bimatoprost on page 133*

Latrodectus antivenin *see antivenin (Latrodectus mactans) on page 84*

Latrodectus mactans antivenin *see antivenin (Latrodectus mactans) on page 84*

Latuda® *see lurasidone on page 542*

Lavacol® [OTC] *see alcohol (ethyl) on page 47*

Lavoclen™-4 *see benzoyl peroxide on page 124*

Lavoclen™-8 *see benzoyl peroxide on page 124*

Lavoclen® Acne Wash Kit *see benzoyl peroxide on page 124*

Laxilose (Can) *see lactulose on page 507*

Lazanda® *see fentanyl on page 371*

***l*-bunolol hydrochloride** *see levobunolol on page 517*

L-carnitine *see* levocarnitine *on page 518*
L-Carnitine® [OTC] *see* levocarnitine *on page 518*
LCD *see* coal tar *on page 227*
LCM *see* lacosamide *on page 505*
L-deoxythymidine *see* telbivudine *on page 847*
L-deprenyl *see* selegiline *on page 806*
LDP-341 *see* bortezomib *on page 139*
LdT *see* telbivudine *on page 847*
LEA29Y *see* belatacept *on page 117*
Lectopam® (Can) *see* bromazepam *(Canada only) on page 142*
Lederle Leucovorin (Can) *see* leucovorin calcium *on page 515*
Leena® *see* ethinyl estradiol and norethindrone *on page 355*

leflunomide (le FLOO noh mide)

U.S. Brand Names Arava®
Canadian Brand Names Apo-Leflunomide®; Arava®; Mylan-Leflunomide; Novo-Leflunomide; PHL-Leflunomide; PMS-Leflunomide; Sandoz-Leflunomide
Therapeutic Category Antiinflammatory Agent
Use Treatment of active rheumatoid arthritis; indicated to reduce signs and symptoms, and to inhibit structural damage and improve physical function
General Dosage Range Dosage adjustment recommended in patients who develop toxicities
Oral: *Adults:* Initial: 100 mg/day for 3 days; Maintenance range: 10-20 mg/day
Dosage Forms
Tablet, oral: 10 mg, 20 mg
Arava®: 10 mg, 20 mg

Legatrin PM® [OTC] *see* acetaminophen and diphenhydramine *on page 27*

lenalidomide (le na LID oh mide)

Medication Safety Issues
Sound-alike/look-alike issues:
Lenalidomide may be confused with thalidomide
High alert medication:
This medication is in a class the Institute for Safe Medication Practices (ISMP) includes among its list of drug classes which have a heightened risk of causing significant patient harm when used in error.
Synonyms CC-5013; IMid-1
U.S. Brand Names Revlimid®
Canadian Brand Names Revlimid®
Therapeutic Category Angiogenesis Inhibitor; Immunosuppressant Agent; Tumor Necrosis Factor (TNF) Blocking Agent
Use Treatment of low- or intermediate-risk myelodysplastic syndrome (MDS) in patients with deletion 5q (del 5q) cytogenetic abnormality with transfusion-dependent anemia (with or without other cytogenetic abnormalities); treatment of multiple myeloma (in combination with dexamethasone) in patients who have received at least one prior therapy
General Dosage Range Dosage adjustment recommended in patients with renal impairment or who develop toxicities
Oral: *Adults:* 10 once daily **or** 25 mg once daily for 21 of 28 days
Dosage Forms
Capsule, oral:
Revlimid®: 5 mg, 10 mg, 15 mg, 25 mg

lepirudin (leh puh ROO din)

Medication Safety Issues
High alert medication:
The Institute for Safe Medication Practices (ISMP) includes this medication among its list of drugs which have a heightened risk of causing significant patient harm when used in error.
Synonyms lepirudin (rDNA); recombinant hirudin
U.S. Brand Names Refludan®

Canadian Brand Names Refludan®

Therapeutic Category Anticoagulant (Other)

Use Indicated for anticoagulation in patients with heparin-induced thrombocytopenia (HIT) and associated thromboembolic disease in order to prevent further thromboembolic complications

General Dosage Range Dosage adjustment recommended in patients with renal impairment

I.V.: *Adults:* Bolus: 0.2-0.4 mg/kg; Infusion: 0.1-0.15 mg/kg/hour (maximum: 0.21 mg/kg/hour)

Dosage Forms

Injection, powder for reconstitution:
Refludan®: 50 mg

lepirudin (rDNA) *see* lepirudin *on page* 514

Lescol® *see* fluvastatin *on page* 394

Lescol® XL *see* fluvastatin *on page* 394

Lessina® *see* ethinyl estradiol and levonorgestrel *on page* 353

Letairis® *see* ambrisentan *on page* 62

letrozole (LET roe zole)

Medication Safety Issues

Sound-alike/look-alike issues:
Femara® may be confused with Famvir®, femhrt®, Provera®
Letrozole may be confused with anastrozole

Synonyms CGS-20267

U.S. Brand Names Femara®

Canadian Brand Names Femara®; MED-Letrozole; PMS-Letrozole; Sandoz-Letrozole

Therapeutic Category Antineoplastic Agent, Hormone (Antiestrogen)

Use For use in postmenopausal women in the adjuvant treatment of hormone receptor-positive early breast cancer, extended adjuvant treatment of early breast cancer after 5 years of tamoxifen, advanced breast cancer with disease progression following antiestrogen therapy, hormone receptor-positive or hormone receptor-unknown, locally-advanced, or first-line (or second-line) treatment of advanced or metastatic breast cancer

General Dosage Range Dosage adjustment recommended in patients with hepatic impairment

Oral: *Adults (postmenopausal females):* 2.5 mg once daily

Dosage Forms

Tablet, oral: 2.5 mg
Femara®: 2.5 mg

leucovorin *see* leucovorin calcium *on page* 515

leucovorin calcium (loo koe VOR in KAL see um)

Medication Safety Issues

Sound-alike/look-alike issues:
Leucovorin may be confused with Leukeran®, Leukine®, LEVOleucovorin
Folinic acid may be confused with folic acid
Folinic acid is an error prone synonym and should not be used

Synonyms 5-formyl tetrahydrofolate; calcium folinate; calcium leucovorin; citrovorum factor; folinate calcium; folinic acid (error prone synonym); leucovorin

Canadian Brand Names Lederle Leucovorin

Therapeutic Category Folic Acid Derivative

Use Antidote for folic acid antagonists (methotrexate, trimethoprim, pyrimethamine) and rescue therapy following high-dose methotrexate; in combination with fluorouracil in the treatment of colon cancer; treatment of megaloblastic anemias when folate is deficient as in infancy, sprue, pregnancy, and nutritional deficiency when oral folate therapy is not possible

General Dosage Range

I.M.: *Children and Adults:* ≤1 mg/day [folate deficient megaloblastic anemia] **or** 15 mg (~10 mg/m^2) every 6 hours for 10 doses [methotrexate rescue dose]

I.V.:
Children: 15 mg (~10 mg/m^2) every 6 hours for 10 doses
Adults: Initial: 15 mg (~10 mg/m^2) every 6 hours for 10 doses [methotrexate rescue dose] **or** 200 mg/m^2 **or** 20 mg/m^2 as a single dose [colorectal cancer]

◀ **Oral:** *Children and Adults:* 5-15 mg/day [weak folic acid antagonist overdose] **or** 15 mg (~10 mg/m^2) every 6 hours for 10 doses [methotrexate rescue dose]

Dosage Forms
Injection, powder for reconstitution: 50 mg, 100 mg, 200 mg, 350 mg
Injection, solution [preservative free]: 10 mg/mL (50 mL)
Tablet, oral: 5 mg, 10 mg, 15 mg, 25 mg

Leukeran® *see* chlorambucil *on page 193*
Leukine® *see* sargramostim *on page 802*

leuprolide (loo PROE lide)

Medication Safety Issues
Sound-alike/look-alike issues:
Lupron® may be confused with Nuprin®
Lupron Depot® (1-month or 3-month formulation) may be confused with Lupron Depot-Ped® (1-month or 3-month formulation)
Lupron Depot-Ped® is available in two formulations, a 1-month formulation and a 3-month formulation. Both formulations offer an 11.25 mg strength which may further add confusion.

Synonyms abbott-43818; leuprolide acetate; leuprorelin acetate; TAP-144

U.S. Brand Names Eligard®; Lupron Depot-Ped®; Lupron Depot®

Canadian Brand Names Eligard®; Lupron®; Lupron® Depot®

Therapeutic Category Antineoplastic Agent; Luteinizing Hormone-Releasing Hormone Analog

Use Palliative treatment of advanced prostate cancer; management of endometriosis; treatment of anemia caused by uterine leiomyomata (fibroids); central precocious puberty

General Dosage Range I.M., SubQ: *Children and Adults:* Dosage varies greatly depending on indication

Product Availability
Lupron Depot-Ped® 3-month formulation: FDA approved August 2011; availability expected August 2011
Lupron Depot-Ped® 3-month formulation will be available in two strengths, 11.25 mg and 30 mg.

Dosage Forms
Injection, powder for reconstitution [preservative free]:
Eligard®: 7.5 mg (monthly), 22.5 mg (3 month), 30 mg (4 month), 45 mg (6 month)
Lupron Depot-Ped®: 7.5 mg (monthly), 11.25 mg (3 month), 11.25 mg (monthly), 15 mg (monthly), 30 mg (3 month)
Lupron Depot®: 3.75 mg (monthly), 7.5 mg (monthly), 11.25 mg (3 month), 22.5 mg (3 month), 30 mg (4 month), 45 mg (6 month)
Injection, solution: 5 mg/mL (2.8 mL)

leuprolide acetate *see* leuprolide *on page 516*
leuprorelin acetate *see* leuprolide *on page 516*
leurocristine sulfate *see* vincristine *on page 915*
Leustatin® *see* cladribine *on page 214*

levalbuterol (leve al BYOO ter ole)

Medication Safety Issues
Sound-alike/look-alike issues:
Xopenex® may be confused with Xanax®

Synonyms levalbuterol hydrochloride; levalbuterol tartrate; R-albuterol

U.S. Brand Names Xopenex HFA™; Xopenex®

Canadian Brand Names Xopenex®

Therapeutic Category Adrenergic Agonist Agent; Beta$_2$-Adrenergic Agonist Agent; Bronchodilator

Use Treatment or prevention of bronchospasm in children and adults with reversible obstructive airway disease

General Dosage Range
Inhalation (metered-dose inhaler): *Children ≥4 years and Adults:* 1-2 puffs every 4-6 hours
Nebulization (solution):
Children ≤4 years: 0.31-1.25 mg every 4-6 hours as needed
Children 5-11 years: 0.31-0.63 mg 3 times/day
Children ≥12 years and Adults: 0.63-1.25 mg every 8 hours as needed
Elderly: Initial: 0.63 mg

Dosage Forms
Aerosol, for oral inhalation:
Xopenex HFA™: 45 mcg/actuation (15 g)
Solution, for nebulization [preservative free]: 1.25 mg/0.5 mL (30s)
Xopenex®: 0.31 mg/3 mL (24s); 0.63 mg/3 mL (24s); 1.25 mg/3 mL (24s)

levalbuterol hydrochloride *see* levalbuterol *on page 516*
levalbuterol tartrate *see* levalbuterol *on page 516*
Levaquin® *see* levofloxacin (systemic) *on page 520*
levarterenol bitartrate *see* norepinephrine *on page 632*
Levate® (Can) *see* amitriptyline *on page 68*
Levatol® *see* penbutolol *on page 683*
Levbid® *see* hyoscyamine *on page 457*
Levemir® *see* insulin detemir *on page 476*
Levemir® FlexPen® *see* insulin detemir *on page 476*

levetiracetam (lee va tye RA se tam)

Medication Safety Issues
Sound-alike/look-alike issues:
Keppra® may be confused with Keflex®, Keppra XR™
LevETIRAcetam may be confused with levOCARNitine, levofloxacin
Potential for dispensing errors between Keppra® and Kaletra® (lopinavir/ritonavir)

Tall-Man levETIRAcetam

U.S. Brand Names Keppra XR™; Keppra®

Canadian Brand Names Apo-Levetiracetam®; CO Levetiracetam; Dom-Levetiracetam; Keppra®; PHL-Levetiracetam; PMS-Levetiracetam; PRO-Levetiracetam

Therapeutic Category Anticonvulsant

Use Adjunctive therapy in the treatment of partial-onset, myoclonic, and/or primary generalized tonic-clonic seizures

General Dosage Range Dosage adjustment recommended in patients with renal impairment
Oral:
Immediate release:
Children 4-15 years: Initial: 10 mg/kg twice daily; Maintenance: 10-30 mg/kg twice daily (maximum: 60 mg/kg/day)
Children ≥12 years: Initial: 500 mg twice daily; Maintenance: 500-1500 mg twice daily (maximum: 3000 mg/day)
Adults: Initial: 500 mg twice daily; Maintenance: 500-1500 mg twice daily (maximum: 3000 mg/day)
Extended release: *Children ≥16 years and Adults:* Initial: 1000 mg once daily; Maintenance: 1000-3000 mg once daily (maximum: 3000 mg/day)
I.V.: *Children ≥16 years and Adults:* Initial: 500 mg twice daily; Maintenance: 500-1500 mg twice daily (maximum: 3000 mg/day)

Dosage Forms
Injection, solution: 100 mg/mL (5 mL)
Keppra®: 100 mg/mL (5 mL)
Solution, oral: 100 mg/mL (5 mL, 118 mL, 472 mL, 473 mL, 480 mL, 500 mL)
Keppra®: 100 mg/mL (480 mL)
Tablet, oral: 250 mg, 500 mg, 750 mg, 1000 mg
Keppra®: 250 mg, 500 mg, 750 mg
Tablet, extended release, oral: 500 mg, 750 mg
Keppra XR™: 500 mg, 750 mg

Levitra® *see* vardenafil *on page 908*

levobunolol (lee voe BYOO noe lole)

Medication Safety Issues
Sound-alike/look-alike issues:
Levobunolol may be confused with levocabastine
Betagan® may be confused with Betadine®, Betoptic® S

Synonyms *l*-bunolol hydrochloride; levobunolol hydrochloride

U.S. Brand Names Betagan®

◄ **Canadian Brand Names** Apo-Levobunolol®; Betagan®; Novo-Levobunolol; Optho-Bunolol®; PMS-Levobunolol; Sandoz-Levobunolol

Therapeutic Category Beta-Adrenergic Blocker

Use To lower intraocular pressure in chronic open-angle glaucoma or ocular hypertension

General Dosage Range Ophthalmic: *Adults:* Instill 1 drop in the affected eye(s) 1-2 times/day

Dosage Forms
Solution, ophthalmic: 0.25% (5 mL, 10 mL); 0.5% (5 mL, 10 mL, 15 mL)
Betagan®: 0.5% (5 mL, 10 mL, 15 mL)

levobunolol hydrochloride *see* levobunolol *on page 517*

levocabastine hydrochloride *see* levocabastine (nasal) *(Canada only) on page 518*

levocabastine hydrochloride *see* levocabastine (ophthalmic) *(Canada only) on page 518*

levocabastine (nasal) *(Canada only)* (LEE voe kab as teen)

Medication Safety Issues
Sound-alike/look-alike issues:
Levocabastine may be confused with levobunolol, levOCARNitine
Livostin® may be confused with lovastatin

Synonyms levocabastine hydrochloride

Canadian Brand Names Livostin®

Therapeutic Category Histamine H_1 Antagonist; Histamine H_1 Antagonist, Second Generation; Piperidine Derivative

Use Symptomatic treatment of allergic rhinitis

General Dosage Range Intranasal: *Children ≥12 years and Adults ≤65 years:* 2 sprays in each nostril 2-4 times/day

Product Availability Not available in U.S.

Dosage Forms - Canada
Microsuspension, intranasal, as hydrochloride [spray]:
Livostin®: 0.05% [50 mcg/spray] (15 mL) [contains benzalkonium chloride]

levocabastine (ophthalmic) *(Canada only)* (LEE voe kab as teen)

Medication Safety Issues
Sound-alike/look-alike issues:
Levocabastine may be confused with levobunolol, levOCARNitine
Livostin® may be confused with lovastatin
International issues:
Livostin [Canada and multiple international markets] may be confused with Limoxin brand name for ambroxol [Indonesia] and amoxicillin [Mexico]; Lovastin brand name for lovastatin [Malaysia, Poland, Singapore]

Synonyms levocabastine hydrochloride

Canadian Brand Names Livostin® Eye Drops

Therapeutic Category Histamine H_1 Antagonist; Histamine H_1 Antagonist, Second Generation; Piperidine Derivative

Use Treatment of seasonal allergic conjunctivitis

General Dosage Range Ophthalmic: *Children ≥12 years and Adults ≤65 years:* Instill 1 drop in affected eye(s) 2-4 times/day

Product Availability Not available in U.S.

Dosage Forms - Canada
Suspension, ophthalmic:
Livostin®: 0.05% (5 mL, 10 mL)

Levocarb CR (Can) *see* carbidopa and levodopa *on page 174*

levocarnitine (lee voe KAR ni teen)

Medication Safety Issues
Sound-alike/look-alike issues:
LevOCARNitine may be confused with levETIRAcetam, levocabastine

Synonyms L-carnitine

Tall-Man levOCARNitine

U.S. Brand Names Carnitine-300 [OTC]; Carnitor®; Carnitor® SF; L-Carnitine® [OTC]
Canadian Brand Names Carnitor®
Therapeutic Category Dietary Supplement
Use
Oral: Primary systemic carnitine deficiency; acute and chronic treatment of patients with an inborn error of metabolism which results in secondary carnitine deficiency
I.V.: Acute and chronic treatment of patients with an inborn error of metabolism which results in secondary carnitine deficiency; prevention and treatment of carnitine deficiency in patients with end-stage renal disease (ESRD) who are undergoing hemodialysis.
General Dosage Range
I.V.:
Children: 50 mg/kg/day in divided doses (maximum: 300 mg/kg/day)
Adults: 50 mg/kg/day (maximum: 300 mg/kg/day) **or** 20 mg/kg after each hemodialysis session
Oral:
Infants and Children: Initial: 50 mg/kg/day; Maintenance: 50-100 mg/kg/day in divided doses (maximum: 3 g/day)
Adults: 990 mg (tablet) 2-3 times/day **or** 1-3 g/day (solution)
Dosage Forms
Capsule, oral:
Carnitine-300 [OTC]: 300 mg
L-Carnitine® [OTC]: 250 mg
Injection, solution [preservative free]: 200 mg/mL (5 mL, 12.5 mL)
Carnitor®: 200 mg/mL (5 mL)
Solution, oral: 100 mg/mL (118 mL, 120 mL)
Carnitor®: 100 mg/mL (118 mL)
Carnitor® SF: 100 mg/mL (118 mL)
Tablet, oral: 330 mg
Carnitor®: 330 mg
L-Carnitine® [OTC]: 500 mg

levocetirizine (LEE vo se TI ra zeen)
Medication Safety Issues
Sound-alike/look-alike issues:
Levocetirizine may be confused with cetirizine
Synonyms levocetirizine dihydrochloride
U.S. Brand Names Xyzal®
Therapeutic Category Antihistamine
Use Relief of symptoms of perennial and seasonal allergic rhinitis; treatment of skin manifestations (uncomplicated) of chronic idiopathic urticaria
General Dosage Range Dosage adjustment recommended in patients with renal impairment
Oral:
Children 6 months to 5 years: 1.25 mg once daily
Children 6-11 years: 2.5 mg once daily
Children ≥12 years and Adults: 2.5-5 mg once daily
Dosage Forms
Solution, oral:
Xyzal®: 0.5 mg/mL (150 mL)
Tablet, oral: 5 mg
Xyzal®: 5 mg

levocetirizine dihydrochloride see levocetirizine on page 519
levodopa and benserazide see benserazide and levodopa (Canada only) on page 120
levodopa and carbidopa see carbidopa and levodopa on page 174

levodopa, carbidopa, and entacapone (lee voe DOE pa, kar bi DOE pa, & en TA ka pone)
Medication Safety Issues
Administration issues:
Strengths listed in Stalevo® brand names correspond to the **levodopa** component of the formulation only. All strengths of Stalevo® contain a levodopa/carbidopa ratio of 4:1 plus entacapone 200 mg.

◀ **Synonyms** carbidopa, entacapone, and levodopa; carbidopa, levodopa, and entacapone; entacapone, carbidopa, and levodopa

U.S. Brand Names Stalevo®

Canadian Brand Names Stalevo®

Therapeutic Category Anti-Parkinson Agent (Dopamine Agonist); Anti-Parkinson Agent, COMT Inhibitor

Use Treatment of idiopathic Parkinson disease

General Dosage Range Oral: *Adults:* 1 tablet (50-200 mg levodopa/12.5-50 mg carbidopa/200 mg entacapone) at each dosing interval (maximum: 1600 mg/day entacapone or 300 mg/day carbidopa)

Dosage Forms

Tablet:

Stalevo®: 50: Levodopa 50 mg, carbidopa 12.5 mg, and entacapone 200 mg; 75: Levodopa 75 mg, carbidopa 18.75 mg, and entacapone 200 mg; 100: Levodopa 100 mg, carbidopa 25 mg, and entacapone 200 mg; 125: Levodopa 125 mg, carbidopa 31.25 mg, and entacapone 200 mg; 150: Levodopa 150 mg, carbidopa 37.5 mg, and entacapone 200 mg; 200: Levodopa 200 mg, carbidopa 50 mg, and entacapone 200 mg

Levo-Dromoran *see levorphanol on page 522*

levofloxacin (systemic) (lee voe FLOKS a sin)

Medication Safety Issues

Sound-alike/look-alike issues:

Levaquin® may be confused with Levoxyl®, Levsin/SL®, Lovenox®

Levofloxacin may be confused with levETIRAcetam, levodopa, Levophed®, levothyroxine

U.S. Brand Names Levaquin®

Canadian Brand Names Levaquin®; Novo-Levofloxacin; PMS-Levofloxacin

Therapeutic Category Antibiotic, Quinolone; Respiratory Fluoroquinolone

Use Treatment of community-acquired pneumonia, including multidrug resistant strains of *S. pneumoniae* (MDRSP); nosocomial pneumonia; chronic bronchitis (acute bacterial exacerbation); acute bacterial sinusitis; prostatitis, urinary tract infection (uncomplicated or complicated); acute pyelonephritis; skin or skin structure infections (uncomplicated or complicated); reduce incidence or disease progression of inhalational anthrax (postexposure)

General Dosage Range Dosage adjustment recommended in patients with renal impairment

I.V., oral:

Children ≥6 months and ≤50 kg: 8 mg/kg every 12 hours (maximum: 250 mg/dose)

Children >50 kg: 500 mg once daily

Adults: 250-750 mg once daily

Dosage Forms

Infusion, premixed in D₅W [preservative free]: 250 mg (50 mL); 500 mg (100 mL); 750 mg (150 mL)

Levaquin®: 250 mg (50 mL); 500 mg (100 mL); 750 mg (150 mL)

Injection, solution [preservative free]:

Levaquin®: 25 mg/mL (20 mL, 30 mL)

Solution, oral: 25 mg/mL (100 mL, 200 mL, 480 mL)

Levaquin®: 25 mg/mL (480 mL)

Tablet, oral: 250 mg, 500 mg, 750 mg

Levaquin®: 250 mg, 500 mg, 750 mg

levofloxacin (ophthalmic) (lee voe FLOKS a sin)

Medication Safety Issues

Sound-alike/look-alike issues:

Levofloxacin may be confused with levETIRAcetam, levodopa, levothyroxine

U.S. Brand Names Iquix®; Quixin®

Therapeutic Category Antibiotic, Ophthalmic; Antibiotic, Quinolone

Use Treatment of bacterial conjunctivitis caused by susceptible organisms (Quixin® 0.5% ophthalmic solution); treatment of corneal ulcer caused by susceptible organisms (Iquix® 1.5% ophthalmic solution)

General Dosage Range Ophthalmic: *Children ≥1 year and Adults:* 1-2 drops every 30 minutes to 6 hours

Dosage Forms

Solution, ophthalmic: 0.5% (5 mL)

Iquix®: 1.5% (5 mL)

Quixin®: 0.5% (5 mL)

levo-folinic acid *see* LEVOleucovorin *on page 521*

LEVOleucovorin (lee voe loo koe VOR in)

Medication Safety Issues
Sound-alike/look-alike issues:
  LEVOleucovorin may be confused with leucovorin calcium, Leukeran®, Leukine®

Synonyms 6S-leucovorin; calcium levoleucovorin; L-leucovorin; levo-folinic acid; levo-leucovorin; levoleucovorin calcium pentahydrate; S-leucovorin

U.S. Brand Names Fusilev™

Therapeutic Category Antidote; Rescue Agent (Chemotherapy)

Use Treatment of advanced, metastatic colorectal cancer (palliative) in combination with fluorouracil; rescue agent after high-dose methotrexate therapy in osteosarcoma; antidote for impaired methotrexate elimination and for inadvertent overdosage of folic acid antagonists

General Dosage Range I.V.: *Children and Adults:* Dosing varies greatly depending on indication

Product Availability
Fusilev™ solution for injection: FDA approved April 2011; availability expected in the third quarter of 2011
Fusilev™ solution for injection is a ready-to-use formulation and will be available in 175 mg/17.5 mL and 250 mg/25 mL presentations.

Dosage Forms
Injection, powder for reconstitution:
  Fusilev™: 50 mg

levo-leucovorin *see* LEVOleucovorin *on page 521*

levoleucovorin calcium pentahydrate *see* LEVOleucovorin *on page 521*

levomefolate calcium, drospirenone, and ethinyl estradiol *see* ethinyl estradiol, drospirenone, and levomefolate *on page 358*

levomefolate, drospirenone, and ethinyl estradiol *see* ethinyl estradiol, drospirenone, and levomefolate *on page 358*

levomepromazine *see* methotrimeprazine *(Canada only) on page 572*

levonordefrin and mepivacaine hydrochloride *see* mepivacaine and levonordefrin *on page 562*

levonorgestrel (LEE voe nor jes trel)

Synonyms LNg 20; Plan B

U.S. Brand Names Mirena®; Next Choice™; Plan B® One Step

Canadian Brand Names Mirena®; Plan B®

Therapeutic Category Contraceptive, Implant (Progestin); Contraceptive, Progestin Only

Use
Intrauterine device (IUD): Prevention of pregnancy; treatment of heavy menstrual bleeding in women who also choose to use an IUD for contraception
Oral: Emergency contraception following unprotected intercourse or possible contraceptive failure
Plan B® One-Step is approved for OTC use by women ≥17 years of age and available by prescription only for women <17 years of age. Next Choice™ (generic of the original Plan-B® 2-dose regimen) is also approved for OTC use by women ≥17 years of age and by prescription only for women <17 years of age.

General Dosage Range
Intrauterine: *Adults:* Insert into uterine cavity, releases 20 mcg/day over 5 years
Oral: *Adults:* 0.75 mg every 12 hours for 2 doses **or** 1.5 mg as a single dose

Dosage Forms
Intrauterine device, intrauterine:
  Mirena®: 52 mg/device
Tablet, oral: 0.75 mg
  Next Choice™: 0.75 mg
  Plan B® One Step: 1.5 mg

levonorgestrel and estradiol *see* estradiol and levonorgestrel *on page 345*

levonorgestrel and ethinyl estradiol *see* ethinyl estradiol and levonorgestrel *on page 353*

Levophed® *see* norepinephrine *on page 632*

Levora® *see* ethinyl estradiol and levonorgestrel *on page 353*

levorphanol (lee VOR fa nole)

Medication Safety Issues

High alert medication:

The Institute for Safe Medication Practices (ISMP) includes this medication among its list of drug classes which have a heightened risk of causing significant patient harm when used in error.

Synonyms Levo-Dromoran; levorphan tartrate; levorphanol tartrate

Therapeutic Category Analgesic, Narcotic

Controlled Substance C-II

Use Relief of moderate-to-severe pain; preoperative sedation/analgesia; management of chronic pain (eg, cancer) requiring opioid therapy

General Dosage Range Dosage adjustment recommended in patients with hepatic impairment

Oral: *Adults:* 2-4 mg every 6-8 hours as needed

Dosage Forms

Tablet, oral: 2 mg

levorphanol tartrate *see* levorphanol *on page* 522
levorphan tartrate *see* levorphanol *on page* 522
Levothroid® *see* levothyroxine *on page* 522

levothyroxine (lee voe thye ROKS een)

Medication Safety Issues

Sound-alike/look-alike issues:

Levothyroxine may be confused with lamoTRIgine, Lanoxin®, levofloxacin, liothyronine

Levoxyl® may be confused with Lanoxin®, Levaquin®, Luvox®

Synthroid® may be confused with Symmetrel

Administration issues:

Significant differences exist between oral and I.V. dosing. Use caution when converting from one route of administration to another.

Other safety concerns:

To avoid errors due to misinterpretation of a decimal point, always express dosage in mcg (**not** mg).

Synonyms *L*-thyroxine sodium; levothyroxine sodium; T_4

U.S. Brand Names Levothroid®; Levoxyl®; Synthroid®; Tirosint®; Unithroid®

Canadian Brand Names Eltroxin®; Euthyrox; Levothyroxine Sodium; Synthroid®

Therapeutic Category Thyroid Product

Use Replacement or supplemental therapy in hypothyroidism; pituitary TSH suppression

General Dosage Range

I.M.: *Children and Adults:* 50% of oral dose

I.V.:

Children: 50% of oral dose

Adults: 50% of oral dose or 200-500 mcg, then 100-300 mcg the next day if needed

Oral:

Children 1-3 months: 10-15 mcg/kg/day

Children 3-6 months: 8-10 mcg/kg/day

Children 6-12 months: 6-8 mcg/kg/day

Children 1-5 years: 5-6 mcg/kg/day

Children 6-12 years: 4-5 mcg/kg/day

Children >12 years: 2-3 mcg/kg/day

Adults: Initial: 12.5-25 mcg/day **or** 1.7 mcg/kg/day (usual doses are ≤200 mcg/day)

Elderly >50 years without cardiac disease **or** *<50 years with cardiac disease:* Initial: 25-50 mcg/day

Elderly >50 years with cardiac disease: Initial: 12.5-25 mcg/day

Dosage Forms

Capsule, soft gelatin, oral:

Tirosint®: 13 mcg, 25 mcg, 50 mcg, 75 mcg, 88 mcg, 100 mcg, 112 mcg, 125 mcg, 137 mcg, 150 mcg

Injection, powder for reconstitution: 200 mcg, 500 mcg

Tablet, oral: 25 mcg, 50 mcg, 75 mcg, 88 mcg, 100 mcg, 112 mcg, 125 mcg, 137 mcg, 150 mcg, 175 mcg, 200 mcg, 300 mcg

    Levothroid®: 25 mcg, 50 mcg, 75 mcg, 88 mcg, 100 mcg, 112 mcg, 125 mcg, 137 mcg, 150 mcg, 175 mcg, 200 mcg, 300 mcg

    Levoxyl®: 25 mcg, 50 mcg, 75 mcg, 88 mcg, 100 mcg, 112 mcg, 125 mcg, 137 mcg, 150 mcg, 175 mcg, 200 mcg

    Synthroid®: 25 mcg, 50 mcg, 75 mcg, 88 mcg, 100 mcg, 112 mcg, 125 mcg, 137 mcg, 150 mcg, 175 mcg, 200 mcg, 300 mcg

    Unithroid®: 25 mcg, 50 mcg, 75 mcg, 88 mcg, 100 mcg, 112 mcg, 125 mcg, 150 mcg, 175 mcg, 200 mcg, 300 mcg

levothyroxine and liothyronine *see* thyroid, desiccated *on page* 865

levothyroxine sodium *see* levothyroxine *on page* 522

Levothyroxine Sodium (Can) *see* levothyroxine *on page* 522

Levoxyl® *see* levothyroxine *on page* 522

Levsin® *see* hyoscyamine *on page* 457

Levsin®/SL *see* hyoscyamine *on page* 457

Lev-Tov [OTC] *see* folic acid, cyanocobalamin, and pyridoxine *on page* 396

Levulan® Kerastick® *see* aminolevulinic acid *on page* 66

levulose, dextrose and phosphoric acid *see* fructose, dextrose, and phosphoric acid *on page* 403

Lexapro® *see* escitalopram *on page* 341

Lexiscan® *see* regadenoson *on page* 772

Lexiva® *see* fosamprenavir *on page* 399

LFA-3/IgG(1) fusion protein, human *see* alefacept *on page* 48

LHRH *see* gonadorelin *(Canada only) on page* 423

***l*-hyoscyamine sulfate** *see* hyoscyamine *on page* 457

Lialda® *see* mesalamine *on page* 564

Librax® [original formulation] *see* clidinium and chlordiazepoxide *on page* 217

Librax® (Can) *see* clidinium and chlordiazepoxide *on page* 217

Librium *see* chlordiazepoxide *on page* 194

Licide® [OTC] *see* pyrethrins and piperonyl butoxide *on page* 756

LidaMantle® *see* lidocaine (topical) *on page* 524

LidaMantle HC® *see* lidocaine and hydrocortisone *on page* 526

LidaMantle HC® Relief Pad™ *see* lidocaine and hydrocortisone *on page* 526

Lidemol® (Can) *see* fluocinonide *on page* 385

Lidex *see* fluocinonide *on page* 385

Lidex® (Can) *see* fluocinonide *on page* 385

lidocaine (systemic) (LYE doe kane)

Medication Safety Issues

High alert medication:
The Institute for Safe Medication Practices (ISMP) includes this medication (epidural administration; I.V. formulation) among its list of drugs which have a heightened risk of causing significant patient harm when used in error.

International issues:
Lidosen [Italy] may be confused with Lincocin brand name for lincomycin [U.S., Canada, and multiple international markets]; Linoten brand name for pamidronate [Spain]; Lodosyn brand name for carbidopa [U.S.]

Synonyms lidocaine hydrochloride; lignocaine hydrochloride

U.S. Brand Names Xylocaine®; Xylocaine® Dental; Xylocaine® MPF

Canadian Brand Names Xylocard®

Therapeutic Category Antiarrhythmic Agent, Class Ib; Local Anesthetic

Use Local and regional anesthesia by infiltration, nerve block, epidural, or spinal techniques; acute treatment of ventricular arrhythmias from myocardial infarction or cardiac manipulation

◀ **General Dosage Range** Dosage adjustment recommended in patients with hepatic impairment.
I.V.:
  Children: Loading dose: 1 mg/kg, may repeat 0.5-1 mg/kg; Infusion: 20-50 mcg/kg/minute
  Adults: Bolus: 1-1.5 mg/kg, may repeat 0.5-0.75 mg/kg up to a total of 3 mg/kg; Infusion: 1-4 mg/minute
Local injection: *Children and Adults:* Maximum: 4.5 mg/kg/dose; do not repeat within 2 hours
Dosage Forms
Infusion, premixed in D$_5$W: 0.4% [4 mg/mL] (250 mL, 500 mL); 0.8% [8 mg/mL] (250 mL, 500 mL)
Injection, solution: 1% [10 mg/mL] (2 mL, 10 mL, 20 mL, 30 mL, 50 mL); 2% [20 mg/mL] (2 mL, 5 mL, 20 mL, 50 mL)
  Xylocaine®: 0.5% [5 mg/mL] (50 mL); 1% [10 mg/mL] (10 mL, 20 mL, 50 mL); 2% [20 mg/mL] (10 mL, 20 mL, 50 mL)
  Xylocaine® Dental: 2% [20 mg/mL] (1.8 mL)
Injection, solution [preservative free]: 0.5% [5 mg/mL] (50 mL); 1% [10 mg/mL] (2 mL, 5 mL, 30 mL); 1.5% [15 mg/mL] (20 mL); 2% [20 mg/mL] (2 mL, 5 mL, 10 mL); 4% [40 mg/mL] (5 mL)
  Xylocaine®: 2% [20 mg/mL] (5 mL)
  Xylocaine® MPF: 0.5% [5 mg/mL] (50 mL); 1% [10 mg/mL] (2 mL, 5 mL, 10 mL, 30 mL); 1.5% [15 mg/mL] (10 mL, 20 mL); 2% [20 mg/mL] (2 mL, 5 mL, 10 mL); 4% [40 mg/mL] (5 mL)
Injection, solution, premixed in D$_{7.5}$W [preservative free]: 5% [50 mg/mL] (2 mL)

lidocaine (ophthalmic) (LYE doe kane)

Synonyms lidocaine hydrochloride; lignocaine hydrochloride
U.S. Brand Names Akten™
Therapeutic Category Local Anesthetic; Local Anesthetic, Ophthalmic
Use To provide local anesthesia to ocular surface during ophthalmologic procedures
General Dosage Range Ophthalmic: *Children and Adults:* 2 drops to ocular surface; may repeat to maintain effect
Dosage Forms
Gel, ophthalmic [preservative free]:
  Akten™: 3.5% (5 mL)

lidocaine (topical) (LYE doe kane)

Synonyms lidocaine hydrochloride; lidocaine patch; lignocaine hydrochloride; Viscous Lidocaine; Xylocaine Viscous
U.S. Brand Names AneCream™ [OTC]; Anestafoam™ [OTC]; Band-Aid® Hurt Free™ Antiseptic Wash [OTC]; Burn Jel Plus [OTC]; Burn Jel® [OTC]; L-M-X® 4 [OTC]; L-M-X® 5 [OTC]; LidaMantle®; Lidoderm®; LTA® 360; Premjact®; Regenecare®; Regenecare® HA [OTC]; Solarcaine® cool aloe Burn Relief [OTC]; Topicaine® [OTC]; Unburn® [OTC]; Xylocaine®
Canadian Brand Names Betacaine®; Lidodan™; Lidoderm®; Maxilene®; Xylocaine®
Therapeutic Category Analgesic, Topical; Local Anesthetic
Use
  Rectal: Temporary relief of pain and itching due to anorectal disorders
  Topical: Local anesthetic for oral mucous membrane; use in laser/cosmetic surgeries; minor burns, cuts, and abrasions of the skin
  Oral topical solution (viscous): Topical anesthesia of irritated oral mucous membranes and pharyngeal tissue
  Patch (Lidoderm®): Relief of allodynia (painful hypersensitivity) and chronic pain in postherpetic neuralgia
General Dosage Range Topical:
  Cream: *Children and Adults:* Dosage varies greatly depending on product
  Gel, ointment, solution: *Adults:* Apply to affected area ≤4 times/day as needed (maximum: 4.5 mg/kg/dose; 300 mg/dose)
  Jelly:
    Children: Maximum: 4.5 mg/kg/dose
    Adults: 3-30 mL (maximum: 30 mL [600 mg]/12-hour period)
  Oral topical solution (viscous):
    Infants and Children <3 years: 1.25 mL applied no more frequently than every 3 hours (maximum: 4 doses per 12-hour period)
    Children ≥3 years: Should not exceed 4.5 mg/kg/dose (or 300 mg/dose); swished in the mouth and spit out no more frequently than every 3 hours

Adults: 15 mL swished in the mouth and spit out or gargled no more frequently than every 3 hours (maximum: 8 doses per 24-hour period)

Patch: *Adults:* Apply up to 3 patches in a single application for up to 12 hours in any 24-hour period

Dosage Forms

Aerosol, topical:
Anestafoam™ [OTC]: 4% (30 g)
Solarcaine® cool aloe Burn Relief [OTC]: 0.5% (127 g)

Cream, rectal:
L-M-X® 5 [OTC]: 5% (15 g, 30 g)

Cream, topical: 0.5% (0.9 g)
AneCream™ [OTC]: 4% (5 g, 15 g, 30 g)
L-M-X® 4 [OTC]: 4% (5 g, 15 g, 30 g)
LidaMantle®: 3% (85 g)

Gel, topical:
Burn Jel Plus [OTC]: 2.5% (118 mL)
Burn Jel® [OTC]: 2% (59 mL, 118 mL); 2% (3.5 g)
Regenecare®: 2% (14 g, 85 g)
Regenecare® HA [OTC]: 2% (85 g)
Solarcaine® cool aloe Burn Relief [OTC]: 0.5% (113 g, 226 g)
Topicaine® [OTC]: 4% (10 g, 30 g, 113 g); 5% (10 g, 30 g, 113 g)
Unburn® [OTC]: 2.5% (59 mL)

Jelly, topical: 2% (5 mL, 30 mL)
Xylocaine®: 2% (5 mL, 30 mL)

Jelly, topical [preservative free]: 2% (5 mL, 10 mL, 20 mL)

Lotion, topical:
LidaMantle®: 3% (177 mL)

Ointment, topical: 5% (30 g, 35.4 g, 50 g)

Patch, topical:
Lidoderm®: 5% (30s)

Solution, topical: 4% [40 mg/mL] (50 mL)
Band-Aid® Hurt Free™ Antiseptic Wash [OTC]: 2% [20 mg/mL] (177 mL)
LTA® 360: 4% [40 mg/mL] (4 mL)
Premjact®: 9.6% (13 mL)
Xylocaine®: 4% (50 mL)

Solution, topical [preservative free]: 4% [40 mg/mL] (4 mL)

Solution, viscous, oral topical: 2% [20 mg/mL] (20 mL, 100 mL, 500 mL)

lidocaine and epinephrine (LYE doe kane & ep i NEF rin)

Synonyms epinephrine and lidocaine

U.S. Brand Names Lignospan® Forte; Lignospan® Standard; Xylocaine® MPF With Epinephrine; Xylocaine® With Epinephrine

Canadian Brand Names Xylocaine® With Epinephrine

Therapeutic Category Local Anesthetic

Use Local infiltration anesthesia; AVS for nerve block

General Dosage Range

Conduction block or infiltration (dental):
Children <12 years: 20-30 mg (1-1.5 mL) of 2% lidocaine with epinephrine 1:100,000 (maximum: 4.5 mg/kg of lidocaine or 100-150 mg as a single dose)
Children ≥12 years and Adults: Do not exceed 7 mg/kg body weight up to a maximum range of 300 mg (usual dental practice) to 500 mg (approved product labeling) of lidocaine hydrochloride and 3 mcg (0.003 mg) of epinephrine/kg of body weight **or** 0.2 mg epinephrine per dental appointment.

Dosage Forms

Injection, solution:
Generics:
0.5% / 1:200,000: Lidocaine hydrochloride 0.5% [5 mg/mL] and epinephrine 1:200,000 (50 mL)
1% / 1:100,000: Lidocaine hydrochloride 1% [10 mg/mL] and epinephrine 1:100,000 (20 mL, 30 mL, 50 mL)
2% / 1:100,000: Lidocaine hydrochloride 2% [20 mg/mL] and epinephrine 1:100,000 (30 mL, 50 mL) ▶

◀ *Brands:*
  Xylocaine® with Epinephrine:
    0.5% / 1:200,000: Lidocaine hydrochloride 0.5% [5 mg/mL] and epinephrine 1:200,000 (50 mL)
    1% / 1:100,000: Lidocaine hydrochloride 1% [10 mg/mL] and epinephrine 1:100,000 (10 mL, 20 mL, 50 mL)
    2% / 1:100,000: Lidocaine hydrochloride 2% [20 mg/mL] and epinephrine 1:100,000 (10 mL, 20 mL, 50 mL)
  Injection, solution [preservative free]:
  Generics:
    1% / 1:200,000: Lidocaine hydrochloride 1% [10 mg/mL] and epinephrine 1:200,000 (30 mL)
    1.5% / 1:200,000: Lidocaine hydrochloride 1.5% [15 mg/mL] and epinephrine 1:200,000 (5 mL, 30 mL)
    2% / 1:200,000: Lidocaine hydrochloride 2% [20 mg/mL] and epinephrine 1:200,000 (20 mL)
  Brands:
  Xylocaine®-MPF with Epinephrine:
    1% / 1:200,000: Lidocaine hydrochloride 1% [10 mg/mL] and epinephrine 1:200,000 (5 mL, 10 mL, 30 mL)
    1.5% / 1:200,000: Lidocaine hydrochloride 1.5% [15 mg/mL] and epinephrine 1:200,000 (5 mL, 10 mL, 30 mL)
    2% / 1:200,000: Lidocaine hydrochloride 2% [20 mg/mL] and epinephrine 1:200,000 (5 mL, 10 mL, 20 mL)
  Injection, solution [for dental use]:
  Generics:
    2% / 1:50,000: Lidocaine hydrochloride 2% [20 mg/mL] and epinephrine 1:50,000 (1.7 mL, 1.8 mL)
    2% / 1:100,000: Lidocaine hydrochloride 2% [20 mg/mL] and epinephrine 1:100,000 (1.7 mL, 1.8 mL)
  Brands:
  Lignospan® Forte: 2% / 1:50,000: Lidocaine hydrochloride 2% [20 mg/mL] and epinephrine 1:50,000 (1.7 mL)
  Lignospan® Standard: 2% / 1:100,000: Lidocaine hydrochloride 2% [20 mg/mL] and epinephrine 1:100,000 (1.7 mL)

lidocaine and hydrocortisone (LYE doe kane & hye droe KOR ti sone)

Synonyms hydrocortisone and lidocaine

U.S. Brand Names AnaMantle HC® Cream; AnaMantle HC® Forte; AnaMantle HC® Gel; LidaMantle HC®; LidaMantle HC® Relief Pad™; LidoCort™; Peranex™ HC; Peranex™ HC Medi-Pad; RectaGel™ HC

Therapeutic Category Anesthetic/Corticosteroid

Use Topical antiinflammatory and anesthetic for skin disorders; rectal for the treatment of hemorrhoids, anal fissures, pruritus ani, or similar conditions

General Dosage Range
  Rectal: *Adults:* 1 applicatorful twice daily
  Topical: *Adults:* Apply 2-3 times/day

Dosage Forms
  Cream, rectal: Lidocaine 3% and hydrocortisone 0.5% (7 g); lidocaine 3% and hydrocortisone 1% (7 g)
    AnaMantle HC® Forte: Lidocaine 3% and hydrocortisone 1% (7 g)
    AnaMantle HC®: Lidocaine 3% and hydrocortisone 0.5% (7 g)
    Peranex™ HC: Lidocaine 2% and hydrocortisone 2% (7 g)
  Cream, topical:
    LidaMantle HC®: Lidocaine 3% and hydrocortisone 0.5% (85 g)
  Gel, rectal: Lidocaine 3% and hydrocortisone 2.5% (7 g)
    AnaMantle HC®, LidoCort™: Lidocaine 3% and hydrocortisone 2.5% (7 g)
    RectaGel™ HC: Lidocaine 2.8% and hydrocortisone 0.55% (20 g)
  Lotion, topical: Lidocaine 3% and hydrocortisone 0.5% (177 mL)
    LidaMantle HC®: Lidocaine 3% and hydrocortisone 0.5% (177 mL)
  Pad, topical:
    LidaMantel HC® Relief Pad™: Lidocaine 2% and hydrocortisone 2% (60s)
    Peranex™ HC Medi-Pad: Lidocaine 3% and hydrocortisone 1% (60s)

lidocaine and prilocaine (LYE doe kane & PRIL oh kane)

Synonyms prilocaine and lidocaine

U.S. Brand Names EMLA®; Oraqix®

Canadian Brand Names EMLA®

Therapeutic Category Analgesic, Topical

Use

Topical anesthetic for use on normal intact skin to provide local analgesia for minor procedures such as I.V. cannulation or venipuncture; has also been used for painful procedures such as lumbar puncture and skin graft harvesting; for superficial minor surgery of genital mucous membranes and as an adjunct for local infiltration anesthesia in genital mucous membranes.

Periodontal gel: Topical anesthetic for use in periodontal pockets during scaling or root planning procedures

General Dosage Range

Periodontal: *Adults:* Maximum recommended dose: 1 treatment session: 5 cartridges (8.5 g)

Topical, cream:

Children 0-3 months or <5 kg: Apply up to 1 g over no more than 10 cm^2 of skin for no longer than 1 hour

Children 3-12 months and >5 kg: Apply up to 2 g total over no more than 20 cm^2 of skin for no longer than 4 hours

Children 1-6 years and >10 kg: Apply up to 10 g total over no more than 100 cm^2 of skin for no longer than 4 hours

Children 7-12 years and >20 kg: Apply up to 20 g total over no more than 200 cm^2 of skin for no longer than 4 hours

Adults: Apply 2-2.5 g per 10-25 cm^2 of skin for at least 1-2 hours **or** 5-10 g for 5-10 minutes

Adults (males): Apply 1 g/10 cm^2 for 15 minutes

Dosage Forms

Cream, topical: Lidocaine 2.5% and prilocaine 2.5% (5 g, 30 g)

EMLA®: Lidocaine 2.5% and prilocaine 2.5% (5 g, 30 g)

Gel, periodontal:

Oraqix®: Lidocaine 2.5% and prilocaine 2.5% (1.7 g)

Dosage Forms - Canada

Patch, transdermal:

EMLA® Patch: Lidocaine 2.5% and prilocaine 2.5% per patch (2s, 20s)

lidocaine and tetracaine (LYE doe kane & TET ra kane)

Medication Safety Issues

Other safety concerns:

Transdermal patch may contain conducting metal (eg, aluminum); remove patch prior to MRI.

Synonyms tetracaine and lidocaine

U.S. Brand Names Synera™

Therapeutic Category Analgesic, Topical; Local Anesthetic

Use Topical anesthetic for use on normal intact skin for minor procedures (eg, I.V. cannulation or venipuncture) and superficial dermatologic procedures

General Dosage Range Topical: *Children ≥3 years and Adults:* Apply patch to intact skin for 20-30 minutes, prior to procedure

Dosage Forms

Patch, transdermal:

Synera™: Lidocaine 70 mg and tetracaine 70 mg (10s)

lidocaine hydrochloride *see* lidocaine (ophthalmic) *on page 524*

lidocaine hydrochloride *see* lidocaine (systemic) *on page 523*

lidocaine hydrochloride *see* lidocaine (topical) *on page 524*

lidocaine patch *see* lidocaine (topical) *on page 524*

LidoCort™ *see* lidocaine and hydrocortisone *on page 526*

Lidodan™ (Can) *see* lidocaine (topical) *on page 524*

Lidoderm® *see* lidocaine (topical) *on page 524*

LID-Pack® (Can) *see* bacitracin and polymyxin B *on page 111*

lignocaine hydrochloride *see* lidocaine (ophthalmic) *on page 524*

lignocaine hydrochloride *see* lidocaine (systemic) *on page 523*

lignocaine hydrochloride *see* lidocaine (topical) *on page 524*

Lignospan® Forte *see* lidocaine and epinephrine *on page 525*

Lignospan® Standard *see* lidocaine and epinephrine *on page 525*

Limbitrol *see* amitriptyline and chlordiazepoxide *on page 68*

Limbrel™ [DSC] *see* flavocoxid *on page 379*

Limbrel 250™ *see* flavocoxid *on page* 379
Limbrel 500™ *see* flavocoxid *on page* 379

linagliptin (lin a GLIP tin)

Synonyms BI-1356; trajenta
U.S. Brand Names Tradjenta™
Canadian Brand Names Trajenta™
Therapeutic Category Antidiabetic Agent, Dipeptidyl Peptidase IV (DPP-IV) Inhibitor
Use Management of type 2 diabetes mellitus (noninsulin dependent, NIDDM) as an adjunct to diet and exercise as monotherapy or in combination with other antidiabetic agents
General Dosage Range Oral: *Adults:* 5 mg once daily
Dosage Forms
   Tablet, oral:
      Tradjenta™: 5 mg

Lin-Amox (Can) *see* amoxicillin *on page* 73
Lin-Buspirone (Can) *see* buspirone *on page* 151
Lincocin® *see* lincomycin *on page* 528

lincomycin (lin koe MYE sin)

Medication Safety Issues
   Sound-alike/look-alike issues:
      Lincocin® may be confused with Cleocin®, Indocin®, Minocin®
   International issues:
      Lincocin [U.S., Canada, and multiple international markets] may be confused with Lidosen brand name for lidocaine [Italy] and Limoxin brand name for ambroxol [Indonesia]; amoxicillin [Mexico]
Synonyms lincomycin hydrochloride
U.S. Brand Names Lincocin®
Canadian Brand Names Lincocin®
Therapeutic Category Antibiotic, Lincosamide
Use Treatment of serious susceptible bacterial infections, mainly those caused by streptococci, pneumococci, and staphylococci resistant to other agents
General Dosage Range Dosage adjustment recommended in patients with renal impairment
   I.M.:
      Children >1 month: 10 mg/kg every 12-24 hours
      Adults: 600 mg every 12-24 hours
   I.V.:
      Children >1 month: 10-20 mg/kg/day divided every 8-12 hours
      Adults: 600 mg to 1 g every 8-12 hours (maximum: 8 g/day)
   Subconjunctival injection: *Adults:* 75 mg
Dosage Forms
   Injection, solution:
      Lincocin®: 300 mg/mL (2 mL, 10 mL)

lincomycin hydrochloride *see* lincomycin *on page* 528

lindane (LIN dane)

Synonyms benzene hexachloride; gamma benzene hexachloride; hexachlorocyclohexane
Canadian Brand Names Hexit™; PMS-Lindane
Therapeutic Category Scabicides/Pediculicides
Use Treatment of *Sarcoptes scabiei* (scabies), *Pediculus capitis* (head lice), and *Phthirus pubis* (crab lice); FDA recommends reserving lindane as a second-line agent or with inadequate response to other therapies
General Dosage Range Topical:
   Lotion: *Children and Adults:* Apply a thin layer; bathe and remove drug after 8-12 hours
   Shampoo: *Children and Adults:* Apply to dry hair (maximum: 60 mL)
Dosage Forms
   Lotion, topical: 1% (60 mL, 480 mL)
   Shampoo, topical: 1% (60 mL, 480 mL)

Linessa® (Can) *see ethinyl estradiol and desogestrel on page 351*

linezolid (li NE zoh lid)

Medication Safety Issues
Sound-alike/look-alike issues:
Zyvox® may be confused with Ziox™, Zosyn®, Zovirax®

U.S. Brand Names Zyvox®

Canadian Brand Names Zyvoxam®

Therapeutic Category Antibiotic, Oxazolidinone

Use Treatment of vancomycin-resistant *Enterococcus faecium* (VRE) infections, nosocomial pneumonia caused by *Staphylococcus aureus* (including MRSA) or *Streptococcus pneumoniae* (including multidrug-resistant strains [MDRSP]), complicated and uncomplicated skin and skin structure infections (including diabetic foot infections without concomitant osteomyelitis), and community-acquired pneumonia caused by susceptible gram-positive organisms

General Dosage Range
I.V.:
Children ≤11 years: 10 mg/kg (maximum dose: 600 mg) every 8 hours
Children ≥12 years and Adults: 600 mg every 12 hours
Oral:
Children <5 years: 10 mg/kg every 8 hours (maximum: 600 mg/dose)
Children 5-11 years: 10 mg/kg every 8-12 hours (maximum: 600 mg/dose)
Children ≥12 years and Adults: 400-600 mg every 12 hours

Dosage Forms
Infusion, premixed:
Zyvox®: 200 mg (100 mL); 600 mg (300 mL)
Powder for suspension, oral:
Zyvox®: 100 mg/5 mL (150 mL)
Tablet, oral:
Zyvox®: 600 mg

Lioresal® *see baclofen on page 112*

Liotec (Can) *see baclofen on page 112*

liothyronine (lye oh THYE roe neen)

Medication Safety Issues
Sound-alike/look-alike issues:
Liothyronine may be confused with levothyroxine
Other safety concerns:
T3 is an error-prone abbreviation (mistaken as acetaminophen and codeine [ie, Tylenol® #3])

Synonyms liothyronine sodium; sodium *L*-triiodothyronine; T_3 sodium (error-prone abbreviation)

U.S. Brand Names Cytomel®; Triostat®

Canadian Brand Names Cytomel®

Therapeutic Category Thyroid Product

Use
Oral: Replacement or supplemental therapy in hypothyroidism; management of nontoxic goiter; a diagnostic aid
I.V.: Treatment of myxedema coma/precoma

General Dosage Range
I.V.: *Adults:* 10-50 mcg/dose
Oral:
Infants: Initial: 5 mcg/day; Usual maintenance dose: 20 mcg/day
Children 1-3 years: Initial: 5 mcg/day; Usual maintenance dose: 50 mcg/day
Children >3 years: Initial: 5 mcg/day; Maintenance: Up to 100 mcg/day
Adults: Initial 5-25 mcg/day; Maintenance range 5-100 mcg/day
Elderly: Initial: 5 mcg/day

Dosage Forms
Injection, solution: 10 mcg/mL (1 mL)
Triostat®: 10 mcg/mL (1 mL)
Tablet, oral: 5 mcg, 25 mcg, 50 mcg
Cytomel®: 5 mcg, 25 mcg, 50 mcg

liothyronine sodium *see liothyronine on page 529*

liotrix (LYE oh triks)

Medication Safety Issues

Sound-alike/look-alike issues:

Liotrix may be confused with Klotrix®

Thyrolar® may be confused with Thyrogen®, Thytropar®

Synonyms T$_3$/T$_4$ liotrix

U.S. Brand Names Thyrolar®

Canadian Brand Names Thyrolar®

Therapeutic Category Thyroid Product

Use

Replacement or supplemental therapy in hypothyroidism (uniform mixture of T$_4$:T$_3$ in 4:1 ratio by weight)

Thyroid-stimulating hormone (TSH) suppressant therapy used in the management of thyroid cancer (levothyroxine is generally recommended for this indication); prevention or treatment of euthyroid goiters (eg, thyroid nodules, subacute or chronic lymphocytic thyroiditis [Hashimoto's], multinodular goiters)

Diagnostic agent in suppression tests to diagnose suspected mild hyperthyroidism or to demonstrate thyroid gland autonomy

General Dosage Range Oral:

Children 0-6 months: Levothyroxine 12.5-25 mcg/Liothyronine 3.1-6.25 mcg once daily

Children 6-12 months: Levothyroxine 25-37.5 mcg/Liothyronine 6.25-9.35 mcg once daily

Children 1-5 years: Levothyroxine 37.5-50 mcg/Liothyronine 9.35-12.5 mcg once daily

Children 6-12 years: Levothyroxine 50-75 mcg/Liothyronine 12.5-18.75 mcg once daily

Children >12 years: Levothyroxine 75 mcg/Liothyronine 18.75 mcg once daily

Adults: Initial: Levothyroxine 25 mcg/Liothyronine 6.25 mcg once daily; Usual maintenance: Levothyroxine 50-100 mcg/Liothyronine 12.5-25 mcg once daily

Elderly: Initial: Levothyroxine 12.5-25 mcg/Liothyronine 3.1-6.25 mcg once daily

Dosage Forms

Tablet, oral:

Thyrolar®:

1/4 [levothyroxine 12.5 mcg and liothyronine 3.1 mcg]

1/2 [levothyroxine 25 mcg and liothyronine 6.25 mcg]

1 [levothyroxine 50 mcg and liothyronine 12.5 mcg]

2 [levothyroxine 100 mcg and liothyronine 25 mcg]

3 [levothyroxine 150 mcg and liothyronine 37.5 mcg]

lipancreatin *see pancrelipase on page 670*

lipase, protease, and amylase *see pancrelipase on page 670*

lipiarrmycin *see fidaxomicin (systemic) on page 377*

Lipidil EZ® (Can) *see fenofibrate on page 369*

Lipidil Micro® (Can) *see fenofibrate on page 369*

Lipidil Supra® (Can) *see fenofibrate on page 369*

Lipitor® *see atorvastatin on page 102*

Lipofen® *see fenofibrate on page 369*

Liposomal Cytarabine *see cytarabine (liposomal) on page 247*

liposomal DAUNOrubicin *see daunorubicin citrate (liposomal) on page 255*

liposomal DOXOrubicin *see doxorubicin (liposomal) on page 311*

Liposyn® II (Can) *see fat emulsion on page 367*

Liposyn® III *see fat emulsion on page 367*

Liqua-Cal [OTC] *see calcium and vitamin D on page 160*

Liquibid® D-R [OTC] *see guaifenesin and phenylephrine on page 428*

Liquibid® PD-R [OTC] *see guaifenesin and phenylephrine on page 428*

liquid antidote *see charcoal on page 191*

Liquid Entero Vu™ *see barium on page 114*

Liquid Polibar® *see barium on page 114*

Liquid Polibar Plus® *see barium on page 114*

Liquifilm® Tears [OTC] *see artificial tears on page 96*

◄ **General Dosage Range** Dosage adjustment recommended in patients with renal impairment
Oral:
  Children ≥6 years: Initial: 0.07 mg/kg once daily (up to 5 mg); Maintenance: Maximum: Doses >0.61 mg/kg or >40 mg have not been evaluated
  Adults: Initial: 2.5-10 mg/day; Maintenance: 10-80 mg/day
  Elderly: Initial: 2.5-5 mg/day (maximum: 40 mg/day)
Dosage Forms
  Tablet, oral: 2.5 mg, 5 mg, 10 mg, 20 mg, 30 mg, 40 mg
  Prinivil®: 5 mg, 10 mg, 20 mg
  Zestril®: 2.5 mg, 5 mg, 10 mg, 20 mg, 30 mg, 40 mg

lisinopril and hydrochlorothiazide (lyse IN oh pril & hye droe klor oh THYE a zide)

Synonyms hydrochlorothiazide and lisinopril
U.S. Brand Names Prinzide®; Zestoretic®
Canadian Brand Names Apo-Lisinopril®/Hctz; Mylan-Lisinopril/Hctz; Novo-Lisinopril/Hctz; Prinzide®; Sandoz-Lisinopril/Hctz; Teva-Lisinopril/Hctz (Type P); Teva-Lisinopril/Hctz (Type Z); Zestoretic®
Therapeutic Category Antihypertensive Agent, Combination
Use Treatment of hypertension
General Dosage Range Oral: *Adults:* Lisinopril 10-80 mg and hydrochlorothiazide 12.5-50 mg once daily
Dosage Forms
  Tablet, oral: 10/12.5: Lisinopril 10 mg and hydrochlorothiazide 12.5 mg; 20/12.5: Lisinopril 20 mg and hydrochlorothiazide 12.5 mg; 20/25: Lisinopril 20 mg and hydrochlorothiazide 25 mg
  Prinzide®:
    10/12.5: Lisinopril 10 mg and hydrochlorothiazide 12.5 mg
    20/12.5: Lisinopril 20 mg and hydrochlorothiazide 12.5 mg
  Zestoretic®:
    10/12.5: Lisinopril 10 mg and hydrochlorothiazide 12.5 mg
    20/12.5: Lisinopril 20 mg and hydrochlorothiazide 12.5 mg
    20/25: Lisinopril 20 mg and hydrochlorothiazide 25 mg

lispro insulin *see* insulin lispro *on page 478*
Lithane™ (Can) *see* lithium *on page 532*

lithium (LITH ee um)

Medication Safety Issues
  Sound-alike/look-alike issues:
    Eskalith® may be confused with Estratest®
    Lithium may be confused with lanthanum
    Lithobid® may be confused with Levbid®, Lithostat®
  Other safety concerns:
    Do not confuse **mEq** (milliequivalent) with **mg** (milligram). **Note:** 300 mg lithium carbonate or citrate contain 8 mEq lithium. Dosage should be written in **mg** (milligrams) to avoid confusion.
    Check prescriptions for unusually high volumes of the syrup for dosing errors.
Synonyms Eskalith; lithium carbonate; lithium citrate
U.S. Brand Names Lithobid®
Canadian Brand Names Apo-Lithium® Carbonate; Apo-Lithium® Carbonate SR; Carbolith™; Duralith®; Euro-Lithium; Lithane™; Lithmax; PHL-Lithium Carbonate; PMS-Lithium Carbonate; PMS-Lithium Citrate
Therapeutic Category Antimanic Agent
Use Management of bipolar disorders; treatment of mania in individuals with bipolar disorder (maintenance treatment prevents or diminishes intensity of subsequent episodes)
General Dosage Range Dosage adjustment recommended in patients with renal impairment
Oral:
  Immediate release:
    Adults: 900-2400 mg/day in 3-4 divided doses
    Elderly: Initial: 300 mg twice daily (maximum: >900-1200 mg/day)
  Extended release: *Adults:* 900-1800 mg/day in 2 divided doses
Dosage Forms
  Capsule, oral: 150 mg, 300 mg, 600 mg
  Solution, oral: 300 mg/5 mL (5 mL, 473 mL, 500 mL)
  Tablet, oral: 300 mg, 600 mg

Tablet, extended release, oral: 300 mg, 450 mg
Lithobid®: 300 mg

lithium carbonate *see* lithium *on page 532*
lithium citrate *see* lithium *on page 532*
Lithmax (Can) *see* lithium *on page 532*
Lithobid® *see* lithium *on page 532*
Lithostat® *see* acetohydroxamic acid *on page 36*
Little Fevers™ [OTC] *see* acetaminophen *on page 23*
Little Noses® Decongestant [OTC] *see* phenylephrine (nasal) *on page 697*
Little Noses® Saline [OTC] *see* sodium chloride *on page 818*
Little Noses® Stuffy Nose Kit [OTC] *see* sodium chloride *on page 818*
Little Phillips'® Milk of Magnesia [OTC] *see* magnesium hydroxide *on page 545*
Little Teethers® [OTC] *see* benzocaine *on page 121*
Little Tummys® Gas Relief [OTC] *see* simethicone *on page 812*
Little Tummys® Laxative [OTC] *see* senna *on page 807*
Livalo® *see* pitavastatin *on page 708*
live attenuated influenza vaccine (LAIV) *see* influenza virus vaccine (live/attenuated) *on page 474*
live smallpox vaccine *see* smallpox vaccine *on page 817*
Livostin® (Can) *see* levocabastine (nasal) *(Canada only) on page 518*
Livostin® Eye Drops (Can) *see* levocabastine (ophthalmic) *(Canada only) on page 518*
L-leucovorin *see* LEVOleucovorin *on page 521*

l-lysine (el LYE seen)

Synonyms l-lysine hydrochloride
U.S. Brand Names Lysinyl [OTC]
Therapeutic Category Dietary Supplement
Use Improves utilization of vegetable proteins; prevention of recurrent herpes simplex infection
General Dosage Range Oral: *Adults:* 334-1500 mg/day
Dosage Forms
 Capsule, oral: 500 mg
  Lysinyl [OTC]: 500 mg
 Powder, oral: (100 g)
  Lysinyl [OTC]: (150 g)
 Tablet, oral: 500 mg, 1000 mg

l-lysine hydrochloride *see* l-lysine *on page 533*
LM3100 *see* plerixafor *on page 710*
LMD® *see* dextran *on page 268*
10% LMD *see* dextran *on page 268*
L-methylfolate *see* methylfolate *on page 576*
L-methylfolate, methylcobalamin, and N-acetylcysteine *see* methylfolate, methylcobalamin, and acetylcysteine *on page 576*
LNg 20 *see* levonorgestrel *on page 521*
Locacorten® Vioform® (Can) *see* clioquinol and flumethasone *(Canada only) on page 219*
Locoid® *see* hydrocortisone (topical) *on page 450*
Locoid Lipocream® *see* hydrocortisone (topical) *on page 450*
Lodine *see* etodolac *on page 360*
Lodosyn® *see* carbidopa *on page 173*

lodoxamide (loe DOKS a mide)

Medication Safety Issues
 International issues:
  Thilomide [Greece, Turkey] may be confused with Thalomid brand name for thalidomide [U.S., Canada]
Synonyms lodoxamide tromethamine
U.S. Brand Names Alomide®
Canadian Brand Names Alomide®

▶

◄ **Therapeutic Category** Mast Cell Stabilizer
Use Treatment of vernal keratoconjunctivitis, vernal conjunctivitis, and vernal keratitis
General Dosage Range Ophthalmic: *Children >2 years and Adults:* Instill 1-2 drops in eye(s) 4 times/day
Dosage Forms
  Solution, ophthalmic:
    Alomide®: 0.1% (10 mL)

Iodoxamide tromethamine *see* lodoxamide *on page 533*
Lodrane® 24 [DSC] *see* brompheniramine *on page 143*
Loestrin™ 1.5/30 (Can) *see* ethinyl estradiol and norethindrone *on page 355*
Loestrin® 21 1.5/30 *see* ethinyl estradiol and norethindrone *on page 355*
Loestrin® 21 1/20 *see* ethinyl estradiol and norethindrone *on page 355*
Loestrin® 24 Fe *see* ethinyl estradiol and norethindrone *on page 355*
Loestrin® Fe 1.5/30 *see* ethinyl estradiol and norethindrone *on page 355*
Loestrin® Fe 1/20 *see* ethinyl estradiol and norethindrone *on page 355*
Lo-Femenal 21 (Can) *see* ethinyl estradiol and norgestrel *on page 357*
Lofibra® *see* fenofibrate *on page 369*
LoHist-12 *see* brompheniramine *on page 143*
LoHist-D *see* chlorpheniramine and pseudoephedrine *on page 199*
L-OHP *see* oxaliplatin *on page 658*
LoKara™ *see* desonide *on page 263*
Lo Loestrin™ Fe *see* ethinyl estradiol and norethindrone *on page 355*
Lomine (Can) *see* dicyclomine *on page 280*
Lomotil® *see* diphenoxylate and atropine *on page 293*

lomustine (loe MUS teen)

Medication Safety Issues
  Sound-alike/look-alike issues:
    Lomustine may be confused with bendamustine, carmustine
  High alert medication:
    The Institute for Safe Medication Practices (ISMP) includes this medication among its list of drug classes which have a heightened risk of causing significant patient harm when used in error.
  Administration issues:
    Lomustine should only be administered as a single dose once every 6 weeks; serious errors have occurred when lomustine was inadvertently administered daily.
Synonyms CCNU; lomustinum
U.S. Brand Names CeeNU®
Canadian Brand Names CeeNU®
Therapeutic Category Antineoplastic Agent
Use Treatment of primary and metastatic brain tumors (after surgery and/or radiation therapy); treatment of relapsed or refractory Hodgkin disease (as part of a combination chemotherapy regimen)
General Dosage Range Dosage adjustment recommended in patients with renal impairment or who develop toxicities
  Oral: *Children and Adults:* 100-130 mg/m^2 as a single dose once every 6 weeks
Dosage Forms
  Capsule, oral:
    CeeNU®: 10 mg, 40 mg, 100 mg

lomustinum *see* lomustine *on page 534*
longastatin *see* octreotide *on page 643*
Loniten® (Can) *see* minoxidil (systemic) *on page 591*
Lo Ovral *see* ethinyl estradiol and norgestrel *on page 357*
Lo/Ovral®-28 *see* ethinyl estradiol and norgestrel *on page 357*
Loperacap (Can) *see* loperamide *on page 535*

loperamide (loe PER a mide)

Medication Safety Issues
Sound-alike/look-alike issues:
Imodium® A-D may be confused with Indocin®

Loperamide may be confused with furosemide

International issues:
Indiaral [France] may be confused with Inderal and Inderal LA brand names for propranolol [U.S., Canada, and multiple international markets]

Lomotil: Brand name for loperamide [Mexico, Philippines], but also the brand name for diphenoxylate [U.S., Canada, and multiple international markets]

Lomotil [Mexico, Phillipines] may be confused with Ludiomil brand name for maprotiline [multiple international markets]

Synonyms loperamide hydrochloride

U.S. Brand Names Anti-Diarrheal [OTC]; Diamode [OTC]; Imodium® A-D for children [OTC]; Imodium® A-D [OTC]

Canadian Brand Names Apo-Loperamide®; Diarr-Eze; Dom-Loperamide; Imodium®; Loperacap; Novo-Loperamide; PMS-Loperamine; Rhoxal-loperamide; Rho®-Loperamine; Riva-Loperamide; Sandoz-Loperamide

Therapeutic Category Antidiarrheal

Use Treatment of chronic diarrhea associated with inflammatory bowel disease; acute nonspecific diarrhea; increased volume of ileostomy discharge

OTC labeling: Control of symptoms of diarrhea, including traveler's diarrhea

General Dosage Range Oral:
Children 2-5 years (13-20 kg): Initial: 1 mg 3 times/day for first 24 hours; Maintenance: 0.1 mg/kg after each loose stool

Children 6-8 years (20-30 kg): Initial: 2 mg twice daily for first 24 hours; Maintenance: 0.1 mg/kg after each loose stool **or** 2 mg after first loose stool, followed by 1 mg after each subsequent stool (maximum: 4 mg/day)

Children 8-12 years (>30 kg): Initial: 2 mg 3 times/day for first 24 hours; Maintenance: 0.1 mg/kg after each loose stool

Children 9-11 years: 2 mg after first loose stool, followed by 1 mg after each subsequent stool (maximum: 6 mg/day)

Children ≥12 years: Initial: 4 mg after first loose stool, followed by 2 mg after each subsequent stool (maximum: 8 mg/day)

Adults: Initial: 4 mg followed by 2 mg after each loose stool (maximum: 8-16 mg/day) **or** 4-8 mg/day in divided doses

Dosage Forms
Caplet, oral: 2 mg

Anti-Diarrheal [OTC]: 2 mg

Diamode [OTC]: 2 mg

Imodium® A-D [OTC]: 2 mg

Capsule, oral: 2 mg

Liquid, oral: 1 mg/5 mL (118 mL, 120 mL)

Anti-Diarrheal [OTC]: 1 mg/5 mL (120 mL)

Imodium® A-D [OTC]: 1 mg/5 mL (60 mL, 120 mL); 1 mg/7.5 mL (120 mL)

Imodium® A-D for children [OTC]: 1 mg/7.5 mL (120 mL)

Solution, oral: 1 mg/5 mL (5 mL, 10 mL, 118 mL, 120 mL)

loperamide and simethicone (loe PER a mide & sye METH i kone)

Synonyms simethicone and loperamide hydrochloride

U.S. Brand Names Imodium® Multi-Symptom Relief [OTC]

Canadian Brand Names Imodium® Advanced Multi-Symptom

Therapeutic Category Antidiarrheal; Antiflatulent

Use Control of symptoms of diarrhea and gas (bloating, pressure, and cramps)

General Dosage Range Oral:
Children 6-8 years (48-59 lbs): 1 caplet/tablet after first loose stool, followed by 1/2 caplet/tablet with each subsequent loose stool (maximum: 2 caplets or tablets/24 hours)

Children 9-11 years (60-95 lbs): 1 caplet/tablet after first loose stool, followed by 1/2 caplet/tablet with each subsequent loose stool (maximum: 3 caplets or tablets/24 hours)

▶

◀ *Children ≥12 years and Adults:* 1 caplet/tablet after each loose stool (maximum: 4 caplets or tablets/24 hours)

Dosage Forms

Caplet:

Imodium® Multi-Symptom Relief: Loperamide hydrochloride 2 mg and simethicone 125 mg

Tablet, chewable:

Imodium® Muliti-Symptom Relief: Loperamide hydrochloride 2 mg and simethicone 125 mg

loperamide hydrochloride *see loperamide on page 535*

Lopid® *see gemfibrozil on page 414*

lopinavir and ritonavir (loe PIN a veer & rit ON uh veer)

Medication Safety Issues

Sound-alike/look-alike issues:

Potential for dispensing errors between Kaletra® and Keppra® (levETIRAcetam)

Administration issues:

Children's doses are based on weight and calculated by milligrams of lopinavir. Care should be taken to accurately calculate the dose. The oral solution contains lopinavir 80 mg and ritonavir 20 mg per one mL. Children <12 years of age (and ≤40 kg) who are not taking certain concomitant antiretroviral medications will receive <5 mL of solution per dose.

Synonyms ritonavir and lopinavir

U.S. Brand Names Kaletra®

Canadian Brand Names Kaletra®

Therapeutic Category Antiretroviral Agent, Nonnucleoside Reverse Transcriptase Inhibitor (NNRTI)

Use Treatment of HIV infection in combination with other antiretroviral agents

General Dosage Range Dosage adjustment recommended in patients on concomitant therapy

Oral:

Children 14 days to 6 months: Lopinavir 16 mg/kg or 300 mg/m^2 twice daily

Children 6 months to 18 years and <15 kg: 12 mg lopinavir/kg twice daily (maximum dose: Lopinavir 400 mg/ritonavir 100 mg)

Children 6 months to 18 years and 15-40 kg: 10 mg lopinavir/kg twice daily (maximum dose: Lopinavir 400 mg/ritonavir 100 mg)

Children 6 months to 18 years and >40 kg: Lopinavir 400 mg/ritonavir 100 mg twice daily

Adults: Lopinavir 400 mg/ritonavir 100 mg twice daily **or** lopinavir 800 mg/ritonavir 200 mg once daily

Dosage Forms

Solution, oral:

Kaletra®: Lopinavir 80 mg and ritonavir 20 mg per mL

Tablet:

Kaletra®:

Lopinavir 100 mg and ritonavir 25 mg

Lopinavir 200 mg and ritonavir 50 mg

Lopressor® *see metoprolol on page 581*

Lopressor HCT® *see metoprolol and hydrochlorothiazide on page 582*

Loprox® *see ciclopirox on page 207*

Loradamed [OTC] *see loratadine on page 536*

loratadine (lor AT a deen)

Medication Safety Issues

Sound-alike/look-alike issues:

Claritin® may be confused with clarithromycin

Claritin® (loratadine) may be confused with Claritin™ Eye (ketotifen)

U.S. Brand Names Alavert® Allergy 24 Hour [OTC]; Alavert® Children's Allergy [OTC]; Claritin® 24 Hour Allergy [OTC]; Claritin® Children's Allergy [OTC]; Claritin® Liqui-Gels® 24 Hour Allergy [OTC]; Claritin® RediTabs® 24 Hour Allergy [OTC]; Loradamed [OTC]; Tavist® ND Allergy [OTC]

Canadian Brand Names Apo-Loratadine®; Claritin®; Claritin® Kids

Therapeutic Category Antihistamine

Use Relief of nasal and nonnasal symptoms of seasonal allergic rhinitis; treatment of chronic idiopathic urticaria

General Dosage Range Dosage adjustment recommended in patients with hepatic or renal impairment
Oral:
Children 2-5 years: 5 mg once daily
Children ≥6 years and Adults: 10 mg once daily
Dosage Forms
Capsule, liquid gel, oral:
Claritin® Liqui-Gels® 24 Hour Allergy [OTC]: 10 mg
Solution, oral: 5 mg/5 mL (120 mL)
Syrup, oral: 5 mg/5 mL (120 mL)
Claritin® Children's Allergy [OTC]: 5 mg/5 mL (60 mL, 120 mL)
Tablet, oral: 10 mg
Alavert® Allergy 24 Hour [OTC]: 10 mg
Claritin® 24 Hour Allergy [OTC]: 10 mg
Loradamed [OTC]: 10 mg
Tavist® ND Allergy [OTC]: 10 mg
Tablet, chewable, oral:
Claritin® Children's Allergy [OTC]: 5 mg
Tablet, orally disintegrating, oral: 10 mg
Alavert® Allergy 24 Hour [OTC]: 10 mg
Alavert® Children's Allergy [OTC]: 10 mg
Claritin® RediTabs® 24 Hour Allergy [OTC]: 10 mg

loratadine and pseudoephedrine (lor AT a deen & soo doe e FED rin)
Medication Safety Issues
Sound-alike/look-alike issues:
Claritin-D® may be confused with Claritin-D® 24
Claritin-D® 24 may be confused with Claritin-D®
Synonyms pseudoephedrine and loratadine
U.S. Brand Names Alavert™ Allergy and Sinus [OTC]; Claritin-D® 12 Hour Allergy & Congestion [OTC]; Claritin-D® 24 Hour Allergy & Congestion [OTC]
Canadian Brand Names Chlor-Tripolon ND®; Claritin® Extra; Claritin® Liberator
Therapeutic Category Antihistamine/Decongestant Combination
Use Temporary relief of symptoms of seasonal allergic rhinitis, other upper respiratory allergies, or the common cold
General Dosage Range Dosage adjustment recommended in patients with renal impairment
Oral: *Children ≥12 years and Adults:* Alavert™ Allergy and Sinus, Claritin-D® 24-Hour: 1 tablet every 24 hours; Claritin-D® 12-Hour: 1 tablet every 12 hours
Dosage Forms
Tablet, extended release: Loratadine 10 mg and pseudoephedrine 240 mg
Alavert™ Allergy and Sinus [OTC]: Loratadine 5 mg and pseudoephedrine 120 mg
Claritin-D® 12 Hour Allergy & Congestion [OTC]: Loratadine 5 mg and pseudoephedrine 120 mg
Claritin-D® 24 Hour Allergy & Congestion [OTC]: Loratadine 10 mg and pseudoephedrine 240 mg

lorazepam (lor A ze pam)
Medication Safety Issues
Sound-alike/look-alike issues:
LORazepam may be confused with ALPRAZolam, clonazePAM, diazepam, KlonoPIN®, Lovaza®, temazepam, zolpidem
Ativan® may be confused with Ambien®, Atarax®, Atgam®, Avitene®
BEERS Criteria medication:
This drug may be inappropriate for use in geriatric patients (high severity risk).
Administration issues:
Injection dosage form contains propylene glycol. Monitor for toxicity when administering continuous lorazepam infusions.
Tall-Man LORazepam
U.S. Brand Names Ativan®; Lorazepam Intensol™
Canadian Brand Names Apo-Lorazepam®; Ativan®; Dom-Lorazepam; Lorazepam Injection, USP; Novo-Lorazem; Nu-Loraz; PHL-Lorazepam; PMS-Lorazepam; PRO-Lorazepam
Therapeutic Category Benzodiazepine
Controlled Substance C-IV

◀ **Use**
Oral: Management of anxiety disorders or short-term (≤4 months) relief of the symptoms of anxiety, anxiety associated with depressive symptoms, or insomnia due to anxiety or transient stress
I.V.: Status epilepticus, amnesia, sedation

General Dosage Range
I.M.:
Children: 0.02-0.09 mg/kg as a single dose
Adults: 0.5-1 mg every 30-60 minutes as needed **or** 0.05 mg/kg as a single dose (maximum: 4 mg/dose)
I.V.: *Children and Adults:* Dosage varies greatly depending on indication
Oral:
Children: 0.02-0.09 mg/kg every 4-8 hours or as a single dose
Adults: Dosage varies greatly depending on indication

Dosage Forms
Injection, solution: 2 mg/mL (1 mL, 10 mL); 4 mg/mL (1 mL, 10 mL)
Ativan®: 2 mg/mL (1 mL, 10 mL); 4 mg/mL (1 mL, 10 mL)
Solution, oral: 2 mg/mL (30 mL)
Lorazepam Intensol™: 2 mg/mL (30 mL)
Tablet, oral: 0.5 mg, 1 mg, 2 mg
Ativan®: 0.5 mg, 1 mg, 2 mg

Lorazepam Injection, USP (Can) *see* lorazepam *on page 537*
Lorazepam Intensol™ *see* lorazepam *on page 537*
Lorcet® 10/650 *see* hydrocodone and acetaminophen *on page 446*
Lorcet® Plus *see* hydrocodone and acetaminophen *on page 446*
Lortab® *see* hydrocodone and acetaminophen *on page 446*
Loryna™ *see* ethinyl estradiol and drospirenone *on page 352*

losartan (loe SAR tan)

Medication Safety Issues
Sound-alike/look-alike issues:
Cozaar® may be confused with Colace®, Coreg®, Hyzaar®, Zocor®
Losartan may be confused with valsartan
Synonyms DuP 753; losartan potassium; MK594
U.S. Brand Names Cozaar®
Canadian Brand Names Cozaar®
Therapeutic Category Angiotensin II Receptor Antagonist
Use Treatment of hypertension (HTN); treatment of diabetic nephropathy in patients with type 2 diabetes mellitus (noninsulin-dependent, NIDDM) and a history of hypertension; stroke risk reduction in patients with HTN and left ventricular hypertrophy (LVH)
General Dosage Range Dosage adjustment recommended in patients with hepatic impairment
Oral:
Children 6-16 years: Initial: 0.7 mg/kg once daily (maximum: 50 mg/day); Maintenance: Maximum: ≤1.4 mg/kg; 100 mg
Adults: Initial: 25-50 mg once daily; Maintenance: 25-100 mg/day in 1-2 divided doses (maximum: 100 mg/day)
Dosage Forms
Tablet, oral: 25 mg, 50 mg, 100 mg
Cozaar®: 25 mg, 50 mg, 100 mg

losartan and hydrochlorothiazide (loe SAR tan & hye droe klor oh THYE a zide)

Medication Safety Issues
Sound-alike/look-alike issues:
Hyzaar® may be confused with Cozaar®
Synonyms hydrochlorothiazide and losartan
U.S. Brand Names Hyzaar®
Canadian Brand Names Hyzaar®; Hyzaar® DS
Therapeutic Category Antihypertensive Agent, Combination

Use Treatment of hypertension; stroke risk reduction in patients with HTN and left ventricular hypertrophy (LVH)

General Dosage Range Oral: *Adults:* Losartan 50-100 mg and hydrochlorothiazide 12.5-50 mg once daily

Dosage Forms
　　Tablet: 50/12.5: Losartan 50 mg and hydrochlorothiazide 12.5 mg; 100/12.5: Losartan 100 mg and hydrochlorothiazide 12.5 mg; 100/25: Losartan 100 mg and hydrochlorothiazide 25 mg
　　Hyzaar®: 50/12.5: Losartan 50 mg and hydrochlorothiazide 12.5 mg; 100/12.5: Losartan 100 mg and hydrochlorothiazide 12.5 mg; 100/25: Losartan 100 mg and hydrochlorothiazide 25 mg

losartan potassium *see losartan on page 538*

LoSeasonique® *see ethinyl estradiol and levonorgestrel on page 353*

Losec® (Can) *see omeprazole on page 649*

Lotemax® *see loteprednol on page 539*

Lotensin® *see benazepril on page 119*

Lotensin HCT® *see benazepril and hydrochlorothiazide on page 119*

loteprednol (loe te PRED nol)

Synonyms loteprednol etabonate

U.S. Brand Names Alrex®; Lotemax®

Canadian Brand Names Alrex®; Lotemax®

Therapeutic Category Corticosteroid, Ophthalmic

Use
Ointment, 0.5% (Lotemax®): Treatment of postoperative inflammation and pain following ocular surgery
Suspension, 0.2% (Alrex®): Temporary relief of signs and symptoms of seasonal allergic conjunctivitis
Suspension, 0.5% (Lotemax®): Inflammatory conditions (treatment of steroid-responsive inflammatory conditions of the palpebral and bulbar conjunctiva, cornea, and anterior segment of the globe such as allergic conjunctivitis, acne rosacea, superficial punctate keratitis, herpes zoster keratitis, iritis, cyclitis, selected infective conjunctivitis, when the inherent hazard of steroid use is accepted to obtain an advisable diminution in edema and inflammation) and treatment of postoperative inflammation following ocular surgery

General Dosage Range Ophthalmic: *Adults:* Ointment: Apply ~1/2 inch ribbon into affected eye(s) 4 times/day; Solution: Instill 1-2 drops into affected eye(s) 4 times/day

Product Availability
Lotemax® 0.5% ointment: FDA approved April 2011; expected availability undetermined
Lotemax® 0.5% ointment is a topical corticosteroid approved for the treatment of postoperative inflammation and pain following ocular surgery.

Dosage Forms
　　Ointment, ophthalmic:
　　　Lotemax®: 0.5% (3.5 g)
　　Suspension, ophthalmic:
　　　Alrex®: 0.2% (5 mL, 10 mL)
　　　Lotemax®: 0.5% (2.5 mL, 5 mL, 10 mL, 15 mL)

loteprednol and tobramycin (loe te PRED nol & toe bra MYE sin)

Synonyms loteprednol etabonate and tobramycin; tobramycin and loteprednol etabonate

U.S. Brand Names Zylet®

Therapeutic Category Antibiotic/Corticosteroid, Ophthalmic

Use Treatment of steroid-responsive ocular inflammatory conditions where either a superficial bacterial ocular infection or the risk of a superficial bacterial ocular infection exists

General Dosage Range Ophthalmic: *Children and Adults:* Instill 1-2 drops into the affected eye(s) every 4-6 hours

Dosage Forms
　　Suspension, ophthalmic [drops]:
　　　Zylet®: Loteprednol 0.5% and tobramycin 0.3% (2.5 mL, 5 mL, 10 mL)

loteprednol etabonate *see loteprednol on page 539*

loteprednol etabonate and tobramycin *see loteprednol and tobramycin on page 539*

Lotrel® *see amlodipine and benazepril on page 70*

Lotriderm® (Can) *see* betamethasone and clotrimazole *on page 130*
Lotrimin AF® [OTC] *see* miconazole (topical) *on page 585*
Lotrimin® AF Athlete's Foot [OTC] *see* clotrimazole (topical) *on page 226*
Lotrimin® AF for Her [OTC] *see* clotrimazole (topical) *on page 226*
Lotrimin® AF Jock Itch [OTC] *see* clotrimazole (topical) *on page 226*
Lotrimin® ultra™ [OTC] *see* butenafine *on page 154*
Lotrisone® *see* betamethasone and clotrimazole *on page 130*
Lotronex® *see* alosetron *on page 55*

lovastatin (LOE va sta tin)

Medication Safety Issues
Sound-alike/look-alike issues:
Lovastatin may be confused with atorvastatin, Leustatin®, Livostin®, Lotensin®, nystatin, pitavastatin
Mevacor® may be confused with Benicar®, Lipitor®, Mivacron®
International issues:
Lovacol [Chile and Finland] may be confused with Levatol brand name for penbutolol [U.S.]
Lovastin [Malaysia, Poland, and Singapore] may be confused with Livostin brand name for levocabastine [multiple international markets]

Synonyms mevinolin; monacolin K
U.S. Brand Names Altoprev®; Mevacor®
Canadian Brand Names Apo-Lovastatin®; CO Lovastatin; Dom-Lovastatin; Gen-Lovastatin; Mevacor®; Mylan-Lovastatin; Novo-Lovastatin; Nu-Lovastatin; PHL-Lovastatin; PMS-Lovastatin; PRO-Lovastatin; RAN™-Lovastatin; ratio-Lovastatin; Riva-Lovastatin; Sandoz-Lovastatin
Therapeutic Category HMG-CoA Reductase Inhibitor
Use
Adjunct to dietary therapy to decrease elevated serum total and LDL-cholesterol concentrations in primary hypercholesterolemia
Primary prevention of coronary artery disease (patients without symptomatic disease with average to moderately elevated total and LDL-cholesterol and below average HDL-cholesterol); slow progression of coronary atherosclerosis in patients with coronary heart disease
Adjunct to dietary therapy in adolescent patients (10-17 years of age, females >1 year postmenarche) with heterozygous familial hypercholesterolemia having LDL >189 mg/dL, **or** LDL >160 mg/dL with positive family history of premature cardiovascular disease (CVD), **or** LDL >160 mg/dL with the presence of at least two other CVD risk factors

General Dosage Range Dosage adjustment recommended in patients with renal impairment or on concomitant therapy
Oral:
Extended release: *Adults:* Initial: 20 mg once daily; Maintenance: 20-60 mg once daily (maximum: 60 mg/day)
Immediate release:
Children 10-17 years: Initial: 10-20 mg once daily; Maintenance: 10-40 mg once daily (maximum: 40 mg/day)
Adults: Initial: 20 mg once daily; Maintenance: 20-80 mg once daily (maximum: 80 mg/day)

Dosage Forms
Tablet, oral: 10 mg, 20 mg, 40 mg
Mevacor®: 20 mg, 40 mg
Tablet, extended release, oral:
Altoprev®: 20 mg, 40 mg, 60 mg

lovastatin and niacin *see* niacin and lovastatin *on page 623*
Lovaza® *see* omega-3-acid ethyl esters *on page 649*
Lovenox® *see* enoxaparin *on page 328*
Lovenox® HP (Can) *see* enoxaparin *on page 328*
low-Molecular-weight iron dextran (INFeD®) *see* iron dextran complex *on page 491*
Low-Ogestrel® *see* ethinyl estradiol and norgestrel *on page 357*
Loxapac® IM (Can) *see* loxapine *on page 541*

loxapine (LOKS a peen)
Medication Safety Issues
Sound-alike/look-alike issues:
Loxitane® may be confused with Lexapro®, Soriatane®
International issues:
Loxitane [U.S.] may be confused with Lexotan which is a brand name for bromazepam [multiple international markets]
Synonyms loxapine succinate; oxilapine succinate
U.S. Brand Names Loxitane®
Canadian Brand Names Apo-Loxapine®; Dom-Loxapine; Loxapac® IM; Nu-Loxapine; PHL-Loxapine; Xylac
Therapeutic Category Antipsychotic Agent, Dibenzoxazepine
Use Management of psychotic disorders
General Dosage Range Oral:
Adults: Initial: 10 mg twice daily; Usual range: 20-100 mg/day in 2-4 divided doses (maximum: 250 mg/day)
Elderly: 20-60 mg/day
Dosage Forms
Capsule, oral: 5 mg, 10 mg, 25 mg, 50 mg
Loxitane®: 5 mg, 10 mg, 25 mg, 50 mg

loxapine succinate *see* loxapine *on page 541*
Loxitane® *see* loxapine *on page 541*
Lozide® (Can) *see* indapamide *on page 470*
Lozi-Flur™ *see* fluoride *on page 386*
Lozol® (Can) *see* indapamide *on page 470*
L-PAM *see* melphalan *on page 556*
L-phenylalanine mustard *see* melphalan *on page 556*
LRH *see* gonadorelin *(Canada only) on page 423*
L-sarcolysin *see* melphalan *on page 556*
LTA® 360 *see* lidocaine (topical) *on page 524*
LTG *see* lamotrigine *on page 509*
L-thyroxine sodium *see* levothyroxine *on page 522*
Lu-26-054 *see* escitalopram *on page 341*

lubiprostone (loo bi PROS tone)
Synonyms RU 0211; SPI 0211
U.S. Brand Names Amitiza®
Therapeutic Category Gastrointestinal Agent, Miscellaneous
Use Treatment of chronic idiopathic constipation; treatment of irritable bowel syndrome with constipation in adult women
General Dosage Range Dosage adjustment recommended in hepatic impairment and in patients who develop toxicities
Oral:
Adults (females): 8 mcg twice daily **or** 24 mcg twice daily
Adults (males): 24 mcg twice daily
Dosage Forms
Capsule, softgel, oral:
Amitiza®: 8 mcg, 24 mcg

Lubriderm® [OTC] *see* lanolin, cetyl alcohol, glycerin, petrolatum, and mineral oil *on page 510*
Lubriderm® Fragrance Free [OTC] *see* lanolin, cetyl alcohol, glycerin, petrolatum, and mineral oil *on page 510*
Lucentis® *see* ranibizumab *on page 767*
Ludiomil *see* maprotiline *on page 549*
Lufyllin® *see* dyphylline *on page 318*
Lufyllin®-GG *see* dyphylline and guaifenesin *on page 318*
lumefantrine and artemether *see* artemether and lumefantrine *on page 94*

Lumigan® *see* bimatoprost *on page 133*
Lumigan® RC (Can) *see* bimatoprost *on page 133*
Lumitene™ [OTC] *see* beta-carotene *on page 128*
Lumizyme® *see* alglucosidase alfa *on page 51*
Lunesta® *see* eszopiclone *on page 350*
LupiCare® Dandruff [OTC] *see* salicylic acid *on page 795*
LupiCare® Psoriasis [OTC] *see* salicylic acid *on page 795*
Lupron® (Can) *see* leuprolide *on page 516*
Lupron Depot® *see* leuprolide *on page 516*
Lupron® Depot® (Can) *see* leuprolide *on page 516*
Lupron Depot-Ped® *see* leuprolide *on page 516*

lurasidone (loo RAS i done)

Medication Safety Issues
Sound-alike/look-alike issues:
Latuda® may be confused with Lantus®
Synonyms lurasidone hydrochloride; SM-13496
U.S. Brand Names Latuda®
Therapeutic Category Antipsychotic Agent, Atypical
Use Treatment of schizophrenia
General Dosage Range Dosage adjustment recommended in patients with hepatic or renal impairment or on concomitant therapy.
Oral: *Adults:* Initial: 40 mg once daily (maximum: 80 mg/day)
Dosage Forms
Tablet, oral:
Latuda®: 40 mg, 80 mg

lurasidone hydrochloride *see* lurasidone *on page 542*
Lusedra™ *see* fospropofol *on page 402*
LuSonal™ [DSC] *see* phenylephrine (systemic) *on page 696*
Lustra® *see* hydroquinone *on page 453*
Lustra-AF® *see* hydroquinone *on page 453*
Lustra-Ultra™ *see* hydroquinone *on page 453*
luteinizing hormone releasing hormone *see* gonadorelin *(Canada only) on page 423*
Lutera® *see* ethinyl estradiol and levonorgestrel *on page 353*
Lutrepulse™ (Can) *see* gonadorelin *(Canada only) on page 423*

lutropin alfa (LOO troe pin AL fa)

Synonyms r-hLH; recombinant human luteinizing hormone
U.S. Brand Names Luveris®
Therapeutic Category Gonadotropin; Ovulation Stimulator
Use Stimulation of follicular development in infertile hypogonadotropic hypogonadal (HH) women with profound luteinizing hormone (LH) deficiency; to be used in combination with follitropin alfa
General Dosage Range SubQ: *Adults (females):* 75 int. units daily (maximum duration: 14 days)
Dosage Forms
Injection, powder for reconstitution:
Luveris®: 75 int. units

Luveris® *see* lutropin alfa *on page 542*
Luvox *see* fluvoxamine *on page 395*
Luvox® (Can) *see* fluvoxamine *on page 395*
Luvox® CR *see* fluvoxamine *on page 395*
Luxiq® *see* betamethasone *on page 129*
LY139603 *see* atomoxetine *on page 101*
LY146032 *see* daptomycin *on page 252*
LY170053 *see* olanzapine *on page 645*
LY-188011 *see* gemcitabine *on page 413*

LY231514 *see* pemetrexed *on page 682*
LY246736 *see* alvimopan *on page 61*
LY248686 *see* duloxetine *on page 316*
LY303366 *see* anidulafungin *on page 79*
LY570310 *see* telaprevir *on page 846*
LY-640315 *see* prasugrel *on page 732*
LY2148568 *see* exenatide *on page 363*
Lybrel® *see* ethinyl estradiol and levonorgestrel *on page 353*
Lyderm® (Can) *see* fluocinonide *on page 385*
Lymphazurin™ *see* isosulfan blue *on page 495*
lymphocyte immune globulin *see* antithymocyte globulin (equine) *on page 83*
lymphocyte mitogenic factor *see* aldesleukin *on page 47*
Lyrica® *see* pregabalin *on page 735*
Lysinyl [OTC] *see* l-lysine *on page 533*
Lysodren® *see* mitotane *on page 593*
Lysteda™ *see* tranexamic acid *on page 881*
Maalox® Advanced Maximum Strength [OTC] *see* aluminum hydroxide, magnesium hydroxide, and simethicone *on page 60*
Maalox® Advanced Maximum Strength [OTC] *see* calcium carbonate and simethicone *on page 162*
Maalox® Advanced Regular Strength [OTC] *see* aluminum hydroxide, magnesium hydroxide, and simethicone *on page 60*
Maalox® Children's [OTC] *see* calcium carbonate *on page 161*
Maalox® Junior Plus Antigas [OTC] *see* calcium carbonate and simethicone *on page 162*
Maalox® Regular Strength [OTC] *see* calcium carbonate *on page 161*
Maalox® Total Relief® [OTC] [DSC] *see* bismuth *on page 135*
MabCampath® (Can) *see* alemtuzumab *on page 48*
Macrobid® *see* nitrofurantoin *on page 629*
Macrodantin® *see* nitrofurantoin *on page 629*
Macugen® *see* pegaptanib *on page 678*

mafenide (MA fe nide)

Synonyms mafenide acetate
U.S. Brand Names Sulfamylon®
Therapeutic Category Antibacterial, Topical
Use
Cream: Adjunctive antibacterial agent in the treatment of second- and third-degree burns
Solution: Adjunctive antibacterial agent for use under moist dressings over meshed autografts on excised burn wounds
General Dosage Range Topical: *Children and Adults:* Apply to a thickness of approximately 1/16" once or twice daily
Dosage Forms
Cream, topical:
Sulfamylon®: 85 mg/g (56.7 g, 113.4 g, 453.6 g)
Powder for solution, topical:
Sulfamylon®: 50 g/packet (5s)

mafenide acetate *see* mafenide *on page 543*
Mag 64™ [OTC] *see* magnesium chloride *on page 544*
Mag-Al [OTC] *see* aluminum hydroxide and magnesium hydroxide *on page 60*

magaldrate and simethicone (MAG al drate & sye METH i kone)

Medication Safety Issues
Sound-alike/look-alike issues:
Riopan Plus® may be confused with Repan®
Synonyms Riopan Plus; simethicone and magaldrate
Therapeutic Category Antacid; Antiflatulent

◄ **Use** Relief of hyperacidity associated with peptic ulcer, gastritis, peptic esophagitis, and hiatal hernia which are accompanied by symptoms of gas

General Dosage Range Oral: *Adults:* 5-10 mL (540-1080 mg magaldrate) between meals and at bedtime

Dosage Forms

Suspension, oral: Magaldrate 540 mg and simethicone 20 mg per 5 mL

Mag-Al Ultimate [OTC] *see* aluminum hydroxide and magnesium hydroxide *on page 60*

mag citrate *see* magnesium citrate *on page 544*

Mag Delay [OTC] *see* magnesium chloride *on page 544*

Mag®-G [OTC] *see* magnesium gluconate *on page 545*

MagGel™ 600 [OTC] *see* magnesium oxide *on page 546*

Maginex™ [OTC] *see* magnesium L-aspartate hydrochloride *on page 546*

Maginex™ DS [OTC] *see* magnesium L-aspartate hydrochloride *on page 546*

MagneBind® 400 Rx *see* magnesium carbonate, calcium carbonate, and folic acid *on page 544*

magnesia magma *see* magnesium hydroxide *on page 545*

magnesium carbonate and aluminum hydroxide *see* aluminum hydroxide and magnesium carbonate *on page 59*

magnesium carbonate, calcium carbonate, and folic acid
(mag NEE zhum KAR bun ate, KAL see um KAR bun ate, & FOE lik AS id)

Synonyms calcium carbonate, folic acid, and magnesium carbonate; folic acid, magnesium carbonate, and calcium carbonate

U.S. Brand Names MagneBind® 400 Rx

Therapeutic Category Calcium Salt; Electrolyte Supplement, Oral; Magnesium Salt; Vitamin; Vitamin, Water Soluble

Use Prevention or treatment of nutritional deficiencies

General Dosage Range Oral: *Adults:* 1-3 tablets 3 times/day

Dosage Forms

Tablet, oral:

MagneBind® 400 Rx: Magnesium carbonate 400 mg, calcium carbonate 200 mg, and folic acid 1 mg

magnesium chloride (mag NEE zhum KLOR ide)

U.S. Brand Names Chloromag®; Mag 64™ [OTC]; Mag Delay [OTC]; Slow-Mag® [OTC]

Therapeutic Category Electrolyte Supplement, Oral

Use Correction or prevention of hypomagnesemia; dietary supplement

General Dosage Range

I.V.:

Children <50 kg: 0.3-0.5 mEq/kg/day

Children >50 kg: 10-30 mEq/day

Adults: 8-24 mEq/day added to TPN

Oral: RDA (elemental magnesium):

Children: 80-240 mg/day

Adults: 360-410 mg/day

Dosage Forms

Injection, solution: 200 mg/mL (50 mL)

Chloromag®: 200 mg/mL (50 mL)

Tablet, delayed release, enteric coated, oral:

Mag 64™ [OTC]: Elemental magnesium 64 mg

Mag Delay [OTC]: Elemental magnesium 64 mg

Tablet, enteric coated, oral:

Slow-Mag® [OTC]: Elemental magnesium 64 mg

magnesium citrate (mag NEE zhum SIT rate)

Synonyms citrate of magnesia; mag citrate

U.S. Brand Names Citroma® [OTC]

Canadian Brand Names Citro-Mag®

Therapeutic Category Laxative

Use Evacuation of bowel prior to certain surgical and diagnostic procedures or overdose situations

General Dosage Range Oral:
Children <6 years: 2-4 mL/kg given once or in divided doses
Children 6-12 years: 100-150 mL given once or in divided doses
Children >12 years and Adults: 150-300 mL given once or in divided doses
Dosage Forms
Solution, oral: 290 mg/5 mL (296 mL, 300 mL)
Citroma® [OTC]: 290 mg/5 mL (296 mL, 340 mL)
Tablet, oral: Elemental magnesium 100 mg

magnesium gluceptate *see* magnesium glucoheptonate *on page 545*

magnesium glucoheptonate (mag NEE zhum gloo koh HEP toh nate)

Synonyms magnesium gluceptate
Canadian Brand Names Magnesium Glucoheptonate
Therapeutic Category Electrolyte Supplement, Parenteral; Magnesium Salt
Use Dietary supplement
General Dosage Range Oral: *Adults:* 1500-3000 mg (75-150 mg elemental magnesium) 1-3 times/day
Product Availability Not available in U.S.
Dosage Forms - Canada
Solution, oral: 100 mg/mL

Magnesium Glucoheptonate (Can) *see* magnesium glucoheptonate *on page 545*

magnesium gluconate (mag NEE zhum GLOO koe nate)

U.S. Brand Names Magonate® [OTC]; Magtrate® [OTC]; Mag®-G [OTC]
Therapeutic Category Electrolyte Supplement, Oral
Use Dietary supplement
General Dosage Range Oral: RDA (elemental magnesium):
Children 1-13 years: 80-240 mg/day
Children ≥14 years and Adults: 310-420 mg/day
Dosage Forms
Liquid, oral:
Magonate® [OTC]: 1000 mg/5 mL (355 mL)
Tablet, oral: 500 mg, 550 mg
Magonate® [OTC]: 500 mg
Magtrate® [OTC]: 500 mg
Mag®-G [OTC]: 500 mg

magnesium hydroxide (mag NEE zhum hye DROKS ide)

Synonyms magnesia magma; milk of magnesia; MOM
U.S. Brand Names Fleet® Pedia-Lax™ Chewable Tablet [OTC]; Little Phillips'® Milk of Magnesia [OTC]; Milk of Magnesia [OTC]; Phillips'® Milk of Magnesia [OTC]
Therapeutic Category Antacid; Electrolyte Supplement, Oral; Laxative
Use Short-term treatment of occasional constipation and symptoms of hyperacidity, laxative; dietary supplement
General Dosage Range Oral:
Children 2-5 years: OTC laxative: Magnesium hydroxide 400 mg/5 mL: 5-15 mL/day
Children 6-11 years: OTC laxative: Magnesium hydroxide 400 mg/5 mL: 15-30 mL/day
Children ≥12 years and Adults: OTC laxative: Magnesium hydroxide 400 mg/5 mL: 30-60 mL/day
Dosage Forms
Suspension, oral: 400 mg/5 mL (30 mL, 473 mL, 3840 mL); 2400 mg/10 mL (10 mL)
Little Phillips'® Milk of Magnesia [OTC]: 800 mg/5 mL (120 mL)
Milk of Magnesia [OTC]: 400 mg/5 mL (360 mL, 480 mL); 800 mg/5 mL (100 mL, 400 mL)
Phillips'® Milk of Magnesia [OTC]: 400 mg/5 mL (120 mL, 240 mL, 360 mL, 780 mL); 800 mg/5 mL (240 mL)
Tablet, chewable, oral:
Fleet® Pedia-Lax™ Chewable Tablet [OTC]: 400 mg
Phillips'® Milk of Magnesia [OTC]: 311 mg

magnesium hydroxide, aluminum hydroxide, and simethicone *see* aluminum hydroxide, magnesium hydroxide, and simethicone *on page 60*

magnesium hydroxide and aluminum hydroxide *see* aluminum hydroxide and magnesium hydroxide *on page 60*

magnesium hydroxide and calcium carbonate *see* calcium carbonate and magnesium hydroxide *on page 162*

magnesium hydroxide and mineral oil (mag NEE zhum hye DROKS ide & MIN er al oyl)

Synonyms Haley's M-O; MOM/mineral oil emulsion

U.S. Brand Names Phillips'® M-O [OTC]

Therapeutic Category Laxative

Use Short-term treatment of occasional constipation

General Dosage Range Oral:
Children 6-11 years: 20-30 mL at bedtime
Children ≥12 years and Adults: 45-60 mL at bedtime

Dosage Forms
Suspension, oral:
Phillips'® M-O [OTC]: Magnesium hydroxide 300 mg and mineral oil 1.25 mL per 5 mL

magnesium hydroxide, famotidine, and calcium carbonate *see* famotidine, calcium carbonate, and magnesium hydroxide *on page 367*

magnesium L-aspartate hydrochloride
(mag NEE zhum el as PAR tate hye droe KLOR ide)

Synonyms MAH

U.S. Brand Names Maginex™ DS [OTC]; Maginex™ [OTC]

Therapeutic Category Electrolyte Supplement, Oral

Use Dietary supplement

General Dosage Range Oral: RDA (elemental magnesium):
Children 1-13 years: 80-240 mg/day
Children ≥14 years and Adults: 310-420 mg/day

Dosage Forms
Granules for solution, oral [preservative free]:
Maginex™ DS [OTC]: 1230 mg/packet (30s)
Tablet, enteric coated, oral [preservative free]:
Maginex™ [OTC]: 615 mg

magnesium oxide (mag NEE zhum OKS ide)

Synonyms mag oxide

U.S. Brand Names Mag-Ox® 400 [OTC]; MagGel™ 600 [OTC]; MAGnesium-Oxide™ [OTC]; Phillips'® Laxative Dietary Supplement Cramp-Free [OTC]; Uro-Mag® [OTC]

Therapeutic Category Antacid; Electrolyte Supplement, Oral; Laxative

Use Electrolyte replacement

General Dosage Range Oral: RDA (elemental magnesium):
Children 1-13 years: 80-240 mg/day
Children ≥14 years and Adults: 310-420 mg/day

Dosage Forms
Caplet, oral: Elemental magnesium 250 mg
Phillips'® Laxative Dietary Supplement Cramp-Free [OTC]: Elemental magnesium 500 mg
Capsule, oral:
Uro-Mag® [OTC]: 140 mg
Capsule, softgel, oral:
MagGel™ 600 [OTC]: 600 mg
Tablet, oral: 400 mg, 500 mg, Elemental magnesium 500 mg
Mag-Ox® 400 [OTC]: 400 mg
MAGnesium-Oxide™ [OTC]: 400 mg

MAGnesium-Oxide™ [OTC] *see* magnesium oxide *on page 546*

magnesium salicylate (mag NEE zhum sa LIS i late)

U.S. Brand Names Doan's® Extra Strength [OTC]; Keygesic [OTC]; Momentum® [OTC]; MST 600

Therapeutic Category Nonsteroidal Antiinflammatory Drug (NSAID)

Use Mild-to-moderate pain, fever, various inflammatory conditions; relief of pain and inflammation of rheumatoid arthritis and osteoarthritis

General Dosage Range Oral: *Children ≥12 years and Adults:*
Doan's® Extra Strength, Momentum®: 2 caplets every 6 hours as needed (maximum: 8 caplets/day)
Keygesic: 1 tablet every 4 hours as needed (maximum: 4 tablets/day)

Dosage Forms
Caplet, oral:
Doan's® Extra Strength [OTC]: 580 mg
Momentum® [OTC]: 580 mg
Tablet, oral:
Keygesic [OTC]: 650 mg
MST 600: 600 mg

magnesium sulfate (mag NEE zhum SUL fate)

Medication Safety Issues
Sound-alike/look-alike issues:
Magnesium sulfate may be confused with manganese sulfate, morphine sulfate
$MgSO_4$ is an error-prone abbreviation (mistaken as morphine sulfate)
High alert medication:
The Institute for Safe Medication Practices (ISMP) includes this medication (I.V. formulation) among its list of drugs which have a heightened risk of causing significant patient harm when used in error.

Synonyms epsom salts; $MgSO_4$ (error-prone abbreviation)

Therapeutic Category Anticonvulsant; Electrolyte Supplement, Oral; Laxative

Use Treatment and prevention of hypomagnesemia; prevention and treatment of seizures in severe preeclampsia or eclampsia, pediatric acute nephritis; torsade de pointes; treatment of cardiac arrhythmias (VT/VF) caused by hypomagnesemia; soaking aid

General Dosage Range
I.V.: *Children and Adults:* Dosage varies greatly depending on indication
Oral: RDA (elemental magnesium):
Children 1-13 years: 80-240 mg/day
Children ≥14 years and Adults: 310-420 mg/day
I.M.: *Adults:* Hypomagnesemia: 1-4 g/day in divided doses
Topical: *Adults:* Soaking aid: Dissolve 2 cupfuls of powder per gallon of warm water

Dosage Forms
Infusion, premixed in D_5W: 10 mg/mL (100 mL)
Infusion, premixed in water for injection: 40 mg/mL (50 mL, 100 mL, 500 mL, 1000 mL); 80 mg/mL (50 mL)
Injection, solution: 500 mg/mL (5 mL, 10 mL, 20 mL, 25 mL, 50 mL)
Injection, solution [preservative free]: 500 mg/mL (2 mL, 5 mL, 10 mL, 20 mL, 50 mL)
Powder, oral/topical: USP: 100% (227 g, 454 g, 1810 g, 2720 g)

magnesium sulfate, potassium sulfate, and sodium sulfate see sodium sulfate, potassium sulfate, and magnesium sulfate on page 824

magnesium sulfate, sodium sulfate, and potassium sulfate see sodium sulfate, potassium sulfate, and magnesium sulfate on page 824

magnesium trisilicate and aluminum hydroxide see aluminum hydroxide and magnesium trisilicate on page 60

Magnevist® see gadopentetate dimeglumine on page 408

Magonate® [OTC] see magnesium gluconate on page 545

Mag-Ox® 400 [OTC] see magnesium oxide on page 546

mag oxide see magnesium oxide on page 546

Magtrate® [OTC] see magnesium gluconate on page 545

MAH see magnesium L-aspartate hydrochloride on page 546

Makena™ see hydroxyprogesterone caproate on page 455

Malarone® see atovaquone and proguanil on page 103

Malarone® Pediatric (Can) see atovaquone and proguanil on page 103

malathion (mal a THYE on)

U.S. Brand Names Ovide®

Therapeutic Category Scabicides/Pediculicides

Use Treatment of head lice and their ova

General Dosage Range Topical: *Children and Adults:* Sprinkle lotion on dry hair, rinse after 8-12 hours; may repeat in 7-9 days

Dosage Forms
Lotion, topical: 0.5% (59 mL)
Ovide®: 0.5% (59 mL)

maltodextrin (mal toe DEK strin)

U.S. Brand Names Carrington® Oral Wound Rinse [OTC]; Multidex® [OTC]

Therapeutic Category Skin and Mucous Membrane Agent

Use Topical: Treatment of infected or noninfected wounds

General Dosage Range
Oral: *Adults:* 1 packet or tablespoonful 3-4 times/day or more if needed
Topical: *Adults:* Apply to wounds with dressing changes

Dosage Forms
Gel, topical [preservative free]:
Multidex® [OTC]: 7.1 mL (7.1 mL); 14.2 mL (14.2 mL); 85.2 mL (85.2 mL)
Powder, topical [preservative free]:
Multidex® [OTC]: 6 g (6 g); 12 g (12 g); 25 g (25 g); 45 g (45 g)
Powder for suspension, oral:
Carrington® Oral Wound Rinse [OTC]: 23 g
Solution, topical [preservative free]:
Multidex® [OTC]: 45 mL (45 mL)

Mandelamine® (Can) *see* methenamine *on page 569*

mandrake *see* podophyllum resin *on page 716*

Manerix® (Can) *see* moclobemide *(Canada only) on page 594*

manganese *see* trace metals *on page 880*

mannitol (MAN i tole)

Medication Safety Issues
Sound-alike/look-alike issues:
Osmitrol® may be confused with esmolol

Synonyms D-mannitol

U.S. Brand Names Aridol™; Osmitrol

Canadian Brand Names Osmitrol®

Therapeutic Category Diuretic, Osmotic

Use
Injection: Reduction of increased intracranial pressure associated with cerebral edema; reduction of increased intraocular pressure; promoting urinary excretion of toxic substances; genitourinary irrigant in transurethral prostatic resection or other transurethral surgical procedures
Note: Although FDA-labeled indications, the use of mannitol for the prevention of acute renal failure and/or promotion of diuresis is not routinely recommended (Kellum, 2008).
Genitourinary irrigation solution: Irrigation in transurethral prostatic resection or other transurethral surgical procedures
Powder for inhalation: Assessment of bronchial hyperresponsiveness

General Dosage Range
Inhalation: *Children ≥6 years and Adults:* 0-635 mg administered in a stepwise fashion until a positive response or the full dose has been administered (whichever comes first)
I.V.: *Adults:* Reduction of intraocular pressure: 1.5-2 g/kg
Transurethral: *Adults:* Use 5% urogenital solution as required for irrigation

Dosage Forms
Injection, solution: 20% [200 mg/mL] (250 mL, 500 mL); 25% [250 mg/mL] (50 mL)
Osmitrol: 5% [50 mg/mL] (1000 mL); 10% [100 mg/mL] (500 mL); 15% [150 mg/mL] (500 mL); 20% [200 mg/mL] (250 mL, 500 mL)
Injection, solution [preservative free]: 25% [250 mg/mL] (50 mL)

Powder, for oral inhalation:
Aridol™: 0 mg (1s) [empty], 5 mg (1s), 10 mg (1s), 20 mg (1s), 40 mg (15s) (19s)
Solution, genitourinary irrigation: 5% [50 mg/mL] (2000 mL)

mantoux *see* tuberculin tests *on page 896*

Mapap® [OTC] *see* acetaminophen *on page 23*

Mapap® Arthritis Pain [OTC] *see* acetaminophen *on page 23*

Mapap® Children's [OTC] *see* acetaminophen *on page 23*

Mapap® Extra Strength [OTC] *see* acetaminophen *on page 23*

Mapap® Infant's [OTC] *see* acetaminophen *on page 23*

Mapap® Junior Rapid Tabs [OTC] *see* acetaminophen *on page 23*

Mapap® Multi-Symptom Cold [OTC] *see* acetaminophen, dextromethorphan, and phenylephrine *on page 32*

Mapap PM [OTC] *see* acetaminophen and diphenhydramine *on page 27*

Mapap® Sinus Congestion and Pain Daytime [OTC] *see* acetaminophen and phenylephrine *on page 28*

Mapezine® (Can) *see* carbamazepine *on page 171*

maprotiline (ma PROE ti leen)

Medication Safety Issues
International issues
Ludiomil [multiple international markets] may be confused with Lamictal brand name for lamotrigine [U.S., Canada, and multiple international markets]; lamotrigine [U.S., Canada, and multiple international markets]; Lomotil brand name for diphenoxylate [U.S, Canada, and multiple international markets] and brand name for loperamide [Mexico, Philippines]
Synonyms Ludiomil; maprotiline hydrochloride
Canadian Brand Names Novo-Maprotiline
Therapeutic Category Antidepressant, Tetracyclic
Use Treatment of major depressive disorder (MDD) or of anxiety associated with depression
General Dosage Range Oral:
Adults: Initial: 75-150 mg once daily; Maintenance: 75-225 mg/day as a single dose or in divided doses
Elderly: Initial: 25 mg/day; Maintenance: 50-75 mg/day
Dosage Forms
Tablet, oral: 25 mg, 50 mg, 75 mg

maprotiline hydrochloride *see* maprotiline *on page 549*

maraviroc (mah RAV er rock)

Synonyms UK-427,857
U.S. Brand Names Selzentry™
Canadian Brand Names Celsentri™
Therapeutic Category Antiretroviral Agent, CCR5 Antagonist
Use Treatment of CCR5-tropic HIV-1 infection, in combination with other antiretroviral agents
General Dosage Range Dosage adjustment recommended in patients with renal impairment or on concomitant therapy
Oral: *Children ≥16 years and Adults:* 300 mg twice daily
Dosage Forms
Tablet, oral:
Selzentry™: 150 mg, 300 mg

Marcaine® *see* bupivacaine *on page 147*

Marcaine® Spinal *see* bupivacaine *on page 147*

Marcaine® with Epinephrine *see* bupivacaine and epinephrine *on page 148*

Mar-Cof® CG *see* guaifenesin and codeine *on page 426*

Margesic *see* butalbital, acetaminophen, and caffeine *on page 152*

Margesic® H *see* hydrocodone and acetaminophen *on page 446*

Marinol® (Can) *see* dronabinol *on page 314*

Mark 1™ *see* atropine and pralidoxime *on page 104*

Marplan® *see* isocarboxazid *on page 492*

Marvelon® (Can) *see* ethinyl estradiol and desogestrel *on page 351*
Matulane® *see* procarbazine *on page 739*
Matzim™ LA *see* diltiazem *on page 286*
3M™ Avagard™ [OTC] *see* chlorhexidine gluconate *on page 194*
Mavik® *see* trandolapril *on page 881*
Maxair® Autohaler® *see* pirbuterol *on page 708*
Maxalt® *see* rizatriptan *on page 787*
Maxalt™ (Can) *see* rizatriptan *on page 787*
Maxalt-MLT® *see* rizatriptan *on page 787*
Maxalt RPD™ (Can) *see* rizatriptan *on page 787*
Maxaron® Forte *see* polysaccharide-iron complex, vitamin B12, and folic acid *on page 721*
Maxibar™ *see* barium *on page 114*
Maxidex® *see* dexamethasone (ophthalmic) *on page 265*
Maxidone® *see* hydrocodone and acetaminophen *on page 446*
Maxifed [OTC] *see* guaifenesin and pseudoephedrine *on page 429*
Maxifed DM *see* guaifenesin, pseudoephedrine, and dextromethorphan *on page 430*
Maxifed DMX *see* guaifenesin, pseudoephedrine, and dextromethorphan *on page 430*
Maxifed-G [OTC] *see* guaifenesin and pseudoephedrine *on page 429*
Maxilene® (Can) *see* lidocaine (topical) *on page 524*
Maximum D3® [OTC] *see* cholecalciferol *on page 204*
Maxiphen [OTC] [DSC] *see* guaifenesin and phenylephrine *on page 428*
Maxiphen DM *see* guaifenesin, dextromethorphan, and phenylephrine *on page 429*
Maxiphen DMX *see* guaifenesin, dextromethorphan, and phenylephrine *on page 429*
Maxipime® *see* cefepime *on page 181*
Maxitrol® *see* neomycin, polymyxin B, and dexamethasone *on page 618*
Maxzide® *see* hydrochlorothiazide and triamterene *on page 446*
Maxzide®-25 *see* hydrochlorothiazide and triamterene *on page 446*
may apple *see* podophyllum resin *on page 716*
3M™ Cavilon™ Antifungal [OTC] *see* miconazole (topical) *on page 585*
MCH *see* collagen hemostat *on page 233*

m-cresyl acetate (em-KREE sil AS e tate)

U.S. Brand Names Cresylate™
Therapeutic Category Otic Agent, Antiinfective
Use Provides an acid medium; for external otitis infections caused by susceptible bacteria or fungus
General Dosage Range Otic: *Children and Adults:* Instill 2-4 drops as required
Dosage Forms
  Solution, otic:
    Cresylate™: 25% (15 mL)

MCT *see* medium chain triglycerides *on page 553*
MCT Oil® [OTC] *see* medium chain triglycerides *on page 553*
MCT Oil® (Can) *see* medium chain triglycerides *on page 553*
MCV *see* meningococcal (groups A / C / Y and W-135) diphtheria conjugate vaccine *on page 558*
MCV4 *see* meningococcal (groups A / C / Y and W-135) diphtheria conjugate vaccine *on page 558*
MD-76®R *see* diatrizoate meglumine and diatrizoate sodium *on page 275*
MD-Gastroview® *see* diatrizoate meglumine and diatrizoate sodium *on page 275*
MDL 73,147EF *see* dolasetron *on page 303*
MDX-010 *see* ipilimumab *on page 488*
MDX-CTLA-4 *see* ipilimumab *on page 488*
ME-609 *see* acyclovir and hydrocortisone *on page 39*

measles, mumps, and rubella virus vaccine

(MEE zels, mumpz & roo BEL a VYE rus vak SEEN)

Medication Safety Issues

Sound-alike/look-alike issues:

MMR (measles, mumps and rubella virus vaccine) may be confused with MMRV (measles, mumps, rubella, and varicella) vaccine

Synonyms MMR; mumps, measles and rubella vaccines; rubella, measles and mumps vaccines

U.S. Brand Names M-M-R® II

Canadian Brand Names M-M-R® II; Priorix™

Therapeutic Category Vaccine, Live Virus

Use Measles, mumps, and rubella prophylaxis

The Advisory Committee on Immunization Practices (ACIP) recommends routine vaccination for the following:

- All children (first dose given at 12-15 months of age)
- Adults born 1957 or later (without evidence of immunity or documentation of vaccination).
- Adults at higher risk for exposure to and transmission of measles mumps and rubella should receive special consideration for vaccination, unless an acceptable evidence of immunity exists. This includes international travelers, persons attending colleges and other post-high school education, persons working in healthcare facilities.

General Dosage Range SubQ:

Children ≥12 months: 0.5 mL

Adults: Born ≥1957 without evidence of immunity: 0.5 mL for 1 or 2 doses

Dosage Forms

Injection, powder for reconstitution [preservative free]:

M-M-R® II: Measles virus ≥1000 $TCID_{50}$, mumps virus ≥20,000 $TCID_{50}$, and rubella virus ≥1000 $TCID_{50}$

measles, mumps, rubella, and varicella virus vaccine

(MEE zels, mumpz, roo BEL a, & var i SEL a VYE rus vak SEEN)

Synonyms MMR-V; MMRV; mumps, rubella, varicella, and measles vaccine; rubella, varicella, measles, and mumps vaccine; varicella, measles, mumps, and rubella vaccine

U.S. Brand Names ProQuad®

Canadian Brand Names Priorix-Tetra™

Therapeutic Category Vaccine, Live Virus

Use To provide simultaneous active immunization against measles, mumps, rubella, and varicella

The Advisory Committee on Immunization Practices (ACIP) recommends routine vaccination against measles, mumps, rubella, and varicella in healthy children 12 months to 12 years of age. For children receiving their first dose at 12-47 months of age, either the MMRV combination vaccine or separate MMR and varicella vaccines can be used. (The ACIP prefers administration of separate MMR and varicella vaccines as the first dose in this age group unless the parent or caregiver expresses preference for the MMRV combination.) For children receiving the first dose at ≥48 months or their second dose at any age, use of MMRV is preferred.

Canadian labeling (not in U.S. labeling): MMRV combination vaccine is approved for use in healthy children 9 months to 6 years; may consider use in healthy children ≤12 years of age based upon prior experience with the separate component (live-attenuated MMR or live-attenuated varicella [OKA-strain]) vaccines.

General Dosage Range SubQ: *Children 12 months to 12 years:* 1 dose (0.5 mL)

Dosage Forms

Injection, powder for reconstitution [preservative free]:

ProQuad®: Measles virus ≥3.00 $\log_{10}$ $TCID_{50}$, mumps virus ≥4.30 $\log_{10}$ $TCID_{50}$, rubella virus ≥3.00 $\log_{10}$ $TCID_{50}$, and varicella virus ≥3.99 $\log_{10}$ PFU

Dosage Forms - Canada

Injection, powder for reconstitution [preservative free]:

Priorix-Tetra™ (CAN): Measles virus ≥3.00 $\log_{10}$ $CCID_{50}$, mumps virus ≥4.4 $\log_{10}$ $CCID_{50}$, rubella virus ≥3.00 $\log_{10}$ $CCID_{50}$, and varicella virus ≥3.3 $\log_{10}$ PFU

Mebaral® [DSC] *see* mephobarbital *on page 561*

Mebaral® (Can) *see* mephobarbital *on page 561*

mebendazole (me BEN da zole)

Medication Safety Issues

Sound-alike/look-alike issues:

Mebendazole may be confused with metroNIDAZOLE

Synonyms Vermox

Canadian Brand Names Vermox®

Therapeutic Category Anthelmintic

Use Treatment of *Enterobius vermicularis* (pinworms), *Trichuris trichiura* (whipworms), *Ascaris lumbricoides* (roundworms), and *Ancylostoma duodenale* or *Necator amiericanus* (hookworms)

General Dosage Range Oral: *Children ≥2 years and Adults:* 100 mg as a single dose **or** twice daily

Dosage Forms

Tablet, chewable, oral: 100 mg

mecasermin (mek a SER min)

Synonyms Iplex; mecasermin (rDNA origin); mecasermin rinfabate; recombinant human insulin-like growth factor-1; rhIGF-1 (mecasermin [Increlex®]); rhIGF-1/rhIGFBP-3 (mecasermin rinfabate [Iplex™])

U.S. Brand Names Increlex®

Therapeutic Category Growth Hormone

Use Treatment of growth failure in children with severe primary insulin-like growth factor-1 deficiency (IGF-1 deficiency; primary IGFD), or with growth hormone (GH) gene deletions who have developed neutralizing antibodies to GH

General Dosage Range SubQ:

Children ≥2 years: Increlex®: Initial: 0.04-0.08 mg/kg twice daily; Maintenance: 0.04-0.12 mg/kg twice daily

Children ≥3 years: Iplex™: Initial: 0.5 mg/kg once daily; Maintenance: 0.5-2 mg/kg once daily

Dosage Forms

Injection, solution:

Increlex®: 10 mg/mL (4 mL)

mecasermin (rDNA origin) *see mecasermin on page 552*

mecasermin rinfabate *see mecasermin on page 552*

mechlorethamine (me klor ETH a meen)

Medication Safety Issues

High alert medication:

The Institute for Safe Medication Practices (ISMP) includes this medication among its list of drugs which have a heightened risk of causing significant patient harm when used in error.

Synonyms chlorethazine; chlorethazine mustard; HN$_2$; mechlorethamine hydrochloride; mustine; nitrogen mustard

U.S. Brand Names Mustargen®

Canadian Brand Names Mustargen®

Therapeutic Category Antineoplastic Agent

Use Hodgkin disease; non-Hodgkin lymphoma; intracavitary injection for treatment of metastatic tumors; pleural and other malignant effusions

General Dosage Range

I.V.: *Adults:* 0.4 mg/kg as a single dose **or** in divided doses of 0.1 mg/kg/day (for 4 days) or 0.2 mg/kg/day (for 2 days) per treatment course

Intracavitary: *Adults:* 0.4 mg/kg as a single dose, although 0.2 mg/kg (10-20 mg) as a single dose has been used by the *intrapericardial* route

Dosage Forms

Injection, powder for reconstitution:

Mustargen®: 10 mg

mechlorethamine hydrochloride *see mechlorethamine on page 552*

meclizine (MEK li zeen)

Medication Safety Issues

Sound-alike/look-alike issues:

Antivert® may be confused with Anzemet®, Axert®

Synonyms meclizine hydrochloride; meclozine hydrochloride

U.S. Brand Names Antivert®; Bonine® [OTC]; Dramamine® Less Drowsy Formula [OTC]; Medi-Meclizine [OTC]; Trav-L-Tabs® [OTC]

Canadian Brand Names Bonamine™; Bonine®

Therapeutic Category Antihistamine

Use Prevention and treatment of symptoms of motion sickness; management of vertigo with diseases affecting the vestibular system

General Dosage Range Oral: *Children >12 years and Adults:* 12.5-50 mg 1 hour before travel, may repeat every 12-24 hours if needed **or** 25-100 mg/day in divided doses

Dosage Forms
Caplet, oral: 12.5 mg
Tablet, oral: 12.5 mg, 25 mg
  Antivert®: 12.5 mg, 25 mg, 50 mg
  Dramamine® Less Drowsy Formula [OTC]: 25 mg
  Medi-Meclizine [OTC]: 25 mg
  Trav-L-Tabs® [OTC]: 25 mg
Tablet, chewable, oral: 25 mg
  Bonine® [OTC]: 25 mg

meclizine hydrochloride see meclizine on page 552

meclofenamate (me kloe fen AM ate)

Synonyms meclofenamate sodium

Canadian Brand Names Meclomen®

Therapeutic Category Analgesic, Nonnarcotic; Nonsteroidal Antiinflammatory Drug (NSAID)

Use Treatment of inflammatory disorders, arthritis, mild-to-moderate pain, dysmenorrhea

General Dosage Range Oral: *Children >14 years and Adults:* 50-100 mg every 4-6 hours (maximum: 400 mg/day)

Dosage Forms
Capsule, oral: 50 mg, 100 mg

meclofenamate sodium see meclofenamate on page 553
Meclomen® (Can) see meclofenamate on page 553
meclozine hydrochloride see meclizine on page 552
Med-Baclofen (Can) see baclofen on page 112
Medent®-PEI [OTC] see guaifenesin and phenylephrine on page 428
Med-Glybe (Can) see glyburide on page 420
medicinal carbon see charcoal on page 191
medicinal charcoal see charcoal on page 191
Medicone® Hemorrhoidal [OTC] see benzocaine on page 121
Medicone® Suppositories [OTC] see phenylephrine (topical) on page 698
Medi-First® Sinus Decongestant [OTC] see phenylephrine (systemic) on page 696
Medi-Meclizine [OTC] see meclizine on page 552
Medi Pads [OTC] see witch hazel on page 923
Medi-Phenyl [OTC] see phenylephrine (systemic) on page 696
Mediproxen [OTC] see naproxen on page 612

medium chain triglycerides (mee DEE um chane trye GLIS er ides)

Synonyms MCT; triglycerides, medium chain

U.S. Brand Names MCT Oil® [OTC]

Canadian Brand Names MCT Oil®

Therapeutic Category Nutritional Supplement

Use Dietary supplement for those who cannot digest long-chain fats; malabsorption associated with disorders such as pancreatic insufficiency, bile salt deficiency, short bowel syndrome, and bacterial overgrowth of the small bowel; induce ketosis as a prevention for seizures

General Dosage Range Oral:
Infants: Initial: 0.5 mL every other feeding, then advance to every feeding, then increase in increments of 0.25-0.5 mL/feeding at intervals of 2-3 days as tolerated

◄ *Children:* 3 tablespoons/day in divided doses **or** ~39 mL with each meal **or** 50% to 70% (800-1120 kcal) of total calories (1600 kcal)

Adults: 3 tablespoons/day in divided doses **or** 15 mL 3-4 times/day

Dosage Forms

Oil, oral:

MCT Oil® [OTC]: 14 g/15 mL (960 mL)

MED-Letrozole (Can) *see* letrozole *on page 515*

Med-Metformin (Can) *see* metformin *on page 566*

Medrol® *see* methylprednisolone *on page 578*

Medrol Dose Pack *see* methylprednisolone *on page 578*

Medrol® Dosepak™ *see* methylprednisolone *on page 578*

Medroxy (Can) *see* medroxyprogesterone *on page 554*

medroxyprogesterone (me DROKS ee proe JES te rone)

Medication Safety Issues

Sound-alike/look-alike issues:

Depo-Provera® may be confused with depo-subQ provera 104™

depo-subQ provera 104™ may be confused with Depo-Provera®

MedroxyPROGESTERone may be confused with hydroxyprogesterone caproate, methylPREDNISolone, methylTESTOSTERone

Provera® may be confused with Covera®, Femara®, Parlodel®, Premarin®, Proscar®, PROzac®

Administration issues:

The injection dosage form is available in different formulations. Carefully review prescriptions to assure the correct formulation and route of administration.

Synonyms acetoxymethylprogesterone; medroxyprogesterone acetate; methylacetoxyprogesterone; MPA

Tall-Man medroxy**PROGESTER**one

U.S. Brand Names Depo-Provera®; Depo-Provera® Contraceptive; depo-subQ provera 104®; Provera®

Canadian Brand Names Alti-MPA; Apo-Medroxy®; Depo-Prevera®; Depo-Provera®; Dom-Medroxyprogesterone; Gen-Medroxy; Medroxy; Medroxyprogesterone Acetate Injectable Suspension USP; Novo-Medrone; PMS-Medroxyprogesterone; Provera-Pak; Provera®; Teva-Medroxyprogesterone

Therapeutic Category Contraceptive, Progestin Only; Progestin

Use Secondary amenorrhea or abnormal uterine bleeding due to hormonal imbalance; reduction of endometrial hyperplasia in nonhysterectomized postmenopausal women receiving conjugated estrogens; prevention of pregnancy; management of endometriosis-associated pain; adjunctive therapy and palliative treatment of recurrent and metastatic endometrial carcinoma

General Dosage Range Dosage adjustment recommended in patients with hepatic impairment.

I.M.:

Adolescents and Adults: Contraception: 150 mg every 3 months

Adults: Endometrial cancer: 400-1000 mg/week

Oral: *Adolescents and Adults:* 5-10 mg once daily

SubQ: *Adolescents and Adults:* 104 mg every 3 months (every 12-14 weeks)

Dosage Forms

Injection, suspension: 150 mg/mL (1 mL)

Depo-Provera®: 400 mg/mL (2.5 mL)

Depo-Provera® Contraceptive: 150 mg/mL (1 mL)

depo-subQ provera 104®: 104 mg/0.65 mL (0.65 mL)

Tablet, oral: 2.5 mg, 5 mg, 10 mg

Provera®: 2.5 mg, 5 mg, 10 mg

medroxyprogesterone acetate *see* medroxyprogesterone *on page 554*

Medroxyprogesterone Acetate Injectable Suspension USP (Can) *see* medroxyprogesterone *on page 554*

medroxyprogesterone and estrogens (conjugated) *see* estrogens (conjugated/equine) and medroxyprogesterone *on page 348*

Med-Salbutamol (Can) *see* albuterol *on page 45*

Med-Sotalol (Can) *see* sotalol *on page 828*

Mefenamic-250 (Can) *see* mefenamic acid *on page 555*

mefenamic acid (me fe NAM ik AS id)

Medication Safety Issues
 Sound-alike/look-alike issues:
   Ponstel® may be confused with Pronestyl®
U.S. Brand Names Ponstel®
Canadian Brand Names Apo-Mefenamic®; Dom-Mefenamic Acid; Mefenamic-250; Nu-Mefenamic; PMS-Mefenamic Acid; Ponstan®
Therapeutic Category Analgesic, Nonnarcotic; Nonsteroidal Antiinflammatory Drug (NSAID)
Use Short-term relief of mild-to-moderate pain including primary dysmenorrhea
General Dosage Range Oral: *Children >14 years and Adults:* Initial: 500 mg, then 250 mg every 4 hours as needed (maximum therapy: 1 week)
Dosage Forms
 Capsule, oral: 250 mg
   Ponstel®: 250 mg

mefloquine (ME floe kwin)

Synonyms mefloquine hydrochloride
Canadian Brand Names Apo-Mefloquine®; Lariam®
Therapeutic Category Antimalarial Agent
Use Treatment of mild-to-moderate acute malarial infections (including treatment of chloroquine-resistant malaria) and prevention of malaria caused by *Plasmodium falciparum* or *P. vivax*
General Dosage Range Oral:
 Children ≥6 months: Prophylaxis: 5 mg/kg/once weekly (maximum: 250 mg/dose); Treatment: 20-25 mg/kg/day in 2 divided doses (maximum: 1250 mg)
 Adults: Prophylaxis: 1 tablet (250 mg) once weekly; Treatment: 5 tablets (1250 mg) as a single dose
Dosage Forms
 Tablet, oral: 250 mg

mefloquine hydrochloride *see* mefloquine *on page* 555
Mefoxin® *see* cefoxitin *on page* 182
Megace® *see* megestrol *on page* 555
Megace® ES *see* megestrol *on page* 555
Megace® OS (Can) *see* megestrol *on page* 555
Megadophilus® [OTC] *see* Lactobacillus *on page* 506

megestrol (me JES trole)

Medication Safety Issues
 Sound-alike/look-alike issues:
   Megace® may be confused with Reglan®
   Megestrol may be confused with mesalamine
Synonyms 5071-1DL(6); megestrol acetate; NSC-71423
U.S. Brand Names Megace®; Megace® ES
Canadian Brand Names Apo-Megestrol®; Megace®; Megace® OS; Nu-Megestrol
Therapeutic Category Antineoplastic Agent; Progestin
Use Palliative treatment of breast and endometrial carcinoma; treatment of anorexia, cachexia, or unexplained significant weight loss in patients with AIDS
General Dosage Range Oral:
 Adults (females): Tablet: 40-320 mg/day in divided doses
 Adults (males/females): Suspension: 400-800 mg/day [Megace®] **or** 625 mg/day [Megace® ES]
Dosage Forms
 Suspension, oral: 40 mg/mL (10 mL, 20 mL, 237 mL, 240 mL, 473 mL, 480 mL)
   Megace®: 40 mg/mL (240 mL)
   Megace® ES: 125 mg/mL (150 mL)
 Tablet, oral: 20 mg, 40 mg

megestrol acetate *see* megestrol *on page* 555
Melanex® [DSC] *see* hydroquinone *on page* 453

meloxicam (mel OKS i kam)

U.S. Brand Names Mobic®

Canadian Brand Names Apo-Meloxicam®; CO Meloxicam; Dom-Meloxicam; Mobicox®; Mobic®; Mylan-Meloxicam; Novo-Meloxicam; PHL-Meloxicam; PMS-Meloxicam; ratio-Meloxicam; Teva-Meloxicam

Therapeutic Category Nonsteroidal Antiinflammatory Drug (NSAID)

Use Relief of signs and symptoms of osteoarthritis, rheumatoid arthritis, and juvenile idiopathic arthritis (JIA)

General Dosage Range Oral:
Children ≥2 years: 0.125 mg/kg/day (maximum: 7.5 mg/day)
Adults: Initial: 7.5 mg once daily; Maintenance: 7.5-15 mg once daily (maximum: 15 mg/day)

Dosage Forms
Suspension, oral: 7.5 mg/5 mL (100 mL)
Mobic®: 7.5 mg/5 mL (100 mL)
Tablet, oral: 7.5 mg, 15 mg
Mobic®: 7.5 mg, 15 mg

Melpaque HP® *see* hydroquinone *on page 453*

melphalan (MEL fa lan)

Medication Safety Issues
Sound-alike/look-alike issues:
Melphalan may be confused with Mephyton®, Myleran®
Alkeran® may be confused with Alferon®, Leukeran®, Myleran®
High alert medication:
This medication is in a class the Institute for Safe Medication Practices (ISMP) includes among its list of drug classes which have a heightened risk of causing significant patient harm when used in error.

Synonyms L-PAM; L-phenylalanine mustard; L-sarcolysin; phenylalanine mustard

U.S. Brand Names Alkeran®

Canadian Brand Names Alkeran®

Therapeutic Category Antineoplastic Agent

Use Palliative treatment of multiple myeloma and nonresectable epithelial ovarian carcinoma

General Dosage Range Dosage adjustment recommended in patients with renal impairment or who develop toxicities
I.V.: *Adults:* 16 mg/m^2 administered at 2-week intervals for 4 doses, then repeat at 4-week intervals
Oral: *Adults:* Dosage varies greatly depending on indication

Dosage Forms
Injection, powder for reconstitution: 50 mg
Alkeran®: 50 mg
Tablet, oral:
Alkeran®: 2 mg

Melquin-3® *see* hydroquinone *on page 453*
Melquin HP® *see* hydroquinone *on page 453*

memantine (me MAN teen)

Medication Safety Issues
Sound-alike/look-alike issues:
Memantine may be confused with mesalamine

Synonyms memantine hydrochloride; Namenda XR

U.S. Brand Names Namenda®

Canadian Brand Names Apo-Memantine; CO Memantine; Ebixa®; PMS-Memantine; ratio-Memantine; Riva-Memantine; Sandoz-Memantine

Therapeutic Category N-Methyl-D-Aspartate Receptor Antagonist

Use Treatment of moderate-to-severe dementia of the Alzheimer type

General Dosage Range Dosage adjustment recommended in patients with renal impairment
Oral: *Adults:* Immediate release: Initial: 5 mg once daily; Target: 20 mg/day in 2 divided doses; Extended release: Initial 7 mg once daily; Target: 28 mg/day

Product Availability
Namenda XR™: FDA approved in June 2010; anticipated availability is currently undetermined
Namenda XR™ is an extended release capsule (once-daily administration) approved for the treatment of moderate-to-severe dementia associated with Alzheimer disease.

Dosage Forms
Combination package, oral:
Namenda®: Tablet: 5 mg (28s) and Tablet: 10 mg (21s)
Solution, oral:
Namenda®: 2 mg/mL (360 mL)
Tablet, oral:
Namenda®: 5 mg, 10 mg

memantine hydrochloride *see* memantine *on page 556*

Menactra® *see* meningococcal (groups A / C / Y and W-135) diphtheria conjugate vaccine *on page 558*

menACWY-D (Menactra®) *see* meningococcal (groups A / C / Y and W-135) diphtheria conjugate vaccine *on page 558*

menACWY-CRM (Menveo®) *see* meningococcal (groups A / C / Y and W-135) diphtheria conjugate vaccine *on page 558*

menCC *see* meningococcal group C-CRM197 conjugate vaccine *(Canada only) on page 557*

menC-CRM197 *see* meningococcal group C-CRM197 conjugate vaccine *(Canada only) on page 557*

Menest® *see* estrogens (esterified) *on page 349*

meningococcal conjugate vaccine *see* meningococcal (groups A / C / Y and W-135) diphtheria conjugate vaccine *on page 558*

meningococcal group C-CRM197 conjugate vaccine *(Canada only)*
(me NIN joe kok al groop see see ahr em wuhn nahyn tee sev uhn KON joo gate vak SEEN)
Synonyms menC-CRM197; menCC
Canadian Brand Names Menjugate®
Therapeutic Category Vaccine
Use To provide active immunization against invasive meningococcal disease caused by *N. meningitidis* serogroup C, in children ≥2 months and adults

The National Advisory Committee on Immunization (NACI) recommendations for persons considered at an increased risk for meningococcal disease:
Chemoprophylaxis and immunoprophylaxis: Selection of meningococcal vaccination to be based upon serogroup(s):
Individuals living in the same household or with close contact (eg, kissing, shared cigarettes, shared eating or drinking utensils) of infected patient
Employees and children of nursery schools or day care
Immunoprophylaxis: Selection of meningococcal vaccination to be based upon serogroup(s):
Adolescents and young adults
Laboratory workers routinely exposed to isolates of *N. meningitidis*
Military recruits
Persons traveling to or who reside in countries where *N. meningitidis* is hyperendemic or epidemic, particularly if contact with local population will be prolonged
Persons with terminal complement component deficiencies
Persons with anatomic or functional asplenia
Note: Use is also recommended during meningococcal outbreaks caused by serogroup C.
Chemoprophylaxis:
Healthcare workers with intensive unprotected contact with infected patients
Airline passengers sitting directly next to an infected patient for duration of at least 8 hours

See NACI guidelines for specific drug treatment at http://www.phac-aspc.gc.ca/naci-ccni
General Dosage Range I.M.:
Infants ≥2-12 months: 0.5 mL as a single dose for a total of 3 doses
Infants ≥4-11 months without prior vaccination: 0.5 mL as a single dose for a total of 2 doses
Children ≥1 year and Adults: 0.5 mL as a single dose
Product Availability Not available in U.S.
Dosage Forms - Canada
Injection, powder for reconstitution:
Menjugate®: 10 mcg of oligosaccharide antigen group C

meningococcal (groups A / C / Y and W-135) diphtheria conjugate vaccine

(me NIN joe kok al groops aye, see, why & dubl yoo won thur tee fyve dif THEER ee a KON joo gate vak SEEN)

Medication Safety Issues

Administration issue:

Menactra® (MCV4) should be administered by intramuscular (I.M.) injection only. Inadvertent subcutaneous (SubQ) administration has been reported; possibly due to confusion of this product with Menomume® (MPSV4), also a meningococcal polysaccharide vaccine, which is administered by the SubQ route.

Synonyms MCV; MCV4; menACWY-CRM (Menveo®); menACWY-D (Menactra®); meningococcal conjugate vaccine

U.S. Brand Names Menactra®; Menveo®

Canadian Brand Names Menactra®; Menveo®

Therapeutic Category Vaccine

Use Provide active immunization of children and adults against invasive meningococcal disease caused by *N. meningitidis* serogroups A, C, Y, and W-135.

The Advisory Committee on Immunization Practices (ACIP) recommends routine vaccination of all persons at age 11 or 12 years of age, followed by a booster at age 16 years of age (CDC, 60[3], 2011). The ACIP also recommends vaccination for:

Children 9 through 23 months of age at increased risk for meningococcal disease (VFC Resolution No 6/11-1). Children at increased risk include:

- Children traveling to or who reside in countries where *N. meningitidis* is hyperendemic or epidemic, particularly if contact with local population will be prolonged
- Children with persistent complement component deficiencies (eg, C5-C9, properidin, factor H, or factor D)
- Children with HIV infection, if another indication for vaccination exists

Persons 2 through 55 years of age at increased risk for meningococcal disease (CDC, 60[3], 2011). Meningococcal conjugate vaccine (MCV4) is preferred for persons aged 2-55 years; meningococcal polysaccharide vaccine (MPSV4) is preferred in adults ≥56 years of age (CDC, 2005). Persons at increased risk include:

- Previously unvaccinated college freshmen living in dormitories
- Microbiologists routinely exposed to isolates of *N. meningitidis*
- Military recruits
- Persons traveling to or who reside in countries where *N. meningitidis* is hyperendemic or epidemic, particularly if contact with local population will be prolonged
- Persons with persistent complement component deficiencies (eg, C5-C9, properidin, factor H, or factor D)
- Persons with anatomic or functional asplenia
- Persons with HIV infection, if another indication for vaccination exists

Use is also recommended during meningococcal outbreaks caused by vaccine preventable serogroups (all recommended age groups) (CDC, 2005; VFC Resolution No. 6/11-1).

General Dosage Range I.M.:

Children 9-23 months (Menactra®): 0.5 mL/dose given as a 2-dose series, 3 months apart

Children ≥2 years and Adults ≤55 years: 0.5 mL as a single dose

Dosage Forms

Injection, solution [preservative free]:

Menactra®: 4 mcg each of polysaccharide antigen groups A, C, Y, and W-135 [bound to diphtheria toxoid 48 mcg] per 0.5 mL

Menveo®: MenA oligosaccharide 10 mcg, MenC oligosaccharide 5 mcg, MenY oligosaccharide 5 mcg, and MenW-135 oligosaccharide 5 mcg [bound to CRM_{197} protein 32.7-64.1 mcg] per 0.5 mL

meningococcal polysaccharide vaccine *see* meningococcal polysaccharide vaccine (groups A / C / Y and W-135) *on page 559*

meningococcal polysaccharide vaccine (groups A / C / Y and W-135)
(me NIN joe kok al pol i SAK a ride vak SEEN groops aye, see, why & dubl yoo won thur tee fyve)

Medication Safety Issues

Administration issue:
Menomune® (MPSV4) should be administered by subcutaneous (SubQ) injection. Menactra® (MCV4), also a meningococcal polysaccharide vaccine, is to be administered by intramuscular (I.M.) injection only.

Synonyms meningococcal polysaccharide vaccine; MPSV; MPSV4

U.S. Brand Names Menomune®-A/C/Y/W-135

Canadian Brand Names Menomune®-A/C/Y/W-135

Therapeutic Category Vaccine, Live Bacteria

Use Provide active immunity to meningococcal serogroups contained in the vaccine

The Advisory Committee on Immunization Practices (ACIP) recommends routine vaccination for persons at increased risk for meningococcal disease. Meningococcal conjugate vaccine (MCV4) is preferred for persons aged 2-55 years; meningococcal polysaccharide vaccine (MPSV4) is preferred in adults ≥56 years of age (CDC, 2005).

Persons at increased risk include:
- Previously unvaccinated college freshmen living in dormitories
- Microbiologists routinely exposed to isolates of *N. meningitidis*
- Military recruits
- Persons traveling to or who reside in countries where *N. meningitidis* is hyperendemic or epidemic, particularly if contact with local population will be prolonged
- Persons with persistent complement component deficiencies (eg, C5-C9, properidin, factor H, or factor D)
- Persons with anatomic or functional asplenia
- Persons with HIV infection

Use is also recommended during meningococcal outbreaks caused by vaccine preventable serogroups.

General Dosage Range SubQ: *Children ≥2 years and Adults:* 0.5 mL as a single dose

Dosage Forms

Injection, powder for reconstitution [MPSV4]:
Menomune®-A/C/Y/W-135: 50 mcg each of polysaccharide antigen groups A, C, Y, and W-135 per 0.5 mL dose

Menjugate® (Can) *see* meningococcal group C-CRM197 conjugate vaccine *(Canada only)* *on page 557*

Menomune®-A/C/Y/W-135 *see* meningococcal polysaccharide vaccine (groups A / C / Y and W-135) *on page 559*

Menopur® *see* menotropins *on page 559*

Menostar® *see* estradiol (systemic) *on page 343*

menotropins (men oh TROE pins)

Medication Safety Issues

Sound-alike/look-alike issues:
Repronex® may be confused with Regranex®

Synonyms hMG; human menopausal gonadotropin

U.S. Brand Names Menopur®; Repronex®

Canadian Brand Names Menopur®; Repronex®

Therapeutic Category Gonadotropin

Use Female:

In conjunction with hCG to induce ovulation and pregnancy in infertile females experiencing oligoanovulation or anovulation when the cause of anovulation is functional and not caused by primary ovarian failure (Repronex®)

Stimulation of multiple follicle development in ovulatory patients as part of an assisted reproductive technology (ART) (Menopur®, Repronex®)

General Dosage Range

I.M.: *Adults:* Repronex®: Initial: 150 int. units **or** 225 int. units daily (maximum: 450 int. units/day; 12 days of therapy)

SubQ: *Adults:* Menopur®: Initial: 225 int. units daily (maximum: 450 int. units/day; 20 days of therapy); Repronex®: Initial: 150 int. units **or** 225 int. units daily (maximum: 450 int. units/day; 12 days of therapy)

◄ **Dosage Forms**
Injection, powder for reconstitution:
Menopur®, Repronex®: Follicle stimulating hormone activity 75 int. units and luteinizing hormone activity 75 int. units

Mentax® *see* butenafine *on page 154*

menthol and methyl salicylate *see* methyl salicylate and menthol *on page 579*

menthol and zinc oxide (topical) (MEN thole & zink OKS ide)

U.S. Brand Names Calmoseptine® [OTC]; Risamine™ [OTC]

Therapeutic Category Protectant, Topical; Topical Skin Product

Use Provides a barrier to protect intact and/or injured skin from moisture, wound or fistula drainage, urine, or feces; diaper rash

General Dosage Range Topical: *Children and Adults:* Apply thin layer 2-4 times/day or after each incontinent episode/diaper change

Dosage Forms
Ointment, topical:
Calmoseptine®: Menthol 0.44% and zinc oxide 20.625% (3.5 g/packet, 75 g, 120 g)
Risamine™: Menthol 0.44% and zinc oxide 20.625% (113 g)

Menveo® *see* meningococcal (groups A / C / Y and W-135) diphtheria conjugate vaccine *on page 558*

mepenzolate (me PEN zoe late)

Medication Safety Issues
Sound-alike/look-alike issues:
Cantil® may be confused with Bentyl®

Synonyms mepenzolate bromide

U.S. Brand Names Cantil®

Canadian Brand Names Cantil®

Therapeutic Category Anticholinergic Agent

Use Adjunctive treatment of peptic ulcer disease

General Dosage Range Oral: *Adults:* 25-50 mg 4 times/day

Dosage Forms
Tablet, oral:
Cantil®: 25 mg

mepenzolate bromide *see* mepenzolate *on page 560*

meperidine (me PER i deen)

Medication Safety Issues
Sound-alike/look-alike issues:
Meperidine may be confused with meprobamate
Demerol® may be confused with Demulen®, Desyrel, dicumarol, Dilaudid®, Dymelor®, Pamelor®

High alert medication:
The Institute for Safe Medication Practices (ISMP) includes this medication among its list of drug classes which have a heightened risk of causing significant patient harm when used in error.

BEERS Criteria medication:
This drug may be inappropriate for use in geriatric patients (high severity risk).

Other safety concerns:
Avoid the use of meperidine for pain control, especially in elderly and renally-compromised patients because of the risk of neurotoxicity (American Pain Society, 2008; Institute for Safe Medication Practices [ISMP], 2007)

Synonyms isonipecaine hydrochloride; meperidine hydrochloride; pethidine hydrochloride

U.S. Brand Names Demerol®

Canadian Brand Names Demerol®

Therapeutic Category Analgesic, Narcotic

Controlled Substance C-II

Use Management of moderate-to-severe pain; adjunct to anesthesia and preoperative sedation

General Dosage Range Dosage adjustment recommended in patients with hepatic impairment
I.M., SubQ:
Children: 1.1-1.8 mg/kg/dose every 3-4 hours as needed (maximum: 50-150 mg/dose) **or** 1.1-2.2 mg/kg given 30-90 minutes before the beginning of anesthesia (maximum: 50-150 mg/dose)
Adults: 50-150 mg every 3-4 hours as needed **or** 50-150 mg given 30-90 minutes before the beginning of anesthesia **or** 50-100 mg when pain becomes regular; may repeat at every 1-3 hours
Elderly: Avoid use
Oral:
Children: 1.1-1.8 mg/kg/dose every 3-4 hours as needed (maximum: 50-150 mg/dose)
Adults: Initial: 50-150 mg every 3-4 hours as needed
Elderly: Avoid use
Dosage Forms
Injection, solution: 10 mg/mL (30 mL, 50 mL, 60 mL); 25 mg/mL (1 mL); 50 mg/mL (1 mL); 100 mg/mL (1 mL)
Demerol®: 25 mg/mL (1 mL); 25 mg/0.5 mL (0.5 mL); 50 mg/mL (1 mL, 1.5 mL, 2 mL, 30 mL); 75 mg/mL (1 mL); 100 mg/mL (1 mL, 20 mL)
Solution, oral: 50 mg/5 mL (500 mL)
Tablet, oral: 50 mg, 100 mg
Demerol®: 50 mg, 100 mg

meperidine hydrochloride *see meperidine on page 560*

mephobarbital (me foe BAR bi tal)
Medication Safety Issues
Sound-alike/look-alike issues:
Mephobarbital may be confused with methocarbamol
Mebaral® may be confused with Medrol®, Mellaril®, TEGretol®
BEERS Criteria medication:
This drug may be inappropriate for use in geriatric patients (high severity risk).
Synonyms methylphenobarbital
U.S. Brand Names Mebaral® [DSC]
Canadian Brand Names Mebaral®
Therapeutic Category Barbiturate
Controlled Substance C-IV
Use Sedative; treatment of grand mal and petit mal epilepsy
General Dosage Range Dosage adjustment recommended in patients with hepatic or renal impairment and on concomitant therapy.
Oral:
Children <5 years: 16-32 mg 3-4 times/day
Children >5 years: 16-64 mg 3-4 times/day
Adults: 96-600 mg/day in 2-4 divided doses
Dosage Forms
Tablet, oral:
Mebaral®: 32 mg, 50 mg, 100 mg

Mephyton® *see phytonadione on page 703*

mepivacaine (me PIV a kane)
Medication Safety Issues
Sound-alike/look-alike issues:
Mepivacaine may be confused with bupivacaine
Polocaine® may be confused with prilocaine
High alert medication:
The Institute for Safe Medication Practices (ISMP) includes this medication (epidural administration) among its list of drug classes which have a heightened risk of causing significant patient harm when used in error.
Synonyms mepivacaine hydrochloride
U.S. Brand Names Carbocaine®; Polocaine®; Polocaine® Dental; Polocaine® MPF; Scandonest® 3% Plain
Canadian Brand Names Carbocaine®; Polocaine®
Therapeutic Category Local Anesthetic

◀ **Use** Local or regional analgesia; anesthesia by local infiltration, peripheral and central neural techniques (epidural and caudal); **not** for use in spinal anesthesia

General Dosage Range

Brachial, cervical, intercostal, pudendal nerve block: *Adults:* 5-40 mL of 1% solution **or** 5-20 mL of 2% solution (maximum: 400 mg)

Caudal and epidural block (preservative free solutions only): *Adults:* 15-30 mL of 1% solution (maximum: 300 mg) **or** 10-25 mL of 1.5% solution (maximum: 375 mg) **or** 10-20 mL of a 2% solution (maximum: 400 mg)

Dental anesthesia: *Adults:* 54 mg (1.8 mL) as a 3% solution (single site) **or** 270 mg (9 mL) as a 3% solution (entire oral cavity) (maximum: 400 mg)

Infiltration: *Adults:* Up to 40 mL of 1% solution (maximum: 400 mg)

Local injection:

Children <3 years or <14 kg: Dose varies; only concentrations less than 2% should be used (maximum: 5-6 mg/kg)

Children ≥3 years or ≥14 kg: Dose varies (maximum: 5-6 mg/kg)

Adults: Dose varies (maximum: 400 mg/dose; 1000 mg/day)

Paracervical block: *Adults:* Up to 20 mL (both sides) of 1% solution (maximum: 200 mg)

Therapeutic block: *Adults:* 1-5 mL of 1% solution (maximum: 50 mg) or 1-5 mL of 2% solution (maximum: 100 mg)

Transvaginal block: *Adults:* Up to 30 mL (both sides) of a 1% solution (maximum: 300 mg)

Dosage Forms

Injection, solution: 3% [30 mg/mL] (1.8 mL)
Carbocaine®: 1% [10 mg/mL] (50 mL); 2% [20 mg/mL] (50 mL); 3% [30 mg/mL] (1.7 mL)
Polocaine®: 1% [10 mg/mL] (50 mL); 2% [20 mg/mL] (50 mL); 1% (10 mg/mL) (50 mL)
Polocaine® Dental: 3% [30 mg/mL] (1.7 mL)
Polocaine® MPF: 2% (20 mg/mL) (20 mL)
Scandonest® 3% Plain: 3% [30 mg/mL] (1.7 mL)

Injection, solution [preservative free]:
Carbocaine®: 1% [10 mg/mL] (30 mL); 1.5% [15 mg/mL] (30 mL); 2% [20 mg/mL] (20 mL)
Polocaine® MPF: 1% [10 mg/mL] (30 mL); 1.5% [15 mg/mL] (30 mL); 2% [20 mg/mL] (20 mL)

mepivacaine and levonordefrin (me PIV a kane & lee voe nor DEF rin)

Synonyms levonordefrin and mepivacaine hydrochloride

U.S. Brand Names Carbocaine® 2% with Neo-Cobefrin®; Polocaine® Dental with Levonordefrin; Scandonest® 2% L

Canadian Brand Names Polocaine® 2% and Levonordefrin 1:20,000

Therapeutic Category Local Anesthetic

General Dosage Range

Infiltration and nerve block (single site): *Children >10 years and Adults:* 36 mg (1.8 mL) of mepivacaine hydrochloride as a 2% solution with levonordefrin 1:20,000

Infiltration and nerve block (entire cavity):

Children ≤10 years: Carefully calculate on basis of patient's weight (maximum: 6.6 mg/kg; 180 mg of mepivacaine as 2% solution with levonordefrin 1:20,000)

Children >10 years and Adults: 180 mg (9 mL) of mepivacaine hydrochloride as 2% solution with levonordefrin 1:20,000 (maximum: 6.6 mg/kg; 400 mg of mepivacaine hydrochloride per appointment)

Dosage Forms

Injection, solution [for dental use]:
Carbocaine® 2% with Neo-Cobefrin®: Mepivacaine 2% and levonordefrin 1:20,000 (1.7 mL)
Polocaine® Dental with Levonordefrin: Mepivacaine 2% and levonordefrin 1:20,000 (1.7 mL)
Scandonest® 2% L: Mepivacaine 2% and levonordefrin 1:20,000 (1.7 mL)

mepivacaine hydrochloride *see* mepivacaine *on page 561*

meprobamate (me proe BA mate)

Medication Safety Issues

Sound-alike/look-alike issues:

Meprobamate may be confused with Mepergan, meperidine

Equanil may be confused with Elavil®

BEERS Criteria medication:

This drug may be inappropriate for use in geriatric patients (high severity risk).

Synonyms Equanil

Canadian Brand Names Novo-Mepro
Therapeutic Category Antianxiety Agent
Controlled Substance C-IV
Use Management of anxiety disorders
General Dosage Range
Oral:
Children 6-12 years: 200-600 mg/day in 2-3 divided doses
Adults: 1200-1600 mg/day in 3-4 divided doses, up to 2400 mg/day
Dosage Forms
Tablet, oral: 200 mg, 400 mg

Mepron® *see* atovaquone *on page 102*

mequinol and tretinoin (ME kwi nole & TRET i noyn)
Synonyms tretinoin and mequinol
U.S. Brand Names Solagé® [DSC]
Canadian Brand Names Solagé®
Therapeutic Category Retinoic Acid Derivative; Vitamin A Derivative; Vitamin, Topical
Use Treatment of solar lentigines; the efficacy of using Solagé® daily for >24 weeks has not been established
General Dosage Range Topical: *Adults:* Apply twice daily

mercaptoethane sulfonate *see* mesna *on page 565*

mercaptopurine (mer kap toe PYOOR een)
Medication Safety Issues
Sound-alike/look-alike issues:
Mercaptopurine may be confused with methotrexate
Purinethol® may be confused with propylthiouracil
High alert medication:
The Institute for Safe Medication Practices (ISMP) includes this medication among its list of drugs which have a heightened risk of causing significant patient harm when used in error.
Other safety concerns:
To avoid potentially serious dosage errors, the terms "6-mercaptopurine" or "6-MP" should be avoided; use of these terms has been associated with sixfold overdosages.
Azathioprine is metabolized to mercaptopurine; concurrent use of these commercially-available products has resulted in profound myelosuppression.
Synonyms 6-mercaptopurine (error-prone abbreviation); 6-MP (error-prone abbreviation); NSC-755
U.S. Brand Names Purinethol®
Canadian Brand Names Purinethol®
Therapeutic Category Antineoplastic Agent
Use Treatment (maintenance and induction) of acute lymphoblastic leukemia (ALL)
General Dosage Range Dosage adjustment recommended in patients on concomitant therapy
Oral:
Children: Induction: 2.5-5 mg/kg/day **or** 70-100 mg/m^2/day given once daily; Maintenance: 1.5-2.5 mg/kg/day **or** 50-75 mg/m^2/day given once daily
Adults: Induction: 2.5-5 mg/kg/day (100-200 mg); Maintenance: 1.5-2.5 mg/kg/day **or** 80-100 mg/m^2/day given once daily
Dosage Forms
Tablet, oral: 50 mg
Purinethol®: 50 mg

6-mercaptopurine (error-prone abbreviation) *see* mercaptopurine *on page 563*
mercapturic acid *see* acetylcysteine *on page 36*
Meridia® [DSC] *see* sibutramine *on page 810*
Meridia® (Can) *see* sibutramine *on page 810*

meropenem (mer oh PEN em)

Medication Safety Issues
Sound-alike/look-alike issues:
Meropenem may be confused with ertapenem, imipenem, metronidazole.

U.S. Brand Names Merrem® I.V.

Canadian Brand Names Merrem®

Therapeutic Category Carbapenem (Antibiotic)

Use
Treatment of intraabdominal infections (complicated appendicitis and peritonitis); treatment of bacterial meningitis in pediatric patients ≥3 months of age caused by *S. pneumoniae*, *H. influenzae*, and *N. meningitidis*; treatment of complicated skin and skin structure infections caused by susceptible organisms

Canadian labeling: Additional indications (not in U.S. labeling): Treatment of lower respiratory tract infections (community-acquired and nosocomial pneumonias), complicated urinary tract infections, gynecologic infections (excluding chlamydia), and septicemia; treatment of bacterial meningitis in adults caused by *S. pneumoniae*, *H. influenzae*, and *N. meningitidis* (use in adult meningitis based on pediatric data)

General Dosage Range Dosage adjustment recommended in patients with renal impairment
I.V.:
Children ≥3 months and <50 kg: 10-40 mg/kg every 8 hours (maximum: 2 g every 8 hours)
Children ≥50 kg and Adults: 500 mg to 2 g every 8 hours

Dosage Forms
Injection, powder for reconstitution: 500 mg, 1 g
Merrem® I.V.: 500 mg, 1 g

Merrem® (Can) *see meropenem on page 564*

Merrem® I.V. *see meropenem on page 564*

Mersyndol® With Codeine (Can) *see acetaminophen, codeine, and doxylamine (Canada only) on page 31*

mesalamine (me SAL a meen)

Medication Safety Issues
Sound-alike/look-alike issues:
Mesalamine may be confused with mecamylamine, megestrol, memantine, metaxalone, methenamine
Apriso™ may be confused with Apri®
Asacol® may be confused with Ansaid®, Os-Cal®, Visicol®
Lialda® may be confused with Aldara®
Pentasa® may be confused with Pancrease®, Pangestyme™

Synonyms 5-aminosalicylic acid; 5-ASA; fisalamine; mesalazine

U.S. Brand Names Apriso™; Asacol®; Asacol® HD; Canasa®; Lialda®; Pentasa®; Rowasa®; sfRowasa™

Canadian Brand Names 5-ASA; Asacol®; Asacol® 800; Mesasal®; Mezavant®; Novo-5 ASA; Novo-5 ASA-ECT; Pentasa®; Salofalk®; Salofalk® 5-ASA

Therapeutic Category 5-Aminosalicylic Acid Derivative

Use
Oral:
Asacol®, Lialda®, Pentasa®: Treatment and maintenance of remission of mildly- to moderately-active ulcerative colitis
Apriso™: Maintenance of remission of ulcerative colitis
Asacol® HD: Treatment of moderately-active ulcerative colitis
Rectal: Treatment of active mild-to-moderate distal ulcerative colitis, proctosigmoiditis, or proctitis

General Dosage Range
Oral: *Adults:*
Capsule: Apriso™: 1.5 g once daily; Pentasa®: 1 g 4 times/day
Tablet: Asacol®: 800 mg 3 times/day or 1.6 g/day in divided doses; Asacol® HD: 1.6 g 3 times/day; Lialda®, Mezavant®: 2.4-4.8 g once daily

Rectal: *Adults:* Retention enema: 60 mL (4 g) at bedtime, retained overnight (~8 hours); Suppository: Insert 1000 mg at bedtime

Dosage Forms
Capsule, controlled release, oral:
Pentasa®: 250 mg, 500 mg
Capsule, delayed and extended release, oral:
Apriso™: 0.375 g
Suppository, rectal:
Canasa®: 1000 mg (30s, 42s)
Suspension, rectal: 4 g/60 mL (7s, 28s)
Rowasa®: 4 g/60 mL (7s, 28s)
sfRowasa™: 4 g/60 mL (7s, 28s)
Tablet, delayed release, enteric coated, oral:
Asacol®: 400 mg
Asacol® HD: 800 mg
Lialda®: 1.2 g
Dosage Forms - Canada
Tablet, delayed and extended release:
Mezavant®: 1.2 g

mesalazine see mesalamine on page 564

Mesasal® (Can) see mesalamine on page 564

M-Eslon® (Can) see morphine (systemic) on page 598

mesna (MES na)
Synonyms mercaptoethane sulfonate; sodium 2-mercaptoethane sulfonate
U.S. Brand Names Mesnex®
Canadian Brand Names Mesna for injection
Therapeutic Category Antidote
Use Preventative agent to reduce the incidence of ifosfamide-induced hemorrhagic cystitis
General Dosage Range
I.V.: *Children and Adults:* 60% of the ifosfamide dose given in 3 divided doses
I.V.,Oral: *Children and Adults:* 100% of the ifosfamide dose, given as 20% I.V., followed by 2 (40% each) doses orally
Dosage Forms
Injection, solution: 100 mg/mL (10 mL)
Mesnex®: 100 mg/mL (10 mL)
Tablet, oral:
Mesnex®: 400 mg
Dosage Forms - Canada
Injection, solution:
Mesna for injection: 100 mg/mL (10 mL)

Mesna for injection (Can) see mesna on page 565

Mesnex® see mesna on page 565

Mestinon® see pyridostigmine on page 757

Mestinon®-SR (Can) see pyridostigmine on page 757

Mestinon® Timespan® see pyridostigmine on page 757

mestranol and norethindrone see norethindrone and mestranol on page 633

Metadate CD® see methylphenidate on page 577

Metadate® ER see methylphenidate on page 577

Metadol™ (Can) see methadone on page 567

Metadol-D™ (Can) see methadone on page 567

Metaglip™ see glipizide and metformin on page 419

123 meta-iodobenzlyguanidine sulfate see iobenguane I 123 on page 483

Metamucil® [OTC] see psyllium on page 755

Metamucil® (Can) see psyllium on page 755

Metamucil® Plus Calcium [OTC] see psyllium on page 755

Metamucil® Smooth Texture [OTC] see psyllium on page 755

metaproterenol (met a proe TER e nol)

Medication Safety Issues
Sound-alike/look-alike issues:
Metaproterenol may be confused with metipranolol, metoprolol
Alupent may be confused with Atrovent®

Synonyms Alupent; metaproterenol sulfate; orciprenaline sulfate

Canadian Brand Names Apo-Orciprenaline®; ratio-Orciprenaline®; Tanta-Orciprenaline®

Therapeutic Category Adrenergic Agonist Agent

Use Bronchodilator in reversible airway obstruction due to asthma or COPD

General Dosage Range Oral:
Children <6 years: 1.3-2.6 mg/kg/day divided every 6-8 hours
Children 6-9 years (or <27 kg): 10 mg/dose 3-4 times/day
Children >9 years (or ≥27 kg) and Adults: 20 mg 3-4 times/day

Dosage Forms
Syrup, oral: 10 mg/5 mL (473 mL)
Tablet, oral: 10 mg, 20 mg

metaproterenol sulfate *see* metaproterenol *on page 566*
Metastron® *see* strontium-89 *on page 831*

metaxalone (me TAKS a lone)

Medication Safety Issues
Sound-alike/look-alike issues:
Metaxalone may be confused with mesalamine, metolazone
Skelaxin® may be confused with Robaxin®
Beers Criteria medication:
This drug may be inappropriate for use in geriatric patients (high severity risk).

U.S. Brand Names Skelaxin®

Canadian Brand Names Skelaxin®

Therapeutic Category Skeletal Muscle Relaxant

Use Relief of discomfort associated with acute, painful musculoskeletal conditions

General Dosage Range Oral: *Children >12 years and Adults:* 800 mg 3-4 times/day

Dosage Forms
Tablet, oral: 800 mg
Skelaxin®: 800 mg

metformin (met FOR min)

Medication Safety Issues
Sound-alike/look-alike issues:
MetFORMIN may be confused with metroNIDAZOLE
Glucophage® may be confused with Glucotrol®, Glutofac®
International issues:
Dianben [Spain] may be confused with Diovan brand name for valsartan [U.S., Canada, and multiple international markets]

Synonyms metformin hydrochloride

Tall-Man metFORMIN

U.S. Brand Names Fortamet®; Glucophage®; Glucophage® XR; Glumetza®; Riomet®

Canadian Brand Names Apo-Metformin®; CO Metformin; Dom-Metformin; Glucophage®; Glumetza®; Glycon; Med-Metformin; Mylan-Metformin; Novo-Metformin; Nu-Metformin; PHL-Metformin; PMS-Metformin; PRO-Metformin; RAN™-Metformin; ratio-Metformin; Riva-Metformin; Sandoz-Metformin FC

Therapeutic Category Antidiabetic Agent, Oral

Use Management of type 2 diabetes mellitus (noninsulin-dependent, NIDDM) when hyperglycemia cannot be managed with diet and exercise alone.

General Dosage Range Oral:
Extended release: Adults: Initial: 500 mg once daily; Maintenance: Up to 2000-2500 mg/day (varies by product) in 1-2 divided doses

Immediate release:
   Children 10-16 years: Initial: 500 mg twice daily; Maintenance: Up to 2000 mg/day in divided doses
   Children >16 years and Adults: Initial: 500 mg twice daily **or** 850 mg once daily; Maintenance: Up to 2000 mg/day in 2 divided doses **or** 2550 mg/day in 3 divided doses

Dosage Forms
   Solution, oral:
      Riomet®: 100 mg/mL (118 mL, 473 mL)
   Tablet, oral: 500 mg, 850 mg, 1000 mg
      Glucophage®: 500 mg, 850 mg, 1000 mg
   Tablet, extended release, oral: 500 mg, 750 mg
      Fortamet®: 500 mg, 1000 mg
      Glucophage® XR: 500 mg, 750 mg
      Glumetza®: 500 mg, 1000 mg

metformin and glipizide *see* glipizide and metformin *on page 419*

metformin and glyburide *see* glyburide and metformin *on page 421*

metformin and repaglinide *see* repaglinide and metformin *on page 774*

metformin and rosiglitazone *see* rosiglitazone and metformin *on page 791*

metformin and saxagliptin *see* saxagliptin and metformin *on page 803*

metformin and sitagliptin *see* sitagliptin and metformin *on page 816*

metformin hydrochloride *see* metformin *on page 566*

metformin hydrochloride and pioglitazone hydrochloride *see* pioglitazone and metformin *on page 706*

metformin hydrochloride and rosiglitazone maleate *see* rosiglitazone and metformin *on page 791*

metformin hydrochloride and saxagliptin *see* saxagliptin and metformin *on page 803*

methacholine (meth a KOLE leen)

Synonyms methacholine chloride

U.S. Brand Names Provocholine®

Canadian Brand Names Methacholine Omega; Provocholine®

Therapeutic Category Diagnostic Agent

Use Diagnosis of bronchial airway hyperactivity

General Dosage Range Inhalation: *Children ≥5 years and Adults:* 5 breaths of each of the following concentrations 0.025 mg/mL, 0.25 mg/mL, 2.5 mg/mL, 10 mg/mL, and 25 mg/mL

Dosage Forms
   Powder for reconstitution, for oral inhalation:
      Provocholine®: 100 mg

methacholine chloride *see* methacholine *on page 567*

Methacholine Omega (Can) *see* methacholine *on page 567*

methadone (METH a done)

Medication Safety Issues
   Sound-alike/look-alike issues:
      Methadone may be confused with dexmethylphenidate, Mephyton®, methylphenidate, Metadate® CD, Metadate® ER, morphine
   High alert medication:
      The Institute for Safe Medication Practices (ISMP) includes this medication among its list of drug classes which have a heightened risk of causing significant patient harm when used in error.

Synonyms methadone hydrochloride

U.S. Brand Names Dolophine®; Methadone Diskets®; Methadone Intensol™; Methadose®

Canadian Brand Names Metadol-D™; Metadol™

Therapeutic Category Analgesic, Narcotic

Controlled Substance C-II

Use Management of moderate-to-severe pain; detoxification and maintenance treatment of opioid addiction as part of an FDA-approved program

◄ **General Dosage Range** Dosage adjustment recommended in patients with renal impairment or who develop toxicities
I.M.:
Adults: Initial: 2.5 mg every 8-12 hours
Elderly: 2.5 mg every 8-12 hours
I.V., SubQ: *Adults:* Initial: 2.5 mg every 8-12 hours
Oral:
Adults: Detoxification: Initial: Up to 40 mg/day; Maintenance: 80-120 mg/day; Pain: 2.5-10 mg every 4-12 hours as needed
Elderly: 2.5 mg every 8-12 hours
Dosage Forms
Injection, solution: 10 mg/mL (20 mL)
Solution, oral: 5 mg/5 mL (500 mL); 10 mg/5 mL (500 mL); 10 mg/mL (946 mL, 960 mL, 1000 mL, 1000s)
Methadone Intensol™: 10 mg/mL (30 mL)
Methadose®: 10 mg/mL (1000 mL)
Tablet, oral: 5 mg, 10 mg
Dolophine®: 5 mg, 10 mg
Tablet, dispersible, oral: 40 mg
Methadone Diskets®: 40 mg
Methadose®: 40 mg

Methadone Diskets® *see* methadone *on page 567*
methadone hydrochloride *see* methadone *on page 567*
Methadone Intensol™ *see* methadone *on page 567*
Methadose® *see* methadone *on page 567*
methaminodiazepoxide hydrochloride *see* chlordiazepoxide *on page 194*

methamphetamine (meth am FET a meen)
Medication Safety Issues
Sound-alike/look-alike issues:
Desoxyn® may be confused with digoxin
BEERS Criteria medication:
This drug may be inappropriate for use in geriatric patients (high severity risk).
Synonyms desoxyephedrine hydrochloride; methamphetamine hydrochloride
U.S. Brand Names Desoxyn®
Canadian Brand Names Desoxyn®
Therapeutic Category Amphetamine
Controlled Substance C-II
Use Treatment of attention-deficit/hyperactivity disorder (ADHD); exogenous obesity (short-term adjunct)

Pharmacotherapy for weight loss is recommended only for obese patients with a body mass index ≥30 kg/m^2, or ≥27 kg/m^2 in the presence of other risk factors such as hypertension, diabetes, and/or dyslipidemia or a high waist circumference; therapy should be used in conjunction with a comprehensive weight management program.
General Dosage Range Oral:
Children ≥6-11 years: Initial: 5 mg 1-2 times/day; Maintenance: 20-25 mg/day
Children ≥12 years and Adults: ADHD: Initial: 5 mg 1-2 times/day; Maintenance: 20-25 mg/day; Obesity: 5 mg before each meal
Dosage Forms
Tablet, oral: 5 mg
Desoxyn®: 5 mg

methamphetamine hydrochloride *see* methamphetamine *on page 568*

methazolamide (meth a ZOE la mide)
Medication Safety Issues
Sound-alike/look-alike issues:
Methazolamide may be confused with methenamine, metolazone
Neptazane™ may be confused with Nesacaine®
U.S. Brand Names Neptazane™

Canadian Brand Names Apo-Methazolamide®

Therapeutic Category Carbonic Anhydrase Inhibitor

Use Treatment of chronic open-angle or secondary glaucoma; short-term therapy of acute angle-closure glaucoma prior to surgery

General Dosage Range Oral: *Adults:* 50-100 mg 2-3 times/day

Dosage Forms
  Tablet, oral: 25 mg, 50 mg
    Neptazane™: 25 mg, 50 mg

methenamine (meth EN a meen)

Medication Safety Issues
  Sound-alike/look-alike issues:
    Hiprex® may be confused with Mirapex®
    Methenamine may be confused with mesalamine, methazolamide, methionine
    Urex may be confused with Eurax®, serax
  International issues:
    Urex: Brand name for methenamine [U.S. (discontinued)], but also the brand name for furosemide [Australia, China, Turkey]
    Urex [U.S. (discontinued)] may be confused with Eurax brand name for crotamitin [U.S., Canada, and multiple international markets]

Synonyms hexamethylenetetramine; methenamine hippurate; methenamine mandelate; Urex

U.S. Brand Names Hiprex®

Canadian Brand Names Dehydral®; Hiprex®; Mandelamine®; Urasal®

Therapeutic Category Antibiotic, Miscellaneous

Use Prophylaxis or suppression of recurrent urinary tract infections; urinary tract discomfort secondary to hypermotility

General Dosage Range Oral:
  Hippurate:
    Children ≥6 years: 0.5-1 g twice daily
    Adults: 1 g twice daily
  Mandelate:
    Children >2-6 years: 50-75 mg/kg/day in 3-4 divided doses **or** 0.25 g/30 lb 4 times/day
    Children 6-12 years: 50-75 mg/kg/day in 3-4 divided doses **or** 0.5 g 4 times/day
    Children >12 years and Adults: 1 g 4 times/day

Dosage Forms
  Tablet, oral: 500 mg, 1 g
    Hiprex®: 1 g

methenamine hippurate *see* methenamine *on page 569*
methenamine mandelate *see* methenamine *on page 569*

methenamine, phenyl salicylate, methylene blue, benzoic acid, and hyoscyamine

(meth EN a meen, fen nil sa LIS i late, METH i leen bloo, ben ZOE ik AS id & hye oh SYE a meen)

Synonyms benzoic acid, hyoscyamine, methenamine, methylene blue, and phenyl salicylate; benzoic acid, methenamine, methylene blue, phenyl salicylate, and hyoscyamine; hyoscyamine, methenamine, benzoic acid, phenyl salicylate, and methylene blue; methylene blue, methenamine, benzoic acid, phenyl salicylate, and hyoscyamine; phenyl salicylate, methenamine, methylene blue, benzoic acid, and hyoscyamine

U.S. Brand Names Prosed®/DS

Therapeutic Category Antibiotic, Miscellaneous

Use Urinary tract discomfort secondary to hypermotility resulting from infection or diagnostic procedures

General Dosage Range Oral: *Adults:* 1 tablet 4 times/day

Dosage Forms
  Tablet, oral:
    Prosed®/DS: Methenamine 81.6 mg, phenyl salicylate 36.2 mg, methylene blue 10.8 mg, benzoic acid 9 mg, hyoscyamine sulfate 0.12 mg

Methergine® *see* methylergonovine *on page 576*

methimazole (meth IM a zole)

Medication Safety Issues

  Sound-alike/look-alike issues:

    Methimazole may be confused with metolazone

Synonyms thiamazole

U.S. Brand Names Tapazole®

Canadian Brand Names Dom-Methimazole; PHL-Methimazole; Tapazole®

Therapeutic Category Antithyroid Agent

Use Treatment of hyperthyroidism; improve hyperthyroidism prior to thyroidectomy or radioactive iodine therapy

General Dosage Range Oral:

  Children: Initial: 0.4 mg/kg/day in 3 divided doses; Maintenance: 0.2 mg/kg/day in 3 divided doses

  Adults: Initial: 15-60 mg/day in 3 divided doses; Maintenance: 5-15 mg/day in 1-3 divided doses

Dosage Forms

  Tablet, oral: 5 mg, 10 mg

  Tapazole®: 5 mg, 10 mg

Methitest™ *see* methyltestosterone *on page* 579

methocarbamol (meth oh KAR ba mole)

Medication Safety Issues

  Sound-alike/look-alike issues:

    Methocarbamol may be confused with mephobarbital

    Robaxin® may be confused with ribavirin, Rubex®, Skelaxin®

  BEERS Criteria medication:

    This drug may be inappropriate for use in geriatric patients (high severity risk).

U.S. Brand Names Robaxin®; Robaxin®-750

Canadian Brand Names Robaxin®

Therapeutic Category Skeletal Muscle Relaxant

Use Adjunctive treatment of muscle spasm associated with acute painful musculoskeletal conditions (eg, tetanus)

General Dosage Range

  I.M.: *Adults:* 1 g every 8 hours (maximum dose: 3 g/day for 3 consecutive days)

  I.V.:

    Children: 15 mg/kg/dose **or** 500 mg/m^2/dose every 6 hours as needed (maximum dose: 1.8 g/m^2/day for 3 consecutive days)

    Adults: 1-3 g every 6 hours **or** 1 g every 8 hours (maximum dose: 3 g/day for 3 consecutive days)

    Oral: *Children ≥16 years and Adults:* Initial: 1.5 g 4 times/day for 2-3 days (maximum: 8 g/day); Maintenance: 4-4.5 g/day in 3-6 divided doses

Dosage Forms

  Injection, solution:

  Robaxin®: 100 mg/mL (10 mL)

  Tablet, oral: 500 mg, 750 mg

  Robaxin®: 500 mg

  Robaxin®-750: 750 mg

methohexital (meth oh HEKS i tal)

Medication Safety Issues

  Sound-alike/look-alike issues:

    Brevital® may be confused with Brevibloc®

  High alert medication:

    The Institute for Safe Medication Practices (ISMP) includes this medication among its list of drugs which have a heightened risk of causing significant patient harm when used in error.

Synonyms methohexital sodium

U.S. Brand Names Brevital® Sodium

Canadian Brand Names Brevital®

Therapeutic Category Barbiturate

Controlled Substance C-IV

Use Induction of anesthesia; procedural sedation

General Dosage Range Dosage adjustment recommended in patients with hepatic impairment
I.M.: *Infants ≥1 month and Children:* Induction: 6.6-10 mg/kg of a 5% solution
I.V.: *Adults:* Induction: 1-1.5 mg/kg
Rectal: *Infants ≥1 month and Children:* Induction: 25 mg/kg of a 1% solution **or** 25 mg/kg of a 10% (100 mg/mL) solution; maximum dose: 500 mg

Dosage Forms
Injection, powder for reconstitution:
Brevital® Sodium: 500 mg, 2.5 g

methohexital sodium *see* methohexital *on page 570*

methotrexate (meth oh TREKS ate)

Medication Safety Issues
Sound-alike/look-alike issues:
Methotrexate may be confused with mercaptopurine, methylPREDNISolone sodium succinate, metolazone, metroNIDAZOLE, mitoXANtrone, PRALAtrexate
High alert medication:
The Institute for Safe Medication Practices (ISMP) includes this medication among its list of drugs which have a heightened risk of causing significant patient harm when used in error.
Administration issues:
Errors have occurred (resulting in death) when methotrexate was administered as "daily" dose instead of the recommended "weekly" dose.

Intrathecal medication safety: The American Society of Clinical Oncology (ASCO)/Oncology Nursing Society (ONS) chemotherapy administration safety standards (Jacobson, 2009) encourage the following safety measures for intrathecal chemotherapy:
• Intrathecal medication should not be prepared during the preparation of any other agents
• After preparation, store in an isolated location or container clearly marked with a label identifying as "intrathecal" use only
• Delivery to the patient should only be with other medications intended for administration into the central nervous system
Other safety concerns:
MTX is an error-prone abbreviation (mistaken as mitoxantrone).
International issues:
Trexall [U.S.] may be confused with Trexol brand name for tamadol [Mexico]; Truxal brand name for chlorprothixene [multiple international markets]
Synonyms amethopterin; methotrexate sodium; methotrexatum; MTX (error-prone abbreviation)
U.S. Brand Names Rheumatrex®; Trexall™
Canadian Brand Names Apo-Methotrexate®; ratio-Methotrexate
Therapeutic Category Antineoplastic Agent
Use
Oncology-related uses: Treatment of trophoblastic neoplasms (gestational choriocarcinoma, chorioadenoma destruens and hydatidiform mole), acute lymphocytic leukemia (ALL), meningeal leukemia, breast cancer, head and neck cancer (epidermoid), cutaneous T-Cell lymphoma (advanced mycosis fungoides), lung cancer (squamous cell and small cell), advanced non-Hodgkin lymphomas (NHL), osteosarcoma
Nononcology uses: Treatment of psoriasis (severe, recalcitrant, disabling) and severe rheumatoid arthritis (RA), including polyarticular-course juvenile idiopathic arthritis (JIA)
General Dosage Range Dosage adjustment recommended in patients with hepatic or renal impairment
I.M., oral:
Children: 5-30 mg/m^2 once weekly or every 2 weeks
Adults: Dosage varies greatly depending on indication
I.V.:
Children: 10-18,000 mg/m^2 bolus dosing or continuous infusion over 6-42 hours
Adults: Dosage varies greatly depending on indication
Intrathecal:
Children <1 year: 6 mg/dose
Children 1 year: 8 mg/dose
Children 2 years: 10 mg/dose
Children ≥3 years and Adults: 12 mg/dose

◄ **Dosage Forms**
  Injection, powder for reconstitution: 1 g
  Injection, solution: 25 mg/mL (2 mL, 10 mL)
  Injection, solution [preservative free]: 25 mg/mL (2 mL, 4 mL, 8 mL, 10 mL, 20 mL, 40 mL, 100 mL)
  Tablet, oral: 2.5 mg
    Rheumatrex®: 2.5 mg
    Trexall™: 5 mg, 7.5 mg, 10 mg, 15 mg

methotrexate sodium *see* methotrexate *on page 571*

methotrexatum *see* methotrexate *on page 571*

methotreximeprazine *(Canada only)* (meth oh trye MEP ra zeen)

Synonyms levomepromazine; methotrimeprazine hydrochloride

Canadian Brand Names Apo-Methoprazine®; Novo-Meprazine; Nozinan®; PMS-Methotrimeprazine

Therapeutic Category Neuroleptic Agent

Use Treatment of schizophrenia; psychosis; manic-depressive syndromes; anxiety or tension disorders; management of pain, including pain caused by neuralgia or cancer; adjunct to general anesthesia; management of nausea and vomiting; sedation

General Dosage Range
I.M.:
  Children: 0.063-0.125 mg/kg/day in 1-3 divided doses
  Adults: 10-25 mg every 8 hours **or** 75-100 mg as a single dose
I.V.:
  Children: 0.063 mg/kg in 250 mL D_5W infused at a rate of 20-40 drops/minute
  Adults: 10-25 mg in 500 mL D_5W infused at a rate of 20-40 drops/minute
Oral:
  Children: 0.25 mg/kg/day in 2-3 divided doses (maximum: 40 mg/day [children <12 years])
  Adults: 6-75 mg/day in 2-3 divided doses (maximum: doses up to 1000 mg/day have been used) **or** 10-25 mg at bedtime

Product Availability Not available in U.S.

Dosage Forms - Canada
Injection, solution:
  Nozinan®: 25 mg/mL (1 mL)
Tablet, oral: 2 mg, 5 mg, 25 mg, 50 mg

methotrimeprazine hydrochloride *see* methotrimeprazine *(Canada only) on page 572*

methoxsalen (systemic) (meth OKS a len)

Medication Safety Issues
Sound-alike/look-alike issues:
  Methoxsalen soft gelatin capsules (Oxsoralen-Ultra®) may be confused with methoxsalen hard gelatin capsules (8-MOP®, Oxsoralen®); bioavailability and photosensitization onset differ between the two products.

Synonyms 8-methoxypsoralen; methoxypsoralen

U.S. Brand Names 8-MOP®; Oxsoralen-Ultra®; Uvadex®

Canadian Brand Names Oxsoralen-Ultra®; Oxsoralen® Capsule; Ultramop™

Therapeutic Category Psoralen

Use
Oral: Symptomatic control of severe, recalcitrant disabling psoriasis; repigmentation of idiopathic vitiligo; palliative treatment of skin manifestations of cutaneous T-cell lymphoma (CTCL)
Extracorporeal: Palliative treatment of skin manifestations of CTCL

General Dosage Range
Extracorporeal: *Adults:* Amount of Uvadex® needed for each treatment may be calculated using the following equation: Treatment volume x 0.017 = mL of Uvadex® needed. Inject this amount into photoactivation bag and administer treatment for 2 consecutive days every 4 weeks for a minimum of 7 treatment cycles; may increase to every 2 weeks (maximum: 20 accelerated therapy cycles)
Oral: *Adults:* Psoriasis: Initial: 10-70 mg; may repeat 2-3 times/week (48 hours between doses); Maintenance: 1 treatment every 1-3 weeks; Vitiligo: 20 mg

Dosage Forms
 Capsule, oral:
  8-MOP®: 10 mg
  Oxsoralen-Ultra®: 10 mg
 Solution, for extracorporeal administration:
  Uvadex®: 20 mcg/mL (10 mL)

methoxsalen (topical) (meth OKS a len)

Synonyms methoxypsoralen
U.S. Brand Names Oxsoralen®
Canadian Brand Names Oxsoralen® Lotion
Therapeutic Category Psoralen
Use Repigmentation of idiopathic vitiligo
General Dosage Range Topical: *Children ≥12 years and Adults:* Lotion is applied by healthcare provider prior to UVA light exposure, usually no more than once weekly
Dosage Forms
 Lotion, topical:
  Oxsoralen®: 1% (29.57 mL)

methoxypsoralen *see* methoxsalen (systemic) *on page 572*
methoxypsoralen *see* methoxsalen (topical) *on page 573*
8-methoxypsoralen *see* methoxsalen (systemic) *on page 572*

methscopolamine (meth skoe POL a meen)

Medication Safety Issues
 International issues:
  Pamine [U.S., Canada] may be confused with Pemine brand name for penicillamine [Italy]
Synonyms methscopolamine bromide
U.S. Brand Names Pamine®; Pamine® Forte
Canadian Brand Names Pamine®
Therapeutic Category Anticholinergic Agent
Use Adjunctive therapy in the treatment of peptic ulcer
General Dosage Range Oral: *Adults:* 2.5-5 mg twice daily
Dosage Forms
 Tablet, oral: 2.5 mg, 5 mg
  Pamine®: 2.5 mg
  Pamine® Forte: 5 mg

methscopolamine and pseudoephedrine *see* pseudoephedrine and methscopolamine *on page 753*
methscopolamine bromide *see* methscopolamine *on page 573*
methscopolamine, chlorpheniramine, and pseudoephedrine *see* chlorpheniramine, pseudoephedrine, and methscopolamine *on page 202*
methscopolamine nitrate, chlorpheniramine maleate, and phenylephrine hydrochloride *see* chlorpheniramine, phenylephrine, and methscopolamine *on page 200*
methscopolamine, pseudoephedrine, and chlorpheniramine *see* chlorpheniramine, pseudoephedrine, and methscopolamine *on page 202*

methsuximide (meth SUKS i mide)

Medication Safety Issues
 Sound-alike/look-alike issues:
  Methsuximide may be confused with ethosuximide
U.S. Brand Names Celontin®
Canadian Brand Names Celontin®
Therapeutic Category Anticonvulsant
Use Control of absence (petit mal) seizures that are refractory to other drugs
General Dosage Range Oral: *Adults:* Initial: 300 mg/day for 1 week; Maintenance: Up to 1.2 g/day in 2-4 divided doses

Dosage Forms
Capsule, oral:
Celontin®: 150 mg, 300 mg

methyclothiazide (meth i kloe THYE a zide)

Medication Safety Issues
Sound-alike/look-alike issues:
Enduron® may be confused with Empirin®, Imuran®, Inderal®
Synonyms Enduron
Therapeutic Category Diuretic, Thiazide
Use Management of mild-to-moderate hypertension; treatment of edema in congestive heart failure and nephrotic syndrome
General Dosage Range Oral: *Adults:* 2.5-10 mg once daily
Dosage Forms
Tablet, oral: 5 mg

methylacetoxyprogesterone *see* medroxyprogesterone *on page 554*

methyl aminolevulinate (METH il a mee noe LEV ue lin ate)

Medication Safety Issues
Sound-alike/look-alike issues:
Methyl aminolevulinate may be confused with aminolevulinic acid
Synonyms methyl aminolevulinate hydrochloride; P-1202
U.S. Brand Names Metvixia™
Canadian Brand Names Metvix®
Therapeutic Category Photosensitizing Agent, Topical; Topical Skin Product
Use Treatment of thin and moderately thick, nonhyperkeratotic, nonpigmented actinic keratoses of the face and scalp; to be used in conjunction with red light illumination
General Dosage Range Topical: *Adults:* Apply up to 1 g once; repeat in 1 week
Dosage Forms
Cream, topical:
Metvixia™: 16.8% (2 g)

methyl aminolevulinate hydrochloride *see* methyl aminolevulinate *on page 574*

methylcellulose (meth il SEL yoo lose)

Medication Safety Issues
Sound-alike/look-alike issues:
Citrucel® may be confused with Citracal®
U.S. Brand Names Citrucel® [OTC]; Soluble Fiber Therapy [OTC]
Therapeutic Category Laxative
Use Adjunct in treatment of constipation
General Dosage Range Oral:
Caplet:
Children 6-11 years: 1 caplet up to 6 times/day (maximum: 6 caplets/day)
Children ≥12 years and Adults: 2 caplets up to 6 times/day (maximum: 12 caplets/day)
Powder:
Children 6-11 years: 1 g (2-2.5 level teaspoons) up to 3 times/day
Children ≥12 years and Adults: 2 g (1 rounded or heaping tablespoon) up to 3 times/day
Dosage Forms
Caplet, oral:
Citrucel® [OTC]: 500 mg
Powder, oral:
Citrucel® [OTC]: 2 g/scoop (454 g, 479 g, 850 g, 907 g, 1190 g, 1843 g)
Soluble Fiber Therapy [OTC]: 2 g/scoop (454 g)

methylcellulose, gelatin, and pectin *see* gelatin, pectin, and methylcellulose *on page 413*
methylcobalamin, acetylcysteine, and methylfolate *see* methylfolate, methylcobalamin, and acetylcysteine *on page 576*

methyldopa (meth il DOE pa)

Medication Safety Issues
  Sound-alike/look-alike issues:
    Methyldopa may be confused with L-dopa, levodopa
  BEERS Criteria medication:
    This drug may be inappropriate for use in geriatric patients (high severity risk).
Synonyms Aldomet; methyldopate hydrochloride
Canadian Brand Names Apo-Methyldopa®; Nu-Medopa
Therapeutic Category Alpha-Adrenergic Blocking Agent
Use Management of moderate-to-severe hypertension
General Dosage Range Dosage adjustment recommended in patients with renal impairment
  I.V.:
    Children: 5-10 mg/kg/dose every 6-8 hours (maximum: 65 mg/kg/day; 3 g/day)
    Adults: 250-500 mg every 6-8 hours (maximum: 1 g every 6 hours)
  Oral:
    Children: Initial: 10 mg/kg/day in 2-4 divided doses; Maintenance: Up to 65 mg/kg/day (maximum: 3 g/day)
    Adults: Initial: 250 mg 2-3 times/day; Maintenance: 250-1000 mg/day in 2 divided doses (maximum: 3 g/day)
    Elderly: Initial: 125 mg 1-2 times/day
Dosage Forms
  Injection, solution: 50 mg/mL (5 mL)
  Tablet, oral: 250 mg, 500 mg

methyldopa and hydrochlorothiazide (meth il DOE pa & hye droe klor oh THYE a zide)

Medication Safety Issues
  Sound-alike/look-alike issues:
    Aldoril® may be confused with Aldoclor®, Aldomet®, Elavil®
  BEERS Criteria medication:
    This drug may be inappropriate for use in geriatric patients (high severity risk).
Synonyms Aldoril; hydrochlorothiazide and methyldopa
Canadian Brand Names Apo-Methazide®
Therapeutic Category Antihypertensive Agent, Combination
Use Management of moderate-to-severe hypertension
General Dosage Range Oral: *Adults:* 1 tablet 2-3 times/day (maximum: 50 mg/day [hydrochlorothiazide]; 3 g/day [methyldopa])
Dosage Forms
  Tablet: Methyldopa 250 mg and hydrochlorothiazide 15 mg; methyldopa 250 mg and hydrochlorothiazide 25 mg

methyldopate hydrochloride *see* methyldopa *on page 575*

methylene blue (METH i leen bloo)

Medication Safety Issues
  Other safety concerns:
    Due to the potential for dosing errors between mg and mL of methylene blue, prescribing and dosing should only be expressed in terms of mg of methylene blue (and not as mL)
    Due to potential toxicity (hemolytic anemia), do not use methylene blue to color enteral feedings to detect aspiration.
Synonyms methylthionine chloride
Therapeutic Category Antidote
Use Antidote for cyanide poisoning and drug-induced methemoglobinemia, indicator dye
General Dosage Range I.V.: *Children and Adults:* 1-2 mg/kg **or** 25-50 mg/m^2 as a single dose; may repeat
Dosage Forms
  Injection, solution: 10 mg/mL (1 mL, 10 mL)

methylene blue, methenamine, benzoic acid, phenyl salicylate, and hyoscyamine *see* methenamine, phenyl salicylate, methylene blue, benzoic acid, and hyoscyamine *on page 569*

methylergometrine maleate *see methylergonovine on page 576*

methylergonovine (meth il er goe NOE veen)

Medication Safety Issues
Sound-alike/look-alike issues:
Methergine® may be confused with Brethine
Methylergonovine and terbutaline parenteral dosage forms look similar. Due to their contrasting indications, use care when administering these agents.

Synonyms methylergometrine maleate; methylergonovine maleate

U.S. Brand Names Methergine®

Canadian Brand Names Methergine®

Therapeutic Category Ergot Alkaloid and Derivative

Use Prevention and treatment of postpartum and postabortion hemorrhage caused by uterine atony or subinvolution

General Dosage Range
I.M., I.V.: *Adults:* 0.2 mg after delivery; may repeat every 2-4 hours
Oral: *Adults:* 0.2 mg 3-4 times/day in the puerperium

Dosage Forms
Injection, solution: 0.2 mg/mL (1 mL)
Methergine®: 0.2 mg/mL (1 mL)
Tablet, oral:
Methergine®: 0.2 mg

methylergonovine maleate *see methylergonovine on page 576*

methylfolate (meth il FO late)

Synonyms 6(S)-5-methyltetrahydrofolate; 6(S)-5-MTHF; L-methylfolate

U.S. Brand Names Deplin™

Therapeutic Category Dietary Supplement

Use Medicinal food for management of patients with low plasma and/or low red blood cell folate

General Dosage Range Oral: *Adults:* 7.5 mg daily

Dosage Forms
Tablet, oral: L-methylfolate 7.5 mg
Deplin™: L-methylfolate 7.5 mg

methylfolate, methylcobalamin, and acetylcysteine
(meth il FO late meth il koe BAL a min & a se teel SIS teen)

Synonyms acetylcysteine, methylcobalamin, and methylfolate; acetylcysteine, methylfolate, and methylcobalamin; L-methylfolate, methylcobalamin, and N-acetylcysteine; methylcobalamin, acetylcysteine, and methylfolate

U.S. Brand Names Cerefolin® NAC

Therapeutic Category Dietary Supplement

Use Medicinal food for use in patients with neurovascular oxidative stress and/or hyperhomocysteinemia

General Dosage Range Oral: *Children ≥12 years and Adults:* 1 caplet daily

Dosage Forms
Caplet, oral:
Cerefolin® NAC: L-methylfolate 5.6 mg, methylcobalamin 2 mg, and N-acetylcysteine 600 mg [gluten free, sugar free]

Methylin® *see methylphenidate on page 577*
Methylin® ER [DSC] *see methylphenidate on page 577*
methylmorphine *see codeine on page 229*

methylnaltrexone (meth il nal TREKS one)

Medication Safety Issues
Sound-alike/look-alike issues:
Methylnaltrexone may be confused with naltrexone

Synonyms methylnaltrexone bromide; N-methylnaltrexone bromide

U.S. Brand Names Relistor®

Canadian Brand Names Relistor®

Therapeutic Category Gastrointestinal Agent, Miscellaneous; Opioid Antagonist, Peripherally-Acting

Use Treatment of opioid-induced constipation in patients with advanced illness receiving palliative care with inadequate response to conventional laxative regimens

General Dosage Range Dosage adjustment recommended in patients with renal impairment

SubQ:
Adults <38 kg and >114 kg: 0.15 mg/kg (round dose up to nearest 0.1 mL of volume) every other day as needed (maximum: 1 dose/24 hours)
Adults 38 to <62 kg: 8 mg every other day as needed (maximum: 1 dose/24 hours)
Adults 62-114 kg: 12 mg every other day as needed (maximum: 1 dose/24 hours)

Dosage Forms

Injection, solution:
Relistor®: 12 mg/0.6 mL (0.6 mL)

methylnaltrexone bromide see methylnaltrexone *on page 576*

methylphenidate (meth il FEN i date)

Medication Safety Issues

Sound-alike/look-alike issues:
Metadate CD® may be confused with Metadate® ER
Metadate® ER may be confused with Metadate CD®, methadone
Methylphenidate may be confused with methadone
Ritalin® may be confused with Ismelin®, Rifadin®, ritodrine
Ritalin LA® may be confused with Ritalin-SR®
Ritalin-SR® may be confused with Ritalin LA®

Synonyms methylphenidate hydrochloride

U.S. Brand Names Concerta®; Daytrana®; Metadate CD®; Metadate® ER; Methylin®; Methylin® ER [DSC]; Ritalin LA®; Ritalin-SR®; Ritalin®

Canadian Brand Names Apo-Methylphenidate®; Apo-Methylphenidate® SR; Biphentin®; Concerta®; Novo-Methylphenidate ER-C; PHL-Methylphenidate; PMS-Methylphenidate; ratio-Methylphenidate; Ritalin®; Ritalin® SR; Sandoz-Methylphenidate SR

Therapeutic Category Central Nervous System Stimulant, Nonamphetamine

Controlled Substance C-II

Use Treatment of attention-deficit/hyperactivity disorder (ADHD); symptomatic management of narcolepsy

General Dosage Range

Oral:
Immediate release:
Children ≥6 years: Initial: 5 mg twice daily; Maintenance: Increase by 5-10 mg/day at weekly intervals (maximum: 60 mg/day)
Adults: ADHD: Initial: 5 mg twice daily; Maintenance: Increase by 5-10 mg/day at weekly intervals (maximum: 60 mg/day); Narcolepsy: 10 mg 2-3 times/day (maximum: 60 mg/day)
Extended release:
Children 6-12 years: Concerta®: 18-54 mg once every morning (maximum: 54 mg/day); Metadate® ER, Methylin® ER, Ritalin® SR: Maximum: 60 mg/day; Metadate CD®, Ritalin LA®: Initial: 20 mg once daily (maximum: 60 mg/day)
Children 13-17 years and Adults: Concerta®: 18-72 mg once every morning (maximum: 72 mg/day); Metadate CD®, Ritalin LA®: Initial: 20 mg once daily (maximum: 60 mg/day)
Transdermal: *Children 6-17 years:* Initial: 10 mg patch once daily

Dosage Forms

Capsule, extended release, oral:
Metadate CD®: 10 mg, 20 mg, 30 mg, 40 mg, 50 mg, 60 mg
Ritalin LA®: 10 mg, 20 mg, 30 mg, 40 mg

Patch, transdermal:
Daytrana®: 10 mg/9 hours (30s); 15 mg/9 hours (30s); 20 mg/9 hours (30s); 30 mg/9 hours (30s)

Solution, oral:
Methylin®: 5 mg/5 mL (500 mL); 10 mg/5 mL (500 mL)

Tablet, oral: 5 mg, 10 mg, 20 mg
Ritalin®: 5 mg, 10 mg, 20 mg

Tablet, chewable, oral:
Methylin®: 2.5 mg, 5 mg, 10 mg

◄ **Tablet, extended release, oral**: 10 mg, 18 mg, 20 mg, 27 mg, 36 mg, 54 mg
   Concerta®: 18 mg, 27 mg, 36 mg, 54 mg
   Metadate® ER: 20 mg
   Tablet, sustained release, oral: 20 mg
   Ritalin-SR®: 20 mg

methylphenidate hydrochloride *see* methylphenidate *on page 577*
methylphenobarbital *see* mephobarbital *on page 561*
methylphenoxy-benzene propanamine *see* atomoxetine *on page 101*
methylphenyl isoxazolyl penicillin *see* oxacillin *on page 658*
methylphytyl napthoquinone *see* phytonadione *on page 703*

methylprednisolone (meth il pred NIS oh lone)

Medication Safety Issues
Sound-alike/look-alike issues:
MethylPREDNISolone may be confused with medroxyPROGESTERone, methotrexate, methylTES-TOSTERone, predniSONE
Depo-Medrol® may be confused with Solu-Medrol®
Medrol® may be confused with Mebaral®
Solu-MEDROL® may be confused with Depo-Medrol®, salmeterol, Solu-CORTEF®
International issues:
Medrol [U.S., Canada, and multiple international markets] may be confused with Medral brand name for omeprazole [Mexico]

Synonyms 6-α-methylprednisolone; Medrol Dose Pack; methylprednisolone acetate; methylprednisolone sodium succinate; Solumedrol

Tall-Man methyl**PREDNIS**olone

U.S. Brand Names A-Methapred®; Depo-Medrol®; Medrol®; Medrol® Dosepak™; Solu-MEDROL®
Canadian Brand Names Depo-Medrol®; Medrol®; Methylprednisolone Acetate; Solu-Medrol®
Therapeutic Category Adrenal Corticosteroid
Use Primarily as an antiinflammatory or immunosuppressant agent in the treatment of a variety of diseases including those of hematologic, allergic, inflammatory, neoplastic, and autoimmune origin. Prevention and treatment of graft-versus-host disease following allogeneic bone marrow transplantation.

General Dosage Range
I.M.:
Acetate: *Adults:* 10-120 mg every 1-2 weeks
Sodium succinate:
   Children: 0.5-1.7 mg/kg/day **or** 5-25 mg/m²/day divided every 6-12 hours; "Pulse" therapy: 15-30 mg/kg/dose given once daily for 3 days
   Adults: 10-80 mg once daily
I.V. (sodium succinate): *Children and Adults:* Dosage varies greatly by indication
Intraarticular (acetate): *Adults:* Administer every 1-5 weeks
   Large joints (eg, knee, ankle): 20-80 mg
   Medium joints (eg, elbow, wrist): 10-40 mg
   Small joints: 4-10 mg
Intralesional (acetate): *Adults:* 20-60 mg every 1-5 weeks
Oral:
   Children: 0.5-1.7 mg/kg/day **or** 5-25 mg/m²/day divided every 6-12 hours; "Pulse" therapy: 15-30 mg/kg/dose once daily for 3 days
   Adults: 2-60 mg/day in 1-4 divided doses

Dosage Forms
Injection, powder for reconstitution: 40 mg, 125 mg, 500 mg, 1 g
   A-Methapred®: 40 mg, 125 mg
   Solu-MEDROL®: 500 mg, 1 g, 2 g
Injection, powder for reconstitution [preservative free]:
   Solu-MEDROL®: 40 mg, 125 mg, 500 mg, 1 g
Injection, suspension: 40 mg/mL (1 mL, 5 mL, 10 mL); 80 mg/mL (1 mL, 5 mL)
   Depo-Medrol®: 20 mg/mL (5 mL); 40 mg/mL (5 mL, 10 mL); 80 mg/mL (5 mL)
Injection, suspension [preservative free]:
   Depo-Medrol®: 40 mg/mL (1 mL); 80 mg/mL (1 mL)
Tablet, oral: 4 mg, 8 mg, 16 mg, 32 mg
   Medrol®: 2 mg, 4 mg, 8 mg, 16 mg, 32 mg
   Medrol® Dosepak™: 4 mg

6-α-methylprednisolone *see* methylprednisolone *on page 578*

methylprednisolone acetate *see* methylprednisolone *on page 578*

Methylprednisolone Acetate (Can) *see* methylprednisolone *on page 578*

methylprednisolone sodium succinate *see* methylprednisolone *on page 578*

4-methylpyrazole *see* fomepizole *on page 398*

methyl salicylate and menthol (METH il sa LIS i late & MEN thol)

Medication Safety Issues
   Other safety concerns:
      Transdermal patch may contain conducting metal (eg, aluminum); remove patch prior to MRI.
Synonyms menthol and methyl salicylate
U.S. Brand Names BenGay® [OTC]; Icy Hot® [OTC]; Salonpas® Arthritis Pain® [OTC]; Salonpas® Pain Relief Patch® [OTC]; Salonpas® [OTC]; Thera-Gesic® Plus [OTC]; Thera-Gesic® [OTC]
Therapeutic Category Analgesic, Topical; Salicylate; Topical Skin Product
Use Temporary relief of minor aches and pains of muscle and joints associated with arthritis, bruises, simple backache, sprains, and strains
General Dosage Range Topical:
   Balm, cream, stick: *Children ≥12 years of age and Adults:* Apply up to 3-4 times/day
   Gel: *Children ≥2 years of age and Adults:* Apply up to 3-4 times/day
   Patch: *Adults:* Apply 1 patch for up to 8-12 hours (maximum: 1 patch/application; 2 patches/24 hours; 3 days of consecutive use)
Dosage Forms
   Balm, topical:
      Icy Hot® Balm [OTC]: Methyl salicylate 29% and menthol 7.6% (99.2 g)
   Cream, topical:
      BenGay® Arthritis Formula [OTC]: Methyl salicylate 30% and menthol 8% (57 g, 113 g)
      BenGay® Greaseless [OTC]: Methyl salicylate 15% and menthol 10% (57 g, 113 g)
      Icy Hot® [OTC]: Methyl salicylate 30% and menthol 10% (35.4 g, 85 g)
      Thera-Gesic® [OTC]: Methyl salicylate 15% and menthol 1% (85 g, 142 g)
      Thera-Gesic® Plus [OTC]: Methyl salicylate 15% and menthol 4% (85 g) [contains aloe]
   Gel, topical:
      Salonpas® [OTC]: Methyl salicylate 15% and menthol 7% (40 g) [contains ethanol]
   Patch, topical:
      Salonpas® Arthritis Pain® [OTC], Salonpas® Pain Relief Patch® [OTC]: Methyl salicylate 10% and menthol 3% (5s)
   Stick, topical:
      Icy Hot® [OTC]: Methyl salicylate 30% and menthol 10% (49 g)

methyltestosterone (meth il tes TOS te rone)

Medication Safety Issues
   Sound-alike/look-alike issues:
      MethylTESTOSTERone may be confused with medroxyPROGESTERone, methylPREDNISolone
      Virilon® may be confused with Verelan®
   Beers Criteria medication:
      This drug may be inappropriate for use in geriatric patients (high severity risk).
Tall-Man methylTESTOSTERone
U.S. Brand Names Android®; Methitest™; Testred®
Therapeutic Category Androgen
Controlled Substance C-III
Use
   Male: Hypogonadism; delayed puberty; impotence and climacteric symptoms
   Female: Palliative treatment of metastatic breast cancer
General Dosage Range
   Oral:
      Adults (female): 50-200 mg/day
      Adults (male): 10-50 mg/day

◀ **Dosage Forms**
Capsule, oral:
Android®: 10 mg
Testred®: 10 mg
Tablet, oral:
Methitest™: 10 mg

methyltestosterone and esterified estrogen *see* estrogens (esterified) and methyltestosterone *on page 349*

methylthionine chloride *see* methylene blue *on page 575*

metipranolol (met i PRAN oh lol)

Medication Safety Issues
Sound-alike/look-alike issues:
Metipranolol may be confused with metaproterenol
International issues:
Betanol [Monaco] may be confused with Beta-Val brand name for betamethasone [U.S.]; Betimol brand name for timolol [U.S., Finland]; Patanol brand name for olopatadine [U.S., Canada, and multiple international markets]

Synonyms metipranolol hydrochloride

U.S. Brand Names OptiPranolol®

Canadian Brand Names OptiPranolol®

Therapeutic Category Beta-Adrenergic Blocker

Use Treatment of chronic open-angle glaucoma or ocular hypertension

General Dosage Range Ophthalmic: *Adults:* Instill 1 drop into affected eye(s) twice daily

Dosage Forms
Solution, ophthalmic: 0.3% (5 mL, 10 mL)
OptiPranolol®: 0.3% (5 mL, 10 mL)

metipranolol hydrochloride *see* metipranolol *on page 580*

metoclopramide (met oh KLOE pra mide)

Medication Safety Issues
Sound-alike/look-alike issues:
Metoclopramide may be confused with metolazone, metoprolol, metroNIDAZOLE
Reglan® may be confused with Megace®, Regonol®, Renagel®

U.S. Brand Names Metozolv™ ODT; Reglan®

Canadian Brand Names Apo-Metoclop®; Metoclopramide Hydrochloride Injection; Metoclopramide Omega; Nu-Metoclopramide; PMS-Metoclopramide

Therapeutic Category Gastrointestinal Agent, Prokinetic

Use
Oral: Symptomatic treatment of diabetic gastroparesis; gastroesophageal reflux
I.V., I.M.: Symptomatic treatment of diabetic gastroparesis; postpyloric placement of enteral feeding tubes; prevention and/or treatment of nausea and vomiting associated with chemotherapy, or postsurgery; to stimulate gastric emptying and intestinal transit of barium during radiological examination of the stomach/small intestine

General Dosage Range Dosage adjustment recommended in patients with renal impairment
I.M.: *Adults:* 10-20 mg as a single dose **or** 10 mg before each meal and at bedtime
I.V.:
Children <6 years: 0.1 mg/kg as a single dose
Children 6-14 years: 2.5-5 mg as a single dose
Children >14 years: 10 mg as a single dose
Adults: 10 mg before each meal and at bedtime **or** 1-2 mg/kg every 2-3 hours (maximum: 5 doses/day) **or** 10 mg as a single dose
Oral: *Adults:* 10-15 mg up to 4 times/day

Dosage Forms
Injection, solution [preservative free]: 5 mg/mL (2 mL, 10 mL, 20 mL, 30 mL)
Reglan®: 5 mg/mL (2 mL, 10 mL, 30 mL)
Solution, oral: 5 mg/5 mL (0.9 mL, 10 mL, 473 mL, 480 mL)

Tablet, oral: 5 mg, 10 mg
  Reglan®: 5 mg, 10 mg
Tablet, orally disintegrating, oral:
  Metozolv™ ODT: 5 mg, 10 mg

Metoclopramide Hydrochloride Injection (Can) *see* metoclopramide *on page* 580
Metoclopramide Omega (Can) *see* metoclopramide *on page* 580

metolazone (me TOLE a zone)
Medication Safety Issues
  Sound-alike/look-alike issues:
    Metolazone may be confused with metaxalone, methazolamide, methimazole, methotrexate, metoclopramide, metoprolol, minoxidil
    Zaroxolyn® may be confused with Zarontin®
U.S. Brand Names Zaroxolyn®
Canadian Brand Names Zaroxolyn®
Therapeutic Category Diuretic, Miscellaneous
Use Management of mild-to-moderate hypertension; treatment of edema in heart failure and nephrotic syndrome, impaired renal function
General Dosage Range Oral: *Adults:* 2.5-20 mg every 24 hours
Dosage Forms
  Tablet, oral: 2.5 mg, 5 mg, 10 mg
    Zaroxolyn®: 2.5 mg, 5 mg

Metopirone® *see* metyrapone *on page* 584

metoprolol (me toe PROE lole)
Medication Safety Issues
  Sound-alike/look-alike issues:
    Lopressor® may be confused with Lyrica®
    Metoprolol may be confused with metaproterenol, metoclopramide, metolazone, misoprostol
    Metoprolol succinate may be confused with metoprolol tartrate
    Toprol-XL® may be confused with TEGretol®, TEGretol®-XR, Topamax®
  High alert medication:
    The Institute for Safe Medication Practices (ISMP) includes this medication among its list of drugs which have a heightened risk of causing significant patient harm when used in error.
  Administration issues:
    Significant differences exist between oral and I.V. dosing. Use caution when converting from one route of administration to another.
Synonyms metoprolol succinate; metoprolol tartrate
U.S. Brand Names Lopressor®; Toprol-XL®
Canadian Brand Names Apo-Metoprolol (Type L®); Apo-Metoprolol SR®; Apo-Metoprolol®; Betaloc®; Dom-Metoprolol; JAMP-Metoprolol-L; Lopressor®; Metoprolol Tartrate Injection, USP; Metoprolol-25; Metoprolol-L; Mylan-Metoprolol (Type L); Nu-Metop; PHL-Metoprolol; PMS-Metoprolol; Riva-Metoprolol; Sandoz-Metoprolol (Type L); Sandoz-Metoprolol SR; Teva-Metoprolol
Therapeutic Category Beta-Adrenergic Blocker
Use Treatment of angina pectoris, hypertension, or hemodynamically-stable acute myocardial infarction
  Extended release: Treatment of angina pectoris or hypertension; to reduce mortality/hospitalization in patients with heart failure (stable NYHA Class II or III) already receiving ACE inhibitors, diuretics, and/or digoxin
General Dosage Range
  I.V.: *Adults:* 1.25-5 mg every 6-12 hours (maximum: 15 mg every 3 hours) **or** 5 mg every 2 minutes for 3 doses (acute MI)
  Oral:
    Extended release:
      Children ≥6 years: 1-2 mg/kg once daily (maximum: 2 mg/kg/day or 200 mg/day)
      Adults: 12.5-200 mg/day (maximum: 400 mg/day)
    Immediate release:
      Children >1 year: 1-6 mg/kg/day divided twice daily (maximum: 200 mg/day)
      Adults: 50-450 mg/day in 2-3 divided doses

◀ **Dosage Forms**
Injection, solution: 1 mg/mL (5 mL)
Lopressor®: 1 mg/mL (5 mL)
Injection, solution [preservative free]: 1 mg/mL (5 mL)
Tablet, oral: 25 mg, 50 mg, 100 mg
Lopressor®: 50 mg, 100 mg
Tablet, extended release, oral: 25 mg, 50 mg, 100 mg, 200 mg
Toprol-XL®: 25 mg, 50 mg, 100 mg, 200 mg

Metoprolol-25 (Can) see metoprolol on page 581
Metoprolol-L (Can) see metoprolol on page 581

metoprolol and hydrochlorothiazide (me toe PROE lole & hye droe klor oh THYE a zide)

Synonyms hydrochlorothiazide and metoprolol; hydrochlorothiazide and metoprolol tartrate; metoprolol tartrate and hydrochlorothiazide
U.S. Brand Names Lopressor HCT®
Therapeutic Category Beta Blocker, Beta-1 Selective; Diuretic, Thiazide
Use Treatment of hypertension (not recommended for initial treatment)
General Dosage Range Oral: *Adults:* Metoprolol 50-100 mg and hydrochlorothiazide 25-50 mg administered daily as single or 2 divided doses (maximum: 50 mg/day [hydrochlorothiazide])
Dosage Forms
Tablet: 50/25: Metoprolol 50 mg and hydrochlorothiazide 25 mg; 100/25: Metoprolol 100 mg and hydrochlorothiazide 25 mg; 100/50: Metoprolol 100 mg and hydrochlorothiazide 50 mg
Lopressor HCT®: 50/25: Metoprolol 50 mg and hydrochlorothiazide 25 mg; 100/25: Metoprolol 100 mg and hydrochlorothiazide 25 mg

metoprolol succinate see metoprolol on page 581
metoprolol tartrate see metoprolol on page 581
metoprolol tartrate and hydrochlorothiazide see metoprolol and hydrochlorothiazide on page 582
Metoprolol Tartrate Injection, USP (Can) see metoprolol on page 581
Metozolv™ ODT see metoclopramide on page 580
MetroCream® see metronidazole (topical) on page 583
MetroGel® see metronidazole (topical) on page 583
Metrogel® (Can) see metronidazole (topical) on page 583
MetroGel® 1% Kit see metronidazole (topical) on page 583
MetroGel-Vaginal® see metronidazole (topical) on page 583
MetroLotion® see metronidazole (topical) on page 583

metronidazole (systemic) (met roe NYE da zole)

Medication Safety Issues
Sound-alike/look-alike issues:
MetroNIDAZOLE may be confused with mebendazole, meropenem, metFORMIN, methotrexate, metoclopramide, miconazole
Synonyms metronidazole hydrochloride
Tall-Man metroNIDAZOLE
U.S. Brand Names Flagyl®; Flagyl® 375; Flagyl® ER
Canadian Brand Names Apo-Metronidazole®; Flagyl®; Florazole® ER
Therapeutic Category Amebicide; Antibiotic, Miscellaneous; Antiprotozoal, Nitroimidazole
Use Treatment of susceptible anaerobic bacterial and protozoal infections in the following conditions: Amebiasis, symptomatic and asymptomatic trichomoniasis; skin and skin structure infections, bone and joint infections, CNS infections, endocarditis, gynecologic infections, intraabdominal infections (as part of combination regimen), respiratory tract infections (lower), systemic anaerobic infections; treatment of antibiotic-associated pseudomembranous colitis (AAPC); as part of a multidrug regimen for *H. pylori* eradication to reduce the risk of duodenal ulcer recurrence; surgical prophylaxis (colorectal)
General Dosage Range Dosage adjustment recommended in patients with hepatic or renal impairment.
I.V.: *Adults:* 500 mg every 6-8 hours (maximum: 4 g/day)
Oral:
Extended release: *Adults:* 750 mg once daily

Regular release:
  Infants and Children: 35-50 mg/kg/day divided every 8 hours
  Adults: 250-750 mg every 6-12 hours (maximum: 4 g/day) **or** 2 g as a single dose
Dosage Forms
  Capsule, oral: 375 mg
    Flagyl® 375: 375 mg
  Infusion, premixed iso-osmotic sodium chloride solution: 500 mg (100 mL)
  Tablet, oral: 250 mg, 500 mg
    Flagyl®: 250 mg, 500 mg
  Tablet, extended release, oral:
    Flagyl® ER: 750 mg

metronidazole (topical) (met roe NYE da zole)

Synonyms metronidazole hydrochloride
Tall-Man metro**NIDAZOLE**
U.S. Brand Names MetroCream®; MetroGel-Vaginal®; MetroGel®; MetroGel® 1% Kit; MetroLotion®; Noritate®; Vandazole®
Canadian Brand Names MetroCream®; Metrogel®; MetroLotion®; Nidagel™; Noritate®; Rosasol®
Therapeutic Category Antibiotic, Topical
Use
Topical: Treatment of inflammatory lesions and erythema of rosacea
Vaginal gel: Bacterial vaginosis
General Dosage Range
  Intravaginal: *Adults:* 1 applicatorful (~37.5 mg metronidazole) intravaginally once or twice daily
  Topical: *Adults:* Apply a thin film to affected area once (1%) or twice (0.75%) daily
Dosage Forms
  Cream, topical: 0.75% (45 g)
    MetroCream®: 0.75% (45 g)
    Noritate®: 1% (60 g)
  Gel, topical: 0.75% (45 g)
    MetroGel®: 1% (60 g)
    MetroGel® 1% Kit: 1% (60 g)
  Gel, vaginal: 0.75% (70 g)
    MetroGel-Vaginal®: 0.75% (70 g)
    Vandazole®: 0.75% (70 g)
  Lotion, topical: 0.75% (59 mL, 60 mL)
    MetroLotion®: 0.75% (59 mL)

metronidazole and nystatin *(Canada only)* (met roe NYE da zole & nye STAT in)

Synonyms nystatin and metronidazole
Canadian Brand Names Flagystatin®
Therapeutic Category Antifungal Agent, Vaginal; Antiprotozoal, Nitroimidazole
Use Treatment of mixed vaginal infection due to *T. vaginalis* and *C. albicans*
General Dosage Range Intravaginal: *Adults:* Insert 1 applicatorful or tablet daily
Product Availability Not available in U.S.
Dosage Forms - Canada
  Cream, vaginal:
    Flagystatin®: Metronidazole 500 mg and nystatin 100,000 units per applicatorful (55 g)
  Tablet, vaginal:
    Flagystatin® Ovule: Metronidazole 500 mg and nystatin 100,000 units (10s)

metronidazole, bismuth subcitrate potassium, and tetracycline *see* bismuth, metronidazole, and tetracycline *on page 136*
metronidazole, bismuth subsalicylate, and tetracycline *see* bismuth, metronidazole, and tetracycline *on page 136*
metronidazole hydrochloride *see* metronidazole (systemic) *on page 582*
metronidazole hydrochloride *see* metronidazole (topical) *on page 583*
Metvix® (Can) *see* methyl aminolevulinate *on page 574*
Metvixia™ *see* methyl aminolevulinate *on page 574*

metyrapone (me TEER a pone)

Medication Safety Issues
Sound-alike/look-alike issues:
Metyrapone may be confused with metyrosine

U.S. Brand Names Metopirone®

Therapeutic Category Diagnostic Agent

Use Diagnostic test for hypothalamic-pituitary ACTH function

General Dosage Range Oral:
Children: 15 mg/kg (minimum: 250 mg; maximum: 750 mg) every 4 hours for 6 doses **or** 30 mg/kg (maximum: 3 g) as a single dose
Adults: 750 mg every 4 hours for 6 doses **or** 30 mg/kg (maximum: 3 g) as a single dose

Dosage Forms
Capsule, oral:
Metopirone®: 250 mg

metyrosine (me TYE roe seen)

Medication Safety Issues
Sound-alike/look-alike issues:
Metyrosine may be confused with metyrapone

Synonyms AMPT; OGMT

U.S. Brand Names Demser®

Canadian Brand Names Demser®

Therapeutic Category Tyrosine Hydroxylase Inhibitor

Use Short-term management of pheochromocytoma before surgery, long-term management when surgery is contraindicated or when chronic malignant pheochromocytoma exists

General Dosage Range Oral: *Children >12 years and Adults:* Initial: 250 mg 4 times/day; Maintenance: 2-3 g/day in 4 divided doses (maximum: 4 g/day)

Dosage Forms
Capsule, oral:
Demser®: 250 mg

Mevacor® *see* lovastatin *on page 540*
mevinolin *see* lovastatin *on page 540*

mexiletine (meks IL e teen)

Canadian Brand Names Novo-Mexiletine

Therapeutic Category Antiarrhythmic Agent, Class I-B

Use Management of serious ventricular arrhythmias; suppression of PVCs

General Dosage Range Dosage adjustment recommended in patients with hepatic impairment
Oral: *Adults:* Initial: 200 mg every 8 hours; Maintenance: 200-300 mg every 8 hours (maximum: 1.2 g/day)

Dosage Forms
Capsule, oral: 150 mg, 200 mg, 250 mg

Mezavant® (Can) *see* mesalamine *on page 564*
MG217® Medicated Tar [OTC] *see* coal tar *on page 227*
MG217® Medicated Tar Extra Strength [OTC] *see* coal tar *on page 227*
MG217® Medicated Tar Intensive Strength [OTC] *see* coal tar *on page 227*
MG217® Sal-Acid [OTC] *see* salicylic acid *on page 795*
MgSO₄ (error-prone abbreviation) *see* magnesium sulfate *on page 547*
Miacalcin® *see* calcitonin *on page 159*
Miacalcin® NS (Can) *see* calcitonin *on page 159*
Mi-Acid [OTC] *see* aluminum hydroxide, magnesium hydroxide, and simethicone *on page 60*
Mi-Acid™ Double Strength [OTC] *see* calcium carbonate and magnesium hydroxide *on page 162*
Mi-Acid Gas Relief [OTC] *see* simethicone *on page 812*
Mi-Acid Maximum Strength [OTC] [DSC] *see* aluminum hydroxide, magnesium hydroxide, and simethicone *on page 60*
Micaderm® [OTC] *see* miconazole (topical) *on page 585*

micafungin (mi ka FUN gin)

Synonyms micafungin sodium

U.S. Brand Names Mycamine®

Canadian Brand Names Mycamine®

Therapeutic Category Antifungal Agent, Parenteral; Drug-induced Neuritis, Treatment Agent

Use Treatment of esophageal candidiasis; *Candida* prophylaxis in patients undergoing hematopoietic stem cell transplant (HSCT); treatment of candidemia, acute disseminated candidiasis, and other *Candida* infections (peritonitis and abscesses)

General Dosage Range I.V.: *Adults:* Prophylaxis: 50 mg daily; Treatment: 100-150 mg daily

Dosage Forms

Injection, powder for reconstitution:
Mycamine®: 50 mg, 100 mg

micafungin sodium *see* micafungin *on page 585*

Micanol® (Can) *see* anthralin *on page 80*

Micardis® *see* telmisartan *on page 848*

Micardis® HCT *see* telmisartan and hydrochlorothiazide *on page 848*

Micardis® Plus (Can) *see* telmisartan and hydrochlorothiazide *on page 848*

Micatin® [OTC] *see* miconazole (topical) *on page 585*

Micatin® (Can) *see* miconazole (topical) *on page 585*

miconazole (oral) (mi KON a zole)

Medication Safety Issues

Sound-alike/look-alike issues:
Miconazole may be confused with metroNIDAZOLE, Micronase®, Micronor®

Synonyms miconazole nitrate

U.S. Brand Names Oravig®

Therapeutic Category Antifungal Agent, Oral Nonabsorbed

Use Treatment of oropharyngeal candidiasis

General Dosage Range Buccal: *Children ≥16 years and Adults:* 50 mg (1 tablet) once daily

Dosage Forms

Tablet, for buccal application:
Oravig®: 50 mg

miconazole (topical) (mi KON a zole)

Medication Safety Issues

Sound-alike/look-alike issues:
Miconazole may be confused with metroNIDAZOLE, Micronase®, Micronor®
Lotrimin® may be confused with Lotrisone®, Otrivin®
Micatin® may be confused with Miacalcin®

Synonyms miconazole nitrate

U.S. Brand Names 3M™ Cavilon™ Antifungal [OTC]; Aloe Vesta® Antifungal [OTC]; Baza® Antifungal [OTC]; Carrington® Antifungal [OTC]; Critic-Aid® Clear AF [OTC]; DermaFungal [OTC]; Dermagran® AF [OTC]; DiabetAid® Antifungal Foot Bath [OTC]; Fungoid® [OTC]; Lotrimin AF® [OTC]; Micaderm® [OTC]; Micatin® [OTC]; Micro-Guard® [OTC]; Miranel AF™ [OTC]; Mitrazol® [OTC]; Monistat® 1 Day or Night [OTC]; Monistat® 1 [OTC]; Monistat® 3 [OTC]; Monistat® 7 [OTC]; Neosporin® AF [OTC]; Podactin Cream [OTC]; Secura® Antifungal Extra Thick [OTC]; Secura® Antifungal Greaseless [OTC]; Ting® Spray Powder [OTC]; Zeasorb®-AF [OTC]

Canadian Brand Names Dermazole; Micatin®; Micozole; Monistat®; Monistat® 3

Therapeutic Category Antifungal Agent

Use Treatment of vulvovaginal candidiasis and a variety of skin and mucous membrane fungal infections

General Dosage Range

Intravaginal: *Children ≥12 years and Adults:* Insert 1 applicatorful or suppository (100 mg or 200 mg) once daily at bedtime **or** insert 1 suppository (1200 mg) as a single dose.

Topical: *Children and Adults:* Apply twice daily **or** dissolve 1 effervescent tablet in ~1 gallon of water and soak feet for 15-30 minutes

◀ **Dosage Forms**
  Aerosol, topical:
    Lotrimin AF® [OTC]: 2% (133 g)
    Micatin® [OTC]: 2% (90 g, 105 mL); 2% (90 g)
    Neosporin® AF [OTC]: 2% (105 mL); 2% (85 g)
    Ting® Spray Powder [OTC]: 2% (128 g)
  Combination package, topical/vaginal: Cream, topical: 2% (9 g) and Suppository, vaginal: 200 mg (3s)
    Monistat® 1 [OTC]: Cream, topical: 2% (9 g) and Insert, vaginal: 1200 mg (1)
    Monistat® 3 [OTC]: Cream, topical: 2% (9 g) and Cream, vaginal: 4% (25 g), Cream, topical: 2% (9 g)
      and Cream, vaginal: 4% (3 x 5 g), Cream, topical: 2% (9 g) and Insert, vaginal: 200 mg (3s)
    Monistat® 7 [OTC]: Cream, topical: 2% (9 g) and Cream, vaginal: 2% (45 g), Cream, topical: 2% (9 g)
      and Cream, vaginal: 2% (7 x 5 g), Cream, topical: 2% (9 g) and Suppository, vaginal: 100 mg (7s)
    Monistat® 1 Day or Night [OTC]: Cream, topical: 2% (9 g) and Insert, vaginal: 1200 mg (1)
  Cream, topical: 2% (15 g, 30 g, 45 g)
    Baza® Antifungal [OTC]: 2% (4 g, 57 g, 142 g)
    Carrington® Antifungal [OTC]: 2% (150 g)
    Micaderm® [OTC]: 2% (30 g)
    Micatin® [OTC]: 2% (14 g)
    Micro-Guard® [OTC]: 2% (60 g)
    Miranel AF™ [OTC]: 2% (28 g)
    3M™ Cavilon™ Antifungal [OTC]: 2% (56 g, 141 g)
    Neosporin® AF [OTC]: 2% (14 g, 15 g)
    Podactin Cream [OTC]: 2% (30 g)
    Secura® Antifungal Extra Thick [OTC]: 2% (97.5 g)
    Secura® Antifungal Greaseless [OTC]: 2% (60 g)
  Cream, vaginal: 2% (45 g)
    Monistat® 7 [OTC]: 2% (45 g)
    Monistat® 3 [OTC]: 4% (15 g, 25 g)
  Gel, topical:
    Zeasorb®-AF [OTC]: 2% (24 g)
  Liquid, topical:
    Lotrimin AF® [OTC]: 2% (150 g)
  Ointment, topical:
    Aloe Vesta® Antifungal [OTC]: 2% (60 g, 150 g)
    Critic-Aid® Clear AF [OTC]: 2% (57 g, 142 g, 300s)
    DermaFungal [OTC]: 2% (120 g)
    Dermagran® AF [OTC]: 2% (120 g)
  Powder, topical:
    Lotrimin AF® [OTC]: 2% (90 g)
    Micro-Guard® [OTC]: 2% (90 g)
    Mitrazol® [OTC]: 2% (30 g)
    Zeasorb®-AF [OTC]: 2% (70 g)
  Suppository, vaginal: 100 mg (7s); 200 mg (3s)
  Tablet for solution, topical:
    DiabetAid® Antifungal Foot Bath [OTC]: 2% (10s)
  Tincture, topical:
    Fungoid® [OTC]: 2% (7.39 mL, 30 mL)

miconazole and zinc oxide (mi KON a zole & zink OKS ide)

Synonyms zinc oxide and miconazole nitrate
U.S. Brand Names Vusion®
Therapeutic Category Antifungal Agent, Topical
Use Adjunctive treatment of diaper dermatitis complicated by *Candida albicans* infection
General Dosage Range Topical: *Children ≥4 weeks:* Apply to affected area with each diaper change
  (maximum therapy: 7 days)
Dosage Forms
  Ointment, topical:
    Vusion®: Miconazole 0.25% and zinc oxide 15% (50 g)

miconazole nitrate *see* miconazole (oral) *on page 585*
miconazole nitrate *see* miconazole (topical) *on page 585*

Micozole (Can) *see* miconazole (topical) *on page 585*
MICRhoGAM® UF Plus *see* Rh$_o$(D) immune globulin *on page 776*
microfibrillar collagen hemostat *see* collagen hemostat *on page 233*
Microgestin® 1.5/30 *see* ethinyl estradiol and norethindrone *on page 355*
Microgestin® 1/20 *see* ethinyl estradiol and norethindrone *on page 355*
Microgestin® Fe 1.5/30 *see* ethinyl estradiol and norethindrone *on page 355*
Microgestin® Fe 1/20 *see* ethinyl estradiol and norethindrone *on page 355*
Micro-Guard® [OTC] *see* miconazole (topical) *on page 585*
microK® *see* potassium chloride *on page 724*
microK® 10 *see* potassium chloride *on page 724*
Micro-K Extencaps® (Can) *see* potassium chloride *on page 724*
Micronase *see* glyburide *on page 420*
Micronor® (Can) *see* norethindrone *on page 633*
Microzide® *see* hydrochlorothiazide *on page 445*
***Micrurus fulvius* antivenin** *see* antivenin *(Micrurus fulvius) on page 84*
Midamor (Can) *see* amiloride *on page 64*

midazolam (MID aye zoe lam)

Medication Safety Issues
Sound-alike/look-alike issues:
Versed may be confused with VePesid®, Vistaril®
High alert medication:
The Institute for Safe Medication Practices (ISMP) includes this medication among its list of drugs which have a heightened risk of causing significant patient harm when used in error.
Synonyms midazolam hydrochloride; Versed
Canadian Brand Names Apo-Midazolam®; Midazolam Injection
Therapeutic Category Benzodiazepine
Controlled Substance C-IV
Use Preoperative sedation; moderate sedation prior to diagnostic or radiographic procedures; ICU sedation (continuous infusion); induction and maintenance of general anesthesia
General Dosage Range
I.M.:
Children: 0.05-0.15 mg/kg 30-60 minutes (maximum: 10 mg total)
Adults: 0.07-0.08 mg/kg 30-60 minutes; Usual dose: 5 mg
I.V.:
Infants <6 months: 0.05-0.2 mg/kg loading dose followed by 0.4-6 mcg/kg/minute infusion
Infants 6 months to Children 5 years: Initial: 0.05-0.1 mg/kg once (maximum: 6 mg or 0.6 mg/kg total) **or** 0.05-0.2 mg/kg loading dose followed by 0.4-6 mcg/kg/minute infusion
Children 6-12 years: 0.025-0.05 mg/kg once (maximum: 10 mg or 0.4 mg/kg total) **or** 0.05-0.2 mg/kg loading dose followed by 0.4-6 mcg/kg/minute infusion
Children 12-16 years: 0.02-0.2 mg/kg once (maximum: 10 mg total) **or** 0.05-0.2 mg/kg loading dose followed by 0.4-6 mcg/kg/minute infusion
Adults: Dosage varies greatly depending on indication
Oral:
Children <6 years: 0.25-0.5 mg/kg as single dose; may require as much as 1 mg/kg (maximum: 20 mg total)
Children 6-16 years: 0.25-0.5 mg/kg as a single dose (maximum: 20 mg total)
Dosage Forms
Injection, solution: 1 mg/mL (2 mL, 5 mL, 10 mL); 5 mg/mL (1 mL, 2 mL, 5 mL, 10 mL)
Injection, solution [preservative free]: 1 mg/mL (2 mL, 5 mL); 5 mg/mL (1 mL, 2 mL)
Syrup, oral: 2 mg/mL (2.5 mL, 118 mL)

midazolam hydrochloride *see* midazolam *on page 587*
Midazolam Injection (Can) *see* midazolam *on page 587*

midodrine (MI doe dreen)

Medication Safety Issues
Sound-alike/look-alike issues:
Midodrine may be confused with Midrin®, minoxidil
ProAmatine® may be confused with protamine

Synonyms midodrine hydrochloride

U.S. Brand Names ProAmatine® [DSC]

Canadian Brand Names Amatine®; Apo-Midodrine®

Therapeutic Category Alpha-Adrenergic Agonist

Use Orphan drug: Treatment of symptomatic orthostatic hypotension

General Dosage Range Dosage adjustment recommended in patients with renal impairment
Oral: Adults: 10 mg 3 times/day (maximum: 40 mg/day)

Dosage Forms
Tablet, oral: 2.5 mg, 5 mg, 10 mg

midodrine hydrochloride *see* midodrine *on page 588*
Midol® Cramps & Body Aches [OTC] *see* ibuprofen *on page 460*
Midol® Extended Relief [OTC] *see* naproxen *on page 612*
Midol® Teen Formula [OTC] *see* acetaminophen and pamabrom *on page 27*
Midrin® [DSC] *see* acetaminophen, isometheptene, and dichloralphenazone *on page 34*
Mifeprex® *see* mifepristone *on page 588*

mifepristone (mi FE pris tone)

Medication Safety Issues
Sound-alike/look-alike issues:
Mifeprex® may be confused with Mirapex®
Mifepristone may be confused with misoprostol
High alert medication:
The Institute for Safe Medication Practices (ISMP) includes this medication among its list of drug classes which have a heightened risk of causing significant patient harm when used in error.

Synonyms RU-38486; RU-486

U.S. Brand Names Mifeprex®

Therapeutic Category Abortifacient; Antineoplastic Agent, Hormone Antagonist; Antiprogestin

Use Medical termination of intrauterine pregnancy, through day 49 of pregnancy. Patients may need treatment with misoprostol and possibly surgery to complete therapy.

General Dosage Range Oral: *Adults:* Day 1: 600 mg (three 200 mg tablets) as a single dose; Day 3: 400 mcg (two 200 mcg tablets) as a single dose if needed

Dosage Forms
Tablet, oral:
Mifeprex®: 200 mg

Migergot® *see* ergotamine and caffeine *on page 337*

miglitol (MIG li tol)

Medication Safety Issues
Sound-alike/look-alike issues:
Glyset® may be confused with Cycloset®

U.S. Brand Names Glyset®

Canadian Brand Names Glyset®

Therapeutic Category Antidiabetic Agent, Oral

Use Type 2 diabetes mellitus (noninsulin-dependent, NIDDM):
Monotherapy as an adjunct to diet to improve glycemic control in patients with type 2 diabetes mellitus (noninsulin-dependent, NIDDM) whose hyperglycemia cannot be managed with diet alone
Combination therapy with a sulfonylurea when diet plus either miglitol or a sulfonylurea alone do not result in adequate glycemic control. The effect of miglitol to enhance glycemic control is additive to that of sulfonylureas when used in combination.

General Dosage Range Oral: *Adults:* Initial: 25 mg 3 times/day; Maintenance: 25-100 mg 3 times/day (maximum: 300 mg/day)

Dosage Forms
Tablet, oral:
Glyset®: 25 mg, 50 mg, 100 mg

miglustat (MIG loo stat)
Medication Safety Issues
International issues:
Zavesca: Brand name for miglustat [U.S., Canada, and multiple international markets], but also brand name for escitalopram [in multiple international markets; ISMP April 21, 2010]
Synonyms OGT-918
U.S. Brand Names Zavesca®
Canadian Brand Names Zavesca®
Therapeutic Category Enzyme Inhibitor
Use Treatment of mild-to-moderate type 1 Gaucher disease when enzyme replacement therapy is not a therapeutic option

Canadian labeling: Additional use (not in U.S. labeling): Treatment to delay the progression of neurological manifestations in Niemann-Pick Type C disease
General Dosage Range Dosage adjustment recommended in patients with renal impairment
Oral: *Adults:* 100 mg 1-3 times/day
Dosage Forms
Capsule, oral:
Zavesca®: 100 mg

Migranal® *see* dihydroergotamine *on page 286*
Mild-C® [OTC] *see* ascorbic acid *on page 96*
milk of magnesia *see* magnesium hydroxide *on page 545*
Milk of Magnesia [OTC] *see* magnesium hydroxide *on page 545*
Millipred™ *see* prednisolone (systemic) *on page 734*

milnacipran (mil NAY ci pran)
Medication Safety Issues
Sound-alike/look-alike issues:
Savella® may be confused with cevimeline, sevelamer
U.S. Brand Names Savella®
Therapeutic Category Antidepressant, Serotonin/Norepinephrine Reuptake Inhibitor
Use Management of fibromyalgia
General Dosage Range Dosage adjustment recommended in patients with renal impairment
Oral: *Adults:* 50 mg twice daily (maximum dose: 200 mg/day)
Dosage Forms
Combination package, oral:
Savella®: Tablet: 12.5 mg (5s), Tablet: 25 mg (8s), and Tablet: 50 mg (42s)
Tablet, oral:
Savella®: 12.5 mg, 25 mg, 50 mg, 100 mg

Milophene® (Can) *see* clomiphene *on page 222*

milrinone (MIL ri none)
Medication Safety Issues
Sound-alike/look-alike issues:
Primacor® may be confused with Primaxin®
High alert medication:
The Institute for Safe Medication Practices (ISMP) includes this medication among its list of drugs which have a heightened risk of causing significant patient harm when used in error.
Synonyms milrinone lactate
Canadian Brand Names Milrinone Lactate Injection; Primacor®
Therapeutic Category Cardiovascular Agent, Other
Use Short-term I.V. therapy of acutely-decompensated heart failure
General Dosage Range Dosage adjustment recommended in patients with renal impairment
I.V.: *Adults:* Loading dose (optional): 50 mcg/kg; Maintenance: 0.375-0.75 mcg/kg/minute

◀ **Dosage Forms**
Infusion, premixed in D₅W: 200 mcg/mL (100 mL, 200 mL)
Injection, solution: 1 mg/mL (10 mL, 20 mL, 50 mL)
Injection, solution [preservative free]: 1 mg/mL (10 mL, 20 mL)

milrinone lactate *see milrinone on page 589*
Milrinone Lactate Injection (Can) *see milrinone on page 589*
Mimvey™ *see estradiol and norethindrone on page 345*
Mimyx® *see emollients on page 325*
mineral oil, petrolatum, lanolin, cetyl alcohol, and glycerin *see lanolin, cetyl alcohol, glycerin, petrolatum, and mineral oil on page 510*
Minestrin™ 1/20 (Can) *see ethinyl estradiol and norethindrone on page 355*
Mini-Prenatal [OTC] *see vitamins (multiple/prenatal) on page 920*
Minipress® *see prazosin on page 733*
Minirin® (Can) *see desmopressin on page 262*
Minitran™ *see nitroglycerin on page 629*
Minocin® *see minocycline on page 590*
Minocin® PAC *see minocycline on page 590*

minocycline (mi noe SYE kleen)

Medication Safety Issues
Sound-alike/look-alike issues:
Dynacin® may be confused with Dyazide®, Dynabac®, DynaCirc®, Dynapen®
Minocin® may be confused with Indocin®, Lincocin®, Minizide®, Mithracin®, niacin

Synonyms minocycline hydrochloride

U.S. Brand Names Minocin®; Minocin® PAC; Solodyn®

Canadian Brand Names Apo-Minocycline®; Arestin Microspheres; Dom-Minocycline; Minocin®; Mylan-Minocycline; Novo-Minocycline; PHL-Minocycline; PMS-Minocycline; ratio-Minocycline; Riva-Minocycline; Sandoz-Minocycline

Therapeutic Category Tetracycline Derivative

Use Treatment of susceptible bacterial infections of both gram-negative and gram-positive organisms; treatment of anthrax (inhalational, cutaneous, and gastrointestinal); moderate-to-severe acne; meningococcal (asymptomatic) carrier state; Rickettsial diseases (including Rocky Mountain spotted fever, Q fever); nongonococcal urethritis, gonorrhea; acute intestinal amebiasis; respiratory tract infection; skin/soft tissue infections; chlamydial infections
Extended release (Solodyn®): Only indicated for treatment of inflammatory lesions of non-nodular moderate-to-severe acne

General Dosage Range Dosage adjustment recommended in patients with renal impairment
I.V.:
Children >8 years: 4 mg/kg initially, followed by 2 mg/kg/dose every 12 hours (maximum: 400 mg/day)
Adults: 200 mg initially, followed by 100 mg every 12 hours (maximum: 400 mg/day)
Oral:
Children >8 years: 4 mg/kg initially, followed by 2 mg/kg/dose every 12 hours
Children ≥12 years: Solodyn®: 45-135 mg once daily (weight-based)
Adults: 200 mg initially, followed by 100 mg every 12 hours **or** 50-100 mg twice daily (acne); Solodyn®: 45-135 mg once daily (weight-based)

Dosage Forms
Capsule, oral: 50 mg, 75 mg, 100 mg
Capsule, pellet filled, oral:
Minocin®: 50 mg, 100 mg
Minocin® PAC: 50 mg, 100 mg
Injection, powder for reconstitution:
Minocin®: 100 mg
Tablet, oral: 50 mg, 75 mg, 100 mg
Tablet, extended release, oral:
Solodyn®: 45 mg, 65 mg, 90 mg, 115 mg, 135 mg

minocycline hydrochloride *see minocycline on page 590*
Min-Ovral® (Can) *see ethinyl estradiol and levonorgestrel on page 353*

minoxidil (systemic) (mi NOKS i dil)

Medication Safety Issues
Sound-alike/look-alike issues:
Loniten® may be confused with Lipitor®
Minoxidil may be confused with metolazone, midodrine, Minipress®, Minocin®, Monopril®, Noxafil®
International issues:
Loniten [Canada and multiple international markets] may be confused with Linoten brand name for pamidronate [Spain]
Noxidil [Thailand] may be confused with Noxafil brand name for posaconazole [U.S. and multiple international markets]
Canadian Brand Names Loniten®
Therapeutic Category Vasodilator, Direct-Acting
Use Management of severe hypertension (usually in combination with a diuretic and beta-blocker)
General Dosage Range Oral:
Children <12 years: Initial: 0.1-0.2 mg/kg once daily (maximum: 5 mg/day); Usual dosage range: 0.25-1 mg/kg/day in 1-2 divided doses (maximum: 50 mg/day)
Children ≥12 years and Adults: Initial: 5 mg once daily; Usual dosage range: 2.5-80 mg/day in 1-2 divided doses (maximum: 100 mg/day)
Elderly: Initial: 2.5 mg once daily
Dosage Forms
Tablet, oral: 2.5 mg, 10 mg

minoxidil (topical) (mi NOKS i dil)

U.S. Brand Names Rogaine® Extra Strength for Men [OTC]; Rogaine® for Men [OTC]; Rogaine® for Women [OTC]
Canadian Brand Names Apo-Gain®; Rogaine®
Therapeutic Category Topical Skin Product
Use Treatment of alopecia androgenetica in males and females
General Dosage Range Topical: *Adults:* Apply twice daily
Dosage Forms
Aerosol, topical:
Rogaine® for Men [OTC]: 5% (60 g)
Solution, topical: 2% (60 mL); 5% (60 mL)
Rogaine® Extra Strength for Men [OTC]: 5% (60 mL)
Rogaine® for Women [OTC]: 2% (60 mL)

Mintab DM [DSC] *see* guaifenesin and dextromethorphan *on page 427*
Mint-Amlodipine (Can) *see* amlodipine *on page 69*
Mint-Atenolol (Can) *see* atenolol *on page 101*
Mint-Cefprozil (Can) *see* cefprozil *on page 183*
Mint-Ciprofloxacin (Can) *see* ciprofloxacin (systemic) *on page 210*
Mint-Citalopram (Can) *see* citalopram *on page 213*
Mint-Lisinopril (Can) *see* lisinopril *on page 531*
Mint-Ondansetron (Can) *see* ondansetron *on page 651*
Mintox Plus [OTC] *see* aluminum hydroxide, magnesium hydroxide, and simethicone *on page 60*
Mint-Pioglitazone (Can) *see* pioglitazone *on page 706*
Mint-Risperidon (Can) *see* risperidone *on page 783*
Mint-Topiramate (Can) *see* topiramate *on page 877*
Miochol®-E *see* acetylcholine *on page 36*
Miostat® *see* carbachol *on page 170*
MiraLAX® [OTC] *see* polyethylene glycol 3350 *on page 718*
Miranel AF™ [OTC] *see* miconazole (topical) *on page 585*
Mirapex® *see* pramipexole *on page 729*
Mirapex® ER® *see* pramipexole *on page 729*
Mircette® *see* ethinyl estradiol and desogestrel *on page 351*
Mirena® *see* levonorgestrel *on page 521*

mirtazapine (mir TAZ a peen)

Medication Safety Issues
Sound-alike/look-alike issues:
Remeron® may be confused with Premarin®, ramelteon, Rozerem®, Zemuron®
International issues:
Avanza [Australia] may be confused with Albenza brand name for albendazole [U.S.]; Avandia brand name for rosiglitazone [U.S., Canada, and multiple international markets]
Remeron [U.S., Canada, and multiple international markets] may be confused with Reneuron which is a brand name for fluoxetine [Spain]

U.S. Brand Names Remeron SolTab®; Remeron®

Canadian Brand Names Apo-Mirtazapine®; CO Mirtazapine; Dom-Mirtazapine; Mylan-Mirtazapine; Novo-Mirtazapine; PHL-Mirtazapine; PMS-Mirtazapine; PRO-Mirtazapine; ratio-Mirtazapine; Remeron®; Remeron® RD; Riva-Mirtazapine; Sandoz-Mirtazapine; Sandoz-Mirtazapine FC; ZYM-Mirtazapine

Therapeutic Category Antidepressant, Alpha-2 Antagonist

Use Treatment of depression

General Dosage Range Oral: *Adults:* Initial: 15 mg nightly; Maintenance: 15-45 mg nightly

Dosage Forms
Tablet, oral: 7.5 mg, 15 mg, 30 mg, 45 mg
Remeron®: 15 mg, 30 mg, 45 mg
Tablet, orally disintegrating, oral: 15 mg, 30 mg, 45 mg
Remeron SolTab®: 15 mg, 30 mg, 45 mg

misoprostol (mye soe PROST ole)

Medication Safety Issues
Sound-alike/look-alike issues:
Cytotec® may be confused with Cytoxan, Sytobex®
Misoprostol may be confused with metoprolol, mifepristone

U.S. Brand Names Cytotec®

Canadian Brand Names Apo-Misoprostol®; Novo-Misoprostol; PMS-Misoprostol

Therapeutic Category Prostaglandin

Use Prevention of NSAID-induced gastric ulcers; medical termination of pregnancy of ≤49 days (in conjunction with mifepristone)

General Dosage Range Oral:
Adults: 100-200 mcg 4 times/day
Elderly: Initial: 100 mcg/day

Dosage Forms
Tablet, oral: 100 mcg, 200 mcg
Cytotec®: 100 mcg, 200 mcg

misoprostol and diclofenac *see* diclofenac and misoprostol *on page* 279

mitomycin (mye toe MYE sin)

Medication Safety Issues
Sound-alike/look-alike issues:
MitoMYcin may be confused with mithramycin, mitotane, mitoXANtrone
High alert medication:
The Institute for Safe Medication Practices (ISMP) includes this medication among its list of drugs which have a heightened risk of causing significant patient harm when used in error.

Synonyms mitomycin-C; mitomycin-X; MTC

Tall-Man mitoMYcin

Canadian Brand Names Mutamycin®

Therapeutic Category Antineoplastic Agent

Use Treatment of adenocarcinoma of stomach or pancreas

General Dosage Range Dosage adjustment recommended in patients with renal impairment
I.V.: *Adults:* 10-20 mg/m^2 every 6-8 weeks

Dosage Forms
Injection, powder for reconstitution: 5 mg, 20 mg, 40 mg

mitomycin-X *see* mitomycin *on page* 592

mitomycin-C *see* mitomycin *on page 592*

mitotane (MYE toe tane)

Medication Safety Issues
Sound-alike/look-alike issues:
Mitotane may be confused with mitoMYcin, mitoXANtrone
High alert medication:
The Institute for Safe Medication Practices (ISMP) includes this medication among its list of drug classes which have a heightened risk of causing significant patient harm when used in error.

Synonyms chloditan; chlodithane; khloditan; mytotan; o,p'-DDD; ortho,para-DDD

U.S. Brand Names Lysodren®

Canadian Brand Names Lysodren®

Therapeutic Category Antineoplastic Agent

Use Treatment of inoperable adrenocortical carcinoma

General Dosage Range Dosage adjustment recommended in patients who develop toxicities
Oral: *Adults:* Initial: 2-6 g/day in divided doses; Maintenance: 9-10 g/day in 3-4 divided doses (maximum: 18 g/day)

Dosage Forms
Tablet, oral:
Lysodren®: 500 mg

mitoxantrone (mye toe ZAN trone)

Medication Safety Issues
Sound-alike/look-alike issues:
MitoXANtrone may be confused with methotrexate, mitoMYcin, mitotane, Mutamycin®
High alert medication:
This medication is in a class the Institute for Safe Medication Practices (ISMP) includes among its list of drug classes which have a heightened risk of causing significant patient harm when used in error.

Synonyms CL-232315; DHAD; DHAQ; dihydroxyanthracenedione; dihydroxyanthracenedione dihydrochloride; mitoxantrone dihydrochloride; mitoxantrone HCl; mitoxantrone hydrochloride; mitozantrone

Tall-Man mitoXANtrone

U.S. Brand Names Novantrone®

Canadian Brand Names Mitoxantrone Injection®; Novantrone®

Therapeutic Category Antineoplastic Agent

Use Treatment of acute nonlymphocytic leukemias (ANLL [includes myelogenous, promyelocytic, monocytic and erythroid leukemias]); advanced hormone-refractory prostate cancer; secondary progressive or relapsing-remitting multiple sclerosis (MS)

General Dosage Range I.V.: *Adults:* 12 mg/m²/day once daily for 2-3 days **or** 12-14 mg/m² every 3 weeks **or** 12 mg/m² every 3 months (multiple sclerosis; maximum lifetime cumulative dose: 140 mg/m²)

Dosage Forms
Injection, solution [preservative free]: 2 mg/mL (10 mL, 12.5 mL, 15 mL, 20 mL)
Novantrone®: 2 mg/mL (10 mL)

mitoxantrone dihydrochloride *see* mitoxantrone *on page 593*
mitoxantrone HCl *see* mitoxantrone *on page 593*
mitoxantrone hydrochloride *see* mitoxantrone *on page 593*
Mitoxantrone Injection® (Can) *see* mitoxantrone *on page 593*
mitozantrone *see* mitoxantrone *on page 593*
Mitrazol® [OTC] *see* miconazole (topical) *on page 585*
MK-217 *see* alendronate *on page 49*
MK383 *see* tirofiban *on page 871*
MK-0431 *see* sitagliptin *on page 815*
MK462 *see* rizatriptan *on page 787*
MK 0517 *see* fosaprepitant *on page 400*
MK-0518 *see* raltegravir *on page 765*
MK594 *see* losartan *on page 538*
MK0826 *see* ertapenem *on page 338*
MK 869 *see* aprepitant *on page 91*

MLN341 *see* bortezomib *on page 139*

MMF *see* mycophenolate *on page 604*

MMR *see* measles, mumps, and rubella virus vaccine *on page 551*

M-M-R® II *see* measles, mumps, and rubella virus vaccine *on page 551*

MMR-V *see* measles, mumps, rubella, and varicella virus vaccine *on page 551*

MMRV *see* measles, mumps, rubella, and varicella virus vaccine *on page 551*

MOAB ABX-EGF *see* panitumumab *on page 672*

MOAB anti-tac *see* daclizumab *on page 249*

MOAB C225 *see* cetuximab *on page 190*

MoAb CD52 *see* alemtuzumab *on page 48*

MOAB-CTLA-4 *see* ipilimumab *on page 488*

MOAB HER2 *see* trastuzumab *on page 882*

Mobic® *see* meloxicam *on page 556*

Mobicox® (Can) *see* meloxicam *on page 556*

Mobisyl® [OTC] *see* trolamine *on page 894*

moclobemide *(Canada only)* (moe KLOE be mide)

Canadian Brand Names Apo-Moclobemide®; Dom-Moclobemide; Manerix®; Novo-Moclobemide; Nu-Moclobemide; PMS-Moclobemide

Therapeutic Category Antidepressant, Monoamine Oxidase Inhibitor

Use Symptomatic relief of depressive illness

General Dosage Range Dosage adjustment recommended in patients with hepatic impairment or on concomitant therapy

Oral: *Adults:* Initial: 300 mg/day in 2 divided doses; Maintenance: Up to 600 mg/day

Product Availability Not available in U.S.

Dosage Forms - Canada

Tablet, oral:

Apo-Moclobemide®, Dom-Moclobemide, Manerix®, Novo-Moclobemide, Nu-Moclobemide, PMS-Moclobemide: 100 mg, 150 mg, 300 mg

modafinil (moe DAF i nil)

U.S. Brand Names Provigil®

Canadian Brand Names Alertec®; Apo-Modafinil®

Therapeutic Category Central Nervous System Stimulant, Nonamphetamine

Controlled Substance C-IV

Use Improve wakefulness in patients with excessive daytime sleepiness associated with narcolepsy and shift work sleep disorder (SWSD); adjunctive therapy for obstructive sleep apnea/hypopnea syndrome (OSAHS)

General Dosage Range Dosage adjustment recommended in patients with hepatic impairment.

Oral: *Adults:* 200 mg once daily (maximum: 400 mg/day)

Dosage Forms

Tablet, oral:

Provigil®: 100 mg, 200 mg

Modecate® (Can) *see* fluphenazine *on page 390*

Modecate® Concentrate (Can) *see* fluphenazine *on page 390*

Modicon® *see* ethinyl estradiol and norethindrone *on page 355*

modified Dakin's solution *see* sodium hypochlorite solution *on page 820*

Moducal® [OTC] *see* glucose polymers *on page 420*

Modulon® (Can) *see* trimebutine *(Canada only) on page 891*

Moduret (Can) *see* amiloride and hydrochlorothiazide *on page 64*

moexipril (mo EKS i pril)

Medication Safety Issues

Sound-alike/look-alike issues:

Moexipril may be confused with Monopril®

Synonyms moexipril hydrochloride

U.S. Brand Names Univasc®
Therapeutic Category Angiotensin-Converting Enzyme (ACE) Inhibitor
Use Treatment of hypertension, alone or in combination with thiazide diuretics
General Dosage Range Dosage adjustment recommended in patients with renal impairment
  Oral: *Adults:* Initial: 3.75-7.5 mg once daily; Maintenance: 7.5-30 mg/day in 1 or 2 divided doses
Dosage Forms
  Tablet, oral: 7.5 mg, 15 mg
  Univasc®: 7.5 mg, 15 mg

moexipril and hydrochlorothiazide (mo EKS i pril & hye droe klor oh THYE a zide)
Synonyms hydrochlorothiazide and moexipril
U.S. Brand Names Uniretic®
Canadian Brand Names Uniretic®
Therapeutic Category Angiotensin-Converting Enzyme (ACE) Inhibitor; Diuretic, Thiazide
Use Treatment of hypertension; not indicated for initial treatment of hypertension
General Dosage Range Oral: *Adults:* 7.5-30 mg of moexipril/day and ≤50 mg hydrochlorothiazide/day in a single or divided dose
Dosage Forms
  Tablet, oral: 7.5/12.5: Moexipril 7.5 mg and hydrochlorothiazide 12.5; 15/12.5: Moexipril 15 mg and hydrochlorothiazide 12.5; 15/25: Moexipril 15 mg and hydrochlorothiazide 25
  Uniretic®: 7.5/12.5: Moexipril 7.5 mg and hydrochlorothiazide 12.5 mg [scored]; 15/12.5: Moexipril 15 mg and hydrochlorothiazide 12.5 mg [scored]; 15/25: Moexipril 15 mg and hydrochlorothiazide 25 mg [scored]

moexipril hydrochloride *see* moexipril *on page 594*
Mogadon (Can) *see* nitrazepam *(Canada only) on page 628*
Moi-Stir® [OTC] *see* saliva substitute *on page 798*
Moisture® Eyes [OTC] *see* artificial tears *on page 96*
Moisture® Eyes PM [OTC] *see* artificial tears *on page 96*
molybdenum *see* trace metals *on page 880*
MOM *see* magnesium hydroxide *on page 545*
Momentum® [OTC] *see* magnesium salicylate *on page 547*

mometasone (oral inhalation) (moe MET a sone)
Synonyms mometasone furoate
U.S. Brand Names Asmanex® Twisthaler®
Therapeutic Category Corticosteroid, Inhalant (Oral)
Use Maintenance treatment of asthma as prophylactic therapy
General Dosage Range Inhalation:
  Children 4-11 years: 110 mcg once daily (maximum: 110 mcg/day)
  Children ≥12 years and Adults: 1-4 inhalations (220-880 mcg) in 1-2 divided doses (maximum: 880 mcg/day)
Dosage Forms
  Powder, for oral inhalation:
  Asmanex® Twisthaler®: 110 mcg (30 units); 220 mcg (14 units, 30 units, 60 units, 120 units)

mometasone (nasal) (moe MET a sone)
Synonyms mometasone furoate
U.S. Brand Names Nasonex®
Canadian Brand Names Nasonex®
Therapeutic Category Corticosteroid, Nasal
Use Treatment of nasal symptoms of seasonal and perennial allergic rhinitis; prevention of nasal symptoms associated with seasonal allergic rhinitis; treatment of nasal polyps in adults

Canadian labeling: Additional use (not in U.S. labeling): Treatment of mild-to-moderate uncomplicated rhinosinusitis or as adjunctive treatment (with antimicrobials) in acute rhinosinusitis

◄ **General Dosage Range Intranasal:**
Children 2-11 years: 1 spray (50 mcg) in each nostril once daily
Children ≥12 years and Adults: 2 sprays (100 mcg) in each nostril once or twice daily
Dosage Forms
Suspension, intranasal:
Nasonex®: 50 mcg/spray (17 g)
Dosage Forms - Canada Excipient information presented when available (limited, particularly for generics); consult specific product labeling.
Suspension, intranasal:
Nasonex®: 50 mcg/spray [delivers 140 sprays]

mometasone (topical) (moe MET a sone)

Medication Safety Issues
Sound-alike/look-alike issues:
Elocon® lotion may be confused with ophthalmic solutions. Manufacturer's labeling emphasizes the product is **NOT** for use in the eyes.
Synonyms mometasone furoate
U.S. Brand Names Elocon®
Canadian Brand Names Elocom®; PMS-Mometasone; ratio-Mometasone; Taro-Mometasone
Therapeutic Category Corticosteroid, Topical
Use Relief of the inflammatory and pruritic manifestations of corticosteroid-responsive dermatoses (medium potency topical corticosteroid)
General Dosage Range Topical:
Cream, ointment: *Children ≥2 years and Adults:* Apply a thin film to affected area once daily
Lotion: *Children ≥12 years and Adults:* Apply a few drops to affected area once daily
Dosage Forms
Cream, topical: 0.1% (15 g, 45 g)
Elocon®: 0.1% (15 g, 45 g)
Lotion, topical: 0.1% (30 mL, 60 mL)
Elocon®: 0.1% (30 mL, 60 mL)
Ointment, topical: 0.1% (15 g, 45 g)
Elocon®: 0.1% (15 g, 45 g)

mometasone and formoterol (moe MET a sone & for MOH te rol)

Synonyms formoterol and mometasone; formoterol and mometasone furoate; formoterol fumarate dihydrate and mometasone
U.S. Brand Names Dulera®
Canadian Brand Names Zenhale™
Therapeutic Category Beta$_2$-Adrenergic Agonist; Beta$_2$-Adrenergic Agonist, Long-Acting; Corticosteroid, Inhalant (Oral)
Use Maintenance treatment of asthma where combination therapy is indicated
General Dosage Range Inhalation: *Children ≥12 years and Adults:* 2 inhalations twice daily (maximum: 4 inhalations/day)
Dosage Forms
Aerosol, for oral inhalation:
Dulera®: Mometasone 100 mcg and formoterol 5 mcg per inhalation (13 g) [120 metered actuations]
Dulera®: Mometasone 200 mcg and formoterol 5 mcg per inhalation (13 g) [120 metered actuations]
Dosage Forms - Canada
Aerosol, for oral inhalation:
Zenhale™: Mometasone furoate 50 mcg and formoterol fumarate dihydrate 5 mcg per inhalation [120 metered actuations]

mometasone furoate *see* mometasone (nasal) *on page 595*
mometasone furoate *see* mometasone (oral inhalation) *on page 595*
mometasone furoate *see* mometasone (topical) *on page 596*
MOM/mineral oil emulsion *see* magnesium hydroxide and mineral oil *on page 546*
monacolin K *see* lovastatin *on page 540*
Monilia skin test *see* Candida albicans (Monilia) *on page 168*
Monistat® (Can) *see* miconazole (topical) *on page 585*

Monistat® 1 [OTC] *see* miconazole (topical) *on page 585*
Monistat® 1 Day or Night [OTC] *see* miconazole (topical) *on page 585*
Monistat® 3 [OTC] *see* miconazole (topical) *on page 585*
Monistat® 3 (Can) *see* miconazole (topical) *on page 585*
Monistat® 7 [OTC] *see* miconazole (topical) *on page 585*

monobenzone (mon oh BEN zone)

Therapeutic Category Topical Skin Product
Use Final depigmentation in extensive vitiligo
General Dosage Range Topical: *Children ≥12 years and Adults:* Initial: Apply 2-3 times/day; once depigmentation obtained apply as needed (usually 2 times/week)

Monocaps [OTC] *see* vitamins (multiple/oral) *on page 919*
Monoclate-P® *see* antihemophilic factor (human) *on page 81*
monoclonal antibody *see* muromonab-CD3 *on page 603*
Monoclonal Antibody 5G1.1 *see* eculizumab *on page 319*
monoclonal antibody ABX-EGF *see* panitumumab *on page 672*
Monoclonal Antibody Anti-C5 *see* eculizumab *on page 319*
monoclonal antibody campath-1H *see* alemtuzumab *on page 48*
monoclonal antibody CD52 *see* alemtuzumab *on page 48*
Monodox® *see* doxycycline *on page 312*
monoethanolamine *see* ethanolamine oleate *on page 351*
Monoket® *see* isosorbide mononitrate *on page 495*
MonoNessa® *see* ethinyl estradiol and norgestimate *on page 357*
Mononine® *see* factor IX *on page 365*
Monopril *see* fosinopril *on page 401*
Monopril® (Can) *see* fosinopril *on page 401*
Monopril-HCT® [DSC] *see* fosinopril and hydrochlorothiazide *on page 401*
Monopril-HCT® (Can) *see* fosinopril and hydrochlorothiazide *on page 401*

montelukast (mon te LOO kast)

Medication Safety Issues
  Sound-alike/look-alike issues:
    Singulair® may be confused with SINEquan®
Synonyms montelukast sodium
U.S. Brand Names Singulair®
Canadian Brand Names Singulair®
Therapeutic Category Leukotriene Receptor Antagonist
Use Prophylaxis and chronic treatment of asthma; relief of symptoms of seasonal allergic rhinitis and perennial allergic rhinitis; prevention of exercise-induced bronchospasm
General Dosage Range Oral:
  Children 6 months-5 years: 4 mg once daily
  Children 6-14 years: 5 mg once daily
  Children ≥15 years and Adults: 10 mg once daily **or** 10 mg 2 hours prior to exercise
Dosage Forms
  Granules, oral:
    Singulair®: 4 mg/packet (30s)
  Tablet, oral:
    Singulair®: 10 mg
  Tablet, chewable, oral:
    Singulair®: 4 mg, 5 mg

montelukast sodium *see* montelukast *on page 597*
Monurol® *see* fosfomycin *on page 400*
8-MOP® *see* methoxsalen (systemic) *on page 572*
MoreDophilus® [OTC] *see* Lactobacillus *on page 506*
morning after pill *see* ethinyl estradiol and norgestrel *on page 357*

morphine (systemic) (MOR feen)

Medication Safety Issues

Sound-alike/look-alike issues:

Morphine may be confused with HYDROmorphone, methadone

Morphine sulfate may be confused with magnesium sulfate

Kadian® may be confused with Kapidex [DSC]

MS Contin® may be confused with OxyCONTIN®

MSO_4 and MS are error-prone abbreviations (mistaken as magnesium sulfate)

AVINza® may be confused with Evista®, INVanz®

Roxanol may be confused with OxyFast®, Roxicet™, Roxicodone®

High alert medication:

The Institute for Safe Medication Practices (ISMP) includes this medication (I.V. formulation) among its list of drug classes which have a heightened risk of causing significant patient harm when used in error.

Other safety concerns:

Use care when prescribing and/or administering morphine solutions. These products are available in different concentrations. Always prescribe dosage in mg; **not** by volume (mL).

Use caution when selecting a morphine formulation for use in neurologic infusion pumps (eg, Medtronic delivery systems). The product should be appropriately labeled as "preservative-free" and suitable for intraspinal use via continuous infusion. In addition, the product should be formulated in a pH range that is compatible with the device operation specifications.

Significant differences exist between oral and I.V. dosing. Use caution when converting from one route of administration to another.

Synonyms MS (error-prone abbreviation and should not be used); MSO_4 (error-prone abbreviation and should not be used); Roxanol

U.S. Brand Names Astramorph®/PF; AVINza®; Duramorph; Infumorph 200; Infumorph 500; Kadian®; MS Contin®; Oramorph® SR

Canadian Brand Names Doloral; Kadian®; M-Eslon®; M.O.S.-SR®; M.O.S.-Sulfate®; M.O.S.® 10; M.O.S.® 20; M.O.S.® 30; Morphine Extra Forte Injection; Morphine Forte Injection; Morphine HP®; Morphine LP® Epidural; Morphine SR; Morphine-EPD; MS Contin SRT; MS Contin®; MS-IR®; Novo-Morphine SR; PMS-Morphine Sulfate SR; ratio-Morphine; ratio-Morphine SR; Sandoz-Morphine SR; Statex®; Teva-Morphine SR

Therapeutic Category Analgesic, Opioid

Controlled Substance C-II

Use Relief of moderate-to-severe acute and chronic pain; relief of pain of myocardial infarction; relief of dyspnea of acute left ventricular failure and pulmonary edema; preanesthetic medication

Infumorph®: Used in continuous microinfusion devices for intrathecal or epidural administration in treatment of intractable chronic pain

Controlled-, extended-, or sustained-release products: Only intended/indicated for use when repeated doses for an extended period of time are required. The 100 mg and 200 mg tablets or capsules of Kadian®, MS Contin®, and morphine sulfate controlled-release tablets and the 60 mg, 90 mg, and 120 mg capsules of Avinza® should only be used in opioid-tolerant patients.

General Dosage Range Dosage adjustment recommended in patients with renal impairment

Epidural: *Adults:* 5 mg (Astromorph/PF™, Duramorph®) as a single dose **or** 1-6 mg bolus followed by 0.1-0.2 mg/hour (maximum: 10 mg/day) **or** continuous microinfusion (Infumorph®): Opioid-naive patients: 3.5-7.5 mg/day; Opioid-tolerant patients: 4.5-30 mg/day

I.M.:

Children >6 months and <50 kg: 0.1-0.2 mg/kg every 3-4 hours as needed

Adults: 5-20 mg every 4 hours as needed

I.T. (I.T. dose is usually 1/10 that of epidural dose): *Adults:* Opioid-naive: 0.2-1 mg/dose as single dose or once daily; Opioid-tolerant: 1-10 mg/day

I.V.:

Children >6 months and <50 kg: 0.1-0.2 mg/kg every 3-4 hours as needed **or** 10-60 mcg/kg/**hour** as a continuous infusion

Adults: 2.5-5 mg every 3-4 hours **or** 0.8-10 mg/hour; Usual range: Up to 80 mg/hour

Adults (mechanically-ventilated): 0.7-10 mg every 1-2 hours as needed **or** 5-35 mg/hour infusion

Oral:

Controlled, extended or sustained release: *Adults:*

Capsules: Established daily dose on prompt-release formulations administered in 1-2 divided doses (every 12 hours)

Tablets: Established daily dose on prompt-release formulations administered in divided doses every 8-12 hours

Immediate release:

Children >6 months and <50 kg: 0.15-0.3 mg/kg every 3-4 hours as needed

Adults: 10-30 mg every 4 hours as needed; **Note:** Much higher doses may be necessary for chronic pain

PCA: *Adults:* Concentration: 1 mg/mL; Demand dose: 0.5-2.5 mg; Lockout interval: 5-10 minutes

Rectal: *Adults:* 10-20 mg every 3-4 hours

SubQ:

Adults: 5-20 mg every 3-4 hours as needed **or** 0.8-10 mg/hour (up to 80 mg/hour) as continuous infusion

Adults (mechanically-ventilated): 0.7-10 mg every 1-2 hours as needed **or** 5-35 mg/hour infusion

Dosage Forms

Capsule, extended release, oral:

AVINza®: 30 mg, 45 mg, 60 mg, 75 mg, 90 mg, 120 mg

Kadian®: 10 mg, 20 mg, 30 mg, 50 mg, 60 mg, 80 mg, 100 mg, 200 mg

Injection, solution: 1 mg/mL (10 mL, 30 mL, 50 mL); 2 mg/mL (1 mL); 4 mg/mL (1 mL); 5 mg/mL (1 mL, 30 mL, 50 mL); 8 mg/mL (1 mL); 10 mg/mL (1 mL, 10 mL); 10 mg/0.7 mL (0.7 mL); 15 mg/mL (1 mL, 20 mL); 25 mg/mL (4 mL, 10 mL, 20 mL); 50 mg/mL (20 mL, 40 mL, 50 mL)

Injection, solution [preservative free]: 0.5 mg/mL (10 mL, 30 mL); 1 mg/mL (10 mL, 30 mL); 5 mg/mL (30 mL); 25 mg/mL (4 mL, 10 mL, 20 mL)

Astramorph®/PF: 0.5 mg/mL (2 mL, 10 mL); 1 mg/mL (2 mL, 10 mL)

Duramorph: 0.5 mg/mL (10 mL); 1 mg/mL (10 mL)

Infumorph 200: 10 mg/mL (20 mL)

Infumorph 500: 25 mg/mL (20 mL)

Solution, oral: 10 mg/5 mL (5 mL, 10 mL, 100 mL, 500 mL); 20 mg/5 mL (100 mL, 500 mL); 100 mg/5 mL (1 mL, 15 mL, 30 mL, 120 mL, 240 mL)

Suppository, rectal: 5 mg (12s); 10 mg (12s); 20 mg (12s); 30 mg (12s)

Tablet, oral: 15 mg, 30 mg

Tablet, controlled release, oral:

MS Contin®: 15 mg, 30 mg, 60 mg, 100 mg, 200 mg

Tablet, extended release, oral: 15 mg, 30 mg, 60 mg, 100 mg, 200 mg

Tablet, sustained release, oral:

Oramorph® SR: 15 mg, 30 mg, 60 mg, 100 mg

Dosage Forms - Canada

Solution, oral:

Doloral: 1 mg/mL; 5 mg/mL [not available in U.S.]

morphine (liposomal) (MOR feen)

Medication Safety Issues

Sound-alike/look-alike issues:

Morphine may be confused with HYDROmorphone

Morphine sulfate may be confused with magnesium sulfate

MSO$_4$ and MS are error-prone abbreviations (mistaken as magnesium sulfate)

Synonyms extended release epidural morphine; MS (error-prone abbreviation and should not be used); MSO$_4$ (error-prone abbreviation and should not be used)

U.S. Brand Names DepoDur®

Therapeutic Category Analgesic, Opioid

Controlled Substance C-II

Use Epidural (lumbar) single-dose management of surgical pain

General Dosage Range Epidural: *Adults:* 10-15 mg as a single dose

Dosage Forms

Injection, extended release liposomal suspension [preservative free]:

DepoDur®: 10 mg/mL (1 mL, 1.5 mL)

morphine and naltrexone (MOR feen & nal TREKS one)

Medication Safety Issues

Sound-alike/look-alike issues:

Morphine may be confused with HYDROmorphone

Morphine sulfate may be confused with magnesium sulfate

Naltrexone may be confused with methylnaltrexone, naloxone

MSO$_4$ and MS are error-prone abbreviations (mistaken as magnesium sulfate)

Synonyms morphine sulfate and naltrexone hydrochloride; MS (error-prone abbreviation and should not be used); MSO_4 (error-prone abbreviation and should not be used); naltrexone and morphine

U.S. Brand Names Embeda™

Therapeutic Category Analgesic, Opioid; Opioid Antagonist

Controlled Substance C-II

Use Relief of moderate-to-severe pain when continual, around-the-clock therapy is needed for an extended period of time

General Dosage Range Oral: *Adults:* Initial: 20 mg/0.8 mg once or twice daily; Maintenance: Adjust based on individual patient requirement

Dosage Forms

Capsule, extended release, oral:
Embeda™ 20/0.8: Morphine 20 mg and naltrexone 0.8 mg
Embeda™ 30/1.2: Morphine 30 mg and naltrexone 1.2 mg
Embeda™ 50/2: Morphine 50 mg and naltrexone 2 mg
Embeda™ 80/3.2: Morphine 80 mg and naltrexone 3.2 mg
Embeda™ 100/4: Morphine 100 mg and naltrexone 4 mg

Morphine-EPD (Can) *see* morphine (systemic) *on page 598*

Morphine Extra Forte Injection (Can) *see* morphine (systemic) *on page 598*

Morphine Forte Injection (Can) *see* morphine (systemic) *on page 598*

Morphine HP® (Can) *see* morphine (systemic) *on page 598*

Morphine LP® Epidural (Can) *see* morphine (systemic) *on page 598*

Morphine SR (Can) *see* morphine (systemic) *on page 598*

morphine sulfate and naltrexone hydrochloride *see* morphine and naltrexone *on page 599*

morrhuate sodium (MOR yoo ate SOW dee um)

Therapeutic Category Sclerosing Agent

Use Treatment of small, uncomplicated varicose veins of the lower extremities

General Dosage Range I.V.: *Adults:* 50-250 mg, repeated at 5- to 7-day intervals

Dosage Forms

Injection, solution: 50 mg/mL (30 mL)

M.O.S.® 10 (Can) *see* morphine (systemic) *on page 598*

M.O.S.® 20 (Can) *see* morphine (systemic) *on page 598*

M.O.S.® 30 (Can) *see* morphine (systemic) *on page 598*

Mosco® Callus & Corn Remover [OTC] *see* salicylic acid *on page 795*

Mosco® One Step Corn Remover [OTC] *see* salicylic acid *on page 795*

M.O.S.-SR® (Can) *see* morphine (systemic) *on page 598*

M.O.S.-Sulfate® (Can) *see* morphine (systemic) *on page 598*

Motofen® *see* difenoxin and atropine *on page 282*

Motrin® Children's [OTC] *see* ibuprofen *on page 460*

Motrin® (Children's) (Can) *see* ibuprofen *on page 460*

Motrin® IB [OTC] *see* ibuprofen *on page 460*

Motrin® IB (Can) *see* ibuprofen *on page 460*

Motrin® Infants' [OTC] *see* ibuprofen *on page 460*

Motrin® Junior [OTC] *see* ibuprofen *on page 460*

Mouthkote® [OTC] *see* saliva substitute *on page 798*

MoviPrep® *see* polyethylene glycol-electrolyte solution *on page 718*

Moxatag™ *see* amoxicillin *on page 73*

Moxeza™ *see* moxifloxacin (ophthalmic) *on page 601*

moxifloxacin (systemic) (moxs i FLOKS a sin)

Medication Safety Issues

Sound-alike/look-alike issues:
Avelox® may be confused with Avonex®

Synonyms moxifloxacin hydrochloride

U.S. Brand Names Avelox®; Avelox® ABC Pack; Avelox® I.V.

Canadian Brand Names Avelox®; Avelox® I.V.

Therapeutic Category Antibiotic, Quinolone; Respiratory Fluoroquinolone

Use Treatment of mild-to-moderate community-acquired pneumonia, including multidrug-resistant *Streptococcus pneumoniae* (MDRSP); acute bacterial exacerbation of chronic bronchitis; acute bacterial sinusitis; complicated and uncomplicated skin and skin structure infections; complicated intraabdominal infections

General Dosage Range I.V., oral: *Adults:* 400 mg every 24 hours

Dosage Forms
Infusion, premixed in sodium chloride 0.8% [preservative free]:
Avelox® I.V.: 400 mg (250 mL)
Tablet, oral:
Avelox®: 400 mg
Avelox® ABC Pack: 400 mg

moxifloxacin (ophthalmic) (moxs i FLOKS a sin)

Medication Safety Issues
International issues:
Vigamox [U.S., Canada, and multiple international markets] may be confused with Fisamox brand name for amoxicillin [Australia]

Synonyms moxifloxacin hydrochloride

U.S. Brand Names Moxeza™; Vigamox®

Canadian Brand Names Vigamox®

Therapeutic Category Antibiotic, Ophthalmic; Antibiotic, Quinolone

Use Treatment of bacterial conjunctivitis caused by susceptible organisms

General Dosage Range Ophthalmic:
Children ≥4 months and Adults: Moxeza™: Instill 1 drop into affected eye(s) 2 times/day
Children ≥1 year and Adults: Vigamox®: Instill 1 drop into affected eye(s) 3 times/day

Dosage Forms
Solution, ophthalmic:
Moxeza™: 0.5% (3 mL)
Vigamox®: 0.5% (3 mL)

moxifloxacin hydrochloride see moxifloxacin (ophthalmic) *on page 601*
moxifloxacin hydrochloride see moxifloxacin (systemic) *on page 600*
Mozobil™ see plerixafor *on page 710*
4-MP see fomepizole *on page 398*
MP-424 see telaprevir *on page 846*
MPA see medroxyprogesterone *on page 554*
MPA see mycophenolate *on page 604*
MPA and estrogens (conjugated) see estrogens (conjugated/equine) and medroxyprogesterone *on page 348*
6-MP (error-prone abbreviation) see mercaptopurine *on page 563*
MPSV see meningococcal polysaccharide vaccine (groups A / C / Y and W-135) *on page 559*
MPSV4 see meningococcal polysaccharide vaccine (groups A / C / Y and W-135) *on page 559*
MRA see tocilizumab *on page 874*
MS Contin® see morphine (systemic) *on page 598*
MS Contin SRT (Can) see morphine (systemic) *on page 598*
MS (error-prone abbreviation and should not be used) see morphine and naltrexone *on page 599*
MS (error-prone abbreviation and should not be used) see morphine (liposomal) *on page 599*
MS (error-prone abbreviation and should not be used) see morphine (systemic) *on page 598*
MS-IR® (Can) see morphine (systemic) *on page 598*
MSO₄ (error-prone abbreviation and should not be used) see morphine and naltrexone *on page 599*
MSO₄ (error-prone abbreviation and should not be used) see morphine (liposomal) *on page 599*
MSO₄ (error-prone abbreviation and should not be used) see morphine (systemic) *on page 598*

MST 600 *see* magnesium salicylate *on page 547*

MTC *see* mitomycin *on page 592*

MTX (error-prone abbreviation) *see* methotrexate *on page 571*

Mucinex® [OTC] *see* guaifenesin *on page 425*

Mucinex® D [OTC] *see* guaifenesin and pseudoephedrine *on page 429*

Mucinex® D Maximum Strength [OTC] *see* guaifenesin and pseudoephedrine *on page 429*

Mucinex® Children's Multi-Symptom Cold [OTC] *see* guaifenesin, dextromethorphan, and phenylephrine *on page 429*

Mucinex® Cold [OTC] *see* guaifenesin and phenylephrine *on page 428*

Mucinex® DM [OTC] *see* guaifenesin and dextromethorphan *on page 427*

Mucinex® DM Maximum Strength [OTC] *see* guaifenesin and dextromethorphan *on page 427*

Mucinex® Kid's [OTC] *see* guaifenesin *on page 425*

Mucinex® Kid's Mini-Melts™ [OTC] *see* guaifenesin *on page 425*

Mucinex® Kid's Cough [OTC] *see* guaifenesin and dextromethorphan *on page 427*

Mucinex® Kid's Cough Mini-Melts™ [OTC] *see* guaifenesin and dextromethorphan *on page 427*

Mucinex® Maximum Strength [OTC] *see* guaifenesin *on page 425*

Mucomyst *see* acetylcysteine *on page 36*

Mucomyst® (Can) *see* acetylcysteine *on page 36*

mucosal barrier gel, oral (myoo KOH sul BAR ee er GEL, OR al)

Synonyms mucosal bioadherent gel

U.S. Brand Names Gelclair®

Therapeutic Category Gastrointestinal Agent, Miscellaneous

Use Management of oral mucosal pain caused by oral mucositis/stomatitis (resulting from chemotherapy or radiation therapy), irritation due to oral surgery, traumatic ulcers caused by braces/ill-fitting dentures or disease, diffuse aphthous ulcers (canker sores)

General Dosage Range Oral: *Adults:* Gargle and spit the mixture of 1 single-use packet (15 mL) and water 3 times/day, or as needed.

Dosage Forms

Gel, oral:

Gelclair®: 15 mL/packet (15s)

mucosal bioadherent gel *see* mucosal barrier gel, oral *on page 602*

Mucus Relief [OTC] *see* guaifenesin *on page 425*

Mucus Relief Sinus [OTC] *see* guaifenesin and phenylephrine *on page 428*

Multaq® *see* dronedarone *on page 314*

Multidex® [OTC] *see* maltodextrin *on page 548*

Multihance® *see* gadobenate dimeglumine *on page 406*

Multihance® Multipack™ *see* gadobenate dimeglumine *on page 406*

Multi-Nate 30 *see* vitamins (multiple/prenatal) *on page 920*

multiple vitamins *see* vitamins (multiple/oral) *on page 919*

Multitrace®-4 *see* trace metals *on page 880*

Multitrace®-4 Concentrate *see* trace metals *on page 880*

Multitrace®-4 Neonatal *see* trace metals *on page 880*

Multitrace®-4 Pediatric *see* trace metals *on page 880*

Multitrace®-5 *see* trace metals *on page 880*

Multitrace®-5 Concentrate *see* trace metals *on page 880*

multivitamins/fluoride *see* vitamins (multiple/pediatric) *on page 920*

mumps, measles and rubella vaccines *see* measles, mumps, and rubella virus vaccine *on page 551*

mumps, rubella, varicella, and measles vaccine *see* measles, mumps, rubella, and varicella virus vaccine *on page 551*

mupirocin (myoo PEER oh sin)

Medication Safety Issues
Sound-alike/look-alike issues:
Bactroban® may be confused with bacitracin, baclofen, Bactrim™

Synonyms mupirocin calcium; pseudomonic acid A
U.S. Brand Names Bactroban Cream®; Bactroban Nasal®; Bactroban®; Centany®; Centany® AT
Canadian Brand Names Bactroban®
Therapeutic Category Antibiotic, Topical
Use
Intranasal: Eradication of nasal colonization with MRSA in adult patients and healthcare workers
Topical: Treatment of impetigo or secondary infected traumatic skin lesions due to *S. aureus* and *S. pyogenes*

General Dosage Range
Intranasal: *Children ≥12 years and Adults:* Approximately one-half of the ointment from the single-use tube should be applied into one nostril and the other half into the other nostril twice daily
Topical: *Children ≥2 months and Adults:* Apply to affected area 3 times/day

Dosage Forms
Cream, topical:
Bactroban Cream®: 2% (15 g, 30 g)
Ointment, intranasal:
Bactroban Nasal®: 2% (1 g)
Ointment, topical: 2% (0.9 g, 15 g, 22 g, 30 g)
Bactroban®: 2% (22 g)
Centany®: 2% (30 g)
Centany® AT: 2% (1s)

mupirocin calcium *see* mupirocin *on page 603*
Murine® Ear [OTC] *see* carbamide peroxide *on page 172*
Murine® Ear Wax Removal Kit [OTC] *see* carbamide peroxide *on page 172*
Murine Tears® [OTC] *see* artificial tears *on page 96*
Murine® Tears Plus [OTC] *see* tetrahydrozoline (ophthalmic) *on page 858*
Muro 128® [OTC] *see* sodium chloride *on page 818*
Murocel® [OTC] *see* artificial tears *on page 96*

muromonab-CD3 (myoo roe MOE nab see dee three)

Synonyms monoclonal antibody; OKT3
U.S. Brand Names Orthoclone OKT® 3 [DSC]
Therapeutic Category Immunosuppressant Agent
Use Treatment of acute allograft rejection in renal transplant patients; treatment of steroid-resistant acute allograft rejection in cardiac or hepatic transplantation
General Dosage Range I.V.:
Children ≤30 kg: 2.5 mg once daily
Children >30 kg and Adults: 5 mg once daily
Product Availability Orthoclone OKT® 3: Due to diminishing use, the manufacturer of muromonab is discontinuing production; supplies are expected to be available through the end of 2010.

Muse® *see* alprostadil *on page 57*
Muse® Pellet (Can) *see* alprostadil *on page 57*
Mustargen® *see* mechlorethamine *on page 552*
mustine *see* mechlorethamine *on page 552*
Mutamycin® (Can) *see* mitomycin *on page 592*
M.V.I.®-12 *see* vitamins (multiple/injectable) *on page 919*
M.V.I. Adult™ *see* vitamins (multiple/injectable) *on page 919*
M.V.I® Pediatric *see* vitamins (multiple/injectable) *on page 919*
Myadec® [OTC] *see* vitamins (multiple/oral) *on page 919*
Myambutol® *see* ethambutol *on page 351*
Mycamine® *see* micafungin *on page 585*
Mycelex *see* clotrimazole (oral) *on page 225*

Mycinettes® [OTC] *see* benzocaine *on page 121*
Mycobutin® *see* rifabutin *on page 779*
Mycocide® NS [OTC] *see* tolnaftate *on page 876*

mycophenolate (mye koe FEN oh late)

Synonyms MMF; MPA; mycophenolate mofetil; mycophenolate sodium; mycophenolic acid
U.S. Brand Names CellCept®; Myfortic®
Canadian Brand Names CellCept®; Myfortic®
Therapeutic Category Immunosuppressant Agent
Use Prophylaxis of organ rejection concomitantly with cyclosporine and corticosteroids in patients receiving allogeneic renal (CellCept®, Myfortic®), cardiac (CellCept®), or hepatic (CellCept®) transplants
General Dosage Range Dosage adjustment recommended in patient with renal impairment and who develop toxicities
I.V.: *Adults:* 1-1.5 g twice daily
Oral:
Cellcept®:
Children (suspension): 600 mg/m²/dose twice daily (maximum: 1 g twice daily)
Children with BSA 1.25-1.5 m²: 750 mg capsule twice daily
Children with BSA >1.5 m²: 1 g capsule or tablet twice daily
Adults: 1-1.5 g twice daily
Myfortic®:
Children with BSA 1.19-1.58 m²: 540 mg twice daily (maximum: 1080 mg/day)
Children with BSA >1.58 m² and Adults: 720 mg twice daily (maximum: 1440 mg/day)
Dosage Forms
Capsule, oral: 250 mg
CellCept®: 250 mg
Injection, powder for reconstitution:
CellCept®: 500 mg
Powder for suspension, oral:
CellCept®: 200 mg/mL (175 mL)
Tablet, oral: 500 mg
CellCept®: 500 mg
Tablet, delayed release, oral:
Myfortic®: 180 mg, 360 mg

mycophenolate mofetil *see* mycophenolate *on page 604*
mycophenolate sodium *see* mycophenolate *on page 604*
mycophenolic acid *see* mycophenolate *on page 604*
Mydfrin® *see* phenylephrine (ophthalmic) *on page 697*
Mydral™ [DSC] *see* tropicamide *on page 895*
Mydriacyl® *see* tropicamide *on page 895*
My First Flintstones™ [OTC] *see* vitamins (multiple/pediatric) *on page 920*
Myfortic® *see* mycophenolate *on page 604*
MyHist-PD *see* chlorpheniramine, pyrilamine, and phenylephrine *on page 202*
MyKidz Iron™ [OTC] *see* vitamins (multiple/pediatric) *on page 920*
MyKidz Iron 10™ [OTC] *see* ferrous sulfate *on page 374*
MyKidz Iron FL™ *see* vitamins (multiple/pediatric) *on page 920*
Mylan-Acebutolol (Can) *see* acebutolol *on page 23*
Mylan-Acebutolol (Type S) (Can) *see* acebutolol *on page 23*
Mylan-Acyclovir (Can) *see* acyclovir (systemic) *on page 39*
Mylan-Alendronate (Can) *see* alendronate *on page 49*
Mylan-Alprazolam (Can) *see* alprazolam *on page 56*
Mylan-Amantadine (Can) *see* amantadine *on page 62*
Mylan-Amiodarone (Can) *see* amiodarone *on page 67*
Mylan-Amlodipine (Can) *see* amlodipine *on page 69*
Mylan-Amoxicillin (Can) *see* amoxicillin *on page 73*
Mylan-Anagrelide (Can) *see* anagrelide *on page 78*
Mylan-Atenolol (Can) *see* atenolol *on page 101*

Mylan-Mirtazapine (Can) *see* mirtazapine *on page 592*
Mylan-Nabumetone (Can) *see* nabumetone *on page 607*
Mylan-Naproxen EC (Can) *see* naproxen *on page 612*
Mylan-Nifedipine Extended Release (Can) *see* nifedipine *on page 626*
Mylan-Nitro Sublingual Spray (Can) *see* nitroglycerin *on page 629*
Mylan-Omeprazole (Can) *see* omeprazole *on page 649*
Mylan-Ondansetron (Can) *see* ondansetron *on page 651*
Mylan-Oxybutynin (Can) *see* oxybutynin *on page 661*
Mylan-Pantoprazole (Can) *see* pantoprazole *on page 672*
Mylan-Paroxetine (Can) *see* paroxetine *on page 676*
Mylan-Pindolol (Can) *see* pindolol *on page 705*
Mylan-Pioglitazone (Can) *see* pioglitazone *on page 706*
Mylan-Pravastatin (Can) *see* pravastatin *on page 732*
Mylan-Propafenone (Can) *see* propafenone *on page 744*
Mylan-Quetiapine (Can) *see* quetiapine *on page 760*
Mylan-Ramipril (Can) *see* ramipril *on page 766*
Mylan-Ranitidine (Can) *see* ranitidine *on page 767*
Mylan-Risperidone (Can) *see* risperidone *on page 783*
Mylan-Rivastigmine (Can) *see* rivastigmine *on page 786*
Mylan-Salbutamol Respirator Solution (Can) *see* albuterol *on page 45*
Mylan-Salbutamol Sterinebs P.F. (Can) *see* albuterol *on page 45*
Mylan-Selegiline (Can) *see* selegiline *on page 806*
Mylan-Sertraline (Can) *see* sertraline *on page 809*
Mylan-Simvastatin (Can) *see* simvastatin *on page 813*
Mylan-Sotalol (Can) *see* sotalol *on page 828*
Mylan-Sumatriptan (Can) *see* sumatriptan *on page 839*
Mylanta™ (Can) *see* aluminum hydroxide and magnesium hydroxide *on page 60*
Mylanta® Classic Maximum Strength Liquid [OTC] *see* aluminum hydroxide, magnesium hydroxide, and simethicone *on page 60*
Mylanta® Classic Regular Strength Liquid [OTC] *see* aluminum hydroxide, magnesium hydroxide, and simethicone *on page 60*
Mylanta® Double Strength (Can) *see* aluminum hydroxide, magnesium hydroxide, and simethicone *on page 60*
Mylanta® Extra Strength (Can) *see* aluminum hydroxide, magnesium hydroxide, and simethicone *on page 60*
Mylanta® Gas Maximum Strength [OTC] *see* simethicone *on page 812*
Mylanta® Gelcaps® [OTC] *see* calcium carbonate and magnesium hydroxide *on page 162*
Mylan-Tamoxifen (Can) *see* tamoxifen *on page 843*
Mylan-Tamsulosin (Can) *see* tamsulosin *on page 843*
Mylanta® Regular Strength (Can) *see* aluminum hydroxide, magnesium hydroxide, and simethicone *on page 60*
Mylanta® Supreme [OTC] *see* calcium carbonate and magnesium hydroxide *on page 162*
Mylanta® Ultra [OTC] *see* calcium carbonate and magnesium hydroxide *on page 162*
Mylan-Terbinafine (Can) *see* terbinafine (systemic) *on page 851*
Mylan-Ticlopidine (Can) *see* ticlopidine *on page 868*
Mylan-Timolol (Can) *see* timolol (ophthalmic) *on page 869*
Mylan-Tizanidine (Can) *see* tizanidine *on page 872*
Mylan-Topiramate (Can) *see* topiramate *on page 877*
Mylan-Trazodone (Can) *see* trazodone *on page 884*
Mylan-Triazolam (Can) *see* triazolam *on page 888*
Mylan-Valacyclovir (Can) *see* valacyclovir *on page 903*
Mylan-Valproic (Can) *see* valproic acid *on page 904*
Mylan-Venlafaxine XR (Can) *see* venlafaxine *on page 911*
Mylan-Verapamil (Can) *see* verapamil *on page 912*

Mylan-Verapamil SR (Can) *see* verapamil *on page 912*
Mylan-Warfarin (Can) *see* warfarin *on page 922*
Mylan-Zolmitriptan (Can) *see* zolmitriptan *on page 933*
Mylan-Zopiclone (Can) *see* zopiclone *(Canada only) on page 934*
Myleran® *see* busulfan *on page 152*
Mylicon® Infants' [OTC] *see* simethicone *on page 812*
Mylotarg *see* gemtuzumab ozogamicin *on page 414*
Myl-Ranitidine (Can) *see* ranitidine *on page 767*
Myobloc® *see* rimabotulinumtoxinB *on page 781*
Myocet™ (Can) *see* doxorubicin (liposomal) *on page 311*
Myochrysine® *see* gold sodium thiomalate *on page 423*
Myoflex® [OTC] *see* trolamine *on page 894*
Myoflex® (Can) *see* trolamine *on page 894*
Myozyme® *see* alglucosidase alfa *on page 51*
Myphetane DX [DSC] *see* brompheniramine, pseudoephedrine, and dextromethorphan *on page 144*
Mysoline® *see* primidone *on page 737*
Mytelase® *see* ambenonium *on page 62*
mytotan *see* mitotane *on page 593*
Mytussin® DAC *see* guaifenesin, pseudoephedrine, and codeine *on page 430*
N-9 *see* nonoxynol 9 *on page 632*
NAAK *see* atropine and pralidoxime *on page 104*
Nabi-HB® *see* hepatitis B immune globulin (human) *on page 438*
nab-paclitaxel *see* paclitaxel (protein bound) *on page 667*

nabumetone (na BYOO me tone)

Synonyms Relafen
Canadian Brand Names Apo-Nabumetone®; Gen-Nabumetone; Mylan-Nabumetone; Novo-Nabumetone; Relafen®; Rhoxal-nabumetone; Sandoz-Nabumetone
Therapeutic Category Analgesic, Nonnarcotic; Nonsteroidal Antiinflammatory Drug (NSAID)
Use Management of osteoarthritis and rheumatoid arthritis
General Dosage Range Dosage adjustment recommended in patients with renal impairment
Oral: *Adults:* 1000 mg/day in 1-2 divided doses (maximum: 2000 mg/day)
Dosage Forms
Tablet, oral: 500 mg, 750 mg

NAC *see* acetylcysteine *on page 36*
N-acetyl-L-cysteine *see* acetylcysteine *on page 36*
N-acetylcysteine *see* acetylcysteine *on page 36*
n-acetyl-p-aminophenol *see* acetaminophen *on page 23*
NaCl *see* sodium chloride *on page 818*

nadolol (NAY doe lol)

Medication Safety Issues
Sound-alike/look-alike issues:
Nadolol may be confused with Mandol®
Corgard® may be confused with Cognex®, Coreg®
U.S. Brand Names Corgard®
Canadian Brand Names Alti-Nadolol; Apo-Nadol®; Corgard®; Novo-Nadolol
Therapeutic Category Beta-Adrenergic Blocker
Use Treatment of hypertension and angina pectoris; prophylaxis of migraine headaches
General Dosage Range Dosage adjustment recommended in patients with renal impairment
Oral:
Adults: Initial: 40 mg once daily; Maintenance: 40-320 mg once daily
Elderly: Initial: 20 mg once daily; Maintenance: 20-240 mg once daily

◄ **Dosage Forms**
Tablet, oral: 20 mg, 40 mg, 80 mg
Corgard®: 20 mg, 40 mg, 80 mg

nadolol and bendroflumethiazide (NAY doe lol & ben droe floo meth EYE a zide)

Synonyms bendroflumethiazide and nadolol

U.S. Brand Names Corzide®

Therapeutic Category Antihypertensive Agent, Combination; Beta-Adrenergic Blocker, Nonselective; Diuretic, Thiazide

Use Treatment of hypertension; combination product should not be used for initial therapy

General Dosage Range Dosage adjustment recommended in patients with renal impairment
Oral: *Adults:* Initial: Nadolol 40 mg and bendroflumethiazide 5 mg once daily; Maintenance: Nadolol 40-80 mg and bendroflumethiazide 5 mg once daily

Dosage Forms
Tablet: Nadolol 40 mg and bendroflumethiazide 5 mg; nadolol 80 mg and bendroflumethiazide 5 mg
Corzide® 40/5: Nadolol 40 mg and bendroflumethiazide 5 mg [scored]
Corzide® 80/5: Nadolol 80 mg and bendroflumethiazide 5 mg [scored]

nadroparin calcium *see* nadroparin *(Canada only) on page 608*

nadroparin *(Canada only)* (nad roe PA rin)

Medication Safety Issues
High alert medication:
This medication is in a class the Institute for Safe Medication Practices (ISMP) includes among its list of drug classes which have a heightened risk of causing significant patient harm when used in error.

Synonyms nadroparin calcium

Canadian Brand Names Fraxiparine™; Fraxiparine™ Forte

Therapeutic Category Low Molecular Weight Heparin

Use Prophylaxis of thromboembolic disorders (particularly deep venous thrombosis and pulmonary embolism) in general and orthopedic surgery; treatment of deep venous thrombosis; prevention of clotting during hemodialysis; treatment of unstable angina and non-Q-wave myocardial infarction

General Dosage Range Dosage varies greatly depending on indication.

Product Availability Not available in U.S.

Dosage Forms - Canada
Injection, solution:
Fraxiparine™: 9500 anti-Xa int. units/mL (0.2 mL, 0.3 mL, 0.4 mL, 0.6 mL, 0.8 mL, 1 mL)
Fraxiparine™ Forte: 19,000 anti-Xa int. units/mL (0.6 mL, 0.8 mL, 1 mL)

nafarelin (naf a REL in)

Medication Safety Issues
Sound-alike/look-alike issues:
Nafarelin may be confused with Anafranil®, enalapril

Synonyms nafarelin acetate

U.S. Brand Names Synarel®

Canadian Brand Names Synarel®

Therapeutic Category Hormone, Posterior Pituitary

Use Treatment of endometriosis, including pain and reduction of lesions; treatment of central precocious puberty (CPP; gonadotropin-dependent precocious puberty) in children of both sexes

General Dosage Range Nasal:
Children: 2 sprays (400 mcg) into each nostril twice daily; may increase to 3 sprays (600 mcg) into alternating nostrils 3 times/day
Adults: 1 spray (200 mcg) in 1-2 nostrils twice daily

Dosage Forms
Solution, intranasal:
Synarel®: 2 mg/mL (8 mL)

nafarelin acetate *see* nafarelin *on page 608*

nafcillin (naf SIL in)

Synonyms ethoxynaphthamido penicillin sodium; nafcillin sodium; Nallpen; sodium nafcillin

Canadian Brand Names Nallpen®; Unipen®

Therapeutic Category Penicillin

Use Treatment of infections such as osteomyelitis, septicemia, endocarditis, and CNS infections caused by susceptible strains of staphylococci species

General Dosage Range

I.M.:
Children: 25 mg/kg twice daily
Adults: 500 mg every 4-6 hours

I.V.:
Children: 50-200 mg/kg/day in divided every 4-6 hours (maximum: 12 g/day)
Adults: 500-2000 mg every 4-6 hours

Dosage Forms
Infusion, premixed iso-osmotic dextrose solution: 1 g (50 mL); 2 g (100 mL)
Injection, powder for reconstitution: 1 g, 2 g, 10 g

nafcillin sodium *see nafcillin on page 609*

naftifine (NAF ti feen)

Synonyms naftifine hydrochloride

U.S. Brand Names Naftin®

Therapeutic Category Antifungal Agent

Use Topical treatment of tinea cruris (jock itch), tinea corporis (ringworm), and tinea pedis (athlete's foot)

General Dosage Range Topical: *Adults:* Apply cream once daily and gel twice daily

Dosage Forms
Cream, topical:
Naftin®: 1% (30 g, 60 g, 90 g)
Gel, topical:
Naftin®: 1% (40 g, 60 g, 90 g)

naftifine hydrochloride *see naftifine on page 609*

Naftin® *see naftifine on page 609*

Naglazyme® *see galsulfase on page 410*

NaHCO₃ *see sodium bicarbonate on page 818*

nalbuphine (NAL byoo feen)

Medication Safety Issues
Sound-alike/look-alike issues:
Nubain may be confused with Navane®, Nebcin®
High alert medication:
The Institute for Safe Medication Practices (ISMP) includes this medication among its list of drug classes which have a heightened risk of causing significant patient harm when used in error.

Synonyms nalbuphine hydrochloride; Nubain

Therapeutic Category Analgesic, Narcotic

Use Relief of moderate-to-severe pain; preoperative analgesia, postoperative and surgical anesthesia, and obstetrical analgesia during labor and delivery

General Dosage Range
I.M., SubQ: *Adults:* 10 mg/70 kg every 3-6 hours (maximum: 20 mg/dose; 160 mg/day)
I.V.: *Adults:* 10 mg/70 kg every 3-6 hours (maximum: 20 mg/dose; 160 mg/day) **or** 0.3-3 mg/kg over 10-15 minutes, then 0.25-0.5 mg/kg as required for anesthesia **or** 2.5-5 mg (1-2 doses)

Dosage Forms
Injection, solution: 10 mg/mL (10 mL); 20 mg/mL (10 mL)
Injection, solution [preservative free]: 10 mg/mL (1 mL); 20 mg/mL (1 mL)

nalbuphine hydrochloride *see nalbuphine on page 609*

Nalcrom® (Can) *see cromolyn (systemic, oral inhalation) on page 238*

Nalex®-A *see chlorpheniramine, phenylephrine, and phenyltoloxamine on page 201*

Nalex A 12 *see chlorpheniramine, pyrilamine, and phenylephrine on page 202*

Nalfon® *see* fenoprofen *on page 370*
Nallpen *see* nafcillin *on page 609*
Nallpen® (Can) *see* nafcillin *on page 609*
N-allylnoroxymorphine hydrochloride *see* naloxone *on page 610*

naloxone (nal OKS one)

Medication Safety Issues
Sound-alike/look-alike issues:
Naloxone may be confused with Lanoxin®, naltrexone
Narcan® may be confused with Marcaine®, Norcuron®
International issues:
Narcan [multiple international markets] may be confused with Marcen brand name for ketazolam [Spain]
Synonyms N-allylnoroxymorphine hydrochloride; naloxone hydrochloride; Narcan
Canadian Brand Names Naloxone Hydrochloride Injection®
Therapeutic Category Antidote
Use Complete or partial reversal of opioid drug effects, including respiratory depression; management of known or suspected opioid overdose; diagnosis of suspected opioid dependence or acute opioid overdose
General Dosage Range I.M., I.V., SubQ, intratracheal:
Birth (including premature infants) to 5 years or ≤20 kg: 0.01 mg/kg **or** 0.1 mg/kg (maximum dose: 2 mg) every 2-3 minutes as needed
Children >5 years or >20 kg: 0.01 mg/kg **or** 2 mg/dose, if no response repeat every 2-3 minutes as needed
Adults: 0.1-2 mg every 2-3 minutes as needed (maximum: 10 mg)
Dosage Forms
Injection, solution: 0.4 mg/mL (1 mL, 10 mL)
Injection, solution [preservative free]: 1 mg/mL (2 mL)

naloxone and buprenorphine *see* buprenorphine and naloxone *on page 149*
naloxone hydrochloride *see* naloxone *on page 610*
naloxone hydrochloride and pentazocine *see* pentazocine and naloxone *on page 687*
naloxone hydrochloride dihydrate and buprenorphine hydrochloride *see* buprenorphine and naloxone *on page 149*
Naloxone Hydrochloride Injection® (Can) *see* naloxone *on page 610*

naltrexone (nal TREKS one)

Medication Safety Issues
Sound-alike/look-alike issues:
Naltrexone may be confused with methylnaltrexone, naloxone
ReVia® may be confused with Revatio®, Revex®
Administration issues:
Vivitrol®: For intramuscular (I.M.) gluteal injection only
Synonyms naltrexone hydrochloride
U.S. Brand Names ReVia®; Vivitrol®
Canadian Brand Names ReVia®
Therapeutic Category Antidote
Use Treatment of ethanol dependence; prevention of relapse in opioid dependent patients, following opioid detoxification
General Dosage Range
I.M.: *Adults:* 380 mg once every 4 weeks
Oral: *Adults:* 25-50 mg once daily
Dosage Forms
Injection, microspheres for suspension, extended release:
Vivitrol®: 380 mg
Tablet, oral: 50 mg
ReVia®: 50 mg

naltrexone and morphine *see* morphine and naltrexone *on page 599*
naltrexone hydrochloride *see* naltrexone *on page 610*

Namenda® *see* memantine *on page 556*
Namenda XR *see* memantine *on page 556*
nanoparticle albumin-bound paclitaxel *see* paclitaxel (protein bound) *on page 667*
NAPA and NABZ *see* sodium phenylacetate and sodium benzoate *on page 822*

naphazoline (nasal) (naf AZ oh leen)

Synonyms naphazoline hydrochloride
U.S. Brand Names Privine® [OTC]
Therapeutic Category Alpha₁ Agonist
Use Temporary relief of nasal congestion associated with the common cold, upper respiratory allergies, or sinusitis
General Dosage Range Intranasal: *Children ≥12 years and Adults:* Instill 1-2 drops or sprays every 6 hours if needed
Dosage Forms
Solution, intranasal:
Privine® [OTC]: 0.05% (20 mL, 25 mL)

naphazoline (ophthalmic) (naf AZ oh leen)

Synonyms naphazoline hydrochloride
U.S. Brand Names AK-Con™; Clear eyes® for Dry Eyes Plus ACR Relief [OTC]; Clear eyes® for Dry Eyes plus Redness Relief [OTC]; Clear eyes® Redness Relief [OTC]; Clear eyes® Seasonal Relief [OTC]
Canadian Brand Names Naphcon Forte®; Vasocon®
Therapeutic Category Alpha₁ Agonist; Ophthalmic Agent, Vasoconstrictor
Use Topical ocular vasoconstrictor; relief of redness of the eye due to minor irritation
General Dosage Range Ophthalmic: *Adults:*
0.1% solution (prescription): 1-2 drops into conjuctival sac every 3-4 hours as needed
0.012% or 0.025% solution (OTC): 1-2 drops into affected eye(s) up to 4 times/day
Dosage Forms
Solution, ophthalmic:
AK-Con™: 0.1% (15 mL)
Clear eyes® for Dry Eyes Plus ACR Relief [OTC]: 0.025% (15 mL)
Clear eyes® for Dry Eyes plus Redness Relief [OTC]: 0.012% (15 mL)
Clear eyes® Redness Relief [OTC]: 0.012% (6 mL, 15 mL, 30 mL)
Clear eyes® Seasonal Relief [OTC]: 0.012% (15 mL, 30 mL)

naphazoline and pheniramine (naf AZ oh leen & fen NIR a meen)

Medication Safety Issues
Sound-alike/look-alike issues:
Visine® may be confused with Visken®
Synonyms pheniramine and naphazoline
U.S. Brand Names Naphcon-A® [OTC]; Opcon-A® [OTC]; Visine-A® [OTC]
Canadian Brand Names Naphcon-A®; Visine® Advanced Allergy
Therapeutic Category Antihistamine/Decongestant Combination
Use Treatment of ocular congestion, irritation, and itching
General Dosage Range Ophthalmic: *Children ≥6 years and Adults:* 1-2 drops up to 4 times/day
Dosage Forms
Solution, ophthalmic:
Naphcon-A® [OTC]: Naphazoline 0.025% and pheniramine 0.3%
Opcon-A® [OTC]: Naphazoline 0.027% and pheniramine 0.3%
Visine-A® [OTC]: Naphazoline 0.025% and pheniramine 0.3%

naphazoline hydrochloride *see* naphazoline (nasal) *on page 611*
naphazoline hydrochloride *see* naphazoline (ophthalmic) *on page 611*
Naphcon-A® [OTC] *see* naphazoline and pheniramine *on page 611*
Naphcon-A® (Can) *see* naphazoline and pheniramine *on page 611*
Naphcon Forte® (Can) *see* naphazoline (ophthalmic) *on page 611*
Naprelan® *see* naproxen *on page 612*

Naprelan™ (Can) *see* naproxen *on page 612*
Naprosyn® *see* naproxen *on page 612*
Naprosyn® E (Can) *see* naproxen *on page 612*
Naprosyn® SR (Can) *see* naproxen *on page 612*

naproxen (na PROKS en)

Medication Safety Issues
Sound-alike/look-alike issues:
Naproxen may be confused with Natacyn®, Nebcin®
Anaprox® may be confused with Anaspaz®, Avapro®
Naprelan® may be confused with Naprosyn®
Naprosyn® may be confused with Naprelan®, Natacyn®, Nebcin®
Beers Criteria medication:
This drug may be inappropriate for use in geriatric patients (high severity risk).
International issues:
Flogen [Mexico] may be confused with Flovent brand name for fluticasone [U.S., Canada]
Flogen [Mexico] may be confused with Floxin brand name for flunarizine [Thailand], norfloxacin [South Africa], ofloxacin [U.S., Canada], and perfloxacin [Philippines]

Synonyms naproxen sodium

U.S. Brand Names Aleve® [OTC]; Anaprox®; Anaprox® DS; EC-Naprosyn®; Mediproxen [OTC]; Midol® Extended Relief [OTC]; Naprelan®; Naprosyn®; Pamprin® Maximum Strength All Day Relief [OTC]

Canadian Brand Names Anaprox®; Anaprox® DS; Apo-Napro-Na DS®; Apo-Napro-Na®; Apo-Naproxen EC®; Apo-Naproxen SR®; Apo-Naproxen®; Mylan-Naproxen EC; Naprelan™; Naprosyn®; Naprosyn® E; Naprosyn® SR; Naproxen Sodium DS; Naproxen-NA; Naproxen-NA DF; PMS-Naproxen; PMS-Naproxen EC; PRO-Naproxen EC; Riva-Naproxen; Riva-Naproxen Sodium; Riva-Naproxen Sodium DS; Teva-Naproxen; Teva-Naproxen EC; Teva-Naproxen Sodium; Teva-Naproxen Sodium DS; Teva-Naproxen SR

Therapeutic Category Analgesic, Nonnarcotic; Antipyretic; Nonsteroidal Antiinflammatory Drug (NSAID)

Use Management of ankylosing spondylitis, osteoarthritis, and rheumatoid disorders (including juvenile idiopathic arthritis [JIA]); acute gout; mild-to-moderate pain; tendonitis; bursitis; dysmenorrhea; fever

General Dosage Range Oral:
Children >2-11 years: 10 mg/kg/day in 2 divided doses (maximum: 10 mg/kg/day)
Children ≥12 years: 10 mg/kg/day in 2 divided doses (maximum: 10 mg/kg/day) **or** 200 mg every 8-12 hours (maximum: 600 mg/day)
Adults: Initial: 200-750 mg as a single dose; Maintenance: 200-500 mg every 6-12 hours (maximum: 1500 mg/day)

Dosage Forms
Caplet, oral: 220 mg
Aleve® [OTC]: 220 mg
Midol® Extended Relief [OTC]: 220 mg
Pamprin® Maximum Strength All Day Relief [OTC]: 220 mg
Capsule, liquid gel, oral:
Aleve® [OTC]: 220 mg
Combination package, oral:
Naprelan®: Day 1-3: Tablet, controlled release: 825 mg [equivalent to naproxen base 750 mg] (6s) [contains sodium 75 mg] and Day 4-10: Tablet, controlled release: 550 mg [equivalent to naproxen base 500 mg] (14s) [contains sodium 50 mg]
Gelcap, oral:
Aleve® [OTC]: 220 mg
Suspension, oral: 125 mg/5 mL (500 mL)
Naprosyn®: 125 mg/5 mL (473 mL)
Tablet, oral: 220 mg, 250 mg, 275 mg, 375 mg, 500 mg, 550 mg
Aleve® [OTC]: 220 mg
Anaprox®: 275 mg
Anaprox® DS: 550 mg
Mediproxen [OTC]: 220 mg
Naprosyn®: 250 mg, 375 mg, 500 mg

Tablet, controlled release, oral:
Naprelan®: 412.5 mg, 550 mg, 825 mg
Tablet, delayed release, enteric coated, oral: 375 mg, 500 mg
EC-Naprosyn®: 375 mg, 500 mg

naproxen and esomeprazole (na PROKS en & es oh ME pray zol)

Medication Safety Issues
Sound-alike/look-alike issues:
Vimovo™ may be confused with Vimpat®
Synonyms esomeprazole and naproxen
U.S. Brand Names Vimovo™
Canadian Brand Names Vimovo™
Therapeutic Category Nonsteroidal Antiinflammatory Drug (NSAID); Proton Pump Inhibitor
Use Reduction of the risk of NSAID-associated gastric ulcers in patients at risk of developing gastric ulcers who require an NSAID for the treatment of rheumatoid arthritis, osteoarthritis, and ankylosing spondylitis
General Dosage Range Oral: *Adults:* 1 tablet (naproxen 375-500 mg/esomeprazole 20 mg) twice daily; Maximum daily dose of esomeprazole: 40 mg/day
Dosage Forms
Tablet, variable release, oral:
Vimovo™: Naproxen [delayed release] 375 mg and esomeprazole [immediate release] 20 mg, Naproxen [delayed release] 500 mg and esomeprazole [immediate release] 20 mg

naproxen and pseudoephedrine (na PROKS en & soo doe e FED rin)

Synonyms naproxen sodium and pseudoephedrine; pseudoephedrine and naproxen
U.S. Brand Names Aleve®-D Sinus & Cold [OTC]; Aleve®-D Sinus & Headache [OTC]; Sudafed® 12 Hour Pressure + Pain [OTC]
Therapeutic Category Decongestant/Analgesic
Use Temporary relief of cold, sinus, and flu symptoms (including nasal congestion, sinus congestion/ pressure, headache, minor body aches and pains, and fever)
General Dosage Range Oral: *Children ≥12 years and Adults:* 1 caplet (naproxen sodium 220 mg/ pseudoephedrine 120 mg) every 12 hours (maximum: 2 caplets/day)
Dosage Forms
Caplet, extended release:
Aleve®-D Sinus & Cold [OTC], Aleve®-D Sinus & Headache [OTC], Sudafed® 12 Hour Pressure + Pain [OTC]: Naproxen sodium 220 mg [equivalent to naproxen 200 mg and sodium 20 mg] and pseudoephedrine hydrochloride 120 mg

naproxen and sumatriptan see sumatriptan and naproxen *on page 839*
Naproxen-NA (Can) see naproxen *on page 612*
Naproxen-NA DF (Can) see naproxen *on page 612*
naproxen sodium see naproxen *on page 612*
naproxen sodium and pseudoephedrine see naproxen and pseudoephedrine *on page 613*
naproxen sodium and sumatriptan see sumatriptan and naproxen *on page 839*
naproxen sodium and sumatriptan succinate see sumatriptan and naproxen *on page 839*
Naproxen Sodium DS (Can) see naproxen *on page 612*

naratriptan (NAR a trip tan)

Medication Safety Issues
Sound-alike/look-alike issues:
Amerge® may be confused with Altace®, Amaryl®
Synonyms naratriptan hydrochloride
U.S. Brand Names Amerge®
Canadian Brand Names Amerge®
Therapeutic Category Antimigraine Agent; Serotonin Agonist
Use Treatment of acute migraine headache with or without aura
General Dosage Range Dosage adjustment recommended in patients with hepatic or renal impairment
Oral: *Adults:* 1-2.5 mg, may repeat after 4 hours (maximum: 5 mg/day)

◀ **Dosage Forms**
Tablet, oral: 1 mg, 2.5 mg
  Amerge®: 1 mg, 2.5 mg

naratriptan hydrochloride *see naratriptan on page 613*
Narcan *see naloxone on page 610*
Nardil® *see phenelzine on page 693*
Naropin® *see ropivacaine on page 790*
Nasacort® AQ *see triamcinolone (nasal) on page 886*
NāSal™ [OTC] *see sodium chloride on page 818*
NasalCrom® [OTC] *see cromolyn (nasal) on page 239*
Nasalide® (Can) *see flunisolide (nasal) on page 384*
Nasal Moist® Saline [OTC] *see sodium chloride on page 818*
Nasal Spray [OTC] [DSC] *see sodium chloride on page 818*
Nascobal® *see cyanocobalamin on page 241*
Nasonex® *see mometasone (nasal) on page 595*
NataChew® [OTC] *see vitamins (multiple/prenatal) on page 920*
Natacyn® *see natamycin on page 614*
NataFort® [OTC] *see vitamins (multiple/prenatal) on page 920*

natalizumab (na ta LIZ u mab)

Synonyms AN100226; anti-4 alpha integrin; IgG4-kappa monoclonal antibody
U.S. Brand Names Tysabri®
Canadian Brand Names Tysabri®
Therapeutic Category Monoclonal Antibody, Selective Adhesion-Molecule Inhibitor
Use Monotherapy for the treatment of relapsing forms of multiple sclerosis; treatment of moderately- to severely-active Crohn disease

Canada labeling: Treatment of relapsing forms of multiple sclerosis
General Dosage Range I.V.: *Adults:* 300 mg every 4 weeks
Dosage Forms
Injection, solution [preservative free]:
  Tysabri®: 300 mg/15 mL (15 mL)

natamycin (na ta MYE sin)

Medication Safety Issues
Sound-alike/look-alike issues:
  Natacyn® may be confused with Naprosyn®
Synonyms pimaricin
U.S. Brand Names Natacyn®
Canadian Brand Names Natacyn®
Therapeutic Category Antifungal Agent
Use Treatment of blepharitis, conjunctivitis, and keratitis caused by susceptible fungi (*Aspergillus, Candida, Cephalosporium, Fusarium,* and *Penicillium*)
General Dosage Range Ophthalmic: *Adults:* Initial: Instill 1 drop in conjunctival sac every 1-2 hours for 3-4 days; Maintenance: 1 drop 4-8 times/day
Dosage Forms
Suspension, ophthalmic:
  Natacyn®: 5% (15 mL)

Natazia™ *see estradiol and dienogest on page 345*

nateglinide (na te GLYE nide)

Medication Safety Issues
High alert medication:
  The Institute for Safe Medication Practices (ISMP) includes this medication among its list of drug classes which have a heightened risk of causing significant patient harm when used in error.
U.S. Brand Names Starlix®

Canadian Brand Names Starlix®

Therapeutic Category Antidiabetic Agent, Oral

Use Management of type 2 diabetes mellitus (noninsulin-dependent, NIDDM) as monotherapy when hyperglycemia cannot be managed by diet and exercise alone; in combination with metformin or a thiazolidinedione to lower blood glucose in patients whose hyperglycemia cannot be controlled by exercise, diet, or a single agent alone

General Dosage Range Oral: *Adults:* 60-120 mg 3 times/day

Dosage Forms

Tablet, oral: 60 mg, 120 mg

Starlix®: 60 mg, 120 mg

Natrecor® *see* nesiritide *on page 620*

natriuretic peptide *see* nesiritide *on page 620*

Natroba™ *see* spinosad *on page 829*

NatrOVA *see* spinosad *on page 829*

Natulan® (Can) *see* procarbazine *on page 739*

Natural Balance Tears [OTC] *see* hydroxypropyl methylcellulose *on page 455*

Natural Fiber Therapy [OTC] *see* psyllium *on page 755*

Natural Fiber Therapy Smooth Texture [OTC] *see* psyllium *on page 755*

natural lung surfactant *see* beractant *on page 127*

Nature's Tears® [OTC] *see* artificial tears *on page 96*

Nature's Tears [OTC] *see* hydroxypropyl methylcellulose *on page 455*

Nature-Throid™ *see* thyroid, desiccated *on page 865*

Nausea Relief [OTC] *see* fructose, dextrose, and phosphoric acid *on page 403*

Nauseatol (Can) *see* dimenhydrinate *on page 288*

Nausetrol® [OTC] *see* fructose, dextrose, and phosphoric acid *on page 403*

Navane® *see* thiothixene *on page 864*

Navelbine® *see* vinorelbine *on page 916*

Na-Zone® [OTC] *see* sodium chloride *on page 818*

N-carbamoyl-L-glutamic acid *see* carglumic acid *on page 176*

N-carbamylglutamate *see* carglumic acid *on page 176*

n-docosanol *see* docosanol *on page 302*

nebivolol (ne BIV oh lole)

Synonyms nebivolol hydrochloride

U.S. Brand Names Bystolic®

Therapeutic Category Beta Blocker, Beta-1 Selective

Use Treatment of hypertension, alone or in combination with other agents

General Dosage Range Dosage adjustment recommended in patients with hepatic or renal impairment

Oral: *Adults:* Initial: 5 mg once daily; Maintenance: 5-40 mg once daily

Dosage Forms

Tablet, oral:

Bystolic®: 2.5 mg, 5 mg, 10 mg, 20 mg

nebivolol hydrochloride *see* nebivolol *on page 615*

Nebupent® *see* pentamidine *on page 686*

Necon® 0.5/35 *see* ethinyl estradiol and norethindrone *on page 355*

Necon® 1/35 *see* ethinyl estradiol and norethindrone *on page 355*

Necon® 1/50 *see* norethindrone and mestranol *on page 633*

Necon® 7/7/7 *see* ethinyl estradiol and norethindrone *on page 355*

Necon® 10/11 *see* ethinyl estradiol and norethindrone *on page 355*

nedocromil (ne doe KROE mil)

Synonyms nedocromil sodium

U.S. Brand Names Alocril®

Canadian Brand Names Alocril®

Therapeutic Category Mast Cell Stabilizer
Use Treatment of itching associated with allergic conjunctivitis
General Dosage Range Ophthalmic: *Children ≥3 years and Adults:* 1-2 drops in each eye twice daily
Dosage Forms
 Solution, ophthalmic:
  Alocril®: 2% (5 mL)

nedocromil sodium *see nedocromil on page 615*
Néevo® *see vitamins (multiple/prenatal) on page 920*
Néevo® DHA *see vitamins (multiple/prenatal) on page 920*

nefazodone (nef AY zoe done)

Medication Safety Issues
 Sound-alike/look-alike issues:
  Serzone® may be confused with selegiline, Serentil®, SEROquel®, sertraline
Synonyms nefazodone hydrochloride; Serzone
Therapeutic Category Antidepressant, Miscellaneous
Use Treatment of depression
General Dosage Range
 Oral:
  Adults: Initial: 200 mg/day in 2 divided doses; Maintenance: 300-600 mg/day in 2 divided doses
  Elderly: Initial: 50 mg twice daily; Maintenance: 200-400 mg/day in 2 divided doses
Dosage Forms
 Tablet, oral: 50 mg, 100 mg, 150 mg, 200 mg, 250 mg

nefazodone hydrochloride *see nefazodone on page 616*

nelarabine (nel AY re been)

Medication Safety Issues
 High alert medication:
  The Institute for Safe Medication Practices (ISMP) includes this medication among its list of drug classes which have a heightened risk of causing significant patient harm when used in error.
Synonyms 2-amino-6-methoxypurine arabinoside; 506U78; GW506U78
U.S. Brand Names Arranon®
Canadian Brand Names Atriance™
Therapeutic Category Antineoplastic Agent, Antimetabolite
Use Treatment of relapsed or refractory T-cell acute lymphoblastic leukemia (ALL) and T-cell lymphoblastic lymphoma
General Dosage Range I.V.:
 Children: 650 mg/m^2/dose on days 1 through 5; repeat every 21 days
 Adults: 1500 mg/m^2/dose on days 1, 3, and 5; repeat every 21 days
Dosage Forms
 Injection, solution:
  Arranon®: 5 mg/mL (50 mL)
Dosage Forms - Canada
 Injection, solution:
  Atriance™: 5 mg/mL (50 mL)

nelfinavir (nel FIN a veer)

Medication Safety Issues
 Sound-alike/look-alike issues:
  Nelfinavir may be confused with nevirapine
  Viracept® may be confused with Viramune®, Viramune® XR™
Synonyms NFV
U.S. Brand Names Viracept®
Canadian Brand Names Viracept®
Therapeutic Category Antiviral Agent
Use In combination with other antiretroviral therapy in the treatment of HIV infection

General Dosage Range Oral:
Children 2-13 years: 45-55 mg/kg twice daily **or** 25-35 mg/kg 3 times/day (maximum: 2500 mg/day)
Adults: 750 mg 3 times/day **or** 1250 mg twice daily
Dosage Forms
Tablet, oral:
Viracept®: 250 mg, 625 mg

Nembutal® *see* pentobarbital *on page 688*
Nembutal® Sodium (Can) *see* pentobarbital *on page 688*
Neo DM *see* brompheniramine, pseudoephedrine, and dextromethorphan *on page 144*
Neo DM [DSC] *see* chlorpheniramine, phenylephrine, and dextromethorphan *on page 200*
Neo-Fradin™ *see* neomycin *on page 617*
Neofrin *see* phenylephrine (ophthalmic) *on page 697*

neomycin (nee oh MYE sin)

Synonyms neomycin sulfate
U.S. Brand Names Neo-Fradin™
Therapeutic Category Aminoglycoside (Antibiotic); Antibiotic, Topical
Use Orally to prepare GI tract for surgery; treatment of diarrhea caused by *E. coli*; adjunct in the treatment of hepatic encephalopathy
General Dosage Range Oral:
Children: Encephalopathy: 50-100 mg/kg/day divided every 6-8 hours **or** 2.5-7 g/m^2/day divided every 4-6 hours (maximum: 12 g/day); Preoperative GI preparation: 75-90 mg/kg/day
Adults: Encephalopathy/hepatic insufficiency: 500 mg to 12 g/day in divided doses every 4-8 hours; Preoperative GI preparation: 1 g for 3-9 doses
Dosage Forms
Solution, oral:
Neo-Fradin™: 125 mg/5 mL (480 mL)
Tablet, oral: 500 mg

neomycin and polymyxin B (nee oh MYE sin & pol i MIKS in bee)

Synonyms polymyxin B and neomycin
U.S. Brand Names Neosporin® G.U. Irrigant
Canadian Brand Names Neosporin® Irrigating Solution
Therapeutic Category Antibiotic, Topical; Genitourinary Irrigant
Use Short-term as a continuous irrigant or rinse in the urinary bladder to prevent bacteriuria and gram-negative rod septicemia associated with the use of indwelling catheters
General Dosage Range Irrigation (bladder): *Children and Adults:* Add 1 mL irrigant to 1 L isotonic saline solution (maximum: Usually no more than 1 L irrigant/day)
Dosage Forms
Solution, irrigation: Neomycin 40 mg and polymyxin B sulfate 200,000 units per 1 mL (1 mL, 20 mL)
Neosporin® G.U. Irrigant: Neomycin 40 mg and polymyxin sulfate B 200,000 units per 1 mL (1 mL, 20 mL)

neomycin, bacitracin, and polymyxin B *see* bacitracin, neomycin, and polymyxin B *on page 111*
neomycin, bacitracin, polymyxin B, and hydrocortisone *see* bacitracin, neomycin, polymyxin B, and hydrocortisone *on page 112*
neomycin, bacitracin, polymyxin B, and pramoxine *see* bacitracin, neomycin, polymyxin B, and pramoxine *on page 112*

neomycin, colistin, hydrocortisone, and thonzonium

(nee oh MYE sin, koe LIS tin, hye droe KOR ti sone, & thon ZOE nee um)

Synonyms colistin, hydrocortisone, neomycin, and thonzonium; hydrocortisone, neomycin, colistin, and thonzonium; thonzonium, neomycin, colistin, and hydrocortisone
U.S. Brand Names Coly-Mycin® S; Cortisporin®-TC
Therapeutic Category Antibiotic/Corticosteroid, Otic
Use Treatment of superficial and susceptible bacterial infections of the external auditory canal; for treatment of susceptible bacterial infections of mastoidectomy and fenestration cavities

◀ **General Dosage Range Otic:**
Children: 3-4 drops in affected ear 3-4 times/day
Adults: 4-5 drops in affected ear 3-4 times/day
Dosage Forms
Suspension, otic [drops]:
Coly-Mycin® S: Neomycin 0.33%, colistin 0.3%, hydrocortisone 1%, and thonzonium 0.05% (5 mL)
Cortisporin®-TC: Neomycin 0.33%, colistin 0.3%, hydrocortisone 1%, and thonzonium 0.05% (10 mL)

neomycin, polymyxin B, and dexamethasone
(nee oh MYE sin, pol i MIKS in bee, & deks a METH a sone)
Synonyms dexamethasone, neomycin, and polymyxin B; polymyxin B, neomycin, and dexamethasone
U.S. Brand Names Maxitrol®; Poly-Dex™ [DSC]
Canadian Brand Names Dioptrol®; Maxitrol®
Therapeutic Category Antibiotic/Corticosteroid, Ophthalmic
Use Steroid-responsive inflammatory ocular conditions in which a corticosteroid is indicated and where bacterial infection or a risk of bacterial infection exists
General Dosage Range Ophthalmic:
Ointment: *Children and Adults:* Place a small amount (~1/2") in the affected eye 3-4 times/day **or** at bedtime
Suspension: *Children and Adults:* Instill 1-2 drops into affected eye(s) every 3-4 hours
Dosage Forms
Ointment, ophthalmic: Neomycin 3.5 mg, polymyxin B 10,000 units, and dexamethasone 0.1% per g (3.5 g)
Maxitrol®: Neomycin 3.5 mg, polymyxin B 10,000 units, and dexamethasone 0.1% per g (3.5 g)
Suspension, ophthalmic: Neomycin 3.5 mg, polymyxin B 10,000 units, and dexamethasone 0.1% per 1 mL (5 mL)
Maxitrol®: Neomycin 3.5 mg, polymyxin B 10,000 units, and dexamethasone 0.1% per 1 mL (5 mL)

neomycin, polymyxin B, and gramicidin
(nee oh MYE sin, pol i MIKS in bee, & gram i SYE din)
Synonyms gramicidin, neomycin, and polymyxin B; polymyxin B, neomycin, and gramicidin
U.S. Brand Names Neosporin® Ophthalmic Solution
Canadian Brand Names Neosporin®; Optimyxin Plus®
Therapeutic Category Antibiotic, Ophthalmic
Use Treatment of superficial ocular infection
General Dosage Range Ophthalmic: *Children and Adults:* Instill 1-2 drops 4-6 times/day
Dosage Forms
Solution, ophthalmic [drops]: Neomycin 1.75 mg, polymyxin B 10,000 units, and gramicidin 0.025 mg per 1 mL (10 mL)
Neosporin® Ophthalmic Solution: Neomycin 1.75 mg, polymyxin B 10,000 units, and gramicidin 0.025 mg per 1 mL (10 mL)

neomycin, polymyxin B, and hydrocortisone
(nee oh MYE sin, pol i MIKS in bee, & hye droe KOR ti sone)
Synonyms hydrocortisone, neomycin, and polymyxin B; polymyxin B, neomycin, and hydrocortisone
U.S. Brand Names Cortisporin®; Cortomycin
Canadian Brand Names Cortimyxin®; Cortisporin® Otic
Therapeutic Category Antibiotic/Corticosteroid, Ophthalmic; Antibiotic/Corticosteroid, Otic; Antibiotic/Corticosteroid, Topical
Use Steroid-responsive inflammatory condition for which a corticosteroid is indicated and where bacterial infection or a risk of bacterial infection exists
General Dosage Range
Ophthalmic: *Adults:* Instill 1-2 drops every 3-4 hours, or more frequently
Otic:
Children ≥2 years: Instill 3 drops into affected ear 3-4 times/day
Children ≥12 years and Adults: Instill 4 drops into affected ear 3-4 times/day
Topical: *Adults:* Apply a thin layer 1-4 times/day

Dosage Forms
Cream, topical:
Cortisporin®: Neomycin 3.5 mg, polymyxin B 10,000 units, and hydrocortisone 5 mg per g (7.5 g)
Solution, otic: Neomycin 3.5 mg, polymyxin B 10,000 units, and hydrocortisone 10 mg per mL (10 mL)
Cortisporin®, Cortomycin: Neomycin 3.5 mg, polymyxin B 10,000 units, and hydrocortisone 10 mg per mL (10 mL)
Suspension, ophthalmic [drops]: Neomycin 3.5 mg, polymyxin B 10,000 units, and hydrocortisone 10 mg per mL (7.5 mL)
Suspension, otic: Neomycin 3.5 mg, polymyxin B 10,000 units, and hydrocortisone 10 mg per mL (10 mL)
Cortomycin: Neomycin 3.5 mg, polymyxin B 10,000 units, and hydrocortisone 10 mg per mL (10 mL)

neomycin, polymyxin B, and prednisolone
(nee oh MYE sin, pol i MIKS in bee, & pred NIS oh lone)
Synonyms polymyxin B, neomycin, and prednisolone; prednisolone, neomycin, and polymyxin B
U.S. Brand Names Poly-Pred®
Therapeutic Category Antibiotic/Corticosteroid, Ophthalmic
Use Steroid-responsive inflammatory ocular condition in which bacterial infection or a risk of bacterial ocular infection exists
General Dosage Range Ophthalmic: *Children and Adults:* Initial: 1-2 drops every 30 minutes; Maintenance: Instill 1-2 drops every 3-4 hours
Dosage Forms
Suspension, ophthalmic [drops]:
Poly-Pred®: Neomycin 0.35%, polymyxin B 10,000 units, and prednisolone acetate 0.5% per 1 mL (5 mL)

neomycin sulfate *see* neomycin *on page 617*
neonatal trace metals *see* trace metals *on page 880*
Neo-Polycin™ *see* bacitracin, neomycin, and polymyxin B *on page 111*
Neo-Polycin™ HC *see* bacitracin, neomycin, polymyxin B, and hydrocortisone *on page 112*
NeoProfen® *see* ibuprofen *on page 460*
Neoral® *see* cyclosporine (systemic) *on page 243*
neosar *see* cyclophosphamide *on page 242*
Neosporin® (Can) *see* neomycin, polymyxin B, and gramicidin *on page 618*
Neosporin® AF [OTC] *see* miconazole (topical) *on page 585*
Neosporin® G.U. Irrigant *see* neomycin and polymyxin B *on page 617*
Neosporin® Irrigating Solution (Can) *see* neomycin and polymyxin B *on page 617*
Neosporin® Neo To Go® [OTC] *see* bacitracin, neomycin, and polymyxin B *on page 111*
Neosporin® Ophthalmic Solution *see* neomycin, polymyxin B, and gramicidin *on page 618*
Neosporin® + Pain Relief Ointment [OTC] *see* bacitracin, neomycin, polymyxin B, and pramoxine *on page 112*
Neosporin® Topical [OTC] *see* bacitracin, neomycin, and polymyxin B *on page 111*

neostigmine (nee oh STIG meen)
Medication Safety Issues
Sound-alike/look-alike issues:
Prostigmin® may be confused with physostigmine
Synonyms neostigmine bromide; neostigmine methylsulfate
U.S. Brand Names Prostigmin®
Canadian Brand Names Prostigmin®
Therapeutic Category Cholinergic Agent
Use Reversal of the effects of nondepolarizing neuromuscular-blocking agents; treatment of myasthenia gravis; prevention and treatment of postoperative bladder distention and urinary retention
General Dosage Range Dosage adjustment recommended in patients with renal impairment
I.M., SubQ:
Children: Myasthenia gravis: Diagnosis: 0.04 mg/kg as a single I.M. dose; Treatment: 0.01-0.04 mg/kg every 2-4 hours

◄ *Adults:*
    Bladder atony: Prevention: 0.25 mg every 4-6 hours; Treatment: 0.5-1 mg every 3 hours for 5 doses after bladder emptied
    Myasthenia gravis: Diagnosis: 0.02 mg/kg as a single I.M. dose; Treatment: 0.5-2.5 mg every 1-3 hours (maximum: 10 mg/day)
I.V.:
    Infants: 0.025-0.1 mg/kg/dose
    Children: 0.01-0.04 mg/kg every 2-4 hours **or** 0.025-0.08 mg/kg/dose
    Adults: 0.5-2.5 mg every 1-3 hours (maximum: 10 mg/day) **or** 0.5-2.5 mg as a single dose (maximum dose: 5 mg)
Oral:
    Children: 2 mg/kg/day divided every 3-4 hours
    Adults: 15 mg/dose every 3-4 hours (maximum: 375 mg/day)
Dosage Forms
    Injection, solution: 0.5 mg/mL (1 mL, 10 mL); 1 mg/mL (10 mL)
    Tablet, oral:
      Prostigmin®: 15 mg

neostigmine bromide *see* neostigmine *on page 619*
neostigmine methylsulfate *see* neostigmine *on page 619*
NeoStrata® HQ (Can) *see* hydroquinone *on page 453*
NeoStrata® HQ Skin Lightening [OTC] *see* hydroquinone *on page 453*
Neo-Synephrine® (Can) *see* phenylephrine (nasal) *on page 697*
Neo-Synephrine® Extra Strength [OTC] *see* phenylephrine (nasal) *on page 697*
Neo-Synephrine® Mild Formula [OTC] *see* phenylephrine (nasal) *on page 697*
Neo-Synephrine® Nighttime12-Hour [OTC] *see* oxymetazoline (nasal) *on page 664*
Neo-Synephrine® Regular Strength [OTC] *see* phenylephrine (nasal) *on page 697*

nepafenac (ne pa FEN ak)
U.S. Brand Names Nevanac®
Canadian Brand Names Nevanac®
Therapeutic Category Nonsteroidal Antiinflammatory Drug (NSAID), Ophthalmic
Use Treatment of pain and inflammation associated with cataract surgery
General Dosage Range Ophthalmic: *Children ≥10 years and Adults:* Instill 1 drop into affected eye(s) 3 times/day
Dosage Forms
    Suspension, ophthalmic:
      Nevanac®: 0.1% (3 mL)

NephrAmine® *see* amino acid injection *on page 65*
Nephro-Calci® [OTC] *see* calcium carbonate *on page 161*
Neptazane™ *see* methazolamide *on page 568*
nerve agent antidote kit *see* atropine and pralidoxime *on page 104*
Nesacaine® *see* chloroprocaine *on page 196*
Nesacaine®-CE (Can) *see* chloroprocaine *on page 196*
Nesacaine®-MPF *see* chloroprocaine *on page 196*

nesiritide (ni SIR i tide)
Medication Safety Issues
    High alert medication:
      The Institute for Safe Medication Practices (ISMP) includes this medication among its list of drugs which have a heightened risk of causing significant patient harm when used in error.
    International issues:
      Natrecor® may be confused with Nitrocor® which is a brand name for nitroglycerin in Chile and Italy
Synonyms B-type natriuretic peptide (human); hBNP; natriuretic peptide
U.S. Brand Names Natrecor®
Canadian Brand Names Natrecor®
Therapeutic Category Natriuretic Peptide, B-type, Human; Vasodilator
Use Treatment of acutely decompensated heart failure (HF) with dyspnea at rest or with minimal activity

General Dosage Range I.V.: *Adults:* Bolus: 2 mcg/kg; Infusion: Initial: 0.01 mcg/kg/minute (maximum: 0.03 mcg/kg/minute)

Dosage Forms
Injection, powder for reconstitution:
Natrecor®: 1.5 mg

NESP see darbepoetin alfa *on page 253*
Neulasta® see pegfilgrastim *on page 679*
Neuleptil® (Can) see periciazine *(Canada only) on page 690*
Neumega® see oprelvekin *on page 653*
Neupogen® see filgrastim *on page 377*
Neurontin® see gabapentin *on page 405*
Neut® see sodium bicarbonate *on page 818*
NeutraCare® see fluoride *on page 386*
NeutraGard® Advanced see fluoride *on page 386*
Neutrahist PDX see chlorpheniramine, pseudoephedrine, and dextromethorphan *on page 201*
Neutrahist Pediatric [OTC] [DSC] see chlorpheniramine and pseudoephedrine *on page 199*
Neutra-Phos see potassium phosphate and sodium phosphate *on page 727*
Neutra-Phos®-K [OTC] [DSC] see potassium phosphate *on page 726*
Neutrogena® Acne Stress Control [OTC] see salicylic acid *on page 795*
Neutrogena® Advanced Solutions™ [OTC] see salicylic acid *on page 795*
Neutrogena® Blackhead Eliminating™ 2-in-1 Foaming Pads [OTC] see salicylic acid *on page 795*
Neutrogena® Blackhead Eliminating™ Daily Scrub [OTC] see salicylic acid *on page 795*
Neutrogena® Blackhead Elinimating™ [OTC] see salicylic acid *on page 795*
Neutrogena® Body Clear® [OTC] see salicylic acid *on page 795*
Neutrogena® Clear Pore™ [OTC] see benzoyl peroxide *on page 124*
Neutrogena® Clear Pore™ Oil-Controlling Astringent [OTC] see salicylic acid *on page 795*
Neutrogena® Maximum Strength T/Sal® [OTC] see salicylic acid *on page 795*
Neutrogena® Oil-Free Acne [OTC] see salicylic acid *on page 795*
Neutrogena® Oil-Free Acne Stress Control [OTC] see salicylic acid *on page 795*
Neutrogena® Oil-Free Acne Wash [OTC] see salicylic acid *on page 795*
Neutrogena® Oil-Free Acne Wash 60 Second Mask Scrub [OTC] see salicylic acid *on page 795*
Neutrogena® Oil-Free Acne Wash Cream Cleanser [OTC] see salicylic acid *on page 795*
Neutrogena® Oil-Free Acne Wash Foam Cleanser [OTC] see salicylic acid *on page 795*
Neutrogena® Oil-Free Anti-Acne [OTC] see salicylic acid *on page 795*
Neutrogena® On The Spot® Acne Treatment [OTC] see benzoyl peroxide *on page 124*
Neutrogena® Rapid Clear® [OTC] see salicylic acid *on page 795*
Neutrogena® Rapid Clear® Acne Defense [OTC] see salicylic acid *on page 795*
Neutrogena® Rapid Clear® Acne Eliminating [OTC] see salicylic acid *on page 795*
Neutrogena® T/Gel® [OTC] see coal tar *on page 227*
Neutrogena® T/Gel® Extra Strength [OTC] see coal tar *on page 227*
Neutrogena® T/Gel® Stubborn Itch Control [OTC] see coal tar *on page 227*
Nevanac® see nepafenac *on page 620*

nevirapine (ne VYE ra peen)
Medication Safety Issues
Sound-alike/look-alike issues:
Nevirapine may be confused with nelfinavir
Viramune®, Viramune® XR™ may be confused with Viracept®
Synonyms NVP
U.S. Brand Names Viramune®; Viramune® XR™
Canadian Brand Names Auro-Nevirapine; Viramune®
Therapeutic Category Antiviral Agent
Use In combination therapy with other antiretroviral agents for the treatment of HIV-1

◀ **General Dosage Range** Dosage adjustment recommended in patients with renal impairment
Oral, immediate release:
Infants and Children <8 years: Initial: 150-200 mg/m^2/dose once daily (maximum: 200 mg/day); Maintenance: 150-200 mg/m^2/dose twice daily (maximum: 400 mg/day).
Children ≥8 years: Initial: 120-150 mg/m^2/dose once daily (maximum: 200 mg/day); Maintenance: 120-150 mg/m^2/dose twice daily (maximum: 400 mg/day)
Adolescents and Adults: Initial: 200 mg once daily; Maintenance: 200 mg twice daily
Oral, extended release: *Adults:* Maintenance: 400 mg once daily

Dosage Forms
Suspension, oral:
Viramune®: 50 mg/5 mL (240 mL)
Tablet, oral:
Viramune®: 200 mg
Tablet, extended release, oral:
Viramune® XR™: 400 mg

NexAVAR® *see* sorafenib *on page 827*

Nexavar® (Can) *see* sorafenib *on page 827*

Nexiclon™ XR *see* clonidine *on page 223*

NexIUM® *see* esomeprazole *on page 342*

Nexium® (Can) *see* esomeprazole *on page 342*

NexIUM® I.V. *see* esomeprazole *on page 342*

Next Choice™ *see* levonorgestrel *on page 521*

Nexterone® *see* amiodarone *on page 67*

NFV *see* nelfinavir *on page 616*

NG-Citalopram (Can) *see* citalopram *on page 213*

NGX-4010 *see* capsaicin *on page 169*

niacin (NYE a sin)

Medication Safety Issues
Sound-alike/look-alike issues:
Niacin may be confused with Minocin®, Niaspan®, Nispan®
Niaspan® may be confused with niacin
Nicobid® may be confused with Nitro-Bid®

Synonyms nicotinic acid; vitamin B$_3$

U.S. Brand Names Niacin-Time® [OTC]; Niacor®; Niaspan®; Slo-Niacin® [OTC]

Canadian Brand Names Niaspan®; Niaspan® FCT; Niodan

Therapeutic Category Vitamin, Water Soluble

Use Treatment of dyslipidemias (Fredrickson types IIa and IIb or primary hypercholesterolemia) as mono- or adjunctive therapy; to lower the risk of recurrent MI in patients with a history of MI and hyperlipidemia; to slow progression or promote regression of coronary artery disease; treatment of hypertriglyceridemia in patients at risk of pancreatitis

General Dosage Range Oral:
Extended release: *Adults:* 500 mg to 2 g once daily
Regular release: *Adults:* 100-250 mg/day in 1-2 divided doses **or** 1.5-6 g/day in 2-3 divided doses (maximum dose: 6 g/day in 3 divided doses)
Sustained release: *Adults:* Usual: 1-2 g/day

Dosage Forms
Caplet, timed release, oral: 500 mg
Capsule, oral: 50 mg, 250 mg
Capsule, extended release, oral: 250 mg, 500 mg
Capsule, timed release, oral: 250 mg, 400 mg, 500 mg
Tablet, oral: 50 mg, 100 mg, 250 mg, 500 mg
Niacor®: 500 mg
Tablet, controlled release, oral:
Slo-Niacin® [OTC]: 250 mg, 500 mg, 750 mg

Tablet, extended release, oral:
Niaspan®: 500 mg, 750 mg, 1000 mg
Tablet, timed release, oral: 250 mg, 500 mg, 750 mg, 1000 mg
Niacin-Time® [OTC]: 500 mg

niacinamide (nye a SIN a mide)

Medication Safety Issues
Sound-alike/look-alike issues:
Niacinamide may be confused with niCARdipine
Synonyms nicotinamide; nicotinic acid amide; vitamin B$_3$
U.S. Brand Names Nicomide-T™ [OTC]
Therapeutic Category Vitamin, Water Soluble
Use
Oral: Prophylaxis and treatment of pellagra
Topical: Improve the appearance of acne and decrease visible inflammation and irritation caused by acne medications
General Dosage Range
Oral:
Children: 10-50 mg every 6 hours
Adults: Initial: 100 mg every 6 hours; Maintenance: 50 mg every 8-12 hours
Topical: *Adults:* Apply to affected area on face twice daily
Dosage Forms
Cream, topical:
Nicomide-T™ [OTC]: 4% (30 g)
Gel, topical:
Nicomide-T™ [OTC]: 4% (30 g)
Tablet, oral: 100 mg, 250 mg, 500 mg

niacin and lovastatin (NYE a sin & LOE va sta tin)

Medication Safety Issues
Sound-alike/look-alike issues:
Advicor® may be confused with Adcirca®, Advair, Altocor™
Synonyms lovastatin and niacin
U.S. Brand Names Advicor®
Canadian Brand Names Advicor®
Therapeutic Category HMG-CoA Reductase Inhibitor; Vitamin, Water Soluble
Use For use when treatment with both extended-release niacin and lovastatin is appropriate in combination with a standard cholesterol-lowering diet:
Extended-release niacin: Adjunctive treatment of dyslipidemias (types IIa and IIb or primary hypercholesterolemia) to lower the risk of recurrent MI and/or slow progression of coronary artery disease, including combination therapy with other antidyslipidemic agents when additional triglyceride-lowering or HDL-increasing effects are desired; treatment of hypertriglyceridemia in patients at risk of pancreatitis
Lovastatin: Treatment of primary hypercholesterolemia (Frederickson types IIa and IIb); primary and secondary prevention of cardiovascular disease
General Dosage Range Oral: *Adults:* Initial: Niacin 500 mg/lovastatin 20 mg at bedtime; Maintenance: Up to niacin 2000 mg/lovastatin 40 mg at bedtime
Dosage Forms
Tablet, variable release:
Advicor®: 500/20: Niacin 500 mg [extended release] and lovastatin 20 mg [immediate release]; 750/20: Niacin 750 mg [extended release] and lovastatin 20 mg [immediate release]; 1000/20: Niacin 1000 mg [extended release] and lovastatin 20 mg [immediate release]; 1000/40: Niacin 1000 mg [extended release] and lovastatin 40 mg [immediate release]

niacin and simvastatin (NYE a sin & sim va STAT in)

Medication Safety Issues
International issue:
Simcor® is also a brand name for simvastatin in Indonesia.
Synonyms simvastatin and niacin

◀ **U.S. Brand Names** Simcor®

Therapeutic Category Antilipemic Agent, HMG-CoA Reductase Inhibitor; Antilipemic Agent, Miscellaneous

Use Reduce total cholesterol, LDL, Apo B, non-HDL, TG, and/or increase HDL in patients with primary hypercholesterolemia, mixed dyslipidemia, or hypertriglyceridemia in combination with standard cholesterol-lowering diet when simvastatin or niacin monotherapy is inadequate

General Dosage Range Oral: *Adults:* Niacin 500-2000 mg/simvastatin 20-40 mg once daily

Dosage Forms

Tablet, variable release, oral:

Simcor®: 500/20: Niacin 500 mg [extended release] and simvastatin 20 mg [immediate release]; 500/40: Niacin 500 mg [extended release] and simvastatin 40 mg [immediate release]; 750/20: Niacin 750 mg [extended release] and simvastatin 20 mg [immediate release]; 1000/20: Niacin 1000 mg [extended release] and simvastatin 20 mg [immediate release]; 1000/40: Niacin 1000 mg [extended release] and simvastatin 40 mg [immediate release]

Niacin-Time® [OTC] *see* niacin *on page 622*

Niacor® *see* niacin *on page 622*

Niaspan® *see* niacin *on page 622*

Niaspan® FCT (Can) *see* niacin *on page 622*

Niastase® (Can) *see* factor VIIa (recombinant) *on page 365*

Niastase® RT (Can) *see* factor VIIa (recombinant) *on page 365*

nicardipine (nye KAR de peen)

Medication Safety Issues

Sound-alike/look-alike issues:

NiCARdipine may be confused with niacinamide, NIFEdipine, niMODipine

Cardene® may be confused with Cardizem®, Cardura®, codeine

Administration issues:

Significant differences exist between oral and I.V. dosing. Use caution when converting from one route of administration to another.

International issues:

Cardene [U.S., Great Britain, Netherlands] may be confused with Cardem brand name for celiprolol [Spain]; Cardin brand name for simvastatin [Poland]

Synonyms nicardipine hydrochloride

Tall-Man niCARdipine

U.S. Brand Names Cardene® I.V.; Cardene® SR

Therapeutic Category Calcium Channel Blocker

Use Chronic stable angina (immediate-release product only); management of hypertension (immediate and sustained release products); parenteral only for short-term use when oral treatment is not feasible

General Dosage Range Dosage adjustment recommended in patients with hepatic or renal impairment

I.V.: *Adults:* Initial: 5 mg/hour; Maintenance: 3-15 mg/hour

Oral:

Immediate release: *Adults:* Initial: 20 mg 3 times/day; Maintenance: 20-40 mg 3 times/day

Sustained release: *Adults:* Initial: 30 mg twice daily; Maintenance: Up to 60 mg twice daily

Dosage Forms

Capsule, oral: 20 mg, 30 mg

Capsule, sustained release, oral:

Cardene® SR: 30 mg, 45 mg, 60 mg

Infusion, premixed iso-osmotic dextrose solution:

Cardene® I.V.: 20 mg (200 mL); 40 mg (200 mL)

Infusion, premixed iso-osmotic sodium chloride solution:

Cardene® I.V.: 20 mg (200 mL); 40 mg (200 mL)

Injection, solution: 2.5 mg/mL (10 mL)

Cardene® I.V.: 2.5 mg/mL (10 mL)

nicardipine hydrochloride *see* nicardipine *on page 624*

Nicoderm® (Can) *see* nicotine *on page 625*

NicoDerm® CQ® [OTC] *see* nicotine *on page 625*

Nicomide-T™ [OTC] *see* niacinamide *on page 623*

Nicorelief [OTC] *see* nicotine *on page 625*

Nicorette® [OTC] *see* nicotine *on page 625*
Nicorette® (Can) *see* nicotine *on page 625*
Nicorette® Plus (Can) *see* nicotine *on page 625*
nicotinamide *see* niacinamide *on page 623*

nicotine (nik oh TEEN)

Medication Safety Issues
  Sound-alike/look-alike issues:
    NicoDerm® may be confused with Nitroderm
    Nicorette® may be confused with Nordette®
  Other safety concerns:
    Transdermal patch may contain conducting metal (eg, aluminum); remove patch prior to MRI.
Synonyms Habitrol; nicotine patch
U.S. Brand Names Commit® [OTC]; NicoDerm® CQ® [OTC]; Nicorelief [OTC]; Nicorette® [OTC]; Nicotrol® Inhaler; Nicotrol® NS; Thrive™ [OTC]
Canadian Brand Names Habitrol®; Nicoderm®; Nicorette®; Nicorette® Plus; Nicotrol®
Therapeutic Category Smoking Deterrent
Use Treatment to aid smoking cessation for the relief of nicotine withdrawal symptoms (including nicotine craving)
General Dosage Range Dosage adjustment recommended for transdermal route in patients on concomitant therapy
  Inhalation:
    Nasal: *Adults:* 1-2 sprays/hour (maximum: 10 sprays/hour; 80 sprays/day)
    Oral: *Adults:* Usually 6 to 16 cartridges per day; best effect was achieved by frequent continuous puffing (20 minutes)
  Oral: *Adults:* 2 mg or 4 mg every 1-2 hours (weeks 1-6); every 2-4 hours (weeks 7-9); and every 4-8 hours (weeks 10-12) (maximum: 24 pieces gum/day; 20 lozenges/day)
  Transdermal:
    Patients smoking >10 cigarettes/day: Begin with **step 1** (21 mg/day) for 6 weeks, followed by **step 2** (14 mg/day) for 2 weeks; finish with **step 3** (7 mg/day) for 2 weeks
    Patients smoking ≤10 cigarettes/day: Begin with **step 2** (14 mg/day) for 6 weeks, followed by **step 3** (7 mg/day) for 2 weeks
Dosage Forms
  Gum, chewing, oral: 2 mg (20s, 40s, 50s, 100s, 108s, 110s); 4 mg (20s, 40s, 48s, 50s, 100s, 108s, 110s)
    Nicorelief [OTC]: 2 mg (50s, 110s); 4 mg (50s, 110s)
    Nicorette® [OTC]: 2 mg (40s, 48s, 50s, 100s, 108s, 110s, 168s, 170s, 192s, 200s, 216s); 4 mg (40s, 48s, 50s, 100s, 108s, 110s, 168s, 170s, 192s, 200s, 216s)
    Thrive™ [OTC]: 2 mg (40s); 4 mg (40s)
  Lozenge, oral:
    Commit® [OTC]: 2 mg (48s, 72s); 4 mg (48s, 72s)
    Nicorette® [OTC]: 4 mg (50s)
  Oral inhalation system, for oral inhalation:
    Nicotrol® Inhaler: 10 mg (10 mL)
  Patch, transdermal: 7 mg/24 hours (7s, 14s, 30s); 14 mg/24 hours (7s, 14s, 30s); 21 mg/24 hours (7s, 14s, 30s)
    NicoDerm® CQ® [OTC]: 7 mg/24 hours (14s); 14 mg/24 hours (14s); 21 mg/24 hours (7s, 14s)
  Solution, intranasal:
    Nicotrol® NS: 10 mg/mL (10 mL)
nicotine patch *see* nicotine *on page 625*
nicotinic acid *see* niacin *on page 622*
nicotinic acid amide *see* niacinamide *on page 623*
Nicotrol® (Can) *see* nicotine *on page 625*
Nicotrol® Inhaler *see* nicotine *on page 625*
Nicotrol® NS *see* nicotine *on page 625*
Nidagel™ (Can) *see* metronidazole (topical) *on page 583*
Nifediac CC® *see* nifedipine *on page 626*
Nifedical XL® *see* nifedipine *on page 626*

nifedipine (nye FED i peen)

Medication Safety Issues

Sound-alike/look-alike issues:

NIFEdipine may be confused with niCARdipine, niMODipine, nisoldipine

Procardia XL® may be confused with Cartia XT®

Beers Criteria medication:

This drug may be inappropriate for use in geriatric patients (high severity risk).

International issues:

Depin [India] may be confused with Depen brand name for penicillamine [U.S.]; Depon brand name for acetaminophen [Greece]; Dipen brand name for diltiazem [Greece]

Nipin [Italy and Singapore] may be confused with Nipent brand name for pentostatin [U.S., Canada, and multiple international markets]

Tall-Man NIFEdipine

U.S. Brand Names Adalat® CC; Afeditab® CR; Nifediac CC®; Nifedical XL®; Procardia XL®; Procardia®

Canadian Brand Names Adalat® XL®; Apo-Nifed PA®; Mylan-Nifedipine Extended Release; Nu-Nifed; Nu-Nifedipine-PA; PMS-Nifedipine

Therapeutic Category Calcium Channel Blocker

Use Management of chronic stable or vasospastic angina; treatment of hypertension (sustained release products only)

General Dosage Range Oral:

Immediate release: *Adults:* Initial: 10 mg 3-4 times/day (maximum: 180 mg/day)

Extended release: *Adults:* Initial: 30 mg once daily; Maintenance: 30-60 mg once daily (maximum: 120-180 mg/day)

Dosage Forms

Capsule, softgel, oral: 10 mg, 20 mg

Procardia®: 10 mg

Tablet, extended release, oral: 30 mg, 60 mg, 90 mg

Adalat® CC: 30 mg, 60 mg, 90 mg

Afeditab® CR: 30 mg, 60 mg

Nifediac CC®: 30 mg, 60 mg, 90 mg

Nifedical XL®: 30 mg, 60 mg

Procardia XL®: 30 mg, 60 mg, 90 mg

Niferex® [OTC] see polysaccharide-iron complex on page 720

Niftolid see flutamide on page 392

Nilandron® see nilutamide on page 627

nilotinib (nye LOE ti nib)

Medication Safety Issues

Sound-alike/look-alike issues:

Nilotinib may be confused with dasatinib, imatinib, nilutamide, SUNItinib, vandetanib

High alert medication:

This medication is in a class the Institute for Safe Medication Practices (ISMP) includes among its list of drug classes which have a heightened risk of causing significant patient harm when used in error.

Synonyms AMN107; nilotinib hydrochloride monohydrate

U.S. Brand Names Tasigna®

Canadian Brand Names Tasigna®

Therapeutic Category Antineoplastic Agent, Tyrosine Kinase Inhibitor

Use Treatment of newly-diagnosed Philadelphia chromosome-positive chronic myelogenous leukemia (Ph+ CML) in chronic phase; treatment of chronic and accelerated phase Ph+ CML (refractory or intolerant to prior therapy, including imatinib)

General Dosage Range Dosage adjustment recommended in patients with hepatic impairment, on concomitant therapy, or who develop toxicities

Oral: *Adults:* 300-400 mg twice daily

Dosage Forms

Capsule, oral:

Tasigna®: 150 mg, 200 mg

nilotinib hydrochloride monohydrate see nilotinib on page 626

nilutamide (ni LOO ta mide)

Medication Safety Issues
Sound-alike/look-alike issues:
Nilutamide may be confused with nilotinib
Synonyms NSC-684588; RU-23908
U.S. Brand Names Nilandron®
Canadian Brand Names Anandron®
Therapeutic Category Antineoplastic Agent
Use Treatment of metastatic prostate cancer (in combination with surgical castration)
General Dosage Range Oral: *Adults:* Initial: 300 mg once daily; Maintenance: 150 mg once daily
Dosage Forms
Tablet, oral:
Nilandron®: 150 mg

Nimbex® *see* cisatracurium *on page 212*

nimodipine (nye MOE di peen)

Medication Safety Issues
Sound-alike/look-alike issues:
NiMODipine may be confused with niCARdipine, NIFEdipine, nisoldipine
Administration issues:
For oral administration only. For patients unable to swallow a capsule, the drug should be dispensed in an oral syringe (preferably amber in color) labeled **"WARNING: For ORAL use only"** or **"Not for I.V. use."** Nimodipine has inadvertently been administered I.V. when withdrawn from capsules into a syringe for subsequent nasogastric tube administration. Severe cardiovascular adverse events, including fatalities, have resulted. Employ precautions against such an event.
Tall-Man niMODipine
Canadian Brand Names Nimotop®
Therapeutic Category Calcium Channel Blocker
Use Vasospasm following subarachnoid hemorrhage from ruptured intracranial aneurysms
General Dosage Range Dosage adjustment recommended in patients with hepatic impairment
Oral: *Adults:* 60 mg every 4 hours
Dosage Forms
Capsule, liquid filled, oral: 30 mg
Capsule, softgel, oral: 30 mg

Nimotop® (Can) *see* nimodipine *on page 627*
Niodan (Can) *see* niacin *on page 622*
Nipent® *see* pentostatin *on page 689*
Nipride® (Can) *see* nitroprusside *on page 630*
Niravam™ *see* alprazolam *on page 56*

nisoldipine (nye SOL di peen)

Medication Safety Issues
Sound-alike/look-alike issues:
Nisoldipine may be confused with NIFEdipine, niMODipine
U.S. Brand Names Sular®
Therapeutic Category Calcium Channel Blocker
Use Management of hypertension, alone or in combination with other antihypertensive agents
General Dosage Range Dosage adjustment recommended in patients with hepatic impairment
Oral:
Adults:
Sular® (Geomatrix® delivery system): Initial: 17 mg once daily; Maintenance: 17-34 mg once daily (maximum: 34 mg/day)
Nisoldipine extended-release (original formulation): Initial: 20 mg once daily; Maintenance: 10-40 mg once daily (maximum: 60 mg/day)
Elderly: Sular® (Geomatrix® delivery system): Initial: 8.5 mg once daily; Nisoldipine extended-release (original formulation): Initial: 10 mg once daily

◄ **Dosage Forms**
Tablet, extended release, oral: 8.5 mg, 17 mg, 20 mg, 25.5 mg, 30 mg, 34 mg, 40 mg
  Sular®: 8.5 mg, 17 mg, 25.5 mg, 34 mg

nitalapram *see* citalopram *on page 213*

nitazoxanide (nye ta ZOX a nide)
Synonyms NTZ
U.S. Brand Names Alinia®
Therapeutic Category Antiprotozoal
Use Treatment of diarrhea caused by *Cryptosporidium parvum* or *Giardia lamblia*
General Dosage Range Oral:
Children 1-3 years: 100 mg every 12 hours
Children 4-11 years: 200 mg every 12 hours
Children ≥12 years and Adults: 500 mg every 12 hours
Dosage Forms
Powder for suspension, oral:
  Alinia®: 100 mg/5 mL (60 mL)
Tablet, oral:
  Alinia®: 500 mg

Nithiodote™ *see* sodium nitrite and sodium thiosulfate *on page 821*

nitisinone (ni TIS i known)
Synonyms NTBC
U.S. Brand Names Orfadin®
Therapeutic Category 4-Hydroxyphenylpyruvate Dioxygenase Inhibitor
Use Treatment of hereditary tyrosinemia type 1 (HT-1) as an adjunct to dietary restriction of tyrosine and phenylalanine
General Dosage Range Oral: *Infants, Children, and Adults:* 1-2 mg/kg/day in 2 divided doses
Dosage Forms
Capsule, oral:
  Orfadin®: 2 mg, 5 mg, 10 mg

Nitoman™ (Can) *see* tetrabenazine *on page 856*
Nitrazadon® (Can) *see* nitrazepam *(Canada only) on page 628*

nitrazepam *(Canada only)* (nye TRA ze pam)
Synonyms nitrozepamum
Canadian Brand Names Apo-Nitrazepam®; Mogadon; Nitrazadon®; Sandoz-Nitrazepam
Therapeutic Category Benzodiazepine
Controlled Substance CDSA IV
Use Short-term management of insomnia; treatment of myoclonic seizures
General Dosage Range Oral:
Children ≤30 kg: 0.3-1 mg/kg/day in 3 divided doses
Adults: 5-10 mg once daily
Elderly: 2.5-5 mg once daily
Product Availability Not available in U.S.
Dosage Forms - Canada
Tablet, oral:
  Apo-Nitrazepam®, Mogadon, Nitrazadon, Nitrazepam (Pro-Doc), Sandoz-Nitrazepam: 5 mg, 10 mg

nitric oxide (NYE trik OKS ide)
U.S. Brand Names INOmax®
Canadian Brand Names INOmax®
Therapeutic Category Vasodilator, Pulmonary
Use Treatment of term and near-term (>34 weeks) neonates with hypoxic respiratory failure associated with pulmonary hypertension; used concurrently with ventilatory support and other agents
General Dosage Range Inhalation: *Neonates (up to 14 days old):* 20 ppm

Dosage Forms
Gas, for inhalation:
INOmax®: 100 ppm (353 L, 1963 L); 800 ppm (353 L, 1963 L)

Nitro-Bid® *see nitroglycerin on page 629*
Nitro-Dur® *see nitroglycerin on page 629*

nitrofurantoin (nye troe fyoor AN toyn)

Medication Safety Issues
Sound alike/look alike issues:
Macrobid® may be confused with microK®, Nitro-Bid®
Nitrofurantoin may be confused with Neurontin®, nitroglycerin
BEERS Criteria medication:
This drug may be inappropriate for use in geriatric patients (high severity risk).

U.S. Brand Names Furadantin®; Macrobid®; Macrodantin®
Canadian Brand Names Apo-Nitrofurantoin®; Macrobid®; Macrodantin®; Novo-Furantoin
Therapeutic Category Antibiotic, Miscellaneous
Use Prevention and treatment of urinary tract infections caused by susceptible strains of *E. coli, S. aureus, Enterococcus, Klebsiella,* and *Enterobacter*
General Dosage Range Oral:
Children >1 month: Furadantin®, Macrodantin®: 5-7 mg/kg/day divided every 6 hours (maximum: 400 mg/day) **or** 1-2 mg/kg/day divided every 12-24 hours (maximum: 100 mg/day)
Children >12 years: Macrobid®: 100 mg twice daily
Adults: Furadantin®, Macrodantin®: 50-100 mg every 6 hours **or** once daily; Macrobid®: 100 mg twice daily
Dosage Forms
Capsule, oral: 50 mg, 100 mg
Macrobid®: 100 mg
Macrodantin®: 25 mg, 50 mg, 100 mg
Suspension, oral: 25 mg/5 mL (230 mL)
Furadantin®: 25 mg/5 mL (230 mL)

nitrogen mustard *see mechlorethamine on page 552*

nitroglycerin (nye troe GLI ser in)

Medication Safety Issues
Sound-alike/look-alike issues:
Nitroglycerin may be confused with nitrofurantoin, nitroprusside
Nitro-Bid® may be confused with Macrobid®, Nicobid®
Nitroderm may be confused with NicoDerm®
Nitrol® may be confused with Nizoral®
Nitrostat® may be confused with Nilstat®, nystatin
Other safety concerns:
Transdermal patch may contain conducting metal (eg, aluminum); remove patch prior to MRI.
International issues:
Nitrocor [Italy, Russia, and Venezuela] may be confused with Natrecor brand name for nesiritide [U.S., Canada, and multiple international markets] and Nutracort brand name for hydrocortisone in the [U.S. and multiple international markets]
Nitro-Dur [U.S., Canada, and multiple international markets] may be confused with Nitrocor [Italy, Russia, and Venezuela]

Synonyms glyceryl trinitrate; nitroglycerol; NTG; Rectiv™; Tridil
U.S. Brand Names Minitran™; Nitro-Bid®; Nitro-Dur®; Nitro-Time®; Nitrolingual®; NitroMist®; Nitrostat®
Canadian Brand Names Minitran™; Mylan-Nitro Sublingual Spray; Nitro-Dur®; Nitroglycerin Injection, USP; Nitrol®; Nitrostat®; Rho®-Nitro Pump Spray; Transderm-Nitro®; Trinipatch®
Therapeutic Category Vasodilator
Use Treatment or prevention of angina pectoris
Intravenous (I.V.) administration: Treatment or prevention of angina pectoris; acute decompensated heart failure (especially when associated with acute myocardial infarction); perioperative hypertension (especially during cardiovascular surgery); induction of intraoperative hypotension
Intra-anal administration (Rectiv™ ointment): Treatment of moderate-to-severe pain associated with chronic anal fissure

◀ **General Dosage Range**
I.V.: *Adults:* Initial: 5 mcg/minute; Maintenance: 20-200 mcg/minute (maximum: 400 mcg/minute)
Intraanal: *Adults:* 1 inch every 12 hours
Oral: *Adults:* 2.5-6.5 mg 3-4 times/day; Maintenance: Up to 26 mg 4 times/day
Sublingual: *Adults:* 0.3-0.6 mg every 5 minutes for maximum of 3 doses in 15 minutes **or** 5-10 minutes prior to activities which may provoke an attack
Topical: *Adults:*
  Ointment: Apply 0.5" to 2" every 6 hours with a daily nitrate-free interval of ~10-12 hours
  Patch: Initial: 0.2-0.4 mg/hour for 12-14 hours/day; Maintenance: 0.2-0.8 mg/hour for 12-14 hours
Translingual: *Adults:* 1-2 sprays under tongue every 3-5 minutes for maximum of 3 doses in 15 minutes **or** 5-10 minutes prior to activities which may provoke an attack

Product Availability
Rectiv™: FDA approved June 2011; availability expected during the first quarter of 2012
Rectiv™ (nitroglycerin 0.4% ointment) is approved for the treatment of moderate-to-severe pain associated with chronic anal fissure.

Dosage Forms
Aerosol, translingual:
  NitroMist®: 0.4 mg/spray (8.5 g)
Capsule, extended release, oral: 2.5 mg, 6.5 mg, 9 mg
  Nitro-Time®: 2.5 mg, 6.5 mg, 9 mg
Infusion, premixed in D₅W: 25 mg (250 mL); 50 mg (250 mL, 500 mL); 100 mg (250 mL)
Injection, solution: 5 mg/mL (5 mL, 10 mL)
Ointment, topical:
  Nitro-Bid®: 2% (1 g, 30 g, 60 g)
Patch, transdermal: 0.1 mg/hr (30s); 0.2 mg/hr (30s); 0.4 mg/hr (30s); 0.6 mg/hr (30s)
  Minitran™: 0.1 mg/hr (30s); 0.2 mg/hr (30s); 0.4 mg/hr (30s); 0.6 mg/hr (30s)
  Nitro-Dur®: 0.1 mg/hr (30s); 0.2 mg/hr (30s); 0.3 mg/hr (30s); 0.4 mg/hr (30s); 0.6 mg/hr (30s); 0.8 mg/hr (30s)
Solution, translingual: 0.4 mg/spray (4.9 g, 12 g)
  Nitrolingual®: 0.4 mg/spray (4.9 g, 12 g)
Tablet, sublingual:
  Nitrostat®: 0.3 mg, 0.4 mg, 0.6 mg

Nitroglycerin Injection, USP (Can) *see nitroglycerin on page 629*
nitroglycerol *see nitroglycerin on page 629*
Nitrol® (Can) *see nitroglycerin on page 629*
Nitrolingual® *see nitroglycerin on page 629*
NitroMist® *see nitroglycerin on page 629*
Nitropress® *see nitroprusside on page 630*

nitroprusside (nye troe PRUS ide)

Medication Safety Issues
Sound-alike/look-alike issues:
  Nitroprusside may be confused with nitroglycerin
High alert medication:
  The Institute for Safe Medication Practices (ISMP) includes this medication among its list of drugs which have a heightened risk of causing significant patient harm when used in error.

Synonyms nitroprusside sodium; sodium nitroferricyanide; sodium nitroprusside

U.S. Brand Names Nitropress®

Canadian Brand Names Nipride®

Therapeutic Category Vasodilator

Use Management of hypertensive crises; acute decompensated heart failure (HF); used for controlled hypotension to reduce bleeding during surgery

General Dosage Range I.V.:
Children: Infusion: Initial: 1 mcg/kg/minute; Usual dose: 3 mcg/kg/minute (maximum: 5 mcg/kg/minute)
Adults: Infusion: Initial: 0.3-0.5 mcg/kg/minute; Usual dose: 3 mcg/kg/minute (maximum: 10 mcg/kg/minute)

Dosage Forms
Injection, solution:
  Nitropress®: 25 mg/mL (2 mL)

nitroprusside sodium *see* nitroprusside *on page 630*
Nitrostat® *see* nitroglycerin *on page 629*
Nitro-Time® *see* nitroglycerin *on page 629*
4′-nitro-3′-trifluoromethylisobutyrantide *see* flutamide *on page 392*

nitrous oxide (NYE trus OKS ide)
Medication Safety Issues
  High alert medication:
    The Institute for Safe Medication Practices (ISMP) includes this medication among its list of drug classes which have a heightened risk of causing significant patient harm when used in error.
Therapeutic Category Anesthetic, Gas
Use Sedation, analgesia, and amnesia; principal adjunct to inhalation and intravenous general anesthesia
General Dosage Range Inhalation: *Children and Adults:* Dental: Concentrations of 25% to 50%; Surgical: Concentrations of 25% to 70%
Dosage Forms
  Supplied in blue cylinders

nitrozepamum *see* nitrazepam *(Canada only) on page 628*
Nix® (Can) *see* permethrin *on page 691*
Nix® Complete Lice Treatment System [OTC] *see* permethrin *on page 691*
Nix® Creme Rinse [OTC] *see* permethrin *on page 691*
Nix® Creme Rinse Lice Treatment [OTC] *see* permethrin *on page 691*
Nix® Lice Control Spray [OTC] *see* permethrin *on page 691*

nizatidine (ni ZA ti deen)
Medication Safety Issues
  Sound-alike/look-alike issues:
    Axid® may be confused with Ansaid®
  International issues:
    Tazac [Australia] may be confused with Tazact brand name for piperacillin/tazobactam [India]; Tiazac brand name for diltiazem [U.S., Canada]
U.S. Brand Names Axid®
Canadian Brand Names Apo-Nizatidine®; Axid®; Gen-Nizatidine; Novo-Nizatidine; Nu-Nizatidine; PMS-Nizatidine
Therapeutic Category Histamine H_2 Antagonist
Use Treatment and maintenance of duodenal ulcer; treatment of benign gastric ulcer; treatment of gastroesophageal reflux disease (GERD)
General Dosage Range Dosage adjustment recommended in patients with renal impairment
  Oral:
    Children ≥12 years: 150 mg twice daily
    Adults: 300 mg/day in 1-2 divided doses **or** 75 mg twice daily (OTC dosing)
Dosage Forms
  Capsule, oral: 150 mg, 300 mg
  Solution, oral: 15 mg/mL (473 mL)
    Axid®: 15 mg/mL (480 mL)

Nizoral® *see* ketoconazole (topical) *on page 500*
Nizoral® A-D [OTC] *see* ketoconazole (topical) *on page 500*
N-methylhydrazine *see* procarbazine *on page 739*
N-methylnaltrexone bromide *see* methylnaltrexone *on page 576*
NN2211 *see* liraglutide *on page 531*
No Doz® Maximum Strength [OTC] *see* caffeine *on page 157*
NoHist [DSC] *see* chlorpheniramine and phenylephrine *on page 198*
NoHist-A *see* chlorpheniramine, phenylephrine, and phenyltoloxamine *on page 201*
NoHist-DMX [DSC] *see* chlorpheniramine, phenylephrine, and dextromethorphan *on page 200*
Nolvadex®-D (Can) *see* tamoxifen *on page 843*

nonoxynol 9 (non OKS i nole nine)

Medication Safety Issues
Sound-alike/look-alike issues:
Delfen® may be confused with Delsym®

Synonyms N-9

U.S. Brand Names Conceptrol® [OTC]; Delfen® [OTC]; Encare® [OTC]; Gynol II® Extra Strength [OTC]; Gynol II® [OTC]; Today® [OTC]; VCF® [OTC]

Therapeutic Category Spermicide

Use Prevention of pregnancy

General Dosage Range Intravaginal: *Adolescents and Adults:* Insert 1 applicatorful, film, suppository, or sponge 10 minutes to 3 hours prior to intercourse

Dosage Forms
Aerosol, vaginal:
Delfen® [OTC]: 12.5% (18 g)
VCF® [OTC]: 12.5% (40 g)
Film, vaginal:
VCF® [OTC]: 28% (3s, 6s, 12s)
Gel, vaginal:
Conceptrol® [OTC]: 4% (2.7 g)
Encare® [OTC]: 4% (2.7 g)
Gynol II® [OTC]: 2% (108 g)
Gynol II® Extra Strength [OTC]: 3% (81 g)
Sponge, vaginal:
Today® [OTC]: 1 g (3s, 12s)
Suppository, vaginal:
Encare® [OTC]: 100 mg (12s, 18s)

Nora-BE® *see* norethindrone *on page 633*
noradrenaline *see* norepinephrine *on page 632*
noradrenaline acid tartrate *see* norepinephrine *on page 632*
Norco® *see* hydrocodone and acetaminophen *on page 446*
Norcuron® (Can) *see* vecuronium *on page 910*
nordeoxyguanosine *see* ganciclovir (ophthalmic) *on page 410*
nordeoxyguanosine *see* ganciclovir (systemic) *on page 410*
Nordette® 28 *see* ethinyl estradiol and levonorgestrel *on page 353*
Norditropin® [DSC] *see* somatropin *on page 826*
Norditropin FlexPro® *see* somatropin *on page 826*
Norditropin® NordiFlex® *see* somatropin *on page 826*
norelgestromin and ethinyl estradiol *see* ethinyl estradiol and norelgestromin *on page 354*
norel® SR *see* acetaminophen, chlorpheniramine, phenylephrine, and phenyltoloxamine *on page 31*

norepinephrine (nor ep i NEF rin)

Medication Safety Issues
Sound-alike/look-alike issues:
Levophed® may be confused with levofloxacin
High alert medication:
The Institute for Safe Medication Practices (ISMP) includes this medication among its list of drugs which have a heightened risk of causing significant patient harm when used in error.

Synonyms levarterenol bitartrate; noradrenaline; noradrenaline acid tartrate; norepinephrine bitartrate

U.S. Brand Names Levophed®

Canadian Brand Names Levophed®

Therapeutic Category Adrenergic Agonist Agent

Use Treatment of shock which persists after adequate fluid volume replacement; severe hypotension

General Dosage Range I.V.:
Children: Initial: 0.05-0.1 mcg/kg/minute; Maintenance: Titrate to desired effect (maximum: 2 mcg/kg/minute)
Adults: Initial: 8-12 mcg/minute; Maintenance: Titrate to desired effect (usual maintenance range: 2-4 mcg/minute)

Dosage Forms
  Injection, solution: 1 mg/mL (4 mL)
    Levophed®: 1 mg/mL (4 mL)

norepinephrine bitartrate *see norepinephrine on page 632*

norethindrone (nor ETH in drone)
Medication Safety Issues
  Sound-alike/look-alike issues:
    Micronor® may be confused with miconazole, Micronase®
Synonyms norethindrone acetate; norethisterone
U.S. Brand Names Aygestin®; Camila®; Errin®; Heather; Jolivette®; Nor-QD®; Nora-BE®; Ortho Micronor®
Canadian Brand Names Micronor®; Norlutate®
Therapeutic Category Contraceptive, Progestin Only; Progestin
Use Treatment of amenorrhea; abnormal uterine bleeding; endometriosis; prevention of pregnancy
General Dosage Range Oral:
  Norethindrone: *Children (postmenarche) and Adults:* 0.35 mg every day
  Norethindrone acetate: *Adolescents and Adults:* 2.5-15 mg once daily for 5-14 days of menstrual cycle
Dosage Forms
  Tablet, oral: 0.35 mg, 5 mg
    Aygestin®: 5 mg
    Camila®: 0.35 mg
    Errin®: 0.35 mg
    Heather: 0.35 mg
    Jolivette®: 0.35 mg
    Nor-QD®: 0.35 mg
    Nora-BE®: 0.35 mg
    Ortho Micronor®: 0.35 mg

norethindrone acetate *see norethindrone on page 633*
norethindrone acetate and ethinyl estradiol *see ethinyl estradiol and norethindrone on page 355*
norethindrone and estradiol *see estradiol and norethindrone on page 345*

norethindrone and mestranol (nor eth IN drone & MES tra nole)
Medication Safety Issues
  Sound-alike/look-alike issues:
    Norinyl® may be confused with Nardil®
Synonyms mestranol and norethindrone; Ortho Novum 1/50
U.S. Brand Names Necon® 1/50; Norinyl® 1+50
Canadian Brand Names Ortho-Novum® 1/50
Therapeutic Category Contraceptive, Oral
Use Prevention of pregnancy
General Dosage Range Oral:
  21-tablet package: *Children (menarche) and Adults:* 1 tablet daily for 21 days, followed by 7 days off
  28-tablet package: *Children (menarche) and Adults:* 1 tablet daily
Dosage Forms
  Tablet, monophasic formulations:
    Necon® 1/50: Norethindrone 1 mg and mestranol 0.05 mg [21 light blue tablets and 7 white inactive tablets] (28s)
    Norinyl® 1+50: Norethindrone 1 mg and mestranol 0.05 mg [21 white tablets and 7 orange inactive tablets] (28s)

norethisterone *see norethindrone on page 633*
Norflex™ *see orphenadrine on page 655*

norfloxacin (nor FLOKS a sin)
Medication Safety Issues
  Sound-alike/look-alike issues:
    Norfloxacin may be confused with Norflex™, Noroxin®

◄   Noroxin® may be confused with Neurontin®, Norflex™, norfloxacin

U.S. Brand Names Noroxin®

Canadian Brand Names Apo-Norflox®; CO Norfloxacin; Norfloxacine®; Novo-Norfloxacin; PMS-Norfloxacin; Riva-Norfloxacin

Therapeutic Category Quinolone

Use Uncomplicated and complicated urinary tract infections caused by susceptible gram-negative and gram-positive bacteria; sexually-transmitted disease (eg, uncomplicated urethral and cervical gonorrhea) caused by *N. gonorrhoeae*; prostatitis due to *E. coli*

    Note: As of April 2007, the CDC no longer recommends the use of fluoroquinolones for the treatment of gonococcal disease.

General Dosage Range Dosage adjustment recommended in patients with renal impairment

    Oral: *Adults:* 400 mg every 12 hours **or** 800 mg as a single dose

Dosage Forms
    Tablet, oral:
        Noroxin®: 400 mg

Norfloxacine® (Can) *see* norfloxacin *on page 633*

Norgesic *see* orphenadrine, aspirin, and caffeine *on page 655*

norgestimate and estradiol *see* estradiol and norgestimate *on page 346*

norgestimate and ethinyl estradiol *see* ethinyl estradiol and norgestimate *on page 357*

norgestrel and ethinyl estradiol *see* ethinyl estradiol and norgestrel *on page 357*

Norinyl® 1+35 *see* ethinyl estradiol and norethindrone *on page 355*

Norinyl® 1+50 *see* norethindrone and mestranol *on page 633*

Noritate® *see* metronidazole (topical) *on page 583*

Norlutate® (Can) *see* norethindrone *on page 633*

normal human serum albumin *see* albumin *on page 44*

normal saline *see* sodium chloride *on page 818*

normal serum albumin (human) *see* albumin *on page 44*

Normlshield® *see* emollients *on page 325*

Normocarb HF® 25 *see* electrolyte solution, renal replacement *on page 323*

Normocarb HF® 35 *see* electrolyte solution, renal replacement *on page 323*

Normodyne® (Can) *see* labetalol *on page 504*

Noroxin® *see* norfloxacin *on page 633*

Norpace® *see* disopyramide *on page 299*

Norpace® CR *see* disopyramide *on page 299*

Norpramin® *see* desipramine *on page 260*

Nor-QD® *see* norethindrone *on page 633*

Nortemp Children's [OTC] *see* acetaminophen *on page 23*

North American antisnake-bite serum, FAB (ovine) *see* crotalidae polyvalent immune FAB (ovine) *on page 239*

North American coral snake antivenin *see* antivenin *(Micrurus fulvius) on page 84*

Nortrel® 0.5/35 *see* ethinyl estradiol and norethindrone *on page 355*

Nortrel® 1/35 *see* ethinyl estradiol and norethindrone *on page 355*

Nortrel® 7/7/7 *see* ethinyl estradiol and norethindrone *on page 355*

nortriptyline (nor TRIP ti leen)

Medication Safety Issues
    Sound-alike/look-alike issues:
        Aventyl® HCl may be confused with Bentyl®
        Nortriptyline may be confused with amitriptyline, desipramine, Norpramin®
        Pamelor® may be confused with Demerol®, Dymelor®, Panlor®, Tambocor™

Synonyms nortriptyline hydrochloride

U.S. Brand Names Pamelor®

Canadian Brand Names Alti-Nortriptyline; Apo-Nortriptyline®; Aventyl®; Gen-Nortriptyline; Norventyl; Novo-Nortriptyline; Nu-Nortriptyline; PMS-Nortriptyline

Therapeutic Category Antidepressant, Tricyclic (Secondary Amine)

Use Treatment of symptoms of depression

General Dosage Range Oral:
Adults: 25 mg 3-4 times/day (maximum: 150 mg/day)
Elderly: Initial: 10-25 mg once daily; Maintenance: 75 mg/day in 1-2 divided doses
Dosage Forms
Capsule, oral: 10 mg, 25 mg, 50 mg, 75 mg
  Pamelor®: 10 mg, 25 mg, 50 mg, 75 mg
Solution, oral: 10 mg/5 mL (473 mL, 480 mL)
  Pamelor®: 10 mg/5 mL (480 mL)

nortriptyline hydrochloride *see* nortriptyline *on page 634*

Norvasc® *see* amlodipine *on page 69*

Norventyl (Can) *see* nortriptyline *on page 634*

Norvir® *see* ritonavir *on page 784*

Norvir® SEC (Can) *see* ritonavir *on page 784*

Nostrilla® [OTC] *see* oxymetazoline (nasal) *on page 664*

Notuss®-DC *see* pseudoephedrine and codeine *on page 752*

NovaFerrum® *see* polysaccharide-iron complex and folic acid *on page 721*

Novahistex® DM Decongestant (Can) *see* pseudoephedrine and dextromethorphan *on page 752*

Novahistex® Expectorant with Decongestant (Can) *see* guaifenesin and pseudoephedrine
  on page 429

Novahistine DH *see* dihydrocodeine, chlorpheniramine, and phenylephrine *on page 285*

Novahistine® DM Decongestant (Can) *see* pseudoephedrine and dextromethorphan *on page 752*

Novamilor (Can) *see* amiloride and hydrochlorothiazide *on page 64*

Novamoxin® (Can) *see* amoxicillin *on page 73*

Novantrone® *see* mitoxantrone *on page 593*

Novarel® *see* chorionic gonadotropin (human) *on page 206*

Novasen (Can) *see* aspirin *on page 98*

novel erythropoiesis-stimulating protein *see* darbepoetin alfa *on page 253*

Novo-5 ASA (Can) *see* mesalamine *on page 564*

Novo-5 ASA-ECT (Can) *see* mesalamine *on page 564*

Novo-Acebutolol (Can) *see* acebutolol *on page 23*

Novo-Acyclovir (Can) *see* acyclovir (systemic) *on page 39*

Novo-Alendronate (Can) *see* alendronate *on page 49*

Novo-Alprazol (Can) *see* alprazolam *on page 56*

Novo-Amiodarone (Can) *see* amiodarone *on page 67*

Novo-Ampicillin (Can) *see* ampicillin *on page 76*

Novo-Atenolthalidone (Can) *see* atenolol and chlorthalidone *on page 101*

Novo-Atorvastatin (Can) *see* atorvastatin *on page 102*

Novo-Azithromycin (Can) *see* azithromycin (systemic) *on page 108*

Novo-AZT (Can) *see* zidovudine *on page 929*

Novo-Baclofen (Can) *see* baclofen *on page 112*

Novo-Benzydamine (Can) *see* benzydamine *(Canada only) on page 126*

Novo-Betahistine (Can) *see* betahistine *(Canada only) on page 128*

Novo-Bicalutamide (Can) *see* bicalutamide *on page 133*

Novo-Bisoprolol (Can) *see* bisoprolol *on page 136*

Novo-Bromazepam (Can) *see* bromazepam *(Canada only) on page 142*

Novo-Bupropion SR (Can) *see* bupropion *on page 150*

Novo-Buspirone (Can) *see* buspirone *on page 151*

Novo-Carvedilol (Can) *see* carvedilol *on page 178*

Novo-Cefaclor (Can) *see* cefaclor *on page 180*

Novo-Cefadroxil (Can) *see* cefadroxil *on page 180*

Novo-Chloroquine (Can) *see* chloroquine *on page 196*

Novo-Chlorpromazine (Can) *see* chlorpromazine *on page 203*

Novo-Cholamine (Can) *see* cholestyramine resin *on page 205*

Novo-Cholamine Light (Can) *see* cholestyramine resin *on page 205*

Novo-Cilazapril (Can) *see* cilazapril *(Canada only) on page 208*
Novo-Cilazapril/HCTZ (Can) *see* cilazapril and hydrochlorothiazide *(Canada only) on page 208*
Novo-Cimetidine (Can) *see* cimetidine *on page 209*
Novo-Ciprofloxacin (Can) *see* ciprofloxacin (systemic) *on page 210*
Novo-Citalopram (Can) *see* citalopram *on page 213*
Novo-Clavamoxin (Can) *see* amoxicillin and clavulanate potassium *on page 74*
Novo-Clindamycin (Can) *see* clindamycin (systemic) *on page 217*
Novo-Clobazam (Can) *see* clobazam *(Canada only) on page 220*
Novo-Clobetasol (Can) *see* clobetasol *on page 220*
Novo-Clonazepam (Can) *see* clonazepam *on page 222*
Novo-Clonidine (Can) *see* clonidine *on page 223*
Novo-Clopate (Can) *see* clorazepate *on page 225*
Novo-Cloxin (Can) *see* cloxacillin *(Canada only) on page 226*
Novo-Cycloprine (Can) *see* cyclobenzaprine *on page 241*
Novo-Cyproterone (Can) *see* cyproterone *(Canada only) on page 245*
Novo-Cyproterone/Ethinyl Estradiol (Can) *see* cyproterone and ethinyl estradiol *(Canada only) on page 245*
Novo-Desmopressin (Can) *see* desmopressin *on page 262*
Novo-Difenac ECT (Can) *see* diclofenac (systemic) *on page 277*
Novo-Difenac K (Can) *see* diclofenac (systemic) *on page 277*
Novo-Difenac-SR (Can) *see* diclofenac (systemic) *on page 277*
Novo-Difenac Suppositories (Can) *see* diclofenac (systemic) *on page 277*
Novo-Diflunisal (Can) *see* diflunisal *on page 282*
Novo-Dimenate (Can) *see* dimenhydrinate *on page 288*
Novo-Dipam (Can) *see* diazepam *on page 276*
Novo-Divalproex (Can) *see* divalproex *on page 300*
Novo-Docusate Calcium (Can) *see* docusate *on page 302*
Novo-Docusate Sodium (Can) *see* docusate *on page 302*
Novo-Doxazosin (Can) *see* doxazosin *on page 308*
Novo-Doxepin (Can) *see* doxepin (systemic) *on page 309*
Novo-Doxylin (Can) *see* doxycycline *on page 312*
Novo-Enalapril (Can) *see* enalapril *on page 326*
Novo-Etidronatecal (Can) *see* etidronate and calcium carbonate *(Canada only) on page 360*
Novo-Famotidine (Can) *see* famotidine *on page 366*
Novo-Fenofibrate (Can) *see* fenofibrate *on page 369*
Novo-Fenofibrate Micronized (Can) *see* fenofibrate *on page 369*
Novo-Fenofibrate-S (Can) *see* fenofibrate *on page 369*
Novo-Fentanyl (Can) *see* fentanyl *on page 371*
Novo-Ferrogluc (Can) *see* ferrous gluconate *on page 373*
Novo-Finasteride (Can) *see* finasteride *on page 378*
Novo-Fluconazole (Can) *see* fluconazole *on page 381*
Novo-Flunarizine (Can) *see* flunarizine *(Canada only) on page 383*
Novo-Fluoxetine (Can) *see* fluoxetine *on page 389*
Novo-Flurprofen (Can) *see* flurbiprofen (systemic) *on page 391*
Novo-Flutamide (Can) *see* flutamide *on page 392*
Novo-Fluvoxamine (Can) *see* fluvoxamine *on page 395*
Novo-Furantoin (Can) *see* nitrofurantoin *on page 629*
Novo-Gemfibrozil (Can) *see* gemfibrozil *on page 414*
Novo-Gesic (Can) *see* acetaminophen *on page 23*
Novo-Gliclazide (Can) *see* gliclazide *(Canada only) on page 417*
Novo-Glimepiride (Can) *see* glimepiride *on page 418*
Novo-Glyburide (Can) *see* glyburide *on page 420*
Novo-Hydrazide (Can) *see* hydrochlorothiazide *on page 445*

Novo-Hydroxyzin (Can) *see* hydroxyzine *on page 456*
Novo-Hylazin (Can) *see* hydralazine *on page 444*
Novo-Indapamide (Can) *see* indapamide *on page 470*
Novo-Ipramide (Can) *see* ipratropium (oral inhalation) *on page 489*
Novo-Ketoconazole (Can) *see* ketoconazole (systemic) *on page 500*
Novo-Ketorolac (Can) *see* ketorolac (systemic) *on page 501*
Novo-Lamotrigine (Can) *see* lamotrigine *on page 509*
Novo-Leflunomide (Can) *see* leflunomide *on page 514*
Novo-Levobunolol (Can) *see* levobunolol *on page 517*
Novo-Levocarbidopa (Can) *see* carbidopa and levodopa *on page 174*
Novo-Levofloxacin (Can) *see* levofloxacin (systemic) *on page 520*
Novo-Lexin (Can) *see* cephalexin *on page 188*
NovoLIN® 70/30 *see* insulin NPH and insulin regular *on page 479*
Novolin® ge 30/70 (Can) *see* insulin NPH and insulin regular *on page 479*
Novolin® ge 40/60 (Can) *see* insulin NPH and insulin regular *on page 479*
Novolin® ge 50/50 (Can) *see* insulin NPH and insulin regular *on page 479*
Novolin® ge NPH (Can) *see* insulin NPH *on page 479*
Novolin® ge Toronto (Can) *see* insulin regular *on page 480*
NovoLIN® N *see* insulin NPH *on page 479*
NovoLIN® R *see* insulin regular *on page 480*
Novo-Lisinopril/Hctz (Can) *see* lisinopril and hydrochlorothiazide *on page 532*
NovoLOG® *see* insulin aspart *on page 475*
NovoLog 70/30 *see* insulin aspart protamine and insulin aspart *on page 476*
NovoLOG® FlexPen® *see* insulin aspart *on page 475*
NovoLOG® Mix 70/30 *see* insulin aspart protamine and insulin aspart *on page 476*
NovoLOG® Mix 70/30 FlexPen® *see* insulin aspart protamine and insulin aspart *on page 476*
NovoLOG® Penfill® *see* insulin aspart *on page 475*
Novo-Loperamide (Can) *see* loperamide *on page 535*
Novo-Lorazem (Can) *see* lorazepam *on page 537*
Novo-Lovastatin (Can) *see* lovastatin *on page 540*
Novo-Maprotiline (Can) *see* maprotiline *on page 549*
Novo-Medrone (Can) *see* medroxyprogesterone *on page 554*
Novo-Meloxicam (Can) *see* meloxicam *on page 556*
Novo-Meprazine (Can) *see* methotrimeprazine *(Canada only) on page 572*
Novo-Mepro (Can) *see* meprobamate *on page 562*
Novo-Metformin (Can) *see* metformin *on page 566*
Novo-Methacin (Can) *see* indomethacin *on page 471*
Novo-Methylphenidate ER-C (Can) *see* methylphenidate *on page 577*
Novo-Mexiletine (Can) *see* mexiletine *on page 584*
Novo-Minocycline (Can) *see* minocycline *on page 590*
Novo-Mirtazapine (Can) *see* mirtazapine *on page 592*
Novo-Misoprostol (Can) *see* misoprostol *on page 592*
NovoMix® 30 (Can) *see* insulin aspart protamine and insulin aspart *on page 476*
Novo-Moclobemide (Can) *see* moclobemide *(Canada only) on page 594*
Novo-Morphine SR (Can) *see* morphine (systemic) *on page 598*
Novo-Nabumetone (Can) *see* nabumetone *on page 607*
Novo-Nadolol (Can) *see* nadolol *on page 607*
Novo-Nizatidine (Can) *see* nizatidine *on page 631*
Novo-Norfloxacin (Can) *see* norfloxacin *on page 633*
Novo-Nortriptyline (Can) *see* nortriptyline *on page 634*
Novo-Ofloxacin (Can) *see* ofloxacin (systemic) *on page 644*
Novo-Oxybutynin (Can) *see* oxybutynin *on page 661*
Novo-Oxycodone Acet (Can) *see* oxycodone and acetaminophen *on page 662*

Novo-Paroxetine (Can) *see* paroxetine *on page 676*
Novo-Pen-VK (Can) *see* penicillin V potassium *on page 686*
Novo-Peridol (Can) *see* haloperidol *on page 434*
Novo-Pheniram (Can) *see* chlorpheniramine *on page 197*
Novo-Pindol (Can) *see* pindolol *on page 705*
Novo-Pioglitazone (Can) *see* pioglitazone *on page 706*
Novo-Pirocam (Can) *see* piroxicam *on page 708*
Novo-Pramine (Can) *see* imipramine *on page 467*
Novo-Pramipexole (Can) *see* pramipexole *on page 729*
Novo-Pranol (Can) *see* propranolol *on page 747*
Novo-Pravastatin (Can) *see* pravastatin *on page 732*
Novo-Prazin (Can) *see* prazosin *on page 733*
Novo-Prednisolone (Can) *see* prednisolone (systemic) *on page 734*
Novo-Prednisone (Can) *see* prednisone *on page 735*
Novo-Profen (Can) *see* ibuprofen *on page 460*
Novo-Propamide (Can) *see* chlorpropamide *on page 203*
Novo-Purol (Can) *see* allopurinol *on page 54*
Novo-Quinidin (Can) *see* quinidine *on page 762*
Novo-Quinine (Can) *see* quinine *on page 762*
Novo-Raloxifene (Can) *see* raloxifene *on page 765*
NovoRapid® (Can) *see* insulin aspart *on page 475*
Novo-Risedronate (Can) *see* risedronate *on page 782*
Novo-Risperidone (Can) *see* risperidone *on page 783*
Novo-Rivastigmine (Can) *see* rivastigmine *on page 786*
Novo-Rythro Estolate (Can) *see* erythromycin (systemic) *on page 339*
Novo-Rythro Ethylsuccinate (Can) *see* erythromycin (systemic) *on page 339*
Novo-Salbutamol HFA (Can) *see* albuterol *on page 45*
Novo-Selegiline (Can) *see* selegiline *on page 806*
Novo-Semide (Can) *see* furosemide *on page 404*
NovoSeven® RT *see* factor VIIa (recombinant) *on page 365*
Novo-Sorbide (Can) *see* isosorbide dinitrate *on page 494*
Novo-Sotalol (Can) *see* sotalol *on page 828*
Novo-Spiroton (Can) *see* spironolactone *on page 829*
Novo-Spirozine (Can) *see* hydrochlorothiazide and spironolactone *on page 446*
Novo-Sucralate (Can) *see* sucralfate *on page 833*
Novo-Sumatriptan (Can) *see* sumatriptan *on page 839*
Novo-Sundac (Can) *see* sulindac *on page 839*
Novo-Temazepam (Can) *see* temazepam *on page 848*
Novo-Theophyl SR (Can) *see* theophylline *on page 860*
Novo-Ticlopidine (Can) *see* ticlopidine *on page 868*
Novo-Timol (Can) *see* timolol (ophthalmic) *on page 869*
Novo-Topiramate (Can) *see* topiramate *on page 877*
Novo-Trazodone (Can) *see* trazodone *on page 884*
Novo-Trifluzine (Can) *see* trifluoperazine *on page 890*
Novo-Trimel (Can) *see* sulfamethoxazole and trimethoprim *on page 836*
Novo-Trimel D.S. (Can) *see* sulfamethoxazole and trimethoprim *on page 836*
Novo-Triptyn (Can) *see* amitriptyline *on page 68*
Novo-Veramil (Can) *see* verapamil *on page 912*
Novo-Veramil SR (Can) *see* verapamil *on page 912*
Novo-Warfarin (Can) *see* warfarin *on page 922*
Novoxapram® (Can) *see* oxazepam *on page 659*
Novo-Zopiclone (Can) *see* zopiclone *(Canada only) on page 934*
Noxafil® *see* posaconazole *on page 722*

Nozinan® (Can) *see* methotrimeprazine *(Canada only) on page 572*
NPH insulin *see* insulin NPH *on page 479*
NPH insulin and regular insulin *see* insulin NPH and insulin regular *on page 479*
Nplate™ *see* romiplostim *on page 789*
NRP104 *see* lisdexamfetamine *on page 531*
NRS® [OTC] *see* oxymetazoline (nasal) *on page 664*
NSC-750 *see* busulfan *on page 152*
NSC-755 *see* mercaptopurine *on page 563*
NSC-13875 *see* altretamine *on page 59*
NSC-71423 *see* megestrol *on page 555*
NSC-89199 *see* estramustine *on page 346*
NSC-105014 *see* cladribine *on page 214*
NSC-147834 *see* flutamide *on page 392*
NSC-218321 *see* pentostatin *on page 689*
NSC606869 *see* clofarabine *on page 221*
NSC-613795 *see* sargramostim *on page 802*
NSC-684588 *see* nilutamide *on page 627*
NSC-697732 *see* daunorubicin citrate (liposomal) *on page 255*
NSC-714371 *see* dalteparin *on page 250*
NSC-725961 *see* pegfilgrastim *on page 679*
NTBC *see* nitisinone *on page 628*
NTG *see* nitroglycerin *on page 629*
N-trifluoroacetyladriamycin-14-valerate *see* valrubicin *on page 905*
NTZ *see* nitazoxanide *on page 628*
Nu-Acebutolol (Can) *see* acebutolol *on page 23*
Nu-Acyclovir (Can) *see* acyclovir (systemic) *on page 39*
Nu-Alpraz (Can) *see* alprazolam *on page 56*
Nu-Amilzide (Can) *see* amiloride and hydrochlorothiazide *on page 64*
Nu-Amoxi (Can) *see* amoxicillin *on page 73*
Nu-Ampi (Can) *see* ampicillin *on page 76*
Nu-Atenol (Can) *see* atenolol *on page 101*
Nu-Baclo (Can) *see* baclofen *on page 112*
Nubain *see* nalbuphine *on page 609*
Nu-Beclomethasone (Can) *see* beclomethasone (nasal) *on page 117*
Nu-Bromazepam (Can) *see* bromazepam *(Canada only) on page 142*
Nu-Buspirone (Can) *see* buspirone *on page 151*
Nu-Capto (Can) *see* captopril *on page 170*
Nu-Carbamazepine (Can) *see* carbamazepine *on page 171*
Nu-Cefaclor (Can) *see* cefaclor *on page 180*
Nu-Cephalex (Can) *see* cephalexin *on page 188*
Nu-Cimet (Can) *see* cimetidine *on page 209*
Nu-Clonazepam (Can) *see* clonazepam *on page 222*
Nu-Clonidine (Can) *see* clonidine *on page 223*
Nu-Cloxi (Can) *see* cloxacillin *(Canada only) on page 226*
Nu-Cotrimox (Can) *see* sulfamethoxazole and trimethoprim *on page 836*
Nu-Cromolyn (Can) *see* cromolyn (systemic, oral inhalation) *on page 238*
Nu-Cyclobenzaprine (Can) *see* cyclobenzaprine *on page 241*
Nucynta® *see* tapentadol *on page 844*
Nucynta™ CR (Can) *see* tapentadol *on page 844*
Nucynta® ER *see* tapentadol *on page 844*
Nu-Desipramine (Can) *see* desipramine *on page 260*
Nu-Diclo (Can) *see* diclofenac (systemic) *on page 277*
Nu-Diclo-SR (Can) *see* diclofenac (systemic) *on page 277*

Nu-Diflunisal (Can) *see* diflunisal *on page 282*
Nu-Diltiaz (Can) *see* diltiazem *on page 286*
Nu-Diltiaz-CD (Can) *see* diltiazem *on page 286*
Nu-Divalproex (Can) *see* divalproex *on page 300*
Nu-Domperidone (Can) *see* domperidone *(Canada only) on page 305*
Nu-Doxycycline (Can) *see* doxycycline *on page 312*
Nuedexta™ *see* dextromethorphan and quinidine *on page 272*
Nu-Erythromycin-S (Can) *see* erythromycin (systemic) *on page 339*
Nu-Famotidine (Can) *see* famotidine *on page 366*
Nu-Fenofibrate (Can) *see* fenofibrate *on page 369*
Nu-Fluoxetine (Can) *see* fluoxetine *on page 389*
Nu-Flurprofen (Can) *see* flurbiprofen (systemic) *on page 391*
Nu-Fluvoxamine (Can) *see* fluvoxamine *on page 395*
Nu-Furosemide (Can) *see* furosemide *on page 404*
Nu-Gemfibrozil (Can) *see* gemfibrozil *on page 414*
Nu-Glyburide (Can) *see* glyburide *on page 420*
Nu-Hydral (Can) *see* hydralazine *on page 444*
Nu-Hydro (Can) *see* hydrochlorothiazide *on page 445*
Nu-Hydroxyzine (Can) *see* hydroxyzine *on page 456*
Nu-Ibuprofen (Can) *see* ibuprofen *on page 460*
Nu-Indapamide (Can) *see* indapamide *on page 470*
Nu-Indo (Can) *see* indomethacin *on page 471*
Nu-Ipratropium (Can) *see* ipratropium (oral inhalation) *on page 489*
Nu-Iron® 150 [OTC] *see* polysaccharide-iron complex *on page 720*
Nu-Ketoprofen (Can) *see* ketoprofen *on page 501*
Nu-Ketoprofen-E (Can) *see* ketoprofen *on page 501*
Nu-Ketorolac (Can) *see* ketorolac (systemic) *on page 501*
Nulecit™ *see* ferric gluconate *on page 372*
Nu-Levocarb (Can) *see* carbidopa and levodopa *on page 174*
Nullo® [OTC] *see* chlorophyll *on page 195*
Nulojix® *see* belatacept *on page 117*
Nu-Loraz (Can) *see* lorazepam *on page 537*
Nu-Lovastatin (Can) *see* lovastatin *on page 540*
Nu-Loxapine (Can) *see* loxapine *on page 541*
NuLYTELY® *see* polyethylene glycol-electrolyte solution *on page 718*
Nu-Medopa (Can) *see* methyldopa *on page 575*
Nu-Mefenamic (Can) *see* mefenamic acid *on page 555*
Nu-Megestrol (Can) *see* megestrol *on page 555*
Nu-Metformin (Can) *see* metformin *on page 566*
Nu-Metoclopramide (Can) *see* metoclopramide *on page 580*
Nu-Metop (Can) *see* metoprolol *on page 581*
Nu-Moclobemide (Can) *see* moclobemide *(Canada only) on page 594*
Numoisyn™ *see* saliva substitute *on page 798*
Nu-Nifed (Can) *see* nifedipine *on page 626*
Nu-Nifedipine-PA (Can) *see* nifedipine *on page 626*
Nu-Nizatidine (Can) *see* nizatidine *on page 631*
Nu-Nortriptyline (Can) *see* nortriptyline *on page 634*
Nu-Oxybutyn (Can) *see* oxybutynin *on page 661*
Nu-Pentoxifylline SR (Can) *see* pentoxifylline *on page 689*
Nu-Pen-VK (Can) *see* penicillin V potassium *on page 686*
Nupercainal® [OTC] *see* dibucaine *on page 277*
Nu-Pindol (Can) *see* pindolol *on page 705*
Nu-Pirox (Can) *see* piroxicam *on page 708*

nystatin (oral) (nye STAT in)

Medication Safety Issues
  Sound-alike/look-alike issues:
    Nystatin may be confused with HMG-CoA reductase inhibitors (also known as "statins"; eg, atorvastatin, fluvastatin, lovastatin, pitavastatin, pravastatin, rosuvastatin, simvastatin), Nitrostat®
U.S. Brand Names Nystat-Rx [DSC]
Canadian Brand Names PMS-Nystatin
Therapeutic Category Antifungal Agent, Oral Nonabsorbed

◄ **Use** Treatment of susceptible cutaneous, mucocutaneous, and oral cavity fungal infections normally caused by the *Candida* species

General Dosage Range Oral:
Premature infants: 100,000 units 4 times/day
Infants: 200,000 units 4 times/day
Children: 400,000-600,000 units 4 times/day
Adults: 400,000-1,000,000 units/day in 3-4 divided doses

Dosage Forms
Powder, for prescription compounding: 50 million units (10 g); 150 million units (30 g); 500 million units (100 g)
Suspension, oral: 100,000 units/mL (5 mL, 60 mL, 240 mL, 473 mL, 480 mL, 3785 mL)
Tablet, oral: 500,000 units

nystatin (topical) (nye STAT in)

Medication Safety Issues
Sound-alike/look-alike issues:
Nystatin may be confused with HMG-CoA reductase inhibitors (also known as "statins"; eg, atorvastatin, fluvastatin, lovastatin, pitavastatin, pravastatin, rosuvastatin, simvastatin), Nitrostat®

U.S. Brand Names Nyamyc®; Nystop®; Pedi-Dri®; Pediaderm™ AF
Canadian Brand Names Candistatin®; Nyaderm
Therapeutic Category Antifungal Agent, Topical; Antifungal Agent, Vaginal
Use Treatment of susceptible cutaneous and mucocutaneous fungal infections normally caused by the *Candida* species

General Dosage Range
Intravaginal: *Adults:* Insert 1 vaginal tablet/day at bedtime
Topical: *Children and Adults:* Apply 2-3 times/day to affected areas

Dosage Forms
Cream, topical: 100,000 units/g (15 g, 30 g)
Pediaderm™ AF: 100,000 units/g (30 g)
Ointment, topical: 100,000 units/g (15 g, 30 g)
Powder, topical: 100,000 units/g (15 g, 30 g, 60 g)
Nyamyc®: 100,000 units/g (15 g, 30 g, 60 g)
Nystop®: 100,000 units/g (15 g, 30 g, 60 g)
Pedi-Dri®: 100,000 units/g (56.7 g)
Tablet, vaginal: 100,000 units

nystatin and metronidazole see metronidazole and nystatin *(Canada only) on page 583*

nystatin and triamcinolone (nye STAT in & trye am SIN oh lone)

Synonyms triamcinolone and nystatin
Therapeutic Category Antifungal/Corticosteroid
Use Treatment of cutaneous candidiasis
General Dosage Range
Topical:
Children: Apply sparingly 2-4 times/day
Adults: Apply sparingly 2-4 times/day
Dosage Forms
Cream: Nystatin 100,000 units and triamcinolone 0.1% (15 g, 30 g, 60 g)
Ointment: Nystatin 100,000 units and triamcinolone 0.1% (15 g, 30 g, 60 g)

Nystat-Rx [DSC] see nystatin (oral) *on page 641*
Nystop® see nystatin (topical) *on page 642*
Nytol® (Can) see diphenhydramine (systemic) *on page 290*
Nytol® Extra Strength (Can) see diphenhydramine (systemic) *on page 290*
Nytol® Quick Caps [OTC] see diphenhydramine (systemic) *on page 290*
Nytol® Quick Gels [OTC] see diphenhydramine (systemic) *on page 290*
Oasis® see saliva substitute *on page 798*
OCBZ see oxcarbazepine *on page 660*
Occlusal™-HP (Can) see salicylic acid *on page 795*

Ocean® [OTC] *see* sodium chloride *on page 818*
Ocean® for Kids [OTC] *see* sodium chloride *on page 818*
Ocella™ *see* ethinyl estradiol and drospirenone *on page 352*
Octagam® *see* immune globulin *on page 468*
Octaplex® (Can) *see* prothrombin complex (human) [(factors II, VII, IX, X), protein C, and protein S] *(Canada only) on page 750*
Octostim® (Can) *see* desmopressin *on page 262*

octreotide (ok TREE oh tide)

Medication Safety Issues
Sound-alike/look-alike issues:
SandoSTATIN® may be confused with SandIMMUNE®, SandoSTATIN LAR®, sargramostim, simvastatin
Synonyms longastatin; octreotide acetate
U.S. Brand Names SandoSTATIN LAR®; SandoSTATIN®
Canadian Brand Names Octreotide Acetate Injection; Octreotide Acetate Omega; Sandostatin LAR®; Sandostatin®
Therapeutic Category Somatostatin Analog
Use Control of symptoms (diarrhea and flushing) in patients with metastatic carcinoid tumors; treatment of watery diarrhea associated with vasoactive intestinal peptide-secreting tumors (VIPomas); treatment of acromegaly
General Dosage Range Dosage adjustment recommended in patients with hepatic or renal impairment
I.M.: *Adults:* Depot: 20 mg every 4 weeks (maximum: 40 mg every 2 weeks)
I.V., SubQ: *Adults:* 50-1500 mcg/day in 2-4 divided doses
Dosage Forms
Injection, microspheres for suspension:
SandoSTATIN LAR®: 10 mg, 20 mg, 30 mg
Injection, solution: 100 mcg/mL (1 mL); 200 mcg/mL (5 mL); 1000 mcg/mL (5 mL)
SandoSTATIN®: 200 mcg/mL (5 mL); 1000 mcg/mL (5 mL)
Injection, solution [preservative free]: 50 mcg/mL (1 mL); 100 mcg/mL (1 mL); 200 mcg/mL (5 mL); 500 mcg/mL (1 mL)
SandoSTATIN®: 50 mcg/mL (1 mL); 100 mcg/mL (1 mL); 500 mcg/mL (1 mL)

octreotide acetate *see* octreotide *on page 643*
Octreotide Acetate Injection (Can) *see* octreotide *on page 643*
Octreotide Acetate Omega (Can) *see* octreotide *on page 643*
Ocudox™ *see* doxycycline *on page 312*
Ocufen® *see* flurbiprofen (ophthalmic) *on page 392*
Ocuflox® *see* ofloxacin (ophthalmic) *on page 644*
OcuNefrin™ [OTC] [DSC] *see* phenylephrine (ophthalmic) *on page 697*
Ocuvite® [OTC] *see* vitamins (multiple/oral) *on page 919*
Ocuvite® Adult 50+ [OTC] *see* vitamins (multiple/oral) *on page 919*
Ocuvite® Extra® [OTC] *see* vitamins (multiple/oral) *on page 919*
Ocuvite® Lutein [OTC] *see* vitamins (multiple/oral) *on page 919*
O-desmethylvenlafaxine *see* desvenlafaxine *on page 264*
ODV *see* desvenlafaxine *on page 264*
Oesclim® (Can) *see* estradiol (systemic) *on page 343*

ofatumumab (oh fa TOOM yoo mab)

Medication Safety Issues
Sound-alike/look-alike issues:
Ofatumumab may be confused with omalizumab
High alert medication:
This medication is in a class the Institute for Safe Medication Practices (ISMP) includes among its list of drug classes which have a heightened risk of causing significant patient harm when used in error.
Synonyms huMax-CD20
U.S. Brand Names Arzerra™
Therapeutic Category Antineoplastic Agent, Monoclonal Antibody; Monoclonal Antibody

◀ **Use** Treatment of refractory chronic lymphocytic leukemia (CLL)

General Dosage Range Dosage adjustment recommended in patients who develop toxicities
I.V.: *Adults:* 300 mg week 1, followed 1 week later by 2000 mg once weekly for 7 doses (doses 2-8), followed 4 weeks later by 2000 mg once every 4 weeks for 4 doses (doses 9-12; for a total of 12 doses)

Dosage Forms
Injection, solution [preservative free]:
Arzerra™: 20 mg/mL (5 mL, 50 mL)

Ofirmev™ *see* acetaminophen *on page 23*

ofloxacin (systemic) (oh FLOKS a sin)

Canadian Brand Names Apo-Oflox®; Novo-Ofloxacin

Therapeutic Category Antibiotic, Quinolone

Use Quinolone antibiotic for the treatment of acute exacerbations of chronic bronchitis, community-acquired pneumonia, skin and skin structure infections (uncomplicated), urethral and cervical gonorrhea (acute, uncomplicated), urethritis and cervicitis (nongonococcal), mixed infections of the urethra and cervix, pelvic inflammatory disease (acute), cystitis (uncomplicated), urinary tract infections (complicated), prostatitis
Note: As of April 2007, the CDC no longer recommends the use of fluoroquinolones for the treatment of gonococcal disease.

General Dosage Range Dosage adjustment recommended in patients with hepatic or renal impairment
Oral: *Adults:* 200-400 mg every 12 hours

Dosage Forms
Tablet, oral: 200 mg, 300 mg, 400 mg

ofloxacin (ophthalmic) (oh FLOKS a sin)

Medication Safety Issues
Sound-alike/look-alike issues:
Ocuflox® may be confused with Occlusal®-HP, Ocufen®

U.S. Brand Names Ocuflox®

Canadian Brand Names Ocuflox®

Therapeutic Category Antibiotic, Ophthalmic; Antibiotic, Quinolone

Use Treatment of superficial ocular infections involving the conjunctiva or cornea due to strains of susceptible organisms

General Dosage Range Ophthalmic: *Children >1 year and Adults:* Initial: 1-2 drops every 30 minutes to 4 hours; Maintenance: 1-2 drops every 4-6 hours

Dosage Forms
Solution, ophthalmic: 0.3% (5 mL, 10 mL)
Ocuflox®: 0.3% (5 mL)

ofloxacin (otic) (oh FLOKS a sin)

Medication Safety Issues
Sound-alike/look-alike issues:
Floxin® may be confused with Flexeril®
International issues:
Floxin: Brand name for ofloxacin [U.S., Canada], but also the brand name for flunarizine [Thailand], norfloxacin [South Africa], and perfloxacin [Philippines]
Floxin® [U.S., Canada] may be confused with Flexin brand name for diclofenac [Argentina], cyclobenzaprine [Chile], and orphenadrine [Israel]; Flogen brand name for naproxen [Mexico]; Fluoxin brand name for fluoxetine [Czech Republic]

Synonyms floxin otic singles

Therapeutic Category Antibiotic, Quinolone

Use Otitis externa, chronic suppurative otitis media, acute otitis media

General Dosage Range
Otic:
Children <6 months: Dosage not established
Children ≥6 months to 12 years: 5 drops daily
Children >12 years: 10 drops once or twice daily
Adults: 10 drops once or twice daily

Dosage Forms
 Solution, otic: 0.3% (5 mL, 10 mL)

Oforta™ *see* fludarabine *on page 382*
Ogen® (Can) *see* estropipate *on page 349*
Ogestrel® *see* ethinyl estradiol and norgestrel *on page 357*
OGMT *see* metyrosine *on page 584*
OGT-918 *see* miglustat *on page 589*
17OHPC *see* hydroxyprogesterone caproate *on page 455*
9-OH-risperidone *see* paliperidone *on page 668*
OKT3 *see* muromonab-CD3 *on page 603*

olanzapine (oh LAN za peen)

Medication Safety Issues
 Sound-alike/look-alike issues:
  OLANZapine may be confused with olsalazine, QUEtiapine
  ZyPREXA® may be confused with CeleXA®, Reprexain™, Zestril®, ZyrTEC®
  ZyPREXA® Zydis® may be confused with Zelapar®, zolpidem
  ZyPREXA® Relprevv™ may be confused with ZyPREXA® IntraMuscular
Synonyms LY170053; olanzapine pamoate
Tall-Man OLANZapine
U.S. Brand Names ZyPREXA®; ZyPREXA® IntraMuscular; ZyPREXA® Relprevv™; ZyPREXA® Zydis®
Canadian Brand Names Apo-Olanzapine®; CO Olanzapine; CO Olanzapine ODT; Olanzapine ODT; PHL-Olanzapine; PHL-Olanzapine ODT; PMS-Olanzapine; PMS-Olanzapine ODT; Riva-Olanzapine; Riva-Olanzapine ODT; Sandoz-Olanzapine; Sandoz-Olanzapine ODT; Teva-Olanzapine; Teva-Olanza-pine OD; Zyprexa®; Zyprexa® Intramuscular; Zyprexa® Zydis®
Therapeutic Category Antipsychotic Agent
Use
 Oral: Treatment of the manifestations of schizophrenia; treatment of acute or mixed mania episodes associated with bipolar I disorder (as monotherapy or in combination with lithium or valproate); maintenance treatment of bipolar disorder; in combination with fluoxetine for treatment-resistant or bipolar I depression
 I.M., extended-release (Zyprexa® Relprevv™): Treatment of schizophrenia
 I.M., short-acting (Zyprexa® IntraMuscular): Treatment of acute agitation associated with schizophrenia and bipolar I mania
General Dosage Range
 I.M.: *Adults:*
  Extended release: 150-300 mg every 2 weeks **or** 300-405 mg every 4 weeks (maximum: 300 mg every 2 weeks; 405 mg every 4 weeks)
  Short-acting: Initial: 10 mg/dose; 2-4 hours between doses (maximum: 30 mg/day)
 Oral:
  Adolescents ≥13 years: Initial: 2.5-5 mg once daily; dosing range: 2.5-20 mg/day
  Adults: Initial: 5-15 mg once daily; Maintenance: 5-20 mg once daily
  Elderly: Initial: 2.5-5 mg/day
Dosage Forms
 Injection, powder for reconstitution:
  ZyPREXA® IntraMuscular: 10 mg
 Injection, powder for suspension, extended release:
  ZyPREXA® Relprevv™: 210 mg, 300 mg, 405 mg
 Tablet, oral:
  ZyPREXA®: 2.5 mg, 5 mg, 7.5 mg, 10 mg, 15 mg, 20 mg
 Tablet, orally disintegrating, oral:
  ZyPREXA® Zydis®: 5 mg, 10 mg, 15 mg, 20 mg

olanzapine and fluoxetine (oh LAN za peen & floo OKS e teen)

Medication Safety Issues
 Sound-alike/look-alike issues:
  Symbyax® may be confused with Cymbalta®
Synonyms fluoxetine and olanzapine; olanzapine and fluoxetine hydrochloride

◀ **U.S. Brand Names** Symbyax®

Therapeutic Category Antidepressant, Selective Serotonin Reuptake Inhibitor; Antipsychotic Agent, Thienobenzodiaepine

Use Treatment of depressive episodes associated with bipolar I disorder; treatment-resistant depression (unresponsive to 2 trials of different antidepressants in the current episode)

General Dosage Range Dosage adjustment recommended in patients with hepatic impairment

Oral:

Adults: Initial: Olanzapine 6 mg and fluoxetine 25 mg once daily; Maintenance: Olanzapine 6-12 mg and fluoxetine 25-50 mg once daily

Elderly >65 years: Initial: Olanzapine 3-6 mg and fluoxetine 25 mg once daily

Dosage Forms

Capsule:

Symbyax®:

3/25: Olanzapine 3 mg and fluoxetine 25 mg

6/25: Olanzapine 6 mg and fluoxetine 25 mg

6/50: Olanzapine 6 mg and fluoxetine 50 mg

12/25: Olanzapine 12 mg and fluoxetine 25 mg

12/50: Olanzapine 12 mg and fluoxetine 50 mg

olanzapine and fluoxetine hydrochloride *see* olanzapine and fluoxetine *on page 645*

Olanzapine ODT (Can) *see* olanzapine *on page 645*

olanzapine pamoate *see* olanzapine *on page 645*

oleovitamin A *see* vitamin A *on page 917*

Oleptro™ *see* trazodone *on page 884*

Olestyr (Can) *see* cholestyramine resin *on page 205*

oleum ricini *see* castor oil *on page 179*

olmesartan (ole me SAR tan)

Medication Safety Issues

Sound-alike/look-alike issues:

Benicar® may be confused with Mevacor®

Synonyms olmesartan medoxomil

U.S. Brand Names Benicar®

Canadian Brand Names Olmetec®

Therapeutic Category Angiotensin II Receptor Antagonist

Use Treatment of hypertension with or without concurrent use of other antihypertensive agents

General Dosage Range Oral:

Children 6-16 years:

20 kg to <35 kg: Initial: 10 mg once daily (maximum: 20 mg once daily)

≥35 kg: Initial: 20 mg once daily (maximum: 40 mg once daily)

Adolescents >16 years and Adults: Initial: 20 mg once daily; Maintenance: 20-40 mg once daily

Elderly: Initial: 5-20 mg once daily

Dosage Forms

Tablet, oral:

Benicar®: 5 mg, 20 mg, 40 mg

olmesartan, amlodipine, and hydrochlorothiazide

(ole me SAR tan, am LOE di peen, & hye droe klor oh THYE a zide)

Synonyms amlodipine besylate, olmesartan medoxomil, and hydrochlorothiazide; amlodipine, hydrochlorothiazide, and olmesartan; hydrochlorothiazide, olmesartan, and amlodipine; olmesartan, hydrochlorothiazide, and amlodipine

U.S. Brand Names Tribenzor™

Therapeutic Category Angiotensin II Receptor Blocker; Calcium Channel Blocker; Calcium Channel Blocker, Dihydropyridine; Diuretic, Thiazide

Use Treatment of hypertension (not for initial therapy)

General Dosage Range Oral: *Adults:* Amlodipine 5-10 mg and olmesartan 20-40 mg and hydrochlorothiazide 12.5-25 mg once daily (maximum: 10 mg/day [amlodipine]; 25 mg/day [hydrochlorothiazide]; 40 mg/day [olmesartan])

Dosage Forms
Tablet, oral:
  Tribenzor™: Olmesartan medoxomil 40 mg, amlodipine 5 mg, and hydrochlorothiazide 25 mg, olmesartan medoxomil 40 mg, amlodipine 10 mg, and hydrochlorothiazide 25 mg, olmesartan medoxomil 20 mg, amlodipine 5 mg, and hydrochlorothiazide 12.5 mg, olmesartan medoxomil 40 mg, amlodipine 5 mg, and hydrochlorothiazide 12.5 mg, olmesartan medoxomil 40 mg, amlodipine 10 mg, and hydrochlorothiazide 12.5 mg

olmesartan and amlodipine *see* amlodipine and olmesartan *on page 70*

olmesartan and hydrochlorothiazide (ole me SAR tan & hye droe klor oh THYE a zide)

Synonyms hydrochlorothiazide and olmesartan medoxomil; olmesartan medoxomil and hydrochlorothiazide
U.S. Brand Names Benicar HCT®
Canadian Brand Names Olmetec Plus®
Therapeutic Category Angiotensin II Receptor Antagonist; Diuretic, Thiazide
Use Treatment of hypertension (not recommended for initial treatment)
General Dosage Range Oral: *Adults:* Olmesartan 20-40 mg and hydrochlorothiazide 12.5-25 mg once daily (maximum: 25 mg/day [hydrochlorothiazide]; 40 mg/day [olmesartan])
Dosage Forms
Tablet:
  Benicar HCT®: 20/12.5: Olmesartan 20 mg and hydrochlorothiazide 12.5 mg; 40/12.5: Olmesartan 40 mg and hydrochlorothiazide 12.5 mg; 40/25: Olmesartan 40 mg and hydrochlorothiazide 25 mg

olmesartan, hydrochlorothiazide, and amlodipine *see* olmesartan, amlodipine, and hydrochlorothiazide *on page 646*
olmesartan medoxomil *see* olmesartan *on page 646*
olmesartan medoxomil and hydrochlorothiazide *see* olmesartan and hydrochlorothiazide *on page 647*
Olmetec® (Can) *see* olmesartan *on page 646*
Olmetec Plus® (Can) *see* olmesartan and hydrochlorothiazide *on page 647*

olopatadine (nasal) (oh la PAT a deen)

Synonyms olopatadine hydrochloride
U.S. Brand Names Patanase®
Therapeutic Category Histamine H_1 Antagonist; Histamine H_1 Antagonist, Second Generation
Use Treatment of the symptoms of seasonal allergic rhinitis
General Dosage Range Intranasal: *Children ≥12 years and Adults:* 2 sprays into each nostril twice daily
Dosage Forms
Solution, intranasal:
  Patanase®: 0.6% (30.5 g)

olopatadine (ophthalmic) (oh la PAT a deen)

Medication Safety Issues
Sound-alike/look-alike issues:
  Patanol® may be confused with Platinol®
International issues:
  Patanol [U.S., Canada, and multiple international markets] may be confused with Bétanol brand name for metipranolol [Monaco]
Synonyms olopatadine hydrochloride
U.S. Brand Names Pataday™; Patanol®
Canadian Brand Names Pataday™; Patanol®
Therapeutic Category Histamine H_1 Antagonist; Histamine H_1 Antagonist, Second Generation
Use Treatment of the signs and symptoms of allergic conjunctivitis
General Dosage Range Ophthalmic: *Children ≥3 years and Adults:* Patanol®: Instill 1 drop into affected eye(s) twice daily; Pataday™: Instill 1 drop into affected eye(s) once daily

◄ **Dosage Forms**
Solution, ophthalmic:
Pataday™: 0.2% (2.5 mL)
Patanol®: 0.1% (5 mL)

olopatadine hydrochloride *see olopatadine (nasal) on page 647*
olopatadine hydrochloride *see olopatadine (ophthalmic) on page 647*

olsalazine (ole SAL a zeen)
Medication Safety Issues
Sound-alike/look-alike issues:
Olsalazine may be confused with OLANZapine
Dipentum® may be confused with Dilantin®
Synonyms olsalazine sodium
U.S. Brand Names Dipentum®
Canadian Brand Names Dipentum®
Therapeutic Category 5-Aminosalicylic Acid Derivative
Use Maintenance of remission of ulcerative colitis in patients intolerant to sulfasalazine
General Dosage Range Oral: *Adults:* 1 g/day in 2 divided doses
Dosage Forms
Capsule, oral:
Dipentum®: 250 mg

olsalazine sodium *see olsalazine on page 648*
Olux® *see clobetasol on page 220*
Olux-E™ *see clobetasol on page 220*
Olux®/Olux-E™ CP [DSC] *see clobetasol on page 220*

omalizumab (oh mah lye ZOO mab)
Medication Safety Issues
Sound-alike/look-alike issues:
Omalizumab may be confused with ofatumumab
Synonyms rhuMAb-E25
U.S. Brand Names Xolair®
Canadian Brand Names Xolair®
Therapeutic Category Monoclonal Antibody
Use Treatment of moderate-to-severe, persistent allergic asthma not adequately controlled with inhaled corticosteroids
General Dosage Range SubQ:
IgE ≥30-100 int. units/mL:
Children ≥12 years and Adults 30-90 kg: 150 mg every 4 weeks
Children ≥12 years and Adults >90-150 kg: 300 mg every 4 weeks
IgE >100-200 int. units/mL:
Children ≥12 years and Adults 30-90 kg: 300 mg every 4 weeks
Children ≥12 years and Adults >90-150 kg: 225 mg every 2 weeks
IgE >200-300 int. units/mL:
Children ≥12 years and Adults 30-60 kg: 300 mg every 4 weeks
Children ≥12 years and Adults >60-90 kg: 225 mg every 2 weeks
Children ≥12 years and Adults >90-150 kg: 300 mg every 2 weeks
IgE >300-400 int. units/mL:
Children ≥12 years and Adults 30-70 kg: 225 mg every 2 weeks
Children ≥12 years and Adults >70-90 kg: 300 mg every 2 weeks
IgE >400-500 int. units/mL:
Children ≥12 years and Adults 30-70 kg: 300 mg every 2 weeks
Children ≥12 years and Adults >70-90 kg: 375 mg every 2 weeks
IgE >500-600 int. units/mL:
Children ≥12 years and Adults 30-60 kg: 300 mg every 2 weeks
Children ≥12 years and Adults >60-70 kg: 375 mg every 2 weeks
IgE >600-700 int. units/mL: *Children ≥12 years and Adults 30-60 kg:* 375 mg every 2 weeks

Dosage Forms
Injection, powder for reconstitution:
Xolair®: 150 mg

omega 3 *see omega-3-acid ethyl esters on page 649*

omega-3-acid ethyl esters (oh MEG a three AS id ETH il ES ters)

Medication Safety Issues
Sound-alike/look-alike issues:
Lovaza® may be confused with LORazepam
Omacor® may be confused with Amicar®
Other safety concerns:
The Institute for Safe Medication Practices (ISMP) reported a case of a foam plastic cup dissolving after contact with the liquid contents from a Lovaza® capsule. ISMP is requesting the manufacturer to add warnings to its labeling and that healthcare providers add Lovaza® to their list of medications to not crush.

Synonyms ethyl esters of omega-3 fatty acids; fish oil; omega 3
U.S. Brand Names Lovaza®
Therapeutic Category Antilipemic Agent, Miscellaneous
Use Lovaza®: Adjunct to diet therapy in the treatment of hypertriglyceridemia (≥500 mg/dL)
Note: A number of OTC formulations containing omega-3 fatty acids are marketed as nutritional supplements; these do not have FDA-approved indications and may not contain the same amounts of the active ingredient.
General Dosage Range Oral: *Adults:* 4 g/day in 1-2 divided doses
Dosage Forms
Capsule, liquid gel, oral:
Lovaza®: 1 g

omeprazole (oh MEP ra zole)

Medication Safety Issues
Sound-alike/look-alike issues:
Omeprazole may be confused with aripiprazole, fomepizole
PriLOSEC® may be confused with Plendil®, Prevacid®, predniSONE, prilocaine, Prinivil®, Proventil®, PROzac®
International issues:
Losec [multiple international markets] may be confused with Lasix, a brand name for furosemide [U.S., Canada, and multiple international markets]
Medral [Mexico] may be confused with Medrol brand name for methylprednisolone [U.S., Canada, and multiple international markets]
Norpramin: Brand name for omeprazole [Spain], but also the brand name for desipramine [U.S., Canada] and enalapril/hydrochlorothiazide [Portugal]
Synonyms omeprazole magnesium
U.S. Brand Names PriLOSEC OTC® [OTC]; PriLOSEC®
Canadian Brand Names Apo-Omeprazole®; Losec®; Mylan-Omeprazole; PMS-Omeprazole; PMS-Omeprazole DR; ratio-Omeprazole; Sandoz-Omeprazole
Therapeutic Category Gastric Acid Secretion Inhibitor
Use Short-term (4-8 weeks) treatment of active duodenal ulcer disease or active benign gastric ulcer; treatment of heartburn and other symptoms associated with gastroesophageal reflux disease (GERD); short-term (4-8 weeks) treatment of endoscopically-diagnosed erosive esophagitis; maintenance healing of erosive esophagitis; long-term treatment of pathological hypersecretory conditions; as part of a multidrug regimen for *H. pylori* eradication to reduce the risk of duodenal ulcer recurrence

OTC labeling: Short-term treatment of frequent, uncomplicated heartburn occurring ≥2 days/week
General Dosage Range Oral:
Children 1-16 years and 5 kg to <10 kg: 5 mg once daily
Children 1-16 years and 10 kg to <20 kg: 10 mg once daily
Children 1-16 years and ≥20 kg: 20 mg once daily
Adults: 20-40 mg/day (may be given in 2 divided doses); doses up to 360 mg/day [pathological hypersecretory syndrome]

◀ **Dosage Forms**
Capsule, delayed release, oral: 10 mg, 20 mg, 40 mg
PriLOSEC®: 10 mg, 20 mg, 40 mg
Granules for suspension, delayed release, oral:
PriLOSEC®: 2.5 mg/packet (30s); 10 mg/packet (30s)
Tablet, delayed release, oral: 20 mg
PriLOSEC OTC® [OTC]: 20 mg

omeprazole and sodium bicarbonate (oh MEP ra zole & SOW dee um bye KAR bun ate)

Medication Safety Issues
Sound-alike/look-alike issues:
Zegerid® may be confused with Zestril®
Synonyms sodium bicarbonate and omeprazole
U.S. Brand Names Zegerid OTC™ [OTC]; Zegerid®
Therapeutic Category Proton Pump Inhibitor; Substituted Benzimidazole
Use Short-term (4-8 weeks) treatment of active duodenal ulcer or active benign gastric ulcer; treatment of heartburn and other symptoms associated with gastroesophageal reflux disease (GERD); short-term (4-8 weeks) treatment of endoscopically-diagnosed erosive esophagitis; maintenance healing of erosive esophagitis; reduction of risk of upper gastrointestinal bleeding in critically-ill patients

OTC labeling: Short-term (2 weeks) treatment of frequent (2 days/week), uncomplicated heartburn
General Dosage Range Oral: *Adults:* 20-40 mg/day in 1-2 divided doses
Dosage Forms
Capsule, oral: Omeprazole 20 mg [immediate release] and sodium bicarbonate 1100 mg; omeprazole 40 mg [immediate release] and sodium bicarbonate 1100 mg
Zegerid®: Omeprazole 20 mg [immediate release] and sodium bicarbonate 1100 mg
Zegerid®: Omeprazole 40 mg [immediate release] and sodium bicarbonate 1100 mg
Zegerid OTC™ [OTC]: Omeprazole 20 mg [immediate release] and sodium bicarbonate 1100 mg
Powder for oral suspension:
Zegerid®: Omeprazole 20 mg and sodium bicarbonate 1680 mg per packet
Zegerid®: Omeprazole 40 mg and sodium bicarbonate 1680 mg per packet

omeprazole magnesium *see* omeprazole *on page 649*
Omnaris™ *see* ciclesonide (nasal) *on page 207*
Omnicef® *see* cefdinir *on page 180*
Omni Gel™ [OTC] *see* fluoride *on page 386*
OMNIhist® II L.A. [DSC] *see* chlorpheniramine, phenylephrine, and methscopolamine *on page 200*
Omnipaque™ (Can) *see* iohexol *on page 485*
Omnipaque™ 140 *see* iohexol *on page 485*
Omnipaque™ 180 *see* iohexol *on page 485*
Omnipaque™ 240 *see* iohexol *on page 485*
Omnipaque™ 300 *see* iohexol *on page 485*
Omnipaque™ 350 *see* iohexol *on page 485*
Omnipred™ *see* prednisolone (ophthalmic) *on page 734*
Omniscan® *see* gadodiamide *on page 407*
Omnitrope® *see* somatropin *on page 826*

onabotulinumtoxinA (oh nuh BOT yoo lin num TOKS in aye)

Medication Safety Issues
Other safety concerns:
Botulinum products are not interchangeable; potency differences may exist between the products.
Synonyms botulinum toxin type A; BTX-A
U.S. Brand Names Botox®; Botox® Cosmetic
Canadian Brand Names Botox®; Botox® Cosmetic
Therapeutic Category Ophthalmic Agent, Toxin
Use Treatment of strabismus and blepharospasm associated with dystonia (including benign essential blepharospasm or VII nerve disorders) in patients ≥12 years of age; treatment of cervical dystonia (spasmodic torticollis) in patients ≥16 years of age; temporary improvement in the appearance of lines/wrinkles of the face (moderate-to-severe glabellar lines associated with corrugator and/or procerus

muscle activity) in adult patients ≤65 years of age; treatment of severe primary axillary hyperhidrosis in adults not adequately controlled with topical treatments; treatment of focal spasticity (specifically upper limb spasticity) in adults; prophylaxis of chronic migraine headache (≥15 days/month with ≥4 hours/day headache duration) in adults

Canadian labeling: Additional use (not in U.S. labeling): Dynamic equinus foot deformity in pediatric cerebral palsy patients; treatment of forehead, lateral canthus, and glabellar lines in adults >65 years of age

General Dosage Range

I.M.: *Children ≥12 years and Adults:* Dosage varies greatly depending on indication

Intradermal: *Adults:* 50 units/axilla evenly distributed into multiple sites (10-15), in 0.1-0.2 mL aliquots, ~1-2 cm apart

Dosage Forms

Injection, powder for reconstitution [preservative free]:
  Botox®: *Clostridium botulinum* type A neurotoxin complex 100 units, *Clostridium botulinum* type A neurotoxin complex 200 units
  Botox® Cosmetic: *Clostridium botulinum* type A neurotoxin complex 100 units

Powder for reconstitution, for injection [preservative free]:
  Botox® Cosmetic: *Clostridium botulinum* type A neurotoxin complex 50 units

Dosage Forms - Canada

Injection, powder for reconstitution [preservative free]:
  Botox®: Botulinum toxin A 50 units, 100 units, 200 units
  Botox Cosmetic®: Botulinum toxin A 50 unit, 100 units, 200 units

OnBrez Breezehaler see indacaterol on page 470

Oncaspar® see pegaspargase on page 678

Oncotice™ (Can) see BCG on page 115

ondansetron (on DAN se tron)

Medication Safety Issues

Sound-alike/look-alike issues:
  Ondansetron may be confused with dolasetron, granisetron, palonosetron
  Zofran® may be confused with Zantac®, Zosyn®

Synonyms GR38032R; ondansetron hydrochloride

U.S. Brand Names Zofran®; Zofran® ODT; Zuplenz®

Canadian Brand Names Apo-Ondansetron®; CO Ondansetron; Dom-Ondansetron; JAMP-Ondansetron; Mint-Ondansetron; Mylan-Ondansetron; Ondansetron Injection; Ondansetron Injection USP; Ondansetron-Odan; Ondansetron-Omega; PHL-Ondansetron; PMS-Ondansetron; RAN™-Ondansetron; ratio-Ondansetron; Sandoz-Ondansetron; Teva-Ondansetron; Zofran®; Zofran® ODT; ZYM-Ondansetron

Therapeutic Category Selective 5-HT$_3$ Receptor Antagonist

Use Prevention of nausea and vomiting associated with moderately- to highly-emetogenic cancer chemotherapy; radiotherapy; prevention of postoperative nausea and vomiting (PONV); treatment of PONV if no prophylactic dose of ondansetron received

General Dosage Range Dosage adjustment recommended in patients with hepatic impairment

I.M.: *Adults:* 4 mg as a single dose

I.V.:
  Infants 1-6 months: 0.1 mg/kg as a single dose
  Children 6 months to 12 years and ≤40 kg: 0.1-0.45 mg/kg as a single dose **or** 0.15 mg/kg/dose for 3 doses
  Children 6 months to 12 years and >40 kg and Children >12 years to 18 years: 0.45 mg/kg **or** 4 mg as a single dose **or** 0.15 mg/kg/dose for 3 doses
  Adults: Dosage varies greatly depending on indication

Oral:
  Children 4-11 years: 4 mg for 3 doses, then 4 mg every 8 hours for 1-2 days
  Children ≥12 years: 24 mg as a single dose **or** 8 mg every 8-12 hours
  Adults: 8-24 mg as a single dose **or** 8 mg every 8-12 hours

Dosage Forms

Film, soluble, oral:
  Zuplenz®: 4 mg (10s); 8 mg (10s)

Infusion, premixed in D$_5$W [preservative free]: 32 mg (50 mL)
  Zofran®: 32 mg (50 mL)

◀ **Infusion, premixed in NS** [preservative free]: 32 mg (50 mL)
Injection, solution: 2 mg/mL (2 mL, 20 mL)
  Zofran®: 2 mg/mL (20 mL)
Injection, solution [preservative free]: 2 mg/mL (2 mL)
Solution, oral: 4 mg/5 mL (5 mL, 50 mL)
  Zofran®: 4 mg/5 mL (50 mL)
Tablet, oral: 4 mg, 8 mg
  Zofran®: 4 mg, 8 mg
Tablet, orally disintegrating, oral: 4 mg, 8 mg
  Zofran® ODT: 4 mg, 8 mg

opium tincture (OH pee um TING chur)

Medication Safety Issues

Sound-alike/look-alike issues:

Opium tincture may be confused with camphorated tincture of opium (paregoric)

High alert medication:

The Institute for Safe Medication Practices (ISMP) includes this medication among its list of drugs which have a heightened risk of causing significant patient harm when used in error.

Administration issues:

Use care when prescribing opium tincture; opium tincture is 25 times more concentrated than paregoric, each undiluted mL of opium tincture contains the equivalent of morphine 10 mg/mL.

If opium tincture is used in neonates, a 25-fold dilution should be prepared (final concentration: 0.4 mg/mL morphine). Of note, paregoric (which contains the equivalent of morphine 0.4 mg/mL) is **not** recommended for use in neonates due to the high alcohol content (~45%) and the presence of other additives; as an alternative to the use of diluted opium tincture or paregoric, ISMP recommends using a diluted preservative free injectable morphine solution orally.

Although historically opium tincture is dosed as mL/kg, the preferred dosing units are **mg**/kg (Levine, 2001). ISMP suggests hospitals evaluate the need for this product at their institution.

Other safety concerns:

DTO is an error-prone abbreviation and should never be used as an abbreviation for opium tincture (also known as *Deodorized* Tincture of Opium) due to potential for being mistaken as *Diluted* Tincture of Opium

Synonyms deodorized tincture of opium (error-prone synonym); DTO (error-prone abbreviation); opium tincture, deodorized; tincture of opium

Therapeutic Category Analgesic, Narcotic

Controlled Substance C-II

Use Treatment of diarrhea in adults

General Dosage Range

Oral: Opium tincture 10% contains morphine 10 mg/mL. Use caution in ordering, dispensing, and/or administering. The following doses are expressed in **mg** (milligram) dosing units of morphine.

Adults: Usual: 6 **mg** of undiluted opium tincture (10 mg/mL) 4 times daily

Dosage Forms

Tincture, oral: Anhydrous morphine 10 mg/mL (120 mL, 480 mL)

opium tincture, deodorized *see* opium tincture *on page 653*

oprelvekin (oh PREL ve kin)

Medication Safety Issues

Sound-alike/look-alike issues:

Oprelvekin may be confused with aldesleukin, Proleukin®

Neumega® may be confused with Neulasta®, Neupogen®

Synonyms IL-11; interleukin-11; recombinant human interleukin-11; recombinant interleukin-11; rhIL-11

U.S. Brand Names Neumega®

Therapeutic Category Platelet Growth Factor

Use Prevention of severe thrombocytopenia; reduce the need for platelet transfusions following myelosuppressive chemotherapy for nonmyeloid malignancy

General Dosage Range Dosage adjustment recommended in patients with renal impairment

SubQ: *Adults:* 50 mcg/kg once daily

Dosage Forms

Injection, powder for reconstitution [preservative free]:

Neumega®: 5 mg

OPT-80 *see* fidaxomicin (systemic) *on page 377*

Optase™ *see* trypsin, balsam Peru, and castor oil *on page 896*

Optho-Bunolol® (Can) *see* levobunolol *on page 517*

Opti-Clear [OTC] *see* tetrahydrozoline (ophthalmic) *on page 858*

Opticrom® (Can) *see* cromolyn (ophthalmic) *on page 239*

OptiMARK® *see* gadoversetamide *on page 408*

Optimyxin® (Can) *see* bacitracin and polymyxin B *on page 111*

Optimyxin Plus® (Can) *see* neomycin, polymyxin B, and gramicidin *on page 618*

OptiNate® *see* vitamins (multiple/prenatal) *on page* 920
OptiPranolol® *see* metipranolol *on page* 580
Optiray® 160 *see* ioversol *on page* 487
Optiray® 240 *see* ioversol *on page* 487
Optiray® 300 *see* ioversol *on page* 487
Optiray® 320 *see* ioversol *on page* 487
Optiray® 350 *see* ioversol *on page* 487
Optivar® *see* azelastine (ophthalmic) *on page* 108
Optive™ [OTC] *see* carboxymethylcellulose *on page* 175
Optivite® P.M.T. [OTC] *see* vitamins (multiple/oral) *on page* 919
Orabase® with Benzocaine [OTC] *see* benzocaine *on page* 121
Oracea® *see* doxycycline *on page* 312
Oracort (Can) *see* triamcinolone (topical) *on page* 887
Orajel® [OTC] *see* benzocaine *on page* 121
Orajel® Baby Daytime and Nighttime [OTC] *see* benzocaine *on page* 121
Orajel® Baby Teething [OTC] *see* benzocaine *on page* 121
Orajel® Baby Teething Nighttime [OTC] *see* benzocaine *on page* 121
Orajel® Cold Sore [OTC] *see* benzocaine *on page* 121
Orajel® Denture Plus [OTC] *see* benzocaine *on page* 121
Orajel® Dry Mouth [OTC] *see* glycerin *on page* 421
Orajel® Maximum Strength [OTC] *see* benzocaine *on page* 121
Orajel® Medicated Mouth Sore [OTC] *see* benzocaine *on page* 121
Orajel® Medicated Toothache [OTC] *see* benzocaine *on page* 121
Orajel® Mouth Sore [OTC] *see* benzocaine *on page* 121
Orajel® Multi-Action Cold Sore [OTC] *see* benzocaine *on page* 121
Orajel® PM Maximum Strength [OTC] *see* benzocaine *on page* 121
Orajel® Ultra Mouth Sore [OTC] *see* benzocaine *on page* 121
Oral Balance® [OTC] *see* saliva substitute *on page* 798
oral cholera vaccine *see* traveler's diarrhea and cholera vaccine *(Canada only) on page* 883
Oralone® *see* triamcinolone (topical) *on page* 887
Oramorph® SR *see* morphine (systemic) *on page* 598
Oranyl [OTC] *see* pseudoephedrine *on page* 751
Orap® *see* pimozide *on page* 704
Orapred® *see* prednisolone (systemic) *on page* 734
Orapred ODT® *see* prednisolone (systemic) *on page* 734
Oraqix® *see* lidocaine and prilocaine *on page* 526
OraVerse™ *see* phentolamine *on page* 696
Oravig® *see* miconazole (oral) *on page* 585
Oraxyl™ *see* doxycycline *on page* 312
Orazinc® 110 [OTC] *see* zinc sulfate *on page* 931
Orazinc® 220 [OTC] *see* zinc sulfate *on page* 931
Orbivan™ *see* butalbital, acetaminophen, and caffeine *on page* 152
orciprenaline sulfate *see* metaproterenol *on page* 566
Orencia® *see* abatacept *on page* 20
Orfadin® *see* nitisinone *on page* 628
ORG 946 *see* rocuronium *on page* 788
Orgalutran® (Can) *see* ganirelix *on page* 411
Organidin® NR [OTC] [DSC] *see* guaifenesin *on page* 425
Orgaran® (Can) *see* danaparoid *(Canada only) on page* 251
ORG NC 45 *see* vecuronium *on page* 910
Orinase *see* tolbutamide *on page* 875

orlistat (OR li stat)

Medication Safety Issues
Sound-alike/look-alike issues:
Xenical® may be confused with Xeloda®
U.S. Brand Names Alli® [OTC]; Xenical®
Canadian Brand Names Xenical®
Therapeutic Category Lipase Inhibitor
Use Management of obesity, including weight loss and weight management, when used in conjunction with a reduced-calorie and low-fat diet; reduce the risk of weight regain after prior weight loss; indicated for obese patients with an initial body mass index (BMI) ≥30 kg/m^2 or ≥27 kg/m^2 in the presence of other risk factors (eg, diabetes, dyslipidemia, hypertension)
General Dosage Range Oral:
Children ≥12 years and Adults: Xenical®: 120 mg 3 times/day
Adults: Alli™ (OTC labeling): 60 mg 3 times/day
Dosage Forms
Capsule, oral:
Alli® [OTC]: 60 mg
Xenical®: 120 mg

Ornex® [OTC] *see* acetaminophen and pseudoephedrine *on page* 29
Ornex® Maximum Strength [OTC] *see* acetaminophen and pseudoephedrine *on page* 29
ORO-Clense (Can) *see* chlorhexidine gluconate *on page* 194
Orphenace® (Can) *see* orphenadrine *on page* 655

orphenadrine (or FEN a dreen)

Medication Safety Issues
Sound-alike/look-alike issues:
Norflex™ may be confused with norfloxacin, Noroxin®
BEERS Criteria medication:
This drug may be inappropriate for use in geriatric patients (high severity risk).
International issues:
Flexin: Brand name for orphenadrine [Israel] but is also the brand name for cyclobenzaprine [Chile] and diclofenac [Argentina]
Flexin [Israel] may be confused with Floxin which is a brand name for flunarizine [Thailand], norfloxacin [South Africa], ofloxacin [U.S., Canada], and perfloxacin [Philippines]; Fluoxin brand name for fluoxetine [Czech Republic]
Synonyms orphenadrine citrate
U.S. Brand Names Norflex™
Canadian Brand Names Norflex™; Orphenace®; Rhoxal-orphendrine
Therapeutic Category Skeletal Muscle Relaxant
Use Treatment of muscle spasm associated with acute painful musculoskeletal conditions
General Dosage Range
I.M., I.V.: *Adults:* 60 mg every 12 hours
Oral: *Adults:* 100 mg twice daily
Dosage Forms
Injection, solution: 30 mg/mL (2 mL)
Norflex™: 30 mg/mL (2 mL)
Tablet, extended release, oral: 100 mg

orphenadrine, aspirin, and caffeine (or FEN a dreen, AS pir in, & KAF een)

Medication Safety Issues
Sound-alike/look-alike issues:
Norgesic™ Forte may be confused with Norgesic 40®
Synonyms aspirin, caffeine, and orphenadrine; aspirin, orphenadrine, and caffeine; caffeine, orphenadrine, and aspirin; Norgesic
Therapeutic Category Analgesic, Nonnarcotic; Skeletal Muscle Relaxant
Use Relief of discomfort associated with skeletal muscular conditions
General Dosage Range Oral: *Adults:* 1-2 tablets 3-4 times/day

◀ **Dosage Forms**
Tablet: Orphenadrine 25 mg, aspirin 385 mg, and caffeine 30 mg; orphenadrine 50 mg, aspirin 770 mg, and caffeine 60 mg

orphenadrine citrate *see* orphenadrine *on page 655*

Orsythia™ *see* ethinyl estradiol and levonorgestrel *on page 353*

Ortho® 0.5/35 (Can) *see* ethinyl estradiol and norethindrone *on page 355*

Ortho® 1/35 (Can) *see* ethinyl estradiol and norethindrone *on page 355*

Ortho® 7/7/7 (Can) *see* ethinyl estradiol and norethindrone *on page 355*

Ortho-Cept® *see* ethinyl estradiol and desogestrel *on page 351*

Orthoclone OKT® 3 [DSC] *see* muromonab-CD3 *on page 603*

Ortho-Cyclen® *see* ethinyl estradiol and norgestimate *on page 357*

Ortho Est *see* estropipate *on page 349*

Ortho Evra® *see* ethinyl estradiol and norelgestromin *on page 354*

Ortho Micronor® *see* norethindrone *on page 633*

Ortho Novum *see* ethinyl estradiol and norethindrone *on page 355*

Ortho-Novum® 1/35 *see* ethinyl estradiol and norethindrone *on page 355*

Ortho Novum 1/50 *see* norethindrone and mestranol *on page 633*

Ortho-Novum® 1/50 (Can) *see* norethindrone and mestranol *on page 633*

Ortho-Novum® 7/7/7 *see* ethinyl estradiol and norethindrone *on page 355*

ortho,para-DDD *see* mitotane *on page 593*

ortho prefest *see* estradiol and norgestimate *on page 346*

Ortho Tri-Cyclen® *see* ethinyl estradiol and norgestimate *on page 357*

Ortho Tri-Cyclen® Lo *see* ethinyl estradiol and norgestimate *on page 357*

Orthovisc® *see* hyaluronate and derivatives *on page 443*

OrthoVisc® (Can) *see* hyaluronate and derivatives *on page 443*

OrthoWash™ *see* fluoride *on page 386*

oscal *see* calcium carbonate *on page 161*

Os-Cal® (Can) *see* calcium carbonate *on page 161*

Os-Cal® 500+D [OTC] *see* calcium and vitamin D *on page 160*

oseltamivir (oh sel TAM i vir)

Medication Safety Issues
Sound-alike/look-alike issues:
Tamiflu® may be confused with Thera-Flu®
Tamiflu® may be confused with Tambocor™
Other safety concerns:
Oseltamivir (Tamiflu®) oral suspension is packaged with an oral syringe. When dispensing commercially prepared oseltamivir oral suspension, verify the intended concentration to be dispensed and the correct dose, dosing instructions, and oral dosing device provided for the patient. Oseltamivir oral suspension is available in a 6 mg/mL concentration. The previous concentration (12 mg/mL) has been discontinued, but may be still be on the market until product expires. The 6 mg/mL concentration is packaged with an oral syringe calibrated in **milliliters** up to a total of 10 mL. The previous, discontinued concentration (12 mg/mL) was packaged with an oral syringe calibrated in mg (30 mg, 45 mg, and 60 mg graduations). **When the oral syringe is dispensed, instructions to the patient should be provided based on these units of measure (ie, mL or mg). Do NOT dispense an oral syringe with units of measure in milligrams when providing oseltamivir suspension for children <1 year of age** instead supply an oral syringe capable of measuring mL doses. Patients should always be provided with a measuring device calibrated the same way as their labeled instructions.

When commercially-prepared oseltamivir oral suspension is not available, an extemporaneously prepared suspension may be compounded to provide a 6 mg/mL concentration (to match the preferred, currently manufactured commercially available oral suspension concentration).
U.S. Brand Names Tamiflu®
Canadian Brand Names Tamiflu®
Therapeutic Category Antiviral Agent, Oral

Use Treatment of uncomplicated acute illness due to influenza (A or B) infection in children ≥1 year of age and adults who have been symptomatic for no more than 2 days; prophylaxis against influenza (A or B) infection in children ≥1 year of age and adults

The Advisory Committee on Immunization Practices (ACIP) recommends that **treatment** be considered for the following:
- Persons with severe, complicated or progressive illness
- Hospitalized persons
- Persons at higher risk for influenza complications:
  - Children <2 years of age (highest risk in children <6 months of age)
  - Adults ≥65 years of age
  - Persons with chronic disorders of the pulmonary (including asthma) or cardiovascular systems (except hypertension)
  - Persons with chronic metabolic diseases (including diabetes mellitus), hepatic disease, renal dysfunction, hematologic disorders (including sickle cell disease), or immunosuppression (including immunosuppression caused by medications or HIV)
  - Persons with neurologic/neuromuscular conditions (including conditions such as spinal cord injuries, seizure disorders, cerebral palsy, stroke, mental retardation, moderate to severe developmental delay, or muscular dystrophy) which may compromise respiratory function, the handling of respiratory secretions, or that can increase the risk of aspiration
  - Pregnant or postpartum women (≤2 weeks after delivery)
  - Persons <19 years of age on long-term aspirin therapy
  - American Indians and Alaskan Natives
  - Persons who are morbidly obese (BMI ≥40)
  - Residents of nursing homes or other chronic care facilities
- Use may also be considered for previously healthy, nonhigh-risk outpatients with confirmed or suspected influenza based on clinical judgment when treatment can be started within 48 hours of illness onset.

The ACIP recommends that **prophylaxis** be considered for the following:
- Postexposure prophylaxis may be considered for family or close contacts of suspected or confirmed cases, who are at higher risk of influenza complications, and who have not been vaccinated against the circulating strain at the time of the exposure.
- Postexposure prophylaxis may be considered for unvaccinated healthcare workers who had occupational exposure without protective equipment.
- Preexposure prophylaxis should only be used for persons at very high risk of influenza complications who cannot be otherwise protected at times of high risk for exposure.
- Prophylaxis should also be administered to all eligible residents of institutions that house patients at high risk when needed to control outbreaks.

The ACIP recommends that treatment and prophylaxis be given to children <1 year of age when indicated.

General Dosage Range Dosage adjustment recommended in patients with renal impairment
Oral:
Children <1 year: 3 mg/kg/dose once daily
Children 1-12 years and ≤15 kg: 30 mg once or twice daily
Children 1-12 years and >15 to ≤23 kg: 45 mg once or twice daily
Children 1-12 years and >23 to ≤40 kg: 60 mg once or twice daily
Children 1-12 years and >40 kg, Children ≥13 years, and Adults: 75 mg once or twice daily

Dosage Forms
Capsule, oral:
Tamiflu®: 30 mg, 45 mg, 75 mg
Powder for suspension, oral:
Tamiflu®: 6 mg/mL (60 mL)

OSI-774 *see* erlotinib *on page* 338

Osmitrol *see* mannitol *on page* 548

Osmitrol® (Can) *see* mannitol *on page* 548

OsmoPrep® *see* sodium phosphates *on page* 823

Osmovist® (Can) *see* iotrolan *(Canada only) on page* 487

Osteocit® (Can) *see* calcium citrate *on page* 163

Ostoforte® (Can) *see* ergocalciferol *on page* 336

OTFC (oral transmucosal fentanyl citrate) *see* fentanyl *on page* 371

Otix® [OTC] *see* carbamide peroxide *on page 172*
Outgro® [OTC] *see* benzocaine *on page 121*
Ovace® *see* sulfacetamide (topical) *on page 835*
Ovace® Plus *see* sulfacetamide (topical) *on page 835*
Ovcon® 35 *see* ethinyl estradiol and norethindrone *on page 355*
Ovcon® 50 *see* ethinyl estradiol and norethindrone *on page 355*
Ovide® *see* malathion *on page 548*
Ovidrel® *see* chorionic gonadotropin (recombinant) *on page 206*
ovine corticotrophin-releasing hormone *see* corticorelin *on page 236*
Ovol® (Can) *see* simethicone *on page 812*
Ovral® (Can) *see* ethinyl estradiol and norgestrel *on page 357*

oxacillin (oks a SIL in)

Synonyms methylphenyl isoxazolyl penicillin; oxacillin sodium
Therapeutic Category Penicillin
Use Treatment of infections such as osteomyelitis, septicemia, endocarditis, and CNS infections caused by susceptible strains of *Staphylococcus*
General Dosage Range I.M., I.V.:
Children: 100-200 mg/kg/day in divided doses every 6 hours (maximum: 12 g/day)
Adults: 250-2000 mg every 4-6 hours
Dosage Forms
Infusion, premixed iso-osmotic solution: 1 g (50 mL); 2 g (50 mL)
Injection, powder for reconstitution: 1 g, 2 g, 10 g

oxacillin sodium *see* oxacillin *on page 658*
oxalatoplatin *see* oxaliplatin *on page 658*
oxalatoplatinum *see* oxaliplatin *on page 658*

oxaliplatin (ox AL i pla tin)

Medication Safety Issues
Sound-alike/look-alike issues:
Oxaliplatin may be confused with Aloxi®, carboplatin, cisplatin
High alert medication:
The Institute for Safe Medication Practices (ISMP) includes this medication among its list of drug classes which have a heightened risk of causing significant patient harm when used in error.
Synonyms diaminocyclohexane oxalatoplatinum; L-OHP; oxalatoplatin; oxalatoplatinum
U.S. Brand Names Eloxatin®
Canadian Brand Names Eloxatin®
Therapeutic Category Antineoplastic Agent, Alkylating Agent
Use Treatment of stage III colon cancer (adjuvant) and advanced colorectal cancer
General Dosage Range Dosage adjustment recommended in patients who develop toxicities
I.V.: *Adults:* 85 mg/m^2 every 2 weeks
Dosage Forms
Injection, powder for reconstitution: 50 mg, 100 mg
Injection, solution: 5 mg/mL (10 mL, 20 mL)
Injection, solution [preservative free]:
Eloxatin®: 5 mg/mL (10 mL, 20 mL, 40 mL)
Dosage Forms - Canada
Injection, powder for reconstitution:
Eloxatin®: 50 mg, 100 mg

Oxandrin® *see* oxandrolone *on page 658*

oxandrolone (oks AN droe lone)

U.S. Brand Names Oxandrin®
Therapeutic Category Androgen
Controlled Substance C-III

Use Adjunctive therapy to promote weight gain after weight loss following extensive surgery, chronic infections, or severe trauma, and in some patients who, without definite pathophysiologic reasons, fail to gain or to maintain normal weight; to offset protein catabolism with prolonged corticosteroid administration; relief of bone pain associated with osteoporosis

General Dosage Range Oral:
Children: ≤0.1 mg/kg/day or ≤0.045 mg/lb/day
Adults: 2.5-20 mg/day in 2-4 divided doses
Elderly: 5 mg twice daily

Dosage Forms
Tablet, oral: 2.5 mg, 10 mg
Oxandrin®: 2.5 mg, 10 mg

oxaprozin (oks a PROE zin)

Medication Safety Issues
Sound-alike/look-alike issues:
Daypro® may be confused with Diupres®
Oxaprozin may be confused with oxazepam
BEERS Criteria medication:
This drug may be inappropriate for use in geriatric patients (high severity risk).

U.S. Brand Names Daypro®

Canadian Brand Names Apo-Oxaprozin®; Daypro®

Therapeutic Category Analgesic, Nonnarcotic; Nonsteroidal Antiinflammatory Drug (NSAID)

Use Acute and long-term use in the management of signs and symptoms of osteoarthritis and rheumatoid arthritis; juvenile idiopathic arthritis (JIA)

General Dosage Range Dosage adjustment recommended in patients with renal impairment
Oral:
Children 6-16 years and 22-31 kg: 600 mg once daily
Children 6-16 years and 32-54 kg: 900 mg once daily
Children 6-16 years and ≥55 kg: 1200 mg once daily
Adults: 600-1800 mg once daily (maximum: 1200 mg/day [<50 kg]; 1800 mg/day or 26 mg/kg/day (whichever lower) [>50 kg])

Dosage Forms
Caplet, oral:
Daypro®: 600 mg
Tablet, oral: 600 mg

oxazepam (oks A ze pam)

Medication Safety Issues
Sound-alike/look-alike issues:
Oxazepam may be confused with oxaprozin, quazepam
Serax may be confused with Eurax®, Urex, ZyrTEC®
BEERS Criteria medication:
This drug may be inappropriate for use in geriatric patients (high severity risk).
International issues:
Murelax [Australia] may be confused with MiraLax brand name for polyethylene glycol 3350 [U.S.]

Synonyms Serax

Canadian Brand Names Apo-Oxazepam®; Bio-Oxazepam; Novoxapram®; Oxpam®; Oxpram®; PMS-Oxazepam; Riva-Oxazepam

Therapeutic Category Anticonvulsant; Benzodiazepine

Controlled Substance C-IV

Use Treatment of anxiety; management of ethanol withdrawal

General Dosage Range Oral:
Adults: 10-30 mg 3-4 times/day
Elderly: Initial: 10 mg 2-3 times/day; Maintenance: 30-45 mg/day

Dosage Forms
Capsule, oral: 10 mg, 15 mg, 30 mg

oxcarbazepine (ox car BAZ e peen)

Medication Safety Issues

Sound-alike/look-alike issues:

OXcarbazepine may be confused with carBAMazepine

Trileptal® may be confused with TriLipix™

Synonyms GP 47680; OCBZ

Tall-Man OXcarbazepine

U.S. Brand Names Trileptal®

Canadian Brand Names Apo-Oxcarbazepine®; Trileptal®

Therapeutic Category Anticonvulsant

Use Monotherapy or adjunctive therapy in the treatment of partial seizures in adults and children ≥4 years of age with epilepsy; adjunctive therapy in the treatment of partial seizures in children ≥2 years of age with epilepsy

General Dosage Range Dosage adjustment recommended in patients with renal impairment

Oral:

Children 2-3 years and <20 kg: Initial: 8-20 mg/kg/day (maximum: 600 mg/day) in 2 divided doses; Maintenance: maximum of 60 mg/kg/day in 2 divided doses

Children 2-3 years and ≥20 kg: Initial: 8-10 mg/kg/day (maximum: 600 mg/day) in 2 divided doses; Maintenance: maximum of 60 mg/kg/day in 2 divided doses

Children 4-16 years and <25 kg: Initial: 8-10 mg/kg/day (maximum: 600 mg/day) in 2 divided doses; Maintenance: up to 900 mg/day

Children 4-16 years and 25-30 kg: Initial: 8-10 mg/kg/day (maximum: 600 mg/day) in 2 divided doses; Maintenance: up to 1200 mg/day

Children 4-16 years and 31-45 kg: Initial: 8-10 mg/kg/day (maximum: 600 mg/day) in 2 divided doses; Maintenance: up to 1500 mg/day

Children 4-16 years and 46-55 kg: Initial: 8-10 mg/kg/day (maximum: 600 mg/day) in 2 divided doses; Maintenance: up to 1800 mg/day

Children 4-16 years and >56 kg: Initial: 8-10 mg/kg/day (maximum: 600 mg/day) in 2 divided doses; Maintenance: up to 2100 mg/day

Children >16 years and Adults: Initial: 300 mg twice daily; Maintenance: 1200-2400 mg/day in 2 divided doses (maximum: 2400 mg/day)

Dosage Forms

Suspension, oral: 300 mg/5 mL (250 mL)

Trileptal®: 300 mg/5 mL (250 mL)

Tablet, oral: 150 mg, 300 mg, 600 mg

Trileptal®: 150 mg, 300 mg, 600 mg

Oxecta™ *see* oxycodone *on page 662*

Oxeze® Turbuhaler® (Can) *see* formoterol *on page 398*

oxiconazole (oks i KON a zole)

Synonyms oxiconazole nitrate

U.S. Brand Names Oxistat®

Canadian Brand Names Oxistat®

Therapeutic Category Antifungal Agent

Use Treatment of tinea pedis (athlete's foot), tinea cruris (jock itch), tinea corporis (ringworm), and tinea (pityriasis) versicolor

General Dosage Range Topical: *Children and Adults:* Apply to affected areas 1-2 times daily

Dosage Forms

Cream, topical:

Oxistat®: 1% (30 g, 60 g)

Lotion, topical:

Oxistat®: 1% (30 mL, 60 mL)

oxiconazole nitrate *see* oxiconazole *on page 660*

oxidized regenerated cellulose *see* cellulose, oxidized regenerated *on page 186*

Oxilan® 300 *see* ioxilan *on page 488*

Oxilan® 350 *see* ioxilan *on page 488*

oxilapine succinate *see* loxapine *on page 541*

Oxipor® VHC [OTC] *see* coal tar *on page 227*
Oxistat® *see* oxiconazole *on page 660*
Oxpam® (Can) *see* oxazepam *on page 659*
oxpentifylline *see* pentoxifylline *on page 689*
Oxpram® (Can) *see* oxazepam *on page 659*
Oxsoralen® *see* methoxsalen (topical) *on page 573*
Oxsoralen® Capsule (Can) *see* methoxsalen (systemic) *on page 572*
Oxsoralen® Lotion (Can) *see* methoxsalen (topical) *on page 573*
Oxsoralen-Ultra® *see* methoxsalen (systemic) *on page 572*
OXY® [OTC] *see* benzoyl peroxide *on page 124*
OXY® [OTC] *see* salicylic acid *on page 795*
oxybate *see* sodium oxybate *on page 822*
OXY® Body Wash [OTC] *see* salicylic acid *on page 795*
Oxybutyn (Can) *see* oxybutynin *on page 661*

oxybutynin (oks i BYOO ti nin)

Medication Safety Issues
Sound-alike/look-alike issues:
Oxybutynin may be confused with OxyCONTIN®
Ditropan may be confused with Detrol®, diazepam, Diprivan®, dithranol
Beers Criteria medication:
This drug may be inappropriate for use in geriatric patients (high severity risk).
Other safety concerns:
Transdermal patch may contain conducting metal (eg, aluminum); remove patch prior to MRI.

Synonyms Ditropan; oxybutynin chloride

U.S. Brand Names Ditropan XL®; Gelnique®; Oxytrol®

Canadian Brand Names Apo-Oxybutynin®; Ditropan XL®; Dom-Oxybutynin; Mylan-Oxybutynin; Novo-Oxybutynin; Nu-Oxybutyn; Oxybutyn; Oxybutynine; Oxytrol®; PHL-Oxybutynin; PMS-Oxybutynin; Riva-Oxybutynin; Uromax®

Therapeutic Category Antispasmodic Agent, Urinary

Use Antispasmodic for neurogenic bladder (urgency, frequency, leakage, urge incontinence, dysuria); extended release formulation also indicated for treatment of symptoms associated with detrusor overactivity due to a neurological condition (eg, spina bifida)

General Dosage Range
Oral:
Extended release:
Children >6 years: 5 mg once daily (maximum: 20 mg/day)
Adults: Initial: 5-10 mg once daily; Maintenance: 5-30 mg once daily (maximum: 30 mg/day)
Regular release:
Children >5 years: 5 mg 2-3 times/day (maximum: 15 mg/day)
Adults: 5 mg 2-4 times/day (maximum: 20 mg/day)
Elderly: 2.5 mg 2-3 times/day
Topical gel: *Adults:* Apply contents of 1 sachet (100 mg/g) once daily
Transdermal: *Adults:* Apply one 3.9 mg/day patch twice weekly

Dosage Forms
Gel, topical:
Gelnique®: 10% (1 g)
Patch, transdermal:
Oxytrol®: 3.9 mg/24 hours (8s)
Syrup, oral: 5 mg/5 mL (5 mL, 473 mL, 480 mL)
Tablet, oral: 5 mg
Tablet, extended release, oral: 5 mg, 10 mg, 15 mg
Ditropan XL®: 5 mg, 10 mg, 15 mg

oxybutynin chloride *see* oxybutynin *on page 661*
Oxybutynine (Can) *see* oxybutynin *on page 661*
OXY® Chill Factor® [OTC] *see* benzoyl peroxide *on page 124*
OXY® Chill Factor® [OTC] *see* salicylic acid *on page 795*

oxychlorosene (oks i KLOR oh seen)

Synonyms oxychlorosene sodium
U.S. Brand Names Clorpactin® WCS-90 [OTC]
Therapeutic Category Antibiotic, Topical
Use Treatment of localized infections
General Dosage Range Topical: *Adults:* Apply by irrigation, instillation, spray, soaks, or wet compresses
Dosage Forms
Powder for solution, topical:
Clorpactin® WCS-90 [OTC]: 2 g/bottle

oxychlorosene sodium *see* oxychlorosene *on page 662*
Oxycocet® (Can) *see* oxycodone and acetaminophen *on page 662*
Oxycodan® (Can) *see* oxycodone and aspirin *on page 664*

oxycodone (oks i KOE done)

Medication Safety Issues
Sound-alike/look-alike issues:
OxyCODONE may be confused with HYDROcodone, OxyCONTIN®, oxymorphone
OxyCONTIN® may be confused with MS Contin®, oxybutynin, oxyCODONE
OxyFast® may be confused with Roxanol
Roxicodone® may be confused with Roxanol
High alert medication:
The Institute for Safe Medication Practices (ISMP) includes this medication among its list of drug classes which have a heightened risk of causing significant patient harm when used in error.
International issues:
Supeudol® [Canada] may be confused with Supadol Mono which is a brand name for acetaminophen in Luxembourg
Synonyms dihydrohydroxycodeinone; Oxecta™; oxycodone hydrochloride
Tall-Man oxyCODONE
U.S. Brand Names OxyCONTIN®; Roxicodone®
Canadian Brand Names Oxy.IR®; OxyContin®; PMS-Oxycodone; Supeudol®
Therapeutic Category Analgesic, Narcotic
Controlled Substance C-II
Use Management of moderate-to-severe pain, normally used in combination with nonopioid analgesics

OxyContin® is indicated for around-the-clock management of moderate-to-severe pain when an analgesic is needed for an extended period of time.
General Dosage Range Dosage adjustment recommended in patients with hepatic impairment or on concomitant therapy
Oral:
Controlled release: *Adults:* 10-160 mg every 12 hours
Immediate release: *Adults:* 5-20 mg every 4-6 hours as needed
Product Availability
Oxecta™: FDA approved June 2011; availability expected late third quarter 2011 or early fourth quarter 2011.
Oxecta™ is an immediate release tablet formulation of oxycodone that uses technology designed to discourage common methods of tampering that may help decrease opioid abuse and misuse.
Dosage Forms
Capsule, oral: 5 mg
Solution, oral: 20 mg/mL (30 mL)
Tablet, oral: 5 mg, 10 mg, 15 mg, 20 mg, 30 mg
Roxicodone®: 5 mg, 15 mg, 30 mg
Tablet, controlled release, oral:
OxyCONTIN®: 10 mg, 15 mg, 20 mg, 30 mg, 40 mg, 60 mg, 80 mg

oxycodone and acetaminophen (oks i KOE done & a seet a MIN oh fen)

Medication Safety Issues
Sound-alike/look-alike issues:
Endocet® may be confused with Indocid®

Percocet® may be confused with Darvocet®, Fioricet®, Percodan®

Roxicet™ may be confused with Roxanol

Tylox® may be confused with Trimox®, Tylenol®, Wymox®, Xanax®

High alert medication:

The Institute for Safe Medication Practices (ISMP) includes this medication among its list of drug classes which have a heightened risk of causing significant patient harm when used in error.

Other safety concerns:

Duplicate therapy issues: This product contains acetaminophen, which may be a component of other combination products. Do not exceed the maximum recommended daily dose of acetaminophen.

Synonyms acetaminophen and oxycodone

U.S. Brand Names Endocet®; Percocet®; Primlev™; Roxicet™; Roxicet™ 5/500; Tylox®

Canadian Brand Names Endocet®; Novo-Oxycodone Acet; Oxycocet®; Percocet®; Percocet®-Demi; PMS-Oxycodone-Acetaminophen

Therapeutic Category Analgesic, Narcotic

Controlled Substance C-II

Use Management of moderate-to-severe pain

General Dosage Range Dosage adjustment recommended in patients with hepatic impairment

Oral:

Acetaminophen:

Children <45 kg: 10-15 mg/kg every 4-6 hours as needed (maximum: 90 mg/kg/day)

Children ≥45 kg: 10-15 mg/kg every 4-6 hours (maximum: 4 g/day)

Adults: 325-650 mg every 4-6 hours (maximum: 4 g/day)

Oxycodone:

Children: 0.05-0.3 mg/kg every 4-6 hours as needed

Adults: 2.5-30 mg/dose every 4-6 hours as needed

Elderly: Initial: 2.5-5 mg every 6 hours as needed

Dosage Forms

Caplet: Oxycodone 5 mg and acetaminophen 500 mg

Roxicet™ 5/500: Oxycodone 5 mg and acetaminophen 500 mg

Capsule: Oxycodone 5 mg and acetaminophen 500 mg

Tylox®: Oxycodone 5 mg and acetaminophen 500 mg

Solution, oral: Oxycodone 5 mg and acetaminophen 325 mg per 5 mL

Roxicet™: Oxycodone 5 mg and acetaminophen 325 mg per 5 mL

Tablet:

Generics:

Oxycodone 2.5 mg and acetaminophen 325 mg

Oxycodone 5 mg and acetaminophen 325 mg

Oxycodone 7.5 mg and acetaminophen 325 mg

Oxycodone 7.5 mg and acetaminophen 500 mg

Oxycodone 10 mg and acetaminophen 325 mg

Oxycodone 10 mg and acetaminophen 650 mg

Brands:

Endocet®:

5/325 [scored]: Oxycodone 5 mg and acetaminophen 325 mg

7.5/325: Oxycodone 7.5 mg and acetaminophen 325 mg

7.5/500: Oxycodone 7.5 mg and acetaminophen 500 mg

10/325: Oxycodone 10 mg and acetaminophen 325 mg

10/650: Oxycodone 10 mg and acetaminophen 650 mg

Percocet®:

2.5/325: Oxycodone 2.5 mg and acetaminophen 325 mg

5/325 [scored]: Oxycodone 5 mg and acetaminophen 325 mg

7.5/325: Oxycodone 7.5 mg and acetaminophen 325 mg

7.5/500: Oxycodone 7.5 mg and acetaminophen 500 mg

10/325: Oxycodone 10 mg and acetaminophen 325 mg

10/650: Oxycodone 10 mg and acetaminophen 650 mg

Primlev™:

5/300: Oxycodone 5 mg and acetaminophen 300 mg

7.5/300: Oxycodone 7.5 mg and acetaminophen 300 mg

10/300: Oxycodone 10 mg and acetaminophen 300 mg

Roxicet™ [scored]: Oxycodone 5 mg and acetaminophen 325 mg

oxycodone and aspirin (oks i KOE done & AS pir in)

Medication Safety Issues
Sound-alike/look-alike issues:
Percodan® may be confused with Decadron®, Percocet®, Percogesic®, Periactin®
High alert medication:
The Institute for Safe Medication Practices (ISMP) includes this medication among its list of drug classes which have a heightened risk of causing significant patient harm when used in error.
Synonyms aspirin and oxycodone
U.S. Brand Names Endodan®; Percodan®
Canadian Brand Names Endodan®; Oxycodan®; Percodan®
Therapeutic Category Analgesic, Narcotic
Controlled Substance C-II
Use Management of moderate- to moderately-severe pain
General Dosage Range Oral:
Children: 0.1-0.2 mg/kg/dose (based on oxycodone content) every 4-6 hours as needed (maximum: 5 mg/dose [oxycodone]; 4 g/day [aspirin])
Adults: 1 tablet every 6 hours as needed (maximum: 4 g/day [aspirin])
Dosage Forms
Tablet: Oxycodone hydrochloride 4.5 mg, oxycodone terephthalate 0.38 mg, and aspirin 325 mg
Endodan®, Percodan®: Oxycodone hydrochloride 4.8355 mg and aspirin 325 mg

oxycodone and ibuprofen (oks i KOE done & eye byoo PROE fen)

Medication Safety Issues
High alert medication:
The Institute for Safe Medication Practices (ISMP) includes this medication among its list of drug classes which have a heightened risk of causing significant patient harm when used in error.
Synonyms ibuprofen and oxycodone
Therapeutic Category Analgesic, Opioid; Nonsteroidal Antiinflammatory Drug (NSAID), Oral
Controlled Substance C-II
Use Short-term (≤7 days) management of acute, moderate-to-severe pain
General Dosage Range Oral: *Adults:* 1 tablet as needed (maximum: 4 tablets/day; 7 days)
Dosage Forms
Tablet: Oxycodone 5 mg and ibuprofen 400 mg

oxycodone hydrochloride *see* oxycodone *on page 662*
OxyCONTIN® *see* oxycodone *on page 662*
OxyContin® (Can) *see* oxycodone *on page 662*
OXY® Daily [OTC] *see* salicylic acid *on page 795*
OXY® Daily Cleansing [OTC] *see* salicylic acid *on page 795*
Oxyderm™ (Can) *see* benzoyl peroxide *on page 124*
OXY® Face Wash [OTC] *see* salicylic acid *on page 795*
Oxy.IR® (Can) *see* oxycodone *on page 662*
OXY® Maximum [OTC] *see* salicylic acid *on page 795*
OXY® Maximum Daily Cleansing [OTC] *see* salicylic acid *on page 795*

oxymetazoline (nasal) (oks i met AZ oh leen)

Medication Safety Issues
Sound-alike/look-alike issues:
Oxymetazoline may be confused with oxymetholone
Afrin® may be confused with aspirin
Afrin® (oxymetazoline) may be confused with Afrin® (saline)
Neo-Synephrine® (oxymetazoline) may be confused with Neo-Synephrine® (phenylephrine, nasal)
Synonyms oxymetazoline hydrochloride
U.S. Brand Names 12 Hour Nasal Relief [OTC]; 4-Way® 12 Hour [OTC]; Afrin® Extra Moisturizing [OTC]; Afrin® Original [OTC]; Afrin® Severe Congestion [OTC]; Afrin® Sinus [OTC]; Dristan® [OTC]; Duramist Plus [OTC]; Neo-Synephrine® Nighttime12-Hour [OTC]; Nostrilla® [OTC]; NRS® [OTC]; Sudafed OM® Sinus Congestion [OTC] [DSC]; Vicks® Sinex® VapoSpray 12-Hour; Vicks® Sinex® VapoSpray 12-Hour UltraFine Mist [OTC]; Vicks® Sinex® VapoSpray Moisturizing 12-Hour UltraFine Mist [OTC]

Canadian Brand Names Claritin® Allergic Decongestant; Dristan® Long Lasting Nasal; Drixoral® Nasal

Therapeutic Category Adrenergic Agonist Agent; Imidazoline Derivative

Use Adjunctive therapy for nasal congestion, associated with acute or chronic rhinitis, the common cold, sinusitis, hay fever, or other allergies

General Dosage Range Intranasal: *Children ≥6 years and Adults:* Instill 2-3 sprays into each nostril twice daily

Dosage Forms
 Solution, intranasal: 0.05% (15 mL, 30 mL)
  12 Hour Nasal Relief [OTC]: 0.05% (15 mL, 30 mL)
  4-Way® 12 Hour [OTC]: 0.05% (15 mL)
  Afrin® Extra Moisturizing [OTC]: 0.05% (15 mL)
  Afrin® Original [OTC]: 0.05% (15 mL, 30 mL)
  Afrin® Severe Congestion [OTC]: 0.05% (15 mL)
  Afrin® Sinus [OTC]: 0.05% (15 mL)
  Dristan® [OTC]: 0.05% (15 mL)
  Duramist Plus [OTC]: 0.05% (15 mL)
  Neo-Synephrine® Nighttime12-Hour [OTC]: 0.05% (15 mL)
  Nostrilla® [OTC]: 0.05% (15 mL)
  NRS® [OTC]: 0.05% (15 mL, 30 mL)
  Vicks® Sinex® VapoSpray 12-Hour: 0.05% (15 mL)
  Vicks® Sinex® VapoSpray 12-Hour UltraFine Mist [OTC]: 0.05% (15 mL)
  Vicks® Sinex® VapoSpray Moisturizing 12-Hour UltraFine Mist [OTC]: 0.05% (15 mL)

oxymetazoline (ophthalmic) (oks i met AZ oh leen)

Medication Safety Issues
 Sound-alike/look-alike issues:
  Oxymetazoline may be confused with oxymetholone
  Visine® may be confused with Visken®

Synonyms oxymetazoline hydrochloride

U.S. Brand Names Visine® L.R.® [OTC]

Therapeutic Category Vasoconstrictor

Use Relief of redness of eye due to minor eye irritations

General Dosage Range Ophthalmic: *Children ≥6 years and Adults:* Instill 1-2 drops in affected eye(s) every 6 hours as needed

Dosage Forms
 Solution, ophthalmic:
  Visine® L.R.® [OTC]: 0.025% (15 mL, 30 mL)

oxymetazoline hydrochloride *see* oxymetazoline (nasal) *on page 664*

oxymetazoline hydrochloride *see* oxymetazoline (ophthalmic) *on page 665*

oxymetholone (oks i METH oh lone)

Medication Safety Issues
 Sound-alike/look-alike issues:
  Oxymetholone may be confused with oxymetazoline, oxymorphone

U.S. Brand Names Anadrol®-50

Therapeutic Category Anabolic Steroid

Controlled Substance C-III

Use Treatment of anemias caused by deficient red cell production

General Dosage Range Oral: *Children and Adults:* 1-5 mg/kg once daily

Dosage Forms
 Tablet, oral:
  Anadrol®-50: 50 mg

oxymorphone (oks i MOR fone)

Medication Safety Issues
Sound-alike/look-alike issues:
Oxymorphone may be confused with oxycodone, oxymetholone
High alert medication:
The Institute for Safe Medication Practices (ISMP) includes this medication among its list of drug classes which have a heightened risk of causing significant patient harm when used in error.

Synonyms oxymorphone hydrochloride
U.S. Brand Names Opana®; Opana® ER
Therapeutic Category Analgesic, Narcotic
Controlled Substance C-II
Use
Parenteral: Management of moderate-to-severe acute pain; relief of anxiety in patients with dyspnea associated with pulmonary edema secondary to acute left ventricular failure
Oral, regular release: Management of moderate-to-severe acute pain
Oral, extended release: Management of moderate-to-severe pain in patients requiring around-the-clock opioid treatment for an extended period of time
General Dosage Range Dosage adjustment recommended in patients with hepatic or renal impairment
I.M., SubQ: *Adults:* Initial: 0.5 mg; Maintenance: 1-1.5 mg every 4-6 hours as needed
I.V.: *Adults:* Initial: 0.5 mg
Oral:
Extended release: *Adults (opioid-naive):* Initial: 5 mg every 12 hours; Maintenance: Titrate upward with 5-10 mg every 12 hours at 3-7 day intervals until desired response
Immediate release: *Adults (opioid-naive):* Initial: 5-20 mg every 4-6 hours; Maintenance: Titrate upward to desired response
Dosage Forms
Injection, solution:
Opana®: 1 mg/mL (1 mL)
Tablet, oral: 5 mg, 10 mg
Opana®: 5 mg, 10 mg
Tablet, extended release, oral: 7.5 mg, 15 mg
Opana® ER: 5 mg, 10 mg, 20 mg, 30 mg, 40 mg

oxymorphone hydrochloride *see* oxymorphone *on page 666*
OXY® Post-Shave [OTC] *see* salicylic acid *on page 795*
OXY® Spot Treatment [OTC] *see* salicylic acid *on page 795*

oxytocin (oks i TOE sin)

Medication Safety Issues
High alert medication:
The Institute for Safe Medication Practices (ISMP) includes this medication among its list of drugs which have a heightened risk of causing significant patient harm when used in error.

Synonyms pit
U.S. Brand Names Pitocin®
Canadian Brand Names Oxytocin for injection
Therapeutic Category Oxytocic Agent
Use Induction of labor in patients with a medical indication; stimulation or reinforcement of labor; adjunctive therapy in management of abortion; to produce uterine contractions during the third stage of labor; control of postpartum bleeding
General Dosage Range
I.M.: *Adults:* Total dose of 10 units after delivery of the placenta
I.V.: *Adults:* Dosage varies greatly depending on indication
Dosage Forms
Injection, solution: 10 units/mL (1 mL, 10 mL, 30 mL)
Pitocin®: 10 units/mL (1 mL, 10 mL)

Oxytocin for injection (Can) *see* oxytocin *on page 666*
Oxytrol® *see* oxybutynin *on page 661*
Oysco D [OTC] *see* calcium and vitamin D *on page 160*

Oysco 500 [OTC] *see* calcium carbonate *on page 161*

Oysco 500+D [OTC] *see* calcium and vitamin D *on page 160*

Oyst-Cal-D [OTC] *see* calcium and vitamin D *on page 160*

Oyst-Cal-D 500 [OTC] *see* calcium and vitamin D *on page 160*

Oystercal™ 500 [OTC] *see* calcium carbonate *on page 161*

Ozurdex® *see* dexamethasone (ophthalmic) *on page 265*

P32 *see* chromic phosphate P 32 *on page 206*

P-071 *see* cetirizine *on page 189*

P-1202 *see* methyl aminolevulinate *on page 574*

Pacerone® *see* amiodarone *on page 67*

Pacis™ (Can) *see* BCG *on page 115*

paclitaxel (pac li TAKS el)

Medication Safety Issues
Sound-alike/look-alike issues:
  PACLitaxel may be confused with DOCEtaxel, PARoxetine, Paxil®
  PACLitaxel (conventional) may be confused with PACLitaxel (protein-bound)
  Taxol® may be confused with Abraxane®, Paxil®, Taxotere®
High alert medication:
  This medication is in a class the Institute for Safe Medication Practices (ISMP) includes among its list of drug classes which have a heightened risk of causing significant patient harm when used in error.

Synonyms Taxol

Tall-Man PACLitaxel

Canadian Brand Names Apo-Paclitaxel®; Paclitaxel For Injection; Taxol®

Therapeutic Category Antineoplastic Agent

Use Treatment of breast, nonsmall cell lung, and ovarian cancers; treatment of AIDS-related Kaposi sarcoma (KS)

General Dosage Range Dosage adjustment recommended in patients with hepatic impairment or who develop toxicities
  I.V.: *Adults:* Dosage varies greatly depending on indication

Dosage Forms
  Injection, solution: 6 mg/mL (5 mL, 16.7 mL, 25 mL, 50 mL)

paclitaxel, albumin-bound *see* paclitaxel (protein bound) *on page 667*

Paclitaxel For Injection (Can) *see* paclitaxel *on page 667*

paclitaxel (protein bound) (pac li TAKS el PROE teen bownd)

Medication Safety Issues
Sound-alike/look-alike issues:
  PACLitaxel may be confused with DOCEtaxel
  PACLitaxel (protein bound) may be confused with PACLitaxel (conventional)
  Abraxane® may be confused with Paxil®, Taxol®, Taxotere®
High alert medication:
  This medication is in a class the Institute for Safe Medication Practices (ISMP) includes among its list of drug classes which have a heightened risk of causing significant patient harm when used in error.

Synonyms ABI-007; albumin-bound paclitaxel; albumin-stabilized nanoparticle paclitaxel; nab-paclitaxel; nanoparticle albumin-bound paclitaxel; paclitaxel, albumin-bound; protein-bound paclitaxel

Tall-Man PACLitaxel

U.S. Brand Names Abraxane®

Canadian Brand Names Abraxane®

Therapeutic Category Antineoplastic Agent, Antimicrotubular; Antineoplastic Agent, Natural Source (Plant) Derivative

Use Treatment of refractory (metastatic) or relapsed (within 6 months of adjuvant therapy) breast cancer

General Dosage Range Dosage adjustment recommended in patients with hepatic impairment or who develop toxicities
  I.V.: *Adults:* 260 mg/m^2 every 3 weeks

◀ **Dosage Forms**
Injection, powder for reconstitution:
Abraxane®: 100 mg

Pacnex™ *see* benzoyl peroxide *on page 124*
Pain-A-Lay® [OTC] *see* phenol *on page 694*
Pain Eze [OTC] *see* acetaminophen *on page 23*
Pain & Fever Children's [OTC] *see* acetaminophen *on page 23*
Pain-Off [OTC] *see* acetaminophen, aspirin, and caffeine *on page 29*
Paire OB™ Plus DHA *see* vitamins (multiple/prenatal) *on page 920*
Palafer® (Can) *see* ferrous fumarate *on page 373*
Palgic® *see* carbinoxamine *on page 174*

palifermin (pal ee FER min)
Synonyms AMJ 9701; rhKGF; rhu keratinocyte growth factor; rHu-KGF
U.S. Brand Names Kepivance®
Canadian Brand Names Kepivance®
Therapeutic Category Keratinocyte Growth Factor
Use Decrease the incidence and severity of severe oral mucositis associated with hematologic malignancies in patients receiving myelotoxic therapy requiring hematopoietic stem cell support
General Dosage Range I.V.: *Adults:* 60 mcg/kg/day for 3 consecutive days before and after myelotoxic therapy
Dosage Forms
Injection, powder for reconstitution [preservative free]:
Kepivance®: 6.25 mg

paliperidone (pal ee PER i done)
Synonyms 9-hydroxy-risperidone; 9-OH-risperidone; paliperidone palmitate
U.S. Brand Names Invega®; Invega® Sustenna®
Canadian Brand Names Invega®; Invega® Sustenna®
Therapeutic Category Antipsychotic Agent, Atypical
Use
Oral: Acute and maintenance treatment of schizophrenia; acute treatment of schizoaffective disorder (monotherapy or adjunctive therapy to mood stabilizers and/or antidepressants)
Injection: Acute and maintenance treatment of schizophrenia
General Dosage Range Dosage adjustment recommended in patients with renal impairment
I.M.: *Adults:* Initial: 234 mg, then 156 mg 1 week later; Maintenance: 39-234 mg/month
Oral: *Adolescents 12-17 years and Adults:* 3-12 mg once daily (maximum: 12 mg/day)
Dosage Forms
Injection, suspension, extended release:
Invega® Sustenna®: 39 mg/0.25 mL (0.25 mL); 78 mg/0.5 mL (0.5 mL); 117 mg/0.75 mL (0.75 mL); 156 mg/mL (1 mL); 234 mg/1.5 mL (1.5 mL)
Tablet, extended release, oral:
Invega®: 1.5 mg, 3 mg, 6 mg, 9 mg
Dosage Forms - Canada
Injection, suspension, extended release:
Invega® Sustenna™: 25 mg/0.25 mL, 50 mg/0.5 mL, 75 mg/0.75 mL, 100mg/1 mL, and 150 mg/1.5 mL

paliperidone palmitate *see* paliperidone *on page 668*

palivizumab (pah li VIZ u mab)
Medication Safety Issues
Sound-alike/look-alike issues:
Synagis® may be confused with Synalgos®-DC, Synvisc®
U.S. Brand Names Synagis®
Canadian Brand Names Synagis®
Therapeutic Category Monoclonal Antibody
Use Prevention of serious lower respiratory tract disease caused by respiratory syncytial virus (RSV) in infants and children at high risk of RSV disease

The American Academy of Pediatrics recommends RSV prophylaxis with palivizumab during RSV season for:
- Infants <3 months of age who were born between 32 and 34 6/7 weeks gestational age and have one of the following:
  - Day care attendance
  - One or more siblings <5 years of age living in the same household
- Infants <6 months of age who were born between 29 and 31 6/7 weeks gestational age
- Infants <12 months of age who were born <28 weeks gestational age
- Infants <12 months of age with congenital airway abnormality or neuromuscular disorder that decreases the ability to manage airway secretions
- Infants and children <24 months of age with chronic lung disease (CLD) necessitating medical therapy within 6 month prior to the beginning of RSV season
- Infants and children ≤24 months of age with congenital heart disease and one of the following:
  - Receiving medication to treat congestive heart failure
  - Moderate-to-severe pulmonary hypertension
  - Cyanotic heart disease

General Dosage Range I.M.: *Children <2 years:* 15 mg/kg monthly

Dosage Forms
Injection, solution [preservative free]:
  Synagis®: 100 mg/mL (0.5 mL, 1 mL)

Palmer's® Skin Success Acne Cleanser [OTC] *see* salicylic acid *on page* 795
Palmer's® Skin Success® Eventone® Fade Cream [OTC] *see* hydroquinone *on page* 453
Palmer's® Skin Success® Eventone® Fade Milk [OTC] *see* hydroquinone *on page* 453
Palmer's® Skin Success® Eventone® Ultra Fade Serum [OTC] *see* hydroquinone *on page* 453
Palmer's® Skin Success Invisible Acne [OTC] *see* benzoyl peroxide *on page* 124

palonosetron (pal oh NOE se tron)

Medication Safety Issues
Sound-alike/look-alike issues:
  Aloxi® may be confused with Eloxatin®, oxaliplatin
  Palonosetron may be confused with dolasetron, granisetron, ondansetron
Synonyms palonosetron hydrochloride; RS-25259; RS-25259-197
U.S. Brand Names Aloxi®
Therapeutic Category Antiemetic; Selective 5-HT$_3$ Receptor Antagonist
Use Prevention of chemotherapy-associated nausea and vomiting; indicated for prevention of acute (highly-emetogenic therapy) as well as acute and delayed (moderately-emetogenic therapy) nausea and vomiting; prevention of postoperative nausea and vomiting (PONV)
General Dosage Range I.V.: *Adults:* 0.25 mg **or** 0.075 mg as a single dose
Dosage Forms
Injection, solution:
  Aloxi®: 0.05 mg/mL (1.5 mL, 5 mL)

palonosetron hydrochloride *see* palonosetron *on page* 669
2-PAM *see* pralidoxime *on page* 729

pamabrom (PAM a brom)

U.S. Brand Names Aqua-Ban® Maximum Strength [OTC]; diurex® Aquagels® [OTC]; diurex® Maximum Relief [OTC]; diurex® [OTC]
Therapeutic Category Diuretic
Use Temporary relief of symptoms associated with premenstrual and menstrual periods (eg, bloating, water-weight gain, swelling, full feeling)
General Dosage Range Oral: *Adults:* 50 mg every 6 hours as needed (maximum: 200 mg/day)
Dosage Forms
Caplet, oral:
  diurex® Maximum Relief [OTC]: 50 mg
Capsule, oral:
  diurex® [OTC]: 50 mg

◀ **Capsule, softgel, oral**:
diurex® Aquagels® [OTC]: 50 mg
Tablet, oral:
Aqua-Ban® Maximum Strength [OTC]: 50 mg

pamabrom and acetaminophen *see* acetaminophen and pamabrom *on page* 27
Pamelor® *see* nortriptyline *on page* 634

pamidronate (pa mi DROE nate)

Medication Safety Issues
Sound-alike/look-alike issues:
Aredia® may be confused with Adriamycin, Meridia®
Pamidronate may be confused with papaverine
International issues:
Linoten [Spain] may be confused with Loniten brand name for minoxidil [Canada and multiple international markets]

Synonyms pamidronate disodium

U.S. Brand Names Aredia®

Canadian Brand Names Aredia®; Pamidronate Disodium Omega; Pamidronate Disodium®; PMS-Pamidronate; Rhoxal-pamidronate

Therapeutic Category Bisphosphonate Derivative

Use Treatment of moderate or severe hypercalcemia associated with malignancy (in conjunction with adequate hydration) with or without bone metastases; treatment of osteolytic bone lesions associated with multiple myeloma or metastatic breast cancer; moderate-to-severe Paget disease of bone

General Dosage Range Dosage adjustment recommended in patients with renal impairment
I.V.: *Adults:* 60-90 mg as a single dose, may repeat every 3-4 weeks **or** 30 mg daily for 3 consecutive days

Dosage Forms
Injection, powder for reconstitution: 30 mg, 90 mg
Aredia®: 30 mg
Injection, solution: 3 mg/mL (10 mL); 6 mg/mL (10 mL); 9 mg/mL (10 mL)
Injection, solution [preservative free]: 3 mg/mL (10 mL); 9 mg/mL (10 mL)

pamidronate disodium *see* pamidronate *on page* 670
Pamidronate Disodium® (Can) *see* pamidronate *on page* 670
Pamidronate Disodium Omega (Can) *see* pamidronate *on page* 670
Pamine® *see* methscopolamine *on page* 573
Pamine® Forte *see* methscopolamine *on page* 573
p-amino-benzenesulfonamide *see* sulfanilamide *on page* 837
p-aminoclonidine *see* apraclonidine *on page* 91
Pamprin® Maximum Strength All Day Relief [OTC] *see* naproxen *on page* 612
Pancof®-EXP *see* dihydrocodeine, pseudoephedrine, and guaifenesin *on page* 285
Pancrease® MT (Can) *see* pancrelipase *on page* 670
pancreatic enzymes *see* pancrelipase *on page* 670
Pancreaze™ *see* pancrelipase *on page* 670

pancrelipase (pan kre LYE pase)

Medication Safety Issues
Sound-alike/look-alike issues:
Pancrelipase may be confused with pancreatin

Synonyms amylase, lipase, and protease; lipancreatin; lipase, protease, and amylase; pancreatic enzymes; protease, lipase, and amylase

U.S. Brand Names Creon®; Pancreaze™; Pancrelipase™; Zenpep™

Canadian Brand Names Cotazym®; Creon®; Pancrease® MT; Ultrase®; Ultrase® MT; Viokase®

Therapeutic Category Enzyme

Use Treatment of exocrine pancreatic insufficiency (EPI) due to conditions such as cystic fibrosis (Creon®, Pancreaze™, Zenpep™); chronic pancreatitis (Creon®); or pancreatectomy (Creon®)

General Dosage Range Oral:
Children ≤1 year: Lipase 2000-4000 units per 120 mL of formula or breast milk
Children >1 and <4 years: Lipase 1000-2500 units/kg/meal; Maximum dose: Lipase 10,000 units/kg/day or lipase 4000 units/g of fat per day
Children ≥4 years and Adults: Lipase 500-2500 units/kg/meal **or** lipase 72,000 units/meal (while consuming ≥100 g of fat per day); Maximum dose: Lipase 10,000 units/kg/day **or** lipase 4000 units/g of fat per day

Dosage Forms
Capsule, delayed release, enteric coated beads [porcine derived]:
Pancrelipase™: Lipase 5000 units, protease 17,000 units, amylase 27,000 units
Zenpep™: Lipase 3000 units, protease 10,000 units, amylase 16,000 units
Zenpep™: Lipase 5000 units, protease 17,000 units, amylase 27,000 units
Zenpep™: Lipase 10,000 units, protease 34,000 units, amylase 55,000 units
Zenpep™: Lipase 15,000 units, protease 51,000 units, amylase 82,000 units
Zenpep™: Lipase 20,000 units, protease 68,000 units, amylase 109,000 units
Capsule, delayed release, enteric coated microspheres [new formulation; porcine derived]:
Creon®: Lipase 3000 units, protease 9500 units, and amylase 15,000 units
Creon®: Lipase 6000 units, protease 19,000 units, and amylase 30,000 units
Creon®: Lipase 12000 units, protease 38,000 units, and amylase 60,000 units
Creon®: Lipase 24,000 units, protease 76,000 units, and amylase 120,000 units
Capsule, delayed release, enteric coated microtablets [porcine derived]:
Pancreaze™: Lipase 4200 units, protease 10,000 units, and amylase 17,500 units
Pancreaze™: Lipase 10,500 units, protease 25,000 units, and amylase 43,750 units
Pancreaze™: Lipase 16,800 units, protease 40,000 units, and amylase 70,000 units
Pancreaze™: Lipase 21,000 units, protease 37,000 units, and amylase 61,000 units

Pancrelipase™ *see pancrelipase on page 670*

pancuronium (pan kyoo ROE nee um)
Medication Safety Issues
Sound-alike/look-alike issues:
Pancuronium may be confused with pipecuronium
High alert medication:
The Institute for Safe Medication Practices (ISMP) includes this medication among its list of drugs which have a heightened risk of causing significant patient harm when used in error.
Other safety concerns:
United States Pharmacopeia (USP) 2006: The Interdisciplinary Safe Medication Use Expert Committee of the USP has recommended the following:
- Hospitals, clinics, and other practice sites should institute special safeguards in the storage, labeling, and use of these agents and should include these safeguards in staff orientation and competency training.
- Healthcare professionals should be on high alert (especially vigilant) whenever a neuromuscular-blocking agent (NMBA) is stocked, ordered, prepared, or administered.

Synonyms pancuronium bromide; Pavulon [DSC]
Canadian Brand Names Pancuronium Bromide®
Therapeutic Category Skeletal Muscle Relaxant
Use Facilitation of endotracheal intubation and relaxation of skeletal muscles during surgery; facilitation of mechanical ventilation in ICU patients; does not relieve pain or produce sedation
General Dosage Range Dosage adjustment recommended in patients with renal impairment
I.V.: *Children >1 month and Adults:*
ICU paralysis: 0.06-0.1 mg/kg bolus followed by 1-2 mcg/kg/minute infusion **or** 0.1-0.2 mg/kg every 1-3 hours
Surgery: Intubation: Initial: 0.06-1 mg/kg **or** 0.05 mg/kg after succinylcholine; Maintenance: 0.01 mg/kg administered 60-100 minutes after initial dose and then every 25-60 minutes
Dosage Forms
Injection, solution: 1 mg/mL (10 mL)

pancuronium bromide *see pancuronium on page 671*
Pancuronium Bromide® (Can) *see pancuronium on page 671*
Pandel® *see hydrocortisone (topical) on page 450*
panglobulin *see immune globulin on page 468*

Panhematin® *see* hemin *on page 435*

panitumumab (pan i TOOM yoo mab)

Synonyms ABX-EGF; MOAB ABX-EGF; monoclonal antibody ABX-EGF; rHuMAb-EGFr

U.S. Brand Names Vectibix®

Canadian Brand Names Vectibix®

Therapeutic Category Antineoplastic Agent, Monoclonal Antibody; Epidermal Growth Factor Receptor (EGFR) Inhibitor

Use Monotherapy in treatment of refractory metastatic colorectal cancer

Note: Subset analyses (retrospective) in metastatic colorectal cancer trials have not shown a benefit with EGFR inhibitor treatment in patients whose tumors have codon 12 or 13 *KRAS* mutations; use is not recommended in these patients.

General Dosage Range Dosage adjustment recommended in patients who develop toxicities

I.V.: *Adults:* 6 mg/kg every 2 weeks

Dosage Forms

Injection, solution [preservative free]:

Vectibix®: 20 mg/mL (5 mL, 20 mL)

Panlor® SS [DSC] *see* acetaminophen, caffeine, and dihydrocodeine *on page 30*

PanOxyl® [OTC] *see* benzoyl peroxide *on page 124*

PanOxyl® (Can) *see* benzoyl peroxide *on page 124*

PanOxyl®-4 [OTC] *see* benzoyl peroxide *on page 124*

PanOxyl®-8 [OTC] *see* benzoyl peroxide *on page 124*

PanOxyl® Aqua Gel [OTC] [DSC] *see* benzoyl peroxide *on page 124*

PanOxyl® Bar [OTC] *see* benzoyl peroxide *on page 124*

Panretin® *see* alitretinoin *on page 53*

Panto-250 [OTC] *see* pantothenic acid *on page 673*

Panto™ I.V. (Can) *see* pantoprazole *on page 672*

Pantoloc® (Can) *see* pantoprazole *on page 672*

pantoprazole (pan TOE pra zole)

Medication Safety Issues

Sound-alike/look-alike issues:

Pantoprazole may be confused with ARIPiprazole

Protonix® may be confused with Lotronex®, Lovenox®, protamine

Administration issues:

Vials containing Protonix® I.V. for injection are not recommended for use with spiked I.V. system adaptors. Nurses and pharmacists have reported breakage of the glass vials during attempts to connect spiked I.V. system adaptors, which may potentially result in injury to healthcare professionals.

International issues:

Protonix [U.S., Canada] may be confused with Pretanix brand name for indapamide [Hungary]

U.S. Brand Names Protonix®; Protonix® I.V.

Canadian Brand Names Apo-Pantoprazole®; CO Pantoprazole; Mylan-Pantoprazole; Pantoloc®; Pantoprazole for Injection; Panto™ I.V.; PMS-Pantoprazole; RAN™-Pantoprazole; ratio-Pantoprazole; Riva-Pantoprazole; Sandoz-Pantoprazole; Tecta™; Teva-Pantoprazole

Therapeutic Category Proton Pump Inhibitor

Use

Oral: Treatment and maintenance of healing of erosive esophagitis associated with GERD; reduction in relapse rates of daytime and nighttime heartburn symptoms in GERD; hypersecretory disorders associated with Zollinger-Ellison syndrome or other GI hypersecretory disorders

I.V.: Short-term treatment (7-10 days) of patients with gastroesophageal reflux disease (GERD) and a history of erosive esophagitis; hypersecretory disorders associated with Zollinger-Ellison syndrome or other neoplastic disorders

General Dosage Range

I.V.: *Adults:* Erosive gastritis: 40 mg once daily; Hypersecretory disorders: 160-240 mg/day in divided doses

Oral: *Adults:* 20-40 mg once or twice daily (maximum: 240 mg/day normally reserved for treatment of hypersecretory conditions)

Dosage Forms
  Granules for suspension, delayed release, enteric coated, oral:
    Protonix®: 40 mg/packet (30s)
  Injection, powder for reconstitution:
    Protonix® I.V.: 40 mg
  Tablet, delayed release, oral: 20 mg, 40 mg
    Protonix®: 20 mg, 40 mg
  Dosage Forms - Canada
  Tablet, enteric coated:
    Pantoloc®: 40 mg

Pantoprazole for Injection (Can) *see* pantoprazole *on page 672*

pantothenic acid (pan toe THEN ik AS id)
Synonyms calcium pantothenate; vitamin B₅
U.S. Brand Names Panto-250 [OTC]
Therapeutic Category Vitamin, Water Soluble
Use Pantothenic acid deficiency
General Dosage Range Oral: *Adults:* 4-7 mg/day
Dosage Forms
  Capsule, oral:
    Panto-250 [OTC]: 250 mg
  Liquid, oral: 200 mg/5 mL (240 mL)
  Tablet, oral: 100 mg, 200 mg, 250 mg, 500 mg
  Tablet, sustained release, oral: 500 mg

pantothenyl alcohol *see* dexpanthenol *on page 267*

papaverine (pa PAV er een)
Medication Safety Issues
  Sound-alike/look-alike issues:
    Papaverine may be confused with pamidronate
Synonyms papaverine hydrochloride; Pavabid [DSC]
Therapeutic Category Vasodilator
Use Oral: Relief of peripheral and cerebral ischemia associated with arterial spasm and myocardial ischemia complicated by arrhythmias
General Dosage Range
  I.M., I.V.:
    Children: 6 mg/kg/day in 4 divided doses
    Adults: 30-65 mg, may repeat every 3 hours
  Oral: *Adults:* 150-300 mg every 12 hours **or** 150 mg every 8 hours
Dosage Forms
  Injection, solution: 30 mg/mL (2 mL, 10 mL)

papaverine hydrochloride *see* papaverine *on page 673*

papillomavirus (types 16, 18) vaccine (human, recombinant)
(pap ih LO ma VYE rus typs SIX teen AYE teen vak SEEN YU man ree KOM be nant)
Medication Safety Issues
  Sound-alike/look-alike issues:
    Papillomavirus vaccine types 16, 18 (Cervarix®) may be confused with Papillomavirus vaccine types 6, 11, 16, 18 (Gardasil®)
    Cervarix® may be confused with Cerebyx®, Celebrex®
Synonyms bivalent human papillomavirus vaccine; GSK-580299; HPV 16/18 L1 VLP/AS04 VAC; HPV vaccine; HPV2; human papillomavirus vaccine; papillomavirus vaccine, recombinant
U.S. Brand Names Cervarix®
Canadian Brand Names Cervarix®
Therapeutic Category Vaccine, Inactivated (Viral)
Use Females 9 through 25 years of age: Prevention of cervical cancer, cervical adenocarcinoma *in situ*, and cervical intraepithelial neoplasia caused by human papillomavirus (HPV) types 16, 18

◀ The Advisory Committee on Immunization Practices (ACIP) recommends routine vaccination for females 11-12 years of age; catch-up vaccination is recommended for females 13-25 years of age.

General Dosage Range I.M.: *Children ≥9 years and Adults ≤25 years (females):* 0.5 mL initial dose, followed by 0.5 mL 1 and 6 months later

Dosage Forms

Injection, suspension [preservative free]:
Cervarix®: HPV 16 L1 protein 20 mcg and HPV 18 L1 protein 20 mcg per 0.5 mL (0.5 mL)

papillomavirus (types 6, 11, 16, 18) vaccine (human, recombinant)
(pap ih LO ma VYE rus typs six e LEV en SIX teen AYE teen vak SEEN YU man ree KOM be nant)

Medication Safety Issues

Sound-alike/look-alike issues:
Papillomavirus vaccine types 6, 11, 16, 18 (Gardasil®) may be confused with Papillomavirus vaccine types 16, 18 (Cervarix®)

Synonyms HPV vaccine; HPV4; human papillomavirus vaccine; papillomavirus vaccine, recombinant; quadrivalent human papillomavirus vaccine

U.S. Brand Names Gardasil®

Canadian Brand Names Gardasil®

Therapeutic Category Vaccine

Use

U.S. labeling:
Females ≥9 years and ≤26 years of age: Prevention of cervical, vulvar, vaginal, and anal cancer caused by HPV types 16 and 18; genital warts caused by HPV types 6 and 11; cervical adenocarcinoma *in situ*, and vulvar, vaginal, cervical, or anal intraepithelial neoplasia caused by HPV types 6, 11, 16, and 18
Males ≥9 years and ≤26 years of age: Prevention of genital warts caused by human papillomavirus (HPV) types 6 and 11; anal cancer caused by HPV types 16 and 18, and anal intraepithelial neoplasia caused by HPV types 6, 11, 16, and 18

Canadian labeling:
Females ≥9 years and ≤26 years of age: Prevention of anal cancer caused by HPV types 16 and 18; anal intraepithelial neoplasia caused by HPV types 6, 11, 16, and 18
Females ≥9 years and ≤45 years of age: Prevention of cervical, vulvar, and vaginal cancer caused by HPV types 16 and 18; genital warts caused by HPV types 6 and 11; cervical adenocarcinoma *in situ*, vulvar, vaginal, or cervical intraepithelial neoplasia caused by HPV types 6, 11, 16, and 18
Males ≥9 years and ≤26 years of age: Prevention of anal cancer caused by HPV types 16 and 18; anal intraepithelial neoplasia caused by HPV types 6, 11, 16, and 18; genital warts caused by HPV types 6 and 11

The Advisory Committee on Immunization Practices (ACIP) recommends routine vaccination for females 11-12 years of age; catch-up vaccination is recommended for females 13-26 years of age; ACIP does not recommend routine use among males; however, eligible males 9-26 years of age may be vaccinated.

General Dosage Range I.M.: *Children ≥9 years and Adults ≤26 years:* 0.5 mL initial dose, followed by 0.5 mL 2 and 6 months later

Dosage Forms

Injection, suspension [preservative free]:
Gardasil®: HPV 6 L1 protein 20 mcg, HPV 11 L1 protein 40 mcg, HPV 16 L1 protein 40 mcg, and HPV 18 L1 protein 20 mcg per 0.5 mL (0.5 mL)

papillomavirus vaccine, recombinant *see* papillomavirus (types 6, 11, 16, 18) vaccine (human, recombinant) *on page 674*

papillomavirus vaccine, recombinant *see* papillomavirus (types 16, 18) vaccine (human, recombinant) *on page 673*

PAR-101 *see* fidaxomicin (systemic) *on page 377*

para-aminosalicylate sodium *see* aminosalicylic acid *on page 67*

paracetamol *see* acetaminophen *on page 23*

Parafon Forte® (Can) *see* chlorzoxazone *on page 204*

Parafon Forte® DSC *see* chlorzoxazone *on page 204*

Paraplatin *see* carboplatin *on page 175*

Paraplatin-AQ (Can) *see* carboplatin *on page 175*

parathyroid hormone (1-34) *see* teriparatide *on page 853*

Parcaine™ *see* proparacaine *on page 745*

Parcopa® *see* carbidopa and levodopa *on page 174*

paregoric (par e GOR ik)

Medication Safety Issues
Sound-alike/look-alike issues:
Camphorated tincture of opium is an error-prone synonym (mistaken as opium tincture)
Paregoric may be confused with Percogesic®
High alert medication:
The Institute for Safe Medication Practices (ISMP) includes this medication among its list of drug classes which have a heightened risk of causing significant patient harm when used in error.
Administration issues:
Use care when prescribing opium tincture; each mL contains the equivalent of morphine 10 mg; paregoric contains the equivalent of morphine 0.4 mg/mL
Synonyms camphorated tincture of opium (error-prone synonym)
Therapeutic Category Analgesic, Narcotic
Controlled Substance C-III
Use Treatment of diarrhea or relief of pain
General Dosage Range Oral:
Children: 0.25-0.5 mL/kg 1-4 times/day
Adults: 5-10 mL 1-4 times/day
Dosage Forms
Liquid, oral: Morphine equivalent 2 mg/5 mL (473 mL)

Paremyd® *see* hydroxyamphetamine and tropicamide *on page 454*

parenteral nutrition *see* total parenteral nutrition *on page 879*

paricalcitol (pah ri KAL si tole)

Medication Safety Issues
Sound-alike/look alike issues:
Paricalcitol may be confused with calcitriol
Zemplar® may be confused with zaleplon, Zelapar®, zolpidem, ZyPREXA® Zydis®
U.S. Brand Names Zemplar®
Canadian Brand Names Zemplar®
Therapeutic Category Vitamin D Analog
Use
I.V.: Prevention and treatment of secondary hyperparathyroidism associated with stage 5 chronic kidney disease (CKD)
Oral: Prevention and treatment of secondary hyperparathyroidism associated with stage 3 and 4 CKD and stage 5 CKD patients on hemodialysis or peritoneal dialysis
General Dosage Range Dosage adjustment recommended in patients with renal impairment
I.V.: *Children ≥5 years and Adults:* 0.04-0.24 mcg/kg (2.8-16.8 mcg) every other day during dialysis
Oral: *Adults:* 1-2 mcg/day **or** 2-4 mcg 3 times/week
Dosage Forms
Capsule, soft gelatin, oral:
Zemplar®: 1 mcg, 2 mcg, 4 mcg
Injection, solution:
Zemplar®: 2 mcg/mL (1 mL); 5 mcg/mL (1 mL, 2 mL)

Pariet® (Can) *see* rabeprazole *on page 763*
pariprazole *see* rabeprazole *on page 763*
Parlodel® *see* bromocriptine *on page 142*
Parlodel® SnapTabs® *see* bromocriptine *on page 142*
Parnate® *see* tranylcypromine *on page 882*

paromomycin (par oh moe MYE sin)

Synonyms paromomycin sulfate
Canadian Brand Names Humatin®
Therapeutic Category Amebicide
Use Treatment of acute and chronic intestinal amebiasis; hepatic coma

◀ **General Dosage Range Oral:** *Children and Adults:* Dosage varies greatly depending on indication
Dosage Forms
   Capsule, oral: 250 mg

paromomycin sulfate *see paromomycin on page 675*

paroxetine (pa ROKS e teen)

Medication Safety Issues
   Sound-alike/look-alike issues:
      PARoxetine may be confused with FLUoxetine, PACLitaxel, piroxicam, pyridoxine
      Paxil® may be confused with Doxil®, paclitaxel, Plavix®, PROzac®, Taxol®

Synonyms paroxetine hydrochloride; paroxetine mesylate

Tall-Man PARoxetine

U.S. Brand Names Paxil CR®; Paxil®; Pexeva®

Canadian Brand Names Apo-Paroxetine®; CO Paroxetine; Dom-Paroxetine; Mylan-Paroxetine; Novo-Paroxetine; Paxil CR®; Paxil®; PHL-Paroxetine; PMS-Paroxetine; ratio-Paroxetine; Riva-paroxetine; Sandoz-Paroxetine; Teva-Paroxetine

Therapeutic Category Antidepressant, Selective Serotonin Reuptake Inhibitor

Use Treatment of major depressive disorder (MDD); treatment of panic disorder with or without agoraphobia; obsessive-compulsive disorder (OCD); social anxiety disorder (social phobia); generalized anxiety disorder (GAD); posttraumatic stress disorder (PTSD); premenstrual dysphoric disorder (PMDD)

General Dosage Range Dosage adjustment recommended in patients with hepatic or renal impairment
Oral:
   Controlled release:
      Adults: Initial: 12.5-25 mg once daily; Maintenance: 12.5-75 mg once daily (maximum: 75 mg/day)
      Elderly: Initial: 12.5 mg once daily; Maintenance: 12.5-50 mg/day (maximum: 50 mg/day)
   Immediate release:
      Adults: Initial: 10-20 mg once daily: Maintenance: 10-60 mg once daily (maximum: 60 mg/day)
      Elderly: Initial: 10 mg once daily; Maintenance: 10-40 mg once daily (maximum: 40 mg/day)

Dosage Forms
   Suspension, oral:
      Paxil®: 10 mg/5 mL (250 mL)
   Tablet, oral: 10 mg, 20 mg, 30 mg, 40 mg
      Paxil®: 10 mg, 20 mg, 30 mg, 40 mg
      Pexeva®: 10 mg, 20 mg, 30 mg, 40 mg
   Tablet, controlled release, enteric coated, oral: 12.5 mg, 25 mg, 37.5 mg
      Paxil CR®: 12.5 mg, 25 mg, 37.5 mg
   Tablet, extended release, enteric coated, oral: 12.5 mg, 25 mg

paroxetine hydrochloride *see paroxetine on page 676*

paroxetine mesylate *see paroxetine on page 676*

Parvolex® (Can) *see acetylcysteine on page 36*

PAS *see aminosalicylic acid on page 67*

Paser® *see aminosalicylic acid on page 67*

Pataday™ *see olopatadine (ophthalmic) on page 647*

Patanase® *see olopatadine (nasal) on page 647*

Patanol® *see olopatadine (ophthalmic) on page 647*

PAT-Galantamine ER (Can) *see galantamine on page 409*

Pathocil® (Can) *see dicloxacillin on page 280*

Pavabid [DSC] *see papaverine on page 673*

Pavulon [DSC] *see pancuronium on page 671*

Paxil® *see paroxetine on page 676*

Paxil CR® *see paroxetine on page 676*

pazopanib (paz OH pa nib)

Medication Safety Issues
   Sound-alike/look-alike issues:
      Pazopanib may be confused with SUNItinib, vandetanib

Votrient™ may be confused with vorinostat

High alert medication:
This medication is in a class the Institute for Safe Medication Practices (ISMP) includes among its list of drug classes which have a heightened risk of causing significant patient harm when used in error.

Synonyms GW786034; pazopanib hydrochloride

U.S. Brand Names Votrient™

Canadian Brand Names Votrient™

Therapeutic Category Antineoplastic Agent, Tyrosine Kinase Inhibitor; Vascular Endothelial Growth Factor (VEGF) Inhibitor

Use Treatment of advanced renal cell cancer (RCC)

General Dosage Range Dosage adjustment recommended in patients with hepatic impairment, on concomitant therapy, or who develop toxicities
Oral: *Adults:* 800 mg once daily

Dosage Forms
Tablet, oral:
Votrient™: 200 mg

pazopanib hydrochloride *see* pazopanib *on page 676*

PCA (error-prone abbreviation) *see* procainamide *on page 739*

PCC *see* factor IX complex (human) *on page 365*

PCE® *see* erythromycin (systemic) *on page 339*

PCEC *see* rabies vaccine *on page 764*

P Chlor GG [DSC] *see* chlorpheniramine, phenylephrine, and guaifenesin *on page 200*

PCV *see* pneumococcal conjugate vaccine (7-valent) *on page 714*

PCV-7 *see* pneumococcal conjugate vaccine (7-valent) *on page 714*

PCV-13 *see* pneumococcal conjugate vaccine (13-valent) *on page 714*

PCV13-CRM(197) *see* pneumococcal conjugate vaccine (13-valent) *on page 714*

PD-Cof [DSC] *see* chlorpheniramine, phenylephrine, and dextromethorphan *on page 200*

PD-Hist-D *see* chlorpheniramine and phenylephrine *on page 198*

PDX *see* pralatrexate *on page 728*

pectin, gelatin, and methylcellulose *see* gelatin, pectin, and methylcellulose *on page 413*

PediaCare® Children's Allergy [OTC] *see* diphenhydramine (systemic) *on page 290*

PediaCare® Children's Decongestant [OTC] *see* phenylephrine (systemic) *on page 696*

PediaCare® Children's Long-Acting Cough [OTC] *see* dextromethorphan *on page 270*

PediaCare® Children's NightTime Cough [OTC] *see* diphenhydramine (systemic) *on page 290*

PediaCare® Children's Multi-Symptom Cold [OTC] *see* dextromethorphan and phenylephrine *on page 271*

Pediacel® (Can) *see* diphtheria and tetanus toxoids, acellular pertussis, poliovirus and *Haemophilus* b conjugate vaccine *on page 295*

Pediaderm™ AF *see* nystatin (topical) *on page 642*

Pediaderm™ HC *see* hydrocortisone (topical) *on page 450*

Pediaderm™ TA *see* triamcinolone (topical) *on page 887*

PediaHist DM *see* brompheniramine, pseudoephedrine, and dextromethorphan *on page 144*

Pediapred® *see* prednisolone (systemic) *on page 734*

Pedia Relief Cough and Cold [OTC] *see* pseudoephedrine and dextromethorphan *on page 752*

Pedia Relief™ Cough-Cold [OTC] *see* chlorpheniramine, pseudoephedrine, and dextromethorphan *on page 201*

Pediarix® *see* diphtheria, tetanus toxoids, acellular pertussis, hepatitis B (recombinant), and poliovirus (inactivated) vaccine *on page 296*

Pediatex® TD *see* triprolidine and pseudoephedrine *on page 893*

Pediatric Digoxin CSD (Can) *see* digoxin *on page 283*

Pediatrix (Can) *see* acetaminophen *on page 23*

Pediazole® (Can) *see* erythromycin and sulfisoxazole *on page 340*

Pedi-Boro® [OTC] *see* aluminum sulfate and calcium acetate *on page 61*

Pedi-Dri® *see* nystatin (topical) *on page 642*

PedvaxHIB® *see* Haemophilus B conjugate vaccine *on page 432*

PEG *see polyethylene glycol 3350 on page 718*
PEG-L-asparaginase *see pegaspargase on page 678*

pegademase (bovine) (peg A de mase BOE vine)

U.S. Brand Names Adagen®
Canadian Brand Names Adagen®
Therapeutic Category Enzyme
Use Enzyme replacement therapy for adenosine deaminase (ADA) deficiency in patients with severe combined immunodeficiency disease (SCID) who are not candidates for or who have failed bone marrow transplant
General Dosage Range I.M.: *Children:* First dose: 10 units/kg; Second dose: 15 units/kg 7 days after first dose; Third dose: 20 units/kg 7 days after second dose; Maintenance: 20 units/kg/week (maximum: 30 units/kg/week)
Dosage Forms
Injection, solution [preservative free]:
Adagen®: 250 units/mL (1.5 mL)

Peganone® *see ethotoin on page 359*

pegaptanib (peg AP ta nib)

Synonyms EYE001; pegaptanib sodium
U.S. Brand Names Macugen®
Canadian Brand Names Macugen®
Therapeutic Category Ophthalmic Agent; Vaccine, Recombinant
Use Treatment of neovascular (wet) age-related macular degeneration (AMD)
General Dosage Range Intravitreous: *Adults:* 0.3 mg into affected eye every 6 weeks
Dosage Forms
Injection, solution [preservative free]:
Macugen®: 0.3 mg/0.09 mL (0.09 mL)

pegaptanib sodium *see pegaptanib on page 678*
PEG-ASP *see pegaspargase on page 678*
PEG-asparaginase *see pegaspargase on page 678*

pegaspargase (peg AS par jase)

Medication Safety Issues
Sound-alike/look-alike issues:
Oncaspar® may be confused with Elspar®
Pegaspargase may be confused with asparaginase
High alert medication:
The Institute for Safe Medication Practices (ISMP) includes this medication among its list of drugs which have a heightened risk of causing significant patient harm when used in error.
Synonyms L-asparaginase with polyethylene glycol; PEG-ASP; PEG-asparaginase; PEG-L-asparaginase; PEGLA; polyethylene glycol-L-asparaginase
U.S. Brand Names Oncaspar®
Therapeutic Category Antineoplastic Agent
Use Treatment of acute lymphocytic leukemia (ALL); treatment of ALL with previous hypersensitivity to native L-asparaginase
General Dosage Range I.M., I.V.: *Children and Adults:* 2500 units/m² every 14 days
Dosage Forms
Injection, solution [preservative free]:
Oncaspar®: 750 int. units/mL (5 mL)

Pegasys® *see peginterferon alfa-2a on page 679*
Pegasys® RBV (Can) *see peginterferon alfa-2a and ribavirin (Canada only) on page 679*
Pegetron® (Can) *see peginterferon alfa-2b and ribavirin (Canada only) on page 681*
Pegetron® RediPen® (Can) *see peginterferon alfa-2b and ribavirin (Canada only) on page 681*

pegfilgrastim (peg fil GRA stim)

Medication Safety Issues
Sound-alike/look-alike issues:
Neulasta® may be confused with Neumega®, Neupogen®, and Lunesta®
Synonyms G-CSF (PEG conjugate); granulocyte colony stimulating factor (PEG conjugate); NSC-725961; pegylated G-CSF; SD/01
U.S. Brand Names Neulasta®
Canadian Brand Names Neulasta®
Therapeutic Category Colony-Stimulating Factor
Use To decrease the incidence of infection, by stimulation of granulocyte production, in patients with nonmyeloid malignancies receiving myelosuppressive therapy associated with a significant risk of febrile neutropenia
General Dosage Range SubQ:
Children: 100 mcg/kg (maximum dose: 6 mg) once per chemotherapy cycle
Adolescents >45 kg and Adults: 6 mg once per chemotherapy cycle
Dosage Forms
Injection, solution [preservative free]:
Neulasta®: 6 mg/0.6 mL (0.6 mL)

PEG-IFN Alfa-2b *see* peginterferon alfa-2b *on page* 680

peginterferon alfa-2a (peg in ter FEER on AL fa too aye)

Synonyms interferon alfa-2a (PEG conjugate); pegylated interferon alfa-2a
U.S. Brand Names Pegasys®
Canadian Brand Names Pegasys®
Therapeutic Category Interferon
Use Treatment of chronic hepatitis C (CHC), alone or in combination with ribavirin, in patients with compensated liver disease and not previously treated with alfa interferons (includes patients with histological evidence of cirrhosis [Child-Pugh class A] and patients with clinically-stable HIV disease); treatment of patients with HBeAg-positive and HBeAg-negative chronic hepatitis B with compensated liver disease and evidence of viral replication and liver inflammation
General Dosage Range Dosage adjustment recommended in patients with hepatic or renal impairment or who develop toxicities
SubQ: *Adults:* 180 mcg once weekly
Dosage Forms
Injection, solution:
Pegasys®: 180 mcg/mL (1 mL); 180 mcg/0.5 mL (0.5 mL)

peginterferon alfa-2a and ribavirin *(Canada only)*
(peg in ter FEER on AL fa too aye & rye ba VYE rin)
Synonyms ribavirin and peginterferon alfa-2a
Canadian Brand Names Pegasys® RBV
Therapeutic Category Antiviral Agent; Interferon
Use Combination therapy for the treatment of chronic hepatitis C (HCV) in patients without cirrhosis and patients with compensated cirrhosis; includes patients coinfected with stable HIV disease
General Dosage Range Dosage adjustment recommended in patients with hepatic or renal impairment or who develop toxicities
SubQ: Peginterferon Alfa-2a: *Adults:* 180 mcg/week
Oral: Ribavirin:
Adults <75kg: 800-1000 mg/day in 2 divided doses
Adults ≥75 kg: 800-1200 mg/day in 2 divided doses
Product Availability Not available in U.S.
Dosage Forms - Canada
Combination package:
Pegasys RBV® [1-week package]:
Tablet, oral: Ribavirin 200 mg (28s)
Injection, solution: Peginterferon alfa-2a: 180 mcg/0.5 mL (0.5 mL) (1s)

◄ Tablet, oral: Ribavirin 200 mg (35s)
Injection, solution: Peginterferon alfa-2a: 180 mcg/0.5 mL (0.5 mL) (1s)

Tablet, oral: Ribavirin 200 mg (42s)
Injection, solution: Peginterferon alfa-2a: 180 mcg/0.5 mL (0.5 mL) (1s)

Pegasys RBV® [1-week package]:
Tablet, oral: Ribavirin 200 mg (28s)
Injection, solution: Peginterferon alfa-2a: 180 mcg/mL (1 mL) (1s)

Tablet, oral: Ribavirin 200 mg (35s)
Injection, solution: Peginterferon alfa-2a: 180 mcg/mL (1 mL) (1s)

Tablet, oral: Ribavirin 200 mg (42s)
Injection, solution: Peginterferon alfa-2a: 180 mcg/mL (1 mL) (1s)

Pegasys RBV® [4-week package]:
Tablet, oral: Ribavirin 200 mg (112s)
Injection, solution: Peginterferon alfa-2a: 180 mcg/0.5 mL (0.5 mL) (4s)

Tablet, oral: Ribavirin 200 mg (140s)
Injection, solution: Peginterferon alfa-2a: 180 mcg/0.5 mL (0.5 mL) (4s)

Tablet, oral: Ribavirin 200 mg (168s)
Injection, solution: Peginterferon alfa-2a: 180 mcg/0.5 mL (0.5 mL) (4s)

Tablet, oral: Ribavirin 200 mg (168s + 28s)
Injection, solution: Peginterferon alfa-2a: 180 mcg/0.5 mL (0.5 mL) (4s)

Pegasys RBV® [4-week package]:
Tablet, oral: Ribavirin 200 mg (112s)
Injection, solution: Peginterferon alfa-2a: 180 mcg/mL (1 mL) (4s)

Tablet, oral: Ribavirin 200 mg (140s)
Injection, solution: Peginterferon alfa-2a: 180 mcg/mL (1 mL) (4s)

Tablet, oral: Ribavirin 200 mg (168s)
Injection, solution: Peginterferon alfa-2a: 180 mcg/mL (1 mL) (4s)

peginterferon alfa-2b (peg in ter FEER on AL fa too bee)

Medication Safety Issues
Sound-alike/look-alike issues:
Peginterferon alfa-2b may be confused with interferon alfa-2a, interferon alfa-2b, interferon alfa-n3, peginterferon alfa-2a

PegIntron® may be confused with Intron® A

International issues:
Peginterferon alfa-2b may be confused with interferon alpha multi-subtype which is available in international markets

Synonyms interferon alfa-2b (PEG conjugate); PEG-IFN Alfa-2b; pegylated interferon alfa-2b; polyethylene glycol interferon alfa-2b

U.S. Brand Names PegIntron®; PegIntron™ Redipen®; Sylatron™

Canadian Brand Names PegIntron®

Therapeutic Category Interferon

Use
PegIntron®: Treatment of chronic hepatitis C (CHC; in combination with ribavirin) in patients who have compensated liver disease; treatment of chronic hepatitis C (as monotherapy) in adult patients with compensated liver disease who have never received alfa interferons

Sylatron™: Adjuvant treatment of melanoma (with microscopic or gross nodal involvement within 84 days of definitive surgical resection, including lymphadenectomy)

General Dosage Range Dosage adjustment recommended in patients with renal impairment or who develop toxicities

SubQ: Melanoma:

Adults: Initial: 6 mcg/kg/week; Maintenance: 3 mcg/kg/week

SubQ: Chronic hepatitis C:

Children ≥3 years: 60 mcg/m^2/week (in combination with ribavirin)

Adults: Peginterferon monotherapy (based on average weekly dose of 1 mcg/kg):
Adults ≤45 kg: 40 mcg once weekly
Adults 46-56 kg: 50 mcg once weekly
Adults 57-72 kg: 64 mcg once weekly
Adults 73-88 kg: 80 mcg once weekly
Adults 89-106 kg: 96 mcg once weekly
Adults 107-136 kg: 120 mcg once weekly
Adults 137-160 kg: 150 mcg once weekly

Adults: Combination therapy with ribavirin (based on average weekly dose of 1.5 mcg/kg):
Adults <40 kg: 50 mcg once weekly (with ribavirin 800 mg/day)
Adults 40-50 kg: 64 mcg once weekly (with ribavirin 800 mg/day)
Adults 51-60 kg: 80 mcg once weekly (with ribavirin 800 mg/day)
Adults 61-65 kg: 96 mcg once weekly (with ribavirin 800 mg/day)
Adults 66-75 kg: 96 mcg once weekly (with ribavirin 1000 mg/day)
Adults 76-80 kg: 120 mcg once weekly (with ribavirin 1000 mg/day)
Adults 81-85 kg: 120 mcg once weekly (with ribavirin 1200 mg/day)
Adults 86-105 kg: 150 mcg once weekly (with ribavirin 1200 mg/day)
Adults >105 kg: 1.5 mcg/kg once weekly (with ribavirin 1400 mg/day)

Dosage Forms
Injection, powder for reconstitution:
Sylatron™: 296 mcg, 444 mcg, 888 mcg
Injection, powder for reconstitution [preservative free]:
PegIntron®: 50 mcg, 80 mcg, 120 mcg, 150 mcg
PegIntron™ Redipen®: 50 mcg, 80 mcg, 120 mcg, 150 mcg

peginterferon alfa-2b and ribavirin *(Canada only)*
(peg in ter FEER on AL fa too bee & rye ba VYE rin)

Synonyms ribavirin and peginterferon alfa-2b

Canadian Brand Names Pegetron®; Pegetron® RediPen®

Therapeutic Category Antiviral Agent; Interferon

Use Combination therapy for the treatment of chronic hepatitis C in patients with compensated liver disease

General Dosage Range Dosage adjustment recommended in patients with hepatic or renal impairment or who develop toxicities

SubQ: Peginterferon Alfa-2b: *Adults:* 1.5 mcg/kg/week
Oral: Ribavirin:
Adults ≤64 kg: 800 mg/day in 2 divided doses
Adults 64-84 kg: 1000 mg/day in 2 divided doses
Adults ≥85 kg: 1200 mg/day in 2 divided doses

Product Availability Not available in U.S.

Dosage Forms - Canada
Combination package:
Pegetron®:
Capsule: Ribavirin 200 mg (56s)
Injection, powder for reconstitution: Peginterferon alfa-2b: 50 mcg/0.5 mL
Pegetron®:
Capsule: Ribavirin 200 mg (56s)
Injection, powder for reconstitution: Peginterferon alfa-2b: 80 mcg/0.5 mL
Pegetron®:
Capsule: Ribavirin 200 mg (70s)
Injection, powder for reconstitution: Peginterferon alfa-2b: 100 mcg/0.5 mL
Pegetron®:
Capsule: Ribavirin 200 mg (70s)
Injection, powder for reconstitution: Peginterferon alfa-2b: 120 mcg/0.5 mL
Pegetron®:
Capsule: Ribavirin 200 mg (84s)
Injection, powder for reconstitution: Peginterferon alfa-2b: 150 mcg/0.5 mL

PegIntron® *see* peginterferon alfa-2b *on page 680*
PegIntron™ Redipen® *see* peginterferon alfa-2b *on page 680*

PEGLA *see pegaspargase on page 678*

pegloticase (peg LOE ti kase)
Synonyms PEG-uricase; pegylated urate oxidase; polyethylene glycol-conjugated uricase; recombinant urate oxidase, pegylated; urate oxidase, pegylated
U.S. Brand Names Krystexxa™
Therapeutic Category Enzyme; Enzyme, Urate-Oxidase (Recombinant)
Use Treatment of chronic gout refractory to conventional therapy
General Dosage Range I.V.: *Adults:* 8 mg every 2 weeks
Dosage Forms
Injection, solution:
Krystexxa™: Uricase protein 8 mg/mL (2 mL)

PegLyte® (Can) *see polyethylene glycol-electrolyte solution on page 718*
PEG-uricase *see pegloticase on page 682*

pegvisomant (peg VI soe mant)
Synonyms B2036-PEG
U.S. Brand Names Somavert®
Canadian Brand Names Somavert®
Therapeutic Category Growth Hormone Receptor Antagonist
Use Treatment of acromegaly in patients resistant to or unable to tolerate other therapies
General Dosage Range SubQ: *Adults:* Initial loading dose: 40 mg; Maintenance: 10-30 mg/day (maximum: 30 mg/day)
Dosage Forms
Injection, powder for reconstitution:
Somavert®: 10 mg, 15 mg, 20 mg

pegylated DOXOrubicin liposomal *see doxorubicin (liposomal) on page 311*
pegylated G-CSF *see pegfilgrastim on page 679*
pegylated interferon alfa-2a *see peginterferon alfa-2a on page 679*
pegylated interferon alfa-2b *see peginterferon alfa-2b on page 680*
pegylated liposomal DOXOrubicin *see doxorubicin (liposomal) on page 311*
pegylated urate oxidase *see pegloticase on page 682*
PE-Hist DM [DSC] *see chlorpheniramine, phenylephrine, and dextromethorphan on page 200*

pemetrexed (pem e TREKS ed)
Medication Safety Issues
Sound-alike/look-alike issues:
PEMEtrexed may be confused with methotrexate, PRALAtrexate
High alert medication:
This medication is in a class the Institute for Safe Medication Practices (ISMP) includes among its list of drug classes which have a heightened risk of causing significant patient harm when used in error.
Synonyms LY231514; pemetrexed disodium
Tall-Man PEMEtrexed
U.S. Brand Names Alimta®
Canadian Brand Names Alimta®
Therapeutic Category Antineoplastic Agent, Antimetabolite; Antineoplastic Agent, Antimetabolite (Antifolate)
Use Treatment of unresectable malignant pleural mesothelioma (in combination with cisplatin); treatment of locally advanced or metastatic nonsquamous nonsmall cell lung cancer (NSCLC; as initial treatment in combination with cisplatin, as single-agent maintenance treatment after 4 cycles of initial platinum-based double therapy, and single-agent treatment after prior chemotherapy)
General Dosage Range Dosage adjustment recommended in patients with hepatic impairment, on concomitant therapy, or who develop toxicities
I.V.: *Adults:* 500 mg/m^2 on day 1 of each 21-day cycle

Dosage Forms
  Injection, powder for reconstitution:
    Alimta®: 100 mg, 500 mg

pemetrexed disodium see pemetrexed on page 682

pemirolast (pe MIR oh last)
  U.S. Brand Names Alamast®
  Canadian Brand Names Alamast®
  Therapeutic Category Mast Cell Stabilizer; Ophthalmic Agent, Miscellaneous
  Use Prevention of itching of the eye due to allergic conjunctivitis
  General Dosage Range Ophthalmic: Children >3 years and Adults: Instill 1-2 drops in affected eye(s) 4 times/day
  Dosage Forms
    Solution, ophthalmic:
      Alamast®: 0.1% (10 mL)

penbutolol (pen BYOO toe lole)
  Medication Safety Issues
    Sound-alike/look-alike issues:
      Levatol® may be confused with Lipitor®
    International issues:
      Levatol [U.S.] may be confused with Lovacol brand name for lovastatin [Chile and Finland]
  Synonyms penbutolol sulfate
  U.S. Brand Names Levatol®
  Canadian Brand Names Levatol®
  Therapeutic Category Beta-Adrenergic Blocker
  Use Treatment of mild-to-moderate arterial hypertension
  General Dosage Range Oral: Adults: Initial: 20 mg once daily; Maintenance: 10-40 mg once daily (maximum: 80 mg/day)
  Dosage Forms
    Tablet, oral:
      Levatol®: 20 mg

penbutolol sulfate see penbutolol on page 683

penciclovir (pen SYE kloe veer)
  Medication Safety Issues
    Sound-alike/look-alike issues:
      Denavir® may be confused with indinavir
  U.S. Brand Names Denavir®
  Therapeutic Category Antiviral Agent
  Use Topical treatment of recurrent herpes simplex labialis (cold sores)
  General Dosage Range Topical: Children ≥12 years and Adults: Apply every 2 hours during waking hours
  Dosage Forms
    Cream, topical:
      Denavir®: 1% (1.5 g, 5 g)

penicillamine (pen i SIL a meen)
  Medication Safety Issues
    Sound-alike/look-alike issues:
      Penicillamine may be confused with penicillin
    International issues:
      Depen [U.S.] may be confused with Depin brand name for nifedipine [India]; Depon brand name for acetaminophen [Greece]; Dipen brand name for diltiazem [Greece]
      Pemine [Italy] may be confused with Pamine brand name for methscopolamine [U.S., Canada]
  Synonyms D-3-mercaptovaline; D-penicillamine; β,β-dimethylcysteine
  U.S. Brand Names Cuprimine®; Depen®

◀ **Canadian Brand Names** Cuprimine®; Depen®

Therapeutic Category Chelating Agent

Use Treatment of Wilson disease, cystinuria; adjunctive treatment of rheumatoid arthritis

General Dosage Range Dosage adjustment recommended in patients with renal impairment

Oral:

Children: 30 mg/kg/day in 4 divided doses

Adults: Dosage varies greatly depending on indication

Dosage Forms

Capsule, oral:

Cuprimine®: 250 mg

Tablet, oral:

Depen®: 250 mg

penicillin G benzathine (pen i SIL in jee BENZ a theen)

Medication Safety Issues

Sound-alike/look-alike issues:

Penicillin may be confused with penicillamine

Bicillin® may be confused with Wycillin®

Administration issues:

Penicillin G benzathine may only be administered by deep intramuscular injection; intravenous administration of penicillin G benzathine has been associated with cardiopulmonary arrest and death.

Other safety concerns:

Bicillin® C-R (penicillin G benzathine and penicillin G procaine) may be confused with Bicillin® L-A (penicillin G benzathine). Penicillin G benzathine is the only product currently approved for the treatment of syphilis. Administration of penicillin G benzathine and penicillin G procaine combination instead of Bicillin® L-A may result in inadequate treatment response.

Synonyms benzathine benzylpenicillin; benzathine penicillin G; benzylpenicillin benzathine

U.S. Brand Names Bicillin® L-A

Canadian Brand Names Bicillin® L-A

Therapeutic Category Penicillin

Use Active against some gram-positive organisms, few gram-negative organisms such as *Neisseria gonorrhoeae*, and some anaerobes and spirochetes; used in the treatment of syphilis; used only for the treatment of mild to moderately-severe upper respiratory tract infections caused by organisms susceptible to low concentrations of penicillin G or for prophylaxis of infections caused by these organisms; primary and secondary prevention of rheumatic fever

General Dosage Range I.M.:

Children ≤27 kg: 600,000 units/dose

Children >27 kg: 1.2 million units/dose

Adults: 1.2-2.4 million units as a single dose

Dosage Forms

Injection, suspension:

Bicillin® L-A: 600,000 units/mL (1 mL, 2 mL, 4 mL)

penicillin G benzathine and penicillin G procaine

(pen i SIL in jee BENZ a theen & pen i SIL in jee PROE kane)

Medication Safety Issues

Sound-alike/look-alike issues:

Penicillin may be confused with penicillamine

Bicillin® may be confused with Wycillin®

Administration issues:

Penicillin G benzathine may only be administered by deep intramuscular injection; intravenous administration of penicillin G benzathine has been associated with cardiopulmonary arrest and death.

Other safety concerns:

Bicillin® C-R (penicillin G benzathine and penicillin G procaine) may be confused with Bicillin® L-A (penicillin G benzathine). Penicillin G benzathine is the only product currently approved for the treatment of syphilis. Administration of penicillin G benzathine and penicillin G procaine combination instead of Bicillin® L-A may result in inadequate treatment response.

Synonyms penicillin G procaine and benzathine combined

U.S. Brand Names Bicillin® C-R; Bicillin® C-R 900/300

Therapeutic Category Penicillin

Use May be used in specific situations in the treatment of streptococcal infections; primary prevention of rheumatic fever

General Dosage Range I.M.:
Children <14 kg: 600,000 units/dose
Children 14-27 kg: 900,000 units to 1.2 million units as a single dose
Children >27 kg and Adults: 2.4 million units/dose

Dosage Forms
Injection, suspension [prefilled syringe]:
Bicillin® C-R: 1,200,000 units: Penicillin G benzathine 600,000 units and penicillin G procaine 600,000 units per 2 mL (2 mL)
Bicillin® C-R 900/300: 1,200,000 units: Penicillin G benzathine 900,000 units and penicillin G procaine 300,000 units per 2 mL (2 mL)

penicillin G (parenteral/aqueous) (pen i SIL in jee, pa REN ter al, AYE kwee us)

Medication Safety Issues
Sound-alike/look-alike issues:
Penicillin may be confused with penicillamine

Synonyms benzylpenicillin potassium; benzylpenicillin sodium; crystalline penicillin; penicillin G potassium; penicillin G sodium

U.S. Brand Names Pfizerpen®

Canadian Brand Names Crystapen®

Therapeutic Category Penicillin

Use Treatment of infections (including sepsis, pneumonia, pericarditis, endocarditis, meningitis, anthrax) caused by susceptible organisms; active against some gram-positive organisms, generally not *Staphylococcus aureus*; some gram-negative organisms such as *Neisseria gonorrhoeae*, and some anaerobes and spirochetes

General Dosage Range Dosage adjustment recommended in patients with renal impairment
I.M., I.V.:
Infants ≥1 month and Children: 100,000-400,000 units/kg/day in divided doses every 4-6 hours (maximum: 24 million units/day)
Adults: 2-30 million units/day in divided doses every 4-6 hours

Dosage Forms
Infusion, premixed iso-osmotic dextrose solution: 1 million units (50 mL); 2 million units (50 mL); 3 million units (50 mL)
Injection, powder for reconstitution: 5 million units, 20 million units
Pfizerpen®: 5 million units, 20 million units

penicillin G potassium *see* penicillin G (parenteral/aqueous) *on page 685*

penicillin G procaine (pen i SIL in jee PROE kane)

Medication Safety Issues
Sound-alike/look-alike issues:
Penicillin G procaine may be confused with penicillin V potassium
Wycillin® may be confused with Bicillin®

Synonyms APPG; aqueous procaine penicillin G; procaine benzylpenicillin; procaine penicillin G; Wycillin [DSC]

Canadian Brand Names Pfizerpen-AS®; Wycillin®

Therapeutic Category Penicillin

Use Treatment of moderately-severe infections due to *Treponema pallidum* and other penicillin G-sensitive microorganisms that are susceptible to low, but prolonged serum penicillin concentrations; anthrax due to *Bacillus anthracis* (postexposure) to reduce the incidence or progression of disease following exposure to aerolized *Bacillus anthracis*

General Dosage Range Dosage adjustment recommended in patients with renal impairment
I.M.:
Children: 25,000-50,000 units/kg/day in divided doses 1-2 times/day (maximum: 4.8 million units/day)
Adults: 0.6-4.8 million units/day in divided doses every 12-24 hours

Dosage Forms
Injection, suspension: 600,000 units/mL (1 mL, 2 mL)

penicillin G procaine and benzathine combined *see* penicillin G benzathine and penicillin G procaine *on page 684*

penicillin G sodium *see* penicillin G (parenteral/aqueous) *on page 685*

penicillin V potassium (pen i SIL in vee poe TASS ee um)

Medication Safety Issues
Sound-alike/look-alike issues:
Penicillin V procaine may be confused with penicillin G potassium

Synonyms pen VK; phenoxymethyl penicillin

Canadian Brand Names Apo-Pen VK®; Novo-Pen-VK; Nu-Pen-VK

Therapeutic Category Penicillin

Use Treatment of infections caused by susceptible organisms involving the respiratory tract, otitis media, sinusitis, skin, and urinary tract; prophylaxis in rheumatic fever

General Dosage Range Dosage adjustment recommended in patients with renal impairment
Oral:
Children <12 years: 25-50 mg/kg/day divided every 6-8 hours (maximum: 3 g/day)
Children ≥12 years and Adults: 125-500 mg every 6-8 hours

Dosage Forms
Powder for solution, oral: 125 mg/5 mL (100 mL, 200 mL); 250 mg/5 mL (100 mL, 200 mL)
Tablet, oral: 250 mg, 500 mg

penicilloyl-polylysine *see* benzylpenicilloyl polylysine *on page 127*

Penlac® *see* ciclopirox *on page 207*

Pennsaid® *see* diclofenac (topical) *on page 279*

Pennsaid® (Can) *see* diclofenac (systemic) *on page 277*

Pentacel® *see* diphtheria and tetanus toxoids, acellular pertussis, poliovirus and *Haemophilus* b conjugate vaccine *on page 295*

pentahydrate *see* sodium thiosulfate *on page 824*

Pentam® 300 *see* pentamidine *on page 686*

pentamidine (pen TAM i deen)

Synonyms pentamidine isethionate

U.S. Brand Names Nebupent®; Pentam® 300

Therapeutic Category Antiprotozoal

Use
I.M., I.V.: Treatment of pneumonia caused by *Pneumocystis jirovecii* pneumonia (PCP)
Inhalation: Prevention of PCP in high-risk, HIV-infected patients either with a history of PCP or with a CD4+ count ≤200/mm³

General Dosage Range Dosage adjustment recommended in patients with renal impairment
I.M.: *Children >4 months and Adults:* 4 mg/kg once daily for 14-21 days
I.V.: *Children >4 months and Adults:* 4 mg/kg once daily for 14-21 days
Inhalation: *Children >16 years and Adults:* 300 mg/dose every 4 weeks

Dosage Forms
Injection, powder for reconstitution:
Pentam® 300: 300 mg
Powder for solution, for nebulization:
Nebupent®: 300 mg

pentamidine isethionate *see* pentamidine *on page 686*

Pentamycetin® (Can) *see* chloramphenicol *on page 193*

Pentasa® *see* mesalamine *on page 564*

pentasodium colistin methanesulfonate *see* colistimethate *on page 232*

Pentaspan® (Can) *see* pentastarch *on page 686*

pentastarch (PEN ta starch)

Synonyms HES; hydroxyethyl starch

Canadian Brand Names Pentaspan®

Therapeutic Category Blood Modifiers

Use Adjunctive treatment in the management of shock

General Dosage Range I.V.: *Adults:* 500-2000 mL/day (maximum daily dose: 28 mL/kg or 2000 mL)

Product Availability Not available in U.S.

Dosage Forms - Canada

Infusion, premixed in NS:

Pentaspan®: 10% (250 mL, 500 mL)

pentavalent human-bovine reassortant rotavirus vaccine (PRV) *see* rotavirus vaccine *on page 792*

pentazocine (pen TAZ oh seen)

Medication Safety Issues

High alert medication:

The Institute for Safe Medication Practices (ISMP) includes this medication among its list of drug classes which have a heightened risk of causing significant patient harm when used in error.

BEERS Criteria medication:

This drug may be inappropriate for use in geriatric patients (high severity risk).

Synonyms pentazocine lactate

U.S. Brand Names Talwin®

Canadian Brand Names Talwin®

Therapeutic Category Analgesic, Narcotic

Controlled Substance C-IV

Use Relief of moderate-to-severe pain; has also been used as a sedative prior to surgery and as a supplement to surgical anesthesia

General Dosage Range Dosage adjustment recommended in patients with renal impairment

I.M.:

Children 1-16 years: 0.5 mg/kg preoperatively

Adults: 30-60 mg every 3-4 hours (maximum: 360 mg/day; 60 mg/dose) **or** 30 mg once

I.V.: *Adults:* 30 mg every 3-4 hours (maximum: 360 mg/day; 30 mg/dose) **or** 20 mg every 2-3 hours as needed (maximum total dose: 60 mg)

SubQ: *Adults:* 30 mg every 3-4 hours (maximum: 360 mg/day; 60 mg/dose)

Dosage Forms

Injection, solution:

Talwin®: 30 mg/mL (1 mL, 10 mL)

pentazocine and acetaminophen (pen TAZ oh seen & a seet a MIN oh fen)

Medication Safety Issues

Sound-alike/look-alike issues:

Talacen may be confused with Tegison®, Timoptic®, Tinactin®

High alert medication:

The Institute for Safe Medication Practices (ISMP) includes this medication among its list of drug classes which have a heightened risk of causing significant patient harm when used in error.

Other safety concerns:

Duplicate therapy issues: This product contains acetaminophen, which may be a component of other combination products. Do not exceed the maximum recommended daily dose of acetaminophen.

Synonyms acetaminophen and pentazocine; pentazocine hydrochloride and acetaminophen; Talacen

Therapeutic Category Analgesic Combination (Opioid)

Controlled Substance C-IV

Use Relief of mild-to-moderate pain

General Dosage Range Oral: *Children ≥12 years and Adults:* One caplet (pentazocine 25 mg/ acetaminophen 650 mg) every 4 hours as needed (maximum: 6 caplets/day)

Dosage Forms

Tablet: Pentazocine 25 mg and acetaminophen 650 mg

pentazocine and naloxone (pen TAZ oh seen & nal OKS one)

Medication Safety Issues

High alert medication:

The Institute for Safe Medication Practices (ISMP) includes this medication among its list of drug classes which have a heightened risk of causing significant patient harm when used in error.

◀ **Synonyms** naloxone hydrochloride and pentazocine; pentazocine hydrochloride and naloxone hydrochloride; Talwin NX

Therapeutic Category Analgesic, Opioid

Controlled Substance C-IV

Use Relief of moderate-to-severe pain; indicated for oral use only

General Dosage Range Dosage adjustment recommended in patients with renal impairment
  Oral: *Children ≥12 years and Adults:* Based upon pentazocine: 50-100 mg every 3-4 hours (maximum: 600 mg/day)

Dosage Forms
  Tablet: Pentazocine 50 mg and naloxone 0.5 mg

pentazocine hydrochloride and acetaminophen *see* pentazocine and acetaminophen *on page 687*

pentazocine hydrochloride and naloxone hydrochloride *see* pentazocine and naloxone *on page 687*

pentazocine lactate *see* pentazocine *on page 687*

pentetate calcium trisodium *see* diethylene triamine penta-acetic acid *on page 281*

pentetate zinc trisodium *see* diethylene triamine penta-acetic acid *on page 281*

pentobarbital (pen toe BAR bi tal)

Medication Safety Issues
  Sound-alike/look-alike issues:
    PENTobarbital may be confused with PHENobarbital
    Nembutal® may be confused with Myambutol®

Synonyms pentobarbital sodium

Tall-Man PENTobarbital

U.S. Brand Names Nembutal®

Canadian Brand Names Nembutal® Sodium

Therapeutic Category Barbiturate

Controlled Substance C-II

Use Sedative/hypnotic; refractory status epilepticus

General Dosage Range
  I.M.:
    Children: 2-6 mg/kg (maximum: 100 mg/dose)
    Adults: 150-200 mg
  I.V.:
    Children:
      Hypnotic/sedative: 1-6 mg/kg
      Refractory status epilepticus: Loading dose: 5-15 mg/kg; Maintenance infusion: 0.5-5 mg/kg/hour
    Adults:
      Hypnotic/sedative: 100 mg; may repeat (maximum total dose: 500 mg)
      Refractory status epilepticus: Loading dose: 10-15 mg/kg; Maintenance infusion: 0.5-10 mg/kg/hour

Dosage Forms
  Injection, solution:
    Nembutal®: 50 mg/mL (20 mL, 50 mL)

pentobarbital sodium *see* pentobarbital *on page 688*

pentosan polysulfate sodium (PEN toe san pol i SUL fate SOW dee um)

Medication Safety Issues
  Sound-alike/look-alike issues:
    Pentosan may be confused with pentostatin
    Elmiron® may be confused with Imuran®

Synonyms PPS

U.S. Brand Names Elmiron®

Canadian Brand Names Elmiron®

Therapeutic Category Analgesic, Urinary

Use Relief of bladder pain or discomfort due to interstitial cystitis

General Dosage Range Oral: *Children ≥16 years and Adults:* 100 mg 3 times/day

Dosage Forms
  Capsule, oral:
    Elmiron®: 100 mg

pentostatin (pen toe STAT in)

Medication Safety Issues
  Sound-alike/look-alike issues:
    Pentostatin may be confused with pentamidine, pentosan
  High alert medication:
    The Institute for Safe Medication Practices (ISMP) includes this medication among its list of drug classes which have a heightened risk of causing significant patient harm when used in error.
  International issues:
    Nipent [U.S., Canada, and multiple international markets] may be confused with Nipin brand name for nifedipine [Italy, Singapore]

Synonyms 2'-deoxycoformycin; co-vidarabine; dCF; deoxycoformycin; NSC-218321

U.S. Brand Names Nipent®

Canadian Brand Names Nipent®

Therapeutic Category Antineoplastic Agent

Use Treatment of hairy cell leukemia

General Dosage Range Dosage adjustment recommended in patients with renal impairment
  I.V.: *Adults:* 4 mg/m^2 every 2 weeks

Dosage Forms
  Injection, powder for reconstitution:
    Nipent®: 10 mg
  Injection, powder for reconstitution [preservative free]: 10 mg

Pentothal® [DSC] *see* thiopental *on page 863*
Pentothal® (Can) *see* thiopental *on page 863*

pentoxifylline (pen toks IF i lin)

Medication Safety Issues
  Sound-alike/look-alike issues:
    Pentoxifylline may be confused with tamoxifen
    TRENtal® may be confused with Bentyl®, TEGretol®, Trandate®

Synonyms oxpentifylline

U.S. Brand Names TRENtal®

Canadian Brand Names Albert® Pentoxifylline; Apo-Pentoxifylline SR®; Nu-Pentoxifylline SR; ratio-Pentoxifylline; Trental®

Therapeutic Category Blood Viscosity Reducer Agent

Use Treatment of intermittent claudication on the basis of chronic occlusive arterial disease of the limbs; may improve function and symptoms, but not intended to replace more definitive therapy

General Dosage Range Dosage adjustment recommended in patients with renal impairment
  Oral: *Adults:* 400 mg 2-3 times/day

Dosage Forms
  Tablet, controlled release, oral:
    TRENtal®: 400 mg
  Tablet, extended release, oral: 400 mg

Pentrax® [OTC] *see* coal tar *on page 227*
pen VK *see* penicillin V potassium *on page 686*
Pepcid® *see* famotidine *on page 366*
Pepcid® AC [OTC] *see* famotidine *on page 366*
Pepcid® AC (Can) *see* famotidine *on page 366*
Pepcid® AC Maximum Strength [OTC] *see* famotidine *on page 366*
Pepcid® Complete® [OTC] *see* famotidine, calcium carbonate, and magnesium hydroxide *on page 367*
Pepcid® I.V. (Can) *see* famotidine *on page 366*
Peptic Relief [OTC] *see* bismuth *on page 135*
Pepto-Bismol® [OTC] *see* bismuth *on page 135*

Pepto-Bismol® Maximum Strength [OTC] *see* bismuth *on page 135*
Pepto Relief [OTC] *see* bismuth *on page 135*
Peranex™ HC *see* lidocaine and hydrocortisone *on page 526*
Peranex™ HC Medi-Pad *see* lidocaine and hydrocortisone *on page 526*
Percocet® *see* oxycodone and acetaminophen *on page 662*
Percocet®-Demi (Can) *see* oxycodone and acetaminophen *on page 662*
Percodan® *see* oxycodone and aspirin *on page 664*
Percogesic® Extra Strength [OTC] *see* acetaminophen and diphenhydramine *on page 27*
Perdiem® Overnight Relief [OTC] *see* senna *on page 807*

perflutren lipid microspheres (per FLOO tren LIP id MIKE roe sfeers)

U.S. Brand Names Definity®
Canadian Brand Names Definity®
Therapeutic Category Diagnostic Agent
Use Opacification of left ventricular chamber and improvement of delineation of the left ventricular endocardial border in patients with suboptimal echocardiograms
General Dosage Range I.V.: *Adults:* Bolus: 10 microliters (µL)/kg of activated product, followed by 10 mL saline flush; may repeat in 30 minutes if needed; Infusion: Initial: 4 mL/minute (or 240 mL/hour) of prepared infusion; titrate to achieve optimal image; Maximum rate: 10 mL/minute (or 600 mL/hour)
Dosage Forms
  Injection, solution [preservative free]:
    Definity®: OFP 6.52 mg/mL and lipid blend 0.75 mg/mL (2 mL)

Perforomist® *see* formoterol *on page 398*
Periactin *see* cyproheptadine *on page 244*

periciazine *(Canada only)* (per ee CYE ah zeen)

Synonyms pericyazine
Canadian Brand Names Neuleptil®
Therapeutic Category Phenothiazine Derivative
Use Adjunctive therapy in selected psychotic patients to control prevailing hostility, impulsivity, or aggression
General Dosage Range Oral:
  Children >5 years: 2.5-10 mg in the morning, followed by 5-30 mg in the evening
  Adults: 5-20 mg in the morning, followed by 10-40 mg in the evening
Product Availability Not available in U.S.
Dosage Forms - Canada
  Capsule, oral:
    Neuleptil®: 5 mg, 10 mg, 20 mg
  Solution, oral [drops]:
    Neuleptil®: 10 mg/mL

Peri-Colace® [OTC] *see* docusate and senna *on page 303*
pericyazine *see* periciazine *(Canada only) on page 690*
Peridex® *see* chlorhexidine gluconate *on page 194*
Peridex® Oral Rinse (Can) *see* chlorhexidine gluconate *on page 194*
perindopril and indapamide *see* perindopril erbumine and indapamide *(Canada only) on page 691*

perindopril erbumine (per IN doe pril er BYOO meen)

U.S. Brand Names Aceon®
Canadian Brand Names Apo-Perindopril®; Coversyl®
Therapeutic Category Miscellaneous Product
Use Treatment of hypertension; reduction of cardiovascular mortality or nonfatal myocardial infarction in patients with stable coronary artery disease

Canadian labeling: Additional use (unlabeled use in U.S.): Treatment of mild-moderate (NYHA I-III) heart failure

General Dosage Range Dosage adjustment recommended in patients with renal impairment
Oral: *Adults:* Initial: 2-4 mg once daily; Maintenance: 4-8 mg/day in 1-2 divided doses (maximum: 16 mg/day)
Dosage Forms
Tablet, oral: 2 mg, 4 mg, 8 mg
Aceon®: 2 mg, 4 mg, 8 mg

perindopril erbumine and indapamide *(Canada only)*
(per IN doe pril er BYOO meen & in DAP a mide)
Synonyms indapamide and perindopril erbumine; perindopril and indapamide
Canadian Brand Names Coversyl® Plus; Coversyl® Plus HD; Coversyl® Plus LD
Therapeutic Category Angiotensin-Converting Enzyme (ACE) Inhibitor; Antihypertensive Agent, Combination; Diuretic, Thiazide-Related
Use Treatment of hypertension
Note: Coversyl® Plus LD may be used as initial treatment; Coversyl® Plus and Coversyl® Plus HD are not indicated for initial treatment of hypertension.
General Dosage Range Oral: *Adults:* Perindopril 2-8 mg/indapamide 0.625-2.5 mg once daily
Product Availability Not available in U.S.
Dosage Forms - Canada
Tablet, oral:
Coversyl® Plus: Perindopril erbumine 4 mg and indapamide 1.25 mg
Coversyl® Plus HD: Perindopril erbumine 8 mg and indapamide 2.5 mg
Coversyl® Plus LD: Perindopril erbumine 2 mg and indapamide 0.625 mg

periochip® *see* chlorhexidine gluconate *on page 194*
PerioGard® [OTC] *see* chlorhexidine gluconate *on page 194*
PerioMed™ *see* fluoride *on page 386*
Periostat® *see* doxycycline *on page 312*
Perlane® *see* hyaluronate and derivatives *on page 443*

permethrin (per METH rin)
Synonyms Elimite
U.S. Brand Names A200® Lice [OTC]; Acticin® [DSC]; Nix® Complete Lice Treatment System [OTC]; Nix® Creme Rinse Lice Treatment [OTC]; Nix® Creme Rinse [OTC]; Nix® Lice Control Spray [OTC]; Rid® [OTC]
Canadian Brand Names Kwellada-P™; Nix®
Therapeutic Category Scabicides/Pediculicides
Use Single-application treatment of infestation with *Pediculus humanus capitis* (head louse) and its nits or *Sarcoptes scabiei* (scabies); indicated for prophylactic use during epidemics of lice
General Dosage Range Topical:
Cream: *Children and Adults:* Apply from head to toe, leave on 8-14 hours before washing off with water; May reapply in 1 week if live mites appear
Liquid (lotion or cream rinse): *Children >2 months and Adults:* Apply a sufficient volume to saturate the hair and scalp, leave on for 10 minutes before rinsing off with water; May reapply in 1 week if lice or nits still present
Dosage Forms
Cream, topical: 5% (60 g)
Liquid, topical:
Nix® Complete Lice Treatment System [OTC]: 1% (1s)
Nix® Creme Rinse [OTC]: 1% (60 mL)
Nix® Creme Rinse Lice Treatment [OTC]: 1% (60 mL)
Nix® Lice Control Spray [OTC]: 0.25% (150 mL)
Lotion, topical: 1% (60 mL)
Solution, topical:
A200® Lice [OTC]: 0.5% (170.1 g)
Rid® [OTC]: 0.5% (150 mL)

perphenazine (per FEN a zeen)

Medication Safety Issues
 Sound-alike/look-alike issues:
  Trilafon® may be confused with Tri-Levlen®
Canadian Brand Names Apo-Perphenazine®
Therapeutic Category Phenothiazine Derivative
Use Treatment of schizophrenia; severe nausea and vomiting
General Dosage Range Oral: *Adults:* 4-16 mg 2-4 times/day (maximum: 64 mg/day)
Dosage Forms
 Tablet, oral: 2 mg, 4 mg, 8 mg, 16 mg

perphenazine and amitriptyline hydrochloride *see* amitriptyline and perphenazine *on page 68*
Persantine® *see* dipyridamole *on page 298*
pertussis, acellular (adsorbed) *see* diphtheria and tetanus toxoids, acellular pertussis, poliovirus and *Haemophilus* b conjugate vaccine *on page 295*
pethidine hydrochloride *see* meperidine *on page 560*
Pexeva® *see* paroxetine *on page 676*
PFA *see* foscarnet *on page 400*
Pfizerpen® *see* penicillin G (parenteral/aqueous) *on page 685*
Pfizerpen-AS® (Can) *see* penicillin G procaine *on page 685*
PGE₁ *see* alprostadil *on page 57*
PGE₂ *see* dinoprostone *on page 289*
PGI₂ *see* epoprostenol *on page 334*
PGX *see* epoprostenol *on page 334*
Pharmorubicin® (Can) *see* epirubicin *on page 333*
Phazyme™ (Can) *see* simethicone *on page 812*
Phazyme® Ultra Strength [OTC] *see* simethicone *on page 812*
Phenabid® [DSC] *see* chlorpheniramine and phenylephrine *on page 198*
Phenadoz® *see* promethazine *on page 742*
Phenagesic [OTC] [DSC] *see* acetaminophen and phenyltoloxamine *on page 28*
Phenaseptic [OTC] *see* phenol *on page 694*
Phenazo™ (Can) *see* phenazopyridine *on page 692*

phenazopyridine (fen az oh PEER i deen)

Medication Safety Issues
 Sound-alike/look-alike issues:
  Phenazopyridine may be confused with phenoxybenzamine
  Pyridium® may be confused with Dyrenium®, Perdiem®, pyridoxine, pyrithione
Synonyms phenazopyridine hydrochloride; phenylazo diamino pyridine hydrochloride
U.S. Brand Names AZO Standard® Maximum Strength [OTC]; AZO Standard® [OTC]; Azo-Gesic™ [OTC]; Baridium [OTC]; Pyridium®; ReAzo [OTC]; UTI Relief® [OTC]
Canadian Brand Names Phenazo™
Therapeutic Category Analgesic, Urinary
Use Symptomatic relief of urinary burning, itching, frequency, and urgency in association with urinary tract infection or following urologic procedures
General Dosage Range Dosage adjustment recommended in patients with renal impairment
 Oral:
  Children: 12 mg/kg/day in 3 divided doses
  Adults: 100-200 mg 3 times/day
Dosage Forms
 Tablet, oral: 100 mg, 200 mg
  AZO Standard® [OTC]: 95 mg
  AZO Standard® Maximum Strength [OTC]: 97.5 mg
  Azo-Gesic™ [OTC]: 95 mg
  Baridium [OTC]: 97.2 mg
  Pyridium®: 100 mg, 200 mg
  ReAzo [OTC]: 95 mg
  UTI Relief® [OTC]: 97.2 mg

phenazopyridine hydrochloride *see phenazopyridine on page 692*

phendimetrazine (fen dye ME tra zeen)

Medication Safety Issues
Sound-alike/look-alike issues:
Bontril PDM® may be confused with Bentyl®
BEERS Criteria medication:
This drug may be inappropriate for use in geriatric patients (high severity risk).
Synonyms phendimetrazine tartrate
U.S. Brand Names Bontril® PDM; Bontril® Slow-Release
Canadian Brand Names Bontril®; Plegine®; Statobex®
Therapeutic Category Anorexiant
Controlled Substance C-III
Use Short-term (few weeks) adjunct in exogenous obesity

Pharmacotherapy for weight loss is recommended only for obese patients with a body mass index ≥30 kg/m^2, or ≥27 kg/m^2 in the presence of other risk factors such as hypertension, diabetes, and/or dyslipidemia or a high waist circumference; therapy should be used in conjunction with a comprehensive weight management program.
General Dosage Range Oral:
Capsule: *Adults:* 105 mg once daily before breakfast
Tablet: *Adults:* 17.5-35 mg 2-3 times/day, 1 hour before meals (maximum: 70 mg 3 times/day)
Dosage Forms
Capsule, slow release, oral: 105 mg
Bontril® Slow-Release: 105 mg
Tablet, oral: 35 mg
Bontril® PDM: 35 mg

phendimetrazine tartrate *see phendimetrazine on page 693*

phenelzine (FEN el zeen)

Medication Safety Issues
Sound-alike/look-alike issues:
Phenelzine may be confused with phenytoin
Nardil® may be confused with Norinyl®
Synonyms phenelzine sulfate
U.S. Brand Names Nardil®
Canadian Brand Names Nardil®
Therapeutic Category Antidepressant, Monoamine Oxidase Inhibitor
Use Symptomatic treatment of atypical, nonendogenous, or neurotic depression
General Dosage Range Oral: *Adults:* Initial: 45 mg/day in 3 divided doses; Maintenance: 15-90 mg/day in 1-3 divided doses
Dosage Forms
Tablet, oral: 15 mg
Nardil®: 15 mg

phenelzine sulfate *see phenelzine on page 693*
Phenergan® *see promethazine on page 742*
pheniramine and naphazoline *see naphazoline and pheniramine on page 611*

phenobarbital (fee noe BAR bi tal)

Medication Safety Issues
Sound-alike/look-alike issues:
PHENobarbital may be confused with PENTobarbital, Phenergan®, phenytoin
Luminal® may be confused with Tuinal®
Synonyms phenobarbital sodium; phenobarbitone; phenylethylmalonylurea
Tall-Man PHENobarbital
Canadian Brand Names PMS-Phenobarbital

Therapeutic Category Anticonvulsant; Barbiturate

Controlled Substance C-IV

Use Management of generalized tonic-clonic (grand mal), status epilepticus, and partial seizures; sedative/hypnotic

Note: Use to treat insomnia is not recommended (Schutte-Rodin, 2008)

General Dosage Range Dosage adjustment recommended in patients with renal impairment

I.M.:
Children: 3-5 mg/kg at bedtime or 1-3 mg/kg 1-1.5 hours before procedure
Adults: Dosage varies greatly depending on indication

I.V.:
Infants: Loading dose: 10-20 mg/kg in a single or divided dose; Maintenance: 5-8 mg/kg/day in 1-2 divided doses
Children: Loading dose: 15-20 mg/kg in a single or divided dose; Maintenance: Dosage varies greatly depending on indication
Adults: Loading dose: 10-20 mg/kg; may repeat dose in 20-minute intervals as needed (maximum total dose: 30 mg/kg); Maintenance: Dosage varies greatly depending on indication

Oral:
Infants: 5-8 mg/kg/day in 1-2 divided doses
Children and Adults: Dosage varies greatly depending on indication

Dosage Forms
Elixir, oral: 20 mg/5 mL (5 mL, 7.5 mL, 15 mL, 473 mL)
Injection, solution: 65 mg/mL (1 mL); 130 mg/mL (1 mL)
Tablet, oral: 15 mg, 30 mg, 60 mg, 100 mg

phenobarbital, hyoscyamine, atropine, and scopolamine *see* hyoscyamine, atropine, scopolamine, and phenobarbital *on page 459*

phenobarbital sodium *see* phenobarbital *on page 693*

phenobarbitone *see* phenobarbital *on page 693*

phenol (FEE nol)

Medication Safety Issues
Sound-alike/look-alike issues:
Cēpastat® may be confused with Capastat®

Synonyms carbolic acid

U.S. Brand Names Castellani Paint Modified [OTC]; Cepastat® Extra Strength [OTC]; Cepastat® [OTC]; Cheracol® Spray [OTC]; Chloraseptic® Kids Sore Throat Spray [OTC]; Chloraseptic® Mouth Pain [OTC]; Chloraseptic® Sore Throat Gargle [OTC]; Chloraseptic® Sore Throat Spray [OTC]; Pain-A-Lay® [OTC]; Phenaseptic [OTC]; Phenol EZ® [OTC]; Ulcerease® [OTC]; Vicks® Formula 44® Sore Throat [OTC]

Canadian Brand Names P & S™ Liquid Phenol

Therapeutic Category Pharmaceutical Aid

Use Relief of sore throat pain, mouth, gum, and throat irritations; antiseptic; topical anesthetic

General Dosage Range
Oral:
Children 2-12 years:
Chloraseptic®: 3 sprays onto throat or affected area; may repeat every 2 hours
Chloraseptic® for Kids: 5 sprays onto throat or affected area; may repeat every 2 hours
Children >3 years: Ulcerease®: Gargle or swish for 15 seconds, then expectorate; may repeat every 2 hours
Children 6-12 years:
Cēpastat® Extra Strength: Up to 1 lozenge every 2 hours as needed (maximum: 10 lozenges/24 hours)
Cēpastat®: Up to 1 lozenge every 2 hours as needed (maximum: 18 lozenges/24 hours)
Pain-A-Lay® Gargle: Using gauze pad, apply 10 mL to affected area, or gargle or swish for 15 seconds, then expectorate
Children ≥12 years and Adults:
Cēpastat® Extra Strength, Cēpastat®: Up to 2 lozenges every 2 hours as needed
Cheracol®, Pain-A-Lay® Spray: Spray directly in throat; rinse for 15 seconds then expectorate; may repeat every 2 hours
Chloraseptic®: 5 sprays onto throat or affected area; may repeat every 2 hours
Chloraseptic® Gargle, Cēpastat® Mouth Pain, Pain-A-Lay® Gargle, Ulcerease®: Gargle or swish for 15 seconds, then expectorate; may repeat every 2 hours

Topical: *Adults:* Apply small amount to affected area 1-3 times/day

Dosage Forms

Lozenge, oral:
  Cepastat® [OTC]: 14.5 mg (18s)
  Cepastat® Extra Strength [OTC]: 29 mg (18s)
Solution, oral: 1.4% (177 mL)
  Cheracol® Spray [OTC]: 1.4% (177 mL)
  Chloraseptic® Kids Sore Throat Spray [OTC]: 0.5% (177 mL)
  Chloraseptic® Mouth Pain [OTC]: 1.4% (29 mL)
  Chloraseptic® Sore Throat Gargle [OTC]: 1.4% (296 mL)
  Chloraseptic® Sore Throat Spray [OTC]: 1.4% (20 mL, 177 mL)
  Pain-A-Lay® [OTC]: 1.4% (177 mL, 236 mL, 532 mL)
  Phenaseptic [OTC]: 1.4% (177 mL)
  Ulcerease® [OTC]: 0.6% (30 mL, 180 mL)
  Vicks® Formula 44® Sore Throat [OTC]: 1.4% (177 mL)
Solution, topical:
  Castellani Paint Modified [OTC]: 1.5% (30 mL)
Swab, topical:
  Phenol EZ® [OTC]: 89% (30s)

phenol and camphor *see* camphor and phenol *on page 167*
Phenol EZ® [OTC] *see* phenol *on page 694*
phenoptin *see* sapropterin *on page 802*

phenoxybenzamine (fen oks ee BEN za meen)

Medication Safety Issues
  Sound-alike/look-alike issues:
    Phenoxybenzamine may be confused with phenazopyridine
Synonyms phenoxybenzamine hydrochloride
U.S. Brand Names Dibenzyline®
Therapeutic Category Alpha-Adrenergic Blocking Agent
Use Symptomatic management of pheochromocytoma
General Dosage Range Oral: *Adults:* Initial: 10 mg twice daily; Maintenance: 10-40 mg 1-3 times/day
  (maximum: 240 mg/day)
Dosage Forms
  Capsule, oral:
    Dibenzyline®: 10 mg

phenoxybenzamine hydrochloride *see* phenoxybenzamine *on page 695*
phenoxymethyl penicillin *see* penicillin V potassium *on page 686*

phentermine (FEN ter meen)

Medication Safety Issues
  Sound-alike/look-alike issues:
    Phentermine may be confused with phentolamine, phenytoin
  BEERS Criteria medication:
    This drug may be inappropriate for use in geriatric patients (high severity risk).
Synonyms phentermine hydrochloride
U.S. Brand Names Adipex-P®
Therapeutic Category Anorexiant
Controlled Substance C-IV
Use Short-term (few weeks) adjunct therapy in obese patients with an initial body mass index (BMI) ≥30
  kg/m^2 or ≥27 kg/m^2 in the presence of other risk factors (eg, diabetes, hyperlipidemia, hypertension);
  therapy should be used in conjunction with a comprehensive weight management program.
General Dosage Range Oral: *Children >16 years and Adults:* 15-37.5 mg/day
Product Availability
  Suprenza™: FDA approved June 2011; expected availability is undetermined.
  Suprenza™ is an oral disintegrating tablet formulation approved as a short-term adjunct in a
  comprehensive weight reduction regimen.

Dosage Forms
Capsule, oral: 15 mg, 30 mg, 37.5 mg
Adipex-P®: 37.5 mg
Tablet, oral: 37.5 mg
Adipex-P®: 37.5 mg

phentermine hydrochloride *see phentermine on page 695*

phentolamine (fen TOLE a meen)

Medication Safety Issues
Sound-alike/look-alike issues:
Phentolamine may be confused with phentermine, Ventolin®
Synonyms phentolamine mesylate; Regitine [DSC]
U.S. Brand Names OraVerse™
Canadian Brand Names Regitine®; Rogitine®
Therapeutic Category Alpha-Adrenergic Blocking Agent; Diagnostic Agent
Use Diagnosis of pheochromocytoma and treatment of hypertension associated with pheochromocytoma or other forms of hypertension caused by excess sympathomimetic amines; treatment of dermal necrosis after extravasation of drugs with alpha-adrenergic effects (ie, dopamine, epinephrine, norepinephrine, phenylephrine)
OraVerse™: Reversal of soft tissue anesthesia and the associated functional deficits resulting from a local dental anesthetic containing a vasoconstrictor
General Dosage Range
I.M., I.V.:
Children: 0.05-0.1 mg/kg/dose as a single dose 1-2 hours before procedure, repeat as needed every 2-4 hours (maximum: 5 mg/dose)
Adults: 5 mg as a single dose 1-2 hours before procedure, may repeat as needed every 2-4 hours **or** 5-20 mg (hypertensive crisis)
Submucosal injection:
Children 15-30 kg and <12 years: 0.2 mg (maximum)
Children >30 kg and <12 years: 0.4 mg (maximum)
Children >30 kg and ≥12 years and Adults: 0.2 mg to 0.8 mg (depending on number of cartridges of anesthesia)
SubQ: *Children and Adults:* Infiltrate area with a small amount (eg, 1 mL) of solution (made by diluting 5-10 mg in 10 mL of NS) within 12 hours of extravasation; in general, do not exceed 0.1-0.2 mg/kg (5 mg total); typically doses of ≤5 mg are effective
Dosage Forms
Injection, powder for reconstitution: 5 mg
Injection, solution [preservative free]:
OraVerse™: 0.4 mg/1.7 mL (1.7 mL)

phentolamine mesylate *see phentolamine on page 696*
phenylalanine mustard *see melphalan on page 556*
phenylazo diamino pyridine hydrochloride *see phenazopyridine on page 692*

phenylephrine (systemic) (fen il EF rin)

Medication Safety Issues
Sound-alike/look-alike issues:
Sudafed PE™ may be confused with Sudafed®
High alert medication:
The Institute for Safe Medication Practices (ISMP) includes this medication among its list of drugs which have a heightened risk of causing significant patient harm when used in error.
Synonyms phenylephrine hydrochloride
U.S. Brand Names LuSonal™ [DSC]; Medi-First® Sinus Decongestant [OTC]; Medi-Phenyl [OTC]; PediaCare® Children's Decongestant [OTC]; Sudafed PE® Children's [OTC]; Sudafed PE® Congestion [OTC]; Sudafed PE™ Nasal Decongestant [OTC]; Sudogest™ PE [OTC]; Triaminic Thin Strips® Children's Cold with Stuffy Nose [OTC]
Therapeutic Category Alpha/Beta Agonist
Use Treatment of hypotension, vascular failure in shock; as a vasoconstrictor in regional analgesia; supraventricular tachycardia (**Note:** Not for routine use in treatment of supraventricular tachycardias); as a decongestant [OTC]

General Dosage Range
I.V.:
Children: Bolus: 5-20 mcg/kg/dose every 10-15 minutes as needed; Infusion: 0.1-0.5 mcg/kg/minute
Adults: Bolus: 100-500 mcg/dose every 10-15 minutes as needed (maximum: 500 mcg); Infusion: Initial: 100-180 mcg/minute
Oral:
Children 4 to <6 years: 2.5 mg every 4 hours as needed for ≤7 days
Children 6 to <12 years: 5 mg every 4 hours as needed for ≤7 days
Children ≥12 years and Adults: 10-20 mg every 4 hours as needed for ≤7 days

Dosage Forms
Injection, solution: 1% [10 mg/mL] (1 mL, 2 mL, 5 mL, 10 mL)
Liquid, oral:
PediaCare® Children's Decongestant [OTC]: 2.5 mg/5 mL (118 mL)
Sudafed PE® Children's [OTC]: 2.5 mg/5 mL (118 mL)
Strip, orally disintegrating, oral:
Triaminic Thin Strips® Children's Cold with Stuffy Nose [OTC]: 2.5 mg (14s)
Tablet, oral:
Medi-First® Sinus Decongestant [OTC]: 10 mg
Medi-Phenyl [OTC]: 5 mg
Sudafed PE® Congestion [OTC]: 10 mg
Sudafed PE™ Nasal Decongestant [OTC]: 10 mg
Sudogest™ PE [OTC]: 10 mg

phenylephrine (nasal) (fen il EF rin)

Medication Safety Issues
Sound-alike/look-alike issues:
Neo-Synephrine® (phenylephrine, nasal) may be confused with Neo-Synephrine® (oxymetazoline)
Synonyms phenylephrine hydrochloride
U.S. Brand Names 4 Way® Fast Acting [OTC]; 4 Way® Menthol [OTC]; Little Noses® Decongestant [OTC]; Neo-Synephrine® Extra Strength [OTC]; Neo-Synephrine® Mild Formula [OTC]; Neo-Synephrine® Regular Strength [OTC]; Rhinall® [OTC]; Vicks® Sinex® VapoSpray™ 4 Hour Decongestant [OTC]
Canadian Brand Names Neo-Synephrine®
Therapeutic Category Alpha/Beta Agonist
Use For OTC use as symptomatic relief of nasal and nasopharyngeal mucosal congestion
General Dosage Range Intranasal:
Children 2-6 years: 0.125% solution: Instill 1 drop in each nostril every 2-4 hours as needed for ≤3 days
Children 6-12 years: 0.25% solution: Instill 2-3 sprays in each nostril every 4 hours as needed for ≤3 days
Children >12 years: 0.25% to 0.5% solution: Instill 2-3 sprays or 2-3 drops in each nostril every 4 hours as needed for ≤3 days
Adults: 0.25% to 1% solution: Instill 2-3 sprays or 2-3 drops in each nostril every 4 hours as needed for ≤3 days

Dosage Forms
Solution, intranasal:
4 Way® Fast Acting [OTC]: 1% (15 mL, 30 mL, 37 mL)
4 Way® Menthol [OTC]: 1% (15 mL, 30 mL)
Little Noses® Decongestant [OTC]: 0.125% (15 mL)
Neo-Synephrine® Extra Strength [OTC]: 1% (15 mL)
Neo-Synephrine® Mild Formula [OTC]: 0.25% (15 mL)
Neo-Synephrine® Regular Strength [OTC]: 0.5% (15 mL)
Rhinall® [OTC]: 0.25% (30 mL, 40 mL)
Vicks® Sinex® VapoSpray™ 4 Hour Decongestant [OTC]: 0.5% (15 mL)

phenylephrine (ophthalmic) (fen il EF rin)

Medication Safety Issues
Sound-alike/look-alike issues:
Mydfrin® may be confused with Midrin®
Synonyms phenylephrine hydrochloride
U.S. Brand Names AK-Dilate™; Altafrin; Mydfrin®; Neofrin; OcuNefrin™ [OTC] [DSC]
Canadian Brand Names Dionephrine®; Mydfrin®

◄ **Therapeutic Category** Alpha/Beta Agonist; Ophthalmic Agent, Antiglaucoma; Ophthalmic Agent, Mydriatic

Use Used as a mydriatic in ophthalmic procedures and treatment of wide-angle glaucoma; OTC use as symptomatic relief of redness of the eye due to irritation

General Dosage Range Ophthalmic:
Infants <1 year: Instill 1 drop of 2.5% solution 15-30 minutes before procedures
Children ≥1 year and Adults: Instill 1 drop of 2.5% or 10% solution; may repeat in 10-60 minutes as needed **or** 1-2 drops of 0.12% solution up to 4 times/day [OTC dosing] (maximum: 72 hours)

Dosage Forms
Solution, ophthalmic: 2.5% (2 mL, 3 mL, 5 mL, 15 mL)
AK-Dilate™: 2.5% (2 mL, 15 mL); 10% (5 mL)
Altafrin: 2.5% (15 mL); 10% (5 mL)
Mydfrin®: 2.5% (3 mL, 5 mL)
Neofrin: 2.5% (15 mL); 10% (5 mL)

phenylephrine (topical) (fen il EF rin)

Synonyms phenylephrine hydrochloride

U.S. Brand Names Anu-Med [OTC]; Formulation R™ [OTC]; Medicone® Suppositories [OTC]; Preparation H® [OTC]; Rectacaine [OTC]; Tronolane® Suppository [OTC]

Therapeutic Category Alpha/Beta Agonist

Use For OTC use as treatment of hemorrhoids

General Dosage Range Rectal: *Children >12 years and Adults:* Ointment: Apply up to 4 times/day; Suppository: Insert 1 up to 4 times/day

Dosage Forms
Ointment, rectal:
Formulation R™ [OTC]: 0.25% (30 g, 60 g)
Preparation H® [OTC]: 0.25% (30 g, 60 g)
Suppository, rectal: 0.25% (12s)
Anu-Med [OTC]: 0.25% (12s)
Medicone® Suppositories [OTC]: 0.25% (12s, 24s)
Preparation H® [OTC]: 0.25% (12s, 24s, 48s)
Rectacaine [OTC]: 0.25% (12s)
Tronolane® Suppository [OTC]: 0.25% (12s, 24s)

phenylephrine, acetaminophen, and dextromethorphan *see* acetaminophen, dextromethorphan, and phenylephrine *on page 32*

phenylephrine and brompheniramine *see* brompheniramine and phenylephrine *on page 143*

phenylephrine and chlorpheniramine *see* chlorpheniramine and phenylephrine *on page 198*

phenylephrine and cyclopentolate *see* cyclopentolate and phenylephrine *on page 242*

phenylephrine and dextromethorphan *see* dextromethorphan and phenylephrine *on page 271*

phenylephrine and diphenhydramine *see* diphenhydramine and phenylephrine *on page 292*

phenylephrine and promethazine *see* promethazine and phenylephrine *on page 744*

phenylephrine and pyrilamine (fen il EF rin & peer IL a meen)

Synonyms pyrilamine tannate and phenylephrine tannate

U.S. Brand Names Aldex®D [DSC]; Ryna-12 S® [DSC]; Ryna®-12 [DSC]

Therapeutic Category Antihistamine; Antihistamine/Decongestant Combination; Sympathomimetic

Use Symptomatic relief of nasal congestion and discharge associated with the common cold, sinusitis, allergic rhinitis, and other respiratory tract conditions

General Dosage Range Oral:
Children 2-6 years: 2.5 mL of the suspension or 1/2 tablet every 12 hours
Children 6-12 years: 5 mL of the suspension or 1/2 to 1 tablet every 12 hours
Children >12 years and Adults: 5-10 mL of the suspension or 1-2 tablets every 12 hours

phenylephrine and zinc sulfate *(Canada only)* (fen il EF rin & zingk SUL fate)

Synonyms zinc sulfate and phenylephrine

Canadian Brand Names Zincfrin®

Therapeutic Category Adrenergic Agonist Agent

Use Soothe, moisturize, and remove redness due to minor eye irritation

General Dosage Range Ophthalmic: *Adults:* Instill 1-2 drops in eye(s) 2-4 times/day as needed

Product Availability Not available in U.S.

Dosage Forms - Canada
  Solution, ophthalmic:
    Zincfrin® [OTC]: Phenylephrine 0.12% and zinc sulfate 0.25% (15 mL)

phenylephrine, chlorpheniramine, acetaminophen, and phenyltoloxamine *see* acetaminophen, chlorpheniramine, phenylephrine, and phenyltoloxamine *on page 31*

phenylephrine, chlorpheniramine, and dextromethorphan *see* chlorpheniramine, phenylephrine, and dextromethorphan *on page 200*

phenylephrine, chlorpheniramine, and dihydrocodeine *see* dihydrocodeine, chlorpheniramine, and phenylephrine *on page 285*

phenylephrine, chlorpheniramine, and guaifenesin *see* chlorpheniramine, phenylephrine, and guaifenesin *on page 200*

phenylephrine, chlorpheniramine, and phenyltoloxamine *see* chlorpheniramine, phenylephrine, and phenyltoloxamine *on page 201*

phenylephrine, chlorpheniramine, and pyrilamine *see* chlorpheniramine, pyrilamine, and phenylephrine *on page 202*

phenylephrine, dextromethorphan, and acetaminophen *see* acetaminophen, dextromethorphan, and phenylephrine *on page 32*

phenylephrine, ephedrine, chlorpheniramine, and carbetapentane *see* chlorpheniramine, ephedrine, phenylephrine, and carbetapentane *on page 199*

phenylephrine hydrochloride *see* phenylephrine (nasal) *on page 697*

phenylephrine hydrochloride *see* phenylephrine (ophthalmic) *on page 697*

phenylephrine hydrochloride *see* phenylephrine (systemic) *on page 696*

phenylephrine hydrochloride *see* phenylephrine (topical) *on page 698*

phenylephrine hydrochloride, acetaminophen, and diphenhydramine *see* acetaminophen, diphenhydramine, and phenylephrine *on page 33*

phenylephrine hydrochloride and acetaminophen *see* acetaminophen and phenylephrine *on page 28*

phenylephrine hydrochloride and diphenhydramine hydrochloride *see* diphenhydramine and phenylephrine *on page 292*

phenylephrine hydrochloride and guaifenesin *see* guaifenesin and phenylephrine *on page 428*

phenylephrine hydrochloride, chlorpheniramine maleate, dextromethorphan hydrobromide, and guaifenesin *see* dextromethorphan, chlorpheniramine, phenylephrine, and guaifenesin *on page 272*

phenylephrine hydrochloride, guaifenesin, and dextromethorphan hydrobromide *see* guaifenesin, dextromethorphan, and phenylephrine *on page 429*

phenylephrine, promethazine, and codeine *see* promethazine, phenylephrine, and codeine *on page 744*

phenylephrine, pyrilamine, and dextromethorphan
(fen il EF rin, peer IL a meen, & deks troe meth OR fan)

Synonyms pyrilamine maleate, dextromethorphan hydrobromide, and phenylephrine hydrochloride

U.S. Brand Names Codal-DM [OTC]

Therapeutic Category Antihistamine; Antihistamine/Decongestant/Antitussive; Antitussive; Sympathomimetic

Use Symptomatic relief of cough, nasal congestion, and discharge associated with the common cold, sinusitis, allergic rhinitis, and other respiratory tract conditions

General Dosage Range Oral:
  Children 6-12 years: (Codal-DM): 5 mL every 4 hours (maximum: 30mL/24 hours)
  Children ≥12 years and Adults: (Codal-DM): 10 mL every 4 hours (maximum: 60 mL/24 hours)

Dosage Forms
  Syrup:
    Codal-DM [OTC]: Phenylephrine 5 mg, pyrilamine 8.33 mg, and dextromethorphan 10 mg per 5 mL (480 mL)

phenylephrine, pyrilamine, and guaifenesin
(fen il EF rin, peer IL a meen, & gwye FEN e sin)

Synonyms guaifenesin, phenylephrine tannate, and pyrilamine tannate; pyrilamine tannate, guaifenesin, and phenylephrine tannate

U.S. Brand Names Ryna-12X® [DSC]

Therapeutic Category Alpha/Beta Agonist; Decongestant; Expectorant; Histamine H$_1$ Antagonist; Histamine H$_1$ Antagonist, First Generation

Use Symptomatic relief of cough, nasal congestion, and discharge associated with the common cold, sinusitis, allergic rhinitis, and other respiratory tract conditions

General Dosage Range Oral:
Children 2-6 years: 2.5-5 mL of the suspension every 12 hours
Children 6-11 years: 5-10 mL of the suspension **or** 1/2 to 1 tablet every 12 hours
Children ≥12 years and Adults: 1-2 tablets every 12 hours

phenylephrine tannate and diphenhydramine tannate *see* diphenhydramine and phenylephrine *on page 292*

phenylephrine tannate, carbetapentane tannate, and pyrilamine tannate *see* carbetapentane, phenylephrine, and pyrilamine *on page 173*

phenylephrine tannate, chlorpheniramine tannate, and methscopolamine nitrate *see* chlorpheniramine, phenylephrine, and methscopolamine *on page 200*

phenylethylmalonylurea *see* phenobarbital *on page 693*

Phenylhistine DH *see* chlorpheniramine, pseudoephedrine, and codeine *on page 201*

phenyl salicylate, methenamine, methylene blue, benzoic acid, and hyoscyamine *see* methenamine, phenyl salicylate, methylene blue, benzoic acid, and hyoscyamine *on page 569*

phenyltoloxamine, chlorpheniramine, and phenylephrine *see* chlorpheniramine, phenylephrine, and phenyltoloxamine *on page 201*

phenyltoloxamine, chlorpheniramine, phenylephrine, and acetaminophen *see* acetaminophen, chlorpheniramine, phenylephrine, and phenyltoloxamine *on page 31*

phenyltoloxamine citrate and acetaminophen *see* acetaminophen and phenyltoloxamine *on page 28*

Phenytek® *see* phenytoin *on page 700*

phenytoin (FEN i toyn)

Medication Safety Issues

Sound-alike/look-alike issues:
Phenytoin may be confused with phenelzine, phentermine, PHENobarbital
Dilantin® may be confused with Dilaudid®, diltiazem, Dipentum®

High alert medication:
The Institute for Safe Medication Practices (ISMP) includes this medication (I.V. formulation) among its list of drug classes which have a heightened risk of causing significant patient harm when used in error.

International issues:
Dilantin [U.S., Canada, and multiple international markets] may be confused with Dolantine brand name for pethidine [Belgium]

Synonyms diphenylhydantoin; DPH; phenytoin sodium; phenytoin sodium, extended; phenytoin sodium, prompt

U.S. Brand Names Dilantin-125®; Dilantin®; Phenytek®

Canadian Brand Names Dilantin®

Therapeutic Category Antiarrhythmic Agent, Class I-B; Hydantoin

Use Management of generalized tonic-clonic (grand mal), complex partial seizures; prevention of seizures following head trauma/neurosurgery

General Dosage Range
I.V.:
Children 6 months to 3 years: Loading dose: 15-20 mg/kg in a single or divided dose; Maintenance: 5-10 mg/kg/day in 2 divided doses
Children 4-6 years: Loading dose: 15-20 mg/kg in a single or divided dose; Maintenance: 5-9 mg/kg/day in 2 divided doses
Children 7-9 years: Loading dose: 15-20 mg/kg in a single or divided dose; Maintenance: 5-8 mg/kg/day in 2 divided doses

Children 10-16 years: Loading dose: 15-20 mg/kg in a single or divided dose; Maintenance: 5-7 mg/kg/day in 2 divided doses

Adolescents >16 years and Adults: Loading dose: 10-25 mg/kg in a single or divided dose; Maintenance: 300 mg/day **or** 5-6 mg/kg/day in 3 divided doses

Oral:

Children: Loading dose: 15-20 mg/kg in divided doses; Maintenance: 4-8 mg/kg/day in divided doses

Adults: Loading dose: 15-20 mg/kg in 3 divided doses every 2-4 hours; Maintenance: 300 mg/day in 1-3 divided doses **or** 5-6 mg/kg/day in 1-3 divided doses **or** 100 mg every 6-8 hours (range: 200-1200 mg/day)

Dosage Forms

Capsule, extended release, oral: 100 mg, 200 mg, 300 mg

Dilantin®: 30 mg, 100 mg

Phenytek®: 200 mg, 300 mg

Injection, solution: 50 mg/mL (2 mL, 5 mL)

Suspension, oral: 100 mg/4 mL (4 mL); 125 mg/5 mL (120 mL, 237 mL, 240 mL)

Dilantin-125®: 125 mg/5 mL (240 mL)

Tablet, chewable, oral:

Dilantin®: 50 mg

phenytoin sodium *see* phenytoin *on page 700*

phenytoin sodium, extended *see* phenytoin *on page 700*

phenytoin sodium, prompt *see* phenytoin *on page 700*

Phillips'® M-O [OTC] *see* magnesium hydroxide and mineral oil *on page 546*

Phillips'® Laxative Dietary Supplement Cramp-Free [OTC] *see* magnesium oxide *on page 546*

Phillips'® Liquid-Gels® [OTC] *see* docusate *on page 302*

Phillips'® Milk of Magnesia [OTC] *see* magnesium hydroxide *on page 545*

Phillips'® Stool Softener Laxative [OTC] *see* docusate *on page 302*

pHisoHex® *see* hexachlorophene *on page 440*

PHL-Alendronate (Can) *see* alendronate *on page 49*

PHL-Amiodarone (Can) *see* amiodarone *on page 67*

PHL-Amlodipine (Can) *see* amlodipine *on page 69*

PHL-Amoxicillin (Can) *see* amoxicillin *on page 73*

PHL-Atenolol (Can) *see* atenolol *on page 101*

PHL-Azithromycin (Can) *see* azithromycin (systemic) *on page 108*

PHL-Baclofen (Can) *see* baclofen *on page 112*

PHL-Bicalutamide (Can) *see* bicalutamide *on page 133*

PHL-Bisoprolol (Can) *see* bisoprolol *on page 136*

PHL-Carvedilol (Can) *see* carvedilol *on page 178*

PHL-Cilazapril (Can) *see* cilazapril (Canada only) *on page 208*

PHL-Ciprofloxacin (Can) *see* ciprofloxacin (systemic) *on page 210*

PHL-Citalopram (Can) *see* citalopram *on page 213*

PHL-Cyclobenzaprine (Can) *see* cyclobenzaprine *on page 241*

PHL-Divalproex (Can) *see* divalproex *on page 300*

PHL-Domperidone (Can) *see* domperidone (Canada only) *on page 305*

PHL-Doxycycline (Can) *see* doxycycline *on page 312*

PHL-Fenofibrate Micro (Can) *see* fenofibrate *on page 369*

PHL-Fenofibrate Supra (Can) *see* fenofibrate *on page 369*

PHL-Fluconazole (Can) *see* fluconazole *on page 381*

PHL-Fluoxetine (Can) *see* fluoxetine *on page 389*

PHL-Gabapentin (Can) *see* gabapentin *on page 405*

PHL-Indapamide (Can) *see* indapamide *on page 470*

PHL-Leflunomide (Can) *see* leflunomide *on page 514*

PHL-Levetiracetam (Can) *see* levetiracetam *on page 517*

PHL-Lithium Carbonate (Can) *see* lithium *on page 532*

PHL-Lorazepam (Can) *see* lorazepam *on page 537*

PHL-Lovastatin (Can) *see* lovastatin *on page 540*

PHL-Loxapine (Can) *see* loxapine *on page 541*
PHL-Meloxicam (Can) *see* meloxicam *on page 556*
PHL-Metformin (Can) *see* metformin *on page 566*
PHL-Methimazole (Can) *see* methimazole *on page 570*
PHL-Methylphenidate (Can) *see* methylphenidate *on page 577*
PHL-Metoprolol (Can) *see* metoprolol *on page 581*
PHL-Minocycline (Can) *see* minocycline *on page 590*
PHL-Mirtazapine (Can) *see* mirtazapine *on page 592*
PHL-Olanzapine (Can) *see* olanzapine *on page 645*
PHL-Olanzapine ODT (Can) *see* olanzapine *on page 645*
PHL-Ondansetron (Can) *see* ondansetron *on page 651*
PHL-Oxybutynin (Can) *see* oxybutynin *on page 661*
PHL-Paroxetine (Can) *see* paroxetine *on page 676*
PHL-Pioglitazone (Can) *see* pioglitazone *on page 706*
PHL-Pramipexole (Can) *see* pramipexole *on page 729*
PHL-Pravastatin (Can) *see* pravastatin *on page 732*
PHL-Procyclidine (Can) *see* procyclidine *(Canada only) on page 741*
PHL-Quetiapine (Can) *see* quetiapine *on page 760*
PHL-Ramipril (Can) *see* ramipril *on page 766*
PHL-Ranitidine (Can) *see* ranitidine *on page 767*
PHL-Risperidone (Can) *see* risperidone *on page 783*
PHL-Salbutamol (Can) *see* albuterol *on page 45*
PHL-Sertraline (Can) *see* sertraline *on page 809*
PHL-Simvastatin (Can) *see* simvastatin *on page 813*
PHL-Sotalol (Can) *see* sotalol *on page 828*
PHL-Sumatriptan (Can) *see* sumatriptan *on page 839*
PHL-Temazepam (Can) *see* temazepam *on page 848*
PHL-Terazosin (Can) *see* terazosin *on page 851*
PHL-Terbinafine (Can) *see* terbinafine *(systemic) on page 851*
PHL-Topiramate (Can) *see* topiramate *on page 877*
PHL-Trazodone (Can) *see* trazodone *on page 884*
PHL-Ursodiol C (Can) *see* ursodiol *on page 902*
PHL-Valacyclovir (Can) *see* valacyclovir *on page 903*
PHL-Valproic Acid (Can) *see* valproic acid *on page 904*
PHL-Valproic Acid E.C. (Can) *see* valproic acid *on page 904*
PHL-Verapamil SR (Can) *see* verapamil *on page 912*
PHL-Zopiclone (Can) *see* zopiclone *(Canada only) on page 934*
Phos-Flur® *see* fluoride *on page 386*
Phos-Flur® Rinse [OTC] *see* fluoride *on page 386*
PhosLo® *see* calcium acetate *on page 160*
Phoslyra™ *see* calcium acetate *on page 160*
Phos-NaK *see* potassium phosphate and sodium phosphate *on page 727*
Phospha 250™ Neutral *see* potassium phosphate and sodium phosphate *on page 727*
phosphate, potassium *see* potassium phosphate *on page 726*
phosphates, sodium *see* sodium phosphates *on page 823*
Phosphocol® P 32 *see* chromic phosphate P 32 *on page 206*
Phospholine Iodide® *see* echothiophate iodide *on page 319*
phosphonoformate *see* foscarnet *on page 400*
phosphonoformic acid *see* foscarnet *on page 400*
phosphorated carbohydrate solution *see* fructose, dextrose, and phosphoric acid *on page 403*
phosphoric acid, levulose and dextrose *see* fructose, dextrose, and phosphoric acid *on page 403*
phosphorus p32 *see* chromic phosphate P 32 *on page 206*
Photofrin® *see* porfimer *on page 722*

Phrenilin® *see* butalbital and acetaminophen *on page 153*
Phrenilin® Forte *see* butalbital and acetaminophen *on page 153*
p-hydroxyampicillin *see* amoxicillin *on page 73*
Phyllocontin® (Can) *see* aminophylline *on page 66*
Phyllocontin®-350 (Can) *see* aminophylline *on page 66*
phylloquinone *see* phytonadione *on page 703*

physostigmine (fye zoe STIG meen)

Medication Safety Issues
Sound-alike/look-alike issues:
Physostigmine may be confused with Prostigmin®, pyridostigmine

Synonyms eserine salicylate; physostigmine salicylate; physostigmine sulfate

Therapeutic Category Cholinesterase Inhibitor

Use Reverse toxic, life-threatening delirium caused by atropine, diphenhydramine, dimenhydrinate, *Atropa belladonna* (deadly nightshade), or jimsonweed (*Datura* spp)

General Dosage Range
I.M.: *Adults:* Initial: 0.5-2 mg, repeat every 20 minutes until response or adverse effects occur; repeat 1-4 mg every 30-60 minutes as life-threatening symptoms recur
I.V.:
Children: 0.01-0.03 mg/kg/dose, may repeat after 5-10 minutes (maximum total dose: 2 mg)
Adults: Initial: 0.5-2 mg, repeat every 20 minutes until response or adverse effects occur; repeat 1-4 mg every 30-60 minutes as life-threatening symptoms recur

Dosage Forms
Injection, solution: 1 mg/mL (2 mL)

physostigmine salicylate *see* physostigmine *on page 703*
physostigmine sulfate *see* physostigmine *on page 703*
phytomenadione *see* phytonadione *on page 703*

phytonadione (fye toe na DYE one)

Medication Safety Issues
Sound-alike/look-alike issues:
Mephyton® may be confused with melphalan, methadone

Synonyms methylphytyl napthoquinone; phylloquinone; phytomenadione; vitamin K_1

U.S. Brand Names Mephyton®

Canadian Brand Names AquaMEPHYTON®; Konakion; Mephyton®

Therapeutic Category Vitamin, Fat Soluble

Use Prevention and treatment of hypoprothrombinemia caused by coumarin derivative-induced or other drug-induced vitamin K deficiency, hypoprothrombinemia caused by malabsorption or inability to synthesize vitamin K; hemorrhagic disease of the newborn

General Dosage Range
I.M.:
Newborns: Prophylaxis: 0.5-1 mg within 1 hour of birth; Treatment: 1 mg/dose/day
Adults: Initial: 2.5-25 mg/dose (usual: 5-10 mg; maximum: 50 mg)
I.V.: *Adults:* Initial: 2.5-25 mg/dose (usual: 5-10 mg; maximum: 50 mg)
Oral:
Children 1-3 years: RDA: 30 mcg/day
Children 4-8 years: RDA: 55 mcg/day
Children 9-13 years: RDA: 60 mcg/day
Children 14-18 years: RDA: 75 mcg/day
Adults: Initial: 2.5-25 mg/dose (usual: 5-10 mg; maximum: 50 mg)
SubQ:
Newborns: 1 mg/dose/day
Adults: Initial: 2.5-25 mg/dose (usual: 5-10 mg; maximum: 50 mg)

Dosage Forms
Injection, aqueous colloidal: 1 mg/0.5 mL (0.5 mL); 10 mg/mL (1 mL)
Injection, aqueous colloidal [preservative free]: 1 mg/0.5 mL (0.5 mL)
Tablet, oral: 100 mcg
Mephyton®: 5 mg

pidorubicin see epirubicin on page 333
pidorubicin hydrochloride see epirubicin on page 333

pilocarpine (systemic) (pye loe KAR peen)

Medication Safety Issues
Sound-alike/look-alike issues:
  Salagen® may be confused with Salacid®, selegiline
Synonyms pilocarpine hydrochloride
U.S. Brand Names Salagen®
Canadian Brand Names Salagen®
Therapeutic Category Cholinergic Agonist
Use Symptomatic treatment of xerostomia caused by salivary gland hypofunction resulting from radiotherapy for cancer of the head and neck or Sjögren syndrome
General Dosage Range Dosage adjustment recommended in patients with hepatic impairment
  Oral: *Adults:* 5 mg 3-4 times/day (maximum: 30 mg/day)
Dosage Forms
  Tablet, oral: 5 mg, 7.5 mg
    Salagen®: 5 mg, 7.5 mg

pilocarpine (ophthalmic) (pye loe KAR peen)

Medication Safety Issues
Sound-alike/look-alike issues:
  Isopto® Carpine may be confused with Isopto® Carbachol
Synonyms pilocarpine hydrochloride
U.S. Brand Names Isopto® Carpine; Pilopine HS®
Canadian Brand Names Diocarpine; Isopto® Carpine; Pilopine HS®
Therapeutic Category Ophthalmic Agent, Antiglaucoma; Ophthalmic Agent, Miotic
Use Management of chronic simple glaucoma, chronic and acute angle-closure glaucoma
General Dosage Range Ophthalmic: *Adults:* Gel: Instill 0.5" ribbon once daily at bedtime; Solution: Instill 1-2 drops up to 6 times/day
Dosage Forms
  Gel, ophthalmic:
    Pilopine HS®: 4% (4 g)
  Solution, ophthalmic: 1% (2 mL, 15 mL); 2% (2 mL, 15 mL); 4% (2 mL, 15 mL)
    Isopto® Carpine: 1% (15 mL); 2% (15 mL); 4% (15 mL)

pilocarpine hydrochloride see pilocarpine (ophthalmic) on page 704
pilocarpine hydrochloride see pilocarpine (systemic) on page 704
Pilopine HS® see pilocarpine (ophthalmic) on page 704
pimaricin see natamycin on page 614

pimecrolimus (pim e KROE li mus)

Medication Safety Issues
Sound-alike/look-alike issues:
  Pimecrolimus may be confused with tacrolimus
U.S. Brand Names Elidel®
Canadian Brand Names Elidel®
Therapeutic Category Immunosuppressant Agent; Topical Skin Product
Use Short-term and intermittent long-term treatment of mild-to-moderate atopic dermatitis in patients not responsive to conventional therapy or when conventional therapy is not appropriate
General Dosage Range Topical: *Children >2 years and Adults:* Apply thin layer to affected area twice daily
Dosage Forms
  Cream, topical:
    Elidel®: 1% (30 g, 60 g, 100 g)

pimozide (PI moe zide)

U.S. Brand Names Orap®

Canadian Brand Names Apo-Pimozide®; Orap®; PMS-Pimozide

Therapeutic Category Neuroleptic Agent

Use Suppression of severe motor and phonic tics in patients with Tourette disorder who have failed to respond satisfactorily to standard treatment

General Dosage Range Dosage adjustment recommended in patients who develop toxicities
Oral:
   Children ≤12 years: Initial: 0.05 mg/kg once daily (preferably bedtime); Maintenance: 2-4 mg once daily (maximum: 10 mg/day [0.2 mg/kg/day])
   Children >12 years and Adults: Initial: 1-2 mg in divided doses; Maintenance: 7-10 mg/day in divided doses (maximum: 10 mg/day [0.2 mg/kg/day])

Dosage Forms
  Tablet, oral:
   Orap®: 1 mg, 2 mg

Pin-X® [OTC] *see* pyrantel pamoate *on page 756*

pinaverium bromide *see* pinaverium *(Canada only) on page 705*

pinaverium *(Canada only)* (pin ah VEER ee um)

Synonyms pinaverium bromide

Canadian Brand Names Dicetel®

Therapeutic Category Calcium Antagonist; Gastrointestinal Agent, Miscellaneous

Use Treatment and relief of symptoms associated with irritable bowel syndrome (IBS); treatment of symptoms related to functional disorders of the biliary tract

General Dosage Range Oral: *Adults:* 50 mg 3 times/day (maximum: 300 mg/day)

Product Availability Not available in U.S.

Dosage Forms - Canada
  Tablet, oral:
   Dicetel®: 50 mg, 100 mg

pindolol (PIN doe lole)

Medication Safety Issues
  Sound-alike/look-alike issues:
   Pindolol may be confused with Parlodel®, Plendil®
   Visken® may be confused with Visine®, Viskazide®

Canadian Brand Names Apo-Pindol®; Dom-Pindolol; Mylan-Pindolol; Novo-Pindol; Nu-Pindol; PMS-Pindolol; Sandoz-Pindolol; Visken®

Therapeutic Category Beta-Adrenergic Blocker

Use Treatment of hypertension, alone or in combination with other agents

General Dosage Range Dosage adjustment recommended in patients with hepatic impairment
Oral:
  Adults: Initial: 5 mg twice daily; Maintenance: 10-40 mg twice daily (maximum: 60 mg/day)
  Elderly: Initial: 5 mg once daily

Dosage Forms
  Tablet, oral: 5 mg, 10 mg

pindolol and hydrochlorothiazide *(Canada only)*
(PIN doe lole & hye droe klor oh THYE a zide)

Medication Safety Issues
  Sound-alike/look-alike issues:
   Viskazide® may be confused with hydrochlorothiazide, Visken®

Synonyms hydrochlorothiazide and pindolol

Canadian Brand Names Viskazide®

Therapeutic Category Beta Blocker With Intrinsic Sympathomimetic Activity; Diuretic, Thiazide

Use Treatment of hypertension; not for initial therapy

General Dosage Range Oral: *Adults:* Usual dose: Pindolol 10-20 mg and hydrochlorothiazide 25-100 mg once daily (maximum daily dose: Pindolol 20 mg/hydrochlorothiazide 100 mg)

Product Availability Not available in U.S.

◀ **Dosage Forms - Canada**
   Tablet, oral:
   Viskazide® 10/25: Pindolol 10 mg and hydrochlorothiazide 25 mg
   Viskazide® 10/50: Pindolol 10 mg and hydrochlorothiazide 50 mg

pink bismuth *see* bismuth *on page* 135

pioglitazone (pye oh GLI ta zone)

Medication Safety Issues
Sound-alike/look-alike issues:
   Actos® may be confused with Actidose®, Actonel®
International issues:
   Tiazac: Brand name for piogitazone [Chile], but also the brand name for diltiazem [U.S, Canada]
U.S. Brand Names Actos®
Canadian Brand Names Accel-Pioglitazone; Actos®; Apo-Pioglitazone®; CO Pioglitazone; Dom-Pioglitazone; JAMP-Pioglitazone; Mint-Pioglitazone; Mylan-Pioglitazone; Novo-Pioglitazone; PHL-Pioglitazone; PMS-Pioglitazone; PRO-Pioglitazone; ratio-Pioglitazone; Sandoz-Pioglitazone; Teva-Pioglitazone; ZYM-Pioglitazone
Therapeutic Category Antidiabetic Agent, Oral; Thiazolidinedione Derivative
Use
   Type 2 diabetes mellitus (noninsulin-dependent, NIDDM), monotherapy: Adjunct to diet and exercise, to improve glycemic control
   Type 2 diabetes mellitus (noninsulin-dependent, NIDDM), combination therapy with sulfonylurea, metformin, or insulin: When diet, exercise, and a single agent alone does not result in adequate glycemic control
General Dosage Range Oral: *Adults:* Initial: 15-30 mg once daily; Maintenance: 15-45 mg once daily (maximum: 45 mg/day)
Dosage Forms
Tablet, oral:
   Actos®: 15 mg, 30 mg, 45 mg

pioglitazone and glimepiride (pye oh GLI ta zone & GLYE me pye ride)

Medication Safety Issues
High alert medication:
   The Institute for Safe Medication Practices (ISMP) includes this medication among its list of drugs which have a heightened risk of causing significant patient harm when used in error.
Synonyms glimepiride and pioglitazone; glimepiride and pioglitazone hydrochloride
U.S. Brand Names Duetact™
Therapeutic Category Antidiabetic Agent, Sulfonylurea; Antidiabetic Agent, Thiazolidinedione; Hypoglycemic Agent, Oral
Use Management of type 2 diabetes mellitus (noninsulin-dependent, NIDDM) as an adjunct to diet and exercise
General Dosage Range Dosage adjustment recommended in patients with renal impairment
Oral:
   Adults:
   Patients inadequately controlled on **glimepiride** alone: Initial dose: Pioglitazone 30 mg and glimepiride 2-4 mg once daily (maximum: 45 mg/day [pioglitazone]; 8 mg/day [glimepiride])
   Patients inadequately controlled on **pioglitazone** alone: Initial dose: Pioglitazone 30 mg and glimepiride 2 mg once daily (maximum: 45 mg/day [pioglitazone]; 8 mg/day [glimepiride])
   Elderly: Initial: Glimepiride 1 mg/day prior to initiating Duetact™
Dosage Forms
Tablet:
   Duetact™: 30 mg/2 mg: Pioglitazone 30 mg and glimepiride 2 mg; 30 mg/4 mg: Pioglitazone 30 mg and glimepiride 4 mg

pioglitazone and metformin (pye oh GLI ta zone & met FOR min)

Synonyms metformin hydrochloride and pioglitazone hydrochloride
U.S. Brand Names Actoplus Met®; Actoplus Met® XR
Therapeutic Category Antidiabetic Agent, Biguanide; Antidiabetic Agent, Thiazolidinedione
Use Management of type 2 diabetes mellitus (noninsulin-dependent, NIDDM)

General Dosage Range Oral: *Adults:*
Immediate release tablet: Pioglitazone 15-45 mg/day and metformin 500-2550 mg/day (maximum: 45 mg/day [pioglitazone]; 2550 mg/day [metformin])
Variable release tablet: Pioglitazone 15-45 mg/day and metformin 1000-2000 mg/day (maximum: 45 mg/day [pioglitazone]; 2000 mg/day [metformin])

Dosage Forms
Tablet, oral:
Actoplus Met®: 15/500: Pioglitazone 15 mg and metformin 500 mg; 15/850: Pioglitazone 15 mg and metformin 850 mg
Tablet, variable release, oral:
Actoplus Met® XR: 15/1000: Pioglitazone 15 mg and metformin 1000 mg; 30/1000: Pioglitazone 30 mg and metformin 1000 mg

piperacillin (pi PER a sil in)

Synonyms piperacillin sodium

Canadian Brand Names Piperacillin for Injection, USP

Therapeutic Category Penicillin

Use Treatment of susceptible infections such as septicemia, acute and chronic respiratory tract infections, skin and soft tissue infections, and urinary tract infections due to susceptible strains of *Pseudomonas*, *Proteus*, and *Escherichia coli* and *Enterobacter*; active against some streptococci and some anaerobic bacteria; febrile neutropenia (as part of combination regimen)

General Dosage Range Dosage adjustment recommended in patients with renal impairment
I.M., I.V.:
Children: 200-300 mg/kg/day in divided doses every 4-6 hours
Adults: 2-4 g/dose every 4-6 hours (maximum: 24 g/day)

Piperacillin and Tazobactam for Injection (Can) *see* piperacillin and tazobactam sodium on page 707

piperacillin and tazobactam sodium (pi PER a sil in & ta zoe BAK tam SOW dee um)

Medication Safety Issues
Sound-alike/look-alike issues:
Zosyn® may be confused with Zofran®, Zyvox®
International issues:
Tazact [India] may be confused with Tazac brand name for nizatidine [Australia]; Tiazac brand name for diltiazem [U.S., Canada]

Synonyms piperacillin sodium and tazobactam sodium; tazobactam and piperacillin

U.S. Brand Names Zosyn®

Canadian Brand Names Piperacillin and Tazobactam for Injection; Tazocin®

Therapeutic Category Penicillin

Use Treatment of moderate-to-severe infections caused by susceptible organisms, including infections of the lower respiratory tract (community-acquired pneumonia, nosocomial pneumonia); urinary tract; uncomplicated and complicated skin and skin structures; gynecologic (endometritis, pelvic inflammatory disease); bone and joint infections; intraabdominal infections (appendicitis with rupture/abscess, peritonitis); and septicemia. Tazobactam expands activity of piperacillin to include beta-lactamase producing strains of *S. aureus*, *H. influenzae*, *Bacteroides*, and other gram-negative bacteria.

General Dosage Range Dosage adjustment recommended in patients with renal impairment
I.V.:
Children 2-8 months: 80 mg/kg every 8 hours
Children ≥9 months and ≤40 kg: 100 mg/kg every 8 hours
Children >40 kg: 4.5 g every 8 hours **or** 3.375 g every 6 hours
Adults: 3.375 g every 6 hours **or** 4.5 g every 6-8 hours (maximum: 18 g/day)

Dosage Forms 8:1 ratio of piperacillin sodium/tazobactam sodium
Infusion [premixed iso-osmotic solution, frozen]:
Zosyn®:
2.25 g: Piperacillin 2 g and tazobactam 0.25 g (50 mL)
3.375 g: Piperacillin 3 g and tazobactam 0.375 g (50 mL)
4.5 g: Piperacillin 4 g and tazobactam 0.5 g (100 mL)

◀ **Injection, powder for reconstitution:** 2.25 g: Piperacillin 2 g and tazobactam 0.25 g; 3.375 g: Piperacillin 3 g and tazobactam 0.375 g; 4.5 g: Piperacillin 4 g and tazobactam 0.5 g; 40.5 g: Piperacillin 36 g and tazobactam 4.5 g

Zosyn®:
2.25 g: Piperacillin 2 g and tazobactam 0.25 g
3.375 g: Piperacillin 3 g and tazobactam 0.375 g
4.5 g: Piperacillin 4 g and tazobactam 0.5 g
40.5 g: Piperacillin 36 g and tazobactam 4.5 g

Piperacillin for Injection, USP (Can) *see* piperacillin *on page 707*
piperacillin sodium *see* piperacillin *on page 707*
piperacillin sodium and tazobactam sodium *see* piperacillin and tazobactam sodium *on page 707*
piperazine estrone sulfate *see* estropipate *on page 349*
piperonyl butoxide and pyrethrins *see* pyrethrins and piperonyl butoxide *on page 756*

pirbuterol (peer BYOO ter ole)

Synonyms pirbuterol acetate
U.S. Brand Names Maxair® Autohaler®
Therapeutic Category Adrenergic Agonist Agent
Use Prevention and treatment of reversible bronchospasm including asthma
General Dosage Range Inhalation: *Children ≥12 years and Adults:* Prevention: 2 inhalations every 4-6 hours; Treatment: 2 inhalations at an interval of at least 1-3 minutes, followed by a third inhalation (maximum: 12 inhalations/day)
Dosage Forms
Aerosol, for oral inhalation:
Maxair® Autohaler®: 200 mcg/actuation (14 g)

pirbuterol acetate *see* pirbuterol *on page 708*

piroxicam (peer OKS i kam)

Medication Safety Issues
Sound-alike/look-alike issues:
Feldene® may be confused with FLUoxetine
Piroxicam may be confused with PARoxetine
BEERS Criteria medication:
This drug may be inappropriate for use in geriatric patients (high severity risk).
International issues:
Flogene [Brazil] may be confused with Florone brand name for diflorasone [Germany, Greece]
U.S. Brand Names Feldene®
Canadian Brand Names Apo-Piroxicam®; Dom-Piroxicam; Gen-Piroxicam; Novo-Pirocam; Nu-Pirox; PMS-Piroxicam; PRO-Piroxicam
Therapeutic Category Analgesic, Nonnarcotic; Nonsteroidal Antiinflammatory Drug (NSAID)
Use Symptomatic treatment of acute and chronic rheumatoid arthritis and osteoarthritis
General Dosage Range Dosage adjustment recommended in patients with hepatic impairment
Oral:
Adults: 10-20 mg once daily (maximum: 20 mg/day: higher doses used with increased frequency of adverse effects)
Elderly: Initial: 10 mg every other day has been used (maximum: 20 mg/day)
Dosage Forms
Capsule, oral: 10 mg, 20 mg
Feldene®: 10 mg, 20 mg

p-isobutylhydratropic acid *see* ibuprofen *on page 460*
pit *see* oxytocin *on page 666*

pitavastatin (pi TA va sta tin)

Medication Safety Issues
Sound-alike/look-alike issues:
Pitavastatin may be confused with atorvastatin, fluvastatin, lovastatin, nystatin, pravastatin, rosuvastatin, simvastatin
Synonyms pitavastatin calcium

U.S. Brand Names Livalo®

Therapeutic Category Antilipemic Agent, HMG-CoA Reductase Inhibitor

Use Adjunct to dietary therapy to reduce elevations in total cholesterol (TC), LDL-C, apolipoprotein B (Apo B), and triglycerides (TG), and to increase low HDL-C in patients with primary hyperlipidemia and mixed dyslipidemia

General Dosage Range Dosage adjustment recommended in patients with renal impairment or on concomitant therapy

Oral: *Adults:* Initial: 2 mg once daily; Maintenance: 2-4 mg once daily (maximum: 4 mg/day)

Dosage Forms
Tablet, oral:
Livalo®: 1 mg, 2 mg, 4 mg

pitavastatin calcium *see* pitavastatin *on page 708*

Pitocin® *see* oxytocin *on page 666*

Pitressin® *see* vasopressin *on page 910*

Pitrex (Can) *see* tolnaftate *on page 876*

pix carbonis *see* coal tar *on page 227*

pizotifen *(Canada only)* (pi ZOE ti fen)

Synonyms pizotifen malate

Canadian Brand Names Sandomigran DS®; Sandomigran®

Therapeutic Category Antimigraine Agent

Use Migraine prophylaxis

General Dosage Range Oral: *Children ≥12 years and Adults:* Initial: 0.5 mg at bedtime; Maintenance: 1-6 mg/day in 1-3 divided doses

Product Availability Not available in U.S.

Dosage Forms - Canada
Tablet:
Sandomigran®: 0.5 mg
Tablet, double strength:
Sandomigran® DS: 1 mg

pizotifen malate *see* pizotifen *(Canada only) on page 709*

Plan B *see* levonorgestrel *on page 521*

Plan B® (Can) *see* levonorgestrel *on page 521*

Plan B® One Step *see* levonorgestrel *on page 521*

plantago seed *see* psyllium *on page 755*

plantain seed *see* psyllium *on page 755*

Plaquenil® *see* hydroxychloroquine *on page 454*

Plasbumin®-5 *see* albumin *on page 44*

Plasbumin®-25 *see* albumin *on page 44*

Plasmanate® *see* plasma protein fraction *on page 709*

plasma protein fraction (PLAS mah PROE teen FRAK shun)

U.S. Brand Names Plasmanate®

Therapeutic Category Blood Product Derivative

Use Plasma volume expansion and maintenance of cardiac output in the treatment of certain types of shock or impending shock

General Dosage Range I.V.: *Adults:* Usual minimum dose: 250-500 mL; adjust dose based on response

Dosage Forms
Injection, solution [preservative free]:
Plasmanate®: 5% (50 mL, 250 mL)

Platinol *see* cisplatin *on page 213*

Platinol-AQ *see* cisplatin *on page 213*

Plavix® *see* clopidogrel *on page 224*

Plegine® (Can) *see* phendimetrazine *on page 693*

Plendil® (Can) *see* felodipine *on page 368*

709

plerixafor (pler IX a fore)
Synonyms AMD3100; LM3100
U.S. Brand Names Mozobil™
Therapeutic Category Hematopoietic Stem Cell Mobilizer
Use Mobilization of hematopoietic stem cells (HSC) for collection and subsequent autologous transplantation (in combination with filgrastim) in patients with non-Hodgkin lymphoma (NHL) and multiple myeloma (MM)
General Dosage Range Dosage adjustment recommended in patients with renal impairment
  SubQ: *Adults:* 0.24 mg/kg/day (maximum dose: 40 mg/day)
Dosage Forms
  Injection, solution [preservative free]:
    Mozobil™: 20 mg/mL (1.2 mL)

Pletal® *see* cilostazol *on page 208*
Plexion® *see* sulfur and sulfacetamide *on page 838*
Plexion SCT® *see* sulfur and sulfacetamide *on page 838*
PLX4032 *see* vemurafenib *on page 911*
PMPA *see* tenofovir *on page 851*
PMS-Adenosine (Can) *see* adenosine *on page 41*
PMS-Alendronate (Can) *see* alendronate *on page 49*
PMS-Alendronate-FC (Can) *see* alendronate *on page 49*
PMS-Amantadine (Can) *see* amantadine *on page 62*
PMS-Amiodarone (Can) *see* amiodarone *on page 67*
PMS-Amitriptyline (Can) *see* amitriptyline *on page 68*
PMS-Amlodipine (Can) *see* amlodipine *on page 69*
PMS-Amoxicillin (Can) *see* amoxicillin *on page 73*
PMS-Anagrelide (Can) *see* anagrelide *on page 78*
PMS-Atenolol (Can) *see* atenolol *on page 101*
PMS-Atorvastatin (Can) *see* atorvastatin *on page 102*
PMS-Azithromycin (Can) *see* azithromycin (systemic) *on page 108*
PMS-Baclofen (Can) *see* baclofen *on page 112*
PMS-Benzydamine (Can) *see* benzydamine *(Canada only) on page 126*
PMS-Bethanechol (Can) *see* bethanechol *on page 131*
PMS-Bicalutamide (Can) *see* bicalutamide *on page 133*
PMS-Bisoprolol (Can) *see* bisoprolol *on page 136*
PMS-Brimonidine Tartrate (Can) *see* brimonidine *on page 141*
PMS-Bromocriptine (Can) *see* bromocriptine *on page 142*
PMS-Bupropion SR (Can) *see* bupropion *on page 150*
PMS-Buspirone (Can) *see* buspirone *on page 151*
PMS-Butorphanol (Can) *see* butorphanol *on page 155*
PMS-Captopril (Can) *see* captopril *on page 170*
PMS-Carbamazepine (Can) *see* carbamazepine *on page 171*
PMS-Carvedilol (Can) *see* carvedilol *on page 178*
PMS-Cefaclor (Can) *see* cefaclor *on page 180*
PMS-Cephalexin (Can) *see* cephalexin *on page 188*
PMS-Cetirizine (Can) *see* cetirizine *on page 189*
PMS-Chloral Hydrate (Can) *see* chloral hydrate *on page 193*
PMS-Cholestyramine (Can) *see* cholestyramine resin *on page 205*
PMS-Cilazapril (Can) *see* cilazapril *(Canada only) on page 208*
PMS-Cimetidine (Can) *see* cimetidine *on page 209*
PMS-Ciprofloxacin (Can) *see* ciprofloxacin (systemic) *on page 210*
PMS-Citalopram (Can) *see* citalopram *on page 213*
PMS-Clarithromycin (Can) *see* clarithromycin *on page 215*
PMS-Clindamycin (Can) *see* clindamycin (systemic) *on page 217*

PMS-Isosorbide (Can) *see* isosorbide dinitrate *on page 494*
PMS-Ketoprofen (Can) *see* ketoprofen *on page 501*
PMS-Ketoprofen-E (Can) *see* ketoprofen *on page 501*
PMS-Lactulose (Can) *see* lactulose *on page 507*
PMS-Lamotrigine (Can) *see* lamotrigine *on page 509*
PMS-Leflunomide (Can) *see* leflunomide *on page 514*
PMS-Letrozole (Can) *see* letrozole *on page 515*
PMS-Levazine (Can) *see* amitriptyline and perphenazine *on page 68*
PMS-Levetiracetam (Can) *see* levetiracetam *on page 517*
PMS-Levobunolol (Can) *see* levobunolol *on page 517*
PMS-Levofloxacin (Can) *see* levofloxacin (systemic) *on page 520*
PMS-Lindane (Can) *see* lindane *on page 528*
PMS-Lisinopril (Can) *see* lisinopril *on page 531*
PMS-Lithium Carbonate (Can) *see* lithium *on page 532*
PMS-Lithium Citrate (Can) *see* lithium *on page 532*
PMS-Loperamine (Can) *see* loperamide *on page 535*
PMS-Lorazepam (Can) *see* lorazepam *on page 537*
PMS-Lovastatin (Can) *see* lovastatin *on page 540*
PMS-Medroxyprogesterone (Can) *see* medroxyprogesterone *on page 554*
PMS-Mefenamic Acid (Can) *see* mefenamic acid *on page 555*
PMS-Meloxicam (Can) *see* meloxicam *on page 556*
PMS-Memantine (Can) *see* memantine *on page 556*
PMS-Metformin (Can) *see* metformin *on page 566*
PMS-Methotrimeprazine (Can) *see* methotrimeprazine *(Canada only) on page 572*
PMS-Methylphenidate (Can) *see* methylphenidate *on page 577*
PMS-Metoclopramide (Can) *see* metoclopramide *on page 580*
PMS-Metoprolol (Can) *see* metoprolol *on page 581*
PMS-Minocycline (Can) *see* minocycline *on page 590*
PMS-Mirtazapine (Can) *see* mirtazapine *on page 592*
PMS-Misoprostol (Can) *see* misoprostol *on page 592*
PMS-Moclobemide (Can) *see* moclobemide *(Canada only) on page 594*
PMS-Mometasone (Can) *see* mometasone (topical) *on page 596*
PMS-Morphine Sulfate SR (Can) *see* morphine (systemic) *on page 598*
PMS-Naproxen (Can) *see* naproxen *on page 612*
PMS-Naproxen EC (Can) *see* naproxen *on page 612*
PMS-Nifedipine (Can) *see* nifedipine *on page 626*
PMS-Nizatidine (Can) *see* nizatidine *on page 631*
PMS-Norfloxacin (Can) *see* norfloxacin *on page 633*
PMS-Nortriptyline (Can) *see* nortriptyline *on page 634*
PMS-Nystatin (Can) *see* nystatin (oral) *on page 641*
PMS-Olanzapine (Can) *see* olanzapine *on page 645*
PMS-Olanzapine ODT (Can) *see* olanzapine *on page 645*
PMS-Omeprazole (Can) *see* omeprazole *on page 649*
PMS-Omeprazole DR (Can) *see* omeprazole *on page 649*
PMS-Ondansetron (Can) *see* ondansetron *on page 651*
PMS-Oxazepam (Can) *see* oxazepam *on page 659*
PMS-Oxybutynin (Can) *see* oxybutynin *on page 661*
PMS-Oxycodone (Can) *see* oxycodone *on page 662*
PMS-Oxycodone-Acetaminophen (Can) *see* oxycodone and acetaminophen *on page 662*
PMS-Pamidronate (Can) *see* pamidronate *on page 670*
PMS-Pantoprazole (Can) *see* pantoprazole *on page 672*
PMS-Paroxetine (Can) *see* paroxetine *on page 676*
PMS-Phenobarbital (Can) *see* phenobarbital *on page 693*

PMS-Pimozide (Can) *see* pimozide *on page 704*
PMS-Pindolol (Can) *see* pindolol *on page 705*
PMS-Pioglitazone (Can) *see* pioglitazone *on page 706*
PMS-Piroxicam (Can) *see* piroxicam *on page 708*
PMS-Polytrimethoprim (Can) *see* trimethoprim and polymyxin B *on page 892*
PMS-Pramipexole (Can) *see* pramipexole *on page 729*
PMS-Pravastatin (Can) *see* pravastatin *on page 732*
PMS-Procyclidine (Can) *see* procyclidine *(Canada only) on page 741*
PMS-Promethazine (Can) *see* promethazine *on page 742*
PMS-Propafenone (Can) *see* propafenone *on page 744*
PMS-Propranolol (Can) *see* propranolol *on page 747*
PMS-Pseudoephedrine (Can) *see* pseudoephedrine *on page 751*
PMS-Quetiapine (Can) *see* quetiapine *on page 760*
PMS-Rabeprazole EC (Can) *see* rabeprazole *on page 763*
PMS-Ramipril (Can) *see* ramipril *on page 766*
PMS-Ramipril HCTZ (Can) *see* ramipril and hydrochlorothiazide *(Canada only) on page 766*
PMS-Ranitidine (Can) *see* ranitidine *on page 767*
PMS-Risedronate (Can) *see* risedronate *on page 782*
PMS-Risperidone (Can) *see* risperidone *on page 783*
PMS-Risperidone ODT (Can) *see* risperidone *on page 783*
PMS-Rivastigmine (Can) *see* rivastigmine *on page 786*
PMS-Ropinirole (Can) *see* ropinirole *on page 790*
PMS-Salbutamol (Can) *see* albuterol *on page 45*
PMS-Sertraline (Can) *see* sertraline *on page 809*
PMS-Simvastatin (Can) *see* simvastatin *on page 813*
PMS-Sodium Cromoglycate (Can) *see* cromolyn (systemic, oral inhalation) *on page 238*
PMS-Sodium Polystyrene Sulfonate (Can) *see* sodium polystyrene sulfonate *on page 823*
PMS-Sotalol (Can) *see* sotalol *on page 828*
PMS-Sucralate (Can) *see* sucralfate *on page 833*
PMS-Sulfacetamide (Can) *see* sulfacetamide (ophthalmic) *on page 835*
PMS-Sumatriptan (Can) *see* sumatriptan *on page 839*
PMS-Tamoxifen (Can) *see* tamoxifen *on page 843*
PMS-Temazepam (Can) *see* temazepam *on page 848*
PMS-Terazosin (Can) *see* terazosin *on page 851*
PMS-Terbinafine (Can) *see* terbinafine (systemic) *on page 851*
PMS-Testosterone (Can) *see* testosterone *on page 854*
PMS-Theophylline (Can) *see* theophylline *on page 860*
PMS-Tiaprofenic (Can) *see* tiaprofenic acid *(Canada only) on page 867*
PMS-Ticlopidine (Can) *see* ticlopidine *on page 868*
PMS-Timolol (Can) *see* timolol (ophthalmic) *on page 869*
PMS-Tobramycin (Can) *see* tobramycin (ophthalmic) *on page 873*
PMS-Topiramate (Can) *see* topiramate *on page 877*
PMS-Trazodone (Can) *see* trazodone *on page 884*
PMS-Trifluoperazine (Can) *see* trifluoperazine *on page 890*
PMS-Trihexyphenidyl (Can) *see* trihexyphenidyl *on page 891*
PMS-Ursodiol C (Can) *see* ursodiol *on page 902*
PMS-Valacyclovir (Can) *see* valacyclovir *on page 903*
PMS-Valproic Acid (Can) *see* valproic acid *on page 904*
PMS-Valproic Acid E.C. (Can) *see* valproic acid *on page 904*
PMS-Vancomycin (Can) *see* vancomycin *on page 906*
PMS-Venlafaxine XR (Can) *see* venlafaxine *on page 911*
PMS-Verapamil SR (Can) *see* verapamil *on page 912*
PMS-Zolmitriptan (Can) *see* zolmitriptan *on page 933*

PMS-Zolmitriptan ODT (Can) *see* zolmitriptan *on page 933*

PMS-Zopiclone (Can) *see* zopiclone *(Canada only) on page 934*

PN *see* total parenteral nutrition *on page 879*

Pneumo 23™ (Can) *see* pneumococcal polysaccharide vaccine (polyvalent) *on page 715*

pneumococcal 7-valent conjugate vaccine *see* pneumococcal conjugate vaccine (7-valent) *on page 714*

pneumococcal conjugate vaccine (7-valent)

(noo moe KOK al KON ju gate vak SEEN, seven vay lent)

Medication Safety Issues

Sound-alike/look-alike issues:

Pneumococcal 7-Valent Conjugate Vaccine (Prevnar®) may be confused with Pneumococcal 13-Valent Conjugate Vaccine (Prevnar 13™) or with Pneumococcal 23-Valent Polysaccharide Vaccine (Pneumovax® 23)

Synonyms diphtheria CRM_{197} protein; PCV; PCV-7; PCV7; pneumococcal 7-valent conjugate vaccine

U.S. Brand Names Prevnar®

Canadian Brand Names Prevnar®

Therapeutic Category Vaccine

Use Note: In March 2010, the Advisory Committee on Immunization Practices (ACIP) released recommendations that pneumococcal 13-valent conjugate vaccine (PCV13; Prevnar 13™) replace pneumococcal 7-valent conjugate vaccine (PCV7; Prevnar®) for all doses for immunization of all children 2-59 months of age. Refer to the pneumococcal conjugate vaccine (13-valent) monograph for additional information.

Immunization of infants and toddlers against *Streptococcus pneumoniae* infection caused by serotypes included in the vaccine

Immunization of infants and toddlers against otitis media caused by serotypes included in the vaccine

The Advisory Committee on Immunization Practices (ACIP) recommends pneumococcal conjugate vaccine (PCV) for routine vaccination of all children 2-59 months and children 60-71 months with underlying medical conditions. PCV13 should be used to complete the vaccination of children who received ≥1 dose of PCV7.

General Dosage Range I.M.: *Infants 2-6 months:* 0.5 mL at approximately 2-month intervals for 3 consecutive doses, followed by a fourth dose of 0.5 mL at 12-15 months of age

Dosage Forms

Injection, suspension:

Prevnar®: 2 mcg of each capsular saccharide for serotypes 4, 9V, 14, 18C, 19F, and 23F, and 4 mcg of serotype 6B per 0.5 mL (0.5 mL)

pneumococcal 13-valent conjugate vaccine *see* pneumococcal conjugate vaccine (13-valent) *on page 714*

pneumococcal conjugate vaccine (13-valent)

(noo moe KOK al KON ju gate vak SEEN, thur TEEN vay lent)

Medication Safety Issues

Sound-alike/look-alike issues:

Pneumococcal 13-Valent Conjugate Vaccine (Prevnar 13™) may be confused with Pneumococcal 7-Valent Conjugate Vaccine (Prevnar®) or with Pneumococcal 23-Valent Polysaccharide Vaccine (Pneumovax® 23)

Synonyms diphtheria CRM_{197} protein; PCV-13; PCV13; PCV13-CRM(197); pneumococcal 13-valent conjugate vaccine

U.S. Brand Names Prevnar 13™

Canadian Brand Names Prevnar 13™

Therapeutic Category Vaccine, Inactivated (Bacterial)

Use

Immunization of infants and children against *Streptococcus pneumoniae* infection caused by serotypes included in the vaccine

Immunization of infants and children against otitis media caused by *Streptococcus pneumoniae* serotypes 4, 6B, 9V, 14, 18C, 19F, and 23F

The Advisory Committee on Immunization Practices (ACIP) recommends routine vaccination for the following:

All children age 2-59 months

Children 60-71 months with underlying medical conditions including: Cochlear implants, functional or anatomic asplenia (includes sickle cell disease and other hemoglobinopathies, congenital or acquired asplenia, or splenic dysfunction); immunocompromising conditions (includes HIV infection, congenital immunodeficiencies [excluding chronic granulomatous disease], chronic renal failure, nephrotic syndrome, diseases associated with immunosuppressive or radiation therapy, solid organ transplant); chronic illnesses (cardiac disease, cerebrospinal fluid leaks, diabetes mellitus, pulmonary disease [excluding asthma unless on high dose oral corticosteroids])

Children who received ≥1 dose of PCV7

Children 6-18 years of age at increased risk for invasive pneumococcal disease due to anatomic or functional asplenia (including sickle cell disease), HIV infection or other immunocompromising conditions, cochlear implant, or cerebrospinal fluid leaks (regardless of prior receipt of PCV7 or PPSV23). Routine use is not recommended for healthy children ≥5 years of age.

General Dosage Range I.M.:

Infants 2-6 months: 0.5 mL at approximately 2-month intervals for 3 consecutive doses, followed by a fourth dose of 0.5 mL at 12-15 months of age

Infants 7-11 months (previously unvaccinated): 0.5 mL for a total of 3 doses, 2 doses at least 4 weeks apart, followed by a third dose at 12-15 months (at least 2 months after second dose)

Children 12-23 months (previously unvaccinated) and Children 24-71 months (previously unvaccinated) with underlying conditions: 0.5 mL for a total of 2 doses, separated by at least 2 months

Healthy Children 24-59 months (previously unvaccinated) and Children 6-18 years at high risk for invasive pneumococcal disease: 0.5 mL as a single dose

Children 14 months-71 months (previously completing vaccination with PCV7): 0.5 mL supplemental dose

Dosage Forms

Injection, suspension:

Prevnar 13™: 2 mcg of each capsular saccharide for serotypes 1, 3, 4, 5, 6A, 7F, 9V, 14, 18C, 19A, 19F, and 23F, and 4 mcg of serotype 6B [bound to diphtheria CRM_{197} protein ~34 mcg] per 0.5 mL (0.5 mL)

pneumococcal polysaccharide vaccine (polyvalent)

(noo moe KOK al pol i SAK a ride vak SEEN, pol i VAY lent)

Medication Safety Issues

Sound-alike/look-alike issues:

Pneumococcal 23-Valent Polysaccharide Vaccine (Pneumovax® 23) may be confused with Pneumococcal 7-Valent Conjugate Vaccine (Prevnar®) or with Pneumococcal 13-Valent Conjugate Vaccine (Prevnar 13™)

Synonyms 23-valent pneumococcal polysaccharide vaccine; 23PS; PPSV; PPSV23; PPV23

U.S. Brand Names Pneumovax® 23

Canadian Brand Names Pneumo 23™; Pneumovax® 23

Therapeutic Category Vaccine, Inactivated Bacteria

Use Immunization against pneumococcal disease caused by serotypes included in the vaccine. Routine vaccination is recommended for persons ≥50 years of age and persons ≥2 years in certain situations.

The Advisory Committee on Immunization Practices (ACIP) recommends routine vaccination for the following:

All immunocompetent patients ≥65 years of age

Patients 2-18 years of age with certain high-risk condition(s):

- Chronic heart disease (particularly cyanotic congenital heart disease and cardiac failure)

- Chronic lung disease (including asthma if treated with high-dose oral corticosteroids)

Patients 2-64 years of age with certain high-risk condition(s):

- Diabetes mellitus

- Cochlear implants

- Cerebrospinal fluid leaks

- Functional or anatomic asplenia (including sickle cell disease and other hemoglobinopathies, splenic dysfunction, or splenectomy)

- Immunocompromising conditions including congenital immunodeficiency (includes B- or T-lymphocyte deficiency, complement deficiencies, and phagocytic disorders [excluding chronic granulomatous disease]); HIV infection; leukemia, lymphoma, Hodgkin disease, multiple myeloma, generalized malignancy; chronic renal failure, nephrotic syndrome; patients requiring treatment with immunosuppressive therapy, including chemotherapy, long-term systemic corticosteroids, or radiation therapy; patients who have received a solid organ transplant

Patients 19-64 years of age with certain high-risk condition(s):
- Chronic heart disease (including heart failure and cardiomyopathy, and excluding hypertension)
- Chronic lung disease (including COPD, emphysema, and asthma)
- Persons who smoke cigarettes
- Alcoholism
- Chronic liver disease (including cirrhosis)

Routine vaccination is not recommended for Alaska Natives or American Indian persons unless they have underlying conditions which are indications for vaccination; in special situations, vaccination may be recommended when living in an area at increased risk of invasive pneumococcal disease.

General Dosage Range I.M., SubQ: *Children ≥2 years and Adults:* 0.5 mL

Dosage Forms
 Injection, solution:
  Pneumovax® 23: 25 mcg each of 23 capsular polysaccharide isolates/0.5 mL (0.5 mL, 2.5 mL)

Pneumovax® 23 *see pneumococcal polysaccharide vaccine (polyvalent) on page 715*
PNU-140690E *see tipranavir on page 871*
Podactin Cream [OTC] *see miconazole (topical) on page 585*
Podactin Powder [OTC] *see tolnaftate on page 876*
Podocon-25® *see podophyllum resin on page 716*
Podofilm® (Can) *see podophyllum resin on page 716*

podofilox (poe DOF il oks)
U.S. Brand Names Condylox®
Canadian Brand Names Condyline™; Wartec®
Therapeutic Category Keratolytic Agent
Use Treatment of external genital warts
General Dosage Range Topical: *Adults:* Apply twice daily for 3 consecutive days, then withhold use for 4 consecutive days; May repeat cycle up to 4 times
Dosage Forms
 Gel, topical:
  Condylox®: 0.5% (3.5 g)
 Solution, topical: 0.5% (3.5 mL)
  Condylox®: 0.5% (3.5 mL)

podophyllin *see podophyllum resin on page 716*

podophyllum resin (po DOF fil um REZ in)
Synonyms mandrake; may apple; podophyllin
U.S. Brand Names Podocon-25®
Canadian Brand Names Podofilm®
Therapeutic Category Keratolytic Agent
Use Topical treatment of soft external genital (venereal) warts (condylomata acuminate); compound benzoin tincture generally is used as the medium for topical application
General Dosage Range Topical: *Children and Adults:* Applied by physician only
Dosage Forms
 Liquid, topical:
  Podocon-25®: 25% (15 mL)

Polibar® ACB *see barium on page 114*

polidocanol (pol i DOE kuh nol)
U.S. Brand Names Asclera™
Therapeutic Category Sclerosing Agent
Use Treatment of small, uncomplicated varicose veins of the lower extremities

General Dosage Range I.V.: *Adults:* 0.1-0.3 mL injection (0.5% or 1% solution) per session (maximum: 10 mL/session)

Dosage Forms
Injection, solution [preservative free]:
Asclera™: 0.5% (2 mL); 1% (2 mL)

poliovirus, inactivated (IPV) *see* diphtheria and tetanus toxoids, acellular pertussis, and poliovirus vaccine *on page 294*

poliovirus, inactivated (IPV) *see* diphtheria and tetanus toxoids, acellular pertussis, poliovirus and *Haemophilus* b conjugate vaccine *on page 295*

poliovirus vaccine (inactivated) (POE lee oh VYE rus vak SEEN, in ak ti VAY ted)

Medication Safety Issues
Administration issues:
Poliovirus vaccine (inactivated) may be confused with tuberculin products. Medication errors have occurred when poliovirus vaccine (IPV) has been inadvertently administered instead of ttuberculin skin tests (PPD). These products are refrigerated and often stored in close proximity to each other.

Synonyms enhanced-potency inactivated poliovirus vaccine; IPV; salk vaccine

U.S. Brand Names IPOL®

Canadian Brand Names Imovax® Polio

Therapeutic Category Vaccine, Live Virus and Inactivated Virus

Use Active immunization against poliomyelitis caused by poliovirus types 1, 2 and 3. **Note:** Combination products containing polio vaccine are also available and may be preferred in certain age groups if recipients are likely to be susceptible to the agents contained within each vaccine.

The Advisory Committee on Immunization Practices (ACIP) recommends routine vaccination for the following:
• All children (first dose given at 2 months of age)

Routine immunization of adults in the United States is generally not recommended. Adults with previous wild poliovirus disease, who have never been immunized, or those who are incompletely immunized may receive inactivated poliovirus vaccine if they fall into one of the following categories:
• Travelers to regions or countries where poliomyelitis is endemic or epidemic
• Healthcare workers in close contact with patients who may be excreting poliovirus
• Laboratory workers handling specimens that may contain poliovirus
• Members of communities or specific population groups with diseases caused by wild poliovirus
• Incompletely vaccinated or unvaccinated adults in a household or with other close contact with children receiving oral poliovirus (may be at increased risk of vaccine associated paralytic poliomyelitis)

General Dosage Range I.M., SubQ:
Children: Primary immunization: Administer three 0.5 mL doses at 2, 4, and 6-18 months of age; do not administer more frequently than 4 weeks apart (preferably given more than 8 weeks apart). Booster dose: 0.5 mL at 4-6 years of age; Minimum interval between booster and previous dose is 6 months.
Adults (previously unvaccinated): Two 0.5 mL doses administered at 1- to 2-month intervals followed by a third dose 6-12 months later.

Dosage Forms
Injection, suspension:
IPOL®: Type 1 poliovirus 40 D-antigen units, type 2 poliovirus 8 D-antigen units, and type 3 poliovirus 32 D-antigen units per 0.5 mL (0.5 mL, 5 mL)

Polocaine® *see* mepivacaine *on page 561*

Polocaine® 2% and Levonordefrin 1:20,000 (Can) *see* mepivacaine and levonordefrin *on page 562*

Polocaine® Dental *see* mepivacaine *on page 561*

Polocaine® Dental with Levonordefrin *see* mepivacaine and levonordefrin *on page 562*

Polocaine® MPF *see* mepivacaine *on page 561*

polycarbophil (pol i KAR boe fil)

U.S. Brand Names Equalactin® [OTC]; Fiber-Lax [OTC]; Fiber-Tabs™ [OTC]; FiberCon® [OTC]; Konsyl® Fiber [OTC]

Therapeutic Category Gastrointestinal Agent, Miscellaneous; Laxative

Use Treatment of constipation or diarrhea

◀ **General Dosage Range Oral:**
Children 6-12 years: 625 mg calcium polycarbophil 1-4 times/day
Children ≥12 years and Adults: 1250 mg calcium polycarbophil 1-4 times/day
Dosage Forms
Caplet, oral: Calcium polycarbophil 625 mg
FiberCon® [OTC]: Calcium polycarbophil 625 mg
Konsyl® Fiber [OTC]: Calcium polycarbophil 625 mg
Captab, oral:
Fiber-Lax [OTC]: Calcium polycarbophil 625 mg
Tablet, oral:
Fiber-Tabs™ [OTC]: Calcium polycarbophil 625 mg
Tablet, chewable, oral:
Equalactin® [OTC]: Calcium polycarbophil 625 mg

Polycin™ *see* bacitracin and polymyxin B *on page* 111
Polycitra *see* citric acid, sodium citrate, and potassium citrate *on page* 214
Polycitra K *see* potassium citrate and citric acid *on page* 725
Polycose® [OTC] *see* glucose polymers *on page* 420
Poly-Dex™ [DSC] *see* neomycin, polymyxin B, and dexamethasone *on page* 618
polyethylene glycol-L-asparaginase *see* pegaspargase *on page* 678

polyethylene glycol 3350 (pol i ETH i leen GLY kol 3350)

Medication Safety Issues
Sound-alike/look-alike issues:
MiraLax™ may be confused with Mirapex®
Polyethylene glycol 3350 may be confused with polyethylene glycol electrolyte solution
International issues:
MiraLax may be confused with Murelax brand name for oxazepam [Australia]
Synonyms PEG
U.S. Brand Names Dulcolax Balance® [OTC]; MiraLAX® [OTC]
Therapeutic Category Laxative, Osmotic
Use Treatment of occasional constipation in adults
General Dosage Range Oral: *Adults:* 17 g of powder (~1 heaping tablespoon) dissolved in 4-8 ounces of beverage once daily (maximum use: 1 week)
Dosage Forms
Powder for solution, oral: 17 g/dose (119 g, 238 g, 255 g, 510 g, 527 g); 17 g/packet (14s, 30s)
Dulcolax Balance® [OTC]: 17 g/dose (119 g, 238 g, 510 g)
MiraLAX® [OTC]: 17 g/dose (119 g, 238 g, 510 g); 17 g/packet (10s)

polyethylene glycol-conjugated uricase *see* pegloticase *on page* 682

polyethylene glycol-electrolyte solution
(pol i ETH i leen GLY kol ee LEK troe lite soe LOO shun)

Medication Safety Issues
Sound-alike/look-alike issues:
GoLYTELY® may be confused with NuLYTELY®
NuLYTELY® may be confused with GoLYTELY®
TriLyte® may be confused with TriLipix™
Synonyms electrolyte lavage solution
U.S. Brand Names Colyte®; GaviLyte™-C; GaviLyte™-G; GaviLyte™-N; GoLYTELY®; MoviPrep®; NuLYTELY®; TriLyte®
Canadian Brand Names Colyte™; Klean-Prep®; PegLyte®
Therapeutic Category Laxative
Use Bowel cleansing prior to GI examination
General Dosage Range
Nasogastric tube:
Children ≥6 months: 25 mL/kg/hour until rectal effluent is clear
Adults: 20-30 mL/minute (1.2-1.8 L/hour) until rectal effluent is clear

Oral:

Children ≥6 months: (GaviLyte™-N, NuLYTELY®, TriLyte®): 25 mL/kg/hour (some studies have used up to 40 mL/kg/hour) for 4-10 hours until rectal effluent is clear (maximum total dose: 4 L)

Adults: CoLyte®, GaviLyte™-C, GaviLyte™-G, GaviLyte™-N, GoLYTELY®, NuLYTELY®, TriLyte®: 240 mL (8 oz) every 10 minutes, until 4 L are consumed or the rectal effluent is clear; MoviPrep®: 240 mL (8 oz) every 15 minutes until 1 L consumed; repeat 1 time

Dosage Forms

Powder, for solution, oral: PEG 3350 240 g, sodium sulfate 22.72 g, sodium bicarbonate 6.72 g, sodium chloride 5.84 g, and potassium 2.98 g; PEG 3350 236 g, sodium sulfate 22.74 g, sodium bicarbonate 6.74 g, sodium chloride 5.86 g, and potassium chloride 2.97 g; PEG 3350 240 g, sodium bicarbonate 5.72 g, sodium chloride 11.2 g, and potassium chloride 1.48 g

Colyte®: PEG 3350 240 g, sodium sulfate 22.72 g, sodium bicarbonate 6.72 g, sodium chloride 5.84 g, and potassium 2.98 g

GaviLyte™-C: PEG 3350 240 g, sodium sulfate 22.72 g, sodium bicarbonate 6.72 g, sodium chloride 5.84 g, and potassium chloride 2.98 g (4000 mL)

GaviLyte™-G: PEG 3350 236 g, sodium sulfate 22.74 g, sodium bicarbonate 6.74 g, sodium chloride 5.86 g, and potassium chloride 2.97 g (4000 mL)

GaviLyte™-N: PEG 3350 420 g, sodium bicarbonate 5.72 g, sodium chloride 11.2 g, and potassium chloride 1.48 g (4000 mL)

GoLYTELY®:
PEG 3350 236 g, sodium sulfate 22.74 g, sodium bicarbonate 6.74 g, sodium chloride 5.86 g, and potassium 2.97 g

PEG 3350 227.1 g, sodium sulfate 21.5 g, sodium bicarbonate 6.36 g, sodium chloride 5.53 g, and potassium 2.82 g per packet (1s)

MoviPrep®: Pouch A: PEG 3350 100g, sodium sulfate 7.5 g, sodium chloride 2.69 g, potassium chloride 1.015 g; Pouch B: Ascorbic acid 4.7 g, sodium ascorbate 5.9 g

NuLYTELY®: PEG 3350 420 g, sodium bicarbonate 5.72 g, sodium chloride 11.2 g, and potassium 1.48 g

TriLyte®: PEG 3350 420 g, sodium bicarbonate 5.72 g, sodium chloride 11.2 g, and potassium 1.48 g

polyethylene glycol-electrolyte solution and bisacodyl
(pol i ETH i leen GLY kol ee LEK troe lite soe LOO shun & bis a KOE dil)

Synonyms bisacodyl and polyethylene glycol-electrolyte solution; electrolyte lavage solution

U.S. Brand Names HalfLytely® and Bisacodyl

Therapeutic Category Laxative, Bowel Evacuant; Laxative, Stimulant

Use Bowel cleansing prior to colonoscopy

General Dosage Range Oral: *Adults:* 5 mg of bisacodyl as a single dose, after bowel movement or 6 hours (whichever occurs first) initiate 8 ounces of polyethylene glycol-electrolyte solution every 10 minutes until 2 L are consumed

Dosage Forms

Kit [each kit contains]:
HalfLytely® and Bisacodyl:
Powder for solution, oral (HalfLytely®): PEG 3350 210 g, sodium bicarbonate 2.86 g, sodium chloride 5.6 g, potassium chloride 0.74 g (2000 mL) [contains 4 flavor packs (each 1 g) cherry, lemon-lime, orange, pineapple flavors]
Tablet, delayed release (Bisacodyl): 5 mg (1s)

polyethylene glycol interferon alfa-2b *see* peginterferon alfa-2b *on page 680*

Poly-Iron 150 [OTC] *see* polysaccharide-iron complex *on page 720*

Poly-Iron 150 Forte *see* polysaccharide-iron complex, vitamin B12, and folic acid *on page 721*

polymyxin B (pol i MIKS in bee)

Medication Safety Issues

High alert medication:
The Institute for Safe Medication Practices (ISMP) includes this medication (intrathecal administration) among its list of drug classes which have a heightened risk of causing significant patient harm when used in error.

Synonyms polymyxin B sulfate

U.S. Brand Names Poly-Rx

Therapeutic Category Antibiotic, Irrigation; Antibiotic, Miscellaneous

◀ **Use** Treatment of acute infections caused by susceptible strains of *Pseudomonas aeruginosa*; used occasionally for gut decontamination; parenteral use of polymyxin B has mainly been replaced by less toxic antibiotics, reserved for life-threatening infections caused by organisms resistant to the preferred drugs (eg, pseudomonal meningitis - intrathecal administration)

General Dosage Range Dosage adjustment recommended in patients with renal impairment

I.M.:
Children <2 years: Up to 40,000 units/kg/day divided every 6 hours
Children ≥2 years and Adults: 25,000-30,000 units/kg/day divided every 4-6 hours (maximum: 2,000,000 units/day)

I.V.:
Children <2 years: Up to 40,000 units/kg/day divided every 12 hours
Children ≥2 years and Adults: 15,000-25,000 units/kg/day divided every 12 hours (maximum: 2,000,000 units/day)

Intrathecal:
Children <2 years: 20,000 units/day for 3-4 days, then 25,000 units every other day
Children ≥2 years and Adults: 50,000 units/day for 3-4 days, then every other day

Irrigation: *Adults:*
Bladder: 20 mg (equal to 200,000 units) added to 1 L of normal saline as continuous irrigant or rinse
Topical: 500,000 units/L of normal saline (maximum: 2 million units/day)

Ophthalmic: *Children ≥2 years and Adults:* Initial: 1-3 drops/hour; Reduce to 1-2 drops 4-6 times/day based on response

Otic: *Children and Adults:* 1-2 drops 3-4 times/day

Dosage Forms
Injection, powder for reconstitution: 500,000 units
Powder, for prescription compounding:
Poly-Rx: 100 million units (13 g)

polymyxin B and bacitracin *see* bacitracin and polymyxin B *on page 111*

polymyxin B and neomycin *see* neomycin and polymyxin B *on page 617*

polymyxin B and trimethoprim *see* trimethoprim and polymyxin B *on page 892*

polymyxin B, bacitracin, and neomycin *see* bacitracin, neomycin, and polymyxin B *on page 111*

polymyxin B, bacitracin, neomycin, and hydrocortisone *see* bacitracin, neomycin, polymyxin B, and hydrocortisone *on page 112*

polymyxin B, neomycin, and dexamethasone *see* neomycin, polymyxin B, and dexamethasone *on page 618*

polymyxin B, neomycin, and gramicidin *see* neomycin, polymyxin B, and gramicidin *on page 618*

polymyxin B, neomycin, and hydrocortisone *see* neomycin, polymyxin B, and hydrocortisone *on page 618*

polymyxin B, neomycin, and prednisolone *see* neomycin, polymyxin B, and prednisolone *on page 619*

polymyxin B, neomycin, bacitracin, and pramoxine *see* bacitracin, neomycin, polymyxin B, and pramoxine *on page 112*

polymyxin B sulfate *see* polymyxin B *on page 719*

polyphenols *see* sinecatechins *on page 814*

polyphenon E *see* sinecatechins *on page 814*

Poly-Pred® *see* neomycin, polymyxin B, and prednisolone *on page 619*

Poly-Rx *see* polymyxin B *on page 719*

Polysaccharide Iron 150 Forte *see* polysaccharide-iron complex, vitamin B12, and folic acid *on page 721*

polysaccharide-iron complex (pol i SAK a ride-EYE ern KOM pleks)

Medication Safety Issues
Sound-alike/look-alike issues:
Niferex® may be confused with Nephrox®

Synonyms iron-polysaccharide complex

U.S. Brand Names Ferrex™ 150 Plus [OTC]; Ferrex™ 150 [OTC]; Niferex® [OTC]; Nu-Iron® 150 [OTC]; Poly-Iron 150 [OTC]; ProFe [OTC]

Therapeutic Category Electrolyte Supplement, Oral

Use Prevention and treatment of iron-deficiency anemias

General Dosage Range Oral:
Children ≥6 years: 50-100 mg once daily or in divided doses
Adults: 100-300 mg/day in 1-2 divided doses
Dosage Forms
Capsule, oral:
Ferrex™ 150 [OTC]: Elemental iron 150 mg
Ferrex™ 150 Plus [OTC]: Elemental iron 150 mg (50 mg as ferrous asparto glycinate)
Niferex® [OTC]: Elemental iron 60 mg
Nu-Iron® 150 [OTC]: Elemental iron 150 mg
Poly-Iron 150 [OTC]: Elemental iron 150 mg
ProFe [OTC]: Elemental iron 180 mg

polysaccharide-iron complex and folic acid
(pol i SAK a ride-EYE ern KOM pleks & FOE lik AS id)
Synonyms folic acid and polysaccharide-iron complex; iron-polysaccharide complex and folic acid
U.S. Brand Names NovaFerrum®
Therapeutic Category Iron Salt
Use Prevention and treatment of iron-deficiency anemias
General Dosage Range Oral: *Children >12 years and Adults:* Iron deficiency: One teaspoonful (5 mL) daily
Dosage Forms
Powder for solution, oral:
NovaFerrum®: Elemental iron 100 mg and folic acid 1 mg per 5 mL (120 mL)

polysaccharide-iron complex, vitamin B12, and folic acid
(pol i SAK a ride-EYE ern KOM pleks, VYE ta min bee twelve & FOE lik AS id)
Synonyms iron-polysaccharide complex, vitamin B12, and folic acid
U.S. Brand Names Ferrex™ 150 Forte; Ferrex™ 150 Forte Plus; Maxaron® Forte; Poly-Iron 150 Forte; Polysaccharide Iron 150 Forte
Therapeutic Category Iron Salt
Use Prevention and treatment of iron-deficiency anemias and/or nutritional megaloblastic anemias
General Dosage Range Oral: *Adults:* 1-2 capsules daily
Dosage Forms
Capsule, oral:
Ferrex™ 150 Forte: Elemental iron 150 mg, cyanocobalamin 25 mcg, and folic acid 1 mg
Ferrex™ 150 Forte Plus: Elemental iron 150 mg (50 mg as ferrous asparto glycinate), cyanocobalamin 25 mcg, and folic acid 1 mg
Maxaron® Forte: Elemental iron 150 mg (80 mg as ferrous bisglycinate), cyanocobalamin 25 mcg, and folic acid 1 mg
Poly-Iron 150 Forte: Elemental iron 150 mg, cyanocobalamin 25 mcg, and folic acid 1 mg
Polysaccharide Iron 150 Forte: Elemental iron 150 mg, cyanocobalamin 25 mcg, and folic acid 1 mg

Polysporin® [OTC] *see* bacitracin and polymyxin B *on page 111*
Polytrim® *see* trimethoprim and polymyxin B *on page 892*
Polytrim™ (Can) *see* trimethoprim and polymyxin B *on page 892*
polyvinyl alcohol *see* artificial tears *on page 96*
polyvinylpyrrolidone with iodine *see* povidone-iodine (ophthalmic) *on page 727*
polyvinylpyrrolidone with iodine *see* povidone-iodine (topical) *on page 727*
Poly-Vi-Sol® [OTC] *see* vitamins (multiple/pediatric) *on page 920*
Poly-Vi-Sol® With Iron [OTC] *see* vitamins (multiple/pediatric) *on page 920*
Ponstan® (Can) *see* mefenamic acid *on page 555*
Ponstel® *see* mefenamic acid *on page 555*
Pontocaine® [DSC] *see* tetracaine (topical) *on page 856*
Pontocaine® (Can) *see* tetracaine (ophthalmic) *on page 856*
Pontocaine® (Can) *see* tetracaine (systemic) *on page 856*
Pontocaine® (Can) *see* tetracaine (topical) *on page 856*

poractant alfa (por AKT ant AL fa)

U.S. Brand Names Curosurf®

Canadian Brand Names Curosurf®

Therapeutic Category Lung Surfactant

Use Treatment of respiratory distress syndrome (RDS) in premature infants

General Dosage Range Intratracheal: *Premature infants:* Initial: 2.5 mL/kg of birth weight, up to 2 subsequent doses of 1.25 mL/kg birth weight can be administered at 12-hour intervals if needed; Maximum total dose: 5 mL/kg

Dosage Forms

Suspension, intratracheal [preservative free]:
Curosurf®: 80 mg/mL (1.5 mL, 3 mL)

porfimer (POR fi mer)

Medication Safety Issues

High alert medication:
This medication is in a class the Institute for Safe Medication Practices (ISMP) includes among its list of drug classes which have a heightened risk of causing significant patient harm when used in error.

Synonyms CL-184116; dihematoporphyrin ether; porfimer sodium

U.S. Brand Names Photofrin®

Canadian Brand Names Photofrin®

Therapeutic Category Antineoplastic Agent

Use Palliation in patients with obstructing (partial or complete) esophageal cancer; treatment of microinvasive endobronchial nonsmall cell lung cancer (NSCLC); reduction of obstruction and palliation in patients with obstructing (partial or complete) NSCLC; ablation of high-grade dysplasia in Barrett esophagus

General Dosage Range I.V.: *Adults:* 2 mg/kg, followed by endoscopic exposure to the appropriate laser light

Dosage Forms

Injection, powder for reconstitution:
Photofrin®: 75 mg

Dosage Forms - Canada

Injection, powder for reconstitution, as sodium:
Photofrin®: 15 mg

porfimer sodium *see* porfimer *on page 722*

Portia® *see* ethinyl estradiol and levonorgestrel *on page 353*

posaconazole (poe sa KON a zole)

Medication Safety Issues

Sound-alike/look-alike issues:
Noxafil® may be confused with minoxidil

International issues:
Noxafil [U.S. and multiple international markets] may be confused with Noxidil brand name for minoxidil [Thailand]

Synonyms SCH 56592

U.S. Brand Names Noxafil®

Canadian Brand Names Posanol™

Therapeutic Category Antifungal Agent, Oral

Use Prophylaxis of invasive *Aspergillus* and *Candida* infections in severely-immunocompromised patients [eg, hematopoietic stem cell transplant (HSCT) recipients with graft-versus-host disease (GVHD) or those with prolonged neutropenia secondary to chemotherapy for hematologic malignancies]; treatment of oropharyngeal candidiasis (including patients refractory to itraconazole and/or fluconazole)

General Dosage Range Oral: *Children ≥13 years and Adults:* 100-800 mg/day; doses >100 mg/day are given in 2-3 divided doses

Dosage Forms

Suspension, oral:
Noxafil®: 40 mg/mL (123 mL)

Posanol™ (Can) *see* posaconazole *on page 722*

Posture® [OTC] *see* calcium phosphate (tribasic) *on page 165*

potassium acetate (poe TASS ee um AS e tate)

Medication Safety Issues
Other safety concerns:
Consider special storage requirements for intravenous potassium salts; I.V. potassium salts have been administered IVP in error, leading to fatal outcomes.
Therapeutic Category Electrolyte Supplement, Oral
Use Potassium deficiency; to avoid chloride when high concentration of potassium is needed, source of bicarbonate
General Dosage Range I.V.:
Children: 2-5 mEq/kg/day; Intermittent infusion: 0.5-1 mEq/kg/dose (maximum: 30 mEq/dose) to infuse at 0.3-0.5 mEq/kg/hour (maximum: 1 mEq/kg/hour)
Adults: 40-100 mEq/day; Intermittent infusion: 5-10 mEq/dose (maximum: 40 mEq/dose) to infuse over 2-3 hours (maximum: 40 mEq over 1 hour)
Dosage Forms
Injection, solution: 2 mEq/mL (20 mL, 50 mL, 100 mL)
Injection, solution [preservative free]: 2 mEq/mL (20 mL, 50 mL, 100 mL); 4 mEq/mL (50 mL)

potassium acid phosphate (poe TASS ee um AS id FOS fate)

U.S. Brand Names K-Phos® Original
Therapeutic Category Urinary Acidifying Agent
Use Acidifies urine and lowers urinary calcium concentration; reduces odor and rash caused by ammoniacal urine; increases the antibacterial activity of methenamine
General Dosage Range Oral: *Adults:* 1000 mg dissolved in 6-8 oz of water 4 times/day
Dosage Forms
Tablet, oral:
K-Phos® Original: 500 mg

potassium bicarbonate (poe TASS ee um bye KAR bun ate)

Therapeutic Category Electrolyte Supplement, Oral
Use Potassium deficiency, hypokalemia
General Dosage Range Oral:
Children: 1-4 mEq/kg/day
Adults: 25 mEq 2-4 times/day
Dosage Forms
Tablet for solution, oral: Potassium 25 mEq

potassium bicarbonate and potassium chloride
(poe TASS ee um bye KAR bun ate & poe TASS ee um KLOR ide)

Synonyms K-Lyte/Cl; potassium bicarbonate and potassium chloride (effervescent)
Therapeutic Category Electrolyte Supplement, Oral
Use Treatment or prevention of hypokalemia
General Dosage Range
Oral:
Children: 1-4 mEq/kg/day in divided doses
Adults: Prevention: 16-24 mEq/day in 2-4 divided doses; Treatment: 40-100 mEq/day in 2-4 divided doses
Dosage Forms
Tablet for solution, oral [effervescent]: Potassium chloride 25 mEq

potassium bicarbonate and potassium chloride (effervescent) *see* potassium bicarbonate and potassium chloride *on page 723*

potassium bicarbonate and potassium citrate
(poe TASS ee um bye KAR bun ate & poe TASS ee um SIT rate)

Medication Safety Issues
Sound-alike/look-alike issues:
Klor-Con® may be confused with Klaron®

◄ **Synonyms** potassium bicarbonate and potassium citrate (effervescent)

U.S. Brand Names Effer-K®; Klor-Con®/EF

Therapeutic Category Electrolyte Supplement, Oral

Use Treatment or prevention of hypokalemia

General Dosage Range
Oral:
Children: 1-4 mEq/kg/day in divided doses
Adults: Prevention: 16-24 mEq/day in 2-4 divided doses; Treatment: 40-100 mEq/day in 2-4 divided doses

Dosage Forms
Tablet for solution, oral [effervescent]:
Effer-K®: Potassium 10 mEq; potassium 20 mEq; potassium 25 mEq
Klor-Con®/EF: Potassium 25 mEq

potassium bicarbonate and potassium citrate (effervescent) *see* potassium bicarbonate and potassium citrate *on page 723*

potassium chloride (poe TASS ee um KLOR ide)

Medication Safety Issues
Sound-alike/look-alike issues:
Kaon-Cl-10® may be confused with kaolin
KCl may be confused with HCl
Klor-Con® may be confused with Klaron®
microK® may be confused with Macrobid®, Micronase®
High alert medication:
The Institute for Safe Medication Practices (ISMP) includes this medication (I.V. formulation) among its list of drugs which have a heightened risk of causing significant patient harm when used in error.
Other safety concerns:
Per JCAHO recommendations, concentrated electrolyte solutions should not be available in patient care areas.
Consider special storage requirements for intravenous potassium salts; I.V. potassium salts have been administered IVP in error, leading to fatal outcomes.

Synonyms KCl; kdur

U.S. Brand Names Epiklor™; Epiklor™/25; K-Tab®; Kaon-CL® 10; Klor-Con®; Klor-Con® 10; Klor-Con® 8; Klor-Con® M10; Klor-Con® M15; Klor-Con® M20; Klor-Con®/25; microK®; microK® 10

Canadian Brand Names Apo-K®; K-10®; K-Dur®; Micro-K Extencaps®; Roychlor®; Slo-Pot; Slow-K®

Therapeutic Category Electrolyte Supplement, Oral

Use Treatment or prevention of hypokalemia

General Dosage Range
I.V.:
Children: Initial: 0.5-1 mEq/kg/dose (maximum dose: 40 mEq); repeat as needed based on lab values
Adults: Intermittent infusion: ≤10 mEq/hour; repeat as needed based on lab values (maximum: 200 mEq/day)
Oral:
Children: 1-2 mEq/kg/day in 1-2 divided doses or as needed based on lab values
Adults: Initial: 6-10 mEq/dose (maximum: 40 mEq/dose); Maintenance: 40-100 mEq/day in divided doses or as needed based on lab values

Dosage Forms
Capsule, extended release, microencapsulated, oral: 8 mEq, 10 mEq
microK®: 8 mEq
microK® 10: 10 mEq
Infusion, premixed in 1/2 NS: 20 mEq (1000 mL)
Infusion, premixed in D_{10} 1/4 NS: 5 mEq (250 mL)
Infusion, premixed in D_5 1/2 NS: 10 mEq (500 mL, 1000 mL); 20 mEq (1000 mL); 30 mEq (1000 mL); 40 mEq (1000 mL)
Infusion, premixed in D_5 1/3 NS: 20 mEq (1000 mL)
Infusion, premixed in D_5 1/4 NS: 5 mEq (250 mL); 10 mEq (500 mL, 1000 mL); 20 mEq (1000 mL); 30 mEq (1000 mL); 40 mEq (1000 mL)
Infusion, premixed in D_5LR: 20 mEq (1000 mL)
Infusion, premixed in D_5NS: 20 mEq (1000 mL); 40 mEq (1000 mL)

Infusion, premixed in D₅W: 20 mEq (500 mL, 1000 mL); 40 mEq (1000 mL)
Infusion, premixed in NS: 20 mEq (1000 mL); 40 mEq (1000 mL)
Infusion, premixed in water for injection: 10 mEq (50 mL, 100 mL); 20 mEq (50 mL, 100 mL); 30 mEq (100 mL); 40 mEq (100 mL)
Injection, solution: 2 mEq/mL (5 mL, 10 mL, 15 mL, 20 mL, 30 mL, 250 mL, 500 mL)
Injection, solution [preservative free]: 2 mEq/mL (5 mL, 10 mL, 15 mL, 20 mL)
Powder for solution, oral:
  Epiklor™: 20 mEq/packet (30s, 100s)
  Epiklor™/25: 25 mEq/packet (30s, 100s)
  Klor-Con®: 20 mEq/packet (30s, 100s)
  Klor-Con®/25: 25 mEq/packet (30s, 100s)
Solution, oral: 20 mEq/15 mL (15 mL, 30 mL, 473 mL, 480 mL); 40 mEq/15 mL (15 mL, 473 mL)
Tablet, extended release, microencapsulated, oral: 8 mEq, 10 mEq, 20 mEq
  Klor-Con® M10: 10 mEq
  Klor-Con® M15: 15 mEq
  Klor-Con® M20: 20 mEq
Tablet, extended release, wax matrix, oral: 8 mEq, 10 mEq
  K-Tab®: 10 mEq
  Kaon-CL® 10: 10 mEq
  Klor-Con® 8: 8 mEq
  Klor-Con® 10: 10 mEq

potassium citrate (poe TASS ee um SIT rate)

Medication Safety Issues
  Sound-alike/look-alike issues:
  Urocit®-K may be confused with Urised®
U.S. Brand Names Urocit®-K
Canadian Brand Names Urocit®-K
Therapeutic Category Alkalinizing Agent
Use Prevention of uric acid nephrolithiasis; prevention of calcium renal stones in patients with hypocitraturia; urinary alkalinizer when sodium citrate is contraindicated
General Dosage Range Oral: *Adults:* 10-20 mEq 3 times/day with meals (maximum: 100 mEq/day)
Dosage Forms
  Tablet, oral: 540 mg, 1080 mg
  Urocit®-K: 540 mg, 1080 mg

potassium citrate and citric acid (poe TASS ee um SIT rate & SI trik AS id)

Synonyms citric acid and potassium citrate; Polycitra K
U.S. Brand Names Cytra-K
Therapeutic Category Alkalinizing Agent
Use Treatment of metabolic acidosis; alkalinizing agent in conditions where long-term maintenance of an alkaline urine is desirable
General Dosage Range Oral:
  Children: 5-15 mL after meals and at bedtime
  Adults: 15-30 mL **or** 1 packet dissolved in water after meals and at bedtime
Dosage Forms Equivalent to potassium 2 mEq/mL and bicarbonate 2 mEq/mL
  Powder for solution, oral:
  Cytra-K: Potassium citrate 3300 mg and citric acid 1002 mg per packet (100s)
  Solution:
  Cytra-K: Potassium citrate 1100 mg and citric acid 334 mg per 5 mL

potassium citrate, citric acid, and sodium citrate *see* citric acid, sodium citrate, and potassium citrate *on page 214*

potassium gluconate (poe TASS ee um GLOO coe nate)

Therapeutic Category Electrolyte Supplement, Oral
Use Treatment or prevention of hypokalemia
General Dosage Range Oral:
  Children: 1-5 mEq/kg/day in 1-4 divided doses
  Adults: 16-100 mEq/day in 1-4 divided doses

◄ **Dosage Forms**
Caplet, oral: 595 mg
Capsule, oral: 99 mg
Tablet, oral: 99 mg, 550 mg, 595 mg
Tablet, timed release, oral: 95 mg

potassium iodide (poe TASS ee um EYE oh dide)
Medication Safety Issues
Sound-alike/look-alike issues:
Potassium iodide products, including saturated solution of potassium iodide (SSKI®) may be confused with potassium iodide and iodine (Strong Iodide Solution or Lugol's solution)
Synonyms KI
U.S. Brand Names iOSAT™ [OTC]; SSKI®; ThyroSafe™; Thyroshield™ [OTC]
Therapeutic Category Antithyroid Agent; Expectorant
Use Expectorant for the symptomatic treatment of chronic pulmonary diseases complicated by mucous; block thyroidal uptake of radioactive isotopes of iodine in a radiation emergency
General Dosage Range Oral:
Infants 1-12 months and Children 1-3 years: Iosat™, ThyroSafe™, ThyroShield™: 32.5 mg once daily
Children 3-18 years: Iosat™, ThyroSafe™, ThyroShield™: 65-130 mg once daily
Adults: Iosat™, ThyroSafe™, ThyroShield™: 130 mg once daily; SSKI®: 300-600 mg (6-12 drops) 3-4 times/day
Dosage Forms
Solution, oral:
SSKI®: 1 g/mL (30 mL, 237 mL)
Thyroshield™ [OTC]: 65 mg/mL (30 mL)
Tablet, oral:
iOSAT™ [OTC]: 130 mg
ThyroSafe™: 65 mg

potassium phosphate (poe TASS ee um FOS fate)
Medication Safety Issues
High alert medication:
The Institute for Safe Medication Practices (ISMP) includes this medication (I.V. formulation) among its list of drugs which have a heightened risk of causing significant patient harm when used in error.
Other safety concerns:
Per JCAHO recommendations, concentrated electrolyte solutions should not be available in patient care areas.
Consider special storage requirements for intravenous potassium salts; I.V. potassium salts have been administered IVP in error, leading to fatal outcomes.
Safe Prescribing: Because inorganic phosphate exists as monobasic and dibasic anions, with the mixture of valences dependent on pH, ordering by mEq amounts is unreliable and may lead to large dosing errors. In addition, I.V. phosphate is available in the sodium and potassium salt; therefore, the content of these cations must be considered when ordering phosphate. The most reliable method of ordering I.V. phosphate is by millimoles, then specifying the potassium or sodium salt. For example, an order for 15 mmol of phosphate as potassium phosphate in one liter of normal saline.
Synonyms phosphate, potassium
U.S. Brand Names Neutra-Phos®-K [OTC] [DSC]
Therapeutic Category Electrolyte Supplement, Oral
Use Treatment and prevention of hypophosphatemia; **Note:** The concomitant amount of potassium must be calculated into the total electrolyte content. For each 1 mmol of phosphate, ~1.5 mEq of potassium will be administered. Therefore, if ordering 30 mmol of potassium phosphate, the patient will receive ~45 mEq of potassium.
General Dosage Range
I.V.:
Children: 0.08-1 mmol phosphate/kg **or** Parenteral nutrition: Infusion: 0.5-2 mmol/kg/24 hours
Adults: 0.08-1 mmol phosphate/kg **or** Parenteral nutrition: Infusion: 20-40 mmol/24 hours
Dosage Forms
Injection, solution: Potassium 4.4 mEq and phosphorus 3 mmol per mL (5 mL, 15 mL, 50 mL)

potassium phosphate and sodium phosphate
(poe TASS ee um FOS fate & SOW dee um FOS fate)

Medication Safety Issues
  Sound-alike/look-alike issues:
   K-Phos® Neutral may be confused with Neutra-Phos-K®
Synonyms Neutra-Phos; sodium phosphate and potassium phosphate
U.S. Brand Names K-Phos® MF; K-Phos® Neutral; K-Phos® No. 2; Phos-NaK; Phospha 250™ Neutral
Therapeutic Category Electrolyte Supplement, Oral
Use Treatment of conditions associated with excessive renal phosphate loss or inadequate GI absorption of phosphate; to acidify the urine to lower calcium concentrations; to increase the antibacterial activity of methenamine; reduce odor and rash caused by ammonia in urine
General Dosage Range Oral: *Children ≥4 years and Adults:* Elemental phosphorus 250 mg 4 times/day after meals and at bedtime
Dosage Forms
  Powder, for oral solution:
   Phos-NaK: Dibasic potassium phosphate, monobasic potassium phosphate, dibasic sodium phosphate, and monobasic sodium phosphate per packet (100s)
  Tablet:
   K-Phos® MF: Potassium phosphate 155 mg and sodium phosphate 350 mg
   K-Phos® Neutral: Monobasic potassium phosphate 155 mg, dibasic sodium phosphate 852 mg, and monobasic sodium phosphate 130 mg
   K-Phos® No. 2: Potassium phosphate 305 mg and sodium phosphate 700 mg
   Phospha 250™ Neutral: Monobasic potassium phosphate 155 mg, dibasic sodium phosphate 852 mg, and monobasic sodium phosphate 130 mg

potassium sulfate, magnesium sulfate, and sodium sulfate *see* sodium sulfate, potassium sulfate, and magnesium sulfate *on page 824*
potassium sulfate, sodium sulfate, and magnesium sulfate *see* sodium sulfate, potassium sulfate, and magnesium sulfate *on page 824*
Potiga™ *see* ezogabine *on page 364*
Povidine™ [OTC] *see* povidone-iodine (topical) *on page 727*

povidone-iodine (ophthalmic) (POE vi done EYE oh dyne)

Medication Safety Issues
  Sound-alike/look-alike issues:
   Betadine® may be confused with Betagan®, betaine
Synonyms polyvinylpyrrolidone with iodine; PVP-I
U.S. Brand Names Betadine®
Therapeutic Category Antiseptic, Ophthalmic
Use Prepping the periocular region (lids, brows, and cheeks) and irrigation of the ocular surface
General Dosage Range Topical: *Adults:* Ophthalmic solution: Eyelids: Apply to area (repeat once); Periocular area: Apply to area (repeat 3 times); Ocular area: Irrigate once
Dosage Forms
  Solution, ophthalmic:
   Betadine®: 5% (30 mL)

povidone-iodine (topical) (POE vi done EYE oh dyne)

Medication Safety Issues
  Sound-alike/look-alike issues:
   Betadine® may be confused with Betagan®, betaine
Synonyms polyvinylpyrrolidone with iodine; PVP-I
U.S. Brand Names Betadine® Swab Aids [OTC]; Betadine® [OTC]; Operand® Povidone-Iodine [OTC]; Povidine™ [OTC]; Summer's Eve® Medicated Douche [OTC]; Vagi-Gard® [OTC]
Canadian Brand Names Betadine®; Proviodine
Therapeutic Category Antiseptic, Topical; Antiseptic, Vaginal; Topical Skin Product
Use External antiseptic with broad microbicidal spectrum for the prevention or treatment of topical infections associated with surgery, burns, minor cuts/scrapes; relief of minor vaginal irritation
General Dosage Range
  Intravaginal: *Adults:* Insert 0.3% solution vaginally once daily

◀ **Topical:** *Adults:* Apply to affected area as needed **or** apply to wet skin or hands, scrub for ~5 minutes, then rinse

Dosage Forms
Gel, topical: 10% (120 mL)
 Operand® Povidone-Iodine [OTC]: 10% (118 mL)
Liquid, topical: 10% (0.65 mL)
Ointment, topical: 10% (1 g, 28 g)
 Povidine™ [OTC]: 10% (30 g)
Pad, topical: 10% (200s)
 Betadine® Swab Aids [OTC]: 10% (100s)
Solution, perineal:
 Operand® Povidone-Iodine [OTC]: 10% (240 mL)
Solution, topical: 7.5% (60 mL, 120 mL); 10% (22 mL, 30 mL, 59 mL, 60 mL, 90 mL, 120 mL, 237 mL, 473 mL, 480 mL, 50s)
 Betadine® [OTC]: 5% (88.7 mL); 10% (15 mL, 120 mL, 237 mL, 473 mL, 960 mL, 3840 mL); 7.5% (118 mL, 473 mL, 960 mL, 3840 mL)
 Operand® Povidone-Iodine [OTC]: 10% (59 mL, 118 mL, 237 mL, 473 mL, 946 mL, 3785 mL); 7.5% (59 mL, 118 mL, 237 mL, 473 mL, 946 mL, 3785 mL)
 Povidine™ [OTC]: 10% (240 mL)
Solution, vaginal:
 Operand® Povidone-Iodine [OTC]: 10% (240 mL)
 Summer's Eve® Medicated Douche [OTC]: 0.3% (135 mL)
 Vagi-Gard® [OTC]: 10% (180 mL, 240 mL)
Swabsticks, topical: 7.5% (50s, 75s, 1000s); 10% (50s, 75s, 1000s)
 Betadine® [OTC]: 10% (150s, 200s)

PPD *see* tuberculin tests *on page 896*
PPI-0903 *see* ceftaroline fosamil *on page 184*
PPI-0903M *see* ceftaroline fosamil *on page 184*
PPL *see* benzylpenicilloyl polylysine *on page 127*
PPS *see* pentosan polysulfate sodium *on page 688*
PPSV *see* pneumococcal polysaccharide vaccine (polyvalent) *on page 715*
PPSV23 *see* pneumococcal polysaccharide vaccine (polyvalent) *on page 715*
PPV23 *see* pneumococcal polysaccharide vaccine (polyvalent) *on page 715*
PR™ *see* emollients *on page 325*
Pradax™ (Can) *see* dabigatran etexilate *on page 248*
Pradaxa® *see* dabigatran etexilate *on page 248*

pralatrexate (pral a TREX ate)

Medication Safety Issues
 Sound-alike/look-alike issues:
 PRALAtrexate may be confused with methotrexate, PEMEtrexed, raltitrexed
 Folotyn® may be confused with Focalin®
 High alert medication:
 This medication is in a class the Institute for Safe Medication Practices (ISMP) includes among its list of drug classes which have a heightened risk of causing significant patient harm when used in error.
Synonyms PDX
Tall-Man PRALAtrexate
U.S. Brand Names Folotyn®
Therapeutic Category Antineoplastic Agent, Antimetabolite (Antifolate)
Use Treatment of relapsed or refractory peripheral T-cell lymphoma (PTCL)
General Dosage Range Dosage adjustment recommended in patients who develop toxicities
 I.V.: *Adults:* 30 mg/m^2 once weekly for 6 weeks of a 7-week treatment cycle
Dosage Forms
 Injection, solution [preservative free]:
 Folotyn®: 20 mg/mL (1 mL, 2 mL)

pralidoxime (pra li DOKS eem)

Medication Safety Issues

Sound-alike/look-alike issues:

Pralidoxime may be confused with pramoxine, pyridoxine

Protopam® may be confused with protamine, Protropin®

Synonyms 2-PAM; 2-pyridine aldoxime methochloride; pralidoxime chloride

U.S. Brand Names Protopam®

Therapeutic Category Antidote

Use Treatment of muscle weakness and/or respiratory depression secondary to poisoning due to organophosphate anticholinesterase pesticides and chemicals (eg, nerve agents); control of overdose of anticholinesterase medications used to treat myasthenia gravis (ambenonium, neostigmine, pyridostigmine)

General Dosage Range Dosage adjustment recommended in patients with renal impairment

I.M.:

Children <40 kg: 15 mg/kg; repeat twice to deliver a total dose of 45 mg/kg

Children ≥40 kg and Adults: 600 mg; repeat twice to deliver a total dose of 1800 mg

I.V.:

Children ≤16 years: Loading dose: 20-50 mg/kg (maximum: 2000 mg/dose); Maintenance infusion: 10-20 mg/kg/hour or repeat bolus of 20-50 mg/kg (maximum: 2000 mg/dose)

Children >16 years and Adults: Loading dose: 1000-2000 mg; Maintenance: Repeat bolus of 1000-2000 mg after 1 hour and every 10-12 hours thereafter, as needed **or** 1000-2000 mg, followed by increments of 250 mg every 5 minutes as needed

Dosage Forms

Injection, powder for reconstitution:

Protopam®: 1 g

Injection, solution: 300 mg/mL (2 mL)

pralidoxime and atropine *see* atropine and pralidoxime *on page 104*

pralidoxime chloride *see* pralidoxime *on page 729*

pramipexole (pra mi PEKS ole)

Medication Safety Issues

Sound-alike/look-alike issues:

Mirapex® may be confused with Hiprex®, Mifeprex®, MiraLax™

Synonyms pramipexole dihydrochloride monohydrate

U.S. Brand Names Mirapex®; Mirapex® ER®

Canadian Brand Names Apo-Pramipexole®; CO Pramipexole; Mirapex®; Novo-Pramipexole; PHL-Pramipexole; PMS-Pramipexole; Sandoz-Pramipexole; Teva-Pramipexole

Therapeutic Category Anti-Parkinson Agent (Dopamine Agonist)

Use

Immediate release: Treatment of the signs and symptoms of idiopathic Parkinson disease; treatment of moderate-to-severe primary Restless Legs Syndrome (RLS)

Extended release: Treatment of the signs and symptoms of idiopathic Parkinson disease

General Dosage Range Dosage adjustment recommended in patients with renal impairment

Oral: Immediate release: *Adults:* Initial: 0.375 mg/day given in 3 divided doses **or** 0.125 mg once daily before bedtime; Maintenance: 1.5-4.5 mg/day in 3 divided doses **or** 0.125-0.5 mg/day

Oral: Extended release: *Adults:* Initial: 0.375-4.5 mg once daily

Dosage Forms

Tablet, oral: 0.125 mg, 0.25 mg, 0.5 mg, 0.75 mg, 1 mg, 1.5 mg

Mirapex®: 0.125 mg, 0.25 mg, 0.5 mg, 0.75 mg, 1 mg, 1.5 mg

Tablet, extended release, oral:

Mirapex® ER®: 0.375 mg, 0.75 mg, 1.5 mg, 2.25 mg, 3 mg, 3.75 mg, 4.5 mg

pramipexole dihydrochloride monohydrate *see* pramipexole *on page 729*

pramlintide (PRAM lin tide)

Medication Safety Issues

High alert medication:

The Institute for Safe Medication Practices (ISMP) includes this medication among its list of drug classes which have a heightened risk of causing significant patient harm when used in error.

Administration issues:

Use caution when drawing up doses from the vial (concentration 600 micrograms (mcg)/mL). Manufacturer recommended dosing ranges from 15 mcg to 120 mcg, which corresponds to injectable volumes of 0.025 mL to 0.2 mL. Patients and healthcare providers should exercise caution when administering this product to avoid inadvertent calculation of the dose based on "units," which could result in a sixfold overdose.

Synonyms pramlintide acetate

U.S. Brand Names SymlinPen®; Symlin® [DSC]

Therapeutic Category Antidiabetic Agent, Oral

Use

Adjunctive treatment with mealtime insulin in type 1 diabetes mellitus (insulin-dependent, IDDM) patients who have failed to achieve desired glucose control despite optimal insulin therapy

Adjunctive treatment with mealtime insulin in type 2 diabetes mellitus (noninsulin-dependent, NIDDM) patients who have failed to achieve desired glucose control despite optimal insulin therapy, with or without concurrent sulfonylurea and/or metformin

General Dosage Range

SubQ:

Children: Dosage not established

Adults:

Type 1 diabetes mellitus (insulin-dependent, IDDM): Initial: 15 mcg immediately prior to meals; Target dose: 30-60 mcg prior to meals; **Note:** Titration is recommended

Type 2 diabetes mellitus (noninsulin-dependent, NIDDM): Initial: 60 mcg immediately prior to meals, after 3-7 days increase to 120 mcg prior to meals

Dosage Forms

Injection, solution:

SymlinPen®: 1000 mcg/mL (1.5 mL, 2.7 mL)

pramlintide acetate *see* pramlintide *on page* 730

Pramosone® *see* pramoxine and hydrocortisone *on page* 731

Pramosone E™ *see* pramoxine and hydrocortisone *on page* 731

Pramox® HC (Can) *see* pramoxine and hydrocortisone *on page* 731

pramoxine (pra MOKS een)

Medication Safety Issues

Sound-alike/look-alike issues:

Pramoxine may be confused with pralidoxime

Anusol® may be confused with Anusol-HC®, Aplisol®, Aquasol®

Synonyms pramoxine hydrochloride

U.S. Brand Names Caladryl® Clear™ [OTC]; Callergy Clear [OTC]; Curasore® [OTC]; Itch-X® [OTC]; Prax® [OTC]; Proctofoam® NS [OTC]; Sarna® Sensitive [OTC]; Sarna® Ultra [OTC]; Soothing Care™ Itch Relief [OTC]; Summer's Eve® Anti-Itch Maximum Strength [OTC]; Tronolane® Cream [OTC]; Tucks® Hemorrhoidal [OTC]

Therapeutic Category Local Anesthetic

Use Temporary relief of pain and itching associated with anogenital pruritus or irritation; dermatosis, minor burns, or hemorrhoids

General Dosage Range Topical: *Adults:* Apply 3-5 times/day to affected area

Dosage Forms

Aerosol, topical: 1% (15 g)

Proctofoam® NS [OTC]: 1% (15 g)

Cloth, topical:

Summer's Eve® Anti-Itch Maximum Strength [OTC]: 1% (12s)

Cream, topical:

Sarna® Ultra [OTC]: 1% (56.6 g)

Tronolane® Cream [OTC]: 1% (30 g, 57 g)

Gel, topical:
  Itch-X® [OTC]: 1% (35.4 g)
  Summer's Eve® Anti-Itch Maximum Strength [OTC]: 1% (30 mL)
Liquid, topical:
  Curasore® [OTC]: 1% (15 mL)
Lotion, topical:
  Caladryl® Clear™ [OTC]: 1% (177 mL)
  Callergy Clear [OTC]: 1% (177 mL)
  Prax® [OTC]: 1% (15 mL, 120 mL, 240 mL)
  Sarna® Sensitive [OTC]: 1% (222 mL)
Ointment, rectal:
  Tucks® Hemorrhoidal [OTC]: 1% (28.3 g)
Solution, topical:
  Itch-X® [OTC]: 1% (60 mL)
  Soothing Care™ Itch Relief [OTC]: 1% (74 mL)

pramoxine and hydrocortisone (pra MOKS een & hye droe KOR ti sone)
Medication Safety Issues
  Sound-alike/look-alike issues:
  Pramosone® may be confused with predniSONE
  Zone-A Forte® may be confused with Zonalon®
Synonyms hydrocortisone and pramoxine; pramoxine hydrochloride and hydrocortisone acetate
U.S. Brand Names Analpram E™; Analpram HC®; Epifoam®; Pramosone E™; Pramosone®; ProCort®; ProctoFoam® HC; Zypram™
Canadian Brand Names Pramox® HC; Proctofoam™-HC
Therapeutic Category Anesthetic/Corticosteroid
Use Relief of inflammatory and pruritic manifestations of corticosteroid-responsive dermatoses
General Dosage Range Rectal, topical: *Adults:* Apply to affected areas 3-4 times/day
Dosage Forms
  Cream, topical: Pramoxine 1% and hydrocortisone 1% (30 g); pramoxine 1% and hydrocortisone 2.5% (4 g, 30 g)
    Analpram Advanced™ Kit: Pramoxine 1% and hydrocortisone 2.5% (1s) [kit includes Analpram HC® cream (4 g x 30), diosmiplex (Vasculera™) tablets, AloeClean™ wipes, and applicators]
    Analpram Advanced™ Kit: Pramoxine 1% and hydrocortisone 2.5% (1s) [kit includes Analpram HC® cream (30 g), diosmiplex (Vasculera™) tablets, AloeClean™ wipes, and applicator]
    Analpram E™: Pramoxine 1% and hydrocortisone 2.5% (4 g, 30 g)
    Analpram HC®: Pramoxine 1% and hydrocortisone 1% (4 g, 30 g); pramoxine 1% and hydrocortisone 2.5% (4 g, 30 g)
    Pramosone®: Pramoxine 1% and hydrocortisone 1% (30 g, 60 g); pramoxine 1% and hydrocortisone 2.5% (30 g, 60 g)
    Pramosone E™: Pramoxine 1% and hydrocortisone 2.5% (30 g, 60 g)
    ProCort®: Pramoxine 1.15% and hydrocortisone 1.85% (60 g)
    Zypram™: Pramoxine 1% and hydrocortisone 2.35% (30 g)
  Foam, rectal:
    ProctoFoam® HC: Pramoxine 1% and hydrocortisone 1% (10 g)
  Foam, topical:
    Epifoam®: Pramoxine 1% and hydrocortisone 1% (10 g)
  Lotion, topical:
    Analpram HC®: Pramoxine 1% and hydrocortisone 2.5% (60 mL)
    Pramosone®: Pramoxine 1% and hydrocortisone 1% (60 mL, 120 mL, 240 mL); pramoxine 1% and hydrocortisone 2.5% (60 mL, 120 mL)
  Ointment, topical:
    Pramosone®: Pramoxine 1% and hydrocortisone 1% (30 g); pramoxine 1% and hydrocortisone 2.5% (30 g)

pramoxine hydrochloride *see* pramoxine *on page 730*
pramoxine hydrochloride and hydrocortisone acetate *see* pramoxine and hydrocortisone *on page 731*
pramoxine, neomycin, bacitracin, and polymyxin B *see* bacitracin, neomycin, polymyxin B, and pramoxine *on page 112*
PrandiMet® *see* repaglinide and metformin *on page 774*

Prandin® *see* repaglinide *on page 773*
Prascion® *see* sulfur and sulfacetamide *on page 838*
Prascion® FC *see* sulfur and sulfacetamide *on page 838*
Prascion® RA *see* sulfur and sulfacetamide *on page 838*

prasugrel (PRA soo grel)

Medication Safety Issues
Sound-alike/look-alike issues:
Prasugrel may be confused with pravastatin, propranolol
Synonyms CS-747; LY-640315; prasugrel hydrochloride
U.S. Brand Names Effient®
Therapeutic Category Antiplatelet Agent
Use Reduces rate of thrombotic cardiovascular events (eg, stent thrombosis) in patients with unstable angina, non-ST-segment elevation MI, or ST-elevation MI (STEMI) managed with percutaneous coronary intervention (PCI)
General Dosage Range Oral: *Adults:* Loading dose: 60 mg; Maintenance dose: 10 mg once daily (in combination with aspirin 81-325 mg/day)
Dosage Forms
Tablet, oral:
Effient®: 5 mg, 10 mg

prasugrel hydrochloride *see* prasugrel *on page 732*
Pravachol® *see* pravastatin *on page 732*

pravastatin (prav a STAT in)

Medication Safety Issues
Sound-alike/look-alike issues:
Pravachol® may be confused with atorvastatin, Prevacid®, Prinivil®, propranolol
Pravastatin may be confused with nystatin, pitavastatin, prasugrel
Synonyms pravastatin sodium
U.S. Brand Names Pravachol®
Canadian Brand Names Apo-Pravastatin®; CO Pravastatin; Dom-Pravastatin; Mylan-Pravastatin; Novo-Pravastatin; Nu-Pravastatin; PHL-Pravastatin; PMS-Pravastatin; Pravachol®; RAN™-Pravastatin; ratio-Pravastatin; Riva-Pravastatin; Sandoz-Pravastatin; ZYM-Pravastatin
Therapeutic Category HMG-CoA Reductase Inhibitor
Use Use with dietary therapy for the following:
Primary prevention of coronary events: In hypercholesterolemic patients without established coronary heart disease to reduce cardiovascular morbidity (myocardial infarction, coronary revascularization procedures) and mortality.
Secondary prevention of cardiovascular events in patients with established coronary heart disease: To slow the progression of coronary atherosclerosis; to reduce cardiovascular morbidity (myocardial infarction, coronary vascular procedures) and to reduce mortality; to reduce the risk of stroke and transient ischemic attacks
Hyperlipidemias: Reduce elevations in total cholesterol, LDL-C, apolipoprotein B, and triglycerides (elevations of 1 or more components are present in Fredrickson type IIa, IIb, III, and IV hyperlipidemias)
Heterozygous familial hypercholesterolemia (HeFH): In pediatric patients, 8-18 years of age, with HeFH having LDL-C ≥190 mg/dL **or** LDL ≥160 mg/dL with positive family history of premature cardiovascular disease (CVD) or 2 or more CVD risk factors in the pediatric patient
General Dosage Range Dosage adjustment recommended in patients with hepatic or renal impairment or on concomitant therapy
Oral:
Children 8-13 years: 20 mg once daily
Children 14-18 years: 40 mg once daily
Adults: Initial: 10-40 mg once daily; Maintenance: 10-80 mg once daily (maximum: 80 mg/day)
Dosage Forms
Tablet, oral: 10 mg, 20 mg, 40 mg, 80 mg
Pravachol®: 10 mg, 20 mg, 40 mg, 80 mg

pravastatin sodium *see* pravastatin *on page 732*
Prax® [OTC] *see* pramoxine *on page 730*

Praxis ASA EC 81 Mg Daily Dose (Can) *see* aspirin *on page 98*

praziquantel (pray zi KWON tel)

U.S. Brand Names Biltricide®

Canadian Brand Names Biltricide®

Therapeutic Category Anthelmintic

Use Treatment of all stages of schistosomiasis caused by all *Schistosoma* species; treatment of infection (clonorchiasis and opisthorchiasis) due to liver flukes

General Dosage Range Oral: *Children ≥4 years and Adults:* 20 mg/kg/dose 2-3 times/day for 1 day at 4- to 6-hour intervals **or** 25 mg/kg 3 times/day for 1 day

Dosage Forms
Tablet, oral:
Biltricide®: 600 mg

prazosin (PRAZ oh sin)

Medication Safety Issues
Sound-alike/look-alike issues:
Prazosin may be confused with predniSONE
International issues:
Prazepam [multiple international markets] may be confused with prazosin

Synonyms furazosin; prazosin hydrochloride

U.S. Brand Names Minipress®

Canadian Brand Names Apo-Prazo®; Minipress®; Novo-Prazin; Nu-Prazo

Therapeutic Category Alpha-Adrenergic Blocking Agent

Use Treatment of hypertension

General Dosage Range Oral: *Adults:* Initial: 1 mg/dose 2-3 times/day; Maintenance: 2-20 mg/day in divided doses 2-3 times/day (maximum: 20 mg/day) (JNC 7)

Dosage Forms
Capsule, oral: 1 mg, 2 mg, 5 mg
Minipress®: 1 mg, 2 mg, 5 mg

prazosin hydrochloride *see* prazosin *on page 733*

PreCare® *see* vitamins (multiple/prenatal) *on page 920*

Precedex® *see* dexmedetomidine *on page 266*

Precose® *see* acarbose *on page 23*

Pred Forte® *see* prednisolone (ophthalmic) *on page 734*

Pred-G® *see* prednisolone and gentamicin *on page 734*

Pred Mild® *see* prednisolone (ophthalmic) *on page 734*

prednicarbate (pred ni KAR bate)

Medication Safety Issues
Sound-alike/look-alike issues:
Dermatop® may be confused with Dimetapp®

U.S. Brand Names Dermatop®

Canadian Brand Names Dermatop®

Therapeutic Category Corticosteroid, Topical

Use Relief of the inflammatory and pruritic manifestations of corticosteroid-responsive dermatoses (medium-potency topical corticosteroid)

General Dosage Range Topical:
Children ≥1 year and Adults: Cream: Apply a thin film to affected area twice daily
Children ≥10 year and Adults: Ointment: Apply a thin film to affected area twice daily

Dosage Forms
Cream, topical: 0.1% (15 g, 60 g)
Dermatop®: 0.1% (60 g)
Ointment, topical: 0.1% (15 g, 60 g)
Dermatop®: 0.1% (60 g)

prednisolone (systemic) (pred NISS oh lone)

Medication Safety Issues
Sound-alike/look-alike issues:
PrednisoLONE may be confused with predniSONE
Pediapred® may be confused with Pediazole®
Prelone® may be confused with Prozac®
Synonyms prednisolone sodium phosphate
Tall-Man prednisoLONE
U.S. Brand Names Flo-Pred™; Millipred™; Orapred ODT®; Orapred®; Pediapred®; Prelone®; Veripred™ 20
Canadian Brand Names Hydeltra T.B.A.®; Novo-Prednisolone; Pediapred®
Therapeutic Category Corticosteroid, Systemic
Use Treatment of endocrine disorders, rheumatic disorders, collagen diseases, allergic states, respiratory diseases, hematologic disorders, neoplastic diseases, edematous states, and gastrointestinal diseases; resolution of acute exacerbations of multiple sclerosis; management of fulminating or disseminated tuberculosis and trichinosis; acute or chronic solid organ rejection
General Dosage Range Oral:
Children: Dosage varies greatly depending on indication
Adults: 5-60 mg/day **or** 200 mg/day for 1 week followed by 80 mg every other day for 1 month
Dosage Forms
Solution, oral: 5 mg/5 mL (5 mL, 10 mL, 20 mL, 118 mL, 120 mL); 15 mg/5 mL (237 mL, 240 mL, 473 mL, 480 mL)
Millipred™: 10 mg/5 mL (237 mL)
Orapred®: 15 mg/5 mL (20 mL, 237 mL)
Pediapred®: 5 mg/5 mL (120 mL)
Veripred™ 20: 20 mg/5 mL (237 mL)
Suspension, oral:
Flo-Pred™: 15 mg/5 mL (52 mL)
Syrup, oral: 15 mg/5 mL (5 mL, 236 mL, 237 mL, 240 mL, 473 mL, 480 mL)
Prelone®: 15 mg/5 mL (240 mL, 480 mL)
Tablet, orally disintegrating, oral:
Orapred ODT®: 10 mg, 15 mg, 30 mg

prednisolone (ophthalmic) (pred NISS oh lone)

Medication Safety Issues
Sound-alike/look-alike issues:
PrednisoLONE may be confused with predniSONE
Synonyms Econopred; prednisolone acetate, ophthalmic; prednisolone sodium phosphate, ophthalmic
Tall-Man prednisoLONE
U.S. Brand Names Omnipred™; Pred Forte®; Pred Mild®
Canadian Brand Names Diopred®; Ophtho-Tate®; Pred Forte®; Pred Mild®
Therapeutic Category Corticosteroid, Ophthalmic
Use Treatment of palpebral and bulbar conjunctivitis; corneal injury from chemical, radiation, thermal burns, or foreign body penetration; steroid-responsive inflammatory ophthalmic diseases
General Dosage Range Ophthalmic: *Children and Adults:* Initial: Instill 1-2 drops into conjunctival sac every hour during day, every 2 hours at night; Maintenance: 1 drop every 4 hours
Dosage Forms
Solution, ophthalmic: 1% (5 mL, 10 mL, 15 mL)
Suspension, ophthalmic: 1% (5 mL, 10 mL, 15 mL)
Omnipred™: 1% (5 mL, 10 mL)
Pred Forte®: 1% (1 mL, 5 mL, 10 mL, 15 mL)
Pred Mild®: 0.12% (5 mL, 10 mL)

prednisolone acetate, ophthalmic *see* prednisolone (ophthalmic) *on page 734*

prednisolone and gentamicin (pred NIS oh lone & jen ta MYE sin)

Synonyms gentamicin and prednisolone
U.S. Brand Names Pred-G®
Therapeutic Category Antibiotic/Corticosteroid, Ophthalmic

Use Treatment of steroid responsive inflammatory conditions and superficial ocular infections due to microorganisms susceptible to gentamicin

General Dosage Range Ophthalmic: *Children and Adults:*
Ointment: Apply 1/2" ribbon in the conjunctival sac 1-3 times/day
Suspension: Initial: 1 drop every hour for 1-2 days; Maintenance: 1 drop 2-4 times/day

Dosage Forms
Ointment, ophthalmic:
Pred-G®: Prednisolone 0.6% and gentamicin 0.3% (3.5 g)

prednisolone and sulfacetamide *see* sulfacetamide and prednisolone *on page 835*

prednisolone, neomycin, and polymyxin B *see* neomycin, polymyxin B, and prednisolone *on page 619*

prednisolone sodium phosphate *see* prednisolone (systemic) *on page 734*

prednisolone sodium phosphate, ophthalmic *see* prednisolone (ophthalmic) *on page 734*

prednisone (PRED ni sone)

Medication Safety Issues
Sound-alike/look-alike issues:
PredniSONE may be confused with methylPREDNISolone, Pramosone®, prazosin, prednisoLONE, PriLOSEC®, primidone, promethazine

Synonyms deltacortisone; deltadehydrocortisone

Tall-Man predni**SONE**

U.S. Brand Names PredniSONE Intensol™

Canadian Brand Names Apo-Prednisone®; Novo-Prednisone; Winpred™

Therapeutic Category Adrenal Corticosteroid

Use Treatment of a variety of diseases, including:
Allergic states (including adjunctive treatment of anaphylaxis)
Autoimmune disorders (including systemic lupus erythematosus [SLE])
Collagen diseases
Dermatologic conditions/diseases
Edematous states (including nephrotic syndrome)
Endocrine disorders
Gastrointestinal diseases
Hematologic disorders (including idiopathic thrombocytopenia purpura [ITP])
Multiple sclerosis exacerbations
Neoplastic diseases
Ophthalmic diseases
Respiratory diseases (including acute asthma exacerbation)
Rheumatic disorders (including rheumatoid arthritis)
Trichinosis with neurologic or myocardial involvement
Tuberculous meningitis

General Dosage Range Oral: *Children:* Initial: 5-60 mg/day

Dosage Forms
Solution, oral: 1 mg/mL (5 mL, 120 mL, 500 mL)
PredniSONE Intensol™: 5 mg/mL (30 mL)
Tablet, oral: 1 mg, 2.5 mg, 5 mg, 10 mg, 20 mg, 50 mg

PredniSONE Intensol™ *see* prednisone *on page 735*

PreferaOB® *see* vitamins (multiple/prenatal) *on page 920*

PreferaOB® + DHA *see* vitamins (multiple/prenatal) *on page 920*

PreferaOB® One™ *see* vitamins (multiple/prenatal) *on page 920*

Prefest™ *see* estradiol and norgestimate *on page 346*

pregabalin (pre GAB a lin)

Medication Safety Issues
Sound-alike/look-alike issues:
Lyrica® may be confused with Lopressor®

Synonyms CI-1008; S-(+)-3-isobutylgaba

U.S. Brand Names Lyrica®

Canadian Brand Names Lyrica®

◀ **Therapeutic Category** Analgesic, Miscellaneous; Anticonvulsant, Miscellaneous

Controlled Substance C-V

Use Management of pain associated with diabetic peripheral neuropathy; management of postherpetic neuralgia; adjunctive therapy for partial-onset seizure disorder in adults; management of fibromyalgia

General Dosage Range Dosage adjustment recommended in patients with renal impairment

  Oral: Adults: Initial: 150 mg/day in 2-3 divided doses; Maintenance: 150-600 mg/day in 2-3 divided doses (maximum: 600 mg/day)

Product Availability Lyrica® oral solution: FDA approved December 2009; anticipated availability is currently undetermined

Dosage Forms

  Capsule, oral:

  Lyrica®: 25 mg, 50 mg, 75 mg, 100 mg, 150 mg, 200 mg, 225 mg, 300 mg

pregnenedione *see* progesterone *on page 741*

Pregnyl® *see* chorionic gonadotropin (human) *on page 206*

Prelone® *see* prednisolone (systemic) *on page 734*

Premarin® *see* estrogens (conjugated/equine, systemic) *on page 347*

Premarin® *see* estrogens (conjugated/equine, topical) *on page 348*

PremaSol™ *see* amino acid injection *on page 65*

Premjact® *see* lidocaine (topical) *on page 524*

Premphase® *see* estrogens (conjugated/equine) and medroxyprogesterone *on page 348*

Premplus® (Can) *see* estrogens (conjugated/equine) and medroxyprogesterone *on page 348*

Prempro® *see* estrogens (conjugated/equine) and medroxyprogesterone *on page 348*

Prenatabs FA *see* vitamins (multiple/prenatal) *on page 920*

Prenatal One Daily [OTC] *see* vitamins (multiple/prenatal) *on page 920*

Prenatal Rx 1 *see* vitamins (multiple/prenatal) *on page 920*

prenatal vitamins *see* vitamins (multiple/prenatal) *on page 920*

Prenatal With Beta Carotene [OTC] *see* vitamins (multiple/prenatal) *on page 920*

Prenate DHA™ *see* vitamins (multiple/prenatal) *on page 920*

Prenate Elite® *see* vitamins (multiple/prenatal) *on page 920*

Prenate Essential™ *see* vitamins (multiple/prenatal) *on page 920*

PreNexa® Premier *see* vitamins (multiple/prenatal) *on page 920*

Preparation H® [OTC] *see* phenylephrine (topical) *on page 698*

Preparation H® Cleansing Pads (Can) *see* witch hazel *on page 923*

Preparation H® Hydrocortisone [OTC] *see* hydrocortisone (topical) *on page 450*

Preparation H® Medicated Wipes [OTC] *see* witch hazel *on page 923*

Pre-Pen® *see* benzylpenicilloyl polylysine *on page 127*

Prepidil® *see* dinoprostone *on page 289*

PreserVision® AREDS [OTC] *see* vitamins (multiple/oral) *on page 919*

PreserVision® Lutein [OTC] *see* vitamins (multiple/oral) *on page 919*

Pressyn® (Can) *see* vasopressin *on page 910*

Pressyn® AR (Can) *see* vasopressin *on page 910*

Pretz® [OTC] *see* sodium chloride *on page 818*

Prevacare® [OTC] *see* alcohol (ethyl) *on page 47*

Prevacid® *see* lansoprazole *on page 511*

Prevacid® 24 HR [OTC] *see* lansoprazole *on page 511*

Prevacid® FasTab (Can) *see* lansoprazole *on page 511*

Prevacid® SoluTab™ *see* lansoprazole *on page 511*

Prevalite® *see* cholestyramine resin *on page 205*

Prevex® B (Can) *see* betamethasone *on page 129*

Prevex® HC (Can) *see* hydrocortisone (topical) *on page 450*

PreviDent® *see* fluoride *on page 386*

PreviDent® 5000 Booster *see* fluoride *on page 386*

PreviDent® 5000 Dry Mouth *see* fluoride *on page 386*

PreviDent® 5000 Plus® *see* fluoride *on page 386*

PreviDent® 5000 Sensitive *see* fluoride *on page 386*
Prevnar® *see* pneumococcal conjugate vaccine (7-valent) *on page 714*
Prevnar 13™ *see* pneumococcal conjugate vaccine (13-valent) *on page 714*
Prevpac® *see* lansoprazole, amoxicillin, and clarithromycin *on page 511*
Prezista® *see* darunavir *on page 254*
Prialt® *see* ziconotide *on page 928*
Priftin® *see* rifapentine *on page 780*

prilocaine (PRIL oh kane)
Medication Safety Issues
  Sound-alike/look-alike issues:
  Prilocaine may be confused with Polocaine®, PriLOSEC®
U.S. Brand Names Citanest® Plain Dental
Canadian Brand Names Citanest® Plain
Therapeutic Category Local Anesthetic
General Dosage Range Dental (infiltration or conduction block):
  Children <10 years: Doses >40 mg (1 mL) as a 4% solution per procedure rarely needed
  Children ≥10 years and Adults: Initial: 40-80 mg (1-2 mL) as a 4% solution, up to a maximum of 400 mg (10 mL) as a 4% solution within a 2-hour period (maximum: 600 mg/dose [per manufacturer])
Dosage Forms
  Injection, solution:
  Citanest® Plain Dental: 4% [40 mg/mL] (1.8 mL)

prilocaine and lidocaine *see* lidocaine and prilocaine *on page 526*
PriLOSEC® *see* omeprazole *on page 649*
PriLOSEC OTC® [OTC] *see* omeprazole *on page 649*
PrimaCare® One *see* vitamins (multiple/prenatal) *on page 920*
primaclone *see* primidone *on page 737*
Primacor® (Can) *see* milrinone *on page 589*

primaquine (PRIM a kween)
Medication Safety Issues
  Sound-alike/look-alike issues:
  Primaquine may be confused with primidone
Synonyms primaquine phosphate; prymaccone
Therapeutic Category Aminoquinoline (Antimalarial)
Use Prevention of relapse of *P. vivax* malaria
General Dosage Range Oral:
  Children: 0.5 mg/kg once daily for 14 days (maximum dose: 30 mg/day); Alternative regimen (recommended for mild G6PD deficiency): 45 mg once weekly for 8 weeks
  Adults: 30 mg once daily for 14 days; Alternative regimen (recommended for mild G6PD deficiency): 45 mg once weekly for 8 weeks
Dosage Forms
  Tablet, oral: 26.3 mg

primaquine phosphate *see* primaquine *on page 737*
Primatene® Mist [OTC] [DSC] *see* epinephrine (systemic, oral inhalation) *on page 331*
Primaxin® I.M. [DSC] *see* imipenem and cilastatin *on page 466*
Primaxin® I.V. *see* imipenem and cilastatin *on page 466*
Primaxin® I.V. Infusion (Can) *see* imipenem and cilastatin *on page 466*
Primene® (Can) *see* amino acid injection *on page 65*

primidone (PRI mi done)
Medication Safety Issues
  Sound-alike/look-alike issues:
  Primidone may be confused with predniSONE, primaquine, pyridoxine
Synonyms desoxyphenobarbital; primaclone
U.S. Brand Names Mysoline®

◀ **Canadian Brand Names** Apo-Primidone®
Therapeutic Category Anticonvulsant; Barbiturate
Use Management of grand mal, psychomotor, and focal seizures
General Dosage Range Dosage adjustment recommended in patients with renal impairment
Oral:
Children <8 years: Initial: 50 mg once daily at bedtime; Maintenance: 375-750 mg/day (10-25 mg/kg/day) in 3-4 divided doses
Children ≥8 years and Adults: Initial: 100-125 mg/day at bedtime; Maintenance: 750-1500 mg/day in 3-4 divided doses (maximum: 2 g/day)
Dosage Forms
Tablet, oral: 50 mg, 250 mg
Mysoline®: 50 mg, 250 mg
Dosage Forms - Canada
Tablet:
Apo-Primidone®: 125 mg, 250 mg

Primlev™ *see* oxycodone and acetaminophen *on page 662*
Primovist (Can) *see* gadoxetate *on page 409*
Primsol® *see* trimethoprim *on page 892*
Prinivil® *see* lisinopril *on page 531*
Prinzide® *see* lisinopril and hydrochlorothiazide *on page 532*
Priorix™ (Can) *see* measles, mumps, and rubella virus vaccine *on page 551*
Priorix-Tetra™ (Can) *see* measles, mumps, rubella, and varicella virus vaccine *on page 551*
PrismaSol *see* electrolyte solution, renal replacement *on page 323*
pristinamycin *see* quinupristin and dalfopristin *on page 763*
Pristiq® *see* desvenlafaxine *on page 264*
Privigen® *see* immune globulin *on page 468*
Privine® [OTC] *see* naphazoline (nasal) *on page 611*
ProAir® HFA *see* albuterol *on page 45*
ProAmatine® [DSC] *see* midodrine *on page 588*
PRO-Amiodarone (Can) *see* amiodarone *on page 67*
PRO-Azithromycin (Can) *see* azithromycin (systemic) *on page 108*

probenecid (proe BEN e sid)

Medication Safety Issues
Sound-alike/look-alike issues:
Probenecid may be confused with Procanbid®
Synonyms Benemid [DSC]
Canadian Brand Names Benuryl™
Therapeutic Category Uricosuric Agent
Use Treatment of hyperuricemia associated with gout or gouty arthritis; prolongation and elevation of beta-lactam plasma levels (eg, uncomplicated gonococcal infection)
General Dosage Range Avoid use if Cl_{cr} <30 mL/minute.
Oral:
Children 2-14 years: Prolong penicillin serum levels: Initial: 25 mg/kg then 40 mg/kg/day given 4 times/day (maximum: 500 mg/dose)
Children >50 kg and Adults:
Gonorrhea, PID: 1 g as a single dose
Gout: Initial: 250 mg twice daily (maximum: 2 g/day)
Neurosyphilis: 500 mg 4 times/day for 10-14 days
Prolong PCN levels: 500 mg 4 times/day
Dosage Forms
Tablet, oral: 500 mg

probenecid and colchicine *see* colchicine and probenecid *on page 231*
PRO-Bicalutamide (Can) *see* bicalutamide *on page 133*
PRO-Bisoprolol (Can) *see* bisoprolol *on page 136*

procainamide (pro KANE a mide)

Medication Safety Issues
Sound-alike/look-alike issues:
Procanbid may be confused with probenecid, Procan SR®
Procan SR® may be confused with procanbid
Pronestyl may be confused with Ponstel®
High alert medication:
The Institute for Safe Medication Practices (ISMP) includes this medication among its list of drugs which have a heightened risk of causing significant patient harm when used in error.
Administration issues:
Procainamide hydrochloride is available in 10 mL vials of 100 mg/mL and in 2 mL vials with 500 mg/mL. Note that **BOTH** vials contain 1 gram of drug; confusing the strengths can lead to massive overdoses or underdoses.
Other safety concerns:
PCA is an error-prone abbreviation (mistaken as patient controlled analgesia)

Synonyms PCA (error-prone abbreviation); procainamide hydrochloride; procaine amide hydrochloride; Procanbid; Pronestyl

Canadian Brand Names Apo-Procainamide®; Procainamide Hydrochloride Injection, USP; Procan SR®

Therapeutic Category Antiarrhythmic Agent, Class I-A

Use
Intravenous: Treatment of life-threatening ventricular arrhythmias
Oral (Canadian labeling; not available in U.S.): Treatment of supraventricular arrhythmias. **Note:** In the treatment of atrial fibrillation, use only when preferred treatment is ineffective or cannot be used. Use in paroxysmal atrial tachycardia when reflex stimulation or other measures are ineffective.

General Dosage Range Dosage adjustment recommended in patients with hepatic or renal impairment
I.M.:
Children: 20-30 mg/kg/day divided every 4-6 hours (maximum: 4 g/day)
Adults: 50 mg/kg/day divided every 3-6 hours **or** 0.5-1 g every 4-8 hours
I.V.:
Children: Loading dose: 3-6 mg/kg/dose over 5 minutes (maximum: 100 mg/dose), may repeat every 5-10 minutes to maximum of 15 mg/kg/load; Infusion: 20-80 mcg/kg/minute (maximum: 2 g/day)
Adults: Loading dose: 15-18 mg/kg administered as slow infusion over 25-30 minutes **or** 100 mg/dose at a rate not to exceed 50 mg/minute repeated every 5 minutes as needed (maximum total dose: 1 g); Infusion: 1-4 mg/minute

Dosage Forms
Injection, solution: 100 mg/mL (10 mL); 500 mg/mL (2 mL)

Dosage Forms - Canada
Tablet, sustained release, oral:
Procan SR®: 250 mg, 500 mg, 750 mg

procainamide hydrochloride *see* procainamide *on page* 739
Procainamide Hydrochloride Injection, USP (Can) *see* procainamide *on page* 739
procaine amide hydrochloride *see* procainamide *on page* 739
procaine benzylpenicillin *see* penicillin G procaine *on page* 685
procaine penicillin G *see* penicillin G procaine *on page* 685
PRO-Calcitonin (Can) *see* calcitonin *on page* 159
Procanbid *see* procainamide *on page* 739
Procan SR® (Can) *see* procainamide *on page* 739

procarbazine (proe KAR ba zeen)

Medication Safety Issues
Sound-alike/look-alike issues:
Procarbazine may be confused with dacarbazine
Matulane® may be confused with Materna®
High alert medication:
The Institute for Safe Medication Practices (ISMP) includes this medication among its list of drugs which have a heightened risk of causing significant patient harm when used in error.

Synonyms benzmethyzin; N-methylhydrazine; procarbazine hydrochloride

U.S. Brand Names Matulane®

◀ **Canadian Brand Names** Matulane®; Natulan®

Therapeutic Category Antineoplastic Agent

Use Treatment of Hodgkin disease

General Dosage Range Dosage adjustment recommended in patients with hepatic impairment

Oral:

Children: 100 mg/m^2/day for 14 days and repeated every 4 weeks

Adults: Initial: 2-4 mg/kg/day in single or divided doses for 7 days, then increase dose to 4-6 mg/kg/day; Maintenance: 1-2 mg/kg/day

Dosage Forms

Capsule, oral:

Matulane®: 50 mg

procarbazine hydrochloride *see* procarbazine *on page 739*

Procardia® *see* nifedipine *on page 626*

Procardia XL® *see* nifedipine *on page 626*

PRO-Cefadroxil (Can) *see* cefadroxil *on page 180*

PRO-Cefuroxime (Can) *see* cefuroxime *on page 185*

ProCentra® *see* dextroamphetamine *on page 268*

procetofene *see* fenofibrate *on page 369*

Prochieve® [DSC] *see* progesterone *on page 741*

prochlorperazine (proe klor PER a zeen)

Medication Safety Issues

Sound-alike/look-alike issues:

Prochlorperazine may be confused with chlorproMAZINE

Compazine® may be confused with Copaxone®, Coumadin®

Other safety concerns:

CPZ (occasional abbreviation for Compazine®) is an error-prone abbreviation (mistaken as chlorpromazine)

Synonyms chlormeprazine; Compazine; prochlorperazine edisylate; prochlorperazine maleate

U.S. Brand Names Compro®

Canadian Brand Names Apo-Prochlorperazine®; Nu-Prochlor; Stemetil®

Therapeutic Category Phenothiazine Derivative

Use Management of nausea and vomiting; psychotic disorders, including schizophrenia and anxiety

General Dosage Range

I.M.:

Children ≥2 years and ≥9 kg: 0.13 mg/kg/dose; change to oral as soon as possible

Adults:

Antiemetic: 5-10 mg every 3-4 hours **or** 5-10 mg as a single dose with surgery, may repeat (maximum: 40 mg/day)

Antipsychotic: Initial: 10-20 mg every 1-4 hours to gain control (more than 3-4 doses are rarely needed); Maintenance: 10-20 mg every 4-6 hours

I.V.: *Adults:* 2.5-10 mg every 3-4 hours as needed (maximum: 40 mg/day) **or** 5-10 mg as a single dose with surgery, may repeat

Oral, rectal:

Children ≥2 years and ≥9 kg: Antiemetic:

>9 kg: 0.4 mg/kg/day in 3-4 divided doses

9-13 kg: 2.5 mg every 12-24 hours as needed (maximum: 7.5 mg/day)

13.1-17 kg: 2.5 mg every 8-12 hours as needed (maximum: 10 mg/day)

17.1-37 kg: 2.5 mg every 8 hours or 5 mg every 12 hours as needed (maximum: 15 mg/day)

Children 2-12 years: Antipsychotic: Initial: 2.5 mg 2-3 times/day; Maintenance: Increase as needed to maximum of 20 mg/day for 2-5 years and 25 mg/day for 6-12 years

Adults:

Antiemetic: 5-10 mg 3-4 times/day (maximum: 40 mg/day)

Antipsychotic: Initial: 5-10 mg 3-4 times/day; Maintenance: Up to 150 mg/day

Nonpsychotic anxiety: 15-20 mg/day in divided doses; do not give doses >20 mg/day or for longer than 12 weeks

Dosage Forms

Injection, solution: 5 mg/mL (2 mL, 10 mL)

Suppository, rectal: 25 mg (12s)
  Compro®: 25 mg (12s)
Tablet, oral: 5 mg, 10 mg

prochlorperazine edisylate *see* prochlorperazine *on page 740*
prochlorperazine maleate *see* prochlorperazine *on page 740*
PRO-Ciprofloxacin (Can) *see* ciprofloxacin (systemic) *on page 210*
PRO-Clonazepam (Can) *see* clonazepam *on page 222*
ProCort® *see* pramoxine and hydrocortisone *on page 731*
Procrit® *see* epoetin alfa *on page 333*
Proctocort® *see* hydrocortisone (topical) *on page 450*
ProctoCream®-HC *see* hydrocortisone (topical) *on page 450*
proctofene *see* fenofibrate *on page 369*
ProctoFoam® HC *see* pramoxine and hydrocortisone *on page 731*
Proctofoam™-HC (Can) *see* pramoxine and hydrocortisone *on page 731*
Proctofoam® NS [OTC] *see* pramoxine *on page 730*
Procto-Pak™ *see* hydrocortisone (topical) *on page 450*
Proctosol-HC® *see* hydrocortisone (topical) *on page 450*
Proctozone-HC 2.5%™ *see* hydrocortisone (topical) *on page 450*

procyclidine *(Canada only)* (proe SYE kli deen)

Synonyms procyclidine hydrochloride
Canadian Brand Names PHL-Procyclidine; PMS-Procyclidine
Therapeutic Category Anti-Parkinson Agent; Anticholinergic Agent
Use Relieves symptoms of parkinsonian syndrome and drug-induced extrapyramidal symptoms
General Dosage Range Oral:
  Adults: Initial: 2.5 mg 3 times/day; Maintenance: Up to 30 mg/day in 3-4 divided doses
  Elderly: Initial: 2.5 mg 1-2 times/day
Product Availability Not available in U.S.
Dosage Forms - Canada
  Tablet, oral: 2.5 mg, 5 mg
  Elixir, oral: 2.5 mg/5 mL

procyclidine hydrochloride *see* procyclidine *(Canada only) on page 741*
Procytox® (Can) *see* cyclophosphamide *on page 242*
PRO-Diclo-Rapide (Can) *see* diclofenac (systemic) *on page 277*
PRO-Doc Limitee Bromazepam (Can) *see* bromazepam *(Canada only) on page 142*
PRO-Enalapril (Can) *see* enalapril *on page 326*
ProFe [OTC] *see* polysaccharide-iron complex *on page 720*
PRO-Feno-Super (Can) *see* fenofibrate *on page 369*
Profilnine® SD *see* factor IX complex (human) *on page 365*
Proflavanol C™ (Can) *see* ascorbic acid *on page 96*
PRO-Fluconazole (Can) *see* fluconazole *on page 381*
PRO-Fluoxetine (Can) *see* fluoxetine *on page 389*
PRO-Gabapentin (Can) *see* gabapentin *on page 405*

progesterone (proe JES ter one)

Synonyms pregnenedione; progestin
U.S. Brand Names Crinone®; Endometrin®; First™-Progesterone VGS 100; First™-Progesterone VGS 200; First™-Progesterone VGS 25; First™-Progesterone VGS 400; First™-Progesterone VGS 50; Prochieve® [DSC]; Prometrium®
Canadian Brand Names Crinone®; Prometrium®
Therapeutic Category Progestin
Use
  Oral: Prevention of endometrial hyperplasia in nonhysterectomized, postmenopausal women who are receiving conjugated estrogen tablets; secondary amenorrhea
  I.M.: Amenorrhea; abnormal uterine bleeding due to hormonal imbalance

◄ Intravaginal gel: Part of assisted reproductive technology (ART) for infertile women with progesterone deficiency; secondary amenorrhea

Vaginal tablet: Part of ART for infertile women with progesterone deficiency

General Dosage Range
I.M.: *Adults (females):* 5-10 mg/day for 6 doses
Intravaginal: *Adults (females):*
ART: 90 mg (8% gel) once or twice daily or 100 mg (vaginal tablet) 2-3 times/day
Secondary amenorrhea: 45 mg (4% gel) every other day, may increase to 90 mg (8% gel) every other day if needed (maximum: 6 doses)
Oral: *Adults (females):*
Amenorrhea: 400 mg once daily in the evening for 10 days
Endometrial hyperplasia prevention: 200 mg once daily in the evening for 12 days sequentially per 28-day cycle

Dosage Forms
Capsule, oral:
Prometrium®: 100 mg, 200 mg
Gel, vaginal:
Crinone®: 4% (1.45 g); 8% (1.45 g)
Injection, oil: 50 mg/mL (10 mL)
Powder, for prescription compounding: USP: 100% (10 g, 25 g, 50 g, 100 g, 1000 g)
Suppository, vaginal:
First™-Progesterone VGS 25: 25 mg (30s)
First™-Progesterone VGS 50: 50 mg (30s)
First™-Progesterone VGS 100: 100 mg (30s)
First™-Progesterone VGS 200: 200 mg (30s)
First™-Progesterone VGS 400: 400 mg (30s)
Tablet, vaginal:
Endometrin®: 100 mg

progestin *see* progesterone *on page 741*
PRO-Glyburide (Can) *see* glyburide *on page 420*
Proglycem® *see* diazoxide *on page 277*
Prograf® *see* tacrolimus (systemic) *on page 842*
proguanil and atovaquone *see* atovaquone and proguanil *on page 103*
proguanil hydrochloride and atovaquone *see* atovaquone and proguanil *on page 103*
ProHance® *see* gadoteridol *on page 408*
ProHance® Multipack™ *see* gadoteridol *on page 408*
PRO-Hydroxyquine (Can) *see* hydroxychloroquine *on page 454*
PRO-Indapamide (Can) *see* indapamide *on page 470*
Pro-Indo (Can) *see* indomethacin *on page 471*
PRO-ISMN (Can) *see* isosorbide mononitrate *on page 495*
Prolastin®-C *see* alpha₁-proteinase inhibitor *on page 55*
Proleukin® *see* aldesleukin *on page 47*
PRO-Levetiracetam (Can) *see* levetiracetam *on page 517*
PRO-Levocarb (Can) *see* carbidopa and levodopa *on page 174*
Prolia® *see* denosumab *on page 259*
PRO-Lisinopril (Can) *see* lisinopril *on page 531*
Prolopa® (Can) *see* benserazide and levodopa *(Canada only) on page 120*
PRO-Lorazepam (Can) *see* lorazepam *on page 537*
PRO-Lovastatin (Can) *see* lovastatin *on page 540*
Promacet *see* butalbital and acetaminophen *on page 153*
Promacta® *see* eltrombopag *on page 324*
PRO-Metformin (Can) *see* metformin *on page 566*

promethazine (proe METH a zeen)
Medication Safety Issues
Sound-alike/look-alike issues:
Promethazine may be confused with chlorproMAZINE, predniSONE, promazine

Phenergan® may be confused with Phenaphen®, PHENobarbital, Phrenilin®, Theragran®

High alert medication:
The Institute for Safe Medication Practices (ISMP) includes this medication (I.V. formulation) among its list of drugs which have a heightened risk of causing significant patient harm when used in error.

Beers Criteria medication:
This drug may be inappropriate for use in geriatric patients (high severity risk).

Administration issues:
To prevent or minimize tissue damage during I.V. administration, the Institute for Safe Medication Practices (ISMP) has the following recommendations:
- Limit concentration available to the 25 mg/mL product
- Consider limiting initial doses to 6.25-12.5 mg
- Further dilute the 25 mg/mL strength into 10-20 mL NS
- Administer through a large bore vein (not hand or wrist)
- Administer via running I.V. line at port farthest from patient's vein
- Consider administering over 10-15 minutes
- Instruct patients to report immediately signs of pain or burning

International issues:
Sominex: Brand name for promethazine in Great Britain, but also is a brand name for diphenhydrAMINE in the U.S.

Synonyms promethazine hydrochloride

U.S. Brand Names Phenadoz®; Phenergan®; Promethegan™

Canadian Brand Names Bioniche Promethazine; Histantil; Phenergan®; PMS-Promethazine

Therapeutic Category Antiemetic; Phenothiazine Derivative

Use Symptomatic treatment of various allergic conditions; antiemetic; motion sickness; sedative; adjunct to postoperative analgesia and anesthesia

General Dosage Range
I.M., I.V.:
Children ≥2 years: 0.25-1 mg/kg 4-6 times/day as needed (maximum: 25 mg/dose; sedation: 50 mg/dose)
Adults: 12.5-75 mg/dose as a single dose **or** 12.5-50 mg every 4-6 hours as needed
Oral, rectal:
Children ≥2 years:
Allergic reactions: 0.1 mg/kg every 6 hours (maximum: 12.5 mg) during the day and 0.5 mg/kg (maximum: 25 mg/dose) at bedtime as needed
Antiemetic: 0.25-1 mg/kg 4-6 times/day as needed (maximum: 25 mg/dose)
Motion sickness: 0.5 mg/kg 30 minutes to 1 hour before departure, then every 12 hours as needed (maximum: 25 mg twice daily)
Sedation: 0.5-1 mg/kg every 6 hours as needed (maximum: 50 mg/dose)
Adults: 6.25-25 mg every 4-8 hours as needed **or** 12.5-50 mg as a single dose **or** 25 mg 30-60 minutes before departure, then every 12 hours as needed

Dosage Forms
Injection, solution: 25 mg/mL (1 mL, 10 mL); 50 mg/mL (1 mL)
Phenergan®: 25 mg/mL (1 mL); 50 mg/mL (1 mL)
Suppository, rectal: 12.5 mg (12s); 25 mg (12s)
Phenadoz®: 12.5 mg (12s); 25 mg (12s)
Promethegan™: 12.5 mg (12s); 25 mg (12s); 50 mg (12s)
Syrup, oral: 6.25 mg/5 mL (118 mL, 473 mL)
Tablet, oral: 12.5 mg, 25 mg, 50 mg

promethazine and codeine (proe METH a zeen & KOE deen)

Synonyms codeine and promethazine

Therapeutic Category Antihistamine/Antitussive

Controlled Substance C-V

Use Temporary relief of coughs and upper respiratory symptoms associated with allergy or the common cold

General Dosage Range Oral:
Children 6-11 years: 2.5-5 mL every 4-6 hours (maximum: 30 mL/day)
Children ≥12 years and Adults: 5 mL every 4-6 hours (maximum: 30 mL/day)

Dosage Forms
Syrup: Promethazine 6.25 mg and codeine 10 mg per 5 mL

promethazine and dextromethorphan (proe METH a zeen & deks troe meth OR fan)

Synonyms dextromethorphan and promethazine

Therapeutic Category Antihistamine/Antitussive

Use Temporary relief of coughs and upper respiratory symptoms associated with allergy or the common cold

General Dosage Range Oral:

Children 2-6 years: 1.25-2.5 mL every 4-6 hours (maximum: 10 mL/day)

Children 6-12 years: 2.5-5 mL every 4-6 hours (maximum: 20 mL/day)

Adults: 5 mL every 4-6 hours (maximum: 30 mL/day)

Dosage Forms

Syrup: Promethazine 6.25 mg and dextromethorphan 15 mg per 5 mL

promethazine and phenylephrine (proe METH a zeen & fen il EF rin)

Synonyms phenylephrine and promethazine

Therapeutic Category Antihistamine/Decongestant Combination

Use Temporary relief of upper respiratory symptoms associated with allergy or the common cold

General Dosage Range Oral:

Children 2-6 years: 1.25-2.5 mL every 4-6 hours (maximum: 7.5 mL/day)

Children 6-12 years: 2.5-5 mL every 4-6 hours (maximum: 30 mL/day)

Children >12 years and Adults: 5 mL every 4-6 hours (maximum: 30 mL/day)

Dosage Forms

Syrup: Promethazine 6.25 mg and phenylephrine 5 mg per 5 mL

promethazine hydrochloride *see* promethazine *on page 742*

promethazine, phenylephrine, and codeine

(proe METH a zeen, fen il EF rin, & KOE deen)

Synonyms codeine, phenylephrine, and promethazine; phenylephrine, promethazine, and codeine

Therapeutic Category Antihistamine/Decongestant/Antitussive

Controlled Substance C-V

Use Temporary relief of coughs and upper respiratory symptoms including nasal congestion associated with allergy or the common cold

General Dosage Range Oral:

Children 6-11 years: 2.5-5 mL every 4-6 hours (maximum: 30 mL/day)

Children ≥12 years and Adults: 5 mL every 4-6 hours (maximum: 30 mL/day)

Dosage Forms

Syrup: Promethazine 6.25 mg, phenylephrine 5 mg, and codeine 10 mg per 5 mL

Promethegan™ *see* promethazine *on page 742*

Prometrium® *see* progesterone *on page 741*

PRO-Mirtazapine (Can) *see* mirtazapine *on page 592*

Promiseb™ *see* emollients *on page 325*

PRO-Naproxen EC (Can) *see* naproxen *on page 612*

Pronestyl *see* procainamide *on page 739*

Pronto® Complete Lice Removal System [OTC] *see* pyrethrins and piperonyl butoxide *on page 756*

Pronto® Lice Control (Can) *see* pyrethrins and piperonyl butoxide *on page 756*

Pronto® Plus Lice Killing Mousse Plus Vitamin E [OTC] *see* pyrethrins and piperonyl butoxide *on page 756*

Pronto® Plus Lice Killing Mousse Shampoo Plus Natural Extracts and Oils [OTC] *see* pyrethrins and piperonyl butoxide *on page 756*

Pronto® Plus Warm Oil Treatment and Conditioner [OTC] *see* pyrethrins and piperonyl butoxide *on page 756*

propafenone (pro PAF en one)

Synonyms propafenone hydrochloride

U.S. Brand Names Rythmol®; Rythmol® SR

Canadian Brand Names Apo-Propafenone®; Mylan-Propafenone; PMS-Propafenone; Rythmol® Gen-Propafenone

Therapeutic Category Antiarrhythmic Agent, Class I-C

Use Treatment of life-threatening ventricular arrhythmias

Rythmol® SR: Maintenance of normal sinus rhythm in patients with symptomatic atrial fibrillation

General Dosage Range Dosage adjustment recommended in patients with hepatic impairment

Oral:

Extended release: *Adults:* Initial: 225 mg every 12 hours; Maintenance: 225-425 mg every 12 hours

Immediate release: *Adults:* Initial: 150 mg every 8 hours; Maintenance: 150-300 mg every 8 hours

Dosage Forms

Capsule, extended release, oral: 225 mg, 325 mg, 425 mg

Rythmol® SR: 225 mg, 325 mg, 425 mg

Tablet, oral: 150 mg, 225 mg, 300 mg

Rythmol®: 150 mg, 225 mg

propafenone hydrochloride *see* propafenone *on page 744*

propantheline (proe PAN the leen)

Medication Safety Issues

BEERS Criteria medication:

This drug may be inappropriate for use in geriatric patients (high severity risk).

Synonyms propantheline bromide

Therapeutic Category Anticholinergic Agent

Use Adjunctive treatment of peptic ulcer

General Dosage Range Oral:

Children: 1-3 mg/kg/day in 3-6 divided doses

Adults: 15 mg 3 times/day and 30 mg at bedtime

Dosage Forms

Tablet, oral: 15 mg

propantheline bromide *see* propantheline *on page 745*

proparacaine (proe PAR a kane)

Medication Safety Issues

Sound-alike/look-alike issues:

Proparacaine may be confused with propoxyphene

Synonyms proparacaine hydrochloride; proxymetacaine

U.S. Brand Names Alcaine®; Parcaine™

Canadian Brand Names Alcaine®; Diocaine®

Therapeutic Category Local Anesthetic

Use Anesthesia for tonometry, gonioscopy; suture removal from cornea; removal of corneal foreign body; cataract extraction, glaucoma surgery; short operative procedure involving the cornea and conjunctiva

General Dosage Range Ophthalmic: *Children and Adults:* Instill 1-2 drops of 0.5% solution in eye once **or** instill 1 drop of 0.5% solution in eye every 5-10 minutes for 5-7 doses

Dosage Forms

Solution, ophthalmic: 0.5% (15 mL)

Alcaine®: 0.5% (15 mL)

Parcaine™: 0.5% (15 mL)

proparacaine and fluorescein (proe PAR a kane & FLURE e seen)

Synonyms fluorescein and proparacaine

U.S. Brand Names Flucaine®

Therapeutic Category Diagnostic Agent; Local Anesthetic

Use Anesthesia for tonometry, gonioscopy; suture removal from cornea; removal of corneal foreign body; cataract extraction, glaucoma surgery

General Dosage Range Ophthalmic: *Children and Adults:* Instill 1 drop in each eye every 5-10 minutes for 5-7 doses **or** instill 1-2 drops in each eye once

◄ **Dosage Forms**
  Solution, ophthalmic: Proparacaine 0.5% and fluorescein 0.25% (5 mL)
  Flucaine®: Proparacaine 0.5% and fluorescein 0.25% (5 mL)

proparacaine hydrochloride *see* proparacaine *on page 745*
Propecia® *see* finasteride *on page 378*
Propine® (Can) *see* dipivefrin *on page 298*
PRO-Pioglitazone (Can) *see* pioglitazone *on page 706*
PRO-Piroxicam (Can) *see* piroxicam *on page 708*

propofol (PROE po fole)

Medication Safety Issues
  Sound-alike/look-alike issues:
    Diprivan® may be confused with Diflucan®, Ditropan
    Propofol may be confused with fospropofol
  High alert medication:
    The Institute for Safe Medication Practices (ISMP) includes this medication among its list of drugs which have a heightened risk of causing significant patient harm when used in error.

U.S. Brand Names Diprivan®

Canadian Brand Names Diprivan®

Therapeutic Category General Anesthetic

Use Induction of anesthesia in patients ≥3 years of age; maintenance of anesthesia in patients >2 months of age; in adults, for monitored anesthesia care sedation during procedures; sedation in intubated, mechanically-ventilated ICU patients

General Dosage Range I.V.: *Children and Adults:* Dosage varies greatly depending on indication

Dosage Forms
  Injection, emulsion: 10 mg/mL (10 mL, 20 mL, 50 mL, 100 mL)
  Diprivan®: 10 mg/mL (20 mL, 50 mL, 100 mL)

propoxyphene (proe POKS i feen)

Medication Safety Issues
  Sound-alike/look-alike issues:
    Propoxyphene may be confused with proparacaine
    Darvon® may be confused with Devrom®, Diovan®
    Darvon-N® may be confused with Darvocet-N®
  High alert medication:
    The Institute for Safe Medication Practices (ISMP) includes this medication among its list of drug classes which have a heightened risk of causing significant patient harm when used in error.
  BEERS Criteria medication:
    This drug may be inappropriate for use in geriatric patients (low severity risk).

Synonyms dextropropoxyphene; propoxyphene hydrochloride; propoxyphene napsylate

U.S. Brand Names Darvon-N® [DSC]; Darvon® [DSC]

Canadian Brand Names 642® Tablet; Darvon-N®

Therapeutic Category Analgesic, Narcotic

Controlled Substance C-IV

Use Management of mild-to-moderate pain

General Dosage Range Oral: *Adults:* Hydrochloride: 65 mg every 4 hours as needed (maximum: 390 mg/day); Napsylate: 100 mg every 4 hours as needed (maximum: 600 mg/day)

propoxyphene and acetaminophen (proe POKS i feen & a seet a MIN oh fen)

Medication Safety Issues
  Sound-alike/look-alike issues:
    Darvocet® may be confused with Percocet®

Darvocet-N® may be confused with Darvon-N®

High alert medication:

The Institute for Safe Medication Practices (ISMP) includes this medication among its list of drug classes which have a heightened risk of causing significant patient harm when used in error.

BEERS Criteria medication:

This drug may be inappropriate for use in geriatric patients (low severity risk).

Other safety concerns:

Duplicate therapy issues: This product contains acetaminophen, which may be a component of other combination products. Do not exceed the maximum recommended daily dose of acetaminophen.

International issues:

Capadex: Brand name for propoxyphene/acetaminophen [Australia, New Zealand] may be confused with Casodex which is a brand name for bicalutamide [U.S, Canada, and multiple international markets]

Synonyms acetaminophen and propoxyphene; propoxyphene hydrochloride and acetaminophen; propoxyphene napsylate and acetaminophen

U.S. Brand Names Balacet 325™ [DSC]; Darvocet A500® [DSC]; Darvocet-N® 100 [DSC]; Darvocet-N® 50 [DSC]

Canadian Brand Names Darvocet-N® 100; Darvocet-N® 50

Therapeutic Category Analgesic, Narcotic

Controlled Substance C-IV

Use Management of mild-to-moderate pain

General Dosage Range Oral:

Propoxyphene hydrochloride and acetaminophen 65/650 mg: *Adults:* 1 tablet every 4 hours as needed (maximum: 4 g/day [acetaminophen]; 390 mg/day propoxyphene hydrochloride])

Propoxyphene napsylate and acetaminophen: *Adults:*

Darvocet A500™, Darvocet-N® 100: 1 tablet every 4 hours as needed (maximum: 4 g/day [acetaminophen]; 600 mg/day [propoxyphene napsylate])

Darvocet-N® 50: 1-2 tablets every 4 hours as needed (maximum: 4 g/day [acetaminophen]; 600 mg/day [propoxyphene napsylate])

Dosage Forms

Tablet:

65/650: Propoxyphene 65 mg and acetaminophen 650 mg; 100/325: Propoxyphene 100 mg and acetaminophen 325 mg; 100/500: Propoxyphene 100 mg and acetaminophen 500 mg; 100/650: Propoxyphene 100 mg and acetaminophen 650 mg

Balacet 325™: Propoxyphene 100 mg and acetaminophen 325 mg

Darvocet A500®: Propoxyphene 100 mg and acetaminophen 500 mg

Darvocet-N® 50: Propoxyphene 50 mg and acetaminophen 325 mg

Darvocet-N® 100: Propoxyphene 100 mg and acetaminophen 650 mg

propoxyphene hydrochloride *see* propoxyphene *on page 746*

propoxyphene hydrochloride and acetaminophen *see* propoxyphene and acetaminophen *on page 746*

propoxyphene napsylate *see* propoxyphene *on page 746*

propoxyphene napsylate and acetaminophen *see* propoxyphene and acetaminophen *on page 746*

propranolol (proe PRAN oh lole)

Medication Safety Issues

Sound-alike/look-alike issues:

Propranolol may be confused with prasugrel, Pravachol®, Propulsid®

Inderal® may be confused with Adderall®, Enduron®, Enduronyl®, Imdur®, Imuran®, Inderide®, Isordil®, Toradol®

◄ Inderal® 40 may be confused with Enduronyl® Forte

High alert medication:
The Institute for Safe Medication Practices (ISMP) includes this medication among its list of drugs which have a heightened risk of causing significant patient harm when used in error.

Administration issues:
Significant differences exist between oral and I.V. dosing. Use caution when converting from one route of administration to another.

International issues:
Inderal [Canada and multiple international markets] and Inderal LA [U.S.] may be confused with Indiaral brand name for loperamide [France]

Synonyms propranolol hydrochloride

U.S. Brand Names Inderal® LA; InnoPran XL®

Canadian Brand Names Apo-Propranolol®; Dom-Propranolol; Inderal®; Inderal® LA; Novo-Pranol; Nu-Propranolol; PMS-Propranolol; Propranolol Hydrochloride Injection, USP

Therapeutic Category Antiarrhythmic Agent, Class II; Beta-Adrenergic Blocker

Use Management of hypertension; angina pectoris; pheochromocytoma; essential tremor; supraventricular arrhythmias (such as atrial fibrillation and flutter, AV nodal reentrant tachycardias), ventricular tachycardias (catecholamine-induced arrhythmias, digoxin toxicity); prevention of myocardial infarction; migraine headache prophylaxis; symptomatic treatment of hypertrophic subaortic stenosis (hypertrophic obstructive cardiomyopathy)

General Dosage Range
I.V.: *Adults:* 1-3 mg, repeat every 2-5 minutes up to a total of 5 mg **or** 0.1 mg/kg divided into 3 equal doses given at 2- to 3-minute intervals; may repeat total dose in 2 minutes if needed
Oral:
Extended release: *Adults:* Initial: 80 mg once daily; Maintenance: 60-320 mg once daily (maximum: 640 mg/day)
Regular release: *Adults:* 30-320 mg/day in 2-4 divided doses (maximum: 640 mg/day)

Dosage Forms
Capsule, extended release, oral: 60 mg, 80 mg, 120 mg, 160 mg
InnoPran XL®: 80 mg, 120 mg
Capsule, sustained release, oral:
Inderal® LA: 60 mg, 80 mg, 120 mg, 160 mg
Injection, solution: 1 mg/mL (1 mL)
Injection, solution [preservative free]: 1 mg/mL (1 mL)
Solution, oral: 4 mg/mL (500 mL); 8 mg/mL (500 mL)
Tablet, oral: 10 mg, 20 mg, 40 mg, 60 mg, 80 mg

propranolol and hydrochlorothiazide (proe PRAN oh lole & hye droe klor oh THYE a zide)
Medication Safety Issues
Sound-alike/look-alike issues:
Inderide® may be confused with Inderal®

Synonyms hydrochlorothiazide and propranolol; Inderide

Therapeutic Category Antihypertensive Agent, Combination

Use Management of hypertension

General Dosage Range Oral: *Adults:* Propranolol 80-160 mg/day and hydrochlorothiazide 12.5-50 mg/day in 2 divided doses

Dosage Forms
Tablet: Propranolol 40 mg and hydrochlorothiazide 25 mg; propranolol 80 mg and hydrochlorothiazide 25 mg

propranolol hydrochloride *see propranolol on page 747*

Propranolol Hydrochloride Injection, USP (Can) *see propranolol on page 747*

Proprinal® [OTC] *see ibuprofen on page 460*

Proprinal® Cold and Sinus [OTC] *see pseudoephedrine and ibuprofen on page 753*

Propulsid® *see cisapride on page 212*

propylene glycol diacetate, acetic acid, and hydrocortisone *see acetic acid, propylene glycol diacetate, and hydrocortisone on page 35*

propylhexedrine (proe pil HEKS e dreen)
U.S. Brand Names Benzedrex® [OTC]

Therapeutic Category Adrenergic Agonist Agent

Use Topical nasal decongestant

General Dosage Range Oral: *Children ≥6 years and Adults:* 2 inhalations in each nostril, not more frequently than every 2 hours

Dosage Forms
  Inhaler, nasal:
    Benzedrex® [OTC]: 0.4-0.5 mg/inhalation (1s)

2-propylpentanoic acid *see* valproic acid *on page 904*

propylthiouracil (proe pil thye oh YOOR a sil)

Medication Safety Issues
  Sound-alike/look-alike issues:
    Propylthiouracil may be confused with Purinethol®
    PTU is an error-prone abbreviation (mistaken as mercaptopurine [Purinethol®; 6-MP])

Synonyms PTU (error-prone abbreviation)

Canadian Brand Names Propyl-Thyracil®

Therapeutic Category Antithyroid Agent

Use Adjunctive therapy in patients intolerant of methimazole to ameliorate hyperthyroidism symptoms in preparation for surgical treatment or radioactive iodine therapy; treatment of hyperthyroidism in patients intolerant of methimazole and not candidates for surgical/radiotherapy

General Dosage Range Oral:
  Children 6-10 years: 50-150 mg/day
  Children >10 years: 150-300 mg/day
  Adults: Initial: 300-900 mg/day in 3 divided doses; Maintenance: 100-150 mg/day

Dosage Forms
  Tablet, oral: 50 mg

Propyl-Thyracil® (Can) *see* propylthiouracil *on page 749*

2-propylvaleric acid *see* valproic acid *on page 904*

ProQuad® *see* measles, mumps, rubella, and varicella virus vaccine *on page 551*

PRO-Quetiapine (Can) *see* quetiapine *on page 760*

PRO-Rabeprazole (Can) *see* rabeprazole *on page 763*

PRO-Risperidone (Can) *see* risperidone *on page 783*

Proscar® *see* finasteride *on page 378*

Prosed®/DS *see* methenamine, phenyl salicylate, methylene blue, benzoic acid, and hyoscyamine *on page 569*

Prosol *see* amino acid injection *on page 65*

ProSom *see* estazolam *on page 343*

PRO-Sotalol (Can) *see* sotalol *on page 828*

prostacyclin *see* epoprostenol *on page 334*

prostacyclin PGI$_2$ *see* iloprost *on page 465*

prostaglandin E$_1$ *see* alprostadil *on page 57*

prostaglandin E$_2$ *see* dinoprostone *on page 289*

prostaglandin F$_2$ *see* carboprost tromethamine *on page 175*

prostate cancer vaccine, cell-based *see* sipuleucel-T *on page 815*

Prostigmin® *see* neostigmine *on page 619*

Prostin E2® *see* dinoprostone *on page 289*

Prostin E$_2$® (Can) *see* dinoprostone *on page 289*

Prostin® VR (Can) *see* alprostadil *on page 57*

Prostin VR Pediatric® *see* alprostadil *on page 57*

protamine sulfate (PROE ta meen SUL fate)

Medication Safety Issues
  Sound-alike/look-alike issues:
    Protamine may be confused with ProAmatine®, Protonix®, Protopam®, Protropin®

Therapeutic Category Antidote

Use Treatment of heparin overdosage; neutralize heparin during surgery or dialysis procedures

◀ **General Dosage Range I.V.:** *Children and Adults:* 1 mg of protamine neutralizes 90 USP units of heparin (lung) and 115 USP units of heparin (intestinal) (maximum dose: 50 mg)
Dosage Forms
Injection, solution [preservative free]: 10 mg/mL (5 mL, 25 mL)

protease, lipase, and amylase *see* pancrelipase *on page 670*
Protection Plus® [OTC] *see* alcohol (ethyl) *on page 47*
protein C *see* protein C concentrate (human) *on page 750*
protein C (activated), human, recombinant *see* drotrecogin alfa *on page 315*
protein-bound paclitaxel *see* paclitaxel (protein bound) *on page 667*

protein C concentrate (human) (PROE teen cee KON suhn trate HYU man)

Medication Safety Issues
  Sound-alike/look-alike issues:
   Ceprotin may be confused with aprotinin, Cipro®
   Protein C concentrate (human) may be confused with activated protein C (human, recombinant) which refers to drotrecogin alfa
Synonyms protein C
U.S. Brand Names Ceprotin
Therapeutic Category Anticoagulant
Use Replacement therapy for severe congenital protein C deficiency for the prevention and/or treatment of venous thromboembolism and purpura fulminans
General Dosage Range I.V.: *Children and Adults:* Initial: 100-120 int. units, followed by 60-80 int. units every 6 hours for 3 doses; maintenance: 45-60 int. units every 6 hours (short-term) or every 12 hours (short-to-long term)
Dosage Forms
  Injection, powder for reconstitution:
   Ceprotin: ~500 int. units, ~1000 int. units

prothrombin complex concentrate *see* factor IX complex (human) *on page 365*
prothrombin complex concentrate *see* prothrombin complex (human) [(factors II, VII, IX, X), protein C, and protein S] *(Canada only) on page 750*

prothrombin complex (human) [(factors II, VII, IX, X), protein C, and protein S] *(Canada only)*

(PRO throm bin KOM pleks HYU man FAK ters too SEV en nyne ten PROE teen cee & PROE teen ess)
Synonyms prothrombin complex concentrate
Canadian Brand Names Octaplex®
Therapeutic Category Hemostatic Agent
Use Prophylaxis (perioperative) and treatment of bleeding due to acquired deficiency (eg, overdose of vitamin K antagonist) of one or more of the prothrombin complex coagulation factors II, VII, IX, and X, when rapid correction of factor deficiency is necessary
General Dosage Range I.V.: *Adults:* Maximum dose not to exceed 120 mL. Approximate doses required for normalization of INR (≤1.2 within 1 hour): Initial INR: 2-2.5: Administer 0.9-1.3 mL/kg; 2.5-3: Administer 1.3-1.6 mL/kg; 3-3.5: Administer 1.6-1.9 mL/kg; >3.5: Administer >1.9 mL/kg
Product Availability Not available in U.S.
Dosage Forms - Canada
  Injection, powder for reconstitution:
   Octaplex®: Human coagulation factor II: 11-38 int. units/mL; factor VII: 9-24 int. units/mL; factor IX: 20-31 int. units/mL; factor X: 18-30 int. units/mL; protein C: 7-31 int. units/mL; protein S: 7-32 int. units/mL (20 mL)

Protonix® *see* pantoprazole *on page 672*
Protonix® I.V. *see* pantoprazole *on page 672*
Protopam® *see* pralidoxime *on page 729*
Protopic® *see* tacrolimus (topical) *on page 842*
PRO-Topiramate (Can) *see* topiramate *on page 877*
Pro-Triazide (Can) *see* hydrochlorothiazide and triamterene *on page 446*

protriptyline (proe TRIP ti leen)

Medication Safety Issues
Sound-alike/look-alike issues:
Vivactil® may be confused with Vyvanse™
Synonyms protriptyline hydrochloride
U.S. Brand Names Vivactil®
Therapeutic Category Antidepressant, Tricyclic (Secondary Amine)
Use Treatment of depression
General Dosage Range Oral:
Adolescents: 15-20 mg/day
Adults: 15-60 mg/day in 3-4 divided doses
Elderly: Initial: 5-10 mg/day; Maintenance: 15-20 mg/day
Dosage Forms
Tablet, oral: 5 mg, 10 mg
Vivactil®: 5 mg, 10 mg

protriptyline hydrochloride *see* protriptyline *on page 751*
PRO-Valacyclovir (Can) *see* valacyclovir *on page 903*
Provenge® *see* sipuleucel-T *on page 815*
Proventil® HFA *see* albuterol *on page 45*
Provera® *see* medroxyprogesterone *on page 554*
Provera-Pak (Can) *see* medroxyprogesterone *on page 554*
PRO-Verapamil SR (Can) *see* verapamil *on page 912*
Provigil® *see* modafinil *on page 594*
Proviodine (Can) *see* povidone-iodine (topical) *on page 727*
Provisc® *see* hyaluronate and derivatives *on page 443*
Provocholine® *see* methacholine *on page 567*
proxymetacaine *see* proparacaine *on page 745*
PROzac® *see* fluoxetine *on page 389*
Prozac® (Can) *see* fluoxetine *on page 389*
PROzac® Weekly™ *see* fluoxetine *on page 389*
PRO-Zopiclone (Can) *see* zopiclone (Canada only) *on page 934*
PRP-OMP *see* Haemophilus B conjugate vaccine *on page 432*
PRP-T *see* Haemophilus B conjugate vaccine *on page 432*
PruClair™ *see* emollients *on page 325*
Prudoxin™ *see* doxepin (topical) *on page 309*
PruMyx™ *see* emollients *on page 325*
prussian blue *see* ferric hexacyanoferrate *on page 373*
PruTect™ *see* emollients *on page 325*
prymaccone *see* primaquine *on page 737*
P&S® [OTC] *see* salicylic acid *on page 795*
23PS *see* pneumococcal polysaccharide vaccine (polyvalent) *on page 715*
PS-341 *see* bortezomib *on page 139*

pseudoephedrine (soo doe e FED rin)

Medication Safety Issues
Sound-alike/look-alike issues:
Sudafed® may be confused with sotalol, Sudafed PE™, Sufenta®
Synonyms d-isoephedrine hydrochloride; pseudoephedrine hydrochloride; pseudoephedrine sulfate; Sudafed
U.S. Brand Names Children's Nasal Decongestant [OTC]; Genaphed™ [OTC] [DSC]; Oranyl [OTC]; Silfedrine Children's [OTC]; Sudafed® 12 Hour [OTC]; Sudafed® 24 Hour [OTC]; Sudafed® Children's [OTC]; Sudafed® Maximum Strength Nasal Decongestant [OTC]; Sudo-Tab® [OTC]; SudoGest 12 Hour [OTC]; SudoGest Children's [OTC]; SudoGest [OTC]

◄ **Canadian Brand Names** Balminil Decongestant; Benylin® D for Infants; Contac® Cold 12 Hour Relief Non Drowsy; Drixoral® ND; Eltor®; PMS-Pseudoephedrine; Pseudofrin; Robidrine®; Sudafed® Decongestant

Therapeutic Category Adrenergic Agonist Agent

Use Temporary symptomatic relief of nasal congestion due to common cold, upper respiratory allergies, and sinusitis; also promotes nasal or sinus drainage

General Dosage Range Oral:
Immediate release:
Children 4-5 years: 15 mg every 4-6 hours (maximum: 60 mg/day)
Children 6-12 years: 30 mg every 4-6 hours (maximum: 120 mg/day)
Adults: 60 mg every 4-6 hours (maximum: 240 mg/day)
Extended release: *Adults:* 120 mg every 12 hours or 240 mg every 24 hours (maximum: 240 mg/day)

Dosage Forms
Caplet, extended release, oral:
Sudafed® 12 Hour [OTC]: 120 mg
Liquid, oral: 30 mg/5 mL (473 mL)
Children's Nasal Decongestant [OTC]: 30 mg/5 mL (118 mL)
Silfedrine Children's [OTC]: 15 mg/5 mL (118 mL, 237 mL)
Sudafed® Children's [OTC]: 15 mg/5 mL (118 mL)
Syrup, oral: 30 mg/5 mL (118 mL)
SudoGest Children's [OTC]: 15 mg/5 mL (118 mL)
Tablet, oral: 30 mg
Oranyl [OTC]: 30 mg
Sudafed® Maximum Strength Nasal Decongestant [OTC]: 30 mg
Sudo-Tab® [OTC]: 30 mg
SudoGest [OTC]: 30 mg, 60 mg
Tablet, extended release, oral:
Sudafed® 24 Hour [OTC]: 240 mg
SudoGest 12 Hour [OTC]: 120 mg

pseudoephedrine, acetaminophen, and chlorpheniramine *see* acetaminophen, chlorpheniramine, and pseudoephedrine *on page 30*

pseudoephedrine and acetaminophen *see* acetaminophen and pseudoephedrine *on page 29*

pseudoephedrine and brompheniramine *see* brompheniramine and pseudoephedrine *on page 144*

pseudoephedrine and carbetapentane *see* carbetapentane and pseudoephedrine *on page 172*

pseudoephedrine and chlorpheniramine *see* chlorpheniramine and pseudoephedrine *on page 199*

pseudoephedrine and codeine (soo doe e FED rin & KOE deen)

Synonyms codeine and pseudoephedrine; codeine phosphate and pseudoephedrine hydrochloride; pseudoephedrine hydrochloride and codeine phosphate

U.S. Brand Names EndaCof-DC; Notuss®-DC

Therapeutic Category Antitussive/Decongestant

Controlled Substance Liquid: C-V

Use Temporary symptomatic relief of congestion and cough due to upper respiratory infections including common cold, bronchitis, sinusitis, and influenza

General Dosage Range Oral:
Children 6-11 years: 2.5-5 mL every 4-6 hours as needed (maximum: 20 mL/24 hours)
Children ≥12 years and Adults: 5-10 mL every 4-6 hours as needed (maximum: 40 mL/24 hours)

Dosage Forms
Liquid, oral:
EndaCof-DC, Notuss®-DC: Pseudoephedrine 30 mg and codeine 10 mg per 5 mL

pseudoephedrine and desloratadine *see* desloratadine and pseudoephedrine *on page 261*

pseudoephedrine and dexbrompheniramine *see* dexbrompheniramine and pseudoephedrine *on page 265*

pseudoephedrine and dextromethorphan (soo doe e FED rin & deks troe meth OR fan)

Synonyms dextromethorphan and pseudoephedrine

U.S. Brand Names Pedia Relief Cough and Cold [OTC]; Sudafed® Children's Cold & Cough [OTC]

Canadian Brand Names Balminil DM D; Benylin® DM-D; Koffex DM-D; Novahistex® DM Decongestant; Novahistine® DM Decongestant; Robitussin® Childrens Cough & Cold

Therapeutic Category Antitussive/Decongestant

Use Temporary symptomatic relief of nasal congestion and cough due to common cold, hay fever, upper respiratory allergies

General Dosage Range Oral:
Children 2-6 years: 15 mg (based on pseudoephedrine) every 4-6 hours (maximum: 60 mg/day)
Children 6-12 years: 30 mg (based on pseudoephedrine) every 4-6 hours (maximum: 120 mg/day)
Children ≥12 years and Adults: 60 mg (based on pseudoephedrine) every 4-6 hours (maximum: 240 mg/day)

Dosage Forms
Liquid:
Sudafed® Children's Cold & Cough [OTC]: Pseudoephedrine 15 mg and dextromethorphan 5 mg per 5 mL
Syrup:
Pedia Relief Cough and Cold [OTC]: Pseudoephedrine 15 mg and dextromethorphan 7.5 mg per 5 mL

pseudoephedrine and fexofenadine *see* fexofenadine and pseudoephedrine *on page 375*

pseudoephedrine and guaifenesin *see* guaifenesin and pseudoephedrine *on page 429*

pseudoephedrine and hydrocodone *see* hydrocodone and pseudoephedrine *on page 449*

pseudoephedrine and ibuprofen (soo doe e FED rin & eye byoo PROE fen)

Synonyms ibuprofen and pseudoephedrine

U.S. Brand Names Advil® Cold & Sinus [OTC]; Proprinal® Cold and Sinus [OTC]

Canadian Brand Names Advil® Cold & Sinus; Advil® Cold & Sinus Daytime; Children's Advil® Cold; Sudafed® Sinus Advance

Therapeutic Category Decongestant/Analgesic

Use For temporary relief of cold, sinus, and flu symptoms (including nasal congestion, sinus pressure, headache, minor body aches and pains, and fever)

General Dosage Range Oral: *Children ≥12 years and Adults:* 1-2 doses (ibuprofen 200 mg and pseudoephedrine 30 mg per dose) every 4-6 hours as needed (maximum: 6 doses/day)

Dosage Forms
Caplet:
Advil® Cold & Sinus [OTC], Proprinal® Cold and Sinus [OTC]: Pseudoephedrine 30 mg and ibuprofen 200 mg
Capsule, liquid filled:
Advil® Cold & Sinus [OTC]: Pseudoephedrine 30 mg and ibuprofen 200 mg

pseudoephedrine and loratadine *see* loratadine and pseudoephedrine *on page 537*

pseudoephedrine and methscopolamine (soo doe e FED rin & meth skoe POL a meen)

Synonyms methscopolamine and pseudoephedrine; pseudoephedrine hydrochloride and methscopolamine nitrate

U.S. Brand Names AlleRx™-D [DSC]

Therapeutic Category Decongestant/Anticholingeric Combination

Use Relief of symptoms of allergic rhinitis, vasomotor rhinitis, sinusitis, and the common cold

General Dosage Range Oral: *Children ≥12 years and Adults:* 1 tablet every 12 hours (maximum: 2 tablets/24 hours)

Dosage Forms
Tablet: Pseudoephedrine hydrochloride 120 mg and methscopolamine nitrate 2.5 mg

pseudoephedrine and naproxen *see* naproxen and pseudoephedrine *on page 613*

pseudoephedrine and triprolidine *see* triprolidine and pseudoephedrine *on page 893*

pseudoephedrine, chlorpheniramine, and acetaminophen *see* acetaminophen, chlorpheniramine, and pseudoephedrine *on page 30*

pseudoephedrine, chlorpheniramine, and codeine *see* chlorpheniramine, pseudoephedrine, and codeine *on page 201*

pseudoephedrine, chlorpheniramine, and dextromethorphan *see* chlorpheniramine, pseudoephedrine, and dextromethorphan *on page 201*

pseudoephedrine, chlorpheniramine, and dihydrocodeine *see* pseudoephedrine, dihydrocodeine, and chlorpheniramine *on page 754*

pseudoephedrine, chlorpheniramine, and ibuprofen *see* ibuprofen, pseudoephedrine, and chlorpheniramine *on page 462*

pseudoephedrine, codeine, and triprolidine *see* triprolidine, pseudoephedrine, and codeine *(Canada only) on page 893*

pseudoephedrine, dextromethorphan, and guaifenesin *see* guaifenesin, pseudoephedrine, and dextromethorphan *on page 430*

pseudoephedrine, dextromethorphan, doxylamine, and acetaminophen *see* acetaminophen, dextromethorphan, doxylamine, and pseudoephedrine *on page 33*

pseudoephedrine, dihydrocodeine, and chlorpheniramine
(soo doe e FED rin, dye hye droe KOE deen, & klor fen IR a meen)

Synonyms chlorpheniramine, dihydrocodeine, and pseudoephedrine; dihydrocodeine bitartrate, pseudoephedrine hydrochloride, and chlorpheniramine maleate; pseudoephedrine, chlorpheniramine, and dihydrocodeine

U.S. Brand Names Coldcough; DiHydro-CP

Therapeutic Category Antihistamine/Decongestant/Antitussive

Controlled Substance C-III

Use Temporary relief of cough, congestion, and sneezing due to colds, respiratory infections, or hay fever

General Dosage Range Oral:
Children 2-6 years: 1.25-2.5 mL every 4-6 hours (maximum: 4 doses/day)
Children 6-12 years: 2.5-5 mL every 4-6 hours (maximum: 4 doses/day)
Children >12 years and Adults: 5-10 mL every 4-6 hours (maximum: 4 doses/day)

Dosage Forms
Syrup:
Coldcough, DiHydro-CP: Pseudoephedrine 15 mg, dihydrocodeine 7.5 mg, and chlorpheniramine 2 mg per 5 mL

pseudoephedrine, guaifenesin, and codeine *see* guaifenesin, pseudoephedrine, and codeine *on page 430*

pseudoephedrine hydrochloride *see* pseudoephedrine *on page 751*

pseudoephedrine hydrochloride and acetaminophen *see* acetaminophen and pseudoephedrine *on page 29*

pseudoephedrine hydrochloride and acrivastine *see* acrivastine and pseudoephedrine *on page 38*

pseudoephedrine hydrochloride and cetirizine hydrochloride *see* cetirizine and pseudoephedrine *on page 189*

pseudoephedrine hydrochloride and codeine phosphate *see* pseudoephedrine and codeine *on page 752*

pseudoephedrine hydrochloride and hydrocodone bitartrate *see* hydrocodone and pseudoephedrine *on page 449*

pseudoephedrine hydrochloride and methscopolamine nitrate *see* pseudoephedrine and methscopolamine *on page 753*

pseudoephedrine hydrochloride, guaifenesin, and dihydrocodeine bitartrate *see* dihydrocodeine, pseudoephedrine, and guaifenesin *on page 285*

pseudoephedrine hydrochloride, hydrocodone bitartrate, and chlorpheniramine maleate *see* hydrocodone, chlorpheniramine, and pseudoephedrine *on page 449*

pseudoephedrine hydrochloride, methscopolamine nitrate, and chlorpheniramine maleate *see* chlorpheniramine, pseudoephedrine, and methscopolamine *on page 202*

pseudoephedrine, hydrocodone, and chlorpheniramine *see* hydrocodone, chlorpheniramine, and pseudoephedrine *on page 449*

pseudoephedrine, methscopolamine, and chlorpheniramine *see* chlorpheniramine, pseudoephedrine, and methscopolamine *on page 202*

pseudoephedrine sulfate *see* pseudoephedrine *on page 751*

pseudoephedrine tannate, dextromethorphan tannate, and brompheniramine tannate *see* brompheniramine, pseudoephedrine, and dextromethorphan *on page 144*

pseudoephedrine, triprolidine, and codeine *see* triprolidine, pseudoephedrine, and codeine *(Canada only) on page 893*

Pseudofrin (Can) *see* pseudoephedrine *on page 751*
pseudomonic acid A *see* mupirocin *on page 603*
P & S™ Liquid Phenol (Can) *see* phenol *on page 694*

psyllium (SIL i yum)

Medication Safety Issues
Sound-alike/look-alike issues:
Fiberall® may be confused with Feverall®
Hydrocil® may be confused with Hydrocet®

Synonyms plantago seed; plantain seed; psyllium husk; psyllium hydrophilic mucilloid

U.S. Brand Names Bulk-K [OTC]; Fiberall® [OTC]; Fibro-Lax [OTC]; Fibro-XL [OTC]; Genfiber™ [OTC] [DSC]; Hydrocil® Instant [OTC]; Konsyl-D™ [OTC]; Konsyl® Easy Mix™ [OTC]; Konsyl® Orange [OTC]; Konsyl® Original [OTC]; Konsyl® [OTC]; Metamucil® Plus Calcium [OTC]; Metamucil® Smooth Texture [OTC]; Metamucil® [OTC]; Natural Fiber Therapy Smooth Texture [OTC]; Natural Fiber Therapy [OTC]; Reguloid [OTC]

Canadian Brand Names Metamucil®

Therapeutic Category Laxative

Use OTC labeling: Dietary fiber supplement; treatment of occasional constipation; reduce risk of coronary heart disease (CHD)

General Dosage Range Oral:
Children 6-11 years: Psyllium 1.25-15 g/day in divided doses
Children ≥12 years and Adults: Psyllium 2.5-30 g/day in divided doses

Dosage Forms
Capsule, oral: 500 mg
  Fibro-XL [OTC]: 0.675 g
  Konsyl® [OTC]: 0.52 g
  Metamucil® [OTC]: 0.52 g
  Metamucil® Plus Calcium [OTC]: 0.52 g
  Reguloid [OTC]: 0.52 g
Powder, oral: (454 g)
  Bulk-K [OTC]: (392 g)
  Fiberall® [OTC]: (454 g)
  Fibro-Lax [OTC]: (140 g, 392 g)
  Hydrocil® Instant [OTC]: (300 g); 3.5 g/packet (30s, 500s)
  Konsyl-D™ [OTC]: (325 g, 397 g, 500 g); 3.4 g/packet (100s, 500s)
  Konsyl® Easy Mix™ [OTC]: (250 g); 6 g/packet (500s)
  Konsyl® Orange [OTC]: (425 g, 538 g); 3.4 g/packet (30s)
  Konsyl® Original [OTC]: (300 g, 450 g); 6 g/packet (30s, 100s, 500s)
  Metamucil® [OTC]: (390 g, 570 g, 870 g, 1254 g)
  Metamucil® Smooth Texture [OTC]: (173 g, 283 g, 288 g, 300 g, 425 g, 432 g, 450 g, 609 g, 660 g, 684 g, 690 g, 912 g, 1020 g, 1368 g); 3.4 g/packet (30s)
  Natural Fiber Therapy [OTC]: (390 g, 539 g)
  Natural Fiber Therapy Smooth Texture [OTC]: (300 g)
  Reguloid [OTC]: (284 g, 369 g, 426 g, 540 g)
Wafer, oral:
  Metamucil® [OTC]: 3.4 g/2 wafers (24s)

psyllium husk *see* psyllium *on page 755*
psyllium hydrophilic mucilloid *see* psyllium *on page 755*
P-Tann [DSC] *see* chlorpheniramine *on page 197*
pteroylglutamic acid *see* folic acid *on page 396*
PTG *see* teniposide *on page 850*
PTU (error-prone abbreviation) *see* propylthiouracil *on page 749*
Pulmicort® (Can) *see* budesonide (systemic, oral inhalation) *on page 145*
Pulmicort Flexhaler® *see* budesonide (systemic, oral inhalation) *on page 145*
Pulmicort Respules® *see* budesonide (systemic, oral inhalation) *on page 145*
Pulmophylline (Can) *see* theophylline *on page 860*
Pulmozyme® *see* dornase alfa *on page 307*
Puregon® (Can) *see* follitropin beta *on page 397*

Purell® [OTC] *see* alcohol (ethyl) *on page 47*

Purell® 2 in 1 [OTC] *see* alcohol (ethyl) *on page 47*

Purell® Lasting Care [OTC] *see* alcohol (ethyl) *on page 47*

Purell® Moisture Therapy [OTC] *see* alcohol (ethyl) *on page 47*

Purell® with Aloe [OTC] *see* alcohol (ethyl) *on page 47*

purified chick embryo cell *see* rabies vaccine *on page 764*

Purinethol® *see* mercaptopurine *on page 563*

PVP-I *see* povidone-iodine (ophthalmic) *on page 727*

PVP-I *see* povidone-iodine (topical) *on page 727*

Pylera™ *see* bismuth, metronidazole, and tetracycline *on page 136*

pyrantel pamoate (pi RAN tel PAM oh ate)

U.S. Brand Names Pin-X® [OTC]; Reese's Pinworm Medicine [OTC]

Canadian Brand Names Combantrin™

Therapeutic Category Anthelmintic

Use Treatment of pinworms (*Enterobius vermicularis*) and roundworms (*Ascaris lumbricoides*)

General Dosage Range Oral: *Children and Adults:* 11 mg/kg as a single dose (maximum: 1 g/dose); repeat in 2 weeks for pinworm (dose is expressed as pyrantel base)

Dosage Forms

Suspension, oral:

Pin-X® [OTC]: 144 mg/mL (30 mL, 60 mL)

Reese's Pinworm Medicine [OTC]: 144 mg/mL (30 mL, 60 mL, 240 mL)

Tablet, chewable, oral:

Pin-X® [OTC]: 720.5 mg

pyrazinamide (peer a ZIN a mide)

Synonyms pyrazinoic acid amide

Canadian Brand Names Tebrazid™

Therapeutic Category Antitubercular Agent

Use Adjunctive treatment of tuberculosis in combination with other antituberculosis agents

General Dosage Range Dosage adjustment recommended in patients with renal impairment

Oral:

Children: 15-30 mg/kg once daily (maximum: 2 g/day) **or** 50 mg/kg/dose twice weekly (maximum: 2 g/dose)

Adults 40-55 kg: 1000 mg once daily **or** 2000 mg twice weekly **or** 1500 mg 3 times/week

Adults 56-75 kg: 1500 mg once daily **or** 3000 mg twice weekly **or** 2500 mg 3 times/week

Adults 76-90 kg: 2000 mg once daily (maximum dose regardless of weight) **or** 4000 mg twice weekly (maximum dose regardless of weight) **or** 3000 mg 3 times/week (maximum dose regardless of weight)

Dosage Forms

Tablet, oral: 500 mg

pyrazinamide, rifampin, and isoniazid *see* rifampin, isoniazid, and pyrazinamide *on page 780*

pyrazinoic acid amide *see* pyrazinamide *on page 756*

pyrethrins and piperonyl butoxide (pye RE thrins & pi PER oh nil byo TOKS ide)

Synonyms piperonyl butoxide and pyrethrins

U.S. Brand Names A-200® Lice Treatment Kit [OTC]; A-200® Maximum Strength [OTC]; Licide® [OTC]; Pronto® Complete Lice Removal System [OTC]; Pronto® Plus Lice Killing Mousse Plus Vitamin E [OTC]; Pronto® Plus Lice Killing Mousse Shampoo Plus Natural Extracts and Oils [OTC]; Pronto® Plus Warm Oil Treatment and Conditioner [OTC]; RID® Maximum Strength [OTC]

Canadian Brand Names Pronto® Lice Control; R & C™ II; R & C™ Shampoo/Conditioner; RID® Mousse

Therapeutic Category Scabicides/Pediculicides

Use Treatment of *Pediculus humanus* infestations (head lice, body lice, pubic lice, and their eggs)

General Dosage Range Topical: *Children and Adults:* Apply to infested area, keep on for 10 minutes, wash, and rinse; may repeat once in a 24-hour period and then again in 7-10 days

Dosage Forms
Kit:
A-200® Lice Treatment Kit [OTC]:
Shampoo: Pyrethrins 0.33% and piperonyl butoxide 4% (120 mL)
Solution: Permethrin 0.5% (180 mL)
Pronto® Complete Lice Removal System [OTC]:
Shampoo: Pyrethrins 0.33% and piperonyl butoxide 4% (60 mL)
Solution, topical: Benzalkonium chloride 0.1% (60 mL)
Oil, topical:
Pronto® Plus Warm Oil Treatment and Conditioner [OTC]: Pyrethrins 0.33% and piperonyl butoxide 4% (36 mL)
Shampoo: Pyrethrins 0.33% and piperonyl butoxide 4% (60 mL, 120 mL)
A-200® Maximum Strength [OTC]: Pyrethrins 0.33% and piperonyl butoxide 4% (60 mL, 120 mL)
Licide® [OTC], Pronto® Plus Lice Killing Mousse Shampoo Plus Vitamin E [OTC]: Pyrethrins 0.33% and piperonyl butoxide 4% (120 mL)
Pronto® Plus Lice Killing Mousse Shampoo Plus Natural Extracts and Oils [OTC]: Pyrethrins 0.33% and piperonyl butoxide 4% (60 mL)
Pronto® Plus Lice Killing Mousse Shampoo Plus Vitamin E [OTC]: Pyrethrins 0.33% and piperonyl butoxide 4% (120 mL)
RID® Maximum Strength [OTC]: Pyrethrins 0.33% and piperonyl butoxide 4% (60 mL, 120 mL, 180 mL, 240 mL)

Pyri-500 [OTC] see pyridoxine on page 758
Pyrichlor PE™ see chlorpheniramine, pyrilamine, and phenylephrine on page 202
2-pyridine aldoxime methochloride see pralidoxime on page 729
Pyridium® see phenazopyridine on page 692

pyridostigmine (peer id oh STIG meen)
Medication Safety Issues
Sound-alike/look-alike issues:
Pyridostigmine may be confused with physostigmine
Mestinon® may be confused with Metatensin®
Regonol® may be confused with Reglan®, Renagel®
Synonyms pyridostigmine bromide
U.S. Brand Names Mestinon®; Mestinon® Timespan®; Regonol®
Canadian Brand Names Mestinon®; Mestinon®-SR
Therapeutic Category Cholinergic Agent
Use Symptomatic treatment of myasthenia gravis; antagonism of nondepolarizing neuromuscular blockers
Military use: Pretreatment for soman nerve gas exposure
General Dosage Range
I.M.:
Children: 0.05-0.15 mg/kg/dose
Adults: ~1/30th of oral dose
I.V.:
Children: 0.05-0.25 mg/kg/dose
Adults: IVP: ~1/30th of oral dose or 0.1-0.25 mg/kg/dose (usual: 10-20 mg); Infusion: 2 mg/hour with gradual titration in increments of 0.5-1 mg/hour (maximum: 4 mg/hour)
Oral:
Immediate release:
Children: 7 mg/kg/day divided into 5-6 doses
Adults: 60-1500 mg/day in 5-6 divided doses (usual: 600 mg/day)
Sustained release: Adults: 180-540 mg once or twice daily (doses separated by at least 6 hours)
Dosage Forms
Injection, solution:
Regonol®: 5 mg/mL (2 mL)
Syrup, oral:
Mestinon®: 60 mg/5 mL (480 mL)
Tablet, oral: 60 mg
Mestinon®: 60 mg
Tablet, sustained release, oral:
Mestinon® Timespan®: 180 mg

pyridostigmine bromide *see* pyridostigmine *on page 757*

pyridoxine (peer i DOKS een)

Medication Safety Issues

Sound-alike/look-alike issues:

Pyridoxine may be confused with paroxetine, pralidoxime, Pyridium®

International issues:

Doxal® [Brazil] may be confused with Doxil® which is a brand name for doxorubicin in the U.S.

Doxal® [Brazil]: Brand name for doxycycline in Austria; brand name for pyridoxine/thiamine combination in Brazil; brand name for doxepin in Finland

Synonyms B6; B_6; pyridoxine hydrochloride; vitamin B_6

U.S. Brand Names Aminoxin® [OTC]; Pyri-500 [OTC]

Therapeutic Category Vitamin, Water Soluble

Use Prevention and treatment of vitamin B_6 deficiency, pyridoxine-dependent seizures in infants

General Dosage Range

I.M., I.V., SubQ: *Infants:* Deficiency: 10-100 mg

Oral:

Infants: Deficiency: 2-100 mg/day

Children: Deficiency: 1.5-25 mg/day; Neuritis: Prophylaxis: 1-2 mg/kg/day; Treatment: 10-50 mg/day

Adults: Deficiency: 10-20 mg/day; Neuritis: Prophylaxis: 25-100 mg/day; Treatment: 100-200 mg/day

Dosage Forms

Capsule, oral: 50 mg, 250 mg

Aminoxin® [OTC]: 20 mg

Injection, solution: 100 mg/mL (1 mL)

Liquid, oral: 200 mg/5 mL (120 mL)

Tablet, oral: 25 mg, 50 mg, 100 mg, 250 mg, 500 mg

Tablet, sustained release, oral:

Pyri-500 [OTC]: 500 mg

pyridoxine and doxylamine *see* doxylamine and pyridoxine *(Canada only) on page 313*

pyridoxine, folic acid, and cyanocobalamin *see* folic acid, cyanocobalamin, and pyridoxine *on page 396*

pyridoxine hydrochloride *see* pyridoxine *on page 758*

pyrilamine, chlorpheniramine, and phenylephrine *see* chlorpheniramine, pyrilamine, and phenylephrine *on page 202*

pyrilamine maleate, dextromethorphan hydrobromide, and phenylephrine hydrochloride *see* phenylephrine, pyrilamine, and dextromethorphan *on page 699*

pyrilamine, phenylephrine, and carbetapentane *see* carbetapentane, phenylephrine, and pyrilamine *on page 173*

pyrilamine tannate and phenylephrine tannate *see* phenylephrine and pyrilamine *on page 698*

pyrilamine tannate, guaifenesin, and phenylephrine tannate *see* phenylephrine, pyrilamine, and guaifenesin *on page 700*

pyrimethamine (peer i METH a meen)

Medication Safety Issues

Sound-alike/look-alike issues:

Daraprim® may be confused with Dantrium®, Daranide®

U.S. Brand Names Daraprim®

Canadian Brand Names Daraprim®

Therapeutic Category Folic Acid Antagonist (Antimalarial)

Use Prophylaxis of malaria due to susceptible strains of plasmodia; used in conjunction with a sulfonamide for the treatment of uncomplicated malaria due to susceptible strains of plasmodia (alternative agent; not preferred therapy); synergistic combination with sulfonamide in treatment of toxoplasmosis

General Dosage Range Oral:

Children <4 years: Malaria prophylaxis: 6.25 mg once weekly (maximum: 25 mg/dose)

Children 4-10 years: Malaria prophylaxis: 12.5 mg once weekly (maximum: 25 mg/dose); Malaria treatment: 25 mg daily

Children >10 years: Malaria prophylaxis: 25 mg once weekly; Malaria treatment: 25 mg daily

Children: Toxoplasmosis treatment: Loading dose: 1 mg/kg/day divided into 2 equal doses for 2-4 days; Maintenance: 0.5 mg/kg/day divided into 2 doses (maximum: 25 mg/day)

Adults: Malaria prophylaxis: 25 mg once weekly; Malaria treatment: 25 mg daily; Toxoplasmosis treatment: Initial: 25-75 mg/day; Maintenance: 12.5-37.5 mg/day

Dosage Forms
Tablet, oral:
Daraprim®: 25 mg

pyrimethamine and sulfadoxine *see* sulfadoxine and pyrimethamine *on page 836*

pyrithione zinc (peer i THYE one zingk)

Medication Safety Issues
Sound-alike/look-alike issues:
Pyrithione may be confused with Pyridium®

U.S. Brand Names BetaMed™ [OTC]; DermaZinc™ [OTC]; DHS™ Zinc [OTC]; Head & Shoulders® Citrus Breeze 2-in-1 [OTC]; Head & Shoulders® Citrus Breeze [OTC]; Head & Shoulders® Classic Clean 2-in-1 [OTC]; Head & Shoulders® Classic Clean [OTC]; Head & Shoulders® Dry Scalp 2-in-1 [OTC]; Head & Shoulders® Dry Scalp Care 2-in-1 [OTC]; Head & Shoulders® Dry Scalp Care [OTC]; Head & Shoulders® Dry Scalp [OTC]; Head & Shoulders® Extra Volume [OTC]; Head & Shoulders® intensive solutions 2 in 1 [OTC]; Head & Shoulders® intensive solutions for dry/damaged hair [OTC]; Head & Shoulders® intensive solutions for fine/oily hair [OTC]; Head & Shoulders® intensive solutions for normal hair [OTC]; Head & Shoulders® Ocean Lift 2-in-1 [OTC]; Head & Shoulders® Ocean Lift [OTC]; Head & Shoulders® Refresh 2-in-1 [OTC]; Head & Shoulders® Refresh [OTC]; Head & Shoulders® Restoring Shine 2 in 1 [OTC]; Head & Shoulders® Restoring Shine [OTC]; Head & Shoulders® Sensitive Care 2 in 1 [OTC]; Head & Shoulders® Sensitive Care [OTC]; Head & Shoulders® Smooth & Silky 2-in-1 [OTC]; Head & Shoulders® Smooth & Silky [OTC]; Selsun® Salon™ Classic [OTC]; Selsun® Salon™ Dandruff 2-in-1 [OTC]; Selsun® Salon™ Dandruff Moisturizing [OTC]; Selsun® Salon™ Dandruff Volumizing [OTC]; Skin Care™ [OTC]; T/Gel® Daily Control 2 in 1 Dandruff Shampoo Plus Conditioner [OTC]; T/Gel® Daily Control Dandruff Shampoo [OTC]; Zincon® [OTC]; ZNP® [OTC]

Therapeutic Category Antiseborrheic Agent, Topical

Use Relieves the itching, irritation, and scalp flaking associated with dandruff and/or seborrheal dermatitis

General Dosage Range Topical: *Adults:* Apply at least twice weekly

Dosage Forms
Bar, topical:
DermaZinc™ [OTC]: 2% (112.5 g)
ZNP® [OTC]: 2% (119 g)
Conditioner, topical:
Head & Shoulders® Classic Clean [OTC]: 0.5% (400 mL)
Head & Shoulders® Dry Scalp Care [OTC]: 0.5% (400 mL)
Cream, topical:
DermaZinc™ [OTC]: 0.25% (120 g)
Lotion, topical:
Skin Care™ [OTC]: 0.25% (120 mL)
Shampoo, topical:
BetaMed™ [OTC]: 2% (480 mL)
DermaZinc™ [OTC]: 2% (240 mL)
DHS™ Zinc [OTC]: 2% (240 mL, 360 mL)
Head & Shoulders® Citrus Breeze [OTC]: 1% (420 mL, 700 mL)
Head & Shoulders® Citrus Breeze 2-in-1 [OTC]: 1% (420 mL)
Head & Shoulders® Classic Clean [OTC]: 1% (50 mL, 420 mL, 700 mL, 1000 mL, 1200 mL)
Head & Shoulders® Classic Clean 2-in-1 [OTC]: 1% (420 mL, 700 mL)
Head & Shoulders® Dry Scalp [OTC]: 1% (420 mL)
Head & Shoulders® Dry Scalp 2-in-1 [OTC]: 1% (420 mL)
Head & Shoulders® Dry Scalp Care [OTC]: 1% (340 mL, 700 mL, 1200 mL)
Head & Shoulders® Dry Scalp Care 2-in-1 [OTC]: 1% (700 mL)
Head & Shoulders® Extra Volume [OTC]: 1% (420 mL, 700 mL)
Head & Shoulders® intensive solutions 2 in 1 [OTC]: 2% (241 mL)
Head & Shoulders® intensive solutions for dry/damaged hair [OTC]: 2% (251 mL)
Head & Shoulders® intensive solutions for fine/oily hair [OTC]: 2% (251 mL)
Head & Shoulders® intensive solutions for normal hair [OTC]: 2% (251 mL)
Head & Shoulders® Ocean Lift [OTC]: 1% (420 mL, 700 mL)
Head & Shoulders® Ocean Lift 2-in-1 [OTC]: 1% (420 mL, 700 mL)

Head & Shoulders® Refresh [OTC]: 1% (420 mL, 700 mL, 1000 mL, 1200 mL)
Head & Shoulders® Refresh 2-in-1 [OTC]: 1% (420 mL)
Head & Shoulders® Restoring Shine [OTC]: 1% (420 mL, 700 mL)
Head & Shoulders® Restoring Shine 2 in 1 [OTC]: 1% (420 mL)
Head & Shoulders® Sensitive Care [OTC]: 1% (420 mL, 700 mL)
Head & Shoulders® Sensitive Care 2 in 1 [OTC]: 1% (420 mL, 700 mL)
Head & Shoulders® Smooth & Silky [OTC]: 1% (420 mL, 700 mL)
Head & Shoulders® Smooth & Silky 2-in-1 [OTC]: 1% (420 mL)
Selsun® Salon™ Classic [OTC]: 1% (384 mL)
Selsun® Salon™ Dandruff 2-in-1 [OTC]: 1% (384 mL)
Selsun® Salon™ Dandruff Moisturizing [OTC]: 1% (384 mL)
Selsun® Salon™ Dandruff Volumizing [OTC]: 1% (384 mL)
T/Gel® Daily Control 2 in 1 Dandruff Shampoo Plus Conditioner [OTC]: 1% (250 mL)
T/Gel® Daily Control Dandruff Shampoo [OTC]: 1% (250 mL)
Zincon® [OTC]: 1% (120 mL, 240 mL)
Solution, topical:
DermaZinc™ [OTC]: 0.25% (120 mL)

QAB149 see indacaterol on page 470

quadrivalent human papillomavirus vaccine see papillomavirus (types 6, 11, 16, 18) vaccine (human, recombinant) on page 674

Qualaquin® see quinine on page 762

Quartuss™ [DSC] see dextromethorphan, chlorpheniramine, phenylephrine, and guaifenesin on page 272

Quasense® see ethinyl estradiol and levonorgestrel on page 353

quaternium-18 bentonite see bentoquatam on page 120

quazepam (KWAZ e pam)
Medication Safety Issues
Sound-alike/look-alike issues:
Quazepam may be confused with oxazepam
Beers Criteria medication:
This drug may be inappropriate for use in geriatric patients (high severity risk).
U.S. Brand Names Doral®
Canadian Brand Names Doral®
Therapeutic Category Benzodiazepine
Controlled Substance C-IV
Use Treatment of insomnia
General Dosage Range Oral:
Adults: 7.5-15 mg at bedtime
Elderly: Initial: 7.5 mg at bedtime
Dosage Forms
Tablet, oral:
Doral®: 15 mg

Quelicin® see succinylcholine on page 832
Questran® see cholestyramine resin on page 205
Questran® Light see cholestyramine resin on page 205
Questran® Light Sugar Free (Can) see cholestyramine resin on page 205

quetiapine (kwe TYE a peen)
Medication Safety Issues
Sound-alike/look-alike issues:
QUEtiapine may be confused with OLANZapine
SEROquel® may be confused with Serentil®, Serzone®, SINEquan®
Synonyms quetiapine fumarate
Tall-Man QUEtiapine
U.S. Brand Names SEROquel XR®; SEROquel®

Canadian Brand Names Apo-Quetiapine®; CO Quetiapine; Dom-Quetiapine; JAMP-Quetiapine; Mylan-Quetiapine; PHL-Quetiapine; PMS-Quetiapine; PRO-Quetiapine; ratio-Quetiapine; Riva-Quetiapine; Sandoz-Quetiapine; Seroquel XR®; Seroquel®; Teva-Quetiapine

Therapeutic Category Antipsychotic Agent

Use Treatment of schizophrenia; treatment of acute manic or mixed episodes associated with bipolar I disorder (as monotherapy or in combination with lithium or divalproex); maintenance treatment of bipolar I disorder (in combination with lithium or divalproex); treatment of acute depressive episodes associated with bipolar disorder; adjunctive treatment of major depressive disorder

General Dosage Range Dosage adjustment recommended in patients with hepatic impairment
Oral:
  Immediate release:
    Children ≥10 years: Initial: 25 mg twice daily; Maintenance: Titrate to 50-800 mg/day
    Adults: Initial: 25-50 mg twice daily; Maintenance: 150-800 mg/day in 2-3 divided doses
    Elderly: Initial: 25 mg/day
  Extended release:
    Adults: Initial: 50-300 mg once daily; Maintenance: Titrate to 150-800 mg/day
    Elderly: Initial: 50 mg/day

Dosage Forms
  Tablet, oral:
    SEROquel®: 25 mg, 50 mg, 100 mg, 200 mg, 300 mg, 400 mg
  Tablet, extended release, oral:
    SEROquel XR®: 50 mg, 150 mg, 200 mg, 300 mg, 400 mg

quetiapine fumarate *see* quetiapine *on page 760*

quinalbarbitone sodium *see* secobarbital *on page 805*

quinapril (KWIN a pril)

Medication Safety Issues
  Sound-alike/look-alike issues:
    Accupril® may be confused with Accolate®, Accutane®, AcipHex®, Monopril®
  International issues:
    Accupril [U.S., Canada] may be confused with Acepril which is a brand name for captopril [Great Britain]; enalapril [Hungary, Switzerland]; lisinopril [Malaysia]

Synonyms quinapril hydrochloride

U.S. Brand Names Accupril®

Canadian Brand Names Accupril®

Therapeutic Category Angiotensin-Converting Enzyme (ACE) Inhibitor

Use Treatment of hypertension; treatment of heart failure

General Dosage Range Dosage adjustment recommended in patients with renal impairment
Oral:
  Adults: Initial: 5-20 mg/day in 1-2 divided doses; Maintenance: 10-40 mg/day in 1-2 divided doses
  Elderly: Initial: 2.5-5 mg/day

Dosage Forms
  Tablet, oral: 5 mg, 10 mg, 20 mg, 40 mg
    Accupril®: 5 mg, 10 mg, 20 mg, 40 mg

quinapril and hydrochlorothiazide (KWIN a pril & hye droe klor oh THYE a zide)

Synonyms hydrochlorothiazide and quinapril; Quinaretic

U.S. Brand Names Accuretic®

Canadian Brand Names Accuretic®

Therapeutic Category Antihypertensive Agent, Combination

Use Treatment of hypertension (not for initial therapy)

General Dosage Range Oral: *Adults:* Initial: 10-20 mg quinapril and 12.5 mg hydrochlorothiazide once daily; Maintenance: 5-40 mg quinapril and 6.25-25 mg hydrochlorothiazide once daily

Dosage Forms
  Tablet: 10/12.5: Quinapril 10 mg and hydrochlorothiazide 12.5 mg; 20/12.5: Quinapril 20 mg and hydrochlorothiazide 12.5 mg; 20/25: Quinapril 20 mg and hydrochlorothiazide 25 mg
    Accuretic®: 10/12.5: Quinapril 10 mg and hydrochlorothiazide 12.5 mg; 20/12.5: Quinapril 20 mg and hydrochlorothiazide 12.5 mg; 20/25: Quinapril 20 mg and hydrochlorothiazide 25 mg

quinapril hydrochloride *see quinapril on page 761*
Quinaretic *see quinapril and hydrochlorothiazide on page 761*
Quinate® (Can) *see quinidine on page 762*

quinidine (KWIN i deen)

Medication Safety Issues
Sound-alike/look-alike issues:
QuiNIDine may be confused with cloNIDine, quiNINE, Quinora®
High alert medication:
The Institute for Safe Medication Practices (ISMP) includes this medication (I.V. formulation) among its list of drug classes which have a heightened risk of causing significant patient harm when used in error.

Synonyms quinidine gluconate; quinidine polygalacturonate; quinidine sulfate

Tall-Man quiNIDine

Canadian Brand Names Apo-Quinidine®; BioQuin® Durules™; Novo-Quinidin; Quinate®

Therapeutic Category Antiarrhythmic Agent, Class I-A

Use
Quinidine gluconate and sulfate salts: Conversion and prevention of relapse into atrial fibrillation and/or flutter; suppression of ventricular arrhythmias. **Note:** Due to proarrhythmic effects, use should be reserved for life-threatening arrhythmias. Moreover, the use of quinidine has largely been replaced by more effective/safer antiarrhythmic agents and/or nonpharmacologic therapies (eg, radiofrequency ablation).
Quinidine gluconate (I.V. formulation): Conversion of atrial fibrillation/flutter and ventricular tachycardia. **Note:** The use of I.V. quinidine gluconate for these indications has been replaced by more effective/ safer antiarrhythmic agents (eg, amiodarone and procainamide).
Quinidine gluconate (I.V. formulation) and quinidine sulfate: Treatment of malaria (*Plasmodium falciparum*)

General Dosage Range Dosages expressed in terms of the salt. Dosage adjustment recommended in patients with renal impairment.
I.V.: Quinidine gluconate: *Children and Adults:* 10 mg/kg bolus followed by 0.02 mg/kg/minute **or** 24 mg/kg bolus followed by 12 mg/kg every 8 hours
Oral:
Immediate release: Quinidine sulfate: *Adults:* Initial: 200-400 mg/dose every 6 hours
Extended release:
  Quinidine gluconate: *Adults:* Initial: 324 mg every 8-12 hours
  Quinidine sulfate: *Adults:* Initial: 300 mg every 8-12 hours

Dosage Forms
Injection, solution: 80 mg/mL (10 mL)
Tablet, oral: 200 mg, 300 mg
Tablet, extended release, oral: 300 mg, 324 mg

quinidine and dextromethorphan *see dextromethorphan and quinidine on page 272*
quinidine gluconate *see quinidine on page 762*
quinidine polygalacturonate *see quinidine on page 762*
quinidine sulfate *see quinidine on page 762*

quinine (KWYE nine)

Medication Safety Issues
Sound-alike/look-alike issues:
QuiNINE may be confused with quiNIDine

Synonyms quinine sulfate

Tall-Man quiNINE

U.S. Brand Names Qualaquin®

Canadian Brand Names Apo-Quinine®; Novo-Quinine; Quinine-Odan

Therapeutic Category Antimalarial Agent

Use In conjunction with other antimalarial agents, treatment of uncomplicated chloroquine-resistant *P. falciparum* malaria

General Dosage Range Dosage adjustment recommended in patients with renal impairment
Oral:
Children: 30 mg/kg/day divided every 8 hours
Adults: 648 mg every 8 hours
Dosage Forms
Capsule, oral:
Qualaquin®: 324 mg

Quinine-Odan (Can) *see* quinine *on page 762*
quinine sulfate *see* quinine *on page 762*
Quinnostik *see* urea *on page 900*
quinol *see* hydroquinone *on page 453*
Quintabs [OTC] *see* vitamins (multiple/oral) *on page 919*
Quintabs-M [OTC] *see* vitamins (multiple/oral) *on page 919*
Quintabs-M Iron-Free [OTC] *see* vitamins (multiple/oral) *on page 919*

quinupristin and dalfopristin (kwi NYOO pris tin & dal FOE pris tin)

Synonyms dalfopristin and quinupristin; pristinamycin; RP-59500
U.S. Brand Names Synercid®
Canadian Brand Names Synercid®
Therapeutic Category Antibiotic, Streptogramin
Use Treatment of complicated skin and skin structure infections caused by methicillin-susceptible *Staphylococcus aureus* or *Streptococcus pyogenes*
General Dosage Range I.V.: *Children ≥12 years and Adults:* 7.5 mg/kg every 12 hours
Dosage Forms
Injection, powder for reconstitution:
Synercid®: 500 mg: Quinupristin 150 mg and dalfopristin 350 mg

Quixin® *see* levofloxacin (ophthalmic) *on page 520*
Qutenza™ *see* capsaicin *on page 169*
QVAR® *see* beclomethasone (oral inhalation) *on page 117*
R & C™ II (Can) *see* pyrethrins and piperonyl butoxide *on page 756*
R & C™ Shampoo/Conditioner (Can) *see* pyrethrins and piperonyl butoxide *on page 756*
R-1569 *see* tocilizumab *on page 874*
RabAvert® *see* rabies vaccine *on page 764*

rabeprazole (ra BEP ra zole)

Medication Safety Issues
Sound-alike/look-alike issues:
AcipHex® may be confused with Acephen®, Accupril®, Aricept®, pHisoHex®
RABEprazole may be confused with ARIPiprazole, donepezil, lansoprazole, omeprazole, raloxifene
Synonyms pariprazole
Tall-Man RABEprazole
U.S. Brand Names AcipHex®
Canadian Brand Names Pariet®; PMS-Rabeprazole EC; PRO-Rabeprazole; Rabeprazole EC; RAN™-Rabeprazole; Riva-Rabeprazole EC; Sandoz-Rabeprazole; Teva-Rabeprazole EC
Therapeutic Category Gastric Acid Secretion Inhibitor
Use Short-term (4-8 weeks) treatment and maintenance of erosive or ulcerative gastroesophageal reflux disease (GERD); symptomatic GERD; short-term (up to 4 weeks) treatment of duodenal ulcers; long-term treatment of pathological hypersecretory conditions, including Zollinger-Ellison syndrome; *H. pylori* eradication (in combination therapy)

Canadian labeling: Additional uses (not in U.S. labeling): Treatment of nonerosive reflux disease (NERD); treatment of gastric ulcers
General Dosage Range Oral:
Children ≥12 years: 20 mg/day
Adults: 10-20 mg once to twice daily **or** 60 mg once daily

◄ **Dosage Forms**
  Tablet, delayed release, enteric coated, oral:
    AcipHex®: 20 mg
Dosage Forms - Canada
  Tablet, delayed release, enteric coated:
    Pariet®: 10 mg, 20 mg

Rabeprazole EC (Can) *see* rabeprazole *on page 763*

rabies immune globulin (human) (RAY beez i MYUN GLOB yoo lin, HYU man)

Synonyms HRIG; RIG
U.S. Brand Names HyperRAB™ S/D; Imogam® Rabies-HT
Canadian Brand Names HyperRAB™ S/D; Imogam® Rabies Pasteurized
Therapeutic Category Immune Globulin
Use Part of postexposure prophylaxis of persons with rabies exposure. Provides passive immunity until active immunity with rabies vaccine is established. Not for use in persons with a history of preexposure vaccination, history of postexposure prophylaxis, or previous vaccination with rabies vaccine and documentation of antibody response.
General Dosage Range Local wound infiltration/I.M.: *Children and Adults:* 20 units/kg in a single dose
Dosage Forms
  Injection, solution [preservative free]:
    HyperRAB™ S/D: 150 int. units/mL (2 mL, 10 mL)
    Imogam® Rabies-HT: 150 int. units/mL (2 mL, 10 mL)

rabies vaccine (RAY beez vak SEEN)

Synonyms HDCV; human diploid cell cultures rabies vaccine; PCEC; purified chick embryo cell
U.S. Brand Names Imovax® Rabies; RabAvert®
Canadian Brand Names Imovax® Rabies; RabAvert®
Therapeutic Category Vaccine, Inactivated Virus
Use Preexposure and postexposure vaccination against rabies

The Advisory Committee on Immunization Practices (ACIP) recommends a primary course of prophylactic immunization (preexposure vaccination) for the following:
  • Persons with continuous risk of infection, including rabies research laboratory and biologics production workers
  • Persons with frequent risk of infection in areas where rabies is enzootic, including rabies diagnostic laboratory workers, cavers, veterinarians and their staff, and animal control and wildlife workers; persons who frequently handle bats
  • Persons with infrequent risk of infection, including veterinarians and animal control staff with terrestrial animals in areas where rabies infection is rare, veterinary students, and travelers visiting areas where rabies is enzootic and immediate access to medical care and biologicals is limited

The ACIP recommends the use of postexposure vaccination for a particular person be assessed by the severity and likelihood versus the actual risk of acquiring rabies. Consideration should include the type of exposure, epidemiology of rabies in the area, species of the animal, circumstances of the incident, and the availability of the exposing animal for observation or rabies testing. Postexposure vaccination is used in both previously vaccinated and previously unvaccinated individuals.
General Dosage Range I.M.: *Children and Adults:* 1 mL
Dosage Forms
  Injection, powder for reconstitution [preservative free]:
    Imovax® Rabies: ≥ 2.5 int. units
    RabAvert®: ≥ 2.5 int. units

racemic epinephrine *see* epinephrine (systemic, oral inhalation) *on page 331*
racepinephrine *see* epinephrine (systemic, oral inhalation) *on page 331*
RAD001 *see* everolimus *on page 362*
Radiogardase® *see* ferric hexacyanoferrate *on page 373*
rAHF *see* antihemophilic factor (recombinant) *on page 81*
R-albuterol *see* levalbuterol *on page 516*
Ralivia™ ER (Can) *see* tramadol *on page 880*

raloxifene (ral OKS i feen)

Medication Safety Issues
  Sound-alike/look-alike issues:
    Evista® may be confused with Avinza™, Eovist®
Synonyms keoxifene hydrochloride; raloxifene hydrochloride
U.S. Brand Names Evista®
Canadian Brand Names Apo-Raloxifene®; Evista®; Novo-Raloxifene
Therapeutic Category Selective Estrogen Receptor Modulator (SERM)
Use Prevention and treatment of osteoporosis in postmenopausal women; risk reduction for invasive breast cancer in postmenopausal women with osteoporosis and in postmenopausal women with high risk for invasive breast cancer
General Dosage Range Oral: *Adults (females):* 60 mg/day
Dosage Forms
  Tablet, oral:
    Evista®: 60 mg

raloxifene hydrochloride see raloxifene *on page 765*

raltegravir (ral TEG ra vir)

Synonyms MK-0518
U.S. Brand Names Isentress®
Canadian Brand Names Isentress®
Therapeutic Category Antiretroviral Agent, Integrase Inhibitor
Use Treatment of HIV-1 infection in combination with other antiretroviral agents
General Dosage Range Dosage adjustment recommended in patients on concomitant therapy
  Oral: *Adolescents ≥16 years and Adults:* 400 mg twice daily
Dosage Forms
  Tablet, oral:
    Isentress®: 400 mg

raltitrexed *(Canada only)* (ral ti TREX ed)

Medication Safety Issues
  Sound-alike/look-alike issues:
    Raltitrexed may be confused with methotrexate, PEMEtrexed, PRALAtrexate
  High alert medication:
    This medication is in a class the Institute for Safe Medication Practices (ISMP) includes among its list of drug classes which have a heightened risk of causing significant patient harm when used in error.
Synonyms D1694; ICI-D1694; raltitrexed disodium; TDX; ZD1694
Canadian Brand Names Tomudex®
Therapeutic Category Antineoplastic Agent
Use Treatment of advanced colorectal cancer
General Dosage Range Dosage adjustment recommended in patients with renal impairment or who develop toxicities
  I.V.: *Adults:* 3 mg/m² every 3 weeks
Product Availability Not available in U.S.
Dosage Forms - Canada
  Injection, powder for reconstitution, as disodium:
    Tomudex®: 2 mg

raltitrexed disodium see raltitrexed *(Canada only) on page 765*

ramelteon (ra MEL tee on)

Medication Safety Issues
  Sound-alike/look-alike issues:
    Ramelteon may be confused with Remeron®
    Rozerem® may be confused with Razadyne®, Remeron®
Synonyms TAK-375
U.S. Brand Names Rozerem™

◀ **Therapeutic Category** Hypnotic, Nonbenzodiazepine

Use Treatment of insomnia characterized by difficulty with sleep onset

General Dosage Range Oral: *Adults:* 8 mg at bedtime

Dosage Forms
Tablet, oral:
Rozerem™: 8 mg

ramipril (RA mi pril)

Medication Safety Issues
Sound-alike/look-alike issues:
Ramipril may be confused with enalapril, Monopril®
Altace® may be confused with alteplase, Amaryl®, Amerge®, Artane®
International issues:
Altace [Canada] may be confused with Altace HCT brand name for ramipril/hydrochlorothiazide [Canada]

U.S. Brand Names Altace®

Canadian Brand Names Altace®; Apo-Ramipril®; CO Ramipril; Dom-Ramipril; JAMP-Ramipril; Mylan-Ramipril; PHL-Ramipril; PMS-Ramipril; RAN™-Ramipril; ratio-Ramipril; Sandoz-Ramipril; Teva-Ramipril

Therapeutic Category Angiotensin-Converting Enzyme (ACE) Inhibitor

Use Treatment of hypertension, alone or in combination with thiazide diuretics; treatment of left ventricular dysfunction after MI; to reduce risk of MI, stroke, and death in patients at increased risk for these events

General Dosage Range Dosage adjustment recommended in patients with renal impairment
Oral: *Adults:* 2.5-20 mg/day (maximum: 20 mg/day)

Dosage Forms
Capsule, oral: 1.25 mg, 2.5 mg, 5 mg, 10 mg
Altace®: 1.25 mg, 2.5 mg, 5 mg, 10 mg

ramipril and felodipine *(Canada only)* (RA mi pril & fe LOE di peen)

Synonyms felodipine and ramipril; ramipril and felodipine ER

Canadian Brand Names Altace® Plus Felodipine

Therapeutic Category Antihypertensive Agent, Combination

Use Treatment of hypertension when combination therapy is appropriate (not for initial therapy)

General Dosage Range Dosage adjustment recommended in patients with hepatic or renal impairment
Oral:
Adults: Ramipril 2.5-10 mg and felodipine ER 2.5-10 mg once daily
Elderly: Initial: Felodipine ER: 2.5 mg daily

Product Availability Not available in U.S.

Dosage Forms - Canada
Tablet, variable release, oral:
Altace® Plus Felodipine 2.5/2.5: Ramipril 2.5 mg [immediate release] and felodipine 2.5 mg [extended release]
Altace® Plus Felodipine 5/5: Ramipril 5 mg [immediate release] and felodipine 5 mg [extended release]

ramipril and felodipine ER *see* ramipril and felodipine *(Canada only) on page 766*

ramipril and hydrochlorothiazide *(Canada only)*
(RA mi pril & hye droe klor oh THYE a zide)

Medication Safety Issues
Sound-alike/look-alike issues:
Altace® HCT may be confused with alteplase, Artane®, Altace®

Synonyms hydrochlorothiazide and ramipril

Canadian Brand Names Altace® HCT; PMS-Ramipril HCTZ

Therapeutic Category Angiotensin-Converting Enzyme (ACE) Inhibitor; Antihypertensive Agent, Combination; Diuretic, Thiazide

Use Treatment of essential hypertension (not for initial therapy)

General Dosage Range Dosage adjustment recommended in patients with renal impairment
Oral: *Adults:* Ramipril 2.5 mg/hydrochlorothiazide 12.5 mg once daily (maximum: Ramipril 10 mg/hydrochlorothiazide 50 mg once daily)

Product Availability Not available in U.S.

Dosage Forms - Canada
  Tablet, oral:
   Altace® HCT: 2.5/12.5: Ramipril 2.5 mg and hydrochlorothiazide 12.5 mg; 5/12.5: Ramipril 5 mg and hydrochlorothiazide 12.5 mg; 5/25: Ramipril 5 mg and hydrochlorothiazide 25 mg; 10/12.5: Ramipril 10 mg and hydrochlorothiazide 12.5 mg;10/25: Ramipril 10 mg and hydrochlorothiazide 25 mg

RAN™-Amlodipine (Can) *see* amlodipine *on page 69*
RAN™-Atenolol (Can) *see* atenolol *on page 101*
RAN™-Atorvastatin (Can) *see* atorvastatin *on page 102*
RAN™-Carvedilol (Can) *see* carvedilol *on page 178*
RAN™-Cefprozil (Can) *see* cefprozil *on page 183*
RAN™-Ciprofloxacin (Can) *see* ciprofloxacin (systemic) *on page 210*
RAN™-Citalo (Can) *see* citalopram *on page 213*
RAN™-Clarithromycin (Can) *see* clarithromycin *on page 215*
RAN™-Domperidone (Can) *see* domperidone *(Canada only) on page 305*
RAN™-Enalapril (Can) *see* enalapril *on page 326*
Ranexa® *see* ranolazine *on page 768*
RAN™-Fentanyl Matrix Patch (Can) *see* fentanyl *on page 371*
RAN™-Fentanyl Transdermal System (Can) *see* fentanyl *on page 371*
RAN™-Fosinopril (Can) *see* fosinopril *on page 401*
RAN™-Gabapentin (Can) *see* gabapentin *on page 405*

ranibizumab (ra ni BIZ oo mab)

Synonyms rhuFabV2
U.S. Brand Names Lucentis®
Canadian Brand Names Lucentis®
Therapeutic Category Monoclonal Antibody; Ophthalmic Agent; Vascular Endothelial Growth Factor (VEGF) Inhibitor
Use Treatment of neovascular (wet) age-related macular degeneration (AMD); treatment of macular edema following retinal vein occlusion (RVO)

Canadian labeling: Additional use (not in in U.S. labeling): Treatment of visual impairment associated with diabetic macular edema (DME)
General Dosage Range Intravitreal: *Adults:* 0.5 mg once every 1-3 months
Dosage Forms
  Injection, solution [preservative free]:
   Lucentis®: 10 mg/mL (0.2 mL)
Dosage Forms - Canada
  Injection, solution [preservative free]:
   Lucentis®: 10 mg/mL (0.3 mL)

RAN™-Imipenem-Cilastatin (Can) *see* imipenem and cilastatin *on page 466*
Ran™-Irbesartan HCTZ (Can) *see* irbesartan and hydrochlorothiazide *on page 490*

ranitidine (ra NI ti deen)

Medication Safety Issues
  Sound-alike/look-alike issues:
   Ranitidine may be confused with amantadine, rimantadine
   Zantac® may be confused with Xanax®, Zarontin®, Zofran®, ZyrTEC®
  International issues:
   Antagon®: Brand name for astemizole in Mexico; brand name for ganirelix in the U.S.
Synonyms ranitidine hydrochloride
U.S. Brand Names Zantac 150® [OTC]; Zantac 75® [OTC]; Zantac®; Zantac® EFFERdose®
Canadian Brand Names Acid Reducer; Apo-Ranitidine®; CO Ranitidine; Dom-Ranitidine; Myl-Ranitidine; Mylan-Ranitidine; Nu-Ranit; PHL-Ranitidine; PMS-Ranitidine; Ranitidine Injection, USP; RAN™-Ranitidine; ratio-Ranitidine; Riva-Ranitidine; Sandoz-Ranitidine; ScheinPharm Ranitidine; Teva-Ranitidine; Zantac 75®; Zantac Maximum Strength Non-Prescription; Zantac®
Therapeutic Category Histamine H_2 Antagonist

◀ **Use**
Zantac®: Short-term and maintenance therapy of duodenal ulcer, gastric ulcer, gastroesophageal reflux disease (GERD), active benign ulcer, erosive esophagitis, and pathological hypersecretory conditions; as part of a multidrug regimen for *H. pylori* eradication to reduce the risk of duodenal ulcer recurrence
Zantac 75® [OTC]: Relief of heartburn, acid indigestion, and sour stomach
General Dosage Range Dosage adjustment recommended in patients with renal impairment
I.M.: *Children >16 years and Adults:* 50 mg every 6-8 hours
I.V.:
Children 1 month to 16 years: 2-4 mg/kg/day divided every 6-8 hours (maximum: 200 mg/day) **or** 1 mg/kg/dose for one dose followed by infusion of 0.08-0.17 mg/kg/hour
Children >16 years and Adults: 50 mg every 6-8 hours **or** Infusion: 6.25 mg/hour **or** 1-2.5 mg/kg/hour
Oral:
Children 1 month to 11 years: 2-4 mg/kg/dose once or twice daily **or** 5-10 mg/kg/day in 2 divided doses (maximum: 300 mg/day)
Children ≥12 to 16 years: 2-4 mg/kg once or twice daily **or** 5-10 mg/kg/day in 2 divided doses (maximum: 300 mg/day); OTC dosing: 75 mg 30-60 minutes before eating or drinking (maximum: 150 mg/day)
Children >16 years and Adults: 150 mg 1-4 times/day **or** 300 mg once daily; OTC dosing: 75 mg 30-60 minutes before eating or drinking (maximum: 150 mg/day)
Dosage Forms
Capsule, oral: 150 mg, 300 mg
Infusion, premixed in 1/2 NS [preservative free]:
Zantac®: 50 mg (50 mL)
Injection, solution: 25 mg/mL (2 mL, 6 mL, 40 mL)
Zantac®: 25 mg/mL (2 mL, 6 mL, 40 mL)
Syrup, oral: 15 mg/mL (5 mL, 10 mL, 120 mL, 473 mL, 480 mL)
Zantac®: 15 mg/mL (480 mL)
Tablet, oral: 75 mg, 150 mg, 300 mg
Zantac 150® [OTC]: 150 mg
Zantac 75® [OTC]: 75 mg
Zantac®: 150 mg, 300 mg
Tablet for solution, oral:
Zantac® EFFERdose®: 25 mg

ranitidine hydrochloride *see ranitidine on page 767*
Ranitidine Injection, USP (Can) *see ranitidine on page 767*
RAN™-Lisinopril (Can) *see lisinopril on page 531*
RAN™-Lovastatin (Can) *see lovastatin on page 540*
RAN™-Metformin (Can) *see metformin on page 566*

ranolazine (ra NOE la zeen)
Medication Safety Issues
Sound-alike/look-alike issues:
Ranexa® may be confused with Celexa®
U.S. Brand Names Ranexa®
Therapeutic Category Cardiovascular Agent, Miscellaneous
Use Treatment of chronic angina
General Dosage Range Dosage adjustment recommended in patients on concomitant therapy
Oral: *Adults:* Initial: 500 mg twice daily; Maintenance: 500-1000 mg twice daily (maximum: 2000 mg/day)
Dosage Forms
Tablet, extended release, oral:
Ranexa®: 500 mg, 1000 mg

RAN™-Ondansetron (Can) *see ondansetron on page 651*
RAN™-Pantoprazole (Can) *see pantoprazole on page 672*
RAN™-Pravastatin (Can) *see pravastatin on page 732*
RAN™-Rabeprazole (Can) *see rabeprazole on page 763*
RAN™-Ramipril (Can) *see ramipril on page 766*
RAN™-Ranitidine (Can) *see ranitidine on page 767*
RAN™-Risperidone (Can) *see risperidone on page 783*

RAN™-Ropinirole (Can) *see* ropinirole *on page 790*
RAN™-Simvastatin (Can) *see* simvastatin *on page 813*
RAN™-Tamsulosin (Can) *see* tamsulosin *on page 843*
Ran-Valsartan (Can) *see* valsartan *on page 905*
RAN™-Zopiclone (Can) *see* zopiclone *(Canada only) on page 934*
Rapaflo® *see* silodosin *on page 811*
Rapamune® *see* sirolimus *on page 815*
rapamycin *see* sirolimus *on page 815*

rasagiline (ra SA ji leen)

Medication Safety Issues
Sound-alike/look-alike issues:
Azilect® may be confused with Aricept®
Synonyms AGN 1135; rasagiline mesylate; TVP-1012
U.S. Brand Names Azilect®
Therapeutic Category Anti-Parkinson Agent, MAO Type B Inhibitor
Use Treatment of idiopathic Parkinson disease (initial monotherapy or as adjunct to levodopa)
General Dosage Range Dosage adjustment recommended in patients with hepatic impairment or on concomitant therapy
Oral: *Adults:* 0.5-1 mg once daily
Dosage Forms
Tablet, oral:
Azilect®: 0.5 mg, 1 mg

rasagiline mesylate *see* rasagiline *on page 769*

rasburicase (ras BYOOR i kayse)

Synonyms recombinant urate oxidase; urate oxidase
U.S. Brand Names Elitek™
Canadian Brand Names Fasturtec®
Therapeutic Category Enzyme
Use Initial management of uric acid levels in patients with leukemia, lymphoma, and solid tumor malignancies receiving chemotherapy expected to result in tumor lysis and elevation of plasma uric acid
General Dosage Range I.V.: *Children and Adults:* 0.2 mg/kg once daily
Dosage Forms
Injection, powder for reconstitution:
Elitek™: 1.5 mg, 7.5 mg

Rasilez® (Can) *see* aliskiren *on page 51*
Rasilez HCT (Can) *see* aliskiren and hydrochlorothiazide *on page 52*
rATG *see* antithymocyte globulin (rabbit) *on page 84*
ratio-Aclavulanate (Can) *see* amoxicillin and clavulanate potassium *on page 74*
ratio-Acyclovir (Can) *see* acyclovir (systemic) *on page 39*
ratio-Alendronate (Can) *see* alendronate *on page 49*
ratio-Amcinonide (Can) *see* amcinonide *on page 63*
ratio-Amiodarone (Can) *see* amiodarone *on page 67*
ratio-Amiodarone I.V. (Can) *see* amiodarone *on page 67*
ratio-Amlodipine (Can) *see* amlodipine *on page 69*
ratio-Atenolol (Can) *see* atenolol *on page 101*
ratio-Atorvastatin (Can) *see* atorvastatin *on page 102*
ratio-Azithromycin (Can) *see* azithromycin (systemic) *on page 108*
ratio-Baclofen (Can) *see* baclofen *on page 112*
ratio-Benzydamine (Can) *see* benzydamine *(Canada only) on page 126*
ratio-Bicalutamide (Can) *see* bicalutamide *on page 133*
ratio-Brimonidine (Can) *see* brimonidine *on page 141*
ratio-Bupropion SR (Can) *see* bupropion *on page 150*
ratio-Buspirone (Can) *see* buspirone *on page 151*

ratio-Carvedilol (Can) *see* carvedilol *on page 178*
ratio-Cefuroxime (Can) *see* cefuroxime *on page 185*
ratio-Ciprofloxacin (Can) *see* ciprofloxacin (systemic) *on page 210*
ratio-Citalopram (Can) *see* citalopram *on page 213*
ratio-Clarithromycin (Can) *see* clarithromycin *on page 215*
ratio-Clindamycin (Can) *see* clindamycin (systemic) *on page 217*
ratio-Clobetasol (Can) *see* clobetasol *on page 220*
ratio-Cotridin (Can) *see* triprolidine, pseudoephedrine, and codeine *(Canada only) on page 893*
ratio-Cyclobenzaprine (Can) *see* cyclobenzaprine *on page 241*
ratio-Diltiazem CD (Can) *see* diltiazem *on page 286*
ratio-Domperidone (Can) *see* domperidone *(Canada only) on page 305*
ratio-Ectosone (Can) *see* betamethasone *on page 129*
ratio-Emtec (Can) *see* acetaminophen and codeine *on page 26*
ratio-Enalapril (Can) *see* enalapril *on page 326*
ratio-Fenofibrate MC (Can) *see* fenofibrate *on page 369*
ratio-Fentanyl (Can) *see* fentanyl *on page 371*
ratio-Finasteride (Can) *see* finasteride *on page 378*
ratio-Fluoxetine (Can) *see* fluoxetine *on page 389*
ratio-Fluticasone (Can) *see* fluticasone (nasal) *on page 393*
ratio-Gabapentin (Can) *see* gabapentin *on page 405*
ratio-Gentamicin (Can) *see* gentamicin (topical) *on page 416*
ratio-Glimepiride (Can) *see* glimepiride *on page 418*
ratio-Glyburide (Can) *see* glyburide *on page 420*
ratio-Indomethacin (Can) *see* indomethacin *on page 471*
ratio-Ipra-Sal (Can) *see* albuterol *on page 45*
ratio-Ipra Sal UDV (Can) *see* ipratropium and albuterol *on page 489*
ratio-Irbesartan (Can) *see* irbesartan *on page 490*
ratio-Irbesartan HCTZ (Can) *see* irbesartan and hydrochlorothiazide *on page 490*
ratio-Ketorolac (Can) *see* ketorolac (ophthalmic) *on page 502*
ratio-Lamotrigine (Can) *see* lamotrigine *on page 509*
ratio-Lenoltec (Can) *see* acetaminophen and codeine *on page 26*
ratio-Lisinopril (Can) *see* lisinopril *on page 531*
ratio-Lisinopril P (Can) *see* lisinopril *on page 531*
ratio-Lisinopril Z (Can) *see* lisinopril *on page 531*
ratio-Lovastatin (Can) *see* lovastatin *on page 540*
ratio-Meloxicam (Can) *see* meloxicam *on page 556*
ratio-Memantine (Can) *see* memantine *on page 556*
ratio-Metformin (Can) *see* metformin *on page 566*
ratio-Methotrexate (Can) *see* methotrexate *on page 571*
ratio-Methylphenidate (Can) *see* methylphenidate *on page 577*
ratio-Minocycline (Can) *see* minocycline *on page 590*
ratio-Mirtazapine (Can) *see* mirtazapine *on page 592*
ratio-Mometasone (Can) *see* mometasone (topical) *on page 596*
ratio-Morphine (Can) *see* morphine (systemic) *on page 598*
ratio-Morphine SR (Can) *see* morphine (systemic) *on page 598*
ratio-Omeprazole (Can) *see* omeprazole *on page 649*
ratio-Ondansetron (Can) *see* ondansetron *on page 651*
ratio-Orciprenaline® (Can) *see* metaproterenol *on page 566*
ratio-Pantoprazole (Can) *see* pantoprazole *on page 672*
ratio-Paroxetine (Can) *see* paroxetine *on page 676*
ratio-Pentoxifylline (Can) *see* pentoxifylline *on page 689*
ratio-Pioglitazone (Can) *see* pioglitazone *on page 706*
ratio-Pravastatin (Can) *see* pravastatin *on page 732*

ratio-Quetiapine (Can) *see* quetiapine *on page 760*
ratio-Ramipril (Can) *see* ramipril *on page 766*
ratio-Ranitidine (Can) *see* ranitidine *on page 767*
ratio-Risedronate (Can) *see* risedronate *on page 782*
ratio-Risperidone (Can) *see* risperidone *on page 783*
ratio-Rivastigmine (Can) *see* rivastigmine *on page 786*
ratio-Salbutamol (Can) *see* albuterol *on page 45*
ratio-Sertraline (Can) *see* sertraline *on page 809*
ratio-Sildenafil R (Can) *see* sildenafil *on page 811*
ratio-Simvastatin (Can) *see* simvastatin *on page 813*
ratio-Sotalol (Can) *see* sotalol *on page 828*
ratio-Sumatriptan (Can) *see* sumatriptan *on page 839*
ratio-Tamsulosin (Can) *see* tamsulosin *on page 843*
ratio-Temazepam (Can) *see* temazepam *on page 848*
ratio-Terazosin (Can) *see* terazosin *on page 851*
ratio-Theo-Bronc (Can) *see* theophylline *on page 860*
ratio-Topilene (Can) *see* betamethasone *on page 129*
ratio-Topiramate (Can) *see* topiramate *on page 877*
ratio-Topisone (Can) *see* betamethasone *on page 129*
ratio-Trazodone (Can) *see* trazodone *on page 884*
ratio-Valproic (Can) *see* valproic acid *on page 904*
ratio-Valproic ECC (Can) *see* valproic acid *on page 904*
ratio-Venlafaxine XR (Can) *see* venlafaxine *on page 911*
ratio-Zopiclone (Can) *see* zopiclone *(Canada only) on page 934*
Razadyne® *see* galantamine *on page 409*
Razadyne® ER *see* galantamine *on page 409*
6R-BH4 *see* sapropterin *on page 802*
RBX-Risperidone (Can) *see* risperidone *on page 783*
Reactine™ (Can) *see* cetirizine *on page 189*
Reactine® Allergy and Sinus (Can) *see* cetirizine and pseudoephedrine *on page 189*
Readi-Cat® *see* barium *on page 114*
Readi-Cat® 2 *see* barium *on page 114*
Rea Lo® 30 [OTC] *see* urea *on page 900*
Rea Lo® 40 *see* urea *on page 900*
ReAzo [OTC] *see* phenazopyridine *on page 692*
Rebetol® *see* ribavirin *on page 777*
Rebif® *see* interferon beta-1a *on page 482*
Reclast® *see* zoledronic acid *on page 932*
Reclipsen® *see* ethinyl estradiol and desogestrel *on page 351*
recombinant α-L-iduronidase (glycosaminoglycan α-L-iduronohydrolase) *see* laronidase *on page 512*
recombinant desulfatohirudin *see* desirudin *on page 261*
recombinant hirudin *see* desirudin *on page 261*
recombinant hirudin *see* lepirudin *on page 514*
recombinant human deoxyribonuclease *see* dornase alfa *on page 307*
recombinant human insulin-like growth factor-1 *see* mecasermin *on page 552*
recombinant human interleukin-2 *see* aldesleukin *on page 47*
recombinant human interleukin-11 *see* oprelvekin *on page 653*
recombinant human luteinizing hormone *see* lutropin alfa *on page 542*
recombinant human parathyroid hormone (1-34) *see* teriparatide *on page 853*
recombinant human platelet-derived growth factor B *see* becaplermin *on page 116*
recombinant human thyrotropin *see* thyrotropin alpha *on page 866*
recombinant interleukin-11 *see* oprelvekin *on page 653*

recombinant N-acetylgalactosamine 4-sulfatase *see* galsulfase *on page 410*
recombinant plasminogen activator *see* reteplase *on page 775*
recombinant urate oxidase *see* rasburicase *on page 769*
recombinant urate oxidase, pegylated *see* pegloticase *on page 682*
Recombinate *see* antihemophilic factor (recombinant) *on page 81*
Recombivax HB® *see* hepatitis B vaccine (recombinant) *on page 438*
Recort [OTC] *see* hydrocortisone (topical) *on page 450*
Recothrom® *see* thrombin (topical) *on page 865*
Rectacaine [OTC] *see* phenylephrine (topical) *on page 698*
RectaGel™ HC *see* lidocaine and hydrocortisone *on page 526*
Rectiv™ *see* nitroglycerin *on page 629*
Red Cross™ Canker Sore [OTC] *see* benzocaine *on page 121*
Reese's Pinworm Medicine [OTC] *see* pyrantel pamoate *on page 756*
Refenesen™ [OTC] *see* guaifenesin *on page 425*
Refenesen™ 400 [OTC] *see* guaifenesin *on page 425*
Refenesen™ DM [OTC] *see* guaifenesin and dextromethorphan *on page 427*
Refenesen™ PE [OTC] *see* guaifenesin and phenylephrine *on page 428*
Refenesen Plus [OTC] *see* guaifenesin and pseudoephedrine *on page 429*
Refissa™ *see* tretinoin (topical) *on page 885*
Refludan® *see* lepirudin *on page 514*
Refresh® [OTC] *see* artificial tears *on page 96*
Refresh Liquigel™ [OTC] *see* carboxymethylcellulose *on page 175*
Refresh Plus® [OTC] *see* artificial tears *on page 96*
Refresh Plus® [OTC] *see* carboxymethylcellulose *on page 175*
Refresh Plus® (Can) *see* carboxymethylcellulose *on page 175*
Refresh Tears® [OTC] *see* artificial tears *on page 96*
Refresh Tears® [OTC] *see* carboxymethylcellulose *on page 175*
Refresh Tears® (Can) *see* carboxymethylcellulose *on page 175*

regadenoson (re ga DEN of son)

Synonyms CVT-3146
U.S. Brand Names Lexiscan®
Therapeutic Category Diagnostic Agent
Use Radionuclide myocardial perfusion imaging (MPI) in patients unable to undergo adequate exercise stress testing
General Dosage Range I.V.: *Adults:* 0.4 mg (5 mL) as a single dose
Dosage Forms
  Injection, solution [preservative free]:
    Lexiscan®: 0.08 mg/mL (5 mL)

Regenecare® *see* lidocaine (topical) *on page 524*
Regenecare® HA [OTC] *see* lidocaine (topical) *on page 524*
Regitine [DSC] *see* phentolamine *on page 696*
Regitine® (Can) *see* phentolamine *on page 696*
Reglan® *see* metoclopramide *on page 580*
Regonol® *see* pyridostigmine *on page 757*
Regranex® *see* becaplermin *on page 116*
regular insulin *see* insulin regular *on page 480*
Regulex® (Can) *see* docusate *on page 302*
Reguloid [OTC] *see* psyllium *on page 755*
Rejuva-A® (Can) *see* tretinoin (topical) *on page 885*
Relafen *see* nabumetone *on page 607*
Relafen® (Can) *see* nabumetone *on page 607*
Relenza® *see* zanamivir *on page 926*
Relief-SF® *see* acetaminophen, chlorpheniramine, and pseudoephedrine *on page 30*

Relistor® *see* methylnaltrexone *on page 576*
Relpax® *see* eletriptan *on page 323*
Remeron® *see* mirtazapine *on page 592*
Remeron® RD (Can) *see* mirtazapine *on page 592*
Remeron SolTab® *see* mirtazapine *on page 592*
Remeven™ *see* urea *on page 900*
Remicade® *see* infliximab *on page 472*

remifentanil (rem i FEN ta nil)

Medication Safety Issues
Sound-alike/look-alike issues:
Remifentanil may be confused with alfentanil
High alert medication:
The Institute for Safe Medication Practices (ISMP) includes this medication among its list of drug classes which have a heightened risk of causing significant patient harm when used in error.

Synonyms GI87084B

U.S. Brand Names Ultiva®

Canadian Brand Names Ultiva®

Therapeutic Category Analgesic, Narcotic

Controlled Substance C-II

Use Analgesic for use during the induction and maintenance of general anesthesia; for continued analgesia into the immediate postoperative period; analgesic component of monitored anesthesia

General Dosage Range I.V.:
Infants Birth to 2 months: Infusion: 0.4-1 mcg/kg/minute; Supplemental bolus dose: ≤1 mcg/kg
Children 1-12 years: Infusion: 0.05-1.3 mcg/kg/minute; Bolus: 1 mcg/kg every 2-5 minutes
Adults: Infusion: 0.025-4 mcg/kg/minute; Bolus: 0.5-1 mcg/kg every 2-5 minutes
Elderly: Doses should be decreased by 50% and titrated

Dosage Forms
Injection, powder for reconstitution:
Ultiva®: 1 mg, 2 mg, 5 mg

Reminyl® (Can) *see* galantamine *on page 409*
Reminyl® ER (Can) *see* galantamine *on page 409*
Remodulin® *see* treprostinil *on page 884*
Renacidin® *see* citric acid, magnesium carbonate, and glucono-delta-lactone *on page 214*
Renagel® *see* sevelamer *on page 809*
renal replacement solution *see* electrolyte solution, renal replacement *on page 323*
Renax® *see* vitamins (multiple/oral) *on page 919*
Renax® 5.5 *see* vitamins (multiple/oral) *on page 919*
Renedil® (Can) *see* felodipine *on page 368*
Renova® *see* tretinoin (topical) *on page 885*
Renvela® *see* sevelamer *on page 809*
Reopro® *see* abciximab *on page 21*
ReoPro® (Can) *see* abciximab *on page 21*

repaglinide (re PAG li nide)

Medication Safety Issues
Sound-alike/look-alike issues:
Prandin® may be confused with Avandia®
High alert medication:
The Institute for Safe Medication Practices (ISMP) includes this medication among its list of drug classes which have a heightened risk of causing significant patient harm when used in error.

U.S. Brand Names Prandin®

Canadian Brand Names GlucoNorm®; Prandin®

Therapeutic Category Hypoglycemic Agent, Oral

Use Management of type 2 diabetes mellitus (noninsulin-dependent, NIDDM) as an adjunct to diet and exercise; may be used in combination with metformin or thiazolidinediones

◄ **General Dosage Range** Dosage adjustment recommended in patients with renal impairment
Oral: *Adults:* Initial: 0.5-2 mg before each meal; Maintenance: 0.5-4 mg before each meal (maximum: 16 mg/day)
Dosage Forms
Tablet, oral:
Prandin®: 0.5 mg, 1 mg, 2 mg

repaglinide and metformin (re PAG li nide & met FOR min)

Medication Safety Issues
Sound-alike/look-alike issues:
PrandiMet® may be confused with Avandamet®, Prandin®
High alert medication:
The Institute for Safe Medication Practices (ISMP) includes this medication among its list of drug classes which have a heightened risk of causing significant patient harm when used in error.
Synonyms metformin and repaglinide; repaglinide and metformin hydrochloride
U.S. Brand Names PrandiMet®
Therapeutic Category Antidiabetic Agent, Biguanide; Antidiabetic Agent, Meglitinide Derivative; Hypoglycemic Agent, Oral
Use Management of type 2 diabetes mellitus (noninsulin-dependent, NIDDM), as an adjunct to diet and exercise, in patients currently receiving or not adequately controlled on metformin and/or a meglitinide
General Dosage Range Oral: *Adults:* Repaglinide 1-2 mg and metformin 500 mg 2-3 times daily with meals (maximum single dose: 4 mg/dose [repaglinide], 1000 mg/dose [metformin]; maximum daily dose: 10 mg/day [repaglinide], 2500 mg/day [metformin])
Dosage Forms
Tablet:
PrandiMet®: 1/500: Repaglinide 1 mg and metformin hydrochloride 500 mg; 2/500: Repaglinide 2 mg and metformin hydrochloride 500 mg

repaglinide and metformin hydrochloride *see* repaglinide and metformin *on page 774*
Repan® *see* butalbital, acetaminophen, and caffeine *on page 152*
Replace [OTC] *see* vitamins (multiple/oral) *on page 919*
Replace Without Iron [OTC] *see* vitamins (multiple/oral) *on page 919*
Replagal™ (Can) *see* agalsidase alfa *(Canada only) on page 43*
Repliva 21/7® *see* vitamins (multiple/oral) *on page 919*
Reprexain™ *see* hydrocodone and ibuprofen *on page 448*
Repronex® *see* menotropins *on page 559*
Requa® Activated Charcoal [OTC] *see* charcoal *on page 191*
Requip® *see* ropinirole *on page 790*
Requip® XL™ *see* ropinirole *on page 790*
Rescon® *see* chlorpheniramine, phenylephrine, and methscopolamine *on page 200*
Rescon DM [OTC] *see* chlorpheniramine, pseudoephedrine, and dextromethorphan *on page 201*
Rescon GG [OTC] *see* guaifenesin and phenylephrine *on page 428*
Rescriptor® *see* delavirdine *on page 257*

reserpine (re SER peen)

Medication Safety Issues
Sound-alike/look-alike issues:
Reserpine may be confused with RisperDAL®, risperiDONE
BEERS Criteria medication:
This drug may be inappropriate for use in geriatric patients (low severity risk).
Therapeutic Category Rauwolfia Alkaloid
Use Management of mild-to-moderate hypertension; treatment of agitated psychotic states (schizophrenia)
General Dosage Range Oral:
Adults: Initial: 0.5 mg once daily; Maintenance: 0.05-0.5 mg once daily
Elderly: Initial: 0.05 mg once daily
Dosage Forms
Tablet, oral: 0.1 mg, 0.25 mg

resistant dextrin *see* wheat dextrin *on page 923*

resistant maltodextrin *see* wheat dextrin *on page 923*
Resonium Calcium® (Can) *see* calcium polystyrene sulfonate *(Canada only) on page 166*
Respa®-BR [DSC] *see* brompheniramine *on page 143*
Respaire®-30 [DSC] *see* guaifenesin and pseudoephedrine *on page 429*
Resperal-DM *see* brompheniramine, pseudoephedrine, and dextromethorphan *on page 144*
Restasis® *see* cyclosporine (ophthalmic) *on page 244*
Restoril™ *see* temazepam *on page 848*
Restylane® *see* hyaluronate and derivatives *on page 443*

retapamulin (re te PAM ue lin)

U.S. Brand Names Altabax™
Therapeutic Category Antibiotic, Pleuromutilin; Antibiotic, Topical
Use Treatment of impetigo caused by susceptible strains of *S. pyogenes* or methicillin-susceptible *S. aureus*
General Dosage Range Topical: *Children ≥9 months and Adults:* Apply to affected area twice daily. Total treatment area should not exceed 2% of total body surface area.
Dosage Forms
  Ointment, topical:
    Altabax™: 1% (15 g)

Retavase® *see* reteplase *on page 775*

reteplase (RE ta plase)

Medication Safety Issues
  High alert medication:
    The Institute for Safe Medication Practices (ISMP) includes this medication (I.V.) among its list of drugs which have a heightened risk of causing significant patient harm when used in error.
Synonyms r-PA; recombinant plasminogen activator
U.S. Brand Names Retavase®
Canadian Brand Names Retavase®
Therapeutic Category Fibrinolytic Agent
Use Management of ST-elevation myocardial infarction (STEMI); improvement of ventricular function; reduction of the incidence of CHF and the reduction of mortality following AMI
  Recommended criteria for treatment: STEMI: Chest pain ≥20 minutes duration, onset of chest pain within 12 hours of treatment (or within prior 12-24 hours in patients with continuing ischemic symptoms), and ST-segment elevation >0.1 mV in at least two contiguous precordial leads or two adjacent limb leads on ECG or new or presumably new left bundle branch block (LBBB)
General Dosage Range I.V.: *Adults:* 10 units; repeat after 30 minutes
Dosage Forms
  Injection, powder for reconstitution [preservative free]:
    Retavase®: 10.4 units

Retigabine (RTG) *see* ezogabine *on page 364*
Retin-A® *see* tretinoin (topical) *on page 885*
Retin-A Micro® *see* tretinoin (topical) *on page 885*
retinoic acid *see* tretinoin (topical) *on page 885*
Retinova® (Can) *see* tretinoin (topical) *on page 885*
Retisert® *see* fluocinolone (ophthalmic) *on page 384*
Retrovir® *see* zidovudine *on page 929*
Retrovir® (AZT™) (Can) *see* zidovudine *on page 929*
Revatio® *see* sildenafil *on page 811*
ReVia® *see* naltrexone *on page 610*
RevitaDERM® 40 *see* urea *on page 900*
Revitalose C-1000® (Can) *see* ascorbic acid *on page 96*
Revlimid® *see* lenalidomide *on page 514*
Revolade® *see* eltrombopag *on page 324*
Revolade™ (Can) *see* eltrombopag *on page 324*

Revonto™ *see* dantrolene *on page 251*
Reyataz® *see* atazanavir *on page 100*
Rezira™ *see* hydrocodone and pseudoephedrine *on page 449*
rFSH-alpha *see* follitropin alfa *on page 397*
rFSH-beta *see* follitropin beta *on page 397*
rFVIIa *see* factor VIIa (recombinant) *on page 365*
RG7024 *see* vemurafenib *on page 911*
R-Gene® 10 *see* arginine *on page 93*
rGM-CSF *see* sargramostim *on page 802*
rhAPC *see* drotrecogin alfa *on page 315*
rhASB *see* galsulfase *on page 410*
rhAT *see* antithrombin III *on page 83*
rhATIII *see* antithrombin III *on page 83*
r-hCG *see* chorionic gonadotropin (recombinant) *on page 206*
rhDNase *see* dornase alfa *on page 307*
Rheumatrex® *see* methotrexate *on page 571*
rhFSH-alpha *see* follitropin alfa *on page 397*
rhFSH-beta *see* follitropin beta *on page 397*
rhGAA *see* alglucosidase alfa *on page 51*
r-h α-GAL *see* agalsidase beta *on page 43*
RhIG *see* Rh$_o$(D) immune globulin *on page 776*
rhIGF-1 (mecasermin [Increlex®]) *see* mecasermin *on page 552*
rhIGF-1/rhIGFBP-3 (mecasermin rinfabate [Iplex™]) *see* mecasermin *on page 552*
rhIL-11 *see* oprelvekin *on page 653*
Rhinacon A *see* chlorpheniramine, phenylephrine, and phenyltoloxamine *on page 201*
Rhinalar® (Can) *see* flunisolide (nasal) *on page 384*
Rhinall® [OTC] *see* phenylephrine (nasal) *on page 697*
Rhinaris® [OTC] *see* sodium chloride *on page 818*
Rhinaris-CS Anti-Allergic Nasal Mist (Can) *see* cromolyn (nasal) *on page 239*
Rhinocort Aqua® *see* budesonide (nasal) *on page 146*
Rhinocort® Aqua™ (Can) *see* budesonide (nasal) *on page 146*
Rhinocort® Turbuhaler® (Can) *see* budesonide (nasal) *on page 146*
RhinoFlex™ *see* acetaminophen and phenyltoloxamine *on page 28*
RhinoFlex™-650 *see* acetaminophen and phenyltoloxamine *on page 28*
r-hirudin *see* desirudin *on page 261*
rhKGF *see* palifermin *on page 668*
r-hLH *see* lutropin alfa *on page 542*
Rho(D) immune globulin (human) *see* Rh$_o$(D) immune globulin *on page 776*
Rho®-Clonazepam (Can) *see* clonazepam *on page 222*

Rh$_o$(D) immune globulin (ar aych oh (dee) i MYUN GLOB yoo lin)

Synonyms RhIG; Rho(D) immune globulin (human); RhoIGIV; RhoIVIM
U.S. Brand Names HyperRHO™ S/D Full Dose; HyperRHO™ S/D Mini-Dose; MICRhoGAM® UF Plus; RhoGAM® UF Plus; Rhophylac®; WinRho® SDF
Canadian Brand Names WinRho® SDF
Therapeutic Category Immune Globulin
Use
  Suppression of Rh isoimmunization: Use in the following situations when an Rh$_o$(D)-negative individual is exposed to Rh$_o$(D)-positive blood: During delivery of an Rh$_o$(D)-positive infant; abortion; amniocentesis; chorionic villus sampling; ruptured tubal pregnancy; abdominal trauma; hydatidiform mole; transplacental hemorrhage. Used when the mother is Rh$_o$(D)-negative, the father of the child is either Rh$_o$(D)-positive or Rh$_o$(D)-unknown, or the baby is either Rh$_o$(D)-positive or Rh$_o$(D)-unknown.
  Transfusion: Suppression of Rh isoimmunization in Rh$_o$(D)-negative individuals transfused with Rh$_o$(D) antigen-positive RBCs or blood components containing Rh$_o$(D) antigen-positive RBCs

Treatment of idiopathic thrombocytopenic purpura (ITP): Used intravenously in the following non-splenectomized Rh$_o$(D)-positive individuals: Children with acute or chronic ITP, adults with chronic ITP, and children and adults with ITP secondary to HIV infection

General Dosage Range I.M., I.V.: *Children and Adults:* Dosage varies greatly depending on indication

Dosage Forms
  Injection, solution [preservative free]:
    HyperRHO™ S/D Full Dose: ≥300 mcg/mL (1 mL)
    HyperRHO™ S/D Mini-Dose: ≥50 mcg/0.17 mL (0.17 mL)
    MICRhoGAM® UF Plus: ~50 mcg/0.75 mL (0.75 mL)
    RhoGAM® UF Plus: ~300 mcg/0.75 mL (0.75 mL)
    Rhophylac®: ≥300 mcg/2 mL (2 mL)
    WinRho® SDF: 300 mcg/~1.3 mL (1.3 mL); 3000 mcg/~13 mL (13 mL); 500 mcg/~2.2 mL (2.2 mL); 1000 mcg/~4.4 mL (4.4 mL)

RhoGAM® UF Plus see Rh$_o$(D) immune globulin on page 776
RhoIGIV see Rh$_o$(D) immune globulin on page 776
RhoIVIM see Rh$_o$(D) immune globulin on page 776
Rho®-Loperamine (Can) see loperamide on page 535
Rho®-Nitro Pump Spray (Can) see nitroglycerin on page 629
Rhophylac® see Rh$_o$(D) immune globulin on page 776
Rhotral (Can) see acebutolol on page 23
Rhotrimine® (Can) see trimipramine on page 892
Rhovane® (Can) see zopiclone (Canada only) on page 934
Rhoxal-cyclosporine (Can) see cyclosporine (systemic) on page 243
Rhoxal-fluvoxamine (Can) see fluvoxamine on page 395
Rhoxal-glimepiride (Can) see glimepiride on page 418
Rhoxal-loperamide (Can) see loperamide on page 535
Rhoxal-nabumetone (Can) see nabumetone on page 607
Rhoxal-orphendrine (Can) see orphenadrine on page 655
Rhoxal-pamidronate (Can) see pamidronate on page 670
Rhoxal-sotalol (Can) see sotalol on page 828
Rhoxal-sumatriptan (Can) see sumatriptan on page 839
Rhoxal-valproic (Can) see valproic acid on page 904
rhPTH(1-34) see teriparatide on page 853
Rh-TSH see thyrotropin alpha on page 866
rHuEPO-α see epoetin alfa on page 333
rhuFabV2 see ranibizumab on page 767
rhu keratinocyte growth factor see palifermin on page 668
rHu-KGF see palifermin on page 668
rhuMAb-E25 see omalizumab on page 648
rHuMAb-EGFr see panitumumab on page 672
rhuMAb HER2 see trastuzumab on page 882
rhuMAb-VEGF see bevacizumab on page 132
RiaSTAP® see fibrinogen concentrate (human) on page 376
Ribasphere® see ribavirin on page 777
Ribasphere® RibaPak® see ribavirin on page 777

ribavirin (rye ba VYE rin)

Medication Safety Issues
  Sound-alike/look-alike issues:
    Ribavirin may be confused with riboflavin, rifampin, Robaxin®
Synonyms RTCA; tribavirin
U.S. Brand Names Copegus®; Rebetol®; Ribasphere®; Ribasphere® RibaPak®; Virazole®
Canadian Brand Names Virazole®
Therapeutic Category Antiviral Agent

◀ **Use**
  Inhalation: Treatment of hospitalized infants and young children with respiratory syncytial virus (RSV) infections; specially indicated for treatment of severe lower respiratory tract RSV infections in patients with an underlying compromising condition (prematurity, cardiopulmonary disease, or immunosuppression)
  Oral capsule:
   In combination with interferon alfa-2b (Intron® A) injection for the treatment of chronic hepatitis C in patients with compensated liver disease who have relapsed after alpha interferon therapy or were previously untreated with alpha interferons
   In combination with peginterferon alfa-2b (PEG-Intron®) injection for the treatment of chronic hepatitis C in patients with compensated liver disease who were previously untreated with alpha interferons
  Oral solution: In combination with interferon alfa 2b (Intron® A) injection for the treatment of chronic hepatitis C in patients with compensated liver disease who were previously untreated with alpha interferons or patients who have relapsed after alpha interferon therapy
  Oral tablet: In combination with peginterferon alfa-2a (Pegasys®) injection for the treatment of chronic hepatitis C in patients with compensated liver disease who were previously untreated with alpha interferons (includes patients with histological evidence of cirrhosis [Child-Pugh class A] and patients with clinically-stable HIV disease)

General Dosage Range Dosage adjustment recommended in patients who develop toxicities
Inhalation: *Children:* 20 mg/mL (6 g in 300 mL) solution; continuous: 12-18 hours/day
Oral:
  Children ≥3 years and ≤25 kg: 15 mg/kg/day in 2 divided doses
  Children ≥3 years and 26-36 kg: 400 mg/day in 2 divided doses
  Children ≥3 years and 37-49 kg: 600 mg/day in 2 divided doses
  Children ≥3 years and 50-61 kg: 800 mg/day in 2 divided doses
  Children ≥3 years and >61 kg to <75 kg: 1000 mg/day in 2 divided doses
  Adults ≤75 kg: 800-1000 mg/day in 2 divided doses
  Adults >75 kg: 800-1200 mg/day in 2 divided doses

Dosage Forms
  Capsule, oral: 200 mg
   Rebetol®: 200 mg
   Ribasphere®: 200 mg
  Combination package, oral:
   Ribasphere® RibaPak®: Tablet: 400 mg (7s) [medium blue tablets] and Tablet: 600 mg (7s) [dark blue tablets] (14s, 56s)
  Powder for solution, for nebulization:
   Virazole®: 6 g
  Solution, oral:
   Rebetol®: 40 mg/mL (100 mL)
  Tablet, oral: 200 mg
   Copegus®: 200 mg
   Ribasphere®: 200 mg, 400 mg, 600 mg
   Ribasphere® RibaPak®: 400 mg, 600 mg

ribavirin and peginterferon alfa-2a *see* peginterferon alfa-2a and ribavirin *(Canada only)* on page 679
ribavirin and peginterferon alfa-2b *see* peginterferon alfa-2b and ribavirin *(Canada only)* on page 681
Ribo-100 [OTC] *see* riboflavin on page 778

riboflavin (RYE boe flay vin)

Medication Safety Issues
  Sound-alike/look-alike issues:
   Riboflavin may be confused with ribavirin
Synonyms lactoflavin; vitamin B$_2$; vitamin G
U.S. Brand Names Ribo-100 [OTC]
Therapeutic Category Vitamin, Water Soluble
Use Prevention of riboflavin deficiency and treatment of ariboflavinosis
General Dosage Range Oral:
  Children: 2.5-10 mg/day in divided doses
  Adults: 5-30 mg/day in divided doses

Dosage Forms
Tablet, oral: 25 mg, 50 mg, 100 mg
Ribo-100 [OTC]: 100 mg

Rid® [OTC] *see* permethrin *on page 691*
Rid-A-Pain Dental [OTC] *see* benzocaine *on page 121*
Ridaura® *see* auranofin *on page 105*
RID® Maximum Strength [OTC] *see* pyrethrins and piperonyl butoxide *on page 756*
RID® Mousse (Can) *see* pyrethrins and piperonyl butoxide *on page 756*

rifabutin (rif a BYOO tin)
Medication Safety Issues
  Sound-alike/look-alike issues:
    Rifabutin may be confused with rifampin
Synonyms ansamycin
U.S. Brand Names Mycobutin®
Canadian Brand Names Mycobutin®
Therapeutic Category Antibiotic, Miscellaneous
Use Prevention of disseminated *Mycobacterium avium* complex (MAC) in patients with advanced HIV infection
General Dosage Range Dosage adjustment recommended in patients with renal impairment or on concomitant therapy
  Oral:
    Children <6 years: 5 mg/kg once daily
    Children ≥6 years and Adults: 300 mg once daily
Dosage Forms
  Capsule, oral:
    Mycobutin®: 150 mg

Rifadin® *see* rifampin *on page 779*
Rifamate® *see* rifampin and isoniazid *on page 779*
rifampicin *see* rifampin *on page 779*

rifampin (rif AM pin)
Medication Safety Issues
  Sound-alike/look-alike issues:
    Rifadin® may be confused with Rifater®, Ritalin®
    Rifampin may be confused with ribavirin, rifabutin, Rifamate®, rifapentine, rifaximin
Synonyms rifampicin
U.S. Brand Names Rifadin®
Canadian Brand Names Rifadin®; Rofact™
Therapeutic Category Antibiotic, Miscellaneous
Use Management of active tuberculosis in combination with other agents; elimination of meningococci from the nasopharynx in asymptomatic carriers
General Dosage Range I.V., oral:
  Children <12 years: 10-20 mg/kg/day in 1-2 divided doses **or** 10-20 mg/kg twice weekly (maximum: 600 mg/day)
  Children ≥12 years and Adults: 10 mg/kg/day **or** 10 mg/kg 2-3 times/week **or** 600 mg every 12-24 hours
Dosage Forms
  Capsule, oral: 150 mg, 300 mg
    Rifadin®: 150 mg, 300 mg
  Injection, powder for reconstitution: 600 mg
    Rifadin®: 600 mg

rifampin and isoniazid (rif AM pin & eye soe NYE a zid)
Medication Safety Issues
  Sound-alike/look-alike issues:
    Rifamate® may be confused with rifampin
Synonyms isoniazid and rifampin

◀ **U.S. Brand Names** IsonaRif™; Rifamate®
Canadian Brand Names Rifamate®
Therapeutic Category Antibiotic, Miscellaneous
Use Management of active tuberculosis; see individual agents for additional information
General Dosage Range Oral: *Adults:* 2 capsules (rifampin 300 mg/isoniazid 150 mg/capsule) once daily
Dosage Forms
Capsule:
IsonaRif™, Rifamate®: 300/150: Rifampin 300 mg and isoniazid 150 mg

rifampin, isoniazid, and pyrazinamide
(rif AM pin, eye soe NYE a zid, & peer a ZIN a mide)
Medication Safety Issues
Sound-alike/look-alike issues:
Rifater® may be confused with Rifadin®
Synonyms isoniazid, pyrazinamide, and rifampin; pyrazinamide, rifampin, and isoniazid
U.S. Brand Names Rifater®
Canadian Brand Names Rifater®
Therapeutic Category Antibiotic, Miscellaneous
Use Initial phase, short-course treatment of pulmonary tuberculosis; see individual agents for additional information
General Dosage Range Oral:
Children ≥15 years and Adults ≤44 kg: 4 tablets (rifampin 120 mg/isoniazid 50 mg/pyrazinamide 300 mg per tablet) once daily
Children ≥15 years and Adults 45-54 kg: 5 tablets (rifampin 120 mg/isoniazid 50 mg/pyrazinamide 300 mg per tablet) once daily
Children ≥15 years and Adults ≥55 kg: 6 tablets (rifampin 120 mg/isoniazid 50 mg/pyrazinamide 300 mg per tablet) once daily
Dosage Forms
Tablet, oral:
Rifater®: Rifampin 120 mg, isoniazid 50 mg, and pyrazinamide 300 mg

rifapentine (rif a PEN teen)
Medication Safety Issues
Sound-alike/look-alike issues:
Rifapentine may be confused with rifampin
U.S. Brand Names Priftin®
Canadian Brand Names Priftin®
Therapeutic Category Antitubercular Agent
Use Treatment of pulmonary tuberculosis; rifapentine must always be used in conjunction with at least one other antituberculosis drug to which the isolate is susceptible; it may also be necessary to add a third agent (either streptomycin or ethambutol) until susceptibility is known.
General Dosage Range Oral: *Adults:* 600 mg once or twice weekly
Dosage Forms
Tablet, oral:
Priftin®: 150 mg

Rifater® *see* rifampin, isoniazid, and pyrazinamide *on page 780*

rifaximin (rif AX i min)
Medication Safety Issues
Sound-alike/look-alike issues:
Rifaximin may be confused with rifampin
U.S. Brand Names Xifaxan®
Therapeutic Category Antibiotic, Miscellaneous
Use Treatment of traveler's diarrhea caused by noninvasive strains of *E. coli*; reduction in the risk of overt hepatic encephalopathy (HE) recurrence
General Dosage Range Oral:
Children ≥12 years: 200 mg 3 times/day
Adults: 200 mg 3 times/day **or** 550 mg 2 times/day

Dosage Forms
  Tablet, oral:
    Xifaxan®: 200 mg, 550 mg

rIFN beta-1a *see* interferon beta-1a *on page 482*
rIFN beta-1b *see* interferon beta-1b *on page 482*
RIG *see* rabies immune globulin (human) *on page 764*

rilonacept (ri LON a sept)

U.S. Brand Names Arcalyst™
Therapeutic Category Interleukin-1 Inhibitor
Use Orphan drug: Treatment of cryopyrin-associated periodic syndromes (CAPS) including familial cold autoinflammatory syndrome (FCAS) and Muckle-Wells syndrome (MWS)
General Dosage Range SubQ:
  Children ≥12 years: Loading dose 4.4 mg/kg (maximum dose: 320 mg); Maintenance dose: 2.2 mg/kg once weekly (maximum dose: 160 mg)
  Adults: Loading dose: 320 mg; Maintenance dose: 160 mg once weekly
Dosage Forms
  Injection, powder for reconstitution:
    Arcalyst™: 220 mg

rilpivirine (ril pi VIR een)

Synonyms TMC278
U.S. Brand Names Edurant™
Therapeutic Category Antiretroviral Agent, Non-nucleoside Reverse Transcriptase Inhibitor (NNRTI)
Use Treatment of HIV-1 infections in combination with at least two other antiretroviral agents
General Dosage Range Oral: *Adults:* 25 mg once daily
Dosage Forms
  Tablet, oral:
    Edurant™: 25 mg

rilpivirine, emtricitabine, and tenofovir *see* emtricitabine, rilpivirine, and tenofovir *on page 326*
Rilutek® *see* riluzole *on page 781*

riluzole (RIL yoo zole)

Synonyms 2-amino-6-trifluoromethoxy-benzothiazole; RP-54274
U.S. Brand Names Rilutek®
Canadian Brand Names Rilutek®
Therapeutic Category Miscellaneous Product
Use Treatment of amyotrophic lateral sclerosis (ALS); riluzole can extend survival or time to tracheostomy
General Dosage Range Oral: *Adults:* 50 mg every 12 hours
Dosage Forms
  Tablet, oral:
    Rilutek®: 50 mg

rimabotulinumtoxinB (rime uh BOT yoo lin num TOKS in bee)

Medication Safety Issues
  Other safety concerns:
    Botulinum products are not interchangeable; potency differences may exist between the products.
Synonyms botulinum toxin type B
U.S. Brand Names Myobloc®
Therapeutic Category Neuromuscular Blocker Agent, Toxin
Use Treatment of cervical dystonia (spasmodic torticollis)
General Dosage Range I.M.: *Adults:* Initial: 2500-5000 units divided among the affected muscles
Dosage Forms
  Injection, solution [preservative free]:
    Myobloc®: 5000 units/mL (0.5 mL, 1 mL, 2 mL)

rimantadine (ri MAN ta deen)

Medication Safety Issues
Sound-alike/look-alike issues:
Rimantadine may be confused with amantadine, ranitidine, Rimactane®
Flumadine® may be confused with fludarabine, flunisolide, flutamide

Synonyms rimantadine hydrochloride

U.S. Brand Names Flumadine®

Canadian Brand Names Flumadine®

Therapeutic Category Antiviral Agent

Use Prophylaxis (adults and children >1 year of age) and treatment (adults) of influenza A viral infection (per manufacturer labeling; also refer to current ACIP guidelines for recommendations during current flu season)

Note: In certain circumstances, the ACIP recommends use of rimantadine in combination with oseltamivir for the treatment or prophylaxis of influenza A infection when resistance to oseltamivir is suspected.

General Dosage Range Dosage adjustment recommended in patients with hepatic or renal impairment
Oral:
Children 1-9 years: 5 mg/kg/day in 1-2 divided doses (maximum: 150 mg/day)
Children ≥10 years and <40 kg: 5 mg/kg/day in 2 divided doses
Children ≥10 years and Adults: 100 mg twice daily
Elderly: 100 mg daily

Dosage Forms
Tablet, oral: 100 mg
Flumadine®: 100 mg

rimantadine hydrochloride *see* rimantadine *on page 782*

rimexolone (ri MEKS oh lone)

Medication Safety Issues
Sound-alike/look-alike issues:
Vexol® may be confused with VoSol®

U.S. Brand Names Vexol®

Canadian Brand Names Vexol®

Therapeutic Category Adrenal Corticosteroid

Use Treatment of inflammation after ocular surgery and the treatment of anterior uveitis

General Dosage Range Ophthalmic: *Adults:* Instill 1-2 drops 4 times/day **or** instill 1-2 drops every 1-2 hours during waking hours

Dosage Forms
Suspension, ophthalmic:
Vexol®: 1% (5 mL, 10 mL)

Rimso-50® *see* dimethyl sulfoxide *on page 288*

Riomet® *see* metformin *on page 566*

Riopan Plus *see* magaldrate and simethicone *on page 543*

Risamine™ [OTC] *see* menthol and zinc oxide (topical) *on page 560*

RisaQuad™ [OTC] *see* Lactobacillus *on page 506*

RisaQuad®-2 [OTC] *see* Lactobacillus *on page 506*

risedronate (ris ED roe nate)

Medication Safety Issues
Sound-alike/look-alike issues:
Actonel® may be confused with Actos®
Risedronate may be confused with alendronate

Synonyms risedronate sodium

U.S. Brand Names Actonel®; Atelvia™

Canadian Brand Names Actonel®; Actonel® DR; Apo-Risedronate®; Dom-Risedronate; Novo-Risedronate; PMS-Risedronate; ratio-Risedronate; Riva-Risedronate; Sandoz-Risedronate; Teva-Risedronate

Therapeutic Category Bisphosphonate Derivative

Use
Actonel®: Treatment of Paget disease of the bone; treatment and prevention of glucocorticoid-induced osteoporosis; treatment and prevention of osteoporosis in postmenopausal women; treatment of osteoporosis in men
Atelvia™: Treatment of osteoporosis in postmenopausal women
General Dosage Range Oral: *Adults:* 5 mg or 30 mg once daily **or** 35 mg once weekly **or** 150 mg once a month
Dosage Forms
Tablet, oral:
Actonel®: 5 mg, 30 mg, 35 mg, 150 mg
Tablet, delayed release, oral:
Atelvia™: 35 mg

risedronate and calcium (ris ED roe nate & KAL see um)
Medication Safety Issues
Sound-alike/look-alike issues:
Actonel® may be confused with Actos®
Synonyms calcium and risedronate; risedronate sodium and calcium carbonate
U.S. Brand Names Actonel® and Calcium
Canadian Brand Names Actonel Plus Calcium
Therapeutic Category Bisphosphonate Derivative; Calcium Salt
Use Treatment and prevention of osteoporosis in postmenopausal women
General Dosage Range Oral: *Adults:* Calcium carbonate: 1250 mg (500 mg elemental calcium) once daily on days 2-7 of 7-day treatment cycle; Risedronate: 35 mg once weekly on day 1 of 7-day treatment cycle
Dosage Forms
Combination package [each package contains]:
Actonel® and Calcium:
Tablet (Actonel®): Risedronate 35 mg (4s)
Tablet: Calcium 1250 mg (24s)

risedronate sodium *see risedronate on page 782*
risedronate sodium and calcium carbonate *see risedronate and calcium on page 783*
RisperDAL® *see risperidone on page 783*
Risperdal® (Can) *see risperidone on page 783*
Risperdal M-Tab *see risperidone on page 783*
RisperDAL® M-Tab® *see risperidone on page 783*
Risperdal® M-Tab® (Can) *see risperidone on page 783*
RisperDAL® Consta® *see risperidone on page 783*
Risperdal® Consta® (Can) *see risperidone on page 783*

risperidone (ris PER i done)
Medication Safety Issues
Sound-alike/look-alike issues:
RisperiDONE may be confused with reserpine, rOPINIRole
RisperDAL® may be confused with lisinopril, reserpine, Restoril™
Synonyms Risperdal M-Tab
Tall-Man risperiDONE
U.S. Brand Names RisperDAL®; RisperDAL® Consta®; RisperDAL® M-Tab®
Canadian Brand Names Apo-Risperidone®; CO Risperidone; Dom-Risperidone; JAMP-Risperidone; Mint-Risperidon; Mylan-Risperidone; Novo-Risperidone; PHL-Risperidone; PMS-Risperidone; PMS-Risperidone ODT; PRO-Risperidone; RAN™-Risperidone; ratio-Risperidone; RBX-Risperidone; Risperdal®; Risperdal® Consta®; Risperdal® M-Tab®; Riva-Risperidone; Sandoz-Risperidone
Therapeutic Category Antipsychotic Agent, Benzisoxazole
Use
Oral: Treatment of schizophrenia; treatment of acute mania or mixed episodes associated with bipolar I disorder (as monotherapy in children or adults, or in combination with lithium or valproate in adults); treatment of irritability/aggression associated with autistic disorder

Injection: Treatment of schizophrenia; maintenance treatment of bipolar I disorder in adults as monotherapy or in combination with lithium or valproate

General Dosage Range Dosage adjustment recommended in patients with hepatic or renal impairment
I.M.:
Adults: 25 mg every 2 weeks (range: 12.5-50 mg every 2 weeks; maximum: 50 mg every 2 weeks)
Elderly: 12.5-25 mg every 2 weeks
Oral:
Children ≥5 years: Autism: Initial: 0.25 mg/day (<20 kg) or 0.5 mg/day (≥20 kg); Maximum dose: 1 mg/day (<20 kg) or 2.5 mg/day (≥20 kg) (3 mg/day in children >45 kg)
Children 10-17 years: Bipolar disorder: Initial: 0.5 mg once daily; Recommended target dose: 2.5 mg/day; dosing range 0.5-6 mg/day
Children: 13-17 years: Schizophrenia: Initial: 0.5 mg once daily; Recommended target dose: 3 mg/day; dosing range 1-6 mg/day
Adults: Initial: 2-3 mg/day in 1-2 divided doses; Maintenance: 1-8 mg/day in 1-2 divided doses
Elderly: Initial: 0.5 mg twice daily

Dosage Forms
Injection, microspheres for reconstitution, extended release:
RisperDAL® Consta®: 12.5 mg, 25 mg, 37.5 mg, 50 mg
Solution, oral: 1 mg/mL (30 mL)
RisperDAL®: 1 mg/mL (30 mL)
Tablet, oral: 0.25 mg, 0.5 mg, 1 mg, 2 mg, 3 mg, 4 mg
RisperDAL®: 0.25 mg, 0.5 mg, 1 mg, 2 mg, 3 mg, 4 mg
Tablet, orally disintegrating, oral: 0.25 mg, 0.5 mg, 1 mg, 2 mg, 3 mg, 4 mg
RisperDAL® M-Tab®: 0.5 mg, 1 mg, 2 mg, 3 mg, 4 mg

Ritalin® *see* methylphenidate *on page 577*
Ritalin LA® *see* methylphenidate *on page 577*
Ritalin-SR® *see* methylphenidate *on page 577*
Ritalin® SR (Can) *see* methylphenidate *on page 577*

ritonavir (ri TOE na veer)

Medication Safety Issues
Sound-alike/look-alike issues:
Ritonavir may be confused with Retrovir®
Norvir® may be confused with Norvasc®

U.S. Brand Names Norvir®

Canadian Brand Names Norvir®; Norvir® SEC

Therapeutic Category Antiviral Agent

Use Treatment of HIV infection; should always be used as part of a multidrug regimen (at least three antiretroviral agents); may be used as a pharmacokinetic "booster" for other protease inhibitors

General Dosage Range Dosage adjustment recommended in patients on concurrent therapy
Oral:
Children >1 month: Initial: 250 mg/m^2 twice daily; Maintenance: 350-400 mg/m^2 twice daily (maximum dose: 1200 mg/day)
Adults: 300-600 mg twice daily (maximum: 1200 mg/day)

Dosage Forms
Capsule, soft gelatin, oral:
Norvir®: 100 mg
Solution, oral:
Norvir®: 80 mg/mL (240 mL)
Tablet, oral:
Norvir®: 100 mg

ritonavir and lopinavir *see* lopinavir and ritonavir *on page 536*
Rituxan® *see* rituximab *on page 784*

rituximab (ri TUK si mab)

Medication Safety Issues
Sound-alike/look-alike issues:
Rituxan® may be confused with Remicade®

RiTUXimab may be confused with brentuximab, bevacizumab, inFLIXimab

High alert medication:
The medication is in a class the Institute for Safe Medication Practices (ISMP) includes among its list of drug classes which have a heightened risk of causing significant patient harm when used in error.

Administration issues:
The rituximab dose for rheumatoid arthritis is a flat dose (1000 mg) and is not based on body surface area (BSA).

Synonyms anti-CD20 monoclonal antibody; C2B8 monoclonal antibody; IDEC-C2B8

Tall-Man riTUXimab

U.S. Brand Names Rituxan®

Canadian Brand Names Rituxan®

Therapeutic Category Antineoplastic Agent

Use
Treatment of CD20-positive non-Hodgkin lymphomas (NHL):
Relapsed or refractory, low-grade or follicular B-cell NHL (as a single agent)
Follicular B-cell NHL, previously untreated (in combination with first-line chemotherapy, and as single-agent maintenance therapy if response to first-line rituximab with chemotherapy)
Nonprogressing, low-grade B-cell NHL (as a single agent after first-line CVP treatment)
Diffuse large B-cell NHL, previously untreated (in combination with CHOP chemotherapy [or other anthracycline-based regimen])
Treatment of CD20-positive chronic lymphocytic leukemia (CLL) (in combination with fludarabine and cyclophosphamide)
Treatment of moderately- to severely-active rheumatoid arthritis (in combination with methotrexate) in adult patients with inadequate response to one or more TNF antagonists
Treatment of Wegener granulomatosis (WG) (in combination with glucocorticoids)
Treatment of microscopic polyangiitis (MPA) (in combination with glucocorticoids)

General Dosage Range I.V.: *Adults:* Dosage varies greatly depending on indication

Dosage Forms
Injection, solution [preservative free]:
Rituxan®: 10 mg/mL (10 mL, 50 mL)

Riva-Alendronate (Can) *see* alendronate *on page 49*
Riva-Amiodarone (Can) *see* amiodarone *on page 67*
Riva-Amlodipine (Can) *see* amlodipine *on page 69*
Riva-Atenolol (Can) *see* atenolol *on page 101*
Riva-Azithromycin (Can) *see* azithromycin (systemic) *on page 108*
Riva-Baclofen (Can) *see* baclofen *on page 112*
Riva-Buspirone (Can) *see* buspirone *on page 151*
Riva-Ciprofloxacin (Can) *see* ciprofloxacin (systemic) *on page 210*
Riva-Citalopram (Can) *see* citalopram *on page 213*
Riva-Clarithromycin (Can) *see* clarithromycin *on page 215*
Riva-Clindamycin (Can) *see* clindamycin (systemic) *on page 217*
Riva-Cycloprine (Can) *see* cyclobenzaprine *on page 241*
Riva-Dicyclomine (Can) *see* dicyclomine *on page 280*
Riva-Enalapril (Can) *see* enalapril *on page 326*
Riva-Fenofibrate Micro (Can) *see* fenofibrate *on page 369*
Riva-Fluconazole (Can) *see* fluconazole *on page 381*
Riva-Fluoxetine (Can) *see* fluoxetine *on page 389*
Riva-Fluvox (Can) *see* fluvoxamine *on page 395*
Riva-Fosinopril (Can) *see* fosinopril *on page 401*
Riva-Gabapentin (Can) *see* gabapentin *on page 405*
Riva-Glyburide (Can) *see* glyburide *on page 420*
Riva-Hydroxyzine (Can) *see* hydroxyzine *on page 456*
Riva-Indapamide (Can) *see* indapamide *on page 470*
Riva-Lisinopril (Can) *see* lisinopril *on page 531*
Riva-Loperamide (Can) *see* loperamide *on page 535*
Riva-Lovastatin (Can) *see* lovastatin *on page 540*

Riva-Memantine (Can) *see* memantine *on page 556*
Riva-Metformin (Can) *see* metformin *on page 566*
Riva-Metoprolol (Can) *see* metoprolol *on page 581*
Riva-Minocycline (Can) *see* minocycline *on page 590*
Riva-Mirtazapine (Can) *see* mirtazapine *on page 592*
Riva-Naproxen (Can) *see* naproxen *on page 612*
Riva-Naproxen Sodium (Can) *see* naproxen *on page 612*
Riva-Naproxen Sodium DS (Can) *see* naproxen *on page 612*
Rivanase AQ (Can) *see* beclomethasone (nasal) *on page 117*
Riva-Norfloxacin (Can) *see* norfloxacin *on page 633*
Riva-Olanzapine (Can) *see* olanzapine *on page 645*
Riva-Olanzapine ODT (Can) *see* olanzapine *on page 645*
Riva-Oxazepam (Can) *see* oxazepam *on page 659*
Riva-Oxybutynin (Can) *see* oxybutynin *on page 661*
Riva-Pantoprazole (Can) *see* pantoprazole *on page 672*
Riva-paroxetine (Can) *see* paroxetine *on page 676*
Riva-Pravastatin (Can) *see* pravastatin *on page 732*
Riva-Quetiapine (Can) *see* quetiapine *on page 760*
Riva-Rabeprazole EC (Can) *see* rabeprazole *on page 763*
Riva-Ranitidine (Can) *see* ranitidine *on page 767*
Riva-Risedronate (Can) *see* risedronate *on page 782*
Riva-Risperidone (Can) *see* risperidone *on page 783*

rivaroxaban (riv a ROX a ban)

Synonyms BAY 59-7939
U.S. Brand Names Xarelto®
Canadian Brand Names Xarelto®
Therapeutic Category Factor Xa Inhibitor
Use Postoperative thromboprophylaxis in patients who have undergone hip or knee replacement surgery
General Dosage Range Oral: *Adults:* 10 mg/day
Dosage Forms
  Tablet, oral:
    Xarelto®: 10 mg

Riva-Sertraline (Can) *see* sertraline *on page 809*
Riva-Simvastatin (Can) *see* simvastatin *on page 813*
Rivasol (Can) *see* zinc sulfate *on page 931*
Rivasone (Can) *see* betamethasone *on page 129*
Riva-Sotalol (Can) *see* sotalol *on page 828*

rivastigmine (ri va STIG meen)

Synonyms ENA 713; rivastigmine tartrate; SDZ ENA 713
U.S. Brand Names Exelon®
Canadian Brand Names Exelon®; Mylan-Rivastigmine; Novo-Rivastigmine; PMS-Rivastigmine; ratio-Rivastigmine; Sandoz-Rivastigmine
Therapeutic Category Acetylcholinesterase Inhibitor; Cholinergic Agent
Use Treatment of mild-to-moderate dementia associated with Alzheimer disease or Parkinson disease
General Dosage Range
  Oral: *Adults:* Initial: 1.5 mg twice daily; Maintenance: 1.5-6 mg twice daily (maximum: 12 mg/day)
  Transdermal patch: *Adults:* Initial: 4.6 mg/24 hours; Maintenance: 9.5 mg/24 hours (maximum dose: 9.5 mg/24 hours)
Dosage Forms
  Capsule, oral: 1.5 mg, 3 mg, 4.5 mg, 6 mg
    Exelon®: 1.5 mg, 3 mg, 4.5 mg, 6 mg
  Patch, transdermal:
    Exelon®: 4.6 mg/24 hours (30s); 9.5 mg/24 hours (30s)

Solution, oral:
  Exelon®: 2 mg/mL (120 mL)

rivastigmine tartrate *see* rivastigmine *on page 786*
Riva-Sumatriptan (Can) *see* sumatriptan *on page 839*
Riva-Terbinafine (Can) *see* terbinafine (systemic) *on page 851*
Riva-Valacyclovir (Can) *see* valacyclovir *on page 903*
Riva-Venlafaxine XR (Can) *see* venlafaxine *on page 911*
Riva-Verapamil SR (Can) *see* verapamil *on page 912*
Riva-Zide (Can) *see* hydrochlorothiazide and triamterene *on page 446*
Riva-Zopiclone (Can) *see* zopiclone *(Canada only) on page 934*
Rivotril® (Can) *see* clonazepam *on page 222*

rizatriptan (rye za TRIP tan)
  Synonyms MK462
  U.S. Brand Names Maxalt-MLT®; Maxalt®
  Canadian Brand Names Maxalt RPD™; Maxalt™
  Therapeutic Category Antimigraine Agent; Serotonin Agonist
  Use Acute treatment of migraine with or without aura
  General Dosage Range Oral: *Adults:* 5-10 mg once, repeat if needed (maximum: 30 mg/day)
  Dosage Forms
  Tablet, oral:
    Maxalt®: 5 mg, 10 mg
  Tablet, orally disintegrating, oral:
    Maxalt-MLT®: 5 mg, 10 mg

rLFN-α2 *see* interferon alfa-2b *on page 481*
R-modafinil *see* armodafinil *on page 94*
Ro 5488 *see* tretinoin (systemic) *on page 885*
RO5185426 *see* vemurafenib *on page 911*
RoActemra® *see* tocilizumab *on page 874*
Robafen [OTC] *see* guaifenesin *on page 425*
Robafen AC *see* guaifenesin and codeine *on page 426*
Robafen CF Cough & Cold [OTC] *see* guaifenesin, dextromethorphan, and phenylephrine
  on page 429
Robafen Cough [OTC] *see* dextromethorphan *on page 270*
Robafen DM [OTC] *see* guaifenesin and dextromethorphan *on page 427*
Robafen DM Clear [OTC] *see* guaifenesin and dextromethorphan *on page 427*
Robaxin® *see* methocarbamol *on page 570*
Robaxin®-750 *see* methocarbamol *on page 570*
Robidrine® (Can) *see* pseudoephedrine *on page 751*
Robinul® *see* glycopyrrolate *on page 422*
Robinul® Forte *see* glycopyrrolate *on page 422*
Robitussin® (Can) *see* guaifenesin *on page 425*
Robitussin AC *see* guaifenesin and codeine *on page 426*
Robitussin® Childrens Cough & Cold (Can) *see* pseudoephedrine and dextromethorphan
  on page 752
Robitussin® Children's Cough & Cold CF [OTC] *see* guaifenesin, dextromethorphan, and
  phenylephrine *on page 429*
Robitussin® Children's Cough Long-Acting [OTC] *see* dextromethorphan *on page 270*
Robitussin® Children's Cough & Cold Long-Acting [OTC] *see* dextromethorphan and
  chlorpheniramine *on page 271*
Robitussin® Cough & Chest Congestion DM [OTC] *see* guaifenesin and dextromethorphan
  on page 427
Robitussin® Cough & Chest Congestion DM Max [OTC] *see* guaifenesin and dextromethorphan
  on page 427

Robitussin® Cough & Chest Congestion Sugar-Free DM [OTC] *see* guaifenesin and dextromethorphan *on page 427*

Robitussin® Cough & Cold CF [OTC] *see* guaifenesin, dextromethorphan, and phenylephrine *on page 429*

Robitussin® Cough & Cold CF Max [OTC] *see* guaifenesin, dextromethorphan, and phenylephrine *on page 429*

Robitussin® Cough & Cold Long-Acting [OTC] *see* dextromethorphan and chlorpheniramine *on page 271*

Robitussin® CoughGels™ Long-Acting [OTC] *see* dextromethorphan *on page 270*

Robitussin® Cough Long Acting [OTC] *see* dextromethorphan *on page 270*

Robitussin® DM (Can) *see* guaifenesin and dextromethorphan *on page 427*

Robitussin® Night Time Cough & Cold [OTC] *see* diphenhydramine and phenylephrine *on page 292*

Rocaltrol® *see* calcitriol *on page 159*

Rocephin® *see* ceftriaxone *on page 185*

rocuronium (roe kyoor OH nee um)

Medication Safety Issues

Sound-alike/look-alike issues:

Zemuron® may be confused with Remeron®

High alert medication:

The Institute for Safe Medication Practices (ISMP) includes this medication among its list of drugs which have a heightened risk of causing significant patient harm when used in error.

Other safety concerns:

United States Pharmacopeia (USP) 2006: The Interdisciplinary Safe Medication Use Expert Committee of the USP has recommended the following:

- Hospitals, clinics, and other practice sites should institute special safeguards in the storage, labeling, and use of these agents and should include these safeguards in staff orientation and competency training.
- Healthcare professionals should be on high alert (especially vigilant) whenever a neuromuscular-blocking agent (NMBA) is stocked, ordered, prepared, or administered.

Synonyms ORG 946; rocuronium bromide

U.S. Brand Names Zemuron®

Canadian Brand Names Rocuronium Bromide Injection; Zemuron®

Therapeutic Category Skeletal Muscle Relaxant

Use Facilitate both rapid sequence and routine endotracheal intubation and to relax skeletal muscles during surgery; to facilitate mechanical ventilation in ICU patients

General Dosage Range I.V.:

Infants ≥28 days and Children: Initial: 0.45-0.6 mg/kg; Maintenance: 0.075-0.15 mg/kg **or** 7-10 **mcg**/kg/minute

Adults: 0.03-1.2 mg/kg; Infusion: 8-12 **mcg**/kg/minute

Dosage Forms

Injection, solution: 10 mg/mL (5 mL, 10 mL)

Zemuron®: 10 mg/mL (5 mL, 10 mL)

Injection, solution [preservative free]: 10 mg/mL (5 mL, 10 mL)

rocuronium bromide *see* rocuronium *on page 788*

Rocuronium Bromide Injection (Can) *see* rocuronium *on page 788*

Rofact™ (Can) *see* rifampin *on page 779*

roflumilast (roe FLUE mi last)

U.S. Brand Names Daliresp™

Canadian Brand Names Daxas™

Therapeutic Category Phosphodiesterase-4 Enzyme Inhibitor

Use Adjunct to bronchodilator therapy in the maintenance treatment of severe chronic obstructive pulmonary disease (COPD) associated with chronic bronchitis

General Dosage Range Oral: *Adults:* 500 mcg once daily

Dosage Forms
Tablet, oral:
Daliresp™: 500 mcg
Dosage Forms - Canada
Tablet, oral:
Daxas™: 500 mcg

Rogaine® (Can) *see* minoxidil (topical) *on page 591*
Rogaine® Extra Strength for Men [OTC] *see* minoxidil (topical) *on page 591*
Rogaine® for Men [OTC] *see* minoxidil (topical) *on page 591*
Rogaine® for Women [OTC] *see* minoxidil (topical) *on page 591*
Rogitine® (Can) *see* phentolamine *on page 696*
Rolaids® [OTC] *see* calcium carbonate and magnesium hydroxide *on page 162*
Rolaids® Extra Strength [OTC] *see* calcium carbonate *on page 161*
Rolaids® Extra Strength [OTC] *see* calcium carbonate and magnesium hydroxide *on page 162*
Rolene (Can) *see* betamethasone *on page 129*
Romazicon® *see* flumazenil *on page 383*

romidepsin (roe mi DEP sin)

Medication Safety Issues
Sound-alike/look-alike issues:
RomiDEPsin may be confused with romiPLOStim
High alert medication:
This medication is in a class the Institute for Safe Medication Practices (ISMP) includes among its list of drug classes which have a heightened risk of causing significant patient harm when used in error.
Synonyms depsipeptide; FK228; FR901228
Tall-Man romiDEPsin
U.S. Brand Names Istodax®
Therapeutic Category Antineoplastic Agent, Histone Deacetylase Inhibitor
Use Treatment of refractory cutaneous T-cell lymphoma (CTCL) and refractory peripheral T-cell lymphoma (PTCL)
General Dosage Range Dosage adjustment recommended in patients who develop toxicities
I.V.: *Adults:* 14 mg/m^2 days 1, 8, and 15 of a 28-day treatment cycle
Dosage Forms
Injection, powder for reconstitution:
Istodax®: 10 mg

romiplostim (roe mi PLOE stim)

Medication Safety Issues
Sound-alike/look-alike issues:
RomiPLOStim may be confused with romiDEPsin
Synonyms AMG 531
Tall-Man romiPLOStim
U.S. Brand Names Nplate™
Canadian Brand Names Nplate™
Therapeutic Category Colony-Stimulating Factor; Thrombopoietic Agent
Use Treatment of thrombocytopenia in patients with chronic immune (idiopathic) thrombocytopenia purpura (ITP) who have had insufficient response to corticosteroids, immune globulin, or splenectomy
General Dosage Range
SubQ:
Children: Dosage not established
Adults: Initial: 1 mcg/kg once weekly; adjust dose by 1 mcg/kg/week to achieve platelet count ≥50,000/mm^3 and reduce the risk of bleeding; Maximum: 10 mcg/kg
Dosage Forms
Injection, powder for reconstitution:
Nplate™: 250 mcg, 500 mcg

ropinirole (roe PIN i role)

Medication Safety Issues
Sound-alike/look-alike issues:
Requip® may be confused with Reglan®
ROPINIRole may be confused with RisperDAL®, risperiDONE, ropivacaine

Synonyms ropinirole hydrochloride

Tall-Man rOPINIRole

U.S. Brand Names Requip®; Requip® XL™

Canadian Brand Names CO Ropinirole; JAMP-Ropinirole; PMS-Ropinirole; RAN™-Ropinirole; Requip®

Therapeutic Category Anti-Parkinson Agent (Dopamine Agonist)

Use Treatment of idiopathic Parkinson disease; in patients with early Parkinson disease who were not receiving concomitant levodopa therapy as well as in patients with advanced disease on concomitant levodopa; treatment of moderate-to-severe primary restless legs syndrome (RLS)

General Dosage Range Oral: *Adults:*
Parkinson:
Immediate release: Initial: 0.25 mg 3 times/day; Maintenance: 0.75-24 mg/day in 3 divided doses
Extended release: Initial: 2 mg once daily; Maintenance: 2-24 mg once daily (maximum: 24 mg/day)
Restless legs: Immediate release: Initial: 0.25 mg prior to bedtime; Maintenance: 0.25-4 mg prior to bedtime

Dosage Forms
Tablet, oral: 0.25 mg, 0.5 mg, 1 mg, 2 mg, 3 mg, 4 mg, 5 mg
Requip®: 0.25 mg, 0.5 mg, 1 mg, 2 mg, 3 mg, 4 mg, 5 mg
Tablet, extended release, oral:
Requip® XL™: 2 mg, 4 mg, 6 mg, 8 mg, 12 mg

ropinirole hydrochloride *see* ropinirole *on page 790*

ropivacaine (roe PIV a kane)

Medication Safety Issues
Sound-alike/look-alike issues:
Ropivacaine may be confused with bupivacaine, rOPINIRole
High alert medication:
The Institute for Safe Medication Practices (ISMP) includes this medication (epidural administration) among its list of drug classes which have a heightened risk of causing significant patient harm when used in error.

Synonyms ropivacaine hydrochloride

U.S. Brand Names Naropin®

Canadian Brand Names Naropin®

Therapeutic Category Local Anesthetic

Use Local anesthetic for use in surgery, postoperative pain management, and obstetrical procedures when local or regional anesthesia is needed

General Dosage Range
Epidural:
Lumbar: *Adults:* 10-30 mL of 0.2% to 1% solution **or** 15-20 mL of 0.75% solution; Infusion: 6-14 mL/hour of 0.2% solution, with incremental injections of 10-15 mL/hour of 0.2% solution
Thoracic: *Adults:* 5-15 mL of 0.5% or 0.75% solution; Infusion: 6-14 mL/hour of 0.2% solution
Field Block: *Adults:* 1-40 mL (5-200 mg) of 0.5% solution
Infiltration: *Adults:* 1-100 mL of 0.2% solution **or** 1-40 mL of 0.5% solution
Nerve Block: *Adults:* Major: 35-50 mL (175-250 mg) of 0.5 % solution **or** 10-40 mL (75-300 mg) of 0.75% solution; Minor: 1-100 mL of 0.2% solution **or** 1-40 mL of 0.5% solution

Dosage Forms
Injection, solution [preservative free]:
Naropin®: 2 mg/mL (10 mL, 20 mL, 100 mL, 200 mL); 5 mg/mL (20 mL, 30 mL); 7.5 mg/mL (20 mL); 10 mg/mL (10 mL, 20 mL)

ropivacaine hydrochloride *see* ropivacaine *on page 790*
Rosanil® *see* sulfur and sulfacetamide *on page 838*
Rosasol® (Can) *see* metronidazole (topical) *on page 583*

rosiglitazone (roh si GLI ta zone)

Medication Safety Issues

Sound-alike/look-alike issues:

Avandia® may be confused with Avalide®, Coumadin®, Prandin®

International issues:

Avandia [U.S., Canada, and multiple international markets] may be confused with Avanza brand name for mirtazapine [Australia]

U.S. Brand Names Avandia®

Canadian Brand Names Avandia®

Therapeutic Category Hypoglycemic Agent, Oral; Thiazolidinedione Derivative

Use Type 2 diabetes mellitus (noninsulin-dependent, NIDDM):

Monotherapy: Improve glycemic control as an adjunct to diet and exercise

Note: Canadian labeling approves use as monotherapy only when metformin is contraindicated or not tolerated.

Combination therapy: **Note:** Use when diet, exercise, and a single agent do not result in adequate glycemic control.

U.S. labeling: In combination with a sulfonylurea, metformin, or sulfonylurea plus metformin

Canadian labeling: In combination with metformin; in combination with a sulfonylurea only when metformin use is contraindicated or not tolerated

General Dosage Range Oral: *Adults:* Initial: 4 mg/day in 1-2 divided doses; Maintenance: 4-8 mg/day in 1-2 divided doses

Dosage Forms

Tablet, oral:

Avandia®: 2 mg, 4 mg, 8 mg

rosiglitazone and glimepiride (roh si GLI ta zone & GLYE me pye ride)

Medication Safety Issues

High alert medication:

The Institute for Safe Medication Practices (ISMP) includes this medication among its list of drugs which have a heightened risk of causing significant patient harm when used in error.

Synonyms glimepiride and rosiglitazone maleate

U.S. Brand Names Avandaryl®

Canadian Brand Names Avandaryl®

Therapeutic Category Antidiabetic Agent, Sulfonylurea; Antidiabetic Agent, Thiazolidinedione

Use Management of type 2 diabetes mellitus (noninsulin-dependent, NIDDM) as an adjunct to diet and exercise

General Dosage Range Dosage adjustment recommended in patients with hepatic or renal impairment

Oral:

Adults: Initial: Rosiglitazone 4 mg and glimepiride 1-2 mg once daily; Maintenance: Rosiglitazone 4-8 mg and glimepiride 1-4 mg once daily

Elderly: Initial: Rosiglitazone 4 mg and glimepiride 1 mg once daily

Dosage Forms

Tablet:

Avandaryl®: 4 mg/1 mg: Rosiglitazone 4 mg and glimepiride 1 mg; 4 mg/2 mg: Rosiglitazone 4 mg and glimepiride 2 mg; 4 mg/4 mg: Rosiglitazone 4 mg and glimepiride 4 mg; 8 mg/2 mg: Rosiglitazone 8 mg and glimepiride 2 mg; 8 mg/4 mg: Rosiglitazone 8 mg and glimepiride 4 mg

rosiglitazone and metformin (roh si GLI ta zone & met FOR min)

Medication Safety Issues

Sound-alike/look-alike issues:

Avandamet® may be confused with Anzemet®

Synonyms metformin and rosiglitazone; metformin hydrochloride and rosiglitazone maleate; rosiglitazone maleate and metformin hydrochloride

U.S. Brand Names Avandamet®

Canadian Brand Names Avandamet®

Therapeutic Category Antidiabetic Agent (Biguanide); Antidiabetic Agent (Thiazolidinedione)

Use Management of type 2 diabetes mellitus (noninsulin-dependent, NIDDM) as an adjunct to diet and exercise in patients where dual rosiglitazone and metformin therapy is appropriate

◄ **General Dosage Range Oral:** *Adults:* Initial: Rosiglitazone 2 mg and metformin 500 mg once or twice daily; may increase by 2 mg/500 mg per day after 4 weeks (maximum: rosiglitazone 8 mg/day; metformin 2000 mg/day)

Dosage Forms
Tablet:
Avandamet®: 2/500: Rosiglitazone 2 mg and metformin 500 mg; 4/500: Rosiglitazone 4 mg and metformin 500 mg; 2/1000: Rosiglitazone 2 mg and metformin 1000 mg; 4/1000: Rosiglitazone 4 mg and metformin 1000 mg

rosiglitazone maleate and metformin hydrochloride *see rosiglitazone and metformin on page 791*

Rosone (Can) *see betamethasone on page 129*

Rosula® *see sulfur and sulfacetamide on page 838*

Rosula® Clarifying *see sulfur and sulfacetamide on page 838*

Rosula® NS *see sulfacetamide (topical) on page 835*

rosuvastatin (roe soo va STAT in)

Medication Safety Issues
Sound-alike/look-alike issues:
Rosuvastatin may be confused with atorvastatin, nystatin, pitavastatin

Synonyms rosuvastatin calcium

U.S. Brand Names Crestor®

Canadian Brand Names Crestor®

Therapeutic Category Antilipemic Agent, HMG-CoA Reductase Inhibitor

Use
Treatment of dyslipidemias:
Used with dietary therapy for hyperlipidemias to reduce elevations in total cholesterol (TC), LDL-C, apolipoprotein B, nonHDL-C, and triglycerides (TG) in patients with primary hypercholesterolemia (elevations of 1 or more components are present in Fredrickson type IIa, IIb, and IV hyperlipidemias); increase HDL-C; treatment of primary dysbetalipoproteinemia (Fredrickson type III hyperlipidemia); treatment of homozygous familial hypercholesterolemia (FH); to slow progression of atherosclerosis as an adjunct to diet to lower TC and LDL-C

Heterozygous familial hypercholesterolemia (HeFH): In adolescent patients (10-17 years of age, females >1 year postmenarche) with HeFH having LDL-C >190 mg/dL or LDL >160 mg/dL with positive family history of premature cardiovascular disease (CVD), or ≥2 other CVD risk factors.

Primary prevention of cardiovascular disease: To reduce the risk of stroke, myocardial infarction, or arterial revascularization procedures in patients without clinically evident coronary heart disease or lipid abnormalities but with all of the following: 1) an increased risk of cardiovascular disease based on age ≥50 years old in men and ≥60 years old in women, 2) hsCRP ≥2 mg/L, and 3) the presence of at least one additional cardiovascular disease risk factor such as hypertension, low HDL-C, smoking, or a family history of premature coronary heart disease.

Secondary prevention of cardiovascular disease: To slow progression of atherosclerosis

General Dosage Range Dosage adjustment recommended in patients with renal impairment, on concomitant therapy, or who develop toxicities

Oral:
Children 10-17 years (females >1 year postmenarche): Initial: 5-20 mg once daily (maximum: 20 mg/day)
Adults: Initial: 5-20 mg once daily; Maintenance: 5-40 mg once daily (maximum: 40 mg/day)

Dosage Forms
Tablet, oral:
Crestor®: 5 mg, 10 mg, 20 mg, 40 mg

rosuvastatin calcium *see rosuvastatin on page 792*

Rotarix® *see rotavirus vaccine on page 792*

RotaTeq® *see rotavirus vaccine on page 792*

rotavirus vaccine (ROE ta vye rus vak SEEN)

Synonyms human rotavirus vaccine, attenuated (HRV); pentavalent human-bovine reassortant rotavirus vaccine (PRV); rotavirus vaccine, pentavalent; RV1 (RotaTeq®); RV5 (Rotarix®)

U.S. Brand Names Rotarix®; RotaTeq®

Canadian Brand Names Rotarix®; RotaTeq®

Therapeutic Category Vaccine

Use Prevention of rotavirus gastroenteritis in infants and children

The Advisory Committee on Immunization Practices (ACIP) recommends routine vaccination of all infants.

General Dosage Range Oral:

Infants 6-24 weeks: Rotarix®: A total of two 1 mL doses administered at 2 and 4 months of age

Infants 6-32 weeks: RotaTeq®: A total of three 2 mL doses given at 2, 4, and 6 months of age

Dosage Forms

Powder, for suspension, oral [preservative free; human derived]:

Rotarix®: G1P[8] ≥10^6 CCID$_{50}$ per 1 mL

Suspension, oral [preservative free]:

RotaTeq®: G1 ≥2.2 x 10^6 infectious units, G2 ≥2.8 x 10^6 infectious units, G3 ≥2.2 x 10^6 infectious units, G4 ≥2 x 10^6 infectious units, and P1A [8] ≥2.3 x 10^6 infectious units per 2 mL (2 mL)

rotavirus vaccine, pentavalent *see rotavirus vaccine on page 792*

Rowasa® *see mesalamine on page 564*

Roxanol *see morphine (systemic) on page 598*

Roxicet™ *see oxycodone and acetaminophen on page 662*

Roxicet™ 5/500 *see oxycodone and acetaminophen on page 662*

Roxicodone® *see oxycodone on page 662*

Roychlor® (Can) *see potassium chloride on page 724*

Rozerem™ *see ramelteon on page 765*

RP-6976 *see docetaxel on page 301*

RP-54274 *see riluzole on page 781*

RP-59500 *see quinupristin and dalfopristin on page 763*

r-PA *see reteplase on page 775*

rPDGF-BB *see becaplermin on page 116*

RPR-116258A *see cabazitaxel on page 156*

(R,R)-formoterol L-tartrate *see arformoterol on page 92*

RS-25259 *see palonosetron on page 669*

RS-25259-197 *see palonosetron on page 669*

R-Tanna *see chlorpheniramine and phenylephrine on page 198*

R-Tanna Pediatric *see chlorpheniramine and phenylephrine on page 198*

RTCA *see ribavirin on page 777*

RU 0211 *see lubiprostone on page 541*

RU-486 *see mifepristone on page 588*

RU-23908 *see nilutamide on page 627*

RU-38486 *see mifepristone on page 588*

rubella, measles and mumps vaccines *see measles, mumps, and rubella virus vaccine on page 551*

rubella, varicella, measles, and mumps vaccine *see measles, mumps, rubella, and varicella virus vaccine on page 551*

rubidomycin hydrochloride *see daunorubicin hydrochloride on page 255*

RUF 331 *see rufinamide on page 793*

rufinamide (roo FIN a mide)

Synonyms CGP 33101; E 2080; RUF 331; xilep

U.S. Brand Names Banzel®

Canadian Brand Names Banzel™

Therapeutic Category Anticonvulsant, Triazole Derivative

Use Adjunctive therapy in the treatment of generalized seizures of Lennox-Gastaut syndrome

General Dosage Range Oral:

Children ≥4 years: Initial: 10 mg/kg/day in 2 equally divided doses (maximum: 45 mg/kg/day or 3200 mg/day)

Adults: Initial: 400-800 mg/day in 2 equally divided doses (maximum: 3200 mg/day)

◄ **Dosage Forms**
  Suspension, oral:
    Banzel®: 40 mg/mL (460 mL)
  Tablet, oral:
    Banzel®: 200 mg, 400 mg
Dosage Forms - Canada
  Tablet, oral:
    Banzel™: 100 mg

Ru-Hist Forte *see* chlorpheniramine, pyrilamine, and phenylephrine *on page 202*

Rulox [OTC] *see* aluminum hydroxide, magnesium hydroxide, and simethicone *on page 60*

RV1 (RotaTeq®) *see* rotavirus vaccine *on page 792*

RV5 (Rotarix®) *see* rotavirus vaccine *on page 792*

Rybix™ ODT *see* tramadol *on page 880*

Rylosol (Can) *see* sotalol *on page 828*

Ryna®-12 [DSC] *see* phenylephrine and pyrilamine *on page 698*

Ryna-12 S® [DSC] *see* phenylephrine and pyrilamine *on page 698*

Ryna-12X® [DSC] *see* phenylephrine, pyrilamine, and guaifenesin *on page 700*

Rynatan® *see* chlorpheniramine and phenylephrine *on page 198*

Rynatan® Pediatric *see* chlorpheniramine and phenylephrine *on page 198*

Rynatuss® *see* chlorpheniramine, ephedrine, phenylephrine, and carbetapentane *on page 199*

Rythmodan® (Can) *see* disopyramide *on page 299*

Rythmodan®-LA (Can) *see* disopyramide *on page 299*

Rythmol® *see* propafenone *on page 744*

Rythmol® Gen-Propafenone (Can) *see* propafenone *on page 744*

Rythmol® SR *see* propafenone *on page 744*

Ryzolt™ *see* tramadol *on page 880*

S2® [OTC] *see* epinephrine (systemic, oral inhalation) *on page 331*

S-(+)-3-isobutylgaba *see* pregabalin *on page 735*

6(S)-5-methyltetrahydrofolate *see* methylfolate *on page 576*

6(S)-5-MTHF *see* methylfolate *on page 576*

S-4661 *see* doripenem *on page 307*

Sabril® *see* vigabatrin *on page 914*

Saccharomyces boulardii (sak roe MYE sees boo LAR dee)

Medication Safety Issues
  International issues:
    Codex: Brand name for *saccharomyces boulardii* [Italy], but also the brand name for acetaminophen/codeine [Brazil]
    Codex [Italy] may be confused with Cedax brand name for ceftibuten [U.S. and multiple international markets]; Clobex® brand name for clobetasol [U.S., Canada, and multiple international markets]
    Precosa [Finland, Sweden] may be confused with Precose brand name for acarbose [U.S., Malaysia]

Synonyms *S. boulardii*; *Saccharomyces boulardii lyo*

U.S. Brand Names Florastor® Kids [OTC]; Florastor® [OTC]

Therapeutic Category Dietary Supplement; Probiotic

Use Promote maintenance of normal microflora in the gastrointestinal tract; used in management of bloating, gas, and diarrhea, particularly to decrease the incidence of diarrhea associated with antibiotic use

General Dosage Range Oral: *Children and Adults:* 250 mg twice daily

Dosage Forms
  Capsule, oral:
    Florastor® [OTC]: S. boulardii lyo 250 mg
  Powder, oral:
    Florastor® Kids [OTC]: S. boulardii lyo 250 mg/packet (10s)

Saccharomyces boulardii lyo see Saccharomyces boulardii on page 794

sacrosidase (sak ROE si dase)

U.S. Brand Names Sucraid®
Canadian Brand Names Sucraid®
Therapeutic Category Enzyme
Use Orphan drug: Oral replacement therapy in sucrase deficiency, as seen in congenital sucrase-isomaltase deficiency (CSID)
General Dosage Range Oral:
Infants and Children ≥5 and <15 kg: 8500 int. units (1 mL) per meal or snack
Children >15 kg and Adults: 17,000 int. units (2 mL) per meal or snack
Dosage Forms
Solution, oral:
Sucraid®: 8500 int. units/mL (118 mL)

Safetussin® CD [OTC] *see* dextromethorphan and phenylephrine *on page 271*
Safe Tussin® DM [OTC] *see* guaifenesin and dextromethorphan *on page 427*
Safyral™ *see* ethinyl estradiol, drospirenone, and levomefolate *on page 358*
SAHA *see* vorinostat *on page 921*
Saizen® *see* somatropin *on page 826*
Salactic® [OTC] *see* salicylic acid *on page 795*
Salagen® *see* pilocarpine (systemic) *on page 704*
Salazopyrin® (Can) *see* sulfasalazine *on page 837*
Salazopyrin En-Tabs® (Can) *see* sulfasalazine *on page 837*
salbutamol *see* albuterol *on page 45*
salbutamol and ipratropium *see* ipratropium and albuterol *on page 489*
salbutamol sulphate *see* albuterol *on page 45*
Salex® *see* salicylic acid *on page 795*
Salflex® (Can) *see* salsalate *on page 799*
salicylazosulfapyridine *see* sulfasalazine *on page 837*

salicylic acid (sal i SIL ik AS id)

Medication Safety Issues
Sound-alike/look-alike issues:
Occlusal®-HP may be confused with Ocuflox®
Other safety concerns:
Transdermal patch may contain conducting metal (eg, aluminum); remove patch prior to MRI.
U.S. Brand Names Aliclen™; Beta Sal® [OTC]; Clean & Clear® Advantage® Acne Cleanser [OTC]; Clean & Clear® Advantage® Acne Spot Treatment [OTC]; Clean & Clear® Advantage® Invisible Acne Patch [OTC]; Clean & Clear® Advantage® Oil-Free Acne [OTC]; Clean & Clear® Blackhead Clearing Daily Cleansing [OTC]; Clean & Clear® Blackhead Clearing Scrub [OTC]; Clean & Clear® Continuous Control® Acne Wash [OTC]; Clean & Clear® Deep Cleaning [OTC]; Clean & Clear® Dual Action Moisturizer [OTC]; Clean & Clear® Invisible Blemish Treatment [OTC]; Compound W® One Step Invisible Strip [OTC]; Compound W® One Step Wart Remover for Feet [OTC]; Compound W® One-Step Wart Remover for Kids [OTC]; Compound W® One-Step Wart Remover [OTC]; Compound W® [OTC]; Curad® Mediplast® [OTC]; Denorex® Extra Strength Protection 2-in-1 [OTC]; Denorex® Extra Strength Protection [OTC]; Dermarest® Psoriasis Medicated Moisturizer [OTC]; Dermarest® Psoriasis Medicated Scalp Treatment [OTC]; Dermarest® Psoriasis Medicated Shampoo/Conditioner [OTC]; Dermarest® Psoriasis Medicated Skin Treatment [OTC]; Dermarest® Psoriasis Overnight Treatment [OTC]; DHS™ Sal [OTC]; Dr. Scholl's® Callus Removers [OTC]; Dr. Scholl's® Clear Away® One Step Wart Remover [OTC]; Dr. Scholl's® Clear Away® Plantar Wart Remover For Feet [OTC]; Dr. Scholl's® Clear Away® Wart Remover Fast-Acting [OTC]; Dr. Scholl's® Clear Away® Wart Remover Invisible Strips [OTC]; Dr. Scholl's® Clear Away® Wart Remover [OTC]; Dr. Scholl's® Corn Removers [OTC]; Dr. Scholl's® Corn/Callus Remover [OTC]; Dr. Scholl's® Extra Thick Corn Removers [OTC]; Dr. Scholl's® Extra-Thick Callus Removers [OTC]; Dr. Scholl's® For Her Corn Removers [OTC]; Dr. Scholl's® OneStep Callus Removers [OTC]; Dr. Scholl's® OneStep Corn Removers [OTC]; Dr. Scholl's® Small Corn Removers [OTC]; Dr. Scholl's® Ultra-Thin Corn Removers [OTC]; DuoFilm® [OTC]; Durasal™; Freezone® [OTC]; Fung-O® [OTC]; Gets-It® [OTC]; Gordofilm [OTC]; Hydrisalic® [OTC]; Ionil Plus® [OTC]; Ionil® [OTC]; Keralyt®; Keralyt® [OTC]; LupiCare® Dandruff [OTC]; LupiCare® Psoriasis [OTC]; MG217® Sal-Acid [OTC]; Mosco® Callus & Corn Remover [OTC]; Mosco® One Step Corn Remover [OTC]; Neutrogena® Acne Stress Control [OTC]; Neutrogena® Advanced Solutions™ [OTC]; Neutrogena® Blackhead

Eliminating™ 2-in-1 Foaming Pads [OTC]; Neutrogena® Blackhead Eliminating™ Daily Scrub [OTC]; Neutrogena® Blackhead Elinimating™ [OTC]; Neutrogena® Body Clear® [OTC]; Neutrogena® Clear Pore™ Oil-Controlling Astringent [OTC]; Neutrogena® Maximum Strength T/Sal® [OTC]; Neutrogena® Oil-Free Acne Stress Control [OTC]; Neutrogena® Oil-Free Acne Wash 60 Second Mask Scrub [OTC]; Neutrogena® Oil-Free Acne Wash Cream Cleanser [OTC]; Neutrogena® Oil-Free Acne Wash Foam Cleanser [OTC]; Neutrogena® Oil-Free Acne Wash [OTC]; Neutrogena® Oil-Free Acne [OTC]; Neutrogena® Oil-Free Anti-Acne [OTC]; Neutrogena® Rapid Clear® Acne Defense [OTC]; Neutrogena® Rapid Clear® Acne Eliminating [OTC]; Neutrogena® Rapid Clear® [OTC]; OXY® Body Wash [OTC]; OXY® Chill Factor® [OTC]; OXY® Daily Cleansing [OTC]; OXY® Daily [OTC]; OXY® Face Wash [OTC]; OXY® Maximum Daily Cleansing [OTC]; OXY® Maximum [OTC]; OXY® Post-Shave [OTC]; OXY® Spot Treatment [OTC]; OXY® [OTC]; P&S® [OTC]; Palmer's® Skin Success Acne Cleanser [OTC]; Sal-Plant® [OTC]; Salactic® [OTC]; Salex®; Salitop™; Salvax; Scalpicin® Anti-Itch [OTC]; Stridex® Essential Care® [OTC]; Stridex® Facewipes To Go® [OTC]; Stridex® Maximum Strength [OTC]; Stridex® Sensitive Skin [OTC]; Thera-Sal [OTC]; Tinamed® Corn and Callus Remover [OTC]; Tinamed® Wart Remover [OTC]; Trans-Ver-Sal® [OTC]; Wart-Off® Maximum Strength [OTC]; Zapzyt® Acne Wash [OTC]; Zapzyt® Pore Treatment [OTC]

Canadian Brand Names Duofilm®; Duoforte® 27; Occlusal™-HP; Sebcur®; Soluver®; Soluver® Plus; Trans-Plantar®; Trans-Ver-Sal®

Therapeutic Category Keratolytic Agent

Use Topically for its keratolytic effect in controlling seborrheic dermatitis or psoriasis of body and scalp, dandruff, and other scaling dermatoses; also used to remove warts, corns, and calluses; acne

General Dosage Range Topical: *Children and Adults:* Dosage varies greatly depending on product

Dosage Forms

Aerosol, topical: 6% (70 g)
  Salvax: 6% (70 g, 200 g)
Bar, topical: 2% (113 g)
  OXY® [OTC]: 0.5% (119 g)
Cloth, topical:
  Neutrogena® Oil-Free Acne Wash [OTC]: 2% (30s)
Cream, topical: 6% (400 g)
  Clean & Clear® Advantage® Acne Cleanser [OTC]: 2% (148 mL)
  Clean & Clear® Advantage® Acne Spot Treatment [OTC]: 2% (22 g)
  Clean & Clear® Blackhead Clearing Scrub [OTC]: 2% (141 g, 226 g)
  Clean & Clear® Dual Action Moisturizer [OTC]: 0.5% (120 mL)
  LupiCare® Psoriasis [OTC]: 2% (227 g)
  Neutrogena® Acne Stress Control [OTC]: 2% (125 g)
  Neutrogena® Oil-Free Acne [OTC]: 2% (125 mL)
  Neutrogena® Oil-Free Acne Stress Control [OTC]: 2% (172 g)
  Neutrogena® Oil-Free Acne Wash Cream Cleanser [OTC]: 2% (200 mL)
  Neutrogena® Oil-Free Anti-Acne [OTC]: 0.5% (50 g)
  Salex®: 6% (454 g)
  Salitop™: 6% (400 g)
Gel, topical:
  Clean & Clear® Advantage® Invisible Acne Patch [OTC]: 2% (1.9 mL)
  Clean & Clear® Invisible Blemish Treatment [OTC]: 2% (22 mL)
  Compound W® [OTC]: 17.6% (7 g)
  Dermarest® Psoriasis Medicated Scalp Treatment [OTC]: 3% (118 mL)
  Dermarest® Psoriasis Medicated Skin Treatment [OTC]: 3% (118 mL)
  Dermarest® Psoriasis Overnight Treatment [OTC]: 3% (56.7 g)
  Hydrisalic® [OTC]: 6% (28 g)
  Keralyt® [OTC]: 3% (30 g); 6% (40 g, 100 g)
  Neutrogena® Advanced Solutions™ [OTC]: 2% (40 g)
  Neutrogena® Oil-Free Acne Wash [OTC]: 2% (177 mL, 296 mL)
  Neutrogena® Rapid Clear® Acne Eliminating [OTC]: 2% (15 mL)
  OXY® [OTC]: 2% (355 mL)
  OXY® Body Wash [OTC]: 2% (355 mL)
  OXY® Chill Factor® [OTC]: 2% (142 g)
  OXY® Face Wash [OTC]: 2% (177 mL)
  OXY® Maximum [OTC]: 2% (142 g)
  OXY® Spot Treatment [OTC]: 1% (14.7 g)

Sal-Plant® [OTC]: 17% (14 g)
Zapzyt® Acne Wash [OTC]: 2% (188.5 g)
Zapzyt® Pore Treatment [OTC]: 2% (22 mL)
Liquid, topical:
Clean & Clear® Advantage® Oil-Free Acne [OTC]: 0.5% (120 mL)
Clean & Clear® Continuous Control® Acne Wash [OTC]: 2% (177 mL)
Clean & Clear® Deep Cleaning [OTC]: 2% (240 mL)
Compound W® [OTC]: 17.6% (9 mL)
Dr. Scholl's® Clear Away® Wart Remover Fast-Acting [OTC]: 17% (9.8 mL)
Dr. Scholl's® Corn/Callus Remover [OTC]: 12.6% (9.8 mL)
DuoFilm® [OTC]: 17% (9.8 mL)
Durasal™: 26% (10 mL)
Freezone® [OTC]: 17.6% (9.3 mL)
Fung-O® [OTC]: 17% (15 mL)
Gets-It® [OTC]: 13.9% (15 mL)
Gordofilm [OTC]: 16.7% (15 mL)
Mosco® Callus & Corn Remover [OTC]: 17.6% (9 mL)
Neutrogena® Blackhead Eliminating™ Daily Scrub [OTC]: 2% (125 mL)
Neutrogena® Body Clear® [OTC]: 2% (250 mL)
Neutrogena® Clear Pore™ Oil-Controlling Astringent [OTC]: 2% (236 mL)
Neutrogena® Oil-Free Acne Stress Control [OTC]: 0.5% (177 mL); 2% (50 mL)
Neutrogena® Oil-Free Acne Wash 60 Second Mask Scrub [OTC]: 1% (170 g)
Neutrogena® Oil-Free Acne Wash Foam Cleanser [OTC]: 2% (150 mL)
Palmer's® Skin Success Acne Cleanser [OTC]: 0.5% (240 mL)
Salactic® [OTC]: 17% (15 mL)
Scalpicin® Anti-Itch [OTC]: 3% (44 mL, 74 mL)
Tinamed® Corn and Callus Remover [OTC]: 17% (15 mL)
Tinamed® Wart Remover [OTC]: 17% (15 mL)
Wart-Off® Maximum Strength [OTC]: 17.5% (14.8 mL)
Lotion, topical: 6% (414 mL, 420 mL)
Dermarest® Psoriasis Medicated Moisturizer [OTC]: 2% (118 mL)
Neutrogena® Rapid Clear® Acne Defense [OTC]: 2% (50 mL)
OXY® Post-Shave [OTC]: 0.5% (50 g)
Salex®: 6% (237 mL)
Salitop™: 6% (414 mL)
Ointment, topical:
MG217® Sal-Acid [OTC]: 3% (57 g)
Pad, topical:
Clean & Clear® Blackhead Clearing Daily Cleansing [OTC]: 1% (70s)
Curad® Mediplast® [OTC]: 40% (25s)
Neutrogena® Blackhead Eliminating™ 2-in-1 Foaming Pads [OTC]: 0.5% (28s)
Neutrogena® Blackhead Elinimating™ [OTC]: 0.5% (28s)
Neutrogena® Rapid Clear® [OTC]: 2% (60s)
OXY® Chill Factor® [OTC]: 2% (90s)
OXY® Daily [OTC]: 0.2% (90s)
OXY® Daily Cleansing [OTC]: 0.5% (90s)
OXY® Maximum Daily Cleansing [OTC]: 2% (55s, 90s)
Stridex® Essential Care® [OTC]: 1% (55s)
Stridex® Facewipes To Go® [OTC]: 0.5% (32s)
Stridex® Maximum Strength [OTC]: 2% (55s, 90s)
Stridex® Sensitive Skin [OTC]: 0.5% (55s, 90s)
Patch, topical:
Compound W® One Step Invisible Strip [OTC]: 14% (14s)
Compound W® One Step Wart Remover for Feet [OTC]: 40% (20s)
Compound W® One-Step Wart Remover [OTC]: 40% (14s)
Compound W® One-Step Wart Remover for Kids [OTC]: 40% (12s)
Dr. Scholl's® Callus Removers [OTC]: 40% (4s)
Dr. Scholl's® Clear Away® One Step Wart Remover [OTC]: 40% (14s)
Dr. Scholl's® Clear Away® Plantar Wart Remover For Feet [OTC]: 40% (24s)
Dr. Scholl's® Clear Away® Wart Remover [OTC]: 40% (18s)
Dr. Scholl's® Clear Away® Wart Remover Invisible Strips [OTC]: 40% (18s)
Dr. Scholl's® Corn Removers [OTC]: 40% (9s)

◄ Dr. Scholl's® Extra Thick Corn Removers [OTC]: 40% (9s)
Dr. Scholl's® Extra-Thick Callus Removers [OTC]: 40% (4s)
Dr. Scholl's® For Her Corn Removers [OTC]: 40% (6s)
Dr. Scholl's® OneStep Callus Removers [OTC]: 40% (4s)
Dr. Scholl's® OneStep Corn Removers [OTC]: 40% (6s)
Dr. Scholl's® Small Corn Removers [OTC]: 40% (9s)
Dr. Scholl's® Ultra-Thin Corn Removers [OTC]: 40% (9s)
Mosco® One Step Corn Remover [OTC]: 40% (8s)
Trans-Ver-Sal® [OTC]: 15% (10s, 12s, 15s, 25s, 40s)

Shampoo, topical: 6% (177 mL)
Aliclen™: 6% (177 mL)
Beta Sal® [OTC]: 3% (480 mL)
Denorex® Extra Strength Protection [OTC]: 3% (118 mL, 355 mL)
DHS™ Sal [OTC]: 3% (120 mL)
Ionil Plus® [OTC]: 2% (240 mL)
Ionil® [OTC]: 2% (120 mL)
LupiCare® Dandruff [OTC]: 2% (237 mL)
LupiCare® Psoriasis [OTC]: 2% (237 mL)
Neutrogena® Maximum Strength T/Sal® [OTC]: 3% (135 mL)
P&S® [OTC]: 2% (118 mL, 236 mL)
Salex®: 6% (177 mL)
Thera-Sal [OTC]: 3% (180 mL)

Shampoo/Conditioner, topical:
Denorex® Extra Strength Protection 2-in-1 [OTC]: 3% (118 mL, 355 mL)
Dermarest® Psoriasis Medicated Shampoo/Conditioner [OTC]: 3% (236 mL)

salicylic acid and coal tar *see* coal tar and salicylic acid *on page* 228

salicylsalicylic acid *see* salsalate *on page* 799

saline *see* sodium chloride *on page* 818

Saline Mist [OTC] *see* sodium chloride *on page* 818

Salitop™ *see* salicylic acid *on page* 795

saliva substitute (sa LYE va SUB stee tute)

Synonyms artificial saliva

U.S. Brand Names Aquoral™; Caphosol®; Entertainer's Secret® [OTC]; Moi-Stir® [OTC]; Mouthkote® [OTC]; Numoisyn™; Oasis®; Oral Balance® [OTC]; SalivaSure™ [OTC]

Therapeutic Category Gastrointestinal Agent, Miscellaneous

Use Relief of dry mouth and throat in xerostomia or hyposalivation; adjunct to standard oral care in relief of symptoms associated with chemotherapy or radiation therapy-induced mucositis

General Dosage Range Oral: *Adults:* Dosage varies greatly depending on product

Dosage Forms

Liquid:
Numoisyn™: Water, sorbitol, linseed extract, *Chondrus crispus*, methylparaben, sodium benzoate, potassium sorbate, dipotassium phosphate, propylparaben
Oral Balance® [OTC]: Water, starch, sunflower oil, propylene glycol, xylitol, glycerine, purified milk extract

Lozenge:
Numoisyn™: Sorbitol 0.3 g/lozenge, polyethylene glycol, malic acid, sodium citrate, calcium phosphate dibasic, hydrogenated cottonseed oil, citric acid, magnesium stearate, silicon dioxide
SalivaSure™ [OTC]: Xylitol, citric acid, apple acid, sodium citrate dihydrate, sodium carboxymethyl-cellulose, dibasic calcium phosphate, silica colloidal, magnesium stearate, stearic acid

Solution, oral:
Caphosol®: Dibasic sodium phosphate 0.032%, monobasic sodium phosphate 0.009%, calcium chloride 0.052%, sodium chloride 0.569%, purified water
Entertainer's Secret® [OTC]: Sodium carboxymethylcellulose, aloe vera gel, glycerin (60 mL)

Solution, oral [mouthwash/gargle]:
Oasis®: Water, glycerin, sorbitol, poloxamer 338, PEG-60, hydrogenated castor oil, copovidone, sodium benzoate, carboxymethycellulose

Solution, oral [spray]:
Aquoral™: Oxidized glycerol triesters and silicon dioxide
Moi-Stir® [OTC]: Water, sorbitol, sodium carboxymethylcellulose, methylparaben, propylparaben, potassium chloride, dibasic sodium phosphate, calcium chloride, magnesium chloride, sodium chloride
Mouthkote® [OTC]: Water, xylitol, sorbitol, yerba santa, citric acid, ascorbic acid, sodium saccharin, sodium benzoate
Oasis®: Glycerin, cetylpyridinium, copovidone

SalivaSure™ [OTC] see saliva substitute *on page 798*

salk vaccine see poliovirus vaccine (inactivated) *on page 717*

salmeterol (sal ME te role)

Medication Safety Issues
Sound-alike/look-alike issues:
Salmeterol may be confused with Salbutamol, Solu-Medrol®
Serevent® may be confused with Atrovent®, Combivent®, Serentil®, sertraline, Sinemet®, Spiriva®, Zoloft®

Synonyms salmeterol xinafoate

U.S. Brand Names Serevent® Diskus®

Canadian Brand Names Serevent® Diskhaler® Disk; Serevent® Diskus®

Therapeutic Category Adrenergic Agonist Agent

Use Maintenance treatment of asthma and prevention of bronchospasm (as concomitant therapy) in patients with reversible obstructive airway disease, including patients with symptoms of nocturnal asthma; prevention of exercise-induced bronchospasm (monotherapy may be indicated in patients without persistent asthma); maintenance treatment of bronchospasm associated with COPD

General Dosage Range Inhalation: *Children ≥4 years and Adults:* 1 inhalation (50 mcg) twice daily

Dosage Forms
Powder, for oral inhalation:
Serevent® Diskus®: 50 mcg (28s, 60s)
Dosage Forms - Canada
Powder for oral inhalation:
Serevent® Diskhaler® Disk: 50 mcg (60s)

salmeterol and fluticasone see fluticasone and salmeterol *on page 394*

salmeterol xinafoate see salmeterol *on page 799*

Salofalk® (Can) see mesalamine *on page 564*

Salofalk® 5-ASA (Can) see mesalamine *on page 564*

Salonpas® [OTC] see methyl salicylate and menthol *on page 579*

Salonpas® Arthritis Pain® [OTC] see methyl salicylate and menthol *on page 579*

Salonpas® Hot [OTC] see capsaicin *on page 169*

Salonpas® Pain Relief Patch® [OTC] see methyl salicylate and menthol *on page 579*

Sal-Plant® [OTC] see salicylic acid *on page 795*

salsalate (SAL sa late)

Medication Safety Issues
Sound-alike/look-alike issues:
Salsalate may be confused with sucralfate, sulfaSALAzine

Synonyms disalicylic acid; salicylsalicylic acid

Canadian Brand Names Amigesic®; Salflex®

Therapeutic Category Analgesic, Nonnarcotic; Antipyretic; Nonsteroidal Antiinflammatory Drug (NSAID)

Use Treatment of rheumatoid arthritis, osteoarthritis, and related rheumatic disorders

General Dosage Range Dosage adjustment recommended in patients with renal impairment
Oral: *Adults:* 3 g/day in 2-3 divided doses
Dosage Forms
Tablet, oral: 500 mg, 750 mg

salt see sodium chloride *on page 818*

salt-poor albumin see albumin *on page 44*

Sal-Tropine™ [DSC] see atropine *on page 103*

Salvax *see* salicylic acid *on page 795*
Samsca™ *see* tolvaptan *on page 877*
Sanctura® *see* trospium *on page 895*
Sanctura® XR *see* trospium *on page 895*
Sancuso® *see* granisetron *on page 424*
SandIMMUNE® *see* cyclosporine (systemic) *on page 243*
Sandimmune® I.V. (Can) *see* cyclosporine (systemic) *on page 243*
Sandomigran® (Can) *see* pizotifen *(Canada only) on page 709*
Sandomigran DS® (Can) *see* pizotifen *(Canada only) on page 709*
SandoSTATIN® *see* octreotide *on page 643*
Sandostatin® (Can) *see* octreotide *on page 643*
SandoSTATIN LAR® *see* octreotide *on page 643*
Sandostatin LAR® (Can) *see* octreotide *on page 643*
Sandoz-Acebutolol (Can) *see* acebutolol *on page 23*
Sandoz-Alendronate (Can) *see* alendronate *on page 49*
Sandoz-Alfuzosin (Can) *see* alfuzosin *on page 50*
Sandoz-Amiodarone (Can) *see* amiodarone *on page 67*
Sandoz Amlodipine (Can) *see* amlodipine *on page 69*
Sandoz-Anagrelide (Can) *see* anagrelide *on page 78*
Sandoz-Atenolol (Can) *see* atenolol *on page 101*
Sandoz-Atorvastatin (Can) *see* atorvastatin *on page 102*
Sandoz-Azithromycin (Can) *see* azithromycin (systemic) *on page 108*
Sandoz-Betaxolol (Can) *see* betaxolol (systemic) *on page 130*
Sandoz-Bicalutamide (Can) *see* bicalutamide *on page 133*
Sandoz-Bisoprolol (Can) *see* bisoprolol *on page 136*
Sandoz-Brimonidine (Can) *see* brimonidine *on page 141*
Sandoz-Bupropion SR (Can) *see* bupropion *on page 150*
Sandoz-Calcitonin (Can) *see* calcitonin *on page 159*
Sandoz-Candesartan (Can) *see* candesartan *on page 167*
Sandoz-Carbamazepine (Can) *see* carbamazepine *on page 171*
Sandoz-Cefprozil (Can) *see* cefprozil *on page 183*
Sandoz-Ciprofloxacin (Can) *see* ciprofloxacin (systemic) *on page 210*
Sandoz-Citalopram (Can) *see* citalopram *on page 213*
Sandoz-Clarithromycin (Can) *see* clarithromycin *on page 215*
Sandoz-Clonazepam (Can) *see* clonazepam *on page 222*
Sandoz-Cyclosporine (Can) *see* cyclosporine (systemic) *on page 243*
Sandoz-Diclofenac (Can) *see* diclofenac (systemic) *on page 277*
Sandoz-Diclofenac Rapide (Can) *see* diclofenac (systemic) *on page 277*
Sandoz-Diclofenac SR (Can) *see* diclofenac (systemic) *on page 277*
Sandoz-Diltiazem CD (Can) *see* diltiazem *on page 286*
Sandoz-Diltiazem T (Can) *see* diltiazem *on page 286*
Sandoz-Dimenhydrinate (Can) *see* dimenhydrinate *on page 288*
Sandoz-Dorzolamide/Timolol (Can) *see* dorzolamide and timolol *on page 308*
Sandoz-Enalapril (Can) *see* enalapril *on page 326*
Sandoz-Estradiol Derm 50 (Can) *see* estradiol (systemic) *on page 343*
Sandoz-Estradiol Derm 75 (Can) *see* estradiol (systemic) *on page 343*
Sandoz-Estradiol Derm 100 (Can) *see* estradiol (systemic) *on page 343*
Sandoz-Famciclovir (Can) *see* famciclovir *on page 366*
Sandoz-Felodipine (Can) *see* felodipine *on page 368*
Sandoz-Fenofibrate S (Can) *see* fenofibrate *on page 369*
Sandoz-Finasteride (Can) *see* finasteride *on page 378*
Sandoz-Fluoxetine (Can) *see* fluoxetine *on page 389*
Sandoz-Fluvoxamine (Can) *see* fluvoxamine *on page 395*

Sandoz-Glimepiride (Can) *see* glimepiride *on page 418*
Sandoz-Glyburide (Can) *see* glyburide *on page 420*
Sandoz-Indomethacin (Can) *see* indomethacin *on page 471*
Sandoz-Irbesartan (Can) *see* irbesartan *on page 490*
Sandoz-Irbesartan HCT (Can) *see* irbesartan and hydrochlorothiazide *on page 490*
Sandoz-Leflunomide (Can) *see* leflunomide *on page 514*
Sandoz-Letrozole (Can) *see* letrozole *on page 515*
Sandoz-Levobunolol (Can) *see* levobunolol *on page 517*
Sandoz-Lisinopril (Can) *see* lisinopril *on page 531*
Sandoz-Lisinopril/Hctz (Can) *see* lisinopril and hydrochlorothiazide *on page 532*
Sandoz-Loperamide (Can) *see* loperamide *on page 535*
Sandoz-Lovastatin (Can) *see* lovastatin *on page 540*
Sandoz-Memantine (Can) *see* memantine *on page 556*
Sandoz-Metformin FC (Can) *see* metformin *on page 566*
Sandoz-Methylphenidate SR (Can) *see* methylphenidate *on page 577*
Sandoz-Metoprolol SR (Can) *see* metoprolol *on page 581*
Sandoz-Metoprolol (Type L) (Can) *see* metoprolol *on page 581*
Sandoz-Minocycline (Can) *see* minocycline *on page 590*
Sandoz-Mirtazapine (Can) *see* mirtazapine *on page 592*
Sandoz-Mirtazapine FC (Can) *see* mirtazapine *on page 592*
Sandoz-Morphine SR (Can) *see* morphine (systemic) *on page 598*
Sandoz-Nabumetone (Can) *see* nabumetone *on page 607*
Sandoz-Nitrazepam (Can) *see* nitrazepam (Canada only) *on page 628*
Sandoz-Olanzapine (Can) *see* olanzapine *on page 645*
Sandoz-Olanzapine ODT (Can) *see* olanzapine *on page 645*
Sandoz-Omeprazole (Can) *see* omeprazole *on page 649*
Sandoz-Ondansetron (Can) *see* ondansetron *on page 651*
Sandoz-Pantoprazole (Can) *see* pantoprazole *on page 672*
Sandoz-Paroxetine (Can) *see* paroxetine *on page 676*
Sandoz-Pindolol (Can) *see* pindolol *on page 705*
Sandoz-Pioglitazone (Can) *see* pioglitazone *on page 706*
Sandoz-Pramipexole (Can) *see* pramipexole *on page 729*
Sandoz-Pravastatin (Can) *see* pravastatin *on page 732*
Sandoz-Quetiapine (Can) *see* quetiapine *on page 760*
Sandoz-Rabeprazole (Can) *see* rabeprazole *on page 763*
Sandoz-Ramipril (Can) *see* ramipril *on page 766*
Sandoz-Ranitidine (Can) *see* ranitidine *on page 767*
Sandoz-Risedronate (Can) *see* risedronate *on page 782*
Sandoz-Risperidone (Can) *see* risperidone *on page 783*
Sandoz-Rivastigmine (Can) *see* rivastigmine *on page 786*
Sandoz-Salbutamol (Can) *see* albuterol *on page 45*
Sandoz-Sertraline (Can) *see* sertraline *on page 809*
Sandoz-Simvastatin (Can) *see* simvastatin *on page 813*
Sandoz-Sotalol (Can) *see* sotalol *on page 828*
Sandoz-Sumatriptan (Can) *see* sumatriptan *on page 839*
Sandoz-Tamsulosin (Can) *see* tamsulosin *on page 843*
Sandoz-Tamsulosin CR (Can) *see* tamsulosin *on page 843*
Sandoz-Terbinafine (Can) *see* terbinafine (systemic) *on page 851*
Sandoz-Ticlopidine (Can) *see* ticlopidine *on page 868*
Sandoz-Timolol (Can) *see* timolol (ophthalmic) *on page 869*
Sandoz-Tobramycin (Can) *see* tobramycin (ophthalmic) *on page 873*
Sandoz-Topiramate (Can) *see* topiramate *on page 877*
Sandoz-Trifluridine (Can) *see* trifluridine *on page 890*

Sandoz-Valproic (Can) *see* valproic acid *on page 904*
Sandoz-Valsartan (Can) *see* valsartan *on page 905*
Sandoz Valsartan HCT (Can) *see* valsartan and hydrochlorothiazide *on page 906*
Sandoz-Venlafaxine XR (Can) *see* venlafaxine *on page 911*
Sandoz-Zolmitriptan (Can) *see* zolmitriptan *on page 933*
Sandoz-Zolmitriptan ODT (Can) *see* zolmitriptan *on page 933*
Sandoz-Zopiclone (Can) *see* zopiclone *(Canada only) on page 934*
Sani-Supp® [OTC] *see* glycerin *on page 421*
Sans Acne® (Can) *see* erythromycin (topical) *on page 340*
Santyl® *see* collagenase (topical) *on page 233*
Saphris® *see* asenapine *on page 97*

sapropterin (sap roe TER in)

Medication Safety Issues
  Sound-alike/look-alike issues:
    Sapropterin may be confused with cyproterone
Synonyms 6R-BH4; phenoptin; sapropterin dihydrochloride
U.S. Brand Names Kuvan™
Therapeutic Category Enzyme Cofactor
Use Adjunct to dietary management in the treatment of tetrahydrobiopterin (BH4) responsive phenylketonuria (PKU)
General Dosage Range Oral: *Children ≥4 years and Adults:* 10 mg/kg once daily; Maintenance range: 5-20 mg/kg/day
Dosage Forms
  Tablet:
    Kuvan™: 100 mg

sapropterin dihydrochloride *see* sapropterin *on page 802*

saquinavir (sa KWIN a veer)

Medication Safety Issues
  Sound-alike/look-alike issues:
    Saquinavir may be confused with SINEquan®
Synonyms saquinavir mesylate
U.S. Brand Names Invirase®
Canadian Brand Names Invirase®
Therapeutic Category Antiviral Agent
Use Treatment of HIV infection; used in combination with at least two other antiretroviral agents
General Dosage Range Dosage adjustment recommended in patients on concomitant therapy
  Oral: *Children >16 years and Adults:* 1000 mg twice daily
Dosage Forms
  Capsule, oral:
    Invirase®: 200 mg
  Tablet, oral:
    Invirase®: 500 mg

saquinavir mesylate *see* saquinavir *on page 802*
Sarafem® *see* fluoxetine *on page 389*

sargramostim (sar GRAM oh stim)

Medication Safety Issues
  Sound-alike/look-alike issues:
    Leukine® may be confused with Leukeran®, leucovorin
Synonyms GM-CSF; granulocyte-macrophage colony-stimulating factor; NSC-613795; rGM-CSF
U.S. Brand Names Leukine®
Canadian Brand Names Leukine®
Therapeutic Category Colony-Stimulating Factor

Use

Acute myelogenous leukemia (AML) following induction chemotherapy in older adults (≥55 years of age) to shorten time to neutrophil recovery and to reduce the incidence of severe and life-threatening infections and infections resulting in death

Bone marrow transplant (allogeneic or autologous) failure or engraftment delay

Myeloid reconstitution after allogeneic bone marrow transplantation

Myeloid reconstitution after autologous bone marrow transplantation: Non-Hodgkin lymphoma (NHL), acute lymphoblastic leukemia (ALL), Hodgkin lymphoma

Peripheral stem cell transplantation: Mobilization and myeloid reconstitution following autologous peripheral stem cell transplantation

General Dosage Range

I.V.: *Children and Adults:* Infusion: 250 mcg/m^2/day (maximum: 500 mcg/m^2/day)

SubQ: *Children and Adults:* 250 mcg/m^2 once daily

Dosage Forms

Injection, powder for reconstitution:
Leukine®: 250 mcg

Injection, solution:
Leukine®: 500 mcg/mL (1 mL)

Sarna® HC (Can) *see* hydrocortisone (topical) *on page 450*

Sarna® Sensitive [OTC] *see* pramoxine *on page 730*

Sarna® Ultra [OTC] *see* pramoxine *on page 730*

Sativex® (Can) *see* tetrahydrocannabinol and cannabidiol *(Canada only) on page 857*

Savella® *see* milnacipran *on page 589*

saxagliptin (sax a GLIP tin)

Medication Safety Issues

Sound-alike/look-alike issues:
Saxagliptin may be confused with sitaGLIPtin, SUMAtriptan

Synonyms BMS-477118

U.S. Brand Names Onglyza™

Canadian Brand Names Onglyza™

Therapeutic Category Antidiabetic Agent, Dipeptidyl Peptidase IV (DPP-IV) Inhibitor

Use Treatment of type 2 diabetes mellitus (noninsulin-dependent, NIDDM) as an adjunct to diet and exercise as monotherapy or in combination therapy with other antidiabetic agents to improve glycemic control

General Dosage Range Dosage adjustment recommended in patients with renal impairment or on concomitant therapy

Oral: *Adults:* 2.5-5 mg once daily

Dosage Forms

Tablet, oral:
Onglyza™: 2.5 mg, 5 mg

saxagliptin and metformin (sax a GLIP tin & met FOR min)

Medication Safety Issues

Sound-alike/look-alike issues:
Saxagliptin and Metformin may be confused with sitaGLIPtin and Metformin

Synonyms metformin and saxagliptin; metformin hydrochloride and saxagliptin; saxagliptin and metformin hydrochloride

U.S. Brand Names Kombiglyze™ XR

Therapeutic Category Antidiabetic Agent, Biguanide; Antidiabetic Agent, Dipeptidyl Peptidase IV (DPP-IV) Inhibitor

Use Management of type 2 diabetes mellitus (noninsulin dependent, NIDDM) as an adjunct to diet and exercise when treatment with both saxagliptin and metformin is appropriate

General Dosage Range Dosage adjustment recommended in patients on concomitant therapy

Oral: *Adults:* Saxagliptin 2.5-5 mg and metformin 500-2000 mg once daily (maximum: 5 mg/day [saxagliptin], 2000 mg/day [metformin])

◀ **Dosage Forms**

Tablet, variable release, oral:

Kombiglyze™ XR 2.5/1000: Saxagliptin 2.5 mg [immediate release] and metformin hydrochloride 1000 mg [extended release]; 5/500: Saxagliptin 5 mg [immediate release] and metformin hydrochloride 500 mg [extended release]; 5/1000: Saxagliptin 5 mg [immediate release] and metformin hydrochloride 1000 mg [extended release]

saxagliptin and metformin hydrochloride *see* saxagliptin and metformin *on page 803*

SB-265805 *see* gemifloxacin *on page 414*

SB-497115 *see* eltrombopag *on page 324*

SB-497115-GR *see* eltrombopag *on page 324*

SB659746-A *see* vilazodone *on page 914*

S. boulardii *see* Saccharomyces boulardii *on page 794*

SC 33428 *see* idarubicin *on page 463*

Scalpana [OTC] *see* hydrocortisone (topical) *on page 450*

Scalpicin® Anti-Itch [OTC] *see* salicylic acid *on page 795*

Scandonest® 2% L *see* mepivacaine and levonordefrin *on page 562*

Scandonest® 3% Plain *see* mepivacaine *on page 561*

SCH 13521 *see* flutamide *on page 392*

SCH 52365 *see* temozolomide *on page 849*

SCH 56592 *see* posaconazole *on page 722*

SCH503034 *see* boceprevir *on page 138*

ScheinPharm Ranitidine (Can) *see* ranitidine *on page 767*

SCIG *see* immune globulin *on page 468*

S-citalopram *see* escitalopram *on page 341*

Sclerosol® *see* talc (sterile) *on page 843*

Scopace™ [DSC] *see* scopolamine (systemic) *on page 804*

scopolamine (systemic) (skoe POL a mee)

Medication Safety Issues

Other safety concerns:

Transdermal patch may contain conducting metal (eg, aluminum); remove patch prior to MRI.

Synonyms hyoscine butylbromide; scopolamine base; scopolamine butylbromide; scopolamine hydrobromide

U.S. Brand Names Scopace™ [DSC]; Transderm Scōp®

Canadian Brand Names Buscopan®; Transderm-V®

Therapeutic Category Anticholinergic Agent

Use

Scopolamine base: Transdermal: Prevention of nausea/vomiting associated with motion sickness and recovery from anesthesia and surgery

Scopolamine hydrobromide:

Injection: Preoperative medication to produce amnesia, sedation, tranquilization, antiemetic effects, and decrease salivary and respiratory secretions

Oral: Symptomatic treatment of postencephalitic parkinsonism and paralysis agitans; in spastic states; inhibits excessive motility and hypertonus of the gastrointestinal tract in such conditions as the irritable colon syndrome, mild dysentery, diverticulitis, pylorospasm, and cardiospasm

Scopolamine butylbromide [not available in the U.S.]: Oral/injection: Treatment of smooth muscle spasm of the genitourinary or gastrointestinal tract; injection may also be used to prior to radiological/diagnostic procedures to prevent spasm

General Dosage Range

I.M., I.V., SubQ:

Children 6 months to 3 years: 0.1-0.15 mg

Children 3-6 years: 0.2-0.3 mg

Adults: 0.3-0.65 mg (single dose) **or** 0.6 mg 3-4 times/day

Oral: *Adults:* 0.4-0.8 mg as a single dose or every 8-12 hours as needed

Transdermal: *Adults:* Apply 1 patch every 3 days as needed

Dosage Forms

Injection, solution: 0.4 mg/mL (1 mL)

Patch, transdermal:
  Transderm Scōp®: 1.5 mg (4s, 10s, 24s)
Dosage Forms - Canada
  Injection, solution:
    Buscopan®: 20 mg/mL
  Tablet:
    Buscopan®: 10 mg

scopolamine (ophthalmic) (skoe POL a meen)

Synonyms hyoscine hydrobromide; scopolamine hydrobromide

U.S. Brand Names Isopto® Hyoscine

Therapeutic Category Anticholinergic Agent; Anticholinergic Agent, Ophthalmic; Ophthalmic Agent, Mydriatic

Use Scopolamine hydrobromide: Produce cycloplegia and mydriasis; treatment of iridocyclitis

General Dosage Range Ophthalmic:
  Children: Instill 1 drop (0.25%) to eye(s) up to 3 times/day
  Adults: Instill 1-2 drops (0.25%) eye(s) up to 4 times/day

Dosage Forms
  Solution, ophthalmic:
    Isopto® Hyoscine: 0.25% (5 mL)

scopolamine base *see* scopolamine (systemic) *on page 804*

scopolamine butylbromide *see* scopolamine (systemic) *on page 804*

scopolamine hydrobromide *see* scopolamine (ophthalmic) *on page 805*

scopolamine hydrobromide *see* scopolamine (systemic) *on page 804*

scopolamine, hyoscyamine, atropine, and phenobarbital *see* hyoscyamine, atropine, scopolamine, and phenobarbital *on page 459*

scorpion antivenin *see Centruroides* immune F(ab')$_2$ (equine) *on page 187*

Scot-Tussin® Diabetes [OTC] *see* dextromethorphan *on page 270*

Scot-Tussin® DM Maximum Strength [OTC] *see* dextromethorphan and chlorpheniramine *on page 271*

Scot-Tussin® Expectorant [OTC] *see* guaifenesin *on page 425*

Scot-Tussin® Senior [OTC] *see* guaifenesin and dextromethorphan *on page 427*

Scytera™ [OTC] *see* coal tar *on page 227*

SD/01 *see* pegfilgrastim *on page 679*

SDX-105 *see* bendamustine *on page 119*

SDZ ENA 713 *see* rivastigmine *on page 786*

Seasonale® *see* ethinyl estradiol and levonorgestrel *on page 353*

Seasonique® *see* ethinyl estradiol and levonorgestrel *on page 353*

Sebcur® (Can) *see* salicylic acid *on page 795*

Sebcur/T® (Can) *see* coal tar and salicylic acid *on page 228*

Sebivo® (Can) *see* telbivudine *on page 847*

Seb-Prev™ *see* sulfacetamide (topical) *on page 835*

secobarbital (see koe BAR bi tal)

Medication Safety Issues
  Sound-alike/look-alike issues:
    Seconal® may be confused with Sectral®
  BEERS Criteria medication:
    This drug may be inappropriate for use in geriatric patients (high severity risk).

Synonyms quinalbarbitone sodium; secobarbital sodium

U.S. Brand Names Seconal®

Therapeutic Category Barbiturate

Controlled Substance C-II

Use Preanesthetic agent; short-term treatment of insomnia

▶

◀ **General Dosage Range Oral:**
  Children: 2-6 mg/kg 1-2 hours before procedure (maximum: 100 mg/dose) **or** 6 mg/kg/day divided every 8 hours
  Adults: 100-200 mg at bedtime **or** 100-300 mg 1-2 hours before procedure
Dosage Forms
  Capsule, oral:
    Seconal®: 100 mg

secobarbital sodium *see* secobarbital *on page 805*
Seconal® *see* secobarbital *on page 805*

secretin (SEE kr tin)
Synonyms secretin, human; secretin, porcine
U.S. Brand Names ChiRhoStim®
Therapeutic Category Diagnostic Agent
Use Secretin-stimulation testing to aid in diagnosis of pancreatic exocrine dysfunction; diagnosis of gastrinoma (Zollinger-Ellison syndrome); facilitation of endoscopic retrograde cholangiopancreatography (ERCP) visualization
General Dosage Range I.V.: *Adults:* Test dose: 0.1 mL (0.2-0.4 mcg); Diagnostic dose: 0.2-0.4 mcg/kg
Dosage Forms
  Injection, powder for reconstitution:
    ChiRhoStim®: 16 mcg

secretin, human *see* secretin *on page 806*
secretin, porcine *see* secretin *on page 806*
Sectral® *see* acebutolol *on page 23*
Secura® Antifungal Extra Thick [OTC] *see* miconazole (topical) *on page 585*
Secura® Antifungal Greaseless [OTC] *see* miconazole (topical) *on page 585*
Sedapap® *see* butalbital and acetaminophen *on page 153*
Selax® (Can) *see* docusate *on page 302*
Select™ 1/35 (Can) *see* ethinyl estradiol and norethindrone *on page 355*
Select-OB™ *see* vitamins (multiple/prenatal) *on page 920*

selegiline (se LE ji leen)
Medication Safety Issues
  Sound-alike/look-alike issues:
    Selegiline may be confused with Salagen®, Serentil®, sertraline, Serzone®, Stelazine®
    Eldepryl® may be confused with Elavil®, enalapril
    Zelapar® may be confused with zaleplon, Zemplar®, zolpidem, ZyPREXA® Zydis®
Synonyms deprenyl; L-deprenyl; selegiline hydrochloride
U.S. Brand Names Eldepryl®; Emsam®; Zelapar®
Canadian Brand Names Apo-Selegiline®; Gen-Selegiline; Mylan-Selegiline; Novo-Selegiline; Nu-Selegiline
Therapeutic Category Anti-Parkinson Agent; Dopaminergic Agent (Anti-Parkinson)
Use Adjunct in the management of parkinsonian patients in which levodopa/carbidopa therapy is deteriorating (oral products); treatment of major depressive disorder (transdermal product)
General Dosage Range
  Oral:
    Capsule/Tablet: *Adults:* 5 mg twice daily
    Disintegrating tablet: *Adults:* Initial: 1.25 mg daily; Maintenance: 1.25-2.5 mg daily (maximum: 2.5 mg daily)
  Transdermal:
    Adults: Initial: 6 mg once daily; Maintenance: 6-12 mg once daily (maximum: 12 mg/day)
    Elderly: 6 mg once daily
Dosage Forms
  Capsule, oral: 5 mg
    Eldepryl®: 5 mg
  Patch, transdermal:
    Emsam®: 6 mg/24 hours (30s); 9 mg/24 hours (30s); 12 mg/24 hours (30s)

Tablet, oral: 5 mg
Tablet, orally disintegrating, oral:
  Zelapar®: 1.25 mg

selegiline hydrochloride *see* selegiline *on page 806*
selenium *see* trace metals *on page 880*

selenium sulfide (se LEE nee um SUL fide)

U.S. Brand Names Dandrex; Head & Shoulders® Intensive Treatment [OTC]; Selseb®; Selsun blue® 2-in-1 Treatment [OTC]; Selsun blue® Daily Treatment [OTC]; Selsun blue® Medicated Treatment [OTC]; Selsun blue® Moisturizing Treatment [OTC]; Tersi

Canadian Brand Names Versel®

Therapeutic Category Antiseborrheic Agent, Topical

Use Treatment of itching and flaking of the scalp associated with dandruff, to control scalp seborrheic dermatitis; treatment of tinea versicolor

General Dosage Range Topical: *Adults:* Foam: Rub into affected skin twice daily; Lotion: Apply to affected area daily; Shampoo: Massage 5-10 mL into wet scalp

Dosage Forms
  Aerosol, topical:
   Tersi: 2.25% (70 g)
  Lotion, topical: 2.5% (118 mL, 120 mL)
  Shampoo, topical: 1% (210 mL)
   Dandrex: 1% (240 mL)
   Head & Shoulders® Intensive Treatment [OTC]: 1% (400 mL, 420 mL)
   Selseb®: 2.25% (180 mL)
   Selsun blue® 2-in-1 Treatment [OTC]: 1% (207 mL, 325 mL)
   Selsun blue® Daily Treatment [OTC]: 1% (207 mL, 325 mL)
   Selsun blue® Medicated Treatment [OTC]: 1% (120 mL, 207 mL, 325 mL)
   Selsun blue® Moisturizing Treatment [OTC]: 1% (207 mL, 325 mL)

Selfemra® [DSC] *see* fluoxetine *on page 389*
Selseb® *see* selenium sulfide *on page 807*
Selsun blue® 2-in-1 Treatment [OTC] *see* selenium sulfide *on page 807*
Selsun blue® Daily Treatment [OTC] *see* selenium sulfide *on page 807*
Selsun blue® Medicated Treatment [OTC] *see* selenium sulfide *on page 807*
Selsun blue® Moisturizing Treatment [OTC] *see* selenium sulfide *on page 807*
Selsun® Salon™ Classic [OTC] *see* pyrithione zinc *on page 759*
Selsun® Salon™ Dandruff 2-in-1 [OTC] *see* pyrithione zinc *on page 759*
Selsun® Salon™ Dandruff Moisturizing [OTC] *see* pyrithione zinc *on page 759*
Selsun® Salon™ Dandruff Volumizing [OTC] *see* pyrithione zinc *on page 759*
Selzentry™ *see* maraviroc *on page 549*
Semprex®-D *see* acrivastine and pseudoephedrine *on page 38*
Senexon [OTC] *see* senna *on page 807*
Senexon-S [OTC] *see* docusate and senna *on page 303*

senna (SEN na)

Medication Safety Issues
  Sound-alike/look-alike issues:
   Perdiem® may be confused with Pyridium®
   Senexon® may be confused with Cenestin®
   Senokot® may be confused with Depakote®

Synonyms sennosides

U.S. Brand Names Black Draught® [OTC]; Evac-U-Gen® [OTC]; ex-lax® Maximum Strength [OTC]; ex-lax® [OTC]; Fleet® Pedia-Lax™ Quick Dissolve [OTC]; Fletcher's® [OTC]; Little Tummys® Laxative [OTC]; Perdiem® Overnight Relief [OTC]; Senexon [OTC]; SennaGen [OTC]; Senokot® [OTC]

Therapeutic Category Laxative

Use Short-term treatment of constipation; evacuate the colon for bowel or rectal examinations

◄ **General Dosage Range Oral:**

Children 2-6 years: Initial: 3.75 mg once daily; Maintenance: 3.75-15 mg/day in 1-2 divided doses (maximum: 15 mg/day) **or** 5-10 mL (33.3 mg/mL) up to twice daily

Children 6-12 years: Initial: 8.6 mg once daily; Maintenance: 8.6-50 mg/day in 1-2 divided doses (maximum: 50 mg/day) **or** 10-30 mL (33.3 mg/mL) up to twice daily

Children ≥12 years and Adults: Initial: 15 mg once daily; Maintenance: 15-100 mg/day in 1-2 divided doses (maximum: 100 mg/day) **or** 130 mg as a single dose

Dosage Forms

Liquid, oral:
Fletcher's® [OTC]: Senna concentrate 33.3 mg/mL (75 mL)
Little Tummys® Laxative [OTC]: Sennosides 8.8 mg/mL (30 mL)
Senexon [OTC]: Sennosides 8.8 mg/5 mL (237 mL)

Strip, orally disintegrating, oral:
Fleet® Pedia-Lax™ Quick Dissolve [OTC]: Sennosides 8.6 mg (12s)

Syrup, oral: Sennosides 8.8 mg/5 mL (237 mL, 240 mL)

Tablet, oral: Sennosides 8.6 mg
ex-lax® [OTC]: Sennosides USP 15 mg
ex-lax® Maximum Strength [OTC]: Sennosides USP 25 mg
Perdiem® Overnight Relief [OTC]: Sennosides USP 15 mg
Senexon [OTC]: Sennosides 8.6 mg
SennaGen [OTC]: Sennosides 8.6 mg
Senokot® [OTC]: Sennosides 8.6 mg

Tablet, chewable, oral:
Black Draught® [OTC]: Sennosides 10 mg
Evac-U-Gen® [OTC]: Sennosides 10 mg
ex-lax® [OTC]: Sennosides USP 15 mg

SEROquel® *see* quetiapine *on page 760*
Seroquel® (Can) *see* quetiapine *on page 760*
SEROquel XR® *see* quetiapine *on page 760*
Seroquel XR® (Can) *see* quetiapine *on page 760*
Serostim® *see* somatropin *on page 826*

sertaconazole (ser ta KOE na zole)

Synonyms sertaconazole nitrate
U.S. Brand Names Ertaczo®
Therapeutic Category Antifungal Agent, Topical
Use Topical treatment of tinea pedis (athlete's foot)
General Dosage Range Topical: *Children ≥12 years and Adults:* Apply twice daily
Dosage Forms
  Cream, topical:
    Ertaczo®: 2% (30 g, 60 g)

sertaconazole nitrate *see* sertaconazole *on page 809*

sertraline (SER tra leen)

Medication Safety Issues
  Sound-alike/look-alike issues:
    Sertraline may be confused with selegiline, Serentil®, Serevent®, Soriatane®
    Zoloft® may be confused with Zocor®
Synonyms sertraline hydrochloride
U.S. Brand Names Zoloft®
Canadian Brand Names Apo-Sertraline®; CO Sertraline; Dom-Sertraline; GD-Sertraline; Mylan-Sertraline; Nu-Sertraline; PHL-Sertraline; PMS-Sertraline; ratio-Sertraline; Riva-Sertraline; Sandoz-Sertraline; Teva-Sertraline; Zoloft®
Therapeutic Category Antidepressant, Selective Serotonin Reuptake Inhibitor
Use Treatment of major depression; obsessive-compulsive disorder (OCD); panic disorder; posttraumatic stress disorder (PTSD); premenstrual dysphoric disorder (PMDD); social anxiety disorder
General Dosage Range Dosage adjustment recommended in patients with hepatic impairment
  Oral:
    Children 6-12 years: Initial: 25 mg once daily; Maintenance: 25-200 mg once daily (maximum: 200 mg/day)
    Children 13-17 years: Initial: 50 mg once daily; Maintenance: 25-200 mg once daily (maximum: 200 mg/day)
    Adults: Initial: 25-50 mg once daily; Maintenance: 50-200 mg once daily (maximum: 200 mg/day)
    Elderly: Initial: 25 mg once daily in the morning; Maintenance: 50-100 mg once daily (maximum: 200 mg/day)
Dosage Forms
  Solution, oral: 20 mg/mL (60 mL)
    Zoloft®: 20 mg/mL (60 mL)
  Tablet, oral: 25 mg, 50 mg, 100 mg
    Zoloft®: 25 mg, 50 mg, 100 mg

sertraline hydrochloride *see* sertraline *on page 809*
Serzone *see* nefazodone *on page 616*

sevelamer (se VEL a mer)

Medication Safety Issues
  Sound-alike/look-alike issues:
    Renagel® may be confused with Reglan®, Regonol®, Renal Caps, Renvela®
    Renvela® may be confused with Reglan®, Regonol®, Renagel®, Renal Caps
    Sevelamer may be confused with Savella®
  International issues:
    Renagel [U.S., Canada, and multiple international markets] may be confused with Remegel brand name for aluminium hydroxide and magnesium carbonate [Netherlands] and for calcium carbonate [Hungary, Great Britain and Ireland] and with Remegel Wind Relief brand name for calcium carbonate and simethicone [Great Britain]

◄ **Synonyms** sevelamer carbonate; sevelamer hydrochloride

U.S. Brand Names Renagel®; Renvela®

Canadian Brand Names Renagel®

Therapeutic Category Phosphate Binder

Use Reduction or control of serum phosphorous in patients with chronic kidney disease on hemodialysis

General Dosage Range Oral: *Adults:* Initial: 800-1600 mg 3 times/day; Maintenance: Up to 2400-14,000 mg/day in 3 divided doses

Dosage Forms

Powder for suspension, oral:

Renvela®: 0.8 g/packet (90s); 2.4 g/packet (90s)

Tablet, oral:

Renagel®: 400 mg, 800 mg

Renvela®: 800 mg

sevelamer carbonate *see* sevelamer *on page 809*

sevelamer hydrochloride *see* sevelamer *on page 809*

sevoflurane (see voe FLOO rane)

Medication Safety Issues

Sound-alike/look-alike issues:

Ultane® may be confused with Ultram®

High alert medication:

The Institute for Safe Medication Practices (ISMP) includes this medication among its list of drug classes which have a heightened risk of causing significant patient harm when used in error.

U.S. Brand Names Sojourn™; Ultane®

Canadian Brand Names Sevorane® AF; Sojourn Sevoflurane

Therapeutic Category General Anesthetic

Use Induction and maintenance of general anesthesia

General Dosage Range Inhalation:

Neonates 0-1 month (full-term): 3.3% in O_2

Infants 1 to <6 months: 3% in O_2

Children 6 months to <3 years: 2.8% in O_2; 2% in 60% N_2O/40% O_2

Children 3-12 years: 2.5% in O_2

Adults 25 years: 2.6% in O_2; 1.4% in 65% N_2O/35% O_2

Adults 40 years: 2.1% in O_2; 1.1% in 65% N_2O/35% O_2

Adults 60 years: 1.7% in O_2; 0.9% in 65% N_2O/35% O_2

Adults 80 years: 1.4% in O_2; 0.7% in 65% N_2O/35% O_2

Dosage Forms

Liquid, for inhalation: 100% (250 mL)

Sojourn™: 100% (250 mL)

Ultane®: 100% (250 mL)

Sevorane® AF (Can) *see* sevoflurane *on page 810*

sfRowasa™ *see* mesalamine *on page 564*

SGN-35 *see* brentuximab vedotin *on page 140*

shingles vaccine *see* zoster vaccine *on page 935*

Sibelium® (Can) *see* flunarizine *(Canada only) on page 383*

sibutramine (si BYOO tra meen)

Medication Safety Issues

Sound-alike/look-alike issues:

Meridia® may be confused with Aredia®

Synonyms sibutramine hydrochloride monohydrate

U.S. Brand Names Meridia® [DSC]

Canadian Brand Names Apo-Sibutramine®; Meridia®

Therapeutic Category Anorexiant

Controlled Substance C-IV

Use Management of obesity in patients with an initial body mass index (BMI) ≥30 kg/m^2 or ≥27 kg/m^2 in the presence of other risk factors (eg, diabetes, hyperlipidemia, hypertension)

General Dosage Range Oral: *Children ≥16 years and Adults:* Initial: 10 mg once daily; Maintenance: 5-15 mg once daily

Dosage Forms
Capsule, oral:
Meridia®: 5 mg, 10 mg, 15 mg

sibutramine hydrochloride monohydrate *see* sibutramine *on page 810*
Sig-Enalapril (Can) *see* enalapril *on page 326*
Silace [OTC] *see* docusate *on page 302*
Siladryl Allergy [OTC] *see* diphenhydramine (systemic) *on page 290*
Silafed [OTC] *see* triprolidine and pseudoephedrine *on page 893*
Silapap Children's [OTC] *see* acetaminophen *on page 23*
Silapap Infant's [OTC] *see* acetaminophen *on page 23*
Sildec PE [DSC] *see* chlorpheniramine and phenylephrine *on page 198*
Sildec PE-DM [DSC] *see* chlorpheniramine, phenylephrine, and dextromethorphan *on page 200*

sildenafil (sil DEN a fil)

Medication Safety Issues
Sound-alike/look-alike issues:
Revatio® may be confused with ReVia®, Revonto™
Sildenafil may be confused with silodosin, tadalafil, vardenafil
Viagra® may be confused with Allegra®, Vaniqa®

Synonyms sildenafil citrate; UK92480
U.S. Brand Names Revatio®; Viagra®
Canadian Brand Names ratio-Sildenafil R; Revatio®; Viagra®
Therapeutic Category Phosphodiesterase (Type 5) Enzyme Inhibitor
Use
Revatio®: Treatment of pulmonary arterial hypertension (PAH) (WHO Group I) to improve exercise ability and delay clinical worsening
Viagra®: Treatment of erectile dysfunction (ED)
General Dosage Range Dosage adjustment recommended in patients with hepatic or renal impairment or on concomitant therapy
I.V.: *Adults:* Revatio®: 10 mg 3 times/day
Oral:
Adults: Revatio®: 20 mg 3 times/day; Viagra®: 25-100 mg once daily
Elderly: Viagra®: Initial: 25 mg
Dosage Forms
Injection, solution:
Revatio®: 0.8 mg/mL (12.5 mL)
Tablet, oral:
Revatio®: 20 mg
Viagra®: 25 mg, 50 mg, 100 mg

sildenafil citrate *see* sildenafil *on page 811*
Silenor® *see* doxepin (systemic) *on page 309*
Silexin [OTC] *see* guaifenesin and dextromethorphan *on page 427*
Silfedrine Children's [OTC] *see* pseudoephedrine *on page 751*

silodosin (SI lo doe sin)

Medication Safety Issues
Sound-alike/look-alike issues:
Rapaflo™ may be confused with Rapamune®, Raptiva®
Silodosin may be confused with sildenafil

Synonyms KMD 3213
U.S. Brand Names Rapaflo®
Therapeutic Category Alpha₁ Blocker
Use Treatment of signs and symptoms of benign prostatic hyperplasia (BPH)
General Dosage Range Dosage adjustment recommended in patients with renal impairment
Oral: *Adults:* Males: 8 mg once daily

▶

◄ **Dosage Forms**
  Capsule, oral:
    Rapaflo®: 4 mg, 8 mg

Silphen [OTC] *see* diphenhydramine (systemic) *on page 290*
Silphen-DM [OTC] *see* dextromethorphan *on page 270*
Siltussin DAS [OTC] [DSC] *see* guaifenesin *on page 425*
Siltussin DM [OTC] *see* guaifenesin and dextromethorphan *on page 427*
Siltussin DM DAS [OTC] *see* guaifenesin and dextromethorphan *on page 427*
Siltussin SA [OTC] *see* guaifenesin *on page 425*
Silvadene® *see* silver sulfadiazine *on page 812*

silver nitrate (SIL ver NYE trate)

Synonyms AgNO$_3$
Therapeutic Category Topical Skin Product
Use Cauterization of wounds and sluggish ulcers, removal of granulation tissue and warts; aseptic prophylaxis of burns
General Dosage Range Topical: *Children and Adults:* Solution: Apply to affected area 2-3 times/day; Sticks: Apply to area to be treated 2-3 times/week
Dosage Forms
  Applicator sticks, topical: Silver nitrate 75% and potassium 25% (6", 12", 18")
  Solution, topical: 0.5% (960 mL); 10% (30 mL); 25% (30 mL); 50% (30 mL)

silver sulfadiazine (SIL ver sul fa DYE a zeen)

U.S. Brand Names Silvadene®; SSD AF®; SSD®; Thermazene®
Canadian Brand Names Flamazine®
Therapeutic Category Antibacterial, Topical
Use Prevention and treatment of infection in second and third degree burns
General Dosage Range Topical: *Children and Adults:* Apply to a thickness of 1/16" once or twice daily
Dosage Forms
  Cream, topical: 1% (20 g, 25 g, 50 g, 85 g, 400 g)
    Silvadene®: 1% (20 g, 50 g, 85 g, 400 g, 1000 g)
    SSD AF®: 1% (50 g, 400 g)
    SSD®: 1% (25 g, 50 g, 85 g, 400 g)
    Thermazene®: 1% (20 g, 50 g, 85 g, 400 g, 1000 g)

Simcor® *see* niacin and simvastatin *on page 623*

simethicone (sye METH i kone)

Medication Safety Issues
  Sound-alike/look-alike issues:
    Simethicone may be confused with cimetidine
    Mylanta® may be confused with Mynatal®
    Mylicon® may be confused with Modicon®, Myleran®
    Phazyme® may be confused with Pherazine®
Synonyms activated dimethicone; activated methylpolysiloxane
U.S. Brand Names Equalizer Gas Relief [OTC]; Gas Free Extra Strength [OTC]; Gas Relief Ultra Strength [OTC]; Gas-X® Children's Tongue Twisters™ [OTC]; Gas-X® Extra Strength [OTC]; Gas-X® Maximum Strength [OTC]; Gas-X® Thin Strips™ [OTC]; Gas-X® [OTC]; Gax-X® Infant [OTC]; Infantaire Gas [OTC]; Infants Gas Relief Drops [OTC]; Little Tummys® Gas Relief [OTC]; Mi-Acid Gas Relief [OTC]; Mylanta® Gas Maximum Strength [OTC]; Mylicon® Infants' [OTC]; Phazyme® Ultra Strength [OTC]
Canadian Brand Names Ovol®; Phazyme™
Therapeutic Category Antiflatulent
Use Postoperative gas pain or for use in endoscopic examination; relief of bloating, pressure, and discomfort of gas
General Dosage Range Oral:
  Infants and Children <2 years or <11 kg: 20 mg 4 times/day, as needed
  Children >2 years or >11 kg: 40 mg 4 times/day, as needed
  Children >12 years and Adults: 40-360 mg after meals and at bedtime, as needed

Dosage Forms

Capsule, softgel, oral:
Gas Free Extra Strength [OTC]: 125 mg
Gas Relief Ultra Strength [OTC]: 180 mg
Gas-X® Extra Strength [OTC]: 125 mg
Gas-X® Maximum Strength [OTC]: 166 mg
Mylanta® Gas Maximum Strength [OTC]: 125 mg
Phazyme® Ultra Strength [OTC]: 180 mg

Strip, orally disintegrating, oral:
Gas-X® Children's Tongue Twisters™ [OTC]: 40 mg (16s)
Gas-X® Thin Strips™ [OTC]: 62.5 mg (18s, 32s)

Suspension, oral: 40 mg/0.6 mL (30 mL)
Equalizer Gas Relief [OTC]: 40 mg/0.6 mL (30 mL)
Gax-X® Infant [OTC]: 40 mg/0.6 mL (30 mL)
Infantaire Gas [OTC]: 40 mg/0.6 mL (30 mL)
Infants Gas Relief Drops [OTC]: 40 mg/0.6 mL (30 mL)
Little Tummys® Gas Relief [OTC]: 40 mg/0.6 mL (30 mL, 45 mL)
Mylicon® Infants' [OTC]: 40 mg/0.6 mL (15 mL, 30 mL)

Tablet, chewable, oral: 80 mg, 125 mg
Gas-X® [OTC]: 80 mg
Gas-X® Extra Strength [OTC]: 125 mg
Mi-Acid Gas Relief [OTC]: 80 mg
Mylanta® Gas Maximum Strength [OTC]: 125 mg

simethicone, aluminum hydroxide, and magnesium hydroxide *see* aluminum hydroxide, magnesium hydroxide, and simethicone *on page 60*

simethicone and calcium carbonate *see* calcium carbonate and simethicone *on page 162*

simethicone and loperamide hydrochloride *see* loperamide and simethicone *on page 535*

simethicone and magaldrate *see* magaldrate and simethicone *on page 543*

Similac® Glucose [OTC] *see* dextrose *on page 273*

Simply Saline® [OTC] *see* sodium chloride *on page 818*

Simply Saline® Baby [OTC] *see* sodium chloride *on page 818*

Simply Saline® Nasal Moist® [OTC] *see* sodium chloride *on page 818*

Simply Sleep® [OTC] *see* diphenhydramine (systemic) *on page 290*

Simply Sleep® (Can) *see* diphenhydramine (systemic) *on page 290*

Simponi® *see* golimumab *on page 423*

Simuc-DM [DSC] *see* guaifenesin and dextromethorphan *on page 427*

Simulect® *see* basiliximab *on page 115*

simvastatin (sim va STAT in)

Medication Safety Issues
Sound-alike/look-alike issues:
Simvastatin may be confused with atorvastatin, nystatin, pitavastatin
Zocor® may be confused with Cozaar®, Lipitor®, Yocon®, Zoloft®, ZyrTEC®
International issues:
Cardin [Poland] may be confused with Cardem brand name for celiprolol [Spain]; Cardene brand name for nicardipine [U.S., Great Britain, Netherlands]

U.S. Brand Names Zocor®

Canadian Brand Names Apo-Simvastatin®; CO Simvastatin; Dom-Simvastatin; JAMP-Simvastatin; Mylan-Simvastatin; Nu-Simvastatin; PHL-Simvastatin; PMS-Simvastatin; RAN™-Simvastatin; ratio-Simvastatin; Riva-Simvastatin; Sandoz-Simvastatin; Taro-Simvastatin; Teva-Simvastatin; Zocor®; ZYM-Simvastatin

Therapeutic Category HMG-CoA Reductase Inhibitor

Use Used with dietary therapy for the following:
Secondary prevention of cardiovascular events in hypercholesterolemic patients with established coronary heart disease (CHD) or at high risk for CHD: To reduce cardiovascular morbidity (myocardial infarction, coronary/noncoronary revascularization procedures) and mortality; to reduce the risk of stroke

◀ Hyperlipidemias: To reduce elevations in total cholesterol (total-C), LDL-C, apolipoprotein B, triglycerides, and VLDL-C, and to increase HDL-C in patients with primary hypercholesterolemia (elevations of 1 or more components are present in Fredrickson type IIa, IIb, III, and IV hyperlipidemias); treatment of homozygous familial hypercholesterolemia

Heterozygous familial hypercholesterolemia (HeFH): In adolescent patients (10-17 years of age, females >1 year postmenarche) with HeFH having LDL-C ≥190 mg/dL **or** LDL-C ≥160 mg/dL with positive family history of premature cardiovascular disease (CVD), or 2 or more CVD risk factors in the adolescent patient

General Dosage Range Dosage adjustment recommended in patients with renal impairment or on concomitant therapy

Oral:

Children 10-17 years (females >1 year postmenarche): Initial: 10 mg once daily; Maintenance: 10-40 mg once daily (maximum: 40 mg/day)

Adults: Initial: 20-40 mg once daily; Maintenance: 5-40 mg once daily (maximum: 40 mg/day)

Dosage Forms

Tablet, oral: 5 mg, 10 mg, 20 mg, 40 mg, 80 mg

Zocor®: 5 mg, 10 mg, 20 mg, 40 mg, 80 mg

simvastatin and ezetimibe *see* ezetimibe and simvastatin *on page 364*

simvastatin and niacin *see* niacin and simvastatin *on page 623*

Sina-12X® [DSC] *see* guaifenesin and phenylephrine *on page 428*

sincalide (SIN ka lide)

Synonyms C8-CCK; OP-CCK

U.S. Brand Names Kinevac®

Therapeutic Category Diagnostic Agent

Use Postevacuation cholecystography; gallbladder bile sampling; stimulate pancreatic secretion for analysis; accelerate the transit of barium through the small bowel

General Dosage Range

I.M.: *Adults:* 0.1 mcg/kg

I.V.: *Adults:* 0.02-0.04 mcg/kg as a single dose; may repeat 0.04 mcg/kg once **or** 0.12 mcg/kg as a single dose

Dosage Forms

Injection, powder for reconstitution:

Kinevac®: 5 mcg

sinecatechins (sin e KAT e kins)

Synonyms catechins; green tea extract; kunecatechins; polyphenols; polyphenon E

U.S. Brand Names Veregen™

Therapeutic Category Immunomodulator, Topical; Topical Skin Product

Use Treatment of external genital and perianal warts secondary to *Condylomata acuminata*

General Dosage Range Topical: *Adults:* Apply a thin layer (~0.5 cm strand) 3 times/day

Dosage Forms

Ointment, topical:

Veregen™: 15% (15 g)

Sinemet® *see* carbidopa and levodopa *on page 174*

Sinemet® CR *see* carbidopa and levodopa *on page 174*

Sinequan® (Can) *see* doxepin (systemic) *on page 309*

Singulair® *see* montelukast *on page 597*

Sinografin® *see* diatrizoate meglumine and iodipamide meglumine *on page 275*

Sinus Pain & Pressure [OTC] *see* acetaminophen and phenylephrine *on page 28*

Sinutab® Non Drowsy (Can) *see* acetaminophen and pseudoephedrine *on page 29*

Sinutab® Sinus [OTC] *see* acetaminophen and phenylephrine *on page 28*

SINUtuss® DM [DSC] *see* guaifenesin, dextromethorphan, and phenylephrine *on page 429*

sipuleucel-T (si pu LOO sel tee)

Medication Safety Issues

Other safety concerns:

For autologous use only; patient identity must be matched to the patient identifiers on the infusion bag and on the "Cell Product Disposition Form" prior to infusion. Healthcare providers should apply universal precautions when handling both the initial leukapheresis product and the activated product.

Synonyms APC8015; prostate cancer vaccine, cell-based

U.S. Brand Names Provenge®

Therapeutic Category Cellular Immunotherapy, Autologous

Use Treatment of metastatic hormone-refractory prostate cancer in patients who are asymptomatic or minimally symptomatic

General Dosage Range I.V.: *Adults (males):* ≥50 million autologous CD54+ cells activated with PAP-GM-CSF; dose administered at ~2 week intervals for a total of 3 doses

Dosage Forms

Infusion, premixed in LR [preservative free]:

Provenge®: ≥50 million autologous CD54$^+$ cells activated with PAP-GM-CSF (250 mL)

Sirdalud® *see* tizanidine *on page 872*

sirolimus (sir OH li mus)

Medication Safety Issues

Sound-alike/look-alike issues:

Rapamune® may be confused with Rapaflo™

Sirolimus may be confused with everolimus, tacrolimus, temsirolimus

Synonyms rapamycin

U.S. Brand Names Rapamune®

Canadian Brand Names Rapamune®

Therapeutic Category Immunosuppressant Agent

Use Prophylaxis of organ rejection in patients receiving renal transplants

General Dosage Range Dosage adjustment recommended in patients with hepatic impairment

Oral:

Children ≥13 years and Adults <40 kg: Low-to-moderate immunologic risk: Loading dose: 3 mg/m^2 on day 1; Maintenance: 1 mg/m^2/day

Children ≥13 years and Adults ≥40 kg: Low-to-moderate immunologic risk: Loading dose: 6 mg on day 1; Maintenance: 2 mg/day (maximum: 40 mg/day)

Adults: High risk: Loading dose: Up to 15 mg on day 1; Maintenance: 5 mg/day (maximum: 40 mg/day)

Dosage Forms

Solution, oral:

Rapamune®: 1 mg/mL (60 mL)

Tablet, oral:

Rapamune®: 0.5 mg, 1 mg, 2 mg

sitagliptin (sit a GLIP tin)

Medication Safety Issues

Sound-alike/look-alike issues:

Januvia® may be confused with Enjuvia™, Janumet®, Jantoven™

SitaGLIPtin may be confused with saxagliptin, SUMAtriptan

Synonyms MK-0431; sitagliptin phosphate

Tall-Man sita**GLIP**tin

U.S. Brand Names Januvia®

Canadian Brand Names Januvia®

Therapeutic Category Antidiabetic Agent, Dipeptidyl Peptidase IV (DPP-IV) Inhibitor

Use Management of type 2 diabetes mellitus (noninsulin-dependent, NIDDM) as an adjunct to diet and exercise as monotherapy or in combination therapy with other antidiabetic agents

General Dosage Range Dosage adjustment recommended in patients with renal impairment

Oral: *Adults:* 100 mg once daily

▶

◀ **Dosage Forms**
Tablet, oral:
Januvia®: 25 mg, 50 mg, 100 mg

sitagliptin and metformin (sit a GLIP tin & met FOR min)

Medication Safety Issues
Sound-alike/look-alike issues:
Janumet® may be confused with Jantoven™, Januvia®

Synonyms metformin and sitagliptin; sitagliptin phosphate and metformin hydrochloride

U.S. Brand Names Janumet®

Canadian Brand Names Janumet®

Therapeutic Category Antidiabetic Agent, Biguanide; Antidiabetic Agent, Dipeptidyl Peptidase IV (DPP-IV) Inhibitor; Hypoglycemic Agent, Oral

Use Management of type 2 diabetes mellitus (noninsulin-dependent, NIDDM) as an adjunct to diet and exercise in patients not adequately controlled on metformin or sitagliptin monotherapy

General Dosage Range Oral: *Adults:* Sitagliptin 50 mg and metformin 500-1000 mg twice daily (maximum: 100 mg/day [sitagliptin], 2000 mg/day [metformin])

Dosage Forms
Tablet, oral:
Janumet®: 50/500: Sitagliptin 50 mg and metformin 500 mg; 50/1000: Sitagliptin 50 mg and metformin 1000 mg

Dosage Forms - Canada
Tablet, oral:
Janumet® 50/850: Sitagliptin 50 mg and metformin 850 mg

sitagliptin phosphate *see* sitagliptin *on page 815*
sitagliptin phosphate and metformin hydrochloride *see* sitagliptin and metformin *on page 816*

sitaxsentan *(Canada only)* (sye TACKS en tan)

Synonyms sitaxsentan sodium

Canadian Brand Names Thelin®

Therapeutic Category Endothelin Antagonist

Use Treatment of primary pulmonary arterial hypertension (PAH) or pulmonary hypertension secondary to connective tissue disease, in World Health Organization (WHO) class III patients unresponsive to conventional therapy; treatment of PAH in WHO class II patients who are unresponsive to conventional therapy and have no alternative treatment options

General Dosage Range Dosage adjustment recommended in patients who develop toxicities
Oral: *Adults:* 100 mg once daily

Product Availability Not available in U.S.

Dosage Forms - Canada
Tablet, oral:
Thelin™: 100 mg

sitaxsentan sodium *see* sitaxsentan *(Canada only) on page 816*
Skeeter Stik® [OTC] *see* benzocaine *on page 121*
Skelaxin® *see* metaxalone *on page 566*
Skelid® *see* tiludronate *on page 868*
SKF 104864 *see* topotecan *on page 878*
SKF 104864-A *see* topotecan *on page 878*
Skin Care™ [OTC] *see* pyrithione zinc *on page 759*
Sleep-ettes D [OTC] *see* diphenhydramine (systemic) *on page 290*
Sleepinal® [OTC] *see* diphenhydramine (systemic) *on page 290*
Sleep-Tabs [OTC] *see* diphenhydramine (systemic) *on page 290*
S-leucovorin *see* LEVOleucovorin *on page 521*
6S-leucovorin *see* LEVOleucovorin *on page 521*
Slo-Niacin® [OTC] *see* niacin *on page 622*
Slo-Pot (Can) *see* potassium chloride *on page 724*
Slow FE® [OTC] *see* ferrous sulfate *on page 374*

Slow-K® (Can) *see* potassium chloride *on page 724*
Slow-Mag® [OTC] *see* magnesium chloride *on page 544*
Slow Release [OTC] *see* ferrous sulfate *on page 374*
SM-13496 *see* lurasidone *on page 542*

smallpox vaccine (SMAL poks vak SEEN)

Synonyms live smallpox vaccine; vaccinia vaccine
U.S. Brand Names ACAM2000®
Therapeutic Category Vaccine
Use Active immunization against vaccinia virus, the causative agent of smallpox in persons determined to be at risk for smallpox infection.

The Advisory Committee on Immunization Practices (ACIP) recommends routine vaccination for the following:
• Laboratory workers at risk of exposure from cultures or contaminated animals which may be a source of vaccinia or related Orthopoxviruses capable of causing infections in humans (monkeypox, cowpox, or variola).
• Consideration may also be given for vaccination of healthcare workers having contact with clinical specimens, contaminated material, or patients receiving vaccinia or recombinant vaccinia viruses.
In a Pre-Event Vaccination Program, the ACIP recommends vaccination for the following:
• Persons designated by authorities to investigate smallpox cases with the likelihood of direct patient contact
• Persons responsible for administering smallpox vaccine
In the event of an intentional release of smallpox virus, the ACIP recommends vaccination for the following:
• Persons exposed to the initial release of the virus
• Persons who had close contact with a confirmed or suspected smallpox patient at any time from the onset of the patient's fever until all scabs have separated
• Healthcare providers involved in evaluation, care, or transport of confirmed or suspected smallpox patients
• Laboratory personnel involved in processing specimens of confirmed or suspected smallpox patients
• Persons likely to have increased contact with infectious materials from smallpox patients
General Dosage Range Percutaneous: *Children ≥12 months and Adults:* ACAM2000®: A single drop of vaccine suspension and 15 needle punctures into superficial skin for both primary vaccination and revaccination
Dosage Forms
Injection, powder for reconstitution [purified monkey cell source]:
ACAM2000®: 1-5 x 10^8 plaque-forming units per mL

smelling salts *see* ammonia spirit (aromatic) *on page 72*
SMX-TMP *see* sulfamethoxazole and trimethoprim *on page 836*
SMZ-TMP *see* sulfamethoxazole and trimethoprim *on page 836*
snake antivenin, FAB (ovine) *see* crotalidae polyvalent immune FAB (ovine) *on page 239*
(+)-(S)-N-methyl-γ-(1-naphthyloxy)-2-thiophenepropylamine hydrochloride *see* duloxetine *on page 316*
sodium 2-mercaptoethane sulfonate *see* mesna *on page 565*
sodium 4-hydroxybutyrate *see* sodium oxybate *on page 822*
sodium L-triiodothyronine *see* liothyronine *on page 529*

sodium acetate (SOW dee um AS e tate)

Therapeutic Category Alkalinizing Agent; Electrolyte Supplement, Oral
Use Sodium source in large volume I.V. fluids to prevent or correct hyponatremia in patients with restricted intake; used to counter acidosis through conversion to bicarbonate
General Dosage Range I.V.:
Children: TPN: 3-4 mEq/kg/24 hours
Adults: TPN: 3-4 mEq/kg/24 hours **or** 25-40 mEq/1000 kcal/24 hours (maximum: 100-150 mEq/24 hours)
Dosage Forms
Injection, solution [preservative free]: 2 mEq/mL (20 mL, 50 mL, 100 mL, 250 mL); 4 mEq/mL (50 mL, 100 mL)

sodium acid carbonate *see* sodium bicarbonate *on page 818*
sodium aurothiomalate *see* gold sodium thiomalate *on page 423*
sodium benzoate and caffeine *see* caffeine *on page 157*
sodium benzoate and sodium phenylacetate *see* sodium phenylacetate and sodium benzoate *on page 822*

sodium bicarbonate (SOW dee um bye KAR bun ate)

Synonyms baking soda; NaHCO$_3$; sodium acid carbonate; sodium hydrogen carbonate

U.S. Brand Names Brioschi® [OTC]; Neut®

Therapeutic Category Alkalinizing Agent; Antacid; Electrolyte Supplement, Oral

Use Management of metabolic acidosis; gastric hyperacidity; as an alkalinization agent for the urine; treatment of hyperkalemia; management of overdose of certain drugs, including tricyclic antidepressants and aspirin

General Dosage Range
I.V.: *Children and Adults:* Dosage varies greatly depending on indication
Oral:
Children: 1-10 mEq/kg/day as a single dose **or** divided every 4-6 hours
Adults <60 years: 0.5-200 mEq/kg/day in 4-5 divided doses **or** 325 mg to 2 g 1-4 times/day (maximum: 16 g [200 mEq] day)
Adults ≥60 years: 0.5-100 mEq/kg/day in 4-6 divided doses **or** 325 mg to 2 g 1-4 times/day (maximum: 8 g [100 mEq] day)

Dosage Forms
Granules for solution, oral:
Brioschi® [OTC]: 2.69 g/capful (120 g, 240 g); 2.69 g/packet (12s)
Injection, solution: 4.2% (10 mL); 8.4% (10 mL, 50 mL, 250 mL, 500 mL)
Neut®: 4% (5 mL)
Injection, solution [preservative free]: 4.2% (5 mL, 10 mL); 7.5% (50 mL); 8.4% (10 mL, 50 mL)
Powder, oral: USP: 100% (120 g, 454 g, 480 g)
Tablet, oral: 325 mg, 650 mg

sodium bicarbonate and omeprazole *see* omeprazole and sodium bicarbonate *on page 650*

sodium chloride (SOW dee um KLOR ide)

Medication Safety Issues
High alert medication:
The Institute for Safe Medication Practices (ISMP) includes this medication (I.V. formulation >0.9% concentration) among its list of drugs which have a heightened risk of causing significant patient harm when used in error.
Other safety concerns:
Per The Joint Commission (TJC) recommendations, concentrated electrolyte solutions (eg, NaCl >0.9%) should not be available in patient care areas.

Inappropriate use of low sodium or sodium-free intravenous fluids (eg, D$_5$W, hypotonic saline) in pediatric patients can lead to significant morbidity and mortality due to hyponatremia (ISMP, 2009).

Synonyms hypertonic saline; NaCl; normal saline; saline; salt

U.S. Brand Names 4-Way® Saline Moisturizing Mist [OTC]; Altachlore [OTC]; Altamist [OTC]; Ayr® Allergy Sinus [OTC]; Ayr® Baby Saline [OTC]; Ayr® Saline No-Drip [OTC]; Ayr® Saline [OTC]; Breathe Free® [OTC]; Deep Sea [OTC]; Entsol® [OTC]; HuMist® for Kids [OTC]; HuMist® [OTC]; Hyper-Sal™; Little Noses® Saline [OTC]; Little Noses® Stuffy Nose Kit [OTC]; Muro 128® [OTC]; Na-Zone® [OTC]; Nasal Moist® Saline [OTC]; Nasal Spray [OTC] [DSC]; NāSal™ [OTC]; Ocean® for Kids [OTC]; Ocean® [OTC]; Pretz® [OTC]; Rhinaris® [OTC]; Saline Mist [OTC]; Simply Saline® Baby [OTC]; Simply Saline® Nasal Moist [OTC]; Simply Saline® [OTC]; Syrex; Wound Wash Saline™ [OTC]

Therapeutic Category Electrolyte Supplement, Oral; Lubricant, Ocular

Use
Parenteral: Restores sodium ion in patients with restricted oral intake (especially hyponatremia states or low salt syndrome).
Concentrated sodium chloride: Additive for parenteral fluid therapy
Hypertonic sodium chloride: For severe hyponatremia and hypochloremia
Hypotonic sodium chloride: Hydrating solution
Normal saline: Restores water/sodium losses
Ophthalmic: Reduces corneal edema

Inhalation: Restores moisture to pulmonary system; loosens and thins congestion caused by colds or allergies; diluent for bronchodilator solutions that require dilution before inhalation
Intranasal: Restores moisture to nasal membranes
Irrigation: Wound cleansing, irrigation, and flushing

General Dosage Range

I.V.: *Children and Adults:* Dosage varies greatly depending on indication
Inhalation: *Children ≥2 years and Adults:* 1-3 sprays (1-3 mL)
Intranasal: *Children ≥2 years and Adults:* 2-3 sprays in each nostril as needed
Irrigation: *Children ≥2 years and Adults:* 1-3 L/day **or** spray affected area
Ophthalmic: *Adults:* Ointment: Apply once or more daily; Solution: Instill 1-2 drops into affected eye(s) every 3-4 hours

Dosage Forms

Aerosol, intranasal [preservative free]:
Entsol® [OTC]: 3% (100 mL)
Gel, intranasal:
Ayr® Saline [OTC]: < 0.5% (14 g)
Ayr® Saline No-Drip [OTC]: < 0.5% (22 mL)
Entsol® [OTC]: 3% (20 g)
Rhinaris® [OTC]: 0.2% (28.4 g)
Simply Saline® Nasal Moist® [OTC]: 0.65% (30 g)
Injection, solution: 0.45% (25 mL, 50 mL, 100 mL, 250 mL, 500 mL, 1000 mL); 0.9% (10 mL, 20 mL, 25 mL, 30 mL, 50 mL, 100 mL, 150 mL, 250 mL, 500 mL, 1000 mL, 1s); 3% (500 mL); 5% (500 mL); 14.6% (20 mL, 40 mL, 250 mL); 23.4% (50 mL, 100 mL, 250 mL)
Injection, solution [preservative free]: 0.9% (1 mL, 2 mL, 2.5 mL, 3 mL, 5 mL, 6 mL, 10 mL, 20 mL, 50 mL, 100 mL, 125 mL); 14.6% (20 mL, 40 mL); 23.4% (30 mL, 100 mL, 200 mL)
Syrex: 0.9% (2.5 mL, 3 mL, 5 mL, 10 mL)
Ointment, ophthalmic: 5% (3.5 g)
Altachlore [OTC]: 5% (3.5 g)
Ointment, ophthalmic [preservative free]:
Muro 128® [OTC]: 5% (3.5 g)
Powder for solution, intranasal [preservative free]:
Entsol® [OTC]: 3% (10s)
Pretz® [OTC]: 1 teaspoon/dose (360 g)
Solution, for blood processing: 0.9% (3000 mL)
Solution, for inhalation [preservative free]: 0.9% (3 mL, 5 mL, 15 mL); 3% (15 mL); 10% (15 mL)
Solution, for irrigation: 0.9% (250 mL, 500 mL, 1000 mL, 1500 mL, 2000 mL, 3000 mL, 4000 mL, 5000 mL)
Solution, for irrigation [preservative free]: 0.9% (250 mL, 500 mL, 1000 mL, 1500 mL, 2000 mL, 3000 mL)
Solution, for nebulization [preservative free]:
Hyper-Sal™: 7% (4 mL)
Solution, intranasal: 0.65% (45 mL, 88 mL)
4-Way® Saline Moisturizing Mist [OTC]: 0.74% (29.6 mL)
Altamist [OTC]: 0.65% (60 mL)
Ayr® Allergy Sinus [OTC]: 2.65% (50 mL)
Ayr® Baby Saline [OTC]: 0.65% (30 mL)
Ayr® Saline [OTC]: 0.65% (50 mL)
Breathe Free® [OTC]: 0.65% (44.3 mL)
Deep Sea [OTC]: 0.65% (45 mL)
Entsol® [OTC]: 3% (30 mL)
HuMist® [OTC]: 0.65% (45 mL)
HuMist® for Kids [OTC]: 0.65% (30 mL)
Little Noses® Saline [OTC]: 0.65% (30 mL)
Little Noses® Stuffy Nose Kit [OTC]: 0.65% (15 mL)
Na-Zone® [OTC]: 0.65% (60 mL)
Nasal Moist® Saline [OTC]: 0.65% (45 mL)
NāSal™ [OTC]: 0.65% (30 mL)
Ocean® [OTC]: 0.65% (45 mL, 473 mL)
Ocean® for Kids [OTC]: 0.65% (37.5 mL)
Pretz® [OTC]: 0.75% (50 mL, 960 mL)
Rhinaris® [OTC]: 0.2% (30 mL)
Saline Mist [OTC]: 0.65% (45 mL)

◀ **Solution, intranasal** [preservative free]:
Entsol® [OTC]: 3% (240 mL)
Pretz® [OTC]: 0.75% (20 mL)
Simply Saline® [OTC]: 0.9% (44 mL, 90 mL); 3% (44 mL)
Simply Saline® Baby [OTC]: 0.9% (45 mL)
Solution, ophthalmic: 5% (15 mL)
Altachlore [OTC]: 5% (15 mL, 30 mL)
Muro 128® [OTC]: 2% (15 mL); 5% (15 mL, 30 mL)
Solution, topical [preservative free]:
Wound Wash Saline™ [OTC]: 0.9% (90 mL, 210 mL)
Swab, intranasal:
Ayr® Saline [OTC]: <0.5% (20s)
Tablet, oral: 1 g
Tablet for solution, topical: 1000 mg

sodium chondroitin sulfate and sodium hyaluronate
(SOW de um kon DROY tin SUL fate & SOW de um hye al yoor ON ate)
Synonyms chondroitin sulfate and sodium hyaluronate; sodium hyaluronate and chondroitin sulfate
U.S. Brand Names DisCoVisc®; Viscoat®
Therapeutic Category Ophthalmic Agent, Viscoelastic
Use Ophthalmic surgical aid in the anterior segment during cataract extraction and intraocular lens implantation
General Dosage Range Ophthalmic: *Adults:* Carefully introduce into anterior chamber during surgery
Dosage Forms
Injection, solution, intraocular:
DisCoVisc®: Sodium chondroitin sulfate ≤4% and sodium hyaluronate ≤1.7% (0.5 mL, 1 mL)
Viscoat®: Sodium chondroitin sulfate ≤4% and sodium hyaluronate ≤3% (0.5 mL, 0.75 mL)

sodium citrate, citric acid, and potassium citrate *see* citric acid, sodium citrate, and potassium citrate *on page 214*
Sodium Diuril® *see* chlorothiazide *on page 197*
Sodium Edecrin® *see* ethacrynic acid *on page 350*
sodium etidronate *see* etidronate *on page 359*
sodium ferric gluconate *see* ferric gluconate *on page 372*
sodium fluorescein *see* fluorescein *on page 386*
sodium fluoride *see* fluoride *on page 386*
sodium fusidate *see* fusidic acid *(Canada only) on page 405*
sodium hyaluronate *see* hyaluronate and derivatives *on page 443*
sodium hyaluronate and chondroitin sulfate *see* sodium chondroitin sulfate and sodium hyaluronate *on page 820*
sodium hydrogen carbonate *see* sodium bicarbonate *on page 818*

sodium hypochlorite solution (SOW dee um hye poe KLOR ite soe LOO shun)
Medication Safety Issues
Administration issues:
A potential for confusion associated with labeling of strengths for Dakin's solution manufactured by Century Pharmaceuticals exists. The labels list strengths as full strength at 0.5%, half strength at 0.25%, and quarter strength at 0.125%. This terminology is confusing to healthcare providers who consider half strength and quarter strength to correspond to 0.5% and 0.25%, respectively. Of note, most hospitals use a modified Dakin's solution of 0.025% for wound care; studies have suggested that concentrations of Dakin's solution >0.025% may potentially be harmful for wound healing.
Synonyms modified Dakin's solution
U.S. Brand Names Dakin's Solution; Di-Dak-Sol
Therapeutic Category Disinfectant
Use Treatment of athlete's foot (0.5%); wound irrigation (0.5%); disinfection of utensils and equipment (5%)
General Dosage Range Topical: *Children and Adults:* Via irrigation: Lightly-to-moderately exudative wounds: Apply once daily; Highly exudative or contaminated wounds: Apply twice daily

Dosage Forms
 Solution, topical:
  Dakin's Solution: 0.125% (473 mL); 0.25% (473 mL); 0.5% (473 mL)
  Di-Dak-Sol: 0.0125% (473 mL)

sodium hyposulfate *see* sodium thiosulfate *on page 824*

sodium lactate (SOW dee um LAK tate)

Therapeutic Category Alkalinizing Agent
Use Source of bicarbonate for prevention and treatment of mild-to-moderate metabolic acidosis
General Dosage Range I.V.: *Adults:* Dosage depends on degree of acidosis
Dosage Forms
 Injection, solution [preservative free]: 560 mg/mL (10 mL)

sodium nafcillin *see* nafcillin *on page 609*

sodium nitrite and sodium thiosulfate
(SOW dee um NYE trite & SOW dee um thye oh SUL fate)

Synonyms sodium thiosulfate and sodium nitrite
U.S. Brand Names Nithiodote™
Therapeutic Category Antidote
Use Acute, life-threatening cyanide poisoning
General Dosage Range
 I.V.:
  Children:
   Sodium nitrite: 6 mg/kg (0.2 mL/kg or 6-8 mL/m^2 of a 3% solution); maximum: 300 mg (10 mL of a 3% solution)
   Sodium thiosulfate: 7 g/m^2 or 250 mg/kg (1 mL/kg or 28-40 mL/m^2 of a 25% solution); maximum: 12.5 g (50 mL of a 25% solution)
  Adults:
   Sodium nitrite: 300 mg (10 mL of a 3% solution)
   Sodium thiosulfate: 12.5 g (50 mL of a 25% solution)
Dosage Forms
 Injection, solution [combination package]:
  Nithiodote™: Sodium nitrite 300 mg/10 mL (10 mL) and sodium thiosulfate 12.5 g/50 mL (50 mL)

sodium nitrite, sodium thiosulfate, and amyl nitrite
(SOW dee um NYE trite, SOW dee um thye oh SUL fate, & AM il NYE trite)

Synonyms amyl nitrite, sodium nitrite, and sodium thiosulfate; cyanide antidote kit; sodium thiosulfate, sodium nitrite, and amyl nitrite
U.S. Brand Names Cyanide Antidote Package
Therapeutic Category Antidote
Use Treatment of cyanide poisoning
General Dosage Range
 I.V.:
  Sodium nitrite: Prior to sodium thiosulfate:
   Children: 6 mg/kg (0.2 mL/kg or 6-8 mL/m^2 of a 3% solution [maximum: 10 mL]); may repeat at $1/2$ the original dose if needed
   Adults: 300 mg (10 mL of a 3% solution); may repeat at $1/2$ the original dose if needed
  Sodium thiosulfate: Given after sodium nitrite:
   Children: 7 g/m^2 (maximum: 12.5 g) over ~10 minutes; may repeat at $1/2$ the original dose if needed
   Adults: 12.5 g over ~10 minutes; may repeat at $1/2$ the original dose if needed
  Inhalation: Amyl nitrite: *Children and Adults:* 0.3 mL ampul crushed every minute and vapor inhaled for 15-30 seconds until I.V. sodium nitrite infusion available
Dosage Forms Kit [each kit contains]:
 Cyanide Antidote Package:
  Injection, solution:
   Sodium nitrite 300 mg/10 mL (2)
   Sodium thiosulfate 12.5 g/50 mL (2)
  Inhalant: Amyl nitrite 0.3 mL (12)

sodium nitroferricyanide *see* nitroprusside *on page 630*
sodium nitroprusside *see* nitroprusside *on page 630*

sodium oxybate (SOW dee um ox i BATE)

Synonyms 4-hydroxybutyrate; gamma hydroxybutyric acid; GHB; oxybate; sodium 4-hydroxybutyrate
U.S. Brand Names Xyrem®
Canadian Brand Names Xyrem®
Therapeutic Category Central Nervous System Depressant
Controlled Substance C-I (illicit use); C-III (medical use)
Use Treatment of cataplexy and daytime sleepiness in patients with narcolepsy
General Dosage Range Dosage adjustment recommended in patients with hepatic impairment
  Oral: *Children ≥16 years and Adults:* Initial: 4.5 g/day in 2 equal doses given at bedtime and 2.5-4 hours later; Maintenance: 4.5-9 g/day (maximum: 9 g/day)
Dosage Forms
  Solution, oral:
  Xyrem®: 500 mg/mL (180 mL)

sodium PAS *see* aminosalicylic acid *on page 67*
sodium-PCA and lactic acid *see* lactic acid *on page 506*

sodium phenylacetate and sodium benzoate
(SOW dee um fen il AS e tate & SOW dee um BENZ oh ate)
Synonyms NAPA and NABZ; sodium benzoate and sodium phenylacetate
U.S. Brand Names Ammonul®
Therapeutic Category Ammonium Detoxicant
Use Adjunct to treatment of acute hyperammonemia and encephalopathy in patients with urea cycle disorders involving partial or complete deficiencies of carbamyl-phosphate synthetase (CPS), ornithine transcarbamoylase (OTC), argininosuccinate lysase (ASL), or argininosuccinate synthetase (ASS); for use with hemodialysis in acute neonatal hyperammonemic coma, moderate-to-severe hyperammonemic encephalopathy and hyperammonemia which fails to respond to initial therapy
General Dosage Range I.V.:
  Children ≤20 kg: Loading dose: Ammonul® 2.5 mL/kg (sodium phenylacetate 250 mg/kg and sodium benzoate 250 mg/kg); Maintenance: Repeat same loading dose over 24 hours
  Children >20 kg and Adults: Loading dose: Ammonul® 55 mL/m^2 (sodium phenylacetate 5.5 g/m^2 and sodium benzoate 5.5 g/m^2); Maintenance: Repeat same loading dose over 24 hours
Dosage Forms
  Injection, solution [concentrate]:
  Ammonul®: Sodium phenylacetate 100 mg and sodium benzoate 100 mg per 1 mL (50 mL)

sodium phenylbutyrate (SOW dee um fen il BYOO ti rate)
Synonyms ammonapse
U.S. Brand Names Buphenyl®
Therapeutic Category Miscellaneous Product
Use Adjunctive therapy in the chronic management of patients with urea cycle disorder involving deficiencies of carbamoylphosphate synthetase, ornithine transcarbamylase, or argininosuccinic acid synthetase
General Dosage Range Oral:
  Children <20 kg: Powder: 450-600 mg/kg/day administered in equally divided amounts with each meal or feeding, 3-6 times daily (maximum: 20 g/day)
  Children ≥20 kg and Adults: 9.9-13 g/m^2/day, administered in equally divided amounts with each meal, 3-6 times daily (maximum: 20 g/day)
Dosage Forms
  Powder for solution, oral:
  Buphenyl®: (250 g)
  Tablet, oral:
  Buphenyl®: 500 mg

sodium phosphate and potassium phosphate *see* potassium phosphate and sodium phosphate *on page 727*

sodium phosphates (SOW dee um FOS fates)

Medication Safety Issues

Sound-alike/look-alike issues:

Visicol® may be confused with Asacol®, VESIcare®

Administration issues:

Enemas and oral solution are available in pediatric and adult sizes; prescribe by "volume" not by "bottle."

Because inorganic phosphate exists as monobasic and dibasic anions, with the mixture of valences dependent on pH, ordering by mEq amounts is unreliable and may lead to large dosing errors. In addition, I.V. phosphate is available in the sodium and potassium salt; therefore, the content of these cations must be considered when ordering phosphate. The most reliable method of ordering I.V. phosphate is by millimoles, then specifying the potassium or sodium salt.

Synonyms phosphates, sodium

U.S. Brand Names Fleet® Enema Extra® [OTC]; Fleet® Enema [OTC]; Fleet® Pedia-Lax™ Enema [OTC]; Fleet® Phospho-soda® EZ-Prep™ [OTC] [DSC]; Fleet® Phospho-soda® [OTC] [DSC]; LaCrosse Complete [OTC]; OsmoPrep®; Visicol®

Canadian Brand Names Fleet Enema®

Therapeutic Category Electrolyte Supplement, Oral; Laxative

Use

Oral, rectal: Short-term treatment of constipation and to evacuate the colon for rectal and bowel exams

I.V.: Source of phosphate in large volume I.V. fluids and parenteral nutrition; treatment and prevention of hypophosphatemia

General Dosage Range

I.V.:

Children: 0.08-1 mmol phosphate/kg **or** Parenteral nutrition infusion: 0.5-2 mmol/kg/24 hours

Adults: 0.08-1 mmol phosphate/kg **or** Parenteral nutrition: Infusion: 20-40 mmol/24 hours

Oral: Solution: Fleet® Phospho-Soda®

Children 5-9 years: 7.5 mL as a single dose (maximum daily dose: 7.5 mL)

Children 10-12 years: 15 mL as a single dose (maximum daily dose: 15 mL)

Children ≥12 years and Adults: 15 mL as a single dose (maximum daily dose: 45 mL)

Rectal:

Children 2-<5 years: One-half contents of one 2.25 oz pediatric enema

Children 5-12 years: Contents of one 2.25 oz pediatric enema; may repeat

Children ≥12 years and Adults: Contents of one 4.5-ounce enema as a single dose; may repeat

Dosage Forms

Injection, solution [concentrate; preservative free]: Phosphorus 3 mmol and sodium 4 mEq per 1 mL (5 mL, 15 mL, 50 mL)

Solution, oral: Monobasic sodium phosphate 2.4 g and dibasic sodium phosphate 0.9 g per 5 mL (45 mL)

Solution, rectal [enema]: Monobasic sodium phosphate 19 g and dibasic sodium phosphate 7 g per 118 mL delivered dose (133 mL)

Fleet® Enema [OTC], LaCrosse Complete [OTC]: Monobasic sodium phosphate 19 g and dibasic sodium phosphate 7 g per 118 mL delivered dose (133 mL)

Fleet® Enema Extra® [OTC]: Monobasic sodium phosphate 19 g and dibasic sodium phosphate 7 g per 197 mL delivered dose (230 mL)

Fleet® Pedia-Lax™ Enema [OTC]: Monobasic sodium phosphate 9.5 g and dibasic sodium phosphate 3.5 g per 59 mL delivered dose (66 mL)

Tablet, oral [scored]:

OsmoPrep®, Visicol®: Monobasic sodium phosphate 1.102 g and dibasic sodium phosphate 0.398 g

sodium polystyrene sulfonate (SOW dee um pol ee STYE reen SUL fon ate)

Medication Safety Issues

Sound-alike/look-alike issues:

Kayexalate® may be confused with Kaopectate®

Sodium polystyrene sulfonate may be confused with calcium polystyrene sulfonate

Administration issues:

Always prescribe either one-time doses or as a specific number of doses (eg, 15 g q6h x 2 doses). Scheduled doses with no dosage limit could be given for days leading to dangerous hypokalemia.

International issues:

Kionex [U.S.] may be confused with Kinex brand name for biperiden [Mexico]

◀ **U.S. Brand Names** Kalexate; Kayexalate®; Kionex®; SPS®

Canadian Brand Names Kayexalate®; PMS-Sodium Polystyrene Sulfonate

Therapeutic Category Antidote

Use Treatment of hyperkalemia

General Dosage Range

Oral:
  Children: 1 g/kg/dose every 6 hours
  Adults: 15 g 1-4 times/day

Rectal:
  Children: 1 g/kg/dose every 2-6 hours
  Adults: 30-50 g every 6 hours

Dosage Forms

Powder for suspension, oral/rectal: (454 g)
  Kalexate: (454 g)
  Kayexalate®: (454 g)
  Kionex®: (454 g)

Suspension, oral/rectal:
  Kionex®: 15 g/60 mL (60 mL, 480 mL)
  SPS®: 15 g/60 mL (60 mL, 120 mL, 473 mL)

Sodium Sulamyd (Can) *see* sulfacetamide (ophthalmic) *on page 835*

sodium sulfacetamide *see* sulfacetamide (ophthalmic) *on page 835*

sodium sulfacetamide *see* sulfacetamide (topical) *on page 835*

sodium sulfacetamide and sulfur *see* sulfur and sulfacetamide *on page 838*

sodium sulfate, magnesium sulfate, and potassium sulfate *see* sodium sulfate, potassium sulfate, and magnesium sulfate *on page 824*

sodium sulfate, potassium sulfate, and magnesium sulfate

(SOW dee um SUL fate, poe TASS ee um SUL fate, & mag NEE zhum SUL fate)

Synonyms magnesium sulfate, potassium sulfate, and sodium sulfate; magnesium sulfate, sodium sulfate, and potassium sulfate; potassium sulfate, magnesium sulfate, and sodium sulfate; potassium sulfate, sodium sulfate, and magnesium sulfate; sodium sulfate, magnesium sulfate, and potassium sulfate

U.S. Brand Names Suprep® Bowel Prep Kit

Therapeutic Category Laxative, Osmotic

Use Bowel cleansing prior to GI examination

General Dosage Range Oral: *Adults:* Contents of 2 bottles diluted as directed prior to colonoscopy; total volume of liquid to be consumed over the course of treatment: 2880 mL

Dosage Forms

Solution, oral:
  Suprep® Bowel Prep Kit: Sodium sulfate 17.5 g, potassium sulfate 3.13 g, and magnesium sulfate 1.6 g per 180 mL (180 mL) [contains sodium benzoate]

sodium tetradecyl (SOW dee um tetra DEK il)

Synonyms sodium tetradecyl sulfate

U.S. Brand Names Sotradecol®

Canadian Brand Names Trombovar®

Therapeutic Category Sclerosing Agent

Use Treatment of small, uncomplicated varicose veins of the lower extremities

General Dosage Range I.V.: *Adults:* 0.5-2 mL in each vein (maximum: 10 mL per treatment session)

Dosage Forms

Injection, solution:
  Sotradecol®: 1% (2 mL); 3% (2 mL)

sodium tetradecyl sulfate *see* sodium tetradecyl *on page 824*

sodium thiosulfate (SOW dee um thye oh SUL fate)

Synonyms disodium thiosulfate pentahydrate; pentahydrate; sodium hyposulfate; sodium thiosulphate; thiosulfuric acid disodium salt

U.S. Brand Names Versiclear™
Therapeutic Category Antidote; Antifungal Agent
Use
Parenteral: Used alone or with sodium nitrite or amyl nitrite in cyanide poisoning; reduce the risk of nephrotoxicity associated with cisplatin therapy; treatment of cyanide poisoning due to nitroprusside
Topical: Treatment of tinea versicolor
General Dosage Range
I.V.:
Children: 7 g/m^2 (maximum dose: 12.5 g) given over 10 minutes; may repeat at ^{1}/$_2$ the original dose if symptoms return **or** 12 g/m^2 over 6 hours or 9 g/m^2 I.V. push followed by 1.2 g/m^2 continuous infusion for 6 hours
Adults: 12.5 g; may repeat at half dose if needed **or** 0.95-1.95 mL/kg (maximum: 50 mL) **or** 12 g/m^2 over 6 hours or 9 g/m^2 I.V. push followed by 1.2 g/m^2 continuous infusion for 6 hours
Topical: *Children and Adults:* Apply a thin layer (20% to 25%) to affected areas twice daily
Dosage Forms
Injection, solution [preservative free]: 100 mg/mL (10 mL); 250 mg/mL (50 mL)
Lotion:
Versiclear™: Sodium thiosulfate 25% and salicylic acid 1% (120 mL)

sodium thiosulfate and sodium nitrite *see* sodium nitrite and sodium thiosulfate *on page 821*
sodium thiosulfate, sodium nitrite, and amyl nitrite *see* sodium nitrite, sodium thiosulfate, and amyl nitrite *on page 821*
sodium thiosulphate *see* sodium thiosulfate *on page 824*
Soflax™ (Can) *see* docusate *on page 302*
Sojourn™ *see* sevoflurane *on page 810*
Sojourn Sevoflurane (Can) *see* sevoflurane *on page 810*
Solagé® [DSC] *see* mequinol and tretinoin *on page 563*
Solagé® (Can) *see* mequinol and tretinoin *on page 563*
Solaquin® (Can) *see* hydroquinone *on page 453*
Solaquin Forte® (Can) *see* hydroquinone *on page 453*
Solaraze® *see* diclofenac (topical) *on page 279*
Solarcaine® cool aloe Burn Relief [OTC] *see* lidocaine (topical) *on page 524*
Solia® [DSC] *see* ethinyl estradiol and desogestrel *on page 351*

solifenacin (sol i FEN a sin)

Medication Safety Issues
Sound-alike/look-alike issues:
VESIcare® may be confused with Vesinoid®,Visicol®
Synonyms solifenacin succinate; YM905
U.S. Brand Names VESIcare®
Therapeutic Category Anticholinergic Agent
Use Treatment of overactive bladder with symptoms of urinary frequency, urgency, or urge incontinence
General Dosage Range Dosage adjustment recommended in patients with hepatic or renal impairment and on concomitant therapy
Oral: *Adults:* 5-10 mg/day
Dosage Forms
Tablet, oral:
VESIcare®: 5 mg, 10 mg

solifenacin succinate *see* solifenacin *on page 825*
Soliris® *see* eculizumab *on page 319*
Solodyn® *see* minocycline *on page 590*
Soluble Fiber Therapy [OTC] *see* methylcellulose *on page 574*
soluble fluorescein *see* fluorescein *on page 386*
Solu-CORTEF® *see* hydrocortisone (systemic) *on page 449*
Solu-Cortef® (Can) *see* hydrocortisone (systemic) *on page 449*
Solugel® (Can) *see* benzoyl peroxide *on page 124*
Solumedrol *see* methylprednisolone *on page 578*

Solu-MEDROL® *see* methylprednisolone *on page 578*

Solu-Medrol® (Can) *see* methylprednisolone *on page 578*

Soluver® (Can) *see* salicylic acid *on page 795*

Soluver® Plus (Can) *see* salicylic acid *on page 795*

Solzira *see* gabapentin enacarbil *on page 406*

Soma® *see* carisoprodol *on page 176*

Soma® Compound *see* carisoprodol and aspirin *on page 177*

soma compound w/codeine *see* carisoprodol, aspirin, and codeine *on page 177*

somatropin (soe ma TROE pin)

Medication Safety Issues

Sound-alike/look-alike issues:

Humatrope® may be confused with homatropine

Somatrem may be confused with somatropin

Somatropin may be confused with homatropine, somatrem, sumatriptan

Synonyms growth hormone, human; hGH; human growth hormone

U.S. Brand Names Genotropin Miniquick®; Genotropin®; Humatrope®; Norditropin FlexPro®; Norditropin® NordiFlex®; Norditropin® [DSC]; Nutropin AQ Pen®; Nutropin AQ®; Nutropin AQ® NuSpin™; Nutropin®; Omnitrope®; Saizen®; Serostim®; Tev-Tropin®; Zorbtive®

Canadian Brand Names Humatrope®; Nutropin®; Nutropin® AQ; Omnitrope®; Saizen®; Serostim®

Therapeutic Category Growth Hormone

Use

Children:

Treatment of growth failure due to inadequate endogenous growth hormone secretion (Genotropin®, Humatrope®, Norditropin®, Nutropin®, Nutropin AQ®, Omnitrope®, Saizen®, Tev-Tropin®)

Treatment of short stature associated with Turner syndrome (Genotropin®, Humatrope®, Norditropin®, Nutropin®, Nutropin AQ®, Omnitrope®)

Treatment of Prader-Willi syndrome (Genotropin®, Omnitrope®)

Treatment of growth failure associated with chronic renal insufficiency (CRI) up until the time of renal transplantation (Nutropin®, Nutropin AQ®)

Treatment of growth failure in children born small for gestational age who fail to manifest catch-up growth by 2 years of age (Genotropin®, Omnitrope®) or by 2-4 years of age (Humatrope®, Norditropin®)

Treatment of idiopathic short stature (nongrowth hormone-deficient short stature) defined by height standard deviation score (SDS) ≤-2.25 and growth rate not likely to attain normal adult height (Genotropin®, Humatrope®, Nutropin®, Nutropin AQ®, Omnitrope®)

Treatment of short stature or growth failure associated with short stature homeobox gene (SHOX) deficiency (Humatrope®)

Treatment of short stature associated with Noonan syndrome (Norditropin®)

Adults:

HIV patients with wasting or cachexia with concomitant antiviral therapy (Serostim®)

Replacement of endogenous growth hormone in patients with adult growth hormone deficiency who meet both of the following criteria (Genotropin®, Humatrope®, Norditropin®, Nutropin®, Nutropin AQ®, Omnitrope®, Saizen®):

Biochemical diagnosis of adult growth hormone deficiency by means of a subnormal response to a standard growth hormone stimulation test (peak growth hormone ≤5 mcg/L). Confirmatory testing may not be required in patients with congenital/genetic growth hormone deficiency or multiple pituitary hormone deficiencies due to organic diseases.

and

Adult-onset: Patients who have adult growth hormone deficiency whether alone or with multiple hormone deficiencies (hypopituitarism) as a result of pituitary disease, hypothalamic disease, surgery, radiation therapy, or trauma

or

Childhood-onset: Patients who were growth hormone deficient during childhood, confirmed as an adult before replacement therapy is initiated

Treatment of short-bowel syndrome (Zorbtive®)

General Dosage Range I.M., SubQ: *Children and Adults:* Dosage varies greatly depending on indication

Dosage Forms
Injection, powder for reconstitution:
Genotropin®: 5.8 mg, 13.8 mg
Humatrope®: 5 mg, 6 mg, 12 mg, 24 mg
Nutropin®: 5 mg, 10 mg
Omnitrope®: 5.8 mg
Saizen®: 5 mg, 8.8 mg
Serostim®: 4 mg, 5 mg, 6 mg
Tev-Tropin®: 5 mg
Zorbtive®: 8.8 mg
Injection, powder for reconstitution [preservative free]:
Genotropin Miniquick®: 0.2 mg, 0.4 mg, 0.6 mg, 0.8 mg, 1 mg, 1.2 mg, 1.4 mg, 1.6 mg, 1.8 mg, 2 mg
Injection, solution:
Norditropin FlexPro®: 5 mg/1.5 mL (1.5 mL); 10 mg/1.5 mL (1.5 mL); 15 mg/1.5 mL (1.5 mL)
Norditropin® NordiFlex®: 30 mg/3 mL (3 mL)
Nutropin AQ Pen®: 10 mg/2 mL (2 mL); 20 mg/2 mL (2 mL)
Nutropin AQ®: 10 mg/2 mL (2 mL)
Nutropin AQ® NuSpin™: 5 mg/2 mL (2 mL); 10 mg/2 mL (2 mL); 20 mg/2 mL (2 mL)
Omnitrope®: 5 mg/1.5 mL (1.5 mL); 10 mg/1.5 mL (1.5 mL)

Somatuline® Autogel® (Can) *see* lanreotide *on page 510*
Somatuline® Depot *see* lanreotide *on page 510*
Somavert® *see* pegvisomant *on page 682*
Sominex® [OTC] *see* diphenhydramine (systemic) *on page 290*
Sominex® (Can) *see* diphenhydramine (systemic) *on page 290*
Sominex® Maximum Strength [OTC] *see* diphenhydramine (systemic) *on page 290*
Somnote® *see* chloral hydrate *on page 193*
Som Pam (Can) *see* flurazepam *on page 391*
Sonata® *see* zaleplon *on page 926*
Soothe® [OTC] *see* artificial tears *on page 96*
Soothing Care™ Itch Relief [OTC] *see* pramoxine *on page 730*

sorafenib (sor AF e nib)

Medication Safety Issues
Sound-alike/look-alike issues:
NexAVAR® may be confused with NexIUM®
SORAfenib may be confused with gefitinib, imatinib, SUNItinib, vandetanib, vemurafenib
High alert medication:
This medication is in a class the Institute for Safe Medication Practices (ISMP) includes among its list of drug classes which have a heightened risk of causing significant patient harm when used in error.
Synonyms BAY 43-9006; sorafenib tosylate
Tall-Man SORAfenib
U.S. Brand Names NexAVAR®
Canadian Brand Names Nexavar®
Therapeutic Category Antineoplastic Agent, Tyrosine Kinase Inhibitor; Vascular Endothelial Growth Factor (VEGF) Inhibitor
Use Treatment of advanced renal cell cancer (RCC); treatment of unresectable hepatocellular cancer (HCC)
General Dosage Range Dosage adjustments recommended in patients with hepatic or renal impairment, on concomitant therapy, or who develop toxicities
Oral: *Adults:* 400 mg twice daily
Dosage Forms
Tablet, oral:
NexAVAR®: 200 mg

sorafenib tosylate *see* sorafenib *on page 827*

sorbitol (SOR bi tole)

Therapeutic Category Genitourinary Irrigant; Laxative

◄ **Use** Genitourinary irrigant in transurethral prostatic resection or other transurethral resection or other transurethral surgical procedures; diuretic; humectant; sweetening agent; hyperosmotic laxative; facilitate the passage of sodium polystyrene sulfonate through the intestinal tract

General Dosage Range

Oral:

Children 2-11 years: 2 mL/kg (70% solution) as a single dose

Children ≥12 years and Adults: 30-150 mL (70% solution) as a single dose

Rectal:

Children 2-11 years: 30-60 mL (25% to 30% solution) as a single dose

Children ≥12 years and Adults: 120 mL (25% to 30% solution) as a single dose

Topical: *Adults:* 3% to 3.3% as a transurethral irrigation

Dosage Forms

Solution, genitourinary irrigation [preservative free]: 3% (3000 mL, 5000 mL); 3.3% (2000 mL, 4000 mL)

Solution, oral: 70% (30 mL, 473 mL, 480 mL, 3840 mL)

Sore Throat Relief [OTC] *see* benzocaine *on page 121*

Soriatane® *see* acitretin *on page 37*

Sorine® *see* sotalol *on page 828*

sotalol (SOE ta lole)

Medication Safety Issues

Sound-alike/look-alike issues:

Sotalol may be confused with Stadol®, Sudafed®

Betapace® may be confused with Betapace AF®

Betapace AF® may be confused with Betapace®

Synonyms sotalol hydrochloride

U.S. Brand Names Betapace AF®; Betapace®; Sorine®

Canadian Brand Names Apo-Sotalol®; CO Sotalol; Dom-Sotalol; Med-Sotalol; Mylan-Sotalol; Novo-Sotalol; Nu-Sotalol; PHL-Sotalol; PMS-Sotalol; PRO-Sotalol; ratio-Sotalol; Rhoxal-sotalol; Riva-Sotalol; Rylosol; Sandoz-Sotalol; ZYM-Sotalol

Therapeutic Category Antiarrhythmic Agent, Class II; Antiarrhythmic Agent, Class III; Beta-Adrenergic Blocker, Nonselective

Use Treatment of documented ventricular arrhythmias (ie, sustained ventricular tachycardia), that in the judgment of the physician are life-threatening; maintenance of normal sinus rhythm in patients with symptomatic atrial fibrillation and atrial flutter who are currently in sinus rhythm. Manufacturer states substitutions should not be made for Betapace AF® since Betapace AF® is distributed with a patient package insert specific for atrial fibrillation/flutter.

Injection: Substitution for oral sotalol in those who are unable to take sotalol orally

General Dosage Range Dosage adjustment recommended in patients with renal impairment or who develop toxicities

I.V.: *Adults:* Initial: 75 mg twice daily; Maintenance: 75-150 mg twice daily (maximum: 300 mg/day)

Oral:

Children ≤2 years: Dosage should be adjusted (decreased) by plotting of the child's age on a logarithmic scale; **Note:** Refer to manufacturer's package labeling

Children >2 years: Initial: 90 mg/m^2/day in 3 divided doses; Maintenance: 90-180 mg/m^2/day in 3 divided doses (maximum: 180 mg/m^2/day)

Adults: Initial: 80 mg twice daily; Maintenance: 240-320 mg/day in 2-3 divided doses (maximum: 320 mg/day)

Dosage Forms

Injection, solution [preservative free]: 15 mg/mL (10 mL)

Tablet, oral: 80 mg, 120 mg, 160 mg, 240 mg

Betapace AF®: 80 mg, 120 mg, 160 mg

Betapace®: 80 mg, 120 mg, 160 mg, 240 mg

Sorine®: 80 mg, 120 mg, 160 mg, 240 mg

sotalol hydrochloride *see* sotalol *on page 828*

Sotradecol® *see* sodium tetradecyl *on page 824*

Sotret® *see* isotretinoin *on page 495*

SourceCF® *see* vitamins (multiple/oral) *on page 919*

SourceCF® [OTC] *see* vitamins (multiple/pediatric) *on page 920*
SPA *see* albumin *on page 44*
SPD417 *see* carbamazepine *on page 171*
Spectracef® *see* cefditoren *on page 181*
SPI 0211 *see* lubiprostone *on page 541*

spinosad (SPIN oh sad)
Synonyms NatrOVA
U.S. Brand Names Natroba™
Therapeutic Category Antiparasitic Agent, Topical; Pediculocide
Use Topical treatment of head lice (*Pediculosis capitis*) infestation in adults and children ≥4 years of age
General Dosage Range Topical: *Children ≥4 years old and Adults:* Apply sufficient amount to cover dry scalp and hair; may repeat in 7 days
Dosage Forms
Suspension, topical:
Natroba™: 0.9% (120 mL)

Spiriva® (Can) *see* tiotropium *on page 871*
Spiriva® HandiHaler® *see* tiotropium *on page 871*

spironolactone (speer on oh LAK tone)
Medication Safety Issues
Sound-alike/look-alike issues:
Aldactone® may be confused with Aldactazide®
International issues:
Aldactone: Brand name for spironolactone [U.S., Canada], but also the brand name for potassium canrenoate [Austria, Czech Republic, Germany, Hungary, Poland]
U.S. Brand Names Aldactone®
Canadian Brand Names Aldactone®; Novo-Spiroton; Teva-Spironolactone
Therapeutic Category Diuretic, Potassium Sparing
Use Management of edema associated with excessive aldosterone excretion; hypertension; primary hyperaldosteronism; hypokalemia; cirrhosis of liver accompanied by edema or ascites; nephrotic syndrome; severe heart failure (NYHA class III-IV) to increase survival and reduce hospitalization when added to standard therapy
General Dosage Range Dosage adjustment recommended in patients with renal impairment
Oral:
Adults: 12.5-400 mg/day in 1-2 divided doses
Elderly: Initial: 25-50 mg/day in 1-2 divided doses
Dosage Forms
Tablet, oral: 25 mg, 50 mg, 100 mg
Aldactone®: 25 mg, 50 mg, 100 mg

spironolactone and hydrochlorothiazide *see* hydrochlorothiazide and spironolactone *on page 446*
SPM 927 *see* lacosamide *on page 505*
Sporanox® *see* itraconazole *on page 496*
Sportscreme® [OTC] *see* trolamine *on page 894*
SPP100 *see* aliskiren *on page 51*
Sprayzoin™ [OTC] *see* benzoin *on page 123*
Sprintec® *see* ethinyl estradiol and norgestimate *on page 357*
Sprix® *see* ketorolac (nasal) *on page 502*
Sprycel® *see* dasatinib *on page 254*
SPS® *see* sodium polystyrene sulfonate *on page 823*
SR33589 *see* dronedarone *on page 314*
Sronyx® *see* ethinyl estradiol and levonorgestrel *on page 353*
SS734 *see* besifloxacin *on page 128*
SSD® *see* silver sulfadiazine *on page 812*
SSD AF® *see* silver sulfadiazine *on page 812*
SSKI® *see* potassium iodide *on page 726*

Stadol *see* butorphanol *on page 155*
Stagesic™ *see* hydrocodone and acetaminophen *on page 446*
Stalevo® *see* levodopa, carbidopa, and entacapone *on page 519*
StanGard® Perio *see* fluoride *on page 386*
stannous fluoride *see* fluoride *on page 386*
Starlix® *see* nateglinide *on page 614*
Statex® (Can) *see* morphine (systemic) *on page 598*
Statobex® (Can) *see* phendimetrazine *on page 693*

stavudine (STAV yoo deen)

Medication Safety Issues
Sound-alike/look-alike issues:
  Zerit® may be confused with Zestril®, Ziac®, ZyrTEC®
Synonyms d4T
U.S. Brand Names Zerit®
Canadian Brand Names Zerit®
Therapeutic Category Antiviral Agent
Use Treatment of HIV infection in combination with other antiretroviral agents
General Dosage Range Dosage adjustment recommended in patients with renal impairment.
Oral:
  Newborns (Birth to 13 days): 0.5 mg/kg every 12 hours
  Children ≥14 days and <30 kg: 1 mg/kg every 12 hours
  Children and Adults 30-59 kg: 30 mg every 12 hours
  Children and Adults ≥60 kg: 40 mg every 12 hours
Dosage Forms
Capsule, oral: 15 mg, 20 mg, 30 mg, 40 mg
  Zerit®: 15 mg, 20 mg, 30 mg, 40 mg
Powder for solution, oral:
  Zerit®: 1 mg/mL (200 mL)

Stavzor™ *see* valproic acid *on page 904*
Staxyn™ *see* vardenafil *on page 908*
Staxyn™ *see* vardenafil *on page 908*
Stelara™ *see* ustekinumab *on page 902*
Stemetil® (Can) *see* prochlorperazine *on page 740*
sterile talc *see* talc (sterile) *on page 843*
Sterile Talc Powder™ *see* talc (sterile) *on page 843*
Sterile Vancomycin Hydrochloride, USP (Can) *see* vancomycin *on page 906*
STI-571 *see* imatinib *on page 465*
Stieprox® (Can) *see* ciclopirox *on page 207*
Stieva-A (Can) *see* tretinoin (topical) *on page 885*
Stimate® *see* desmopressin *on page 262*
Sting-Kill® [OTC] *see* benzocaine *on page 121*
St Joseph® Adult Aspirin [OTC] *see* aspirin *on page 98*
Stop® *see* fluoride *on page 386*
Strattera® *see* atomoxetine *on page 101*

streptomycin (strep toe MYE sin)

Medication Safety Issues
Sound-alike/look-alike issues:
  Streptomycin may be confused with streptozocin
Synonyms streptomycin sulfate
Therapeutic Category Antibiotic, Aminoglycoside; Antitubercular Agent
Use Part of combination therapy of active tuberculosis; used in combination with other agents for treatment of streptococcal or enterococcal endocarditis, mycobacterial infections, plague, tularemia, and brucellosis

General Dosage Range Dosage adjustment recommended in patients with renal impairment
I.M.:
  Children: 20-40 mg/kg given daily or 2-3 times/week (maximum: 1 g/day)
  Adults: Tuberculosis: 15 mg/kg/day **or** 25-30 mg/kg 2-3 times/week; Other indications: 1-4 g/day in 2 divided doses
  Elderly: 10 mg/kg/day (maximum: 750 mg/day)
I.V.:
  Children: 20-40 mg/kg/day **or** 20-40 mg/kg twice weekly **or** 25-30 mg/kg 3 times/week (maximum: 1 g/day)
  Adults: 1-4 g/day in 2 divided doses
Dosage Forms
  Injection, powder for reconstitution: 1 g

streptomycin sulfate *see* streptomycin *on page 830*

streptozocin (strep toe ZOE sin)
Medication Safety Issues
  Sound-alike/look-alike issues:
    Streptozocin may be confused with streptomycin
  High alert medication:
    The Institute for Safe Medication Practices (ISMP) includes this medication among its list of drugs which have a heightened risk of causing significant patient harm when used in error.
U.S. Brand Names Zanosar®
Canadian Brand Names Zanosar®
Therapeutic Category Antineoplastic Agent
Use Treatment of metastatic islet cell carcinoma of the pancreas
General Dosage Range Dosage adjustment recommended in patients with renal impairment
  I.V.: *Children and Adults:* 1-1.5 g/m^2 weekly for 6 weeks followed by a 4-week rest period **or** 0.5-1 g/m^2 for 5 consecutive days as combination therapy followed by a 4- to 6-week rest period
Dosage Forms
  Injection, powder for reconstitution:
    Zanosar®: 1 g

Striant® *see* testosterone *on page 854*
Stridex® Essential Care® [OTC] *see* salicylic acid *on page 795*
Stridex® Facewipes To Go® [OTC] *see* salicylic acid *on page 795*
Stridex® Maximum Strength [OTC] *see* salicylic acid *on page 795*
Stridex® Sensitive Skin [OTC] *see* salicylic acid *on page 795*
Strifon Forte® (Can) *see* chlorzoxazone *on page 204*
Stromectol® *see* ivermectin *on page 497*
strontium-89 chloride *see* strontium-89 *on page 831*

strontium-89 (STRON shee um atey nine)
Synonyms strontium-89 chloride
U.S. Brand Names Metastron®
Canadian Brand Names Metastron®
Therapeutic Category Radiopharmaceutical
Use Relief of bone pain in patients with skeletal metastases
General Dosage Range I.V.: *Adults:* 148 megabecquerel (4 millicurie) **or** 1.5-2.2 megabecquerel (40-60 microcurie)/kg
Dosage Forms
  Injection, solution [preservative free]:
    Metastron®: 1 mCi/mL (4 mL)

Strovite® *see* vitamins (multiple/oral) *on page 919*
Strovite® Advance *see* vitamins (multiple/oral) *on page 919*
Strovite® Forte *see* vitamins (multiple/oral) *on page 919*
Strovite® Plus *see* vitamins (multiple/oral) *on page 919*
Stuart Prenatal® [OTC] *see* vitamins (multiple/prenatal) *on page 920*

SU011248 *see* sunitinib *on page 840*
suberoylanilide hydroxamic acid *see* vorinostat *on page 921*
Suboxone® *see* buprenorphine and naloxone *on page 149*
Subutex® *see* buprenorphine *on page 149*

succimer (SUKS si mer)
Synonyms DMSA
U.S. Brand Names Chemet®
Canadian Brand Names Chemet®
Therapeutic Category Chelating Agent
Use Treatment of lead poisoning in children with serum lead levels >45 mcg/dL
General Dosage Range Oral: *Children and Adults:* 10 mg/kg (or 350 mg/m²/dose) every 8-12 hours (maximum: 500 mg/dose)
Dosage Forms
Capsule, oral:
Chemet®: 100 mg

succinylcholine (suks in il KOE leen)
Medication Safety Issues
High alert medication:
The Institute for Safe Medication Practices (ISMP) includes this medication among its list of drugs which have a heightened risk of causing significant patient harm when used in error.
Other safety concerns:
United States Pharmacopeia (USP) 2006: The Interdisciplinary Safe Medication Use Expert Committee of the USP has recommended the following:
- Hospitals, clinics, and other practice sites should institute special safeguards in the storage, labeling, and use of these agents and should include these safeguards in staff orientation and competency training.
- Healthcare professionals should be on high alert (especially vigilant) whenever a neuromuscular-blocking agent (NMBA) is stocked, ordered, prepared, or administered.
International issues:
Quelicin [U.S., Brazil, Canada, Indonesia] may be confused with Keflin, a brand name for cefalotin [Argentina, Brazil, Mexico, Netherlands, Norway]
Synonyms succinylcholine chloride; suxamethonium chloride
U.S. Brand Names Anectine®; Quelicin®
Canadian Brand Names Quelicin®
Therapeutic Category Skeletal Muscle Relaxant
Use To facilitate both rapid sequence and routine endotracheal intubation and to relax skeletal muscles during surgery
Note: Does not relieve pain or produce sedation
General Dosage Range Dosage adjustment recommended in patients with renal or hepatic impairment
I.M.: *Children and Adults:* Up to 3-4 mg/kg (maximum: 150 mg total dose)
I.V.:
Smaller Children: Intermittent: Initial: 2 mg/kg/dose; Maintenance: 0.3-0.6 mg/kg/dose every 5-10 minutes as needed
Older Children and Adolescents: Intermittent: Initial: 1 mg/kg/dose; Maintenance: 0.3-0.6 mg/kg every 5-10 minutes as needed
Adults: Intubation: 0.6 mg/kg (range: 0.3-1.1 mg/kg); Rapid sequence intubation: 1-1.5 mg/kg
Dosage Forms
Injection, solution:
Anectine®: 20 mg/mL (10 mL)
Quelicin®: 20 mg/mL (10 mL)
Injection, solution [preservative free]:
Quelicin®: 100 mg/mL (10 mL)

succinylcholine chloride *see* succinylcholine *on page 832*
Suclor™ [DSC] *see* chlorpheniramine and pseudoephedrine *on page 199*
Sucraid® *see* sacrosidase *on page 795*

sucralfate (soo KRAL fate)

Medication Safety Issues
Sound-alike/look-alike issues:
Sucralfate may be confused with salsalate
Carafate® may be confused with Cafergot®

Synonyms aluminum sucrose sulfate, basic

U.S. Brand Names Carafate®

Canadian Brand Names Apo-Sucralfate; Dom-Sucralfate; Novo-Sucralate; Nu-Sucralate; PMS-Sucralate; Sucralfate-1; Sulcrate®; Sulcrate® Suspension Plus; Teva-Sucralfate

Therapeutic Category Gastrointestinal Agent, Gastric or Duodenal Ulcer Treatment

Use Short-term (≤8 weeks) management of duodenal ulcers; maintenance therapy for duodenal ulcers

General Dosage Range Oral: *Adults:* 1 g 2-4 times/day

Dosage Forms
Suspension, oral: 1 g/10 mL (10 mL)
Carafate®: 1 g/10 mL (420 mL)
Tablet, oral: 1 g
Carafate®: 1 g

Sucralfate-1 (Can) see sucralfate *on page 833*
Sucrets® Children's [OTC] see dyclonine *on page 317*
Sucrets® Maximum Strength [OTC] see dyclonine *on page 317*
Sucrets® Original [OTC] see hexylresorcinol *on page 440*
Sucrets® Regular Strength [OTC] see dyclonine *on page 317*
Sudafed see pseudoephedrine *on page 751*
Sudafed® 12 Hour [OTC] see pseudoephedrine *on page 751*
Sudafed® 12 Hour Pressure + Pain [OTC] see naproxen and pseudoephedrine *on page 613*
Sudafed® 24 Hour [OTC] see pseudoephedrine *on page 751*
Sudafed® Children's [OTC] see pseudoephedrine *on page 751*
Sudafed® Children's Cold & Cough [OTC] see pseudoephedrine and dextromethorphan *on page 752*
Sudafed® Decongestant (Can) see pseudoephedrine *on page 751*
Sudafed® Head Cold and Sinus Extra Strength (Can) see acetaminophen and pseudoephedrine *on page 29*
Sudafed® Maximum Strength Nasal Decongestant [OTC] see pseudoephedrine *on page 751*
Sudafed OM® Sinus Congestion [OTC] [DSC] see oxymetazoline (nasal) *on page 664*
Sudafed PE® Children's [OTC] see phenylephrine (systemic) *on page 696*
Sudafed PE® Children's Cold & Cough [OTC] see dextromethorphan and phenylephrine *on page 271*
Sudafed PE® Congestion [OTC] see phenylephrine (systemic) *on page 696*
Sudafed PE™ Nasal Decongestant [OTC] see phenylephrine (systemic) *on page 696*
Sudafed PE® Nighttime Cold [OTC] see acetaminophen, diphenhydramine, and phenylephrine *on page 33*
Sudafed PE® Non-Drying Sinus [OTC] see guaifenesin and phenylephrine *on page 428*
Sudafed PE® Pressure + Pain [OTC] see acetaminophen and phenylephrine *on page 28*
Sudafed PE® Severe Cold [OTC] see acetaminophen, diphenhydramine, and phenylephrine *on page 33*
Sudafed PE® Sinus + Allergy [OTC] see chlorpheniramine and phenylephrine *on page 198*
Sudafed® Sinus Advance (Can) see pseudoephedrine and ibuprofen *on page 753*
SudaHist® [DSC] see chlorpheniramine and pseudoephedrine *on page 199*
SudaTex-G [OTC] see guaifenesin and pseudoephedrine *on page 429*
SudoGest [OTC] see pseudoephedrine *on page 751*
SudoGest 12 Hour [OTC] see pseudoephedrine *on page 751*
SudoGest Children's [OTC] see pseudoephedrine *on page 751*
Sudogest™ PE [OTC] see phenylephrine (systemic) *on page 696*
Sudo-Tab® [OTC] see pseudoephedrine *on page 751*
Sufenta® see sufentanil *on page 834*

sufentanil (soo FEN ta nil)

Medication Safety Issues
Sound-alike/look-alike issues:
SUFentanil may be confused with alfentanil, fentaNYL
Sufenta® may be confused with Alfenta®, Sudafed®, Survanta®
High alert medication:
The Institute for Safe Medication Practices (ISMP) includes this medication among its list of drugs which have a heightened risk of causing significant patient harm when used in error.
Synonyms sufentanil citrate
Tall-Man SUFentanil
U.S. Brand Names Sufenta®
Canadian Brand Names Sufentanil Citrate Injection, USP; Sufenta®
Therapeutic Category Analgesic, Narcotic; General Anesthetic
Controlled Substance C-II
Use Analgesic supplement in maintenance of general anesthesia; epidural analgesic in conjunction with a local anesthetic
General Dosage Range
I.V.:
Children 2-12 years: 10-25 mcg/kg with 100% O_2; Maintenance: Up to 1-2 mcg/kg total dose
Adults: 1-2 mcg/kg with N_2O/O_2; Maintenance: 5-20 mcg/kg as needed
Epidural: *Adults:* 10-15 mcg (maximum: 3 doses)
Dosage Forms
Injection, solution [preservative free]: 50 mcg/mL (1 mL, 2 mL, 5 mL)
Sufenta®: 50 mcg/mL (1 mL, 2 mL, 5 mL)

sufentanil citrate *see* sufentanil *on page 834*
Sufentanil Citrate Injection, USP (Can) *see* sufentanil *on page 834*
sulamyd *see* sulfacetamide (ophthalmic) *on page 835*
sulamyd *see* sulfacetamide (topical) *on page 835*
Sular® *see* nisoldipine *on page 627*
sulbactam and ampicillin *see* ampicillin and sulbactam *on page 77*

sulconazole (sul KON a zole)

Synonyms sulconazole nitrate
U.S. Brand Names Exelderm®
Canadian Brand Names Exelderm®
Therapeutic Category Antifungal Agent
Use Treatment of superficial fungal infections of the skin, including tinea cruris (jock itch), tinea corporis (ringworm), tinea versicolor, and tinea pedis (athlete's foot, cream only)
General Dosage Range Topical: *Adults:* Apply a small amount to affected area once or twice daily
Dosage Forms
Cream, topical:
Exelderm®: 1% (15 g, 30 g, 60 g)
Solution, topical:
Exelderm®: 1% (30 mL)

sulconazole nitrate *see* sulconazole *on page 834*
Sulcrate® (Can) *see* sucralfate *on page 833*
Sulcrate® Suspension Plus (Can) *see* sucralfate *on page 833*

sulfabenzamide, sulfacetamide, and sulfathiazole
(sul fa BENZ a mide, sul fa SEE ta mide, & sul fa THYE a zole)

Synonyms triple sulfa
U.S. Brand Names V.V.S.®
Therapeutic Category Antibiotic, Vaginal
Use Treatment of *Haemophilus vaginalis* vaginitis
General Dosage Range Intravaginal: *Adults:* Insert ¼ to 1 applicatorful twice daily

Dosage Forms
Cream, vaginal: Sulfabenzamide 3.7%, sulfacetamide 2.86%, and sulfathiazole 3.42% (78 g with applicator)
V.V.S.®: Sulfabenzamide 3.7%, sulfacetamide 2.86%, and sulfathiazole 3.42% (78 g with applicator)

sulfacetamide (ophthalmic) (sul fa SEE ta mide)
Medication Safety Issues
Sound-alike/look-alike issues:
Bleph®-10 may be confused with Blephamide®
Synonyms sodium sulfacetamide; sulamyd
U.S. Brand Names Bleph®-10; Sulfamide
Canadian Brand Names AK Sulf Liq; Bleph 10 DPS; Diosulf™; PMS-Sulfacetamide; Sodium Sulamyd
Therapeutic Category Antibiotic, Ophthalmic
Use Treatment and prophylaxis of conjunctivitis due to susceptible organisms; corneal ulcers; adjunctive treatment with systemic sulfonamides for therapy of trachoma
General Dosage Range Ophthalmic: *Children >2 months and Adults:* Solution: Instill 1-2 drops up to every 2-3 hours
Dosage Forms
Solution, ophthalmic: 10% (15 mL)
Bleph®-10: 10% (5 mL)
Sulfamide: 10% (15 mL)

sulfacetamide (topical) (sul fa SEE ta mide)
Medication Safety Issues
Sound-alike/look-alike issues:
Klaron® may be confused with Klor-Con®
Synonyms sodium sulfacetamide; sulamyd; sulfacetamide sodium
U.S. Brand Names Carmol® Scalp Treatment; Klaron®; Ovace®; Ovace® Plus; Rosula® NS; Seb-Prev™
Canadian Brand Names Sulfacet-R
Therapeutic Category Acne Products; Antibiotic, Sulfonamide Derivative; Topical Skin Product, Acne
Use Scaling dermatosis (seborrheic); bacterial infections of the skin; acne vulgaris
General Dosage Range Topical: *Children >12 years and Adults:* Apply thin film to affected area 1-4 times/day
Dosage Forms
Aerosol, topical:
Ovace®: 10% (70 g)
Lotion, topical: 10% (118 mL)
Carmol® Scalp Treatment: 10% (85 g)
Klaron®: 10% (118 mL)
Ovace®: 10% (180 mL, 360 mL)
Ovace® Plus: 10% (480 mL)
Pad, topical: 10% (30s)
Rosula® NS: 10% (30s)
Soap, topical:
Seb-Prev™: 10% (170 mL, 340 mL)
Suspension, topical: 10% (118 mL)

sulfacetamide and prednisolone (sul fa SEE ta mide & pred NIS oh lone)
Medication Safety Issues
Sound-alike/look-alike issues:
Blephamide® may be confused with Bleph®-10
Synonyms prednisolone and sulfacetamide
U.S. Brand Names Blephamide®
Canadian Brand Names AK Cide Oph; Blephamide®; Dioptimyd®
Therapeutic Category Antibiotic/Corticosteroid, Ophthalmic
Use Steroid-responsive inflammatory ocular conditions in which a corticosteroid is indicated and where infection is present or there is a risk of infection

▶

◀ **General Dosage Range Ophthalmic:** *Children ≥6 years and Adults:*
  Ointment: Apply ~¹/₂" ribbon 3-4 times/day and 1-2 times at night
  Solution, suspension: Instill 2 drops every 4 hours
Dosage Forms
  Ointment, ophthalmic:
    Blephamide®: Sulfacetamide 10% and prednisolone 0.2% (3.5 g)
  Solution, ophthalmic: Sulfacetamide 10% and prednisolone 0.25% (5 mL, 10 mL)
  Suspension, ophthalmic:
    Blephamide®: Sulfacetamide 10% and prednisolone 0.2% (5 mL, 10 mL)

sulfacetamide and sulfur *see sulfur and sulfacetamide on page 838*
sulfacetamide sodium *see sulfacetamide (topical) on page 835*
Sulfacet-R® *see sulfur and sulfacetamide on page 838*
Sulfacet-R (Can) *see sulfacetamide (topical) on page 835*

sulfadiazine (sul fa DYE a zeen)
Medication Safety Issues
  Sound-alike/look-alike issues:
    SulfADIAZINE may be confused with sulfaSALAzine, sulfiSOXAZOLE
Tall-Man sulf**ADIAZINE**
Therapeutic Category Sulfonamide
Use Treatment of the following conditions (per product labeling): Chancroid, trachoma, inclusion conjunctivitis, nocardiosis, urinary tract infections, toxoplasmosis encephalitis, malaria, meningococcal meningitis, acute otitis media, rheumatic fever (prophylaxis), meningitis (adjunctive)

  Refer to current guidelines for appropriate use.
General Dosage Range Oral:
  Children >2 months: Initial: 75 mg/kg; Maintenance: 150 mg/kg /day (maximum: 6 g/24 hours)
  Children <30 kg and Adults <30 kg: 0.5 g/day (rheumatic fever prophylaxis)
  Children ≥30 kg and Adults ≥30 kg: 1 g/day (rheumatic fever prophylaxis)
  Adults: 2-4 g/day in divided doses
Dosage Forms
  Tablet, oral: 500 mg

sulfadoxine and pyrimethamine (sul fa DOKS een & peer i METH a meen)
Synonyms pyrimethamine and sulfadoxine
U.S. Brand Names Fansidar® [DSC]
Therapeutic Category Antimalarial Agent
Use Treatment of *Plasmodium falciparum* malaria in patients in whom chloroquine resistance is suspected; malaria prophylaxis for travelers to areas where chloroquine-resistant malaria is endemic
General Dosage Range Oral:
  Children 2-11 months: ¹/₄ tablet as a single dose
  Children 1-3 years: ¹/₂ tablet as a single dose
  Children 4-8 years: 1 tablet as a single dose
  Children 9-14 years: 2 tablets as a single dose
  Children >14 years and Adults: 3 tablets as a single dose

sulfamethoxazole and trimethoprim (sul fa meth OKS a zole & trye METH oh prim)
Medication Safety Issues
  Sound-alike/look-alike issues:
    Bactrim™ may be confused with bacitracin, Bactine®, Bactroban®
    Co-trimoxazole may be confused with clotrimazole
    Septra® may be confused with Ceptaz®, Sectral®
    Septra® DS may be confused with Semprex®-D
Synonyms co-trimoxazole; SMX-TMP; SMZ-TMP; Sulfatrim; TMP-SMX; TMP-SMZ; trimethoprim and sulfamethoxazole
U.S. Brand Names Bactrim™; Bactrim™ DS; Septra® DS; Septra® [DSC]
Canadian Brand Names Apo-Sulfatrim®; Apo-Sulfatrim® DS; Apo-Sulfatrim® Pediatric; Novo-Trimel; Novo-Trimel D.S.; Nu-Cotrimox; Septra® Injection
Therapeutic Category Sulfonamide

Use

Oral treatment of urinary tract infections due to *E. coli, Klebsiella* and *Enterobacter* sp, *M. morganii, P. mirabilis* and *P. vulgaris*; acute otitis media in children; acute exacerbations of chronic bronchitis in adults due to susceptible strains of *H. influenzae* or *S. pneumoniae*; treatment and prophylaxis of *Pneumocystis jirovecii* pneumonia (PCP); traveler's diarrhea due to enterotoxigenic *E. coli*; treatment of enteritis caused by *Shigella flexneri* or *Shigella sonnei*

I.V. treatment of severe or complicated infections when oral therapy is not feasible, for documented PCP, empiric treatment of PCP in immune compromised patients; treatment of documented or suspected shigellosis, typhoid fever, *Nocardia asteroides* infection, or other infections caused by susceptible bacteria

General Dosage Range Dosage adjustment recommended in patients with renal impairment

I.V.: *Children >2 months and Adults:* 8-20 mg TMP/kg/day divided every 6-12 hours

Oral:

Children >2 months: 6-20 mg TMP/kg/day divided every 6-12 hours **or** 150 mg TMP/m^2/day in divided doses every 12-24 hours for 3-7 days/week (maximum: sulfamethoxazole 1600 mg/day; trimethoprim 320 mg/day)

Adults: 1 or 2 double-strength tablets (sulfamethoxazole 800-1600 mg; trimethoprim 160-320 mg) every 12-24 hours **or** 15-20 mg TMP/kg/day in 3-4 divided doses

Dosage Forms The 5:1 ratio (SMX:TMP) remains constant in all dosage forms.

Injection, solution: Sulfamethoxazole 80 mg and trimethoprim 16 mg per mL (5 mL, 10 mL, 30 mL)

Suspension, oral: Sulfamethoxazole 200 mg and trimethoprim 40 mg per 5 mL

Tablet: Sulfamethoxazole 400 mg and trimethoprim 80 mg

Bactrim™: Sulfamethoxazole 400 mg and trimethoprim 80 mg

Tablet, double-strength: Sulfamethoxazole 800 mg and trimethoprim 160 mg

Bactrim™ DS, Septra® DS: Sulfamethoxazole 800 mg and trimethoprim 160 mg

Sulfamide *see* sulfacetamide (ophthalmic) *on page 835*

Sulfamylon® *see* mafenide *on page 543*

sulfanilamide (sul fa NIL a mide)

Synonyms p-amino-benzenesulfonamide

U.S. Brand Names AVC™

Therapeutic Category Antifungal Agent, Vaginal

Use Treatment of vulvovaginitis caused by *Candida albicans*

General Dosage Range Intravaginal: *Adults:* 1 applicatorful once or twice daily

Dosage Forms

Cream, vaginal:

AVC™: 15% (120 g)

sulfasalazine (sul fa SAL a zeen)

Medication Safety Issues

Sound-alike/look-alike issues:

SulfaSALAzine may be confused with salsalate, sulfADIAZINE, sulfiSOXAZOLE

Azulfidine® may be confused with Augmentin®, azaTHIOprine

Synonyms salicylazosulfapyridine

Tall-Man sulfaSALAzine

U.S. Brand Names Azulfidine EN-tabs®; Azulfidine®

Canadian Brand Names Alti-Sulfasalazine; Salazopyrin En-Tabs®; Salazopyrin®

Therapeutic Category 5-Aminosalicylic Acid Derivative

Use Treatment of mild-to-moderate ulcerative colitis or as adjunctive therapy in severe ulcerative colitis; enteric coated tablets are also used for rheumatoid arthritis (including juvenile idiopathic arthritis [JIA]) in patients who inadequately respond to analgesics and NSAIDs

General Dosage Range Oral:

Delayed release:

Children ≥6 years: Initial: 1/4 to 1/3 of expected maintenance dose; Maintenance: 30-50 mg/kg/day in 2 divided doses (maximum: 2 g/day)

Adults: Initial: 0.5-1 g/day; Maintenance: 2 g/day in 2 divided doses (maximum: 3 g/day)

◀ Immediate release:
Children ≥6 years: Initial: 40-60 mg/kg/day in 3-6 divided doses; Maintenance: 30 mg/kg/day in 4 divided doses
Adults: Initial: 3-4 g/day in evenly divided doses at ≤8-hour intervals; Maintenance: 2 g/day in divided doses at ≤8-hour intervals

Dosage Forms
Tablet, oral: 500 mg
Azulfidine®: 500 mg
Tablet, delayed release, enteric coated, oral: 500 mg
Azulfidine EN-tabs®: 500 mg

Sulfatol® *see sulfur and sulfacetamide on page 838*
Sulfatol C™ *see sulfur and sulfacetamide on page 838*
Sulfatol®-M [DSC] *see sulfur and sulfacetamide on page 838*
Sulfatol SS™ *see sulfur and sulfacetamide on page 838*
Sulfatrim *see sulfamethoxazole and trimethoprim on page 836*
sulfisoxazole and erythromycin *see erythromycin and sulfisoxazole on page 340*

sulfur and sulfacetamide (SUL fur & sul fa SEE ta mide)

Synonyms sodium sulfacetamide and sulfur; sulfacetamide and sulfur; sulfur and sulfacetamide sodium
U.S. Brand Names AVAR™; AVAR™ LS; AVAR™-e; AVAR™-e Green; AVAR™-e LS; BP Cleansing Wash; BP10-1; Clarifoam™ EF; Clenia™; Plexion SCT®; Plexion®; Prascion®; Prascion® FC; Prascion® RA; Rosanil®; Rosula®; Rosula® Clarifying; Sulfacet-R®; Sulfatol C™; Sulfatol SS™; Sulfatol®; Sulfatol®-M [DSC]; Sumaxin™
Canadian Brand Names Sulfacet-R®
Therapeutic Category Antiseborrheic Agent, Topical
Use Aid in the treatment of acne vulgaris, acne rosacea, and seborrheic dermatitis
General Dosage Range Topical: *Children ≥12 years and Adults:* Apply a thin film 1-3 times/day
Dosage Forms
Aerosol, topical [foam]:
Clarifoam™ EF: Sulfur 5% and sulfacetamide 10% (60 g)
Cleanser, topical:
AVAR™: Sulfur 5% and sulfacetamide 10% (228 g)
AVAR™ LS: Sulfur 2% and sulfacetamide 10% (226.8 g)
Plexion®, Prascion®: Sulfur 5% and sulfacetamide 10% (170 g, 340 g)
Rosanil®: Sulfur 5% and sulfacetamide 10% (170 g, 390 g)
Rosula®: Sulfur 5% and sulfacetamide 10% (355 mL)
Cleanser, topical [emulsion-based]:
Sulfatol®: Sulfur 5% and sulfacetamide 10% (355 mL)
Cream, topical:
AVAR™-e, AVAR™-e Green, Prascion® RA: Sulfur 5% and sulfacetamide 10% (45 g)
AVAR™-e LS, Sulfatol SS™: Sulfur 2% and sulfacetamide 10% (45 g)
Clenia™, Sulfatol C™: Sulfur 5% and sulfacetamide 10% (28 g)
Plexion SCT®: Sulfur 5% and sulfacetamide 10% (120 g)
Gel, topical:
Rosula®: Sulfur 5% and sulfacetamide 10% (45 g)
Gel, topical [emulsion-based]:
Sulfatol®: Sulfur 5% and sulfacetamide 10% (45 mL)
Lotion, topical: Sulfur 5% and sulfacetamide 10% (25 g, 30 g, 45 g, 60 g)
Sulfacaet-R®: Sulfur 5% and sulfacetamide 10% (25 g)
Pad, topical [cleansing cloth]: Sulfur 4% and sulfacetamide sodium 10% (60s)
Plexion®, Prascion® FC: Sulfur 5% and sulfacetamide 10% (30s, 60s)
Sumaxin™: Sulfur 4% and sulfacetamide 10% (60s)
Suspension, topical: Sulfur 5% and sulfacetamide 10% (30 g)
Wash, topical: Sulfur 5% and sulfacetamide 10% (170 g, 340 g)
BP10-1: Sulfur 1% and sulfacetamide sodium 10% (170 g)
BP Cleansing Wash, Clenia™: Sulfur 5% and sulfacetamide 10% (170 g, 340 g)
Wash, topical [emulsion-based]:
Rosula® Clarifying: Sulfur 4% and sulfacetamide 10% (473 mL)

sulfur and sulfacetamide sodium *see sulfur and sulfacetamide on page 838*

sulindac (SUL in dak)

Medication Safety Issues
Sound-alike/look-alike issues:
Clinoril® may be confused with Cleocin®, Clozaril®

U.S. Brand Names Clinoril®

Canadian Brand Names Apo-Sulin®; Novo-Sundac; Nu-Sulindac; Nu-Sundac; Teva-Sulindac

Therapeutic Category Analgesic, Nonnarcotic; Nonsteroidal Antiinflammatory Drug (NSAID)

Use Management of inflammatory diseases including osteoarthritis, rheumatoid arthritis, acute gouty arthritis, ankylosing spondylitis, acute painful shoulder (bursitis/tendonitis)

General Dosage Range Dosage adjustment recommended in patients with hepatic impairment
Oral: *Adults:* 150-200 mg twice daily (maximum: 400 mg/day)

Dosage Forms
Tablet, oral: 150 mg, 200 mg
Clinoril®: 200 mg

sumatriptan (soo ma TRIP tan)

Medication Safety Issues
Sound-alike/look-alike issues:
SUMAtriptan may be confused with saxagliptin, sitaGLIPtin, somatropin, ZOLMitriptan

Synonyms sumatriptan succinate

Tall-Man SUMAtriptan

U.S. Brand Names Alsuma™; Imitrex®; Sumavel™ DosePro™

Canadian Brand Names Apo-Sumatriptan®; CO Sumatriptan; Dom-Sumatriptan; Gen-Sumatriptan; Imitrex®; Imitrex® DF; Imitrex® Injection; Imitrex® Nasal Spray; Mylan-Sumatriptan; Novo-Sumatriptan; PHL-Sumatriptan; PMS-Sumatriptan; ratio-Sumatriptan; Rhoxal-sumatriptan; Riva-Sumatriptan; Sandoz-Sumatriptan; Sumatriptan Injection; Sumatriptan Sun Injection; Sumatryx; Teva-Sumatriptan; Teva-Sumatriptan DF

Therapeutic Category Antimigraine Agent

Use
Intranasal, Oral, SubQ: Acute treatment of migraine with or without aura
SubQ: Acute treatment of cluster headache episodes

General Dosage Range Dosage adjustment recommended for oral route in patients with hepatic impairment
Intranasal: *Adults:* 5-20 mg in one nostril as a single dose (may divide dose into both nostrils); may repeat after 2 hours (maximum: 40 mg/day)
Oral: *Adults:* 25-100 mg as a single dose; may repeat after 2 hours (maximum: 200 mg/day)
SubQ: *Adults:* Initial: Up to 6 mg; may repeat if needed ≥1 hour after initial dose (maximum: Two 6 mg injections per 24-hour period)

Dosage Forms
Injection, solution: 4 mg/0.5 mL (0.5 mL); 6 mg/0.5 mL (0.5 mL)
Alsuma™: 6 mg/0.5 mL (0.5 mL)
Imitrex®: 4 mg/0.5 mL (0.5 mL); 6 mg/0.5 mL (0.5 mL)
Sumavel™ DosePro™: 6 mg/0.5 mL (0.5 mL)
Injection, solution [preservative free]: 6 mg/0.5 mL (0.5 mL)
Solution, intranasal: 5 mg/0.1 mL (6s); 20 mg/0.1 mL (6s)
Imitrex®: 5 mg/0.1 mL (6s); 20 mg/0.1 mL (6s)
Tablet, oral: 25 mg, 50 mg, 100 mg
Imitrex®: 25 mg, 50 mg, 100 mg

sumatriptan and naproxen (soo ma TRIP tan & na PROKS en)

Medication Safety Issues
Sound-alike/look-alike issues:
Naproxen may be confused with Natacyn®, Nebcin®, neomycin, niacin
SUMAtriptan may be confused with somatropin, ZOLMitriptan
Treximet™ may be confused with Trexall™

Synonyms naproxen and sumatriptan; naproxen sodium and sumatriptan; naproxen sodium and sumatriptan succinate; sumatriptan succinate and naproxen; sumatriptan succinate and naproxen sodium

U.S. Brand Names Treximet™

◄ **Therapeutic Category** Antimigraine Agent; Nonsteroidal Antiinflammatory Drug (NSAID); Serotonin 5-HT$_{1B, 1D}$ Receptor Agonist

Use Acute treatment of migraine with or without aura

General Dosage Range Oral: *Adults:* 1 tablet (sumatriptan 85 mg and naproxen 500 mg); may repeat in 2 hours if needed (maximum: 2 tablets/24 hours)

Dosage Forms
Tablet:
Treximet™ 85/500: Sumatriptan 85 mg and naproxen sodium 500 mg

Sumatriptan Injection (Can) *see* sumatriptan *on page 839*
sumatriptan succinate *see* sumatriptan *on page 839*
sumatriptan succinate and naproxen *see* sumatriptan and naproxen *on page 839*
sumatriptan succinate and naproxen sodium *see* sumatriptan and naproxen *on page 839*
Sumatriptan Sun Injection (Can) *see* sumatriptan *on page 839*
Sumatryx (Can) *see* sumatriptan *on page 839*
Sumavel™ DosePro™ *see* sumatriptan *on page 839*
Sumaxin™ *see* sulfur and sulfacetamide *on page 838*
Summer's Eve® Anti-Itch Maximum Strength [OTC] *see* pramoxine *on page 730*
Summer's Eve® Medicated Douche [OTC] *see* povidone-iodine (topical) *on page 727*
Sun-Benz® (Can) *see* benzydamine *(Canada only) on page 126*

sunitinib (su NIT e nib)

Medication Safety Issues
Sound-alike/look-alike issues:
SUNItinib may be confused with dasatinib, erlotinib, gefitinib, imatinib, lapatinib, nilotinib, pazopanib, SORAfenib, vandetanib
High alert medication:
This medication is in a class the Institute for Safe Medication Practices (ISMP) includes among its list of drug classes which have a heightened risk of causing significant patient harm when used in error.
Administration issues:
Dosing schedules vary by indication; some treatment regimens are continuous daily dosing; other treatment schedules are daily dosing for 4 weeks of a 6 week cycle (4 weeks on, 2 weeks off)
Synonyms SU011248; SU11248; sunitinib malate
Tall-Man SUNItinib
U.S. Brand Names Sutent®
Canadian Brand Names Sutent®
Therapeutic Category Antineoplastic Agent, Tyrosine Kinase Inhibitor; Vascular Endothelial Growth Factor (VEGF) Inhibitor
Use Treatment of gastrointestinal stromal tumor (GIST) intolerant to or with disease progression on imatinib; treatment of advanced renal cell cancer (RCC); treatment of advanced, metastatic or unresectable pancreatic neuroendocrine tumors (PNET)
General Dosage Range Dosage adjustment recommended in patients with renal impairment, on concomitant therapy, or who develop toxicities
Oral: *Adults:* 50 mg once daily for 4 weeks of a 6-week treatment cycle **or** 37.5 mg once daily, continuous daily dosing
Dosage Forms
Capsule, oral:
Sutent®: 12.5 mg, 25 mg, 50 mg

sunitinib malate *see* sunitinib *on page 840*
Supartz® *see* hyaluronate and derivatives *on page 443*
Super Calcium 600 [OTC] *see* calcium carbonate *on page 161*
Superdophilus® [OTC] *see* Lactobacillus *on page 506*
Supeudol® (Can) *see* oxycodone *on page 662*
Suplasyn® (Can) *see* hyaluronate and derivatives *on page 443*
Suprane® *see* desflurane *on page 260*
Suprefact® (Can) *see* buserelin *(Canada only) on page 151*
Suprefact® Depot (Can) *see* buserelin *(Canada only) on page 151*

Suprep® Bowel Prep Kit see sodium sulfate, potassium sulfate, and magnesium sulfate on page 824
Surgicel® see cellulose, oxidized regenerated on page 186
Surgicel® Fibrillar see cellulose, oxidized regenerated on page 186
Surgicel® NuKnit see cellulose, oxidized regenerated on page 186
Surmontil® see trimipramine on page 892
Survanta® see beractant on page 127
Sustiva® see efavirenz on page 321
Sutent® see sunitinib on page 840
Su-Tuss DM [DSC] see guaifenesin and dextromethorphan on page 427
suxamethonium chloride see succinylcholine on page 832
Sween Cream® [OTC] see vitamin A and vitamin D on page 917
Syeda™ see ethinyl estradiol and drospirenone on page 352
Sylatron™ see peginterferon alfa-2b on page 680
Symax® DuoTab see hyoscyamine on page 457
Symax® FasTab see hyoscyamine on page 457
Symax® SL see hyoscyamine on page 457
Symax® SR see hyoscyamine on page 457
Symbicort® see budesonide and formoterol on page 146
Symbyax® see olanzapine and fluoxetine on page 645
Symlin® [DSC] see pramlintide on page 730
SymlinPen® see pramlintide on page 730
Symmetrel see amantadine on page 62
Symmetrel® (Can) see amantadine on page 62
synacthen see cosyntropin on page 237
Synagis® see palivizumab on page 668
Synalar® (Can) see fluocinolone (topical) on page 384
Synalgos®-DC see dihydrocodeine, aspirin, and caffeine on page 285
Synarel® see nafarelin on page 608
Synera™ see lidocaine and tetracaine on page 527
Synercid® see quinupristin and dalfopristin on page 763
Synphasic® (Can) see ethinyl estradiol and norethindrone on page 355
Synthroid® see levothyroxine on page 522
Synvisc® see hyaluronate and derivatives on page 443
Synvisc-One® see hyaluronate and derivatives on page 443
Syprine® see trientine on page 889
Syrex see sodium chloride on page 818
SyringeAvitene™ see collagen hemostat on page 233
syrup of ipecac see ipecac syrup on page 488
Systane® [OTC] see artificial tears on page 96
Systane® Free [OTC] see artificial tears on page 96
T$_3$ sodium (error-prone abbreviation) see liothyronine on page 529
T$_3$/T$_4$ liotrix see liotrix on page 530
T$_4$ see levothyroxine on page 522
T-20 see enfuvirtide on page 328
T-91825 see ceftaroline fosamil on page 184
642® Tablet (Can) see propoxyphene on page 746
Tabloid® see thioguanine on page 862
TachoSil® see fibrin sealant on page 376
Taclonex® see calcipotriene and betamethasone on page 158
Taclonex Scalp® see calcipotriene and betamethasone on page 158

tacrolimus (systemic) (ta KROE li mus)

Medication Safety Issues
Sound-alike/look-alike issues:
Prograf® may be confused with Gengraf®, PROzac®
Tacrolimus may be confused with everolimus, pimecrolimus, sirolimus, temsirolimus

Synonyms FK506

U.S. Brand Names Prograf®

Canadian Brand Names Advagraf™; Prograf®

Therapeutic Category Calcineurin Inhibitor; Immunosuppressant Agent

Use Prevention of organ rejection in heart, kidney, or liver transplant recipients

General Dosage Range
I.V.:
Children: 0.03-0.05 mg/kg/day as a continuous infusion
Adults: 0.01-0.05 mg/kg/day as a continuous infusion
Oral:
Children: 0.15-0.2 mg/kg/day in divided doses every 12 hours
Adults: 0.075-0.2 mg/kg/day in divided doses every 12 hours

Dosage Forms
Capsule, oral: 0.5 mg, 1 mg, 5 mg
Prograf®: 0.5 mg, 1 mg, 5 mg
Injection, solution:
Prograf®: 5 mg/mL (1 mL)

tacrolimus (topical) (ta KROE li mus)

Medication Safety Issues
Sound-alike/look-alike issues:
Tacrolimus may be confused with everolimus, pimecrolimus, sirolimus, temsirolimus

U.S. Brand Names Protopic®

Canadian Brand Names Protopic®

Therapeutic Category Calcineurin Inhibitor; Topical Skin Product

Use Moderate-to-severe atopic dermatitis in immunocompetent patients not responsive to conventional therapy or when conventional therapy is not appropriate

Canadian labeling: Additional use (not in U.S. labeling): Maintenance therapy to prevent flares and extend flare-free intervals in patients with moderate-to-severe atopic dermatitis who are responsive to initial therapy and experiencing ≥5 flares per year

General Dosage Range Topical:
Children ≥2-15 years: Apply thin layer of 0.03% to affected area twice daily
Children >15 years and Adults: Apply thin layer of 0.03% or 0.1% to affected area twice daily

Dosage Forms
Ointment, topical:
Protopic®: 0.03% (30 g, 60 g, 100 g); 0.1% (30 g, 60 g, 100 g)

Tactuo™ (Can) *see* adapalene and benzoyl peroxide *on page 40*

tadalafil (tah DA la fil)

Medication Safety Issues
Sound-alike/look-alike issues:
Tadalafil may be confused with sildenafil, vardenafil
Adcirca® may be confused with Advair® Diskus®, Advair® HFA, Advicor®

Synonyms GF196960

U.S. Brand Names Adcirca®; Cialis®

Canadian Brand Names Adcirca®; Cialis®

Therapeutic Category Phosphodiesterase (Type 5) Enzyme Inhibitor

Use
Adcirca®: Treatment of pulmonary arterial hypertension (PAH) (WHO Group I) to improve exercise ability
Cialis®: Treatment of erectile dysfunction (ED)

General Dosage Range Dosage adjustment recommended in patient with hepatic or renal impairment or on concomitant therapy

Oral: *Adults:* Erectile dysfunction: As-needed dosing: 5-20 mg prior to anticipated sexual activity as a single dose (maximum: 1 dose/day); Once-daily dosing: 2.5-5 mg once daily; Pulmonary arterial hypertension: 40 mg once daily

Dosage Forms
  Tablet, oral:
    Adcirca®: 20 mg
    Cialis®: 2.5 mg, 5 mg, 10 mg, 20 mg

Tagamet® HB (Can) *see* cimetidine *on page 209*
Tagamet HB 200® [OTC] *see* cimetidine *on page 209*
Tagitol™ V *see* barium *on page 114*
TAK-375 *see* ramelteon *on page 765*
TAK-390MR *see* dexlansoprazole *on page 266*
TAK-599 *see* ceftaroline fosamil *on page 184*
Talacen *see* pentazocine and acetaminophen *on page 687*
talc *see* talc (sterile) *on page 843*
talc for pleurodesis *see* talc (sterile) *on page 843*

talc (sterile) (talk STARE il)

Synonyms intrapleural talc; sterile talc; talc; talc for pleurodesis
U.S. Brand Names Sclerosol®; Sterile Talc Powder™
Therapeutic Category Sclerosing Agent
Use Prevention of recurrence of malignant pleural effusion in symptomatic patients
General Dosage Range Intrapleural: *Adults:* Aerosol: 4-8 g (1-2 cans) as a single dose; Instillation: 5 g
Dosage Forms
  Aerosol, intrapleural:
    Sclerosol®: 4 g (4 g)
  Powder, intrapleural:
    Sterile Talc Powder™: USP: 100% (5 g)

Talwin® *see* pentazocine *on page 687*
Talwin NX *see* pentazocine and naloxone *on page 687*
Tambocor™ *see* flecainide *on page 379*
Tamiflu® *see* oseltamivir *on page 656*

tamoxifen (ta MOKS i fen)

Medication Safety Issues
  Sound-alike/look-alike issues:
    Tamoxifen may be confused with pentoxifylline, Tambocor™, tamsulosin, temazepam
Synonyms ICI-46474; tamoxifen citras; tamoxifen citrate
Canadian Brand Names Apo-Tamox®; Mylan-Tamoxifen; Nolvadex®-D; PMS-Tamoxifen; Teva-Tamoxifen
Therapeutic Category Antineoplastic Agent
Use Treatment of metastatic (female and male) breast cancer; adjuvant treatment of breast cancer after primary treatment with surgery and radiation; reduce risk of invasive breast cancer in women with ductal carcinoma *in situ* (DCIS) after surgery and radiation; reduce the incidence of breast cancer in women at high risk
General Dosage Range Oral: *Adults:* 20-40 mg/day
Dosage Forms
  Tablet, oral: 10 mg, 20 mg

tamoxifen citras *see* tamoxifen *on page 843*
tamoxifen citrate *see* tamoxifen *on page 843*

tamsulosin (tam SOO loe sin)

Medication Safety Issues
  Sound-alike/look-alike issues:
    Flomax® may be confused with Flonase®, Flovent®, Foltx®, Fosamax®

Tamsulosin may be confused with tacrolimus, tamoxifen, terazosin

International issues:

Flomax [U.S., Canada, and multiple international markets] may be confused with Flomox brand name for cefcapene [Japan] and Volmax brand name for salbutamol [multiple international markets]

Flomax: Brand name for tamsulosin [U.S., Canada, and multiple international markets], but also the brand name for morniflumate [Italy]

Synonyms tamsulosin hydrochloride

U.S. Brand Names Flomax®

Canadian Brand Names Flomax® CR; JAMP-Tamsulosin; Mylan-Tamsulosin; RAN™-Tamsulosin; ratio-Tamsulosin; Sandoz-Tamsulosin; Sandoz-Tamsulosin CR; Teva-Tamsulosin

Therapeutic Category Alpha-Adrenergic Blocking Agent

Use Treatment of signs and symptoms of benign prostatic hyperplasia (BPH)

General Dosage Range Oral: *Adults:* Initial: 0.4 mg once daily; Maintenance: 0.4-0.8 mg once daily

Dosage Forms

Capsule, oral: 0.4 mg
  Flomax®: 0.4 mg
Tablet, oral: 0.4 mg

tamsulosin and dutasteride see dutasteride and tamsulosin *on page 317*

tamsulosin hydrochloride see tamsulosin *on page 843*

tamsulosin hydrochloride and dutasteride see dutasteride and tamsulosin *on page 317*

Tanac® [OTC] see benzocaine *on page 121*

TanaCof-XR [DSC] see brompheniramine *on page 143*

Tanafed DMX™ see chlorpheniramine, pseudoephedrine, and dextromethorphan *on page 201*

Tandem® DHA see vitamins (multiple/prenatal) *on page 920*

Tandem® OB see vitamins (multiple/prenatal) *on page 920*

Tanta-Orciprenaline® (Can) see metaproterenol *on page 566*

Tantum® (Can) see benzydamine *(Canada only) on page 126*

TAP-144 see leuprolide *on page 516*

Tapazole® see methimazole *on page 570*

tapentadol (ta PEN ta dol)

Medication Safety Issues
Sound-alike/look-alike issues:
Tapentadol may be confused with traMADol

Synonyms CG5503; tapentadol hydrochloride

U.S. Brand Names Nucynta®; Nucynta® ER

Canadian Brand Names Nucynta™ CR

Therapeutic Category Analgesic, Opioid

Controlled Substance C-II

Use
Immediate release formulation: Relief of moderate-to-severe acute pain
Long acting formulations: Relief of moderate-to-severe chronic pain when continuous, around-the-clock analgesia is necessary for an extended period of time

General Dosage Range Dosage adjustment recommended in patients with hepatic impairment

Oral:
Immediate release: *Adults:* 50-100 mg every 4-6 hours as needed (maximum: 700 mg/day on day 1; 600 mg/day subsequent days)
Extended release: *Adults:* 50-250 mg twice daily (maximum: 500 mg/day)

Dosage Forms
Tablet, oral:
Nucynta®: 50 mg, 75 mg, 100 mg
Tablet, extended release, oral:
Nucynta® ER: 50 mg, 100 mg, 150 mg, 200 mg, 250 mg

Dosage Forms - Canada
Tablet, controlled release, oral:
Nucynta™ CR: 50 mg, 100 mg, 150 mg, 200 mg, 250 mg

tapentadol hydrochloride see tapentadol *on page 844*

Tarceva® *see* erlotinib *on page 338*
Targel® (Can) *see* coal tar *on page 227*
Targretin® *see* bexarotene (systemic) *on page 132*
Targretin® *see* bexarotene (topical) *on page 132*
Tarka® *see* trandolapril and verapamil *on page 881*
Taro-Amcinonide (Can) *see* amcinonide *on page 63*
Taro-Carbamazepine Chewable (Can) *see* carbamazepine *on page 171*
Taro-Ciprofloxacin (Can) *see* ciprofloxacin (systemic) *on page 210*
Taro-Clindamycin (Can) *see* clindamycin (topical) *on page 218*
Taro-Clobetasol (Can) *see* clobetasol *on page 220*
Taro-Desoximetasone (Can) *see* desoximetasone *on page 263*
Taro-Enalapril (Can) *see* enalapril *on page 326*
Taro-Fluconazole (Can) *see* fluconazole *on page 381*
Taro-Mometasone (Can) *see* mometasone (topical) *on page 596*
Taro-Simvastatin (Can) *see* simvastatin *on page 813*
Taro-Sone (Can) *see* betamethasone *on page 129*
Taro-Warfarin (Can) *see* warfarin *on page 922*
Tarsum® [OTC] *see* coal tar and salicylic acid *on page 228*
Tasigna® *see* nilotinib *on page 626*
Tasmar® *see* tolcapone *on page 875*
Tavist® Allergy [OTC] *see* clemastine *on page 216*
Tavist® ND Allergy [OTC] *see* loratadine *on page 536*
Taxol *see* paclitaxel *on page 667*
Taxol® (Can) *see* paclitaxel *on page 667*
Taxotere® *see* docetaxel *on page 301*

tazarotene (taz AR oh teen)
U.S. Brand Names Avage®; Tazorac®
Canadian Brand Names Tazorac®
Therapeutic Category Keratolytic Agent
Use Topical treatment of facial acne vulgaris; topical treatment of stable plaque psoriasis; mitigation (palliation) of facial skin wrinkling, facial mottled hyper-/hypopigmentation, and benign facial lentigines
General Dosage Range Topical: *Children ≥12 years and Adults:* Apply a pea-sized amount or thin film **or** 2 mg/cm^2 once daily
Dosage Forms
  Cream, topical:
    Avage®: 0.1% (30 g)
    Tazorac®: 0.05% (30 g, 60 g); 0.1% (30 g, 60 g)
  Gel, topical:
    Tazorac®: 0.05% (30 g, 100 g); 0.1% (30 g, 100 g)

Tazicef® *see* ceftazidime *on page 184*
tazobactam and piperacillin *see* piperacillin and tazobactam sodium *on page 707*
Tazocin® (Can) *see* piperacillin and tazobactam sodium *on page 707*
Tazorac® *see* tazarotene *on page 845*
Taztia XT® *see* diltiazem *on page 286*
TBC *see* trypsin, balsam Peru, and castor oil *on page 896*
TB skin test *see* tuberculin tests *on page 896*
3TC *see* lamivudine *on page 508*
3TC® (Can) *see* lamivudine *on page 508*
3TC, abacavir, and zidovudine *see* abacavir, lamivudine, and zidovudine *on page 20*
T-cell growth factor *see* aldesleukin *on page 47*
TCGF *see* aldesleukin *on page 47*
TCN *see* tetracycline *on page 857*
Td *see* diphtheria and tetanus toxoid *on page 293*

TD-6424 *see* telavancin *on page 847*

Td Adsorbed (Can) *see* diphtheria and tetanus toxoid *on page 293*

Tdap *see* diphtheria, tetanus toxoids, and acellular pertussis vaccine *on page 296*

TDF *see* tenofovir *on page 851*

TDX *see* raltitrexed *(Canada only) on page 765*

Teardrops® (Can) *see* artificial tears *on page 96*

Teargen® [OTC] *see* artificial tears *on page 96*

Teargen® II [OTC] *see* artificial tears *on page 96*

Tearisol® [OTC] *see* artificial tears *on page 96*

Tears Again® [OTC] *see* artificial tears *on page 96*

Tears Again® MC Gel Drops™ [OTC] *see* hydroxypropyl methylcellulose *on page 455*

Tears Again® Gel Drops™ [OTC] [DSC] *see* carboxymethylcellulose *on page 175*

Tears Again® Night & Day™ [OTC] *see* carboxymethylcellulose *on page 175*

Tears Naturale® [OTC] *see* artificial tears *on page 96*

Tears Naturale® II [OTC] *see* artificial tears *on page 96*

Tears Naturale® Free [OTC] *see* artificial tears *on page 96*

Tears Plus® [OTC] *see* artificial tears *on page 96*

Tears Renewed® [OTC] *see* artificial tears *on page 96*

TEAS *see* trolamine *on page 894*

Tebrazid™ (Can) *see* pyrazinamide *on page 756*

Tecnal C 1/2 (Can) *see* butalbital, aspirin, caffeine, and codeine *on page 154*

Tecnal C 1/4 (Can) *see* butalbital, aspirin, caffeine, and codeine *on page 154*

Tecta™ (Can) *see* pantoprazole *on page 672*

Teflaro™ *see* ceftaroline fosamil *on page 184*

tegaserod (teg a SER od)

Synonyms HTF919; tegaserod maleate

U.S. Brand Names Zelnorm®

Canadian Brand Names Zelnorm® [DSC]

Therapeutic Category Serotonin 5-HT$_4$ Receptor Agonist

Use Emergency treatment of irritable bowel syndrome with constipation (IBS-C) and chronic idiopathic constipation (CIC) in women (<55 years of age) in which no alternative therapy exists

General Dosage Range Oral: *Adults (females <55 years of age):* 6 mg twice daily

Dosage Forms
Tablet, oral:
Zelnorm®: 2 mg, 6 mg

tegaserod maleate *see* tegaserod *on page 846*

TEGretol® *see* carbamazepine *on page 171*

Tegretol® (Can) *see* carbamazepine *on page 171*

TEGretol®-XR *see* carbamazepine *on page 171*

TEI-6720 *see* febuxostat *on page 368*

Tekamlo™ *see* aliskiren and amlodipine *on page 52*

Tekturna® *see* aliskiren *on page 51*

Tekturna HCT® *see* aliskiren and hydrochlorothiazide *on page 52*

telaprevir (tel A pre vir)

Synonyms LY570310; MP-424; MP424; VRT111950; VX-950; VX950

U.S. Brand Names Incivek™

Therapeutic Category Antiviral Agent; Protease Inhibitor

Use Treatment of chronic hepatitis C (CHC) genotype 1 (in combination with peginterferon alfa and ribavirin) in adult patients with compensated liver disease (including cirrhosis) who are treatment naive or who have received previous interferon-based treatment, including null or partial responders, and treatment relapsers.

General Dosage Range Oral: Adults: 750 mg 3 times/day

Dosage Forms
Tablet, oral:
Incivek™: 375 mg

telavancin (tel a VAN sin)

Medication Safety Issues
Sound-alike/look-alike issues:
Telavancin may be confused with telithromycin
Vibativ™ may be confused with Viactiv®, Vibramycin®, vigabatrin
Synonyms TD-6424; telavancin hydrochloride
U.S. Brand Names Vibativ™
Therapeutic Category Antibiotic, Miscellaneous
Use Treatment of complicated skin and skin structure infections caused by susceptible gram-positive organisms including methicillin-susceptible or -resistant *Staphylococcus aureus*, vancomycin-susceptible *Enterococcus faecalis*, and *Streptococcus pyogenes*, *Streptococcus agalactiae*, or *Streptococcus anginosus* group
General Dosage Range Dosage adjustment recommended in patients with renal impairment
I.V.: *Adults:* 10 mg/kg every 24 hours
Dosage Forms
Injection, powder for reconstitution:
Vibativ™: 250 mg, 750 mg

telavancin hydrochloride *see* telavancin *on page 847*

telbivudine (tel BI vyoo deen)

Synonyms L-deoxythymidine; LdT
U.S. Brand Names Tyzeka®
Canadian Brand Names Sebivo®
Therapeutic Category Antiretroviral Agent, Reverse Transcriptase Inhibitor (Nucleoside)
Use Treatment of chronic hepatitis B with evidence of viral replication and either persistent transaminase elevations or histologically-active disease
General Dosage Range Dosage adjustment recommended in patients with renal impairment
Oral: *Children ≥16 years and Adults:* 600 mg once daily
Product Availability Tyzeka® oral solution: FDA approved April 2009; anticipated availability is currently undetermined
Dosage Forms
Tablet, oral:
Tyzeka®: 600 mg

Teldrin® HBP [OTC] *see* chlorpheniramine *on page 197*

telithromycin (tel ith roe MYE sin)

Medication Safety Issues
Sound-alike/look-alike issues:
Telithromycin may be confused with telavancin
Synonyms HMR 3647
U.S. Brand Names Ketek®
Canadian Brand Names Ketek®
Therapeutic Category Antibiotic, Ketolide
Use Treatment of community-acquired pneumonia (mild-to-moderate) caused by susceptible strains of *Streptococcus pneumoniae* (including multidrug-resistant isolates), *Haemophilus influenzae*, *Chlamydophila pneumoniae*, *Moraxella catarrhalis*, and *Mycoplasma pneumoniae*
General Dosage Range Dosage adjustment recommended in patients with renal impairment
Oral: *Adults:* 800 mg once daily
Dosage Forms
Tablet, oral:
Ketek®: 300 mg, 400 mg

Dosage Forms - Canada
    Tablet:
      Ketek®: 400 mg

telmisartan (tel mi SAR tan)
U.S. Brand Names Micardis®
Canadian Brand Names Micardis®
Therapeutic Category Angiotensin II Receptor Antagonist
Use Treatment of hypertension (may be used alone or in combination with other antihypertensive agents); cardiovascular risk reduction in patients ≥55 years of age unable to take ACE inhibitors and who are at high risk of major cardiovascular events (eg, MI, stroke, death)
General Dosage Range Oral:
    Adults: Initial: 40-80 mg once daily; Maintenance: 20-80 mg/day once daily
    Elderly: Initial: 20-80 mg once daily
Dosage Forms
    Tablet, oral:
      Micardis®: 20 mg, 40 mg, 80 mg

telmisartan and amlodipine (tel mi SAR tan & am LOE di peen)
Synonyms amlodipine and telmisartan; amlodipine besylate and telmisartan
U.S. Brand Names Twynsta®
Therapeutic Category Angiotensin II Receptor Blocker; Calcium Channel Blocker; Calcium Channel Blocker, Dihydropyridine
Use Treatment of hypertension, including initial treatment in patients who will require multiple antihypertensives for adequate control
General Dosage Range Oral: *Adults:* Amlodipine 5-10 mg and telmisartan 40-80 mg once daily (maximum: 10 mg/day [amlodipine]; 80 mg/day [telmisartan])
Dosage Forms
    Tablet, oral:
      Twynsta® 40/5: Telmisartan 40 mg and amlodipine 5 mg; Twynsta® 40/10: telmisartan 40 mg and amlodipine 10 mg; Twynsta® 80/5: telmisartan 80 mg and amlodipine 5 mg; Twynsta® 80/10: telmisartan 80 mg and amlodipine10 mg

telmisartan and hydrochlorothiazide (tel mi SAR tan & hye droe klor oh THYE a zide)
Synonyms hydrochlorothiazide and telmisartan
U.S. Brand Names Micardis® HCT
Canadian Brand Names Micardis® Plus
Therapeutic Category Antihypertensive Agent, Combination
Use Treatment of hypertension; combination product should not be used for initial therapy
General Dosage Range Oral: *Adults:* Initial: Telmisartan 80 mg and hydrochlorothiazide 12.5-25 mg once daily; Maintenance: Telmisartan 80-160 mg and hydrochlorothiazide 12.5-25 mg once daily
Dosage Forms
    Tablet, oral:
      Micardis® HCT: 40/12.5: Telmisartan 40 mg and hydrochlorothiazide 12.5 mg; 80/12.5: Telmisartan 80 mg and hydrochlorothiazide 12.5 mg; 80/25: Telmisartan 80 mg and hydrochlorothiazide 25 mg
Dosage Forms - Canada
    Tablet, oral:
      Micardis® Plus: 80/25: Telmisartan 80 mg and hydrochlorothiazide 25 mg

Telzir® (Can) *see* fosamprenavir *on page 399*

temazepam (te MAZ e pam)
Medication Safety Issues
    Sound-alike/look-alike issues:
      Temazepam may be confused with flurazepam, LORazepam, tamoxifen
      Restoril™ may be confused with, RisperDAL®, Vistaril®, Zestril®
    BEERS Criteria medication:
      This drug may be inappropriate for use in geriatric patients (high severity risk).
U.S. Brand Names Restoril™

Canadian Brand Names Apo-Temazepam®; CO Temazepam; Dom-Temazepam; Gen-Temazepam; Novo-Temazepam; Nu-Temazepam; PHL-Temazepam; PMS-Temazepam; ratio-Temazepam; Restoril™

Therapeutic Category Benzodiazepine

Controlled Substance C-IV

Use Short-term treatment of insomnia

General Dosage Range Oral:
Adults: 7.5-30 mg at bedtime
Elderly: Initial: 7.5 mg at bedtime

Dosage Forms
Capsule, oral: 7.5 mg, 15 mg, 22.5 mg, 30 mg
Restoril™: 7.5 mg, 15 mg, 22.5 mg, 30 mg

Temodal® (Can) *see* temozolomide *on page 849*

Temodar® *see* temozolomide *on page 849*

Temovate® *see* clobetasol *on page 220*

Temovate E® *see* clobetasol *on page 220*

temozolomide (te moe ZOE loe mide)

Medication Safety Issues
Sound-alike/look-alike issues:
Temodar® may be confused with Tambocor®
Temozolomide may be confused with temsirolimus
High alert medication:
This medication is in a class the Institute for Safe Medication Practices (ISMP) includes among its list of drug classes which have a heightened risk of causing significant patient harm when used in error.

Synonyms SCH 52365; TMZ

U.S. Brand Names Temodar®

Canadian Brand Names Temodal®

Therapeutic Category Antineoplastic Agent, Alkylating Agent

Use Treatment of newly-diagnosed glioblastoma multiforme (initially in combination with radiotherapy, then as maintenance treatment); treatment of refractory anaplastic astrocytoma

Canadian labeling (not an approved indication in the U.S.): Treatment of recurrent or progressive glioblastoma multiforme

General Dosage Range Dosage adjustment recommended in patients who develop toxicities.
I.V., Oral: *Adults:* Dosage varies greatly depending on indication

Dosage Forms
Capsule, oral:
Temodar®: 5 mg, 20 mg, 100 mg, 140 mg, 180 mg, 250 mg
Injection, powder for reconstitution:
Temodar®: 100 mg

Tempra® (Can) *see* acetaminophen *on page 23*

temsirolimus (tem sir OH li mus)

Medication Safety Issues
Sound-alike/look-alike issues:
Temsirolimus may be confused with everolimus, sirolimus, tacrolimus, temozolomide, tesamorelin
High alert medication:
This medication is in a class the Institute for Safe Medication Practices (ISMP) includes among its list of drug classes which have a heightened risk of causing significant patient harm when used in error.
Administration issues:
Temsirolimus requires a two-step dilution process prior to administration. Dilute initially to 10 mg/mL (with provided diluent), then further dilute for infusion in 250 mL sodium chloride 0.9%. Errors have occurred due to improper preparation.
Temsirolimus, for the treatment of advanced renal cell cancer, is a flat dose (25 mg) and is not based on body surface area (BSA).

Synonyms CCI-779

U.S. Brand Names Torisel®

Canadian Brand Names Torisel®

Therapeutic Category Antineoplastic Agent, mTOR Kinase Inhibitor

Use Treatment of advanced renal cell cancer (RCC)

General Dosage Range Dosage adjustment recommended in patients with hepatic impairment, on concomitant therapy, or who develop toxicities

I.V.: *Adults:* 25 mg once weekly

Dosage Forms

Injection, solution:

Torisel®: 25 mg/mL (1.2 mL)

Tenar™ PSE [DSC] *see* guaifenesin and pseudoephedrine *on page 429*

teniposide (ten i POE side)

tenecteplase (ten EK te plase)

Medication Safety Issues

Sound-alike/look-alike issues:

TNKase® may be confused with Activase®, t-PA

TNK (occasional abbreviation for TNKase®) is an error-prone abbreviation (mistaken as TPA)

High alert medication:

The Institute for Safe Medication Practices (ISMP) includes this medication (I.V.) among its list of drugs which have a heightened risk of causing significant patient harm when used in error.

U.S. Brand Names TNKase®

Canadian Brand Names TNKase®

Therapeutic Category Thrombolytic Agent

Use Thrombolytic agent used in the management of ST-elevation myocardial infarction (STEMI) for the lysis of thrombi in the coronary vasculature to restore perfusion and reduce mortality.

Recommended criteria for treatment: STEMI: Chest pain ≥20 minutes duration, onset of chest pain within 12 hours of treatment (or within prior 12-24 hours in patients with continuing ischemic symptoms), and S-T segment elevation >0.1 mV in at least two contiguous precordial leads or two adjacent limb leads on ECG or new or presumably new left bundle branch block (LBBB)

General Dosage Range I.V.:

Adults <60 kg: 30 mg as a single dose

Adults ≥60 to <70 kg: 35 mg as a single dose

Adults ≥70 to <80 kg: 40 mg as a single dose

Adults ≥80 to <90 kg: 45 mg as a single dose

Adults ≥90 kg: 50 mg as a single dose

Dosage Forms

Injection, powder for reconstitution:

TNKase®: 50 mg

Tenex® *see* guanfacine *on page 431*

teniposide (ten i POE side)

Medication Safety Issues

Sound-alike/look-alike issues:

Teniposide may be confused with etoposide

High alert medication:

This medication is in a class the Institute for Safe Medication Practices (ISMP) includes among its list of drug classes which have a heightened risk of causing significant patient harm when used in error.

Synonyms EPT; PTG; VM-26

U.S. Brand Names Vumon®

Canadian Brand Names Vumon®

Therapeutic Category Antineoplastic Agent

Use Treatment of refractory childhood acute lymphoblastic leukemia (ALL) in combination with other chemotherapy

General Dosage Range I.V.: *Children:* 165 mg/m^2 twice weekly for 8-9 doses **or** 250 mg/m^2 weekly for 4-8 weeks

Dosage Forms

Injection, solution:

Vumon®: 10 mg/mL (5 mL)

tenofovir (te NOE fo veer)

Synonyms PMPA; TDF; tenofovir disoproxil fumarate
U.S. Brand Names Viread®
Canadian Brand Names Viread®
Therapeutic Category Antiretroviral Agent, Reverse Transcriptase Inhibitor (Nucleotide)
Use Management of HIV infections in combination with at least two other antiretroviral agents; treatment of chronic hepatitis B virus (HBV) in patients with compensated or decompensated liver disease
General Dosage Range Dosage adjustment recommended in patients with renal impairment
  Oral: *Children ≥12 years and ≥35 kg and Adults:* 300 mg once daily
Dosage Forms
  Tablet, oral:
    Viread®: 300 mg

tenofovir and emtricitabine *see* emtricitabine and tenofovir *on page 326*
tenofovir disoproxil fumarate *see* tenofovir *on page 851*
tenofovir disoproxil fumarate, efavirenz, and emtricitabine *see* efavirenz, emtricitabine, and tenofovir *on page 321*
tenofovir, emtricitabine, and rilpivirine *see* emtricitabine, rilpivirine, and tenofovir *on page 326*
Tenoretic® *see* atenolol and chlorthalidone *on page 101*
Tenormin® *see* atenolol *on page 101*
Tensilon® (Can) *see* edrophonium *on page 320*
Tenuate® (Can) *see* diethylpropion *on page 281*
Tenuate® Dospan® (Can) *see* diethylpropion *on page 281*
Tera-Gel™ [OTC] *see* coal tar *on page 227*
Terazol® (Can) *see* terconazole *on page 853*
Terazol® 3 *see* terconazole *on page 853*
Terazol® 7 *see* terconazole *on page 853*

terazosin (ter AY zoe sin)

Synonyms Hytrin
Canadian Brand Names Apo-Terazosin®; Dom-Terazosin; Hytrin®; Nu-Terazosin; PHL-Terazosin; PMS-Terazosin; ratio-Terazosin; Teva-Terazosin
Therapeutic Category Alpha-Adrenergic Blocking Agent
Use Management of mild-to-moderate hypertension; alone or in combination with other agents such as diuretics or beta-blockers; benign prostate hyperplasia (BPH)
General Dosage Range Dosage adjustment recommended in patients on concomitant therapy
  Oral: *Adults:* Initial: 1 mg at bedtime; Maintenance: 1-20 mg once daily (maximum: 20 mg/day)
Dosage Forms
  Capsule, oral: 1 mg, 2 mg, 5 mg, 10 mg

terbinafine (systemic) (TER bin a feen)

Medication Safety Issues
  Sound-alike/look-alike issues:
    Terbinafine may be confused with terbutaline
    LamISIL® may be confused with LaMICtal®, Lomotil®
Synonyms terbinafine hydrochloride
U.S. Brand Names LamISIL®; Terbinex™
Canadian Brand Names Apo-Terbinafine®; Auro-Terbinafine; CO Terbinafine; Dom-Terbinafine; JAMP-Terbinafine; Lamisil®; Mylan-Terbinafine; Nu-Terbinafine; PHL-Terbinafine; PMS-Terbinafine; Riva-Terbinafine; Sandoz-Terbinafine; Teva-Terbinafine
Therapeutic Category Antifungal Agent, Oral
Use Active against most strains of *Trichophyton mentagrophytes, Trichophyton rubrum*; may be effective for infections of *Microsporum gypseum* and *M. nanum, Trichophyton verrucosum, Epidermophyton floccosum, Candida albicans*, and *Scopulariopsis brevicaulis*

Onychomycosis of the toenail or fingernail due to susceptible dermatophytes; treatment of tinea capitis

◀ **General Dosage Range**
Oral granules: *Children ≥4 years:*
<25 kg: 125 mg once daily for 6 weeks
25-35 kg: 187.5 mg once daily for 6 weeks
>35 kg: 250 mg once daily for 6 weeks
Oral tablet: *Adults:* 250-500 mg daily in 1-2 divided doses

Dosage Forms
Granules, oral:
LamISIL®: 125 mg/packet (14s, 42s); 187.5 mg/packet (14s, 42s)
Tablet, oral: 250 mg
LamISIL®: 250 mg
Terbinex™: 250 mg

terbinafine (topical) (TER bin a feen)

Medication Safety Issues
Sound-alike/look-alike issues:
Terbinafine may be confused with terbutaline

Synonyms terbinafine hydrochloride

U.S. Brand Names LamISIL AT® [OTC]

Canadian Brand Names Lamisil®

Therapeutic Category Antifungal Agent, Topical

Use Antifungal for the treatment of tinea pedis (athlete's foot), tinea cruris (jock itch), and tinea corporis (ringworm) [OTC/prescription formulations]; tinea versicolor [prescription formulations]

General Dosage Range Topical: *Children ≥12 years and Adults:* Apply to affected area once or twice daily

Dosage Forms
Cream, topical: 1% (12 g, 15 g, 24 g, 30 g)
LamISIL AT® [OTC]: 1% (12 g, 15 g, 24 g, 30 g, 36 g)
Gel, topical:
LamISIL AT® [OTC]: 1% (6 g, 12 g)
Solution, topical:
LamISIL AT® [OTC]: 1% (30 mL)

Dosage Forms - Canada
Cream, topical:
Lamisil®: 1% (15 g, 30 g)
Solution, topical [spray]:
Lamisil®: 1% (30 mL)

terbinafine hydrochloride *see* terbinafine (systemic) *on page 851*
terbinafine hydrochloride *see* terbinafine (topical) *on page 852*
Terbinex™ *see* terbinafine (systemic) *on page 851*

terbutaline (ter BYOO ta leen)

Medication Safety Issues
Sound-alike/look-alike issues:
Brethine may be confused with Methergine®
Terbutaline may be confused with terbinafine, TOLBUTamide
Terbutaline and methylergonovine parenteral dosage forms look similar. Due to their contrasting indications, use care when administering these agents.

Synonyms Brethaire [DSC]; brethine; Bricanyl [DSC]

Canadian Brand Names Bricanyl®

Therapeutic Category Adrenergic Agonist Agent

Use Bronchodilator in reversible airway obstruction and bronchial asthma

General Dosage Range Dosage adjustment recommended in patients with renal impairment
Oral:
Children 12-15 years: 2.5 mg every 6 hours 3 times/day (maximum: 7.5 mg/day)
Children >15 years and Adults: 2.5-5 mg every 6 hours 3 times/day (maximum: 15 mg/day)

SubQ:
Children <12 years: 0.005-0.01 mg/kg/dose to a maximum of 0.4 mg/dose; may repeat in 15-20 minutes
Children ≥12 years and Adults: 0.25 mg/dose; may repeat in 15-30 minutes (maximum: 0.5 mg/4-hour period)

Dosage Forms
Injection, solution: 1 mg/mL (1 mL)
Tablet, oral: 2.5 mg, 5 mg
Dosage Forms - Canada
Powder for oral inhalation:
Bricanyl® Turbuhaler: 500 mcg/actuation [50 or 200 metered actuations]

terconazole (ter KONE a zole)

Medication Safety Issues
Sound-alike/look-alike issues:
Terconazole may be confused with tioconazole
International issues:
Terazol [U.S., Canada] may be confused with Theradol brand name for tramadol [Netherlands]
Synonyms triaconazole
U.S. Brand Names Terazol® 3; Terazol® 7; Zazole™ [DSC]
Canadian Brand Names Terazol®
Therapeutic Category Antifungal Agent
Use Local treatment of vulvovaginal candidiasis
General Dosage Range Intravaginal: *Adults:* Insert 1 applicatorful or suppository at bedtime
Dosage Forms
Cream, vaginal: 0.4% (45 g); 0.8% (20 g)
Terazol® 7: 0.4% (45 g)
Terazol® 3: 0.8% (20 g)
Suppository, vaginal: 80 mg (3s)
Terazol® 3: 80 mg (3s)

Terfluzine (Can) *see* trifluoperazine *on page 890*

teriparatide (ter i PAR a tide)

Synonyms parathyroid hormone (1-34); recombinant human parathyroid hormone (1-34); rhPTH(1-34)
U.S. Brand Names Forteo®
Canadian Brand Names Forteo®
Therapeutic Category Diagnostic Agent
Use Treatment of osteoporosis in postmenopausal women at high risk of fracture; treatment of primary or hypogonadal osteoporosis in men at high risk of fracture; treatment of glucocorticoid-induced osteoporosis in men and women at high risk for fracture
General Dosage Range SubQ: *Adults:* 20 mcg once daily
Dosage Forms
Injection, solution:
Forteo®: 250 mcg/mL (2.4 mL)
Dosage Forms - Canada
Injection, solution:
Forteo®: 250 mcg/mL (3 mL)

Terrell™ *see* isoflurane *on page 493*
Tersi *see* selenium sulfide *on page 807*

tesamorelin (tes a moe REL in)

Medication Safety Issues
Sound-alike/look-alike issues:
Tesamorelin may be confused with temsirolimus
Synonyms tesamorelin acetate; TH9507
U.S. Brand Names Egrifta™
Therapeutic Category Growth Hormone Releasing Factor
Use Reduction of excess abdominal fat in HIV-infected patients with lipodystrophy

◀ **General Dosage Range SubQ:** *Adults:* 2 mg once daily
Dosage Forms
Injection, powder for reconstitution:
Egrifta™: 1 mg

tesamorelin acetate *see tesamorelin on page 853*
TESPA *see thiotepa on page 864*
Tessalon® *see benzonatate on page 124*
tessalon perles *see benzonatate on page 124*
Testim® *see testosterone on page 854*
Testopel® *see testosterone on page 854*

testosterone (tes TOS ter one)

Medication Safety Issues
Sound-alike/look-alike issues:
Testosterone may be confused with testolactone
Testoderm® may be confused with Estraderm®
AndroGel® 1% may be confused with AndroGel® 1.62%
Other safety concerns:
Transdermal patch may contain conducting metal (eg, aluminum); remove patch prior to MRI.
Synonyms testosterone cypionate; testosterone enanthate
U.S. Brand Names Androderm®; AndroGel®; Axiron®; Delatestryl®; Depo®-Testosterone; First®-Testosterone; First®-Testosterone MC; Fortesta™; Striant®; Testim®; Testopel®
Canadian Brand Names Andriol®; Androderm®; AndroGel®; Andropository; Delatestryl®; Depotest® 100; Everone® 200; PMS-Testosterone; Testim®
Therapeutic Category Androgen
Controlled Substance C-III
Use
Injection: Androgen replacement therapy in the treatment of delayed male puberty; male hypogonadism (primary or hypogonadotropic); inoperable metastatic female breast cancer (enanthate only)
Pellet: Androgen replacement therapy in the treatment of delayed male puberty; male hypogonadism (primary or hypogonadotropic)
Buccal system, topical gel, topical solution, transdermal system: Male hypogonadism (primary or hypogonadotropic)
Capsule (not available in U.S.): Conditions associated with a deficiency or absence of endogenous testosterone
General Dosage Range
Buccal: *Adults (males):* 30 mg every 12 hours
I.M.: *Adolescents and Adults (males):* 50-400 mg every 2-4 weeks
SubQ: *Adolescents and Adults (males):* 150-450 mg every 3-6 months
Transdermal: *Adults (males):* Androderm®: Apply 2.5-7.5 mg/day; AndroGel® 1%, Testim®: 5-10 g (50-100 mg testosterone) applied once daily (maximum: 10 g/day); AndroGel® 1.62%: Apply 20.25-81 mg/day; Axiron®: Apply 30-120 mg/day; Fortesta™: Apply 10-70 mg/day
Dosage Forms
Cream, topical:
First®-Testosterone MC: 2% (60 g)
Gel, topical:
AndroGel®: 1% [5 g gel/packet] (30s); 1% [2.5 g gel/packet] (30s); 1% [1.25 g gel/actuation] (75 g); 1.62% [1.25 g gel/actuation] (75 g)
Fortesta™: 10 mg/actuation (60 g)
Testim®: 1% [5 g gel/tube] (30s)
Implant, subcutaneous:
Testopel®: 75 mg (10s, 24s, 100s)
Injection, oil: 100 mg/mL (10 mL); 200 mg/mL (1 mL, 5 mL, 10 mL)
Delatestryl®: 200 mg/mL (5 mL)
Depo®-Testosterone: 100 mg/mL (10 mL); 200 mg/mL (1 mL, 10 mL)
Mucoadhesive, for buccal application:
Striant®: 30 mg (60s)
Ointment, topical:
First®-Testosterone: 2% (60 g)

Patch, transdermal:
Androderm®: 2.5 mg/24 hours (60s); 5 mg/24 hours (30s)
Powder, for prescription compounding: USP: 100% (5 g, 25 g)
Solution, topical:
Axiron®: 30 mg/actuation (110 mL)
Dosage Forms - Canada
Capsule, gelatin:
Andriol™: 40 mg (10s)

testosterone cypionate *see* testosterone *on page* *854*
testosterone enanthate *see* testosterone *on page* *854*
Testred® *see* methyltestosterone *on page* *579*
tetanus and diphtheria toxoid *see* diphtheria and tetanus toxoid *on page* *293*

tetanus immune globulin (human) (TET a nus i MYUN GLOB yoo lin HYU man)

Synonyms TIG
U.S. Brand Names HyperTET™ S/D
Canadian Brand Names HyperTET™ S/D
Therapeutic Category Immune Globulin
Use Prophylaxis against tetanus following injury in patients where immunization status is not known or uncertain
The Advisory Committee on Immunization Practices (ACIP) recommends passive immunization with TIG for the following:
• Persons with a wound that is not clean or minor and in whom contraindications to a tetanus-toxoid containing vaccine exist and they have not completed a primary series of tetanus toxoid immunization.
• Persons who are wounded in bombings or similar mass casualty events who have penetrating injuries or nonintact skin exposure and who cannot confirm receipt of a tetanus booster within the previous 5 years. In case of shortage, use should be reserved for persons ≥60 years of age.
General Dosage Range I.M.:
Children <7 years: Prophylaxis: 4 units/kg
Children ≥7 years: Prophylaxis: 250 units
Children: Treatment: 500-6000 units
Adults: Prophylaxis: 250 units; Treatment: 500-6000 units
Dosage Forms
Injection, solution [preservative free]:
HyperTET™ S/D: 250 units/mL (~1 mL)

tetanus toxoid *see* diphtheria and tetanus toxoids, acellular pertussis, poliovirus and *Haemophilus* b conjugate vaccine *on page* *295*

tetanus toxoid (adsorbed) (TET a nus TOKS oyd, ad SORBED)

Medication Safety Issues
Sound-alike/look-alike issues:
Tetanus toxoid products may be confused with influenza virus vaccine and tuberculin products. Medication errors have occurred when tetanus toxoid products have been inadvertently administered instead of tuberculin skin tests (PPD) and influenza virus vaccine. These products are refrigerated and often stored in close proximity to each other.
Synonyms TT
Therapeutic Category Toxoid
Use Active immunization against tetanus when combination antigen preparations are not indicated; tetanus prophylaxis in wound management. **Note:** Tetanus and diphtheria toxoids for adult use (Td) is the preferred immunizing agent for most adults and for children after their seventh birthday. Young children should receive trivalent DTaP (diphtheria/tetanus/acellular pertussis) as part of their childhood immunization program, unless pertussis is contraindicated, then DT is warranted.
General Dosage Range I.M.: *Children ≥7 years and Adults:* Initial: 0.5 mL; repeat at 4-8 weeks after first dose and 6-12 months after second dose
Dosage Forms
Injection, suspension: 5 Lf units/0.5 mL (0.5 mL, 5 mL)

tetanus toxoid, reduced diphtheria toxoid, and acellular pertussis, adsorbed *see* diphtheria, tetanus toxoids, and acellular pertussis vaccine *on page* *296*

Tetcaine *see* tetracaine (ophthalmic) *on page 856*

tetrabenazine (tet ra BEN a zeen)

U.S. Brand Names Xenazine®

Canadian Brand Names Nitoman™

Therapeutic Category Monoamine Depleting Agent

Use Treatment of chorea associated with Huntington disease

Canadian labeling: Treatment of hyperkinetic movement disorders, including Huntington chorea, hemiballismus, senile chorea, Tourette syndrome, and tardive dyskinesia

General Dosage Range Dosage adjustment recommended in patients on concomitant therapy or who develop toxicities

Oral: *Adults:* 12.5 mg once daily; Maintenance: 25-100 mg/day in 2-3 divided doses

Dosage Forms

Tablet, oral:

Xenazine®: 12.5 mg, 25 mg

Dosage Forms - Canada

Tablet:

Nitoman™: 25 mg

tetracaine (systemic) (TET ra kane)

Synonyms amethocaine hydrochloride; tetracaine hydrochloride

Canadian Brand Names Pontocaine®

Therapeutic Category Local Anesthetic

Use Spinal anesthesia

General Dosage Range Subarachnoid injection: *Adults:* 2-15 mg (maximum: 20 mg)

Dosage Forms

Injection, solution [preservative free]: 1% [10 mg/mL] (2 mL)

tetracaine (ophthalmic) (TET ra kane)

Synonyms amethocaine hydrochloride; tetracaine hydrochloride

U.S. Brand Names Altacaine; Tetcaine; TetraVisc™; TetraVisc™ FORTE

Canadian Brand Names Pontocaine®

Therapeutic Category Local Anesthetic

Use Local anesthesia for various ophthalmic procedures of short duration (eg, tonometry, gonioscopy); minor ophthalmic surgical procedures (eg, removal of corneal foreign bodies, suture removal); and for various diagnostic purposes (eg, conjunctival scrapings)

General Dosage Range Ophthalmic: *Adults:* Instill 1-2 drops into eye(s); may repeat every 5-10 minutes; do not exceed 5 doses

Dosage Forms

Solution, ophthalmic: 0.5% [5 mg/mL] (2 mL, 15 mL)

Altacaine: 0.5% [5 mg/mL] (15 mL, 30 mL)

Tetcaine: 0.5% [5 mg/mL] (15 mL)

TetraVisc™: 0.5% [5 mg/mL] (0.6 mL, 5 mL)

TetraVisc™ FORTE: 0.5% [5 mg/mL] (0.6 mL, 5 mL)

tetracaine (topical) (TET ra kane)

Synonyms amethocaine hydrochloride; tetracaine hydrochloride

U.S. Brand Names Pontocaine® [DSC]

Canadian Brand Names Ametop™; Pontocaine®

Therapeutic Category Local Anesthetic

Use Applied to nose and throat for diagnostic procedures

General Dosage Range Topical: *Adults:* 0.25% or 0.5% by direct application or nebulization (maximum: 20 mg total)

Dosage Forms

Solution, topical:

Pontocaine®: 2% [20 mg/mL] (30 mL, 118 mL)

tetracaine and lidocaine *see* lidocaine and tetracaine *on page 527*

tetracaine, benzocaine, and butamben *see* benzocaine, butamben, and tetracaine *on page 123*
tetracaine hydrochloride *see* tetracaine (ophthalmic) *on page 856*
tetracaine hydrochloride *see* tetracaine (systemic) *on page 856*
tetracaine hydrochloride *see* tetracaine (topical) *on page 856*
tetracosactide *see* cosyntropin *on page 237*

tetracycline (tet ra SYE kleen)

Medication Safety Issues
Sound-alike/look-alike issues:
  Tetracycline may be confused with tetradecyl sulfate
  Achromycin may be confused with actinomycin, Adriamycin PFS®
Synonyms achromycin; TCN; tetracycline hydrochloride
Canadian Brand Names Apo-Tetra®; Nu-Tetra
Therapeutic Category Tetracycline Derivative
Use Treatment of susceptible bacterial infections of both gram-positive and gram-negative organisms; also infections due to *Mycoplasma, Chlamydia,* and *Rickettsia*; indicated for acne, exacerbations of chronic bronchitis, and treatment of gonorrhea and syphilis in patients who are allergic to penicillin; as part of a multidrug regimen for *H. pylori* eradication to reduce the risk of duodenal ulcer recurrence
General Dosage Range Dosage adjustment recommended in patients with renal impairment
Oral:
  Children >8 years: 25-50 mg/kg/day divided every 6 hours
  Adults: 250-500 mg 2-4 times/day
Dosage Forms
Capsule, oral: 250 mg, 500 mg

tetracycline hydrochloride *see* tetracycline *on page 857*
tetracycline, metronidazole, and bismuth subcitrate potassium *see* bismuth, metronidazole, and tetracycline *on page 136*
tetracycline, metronidazole, and bismuth subsalicylate *see* bismuth, metronidazole, and tetracycline *on page 136*
tetrahydrocannabinol *see* dronabinol *on page 314*

tetrahydrocannabinol and cannabidiol *(Canada only)*
(TET ra hye droe can NAB e nol & can nab e DYE ol)
Synonyms cannabidiol and tetrahydrocannabinol; delta-9-tetrahydrocannabinol and cannabinol; GW-1000-02; THC and CBD
Canadian Brand Names Sativex®
Therapeutic Category Analgesic, Miscellaneous
Controlled Substance CDSA-II
Use Adjunctive treatment of neuropathic pain or spasticity in multiple sclerosis; adjunctive treatment of moderate-to-severe pain in advanced cancer
General Dosage Range Dosage adjustment recommended in patients who develop toxicities
Buccal: *Adults:* Initial: 1 spray twice daily; Maintenance: Usual maximum: 12 sprays/day
Product Availability Not available in U.S.
Dosage Forms - Canada
Solution, buccal [spray]:
  Sativex®: Delta-9 tetrahydrocannabinol 27 mg/mL and cannabidiol 25 mg/mL (5.5 mL)

tetrahydrozoline (nasal) (tet ra hye DROZ a leen)
Synonyms tetrahydrozoline hydrochloride; tetryzoline
U.S. Brand Names Tyzine®; Tyzine® Pediatric
Therapeutic Category Adrenergic Agonist Agent; Imidazoline Derivative
Use Symptomatic relief of nasal congestion
General Dosage Range Intranasal:
  Children 2-6 years: Instill 2-3 drops (0.05%) into each nostril every 4-6 hours as needed (maximum: Every 3 hours)
  Children >6 years and Adults: Instill 2-4 drops (0.1%) **or** 3-4 sprays (0.1%) into each nostril every 3-4 hours as needed (maximum: Every 3 hours)

▶

◀ **Dosage Forms**
Solution, intranasal:
Tyzine®: 0.1% (15 mL, 30 mL)
Tyzine® Pediatric: 0.05% (15 mL)

tetrahydrozoline (ophthalmic) (tet ra hye DROZ a leen)

Medication Safety Issues
Sound-alike/look-alike issues:
Visine® may be confused with Visken®
Synonyms tetrahydrozoline hydrochloride; tetryzoline
U.S. Brand Names Murine® Tears Plus [OTC]; Opti-Clear [OTC]; Visine® Advanced Relief [OTC]; Visine® Original [OTC]
Therapeutic Category Adrenergic Agonist Agent; Imidazoline Derivative; Ophthalmic Agent, Vasoconstrictor
Use Symptomatic relief of conjunctival congestion
General Dosage Range Ophthalmic: *Adults:* Instill 1-2 drops in each eye 2-4 times/day
Dosage Forms
Solution, ophthalmic: 0.05% (15 mL)
Murine® Tears Plus [OTC]: 0.05% (15 mL)
Opti-Clear [OTC]: 0.05% (15 mL)
Visine® Advanced Relief [OTC]: 0.05% (15 mL, 30 mL)
Visine® Original [OTC]: 0.05% (15 mL, 30 mL)

tetrahydrozoline hydrochloride *see* tetrahydrozoline (nasal) *on page 857*
tetrahydrozoline hydrochloride *see* tetrahydrozoline (ophthalmic) *on page 858*
tetraiodothyronine and triiodothyronine *see* thyroid, desiccated *on page 865*
2,2,2-tetramine *see* trientine *on page 889*

tetrastarch (TET ra starch)

Synonyms HES; HES 130/0.4; hydroxyethyl starch
U.S. Brand Names Voluven®
Canadian Brand Names Voluven®
Therapeutic Category Plasma Volume Expander, Colloid
Use Blood volume expander used in treatment and prevention of hypovolemia
General Dosage Range I.V. infusion:
Children <2 years: Average dose: 7-25 mL/kg
Children >12 years and Adults: Maximum dose: 50 mL/kg/day (or up to 3500 mL in a 70 kg patient)
Dosage Forms
Infusion, premixed in NS:
Voluven®: 6% (500 mL)

Tetra Tannate Pediatric [DSC] *see* chlorpheniramine, ephedrine, phenylephrine, and carbetapentane *on page 199*
TetraVisc™ *see* tetracaine (ophthalmic) *on page 856*
TetraVisc™ FORTE *see* tetracaine (ophthalmic) *on page 856*
tetryzoline *see* tetrahydrozoline (nasal) *on page 857*
tetryzoline *see* tetrahydrozoline (ophthalmic) *on page 858*
Teva-Acebutolol (Can) *see* acebutolol *on page 23*
Teva-Acyclovir (Can) *see* acyclovir (systemic) *on page 39*
Teva-Alendronate (Can) *see* alendronate *on page 49*
Teva-Alfuzosin PR (Can) *see* alfuzosin *on page 50*
Teva-Alprazolam (Can) *see* alprazolam *on page 56*
Teva-Amiodarone (Can) *see* amiodarone *on page 67*
Teva-Amlodipine (Can) *see* amlodipine *on page 69*
Teva-Atenolol (Can) *see* atenolol *on page 101*
Teva-Atenolol Chlorthalidone (Can) *see* atenolol and chlorthalidone *on page 101*
Teva-Azathioprine (Can) *see* azathioprine *on page 107*
Teva-Captopril (Can) *see* captopril *on page 170*

Teva-Theophylline SR (Can) *see* theophylline *on page 860*

Teva-Tiaprofenic Acid (Can) *see* tiaprofenic acid *(Canada only) on page 867*

Teva-Ticlopidine (Can) *see* ticlopidine *on page 868*

Teva-Timolol (Can) *see* timolol (systemic) *on page 868*

Teva-Trazodone (Can) *see* trazodone *on page 884*

Teva-Triamterene HCTZ (Can) *see* hydrochlorothiazide and triamterene *on page 446*

Teva-Valsartan (Can) *see* valsartan *on page 905*

Teva-Valsartan HCTZ (Can) *see* valsartan and hydrochlorothiazide *on page 906*

Teva-Venlafaxine XR (Can) *see* venlafaxine *on page 911*

Teva-Zolmitriptan (Can) *see* zolmitriptan *on page 933*

Teva-Zolmitriptan OD (Can) *see* zolmitriptan *on page 933*

Teveten® *see* eprosartan *on page 335*

Teveten® HCT *see* eprosartan and hydrochlorothiazide *on page 335*

Teveten® Plus (Can) *see* eprosartan and hydrochlorothiazide *on page 335*

Tev-Tropin® *see* somatropin *on page 826*

Texacort® *see* hydrocortisone (topical) *on page 450*

TG *see* thioguanine *on page 862*

T/Gel® Daily Control 2 in 1 Dandruff Shampoo Plus Conditioner [OTC] *see* pyrithione zinc *on page 759*

T/Gel® Daily Control Dandruff Shampoo [OTC] *see* pyrithione zinc *on page 759*

6-TG (error-prone abbreviation) *see* thioguanine *on page 862*

TH9507 *see* tesamorelin *on page 853*

thalidomide (tha LI doe mide)

Medication Safety Issues
Sound-alike/look-alike issues:
Thalidomide may be confused with flutamide, lenalidomide
Thalomid® may be confused with thiamine
High alert medication:
This medication is in a class the Institute for Safe Medication Practices (ISMP) includes among its list of drugs which have a heightened risk of causing significant patient harm when used in error.
International issues:
Thalomid [U.S., Canada] may be confused with Thilomide brand name for Iodoxamide [Greece, Turkey]
U.S. Brand Names Thalomid®
Canadian Brand Names Thalomid®
Therapeutic Category Immunosuppressant Agent
Use Treatment of newly-diagnosed multiple myeloma; treatment and maintenance of cutaneous manifestations of erythema nodosum leprosum (ENL)
General Dosage Range Dosage adjustment recommended in patients who develop toxicities
Oral: *Children ≥12 years and Adults:* Initial: 100-300 mg once daily (maximum: 400 mg/day)
Dosage Forms
Capsule, oral:
Thalomid®: 50 mg, 100 mg, 150 mg, 200 mg

Thalitone® *see* chlorthalidone *on page 204*

Thalomid® *see* thalidomide *on page 860*

THAM® *see* tromethamine *on page 895*

THC *see* dronabinol *on page 314*

THC and CBD *see* tetrahydrocannabinol and cannabidiol *(Canada only) on page 857*

Thelin® (Can) *see* sitaxsentan *(Canada only) on page 816*

Theo-24® *see* theophylline *on page 860*

Theochron® SR (Can) *see* theophylline *on page 860*

Theo ER (Can) *see* theophylline *on page 860*

Theolair (Can) *see* theophylline *on page 860*

theophylline (thee OFF i lin)

Synonyms theophylline anhydrous

U.S. Brand Names Elixophyllin® Elixir; Theo-24®

Canadian Brand Names Apo-Theo LA®; Novo-Theophyl SR; PMS-Theophylline; Pulmophylline; ratio-Theo-Bronc; Teva-Theophylline SR; Theo ER; Theochron® SR; Theolair; Uniphyl

Therapeutic Category Theophylline Derivative

Use Treatment of symptoms and reversible airway obstruction due to chronic asthma, or other chronic lung diseases

Note: The Global Initiative for Asthma Guidelines (2009) and the National Heart, Lung and Blood Institute Guidelines (2007) do not recommend oral theophylline as a long-term control medication for asthma in children ≤5 years of age; use has been shown to be effective as an add-on (but not preferred) agent in older children and adults with severe asthma treated with inhaled or oral glucocorticoids. The guidelines do not recommend theophylline for the treatment of exacerbations of asthma.

The Global Initiative for Chronic Obstructive Lung Disease Guidelines (2009) suggest that while higher doses of slow release formulations of theophylline have been proven to be effective for use in COPD, it is not a preferred agent due to its potential for toxicity.

General Dosage Range

I.V.:

Infants 6-52 weeks: mg/kg/hour = (0.008) (age in weeks) + 0.21

Children 1-9 years: 0.8 mg/kg/hour

Children 9-12 years and Adolescents 12-16 years (cigarette or marijuana smokers): 0.7 mg/kg/hour

Adolescents 12-16 years (nonsmokers): 0.5 mg/kg/hour; maximum 900 mg/day unless serum levels indicate need for larger dose

Adults 16-60 years (otherwise healthy, nonsmokers): 0.4 mg/kg/hour; maximum 900 mg/day unless serum levels indicate need for larger dose

Adults >60 years: 0.3 mg/kg/hour; maximum 400 mg/day unless serum levels indicate need for larger dose

Oral solution:

Full-term Infants and Infants <26 weeks: Total daily dose (mg) = [(0.2 x age in weeks) +5] x (weight in kg); divide dose into 3 equal amounts and administer at 8-hour intervals

Full-term Infants and Infants ≥26 weeks and <52 weeks: Total daily dose (mg) = [(0.2 x age in weeks) +5] x (weight in kg); divide dose into 4 equal amounts and administer at 6-hour intervals

Children ≥1 year and <45 kg: Initial: 10-14 mg/kg/day in divided doses (maximum dose: 300 mg/day); titrate to maintenance dose: 20 mg/kg/day in divided doses every 4-6 hours (maximum dose: 600 mg/day)

Children >45 kg and Adults: Initial: 300 mg/day in divided doses; titrate to maintenance dose: 600 mg/day in divided doses every 6-8 hours

Oral extended release formulations:

Children ≥1 year and <45 kg: Initial: 10-14 mg/kg once daily (maximum dose: 300 mg/day); titrate to maintenance dose: 20 mg/kg once daily (maximum dose: 600 mg/day)

Children >45 kg and Adults: 300-600 mg once daily

Dosage Forms

Capsule, extended release, oral: Theo-24®: 100 mg, 200 mg, 300 mg, 400 mg

Infusion, premixed in D$_5$W: 400 mg (100 mL, 250 mL, 500 mL, 1000 mL); 800 mg (250 mL, 500 mL, 1000 mL)

Solution, oral: 80 mg/15 mL (15 mL)
Elixophyllin® Elixir: 80 mg/15 mL (473 mL)

Tablet, extended release, oral: 100 mg, 200 mg, 300 mg, 400 mg, 450 mg, 600 mg

theophylline anhydrous *see* theophylline *on page 860*

theophylline ethylenediamine *see* aminophylline *on page 66*

TheraCys® *see* BCG *on page 115*

Theraflu® Daytime Severe Cold & Cough [OTC] *see* acetaminophen, dextromethorphan, and phenylephrine *on page 32*

Theraflu® Nighttime Severe Cold & Cough [OTC] *see* acetaminophen, diphenhydramine, and phenylephrine *on page 33*

Theraflu® Sugar-Free Nighttime Severe Cold & Cough [OTC] *see* acetaminophen, diphenhydramine, and phenylephrine *on page 33*

Theraflu® Thin Strips® Multi Symptom [OTC] *see* diphenhydramine (systemic) *on page 290*

Theraflu Warming Relief® Daytime Multi-Symptom Cold [OTC] *see* acetaminophen, dextromethorphan, and phenylephrine *on page 32*

Theraflu Warming Relief® Daytime Severe Cold & Cough [OTC] *see* acetaminophen, dextromethorphan, and phenylephrine *on page 32*

Theraflu® Warming Relief ™ Flu & Sore Throat [OTC] *see* acetaminophen, diphenhydramine, and phenylephrine *on page 33*

Theraflu® Warming Relief™ Nighttime Severe Cold & Cough [OTC] *see* acetaminophen, diphenhydramine, and phenylephrine *on page 33*

Thera-Gel [OTC] *see* coal tar *on page 227*

Thera-Gesic® [OTC] *see* methyl salicylate and menthol *on page 579*

Thera-Gesic® Plus [OTC] *see* methyl salicylate and menthol *on page 579*

therapeutic multivitamins *see* vitamins (multiple/oral) *on page 919*

Thera-Sal [OTC] *see* salicylic acid *on page 795*

Theratears® [OTC] *see* carboxymethylcellulose *on page 175*

Thermazene® *see* silver sulfadiazine *on page 812*

thiamazole *see* methimazole *on page 570*

thiamin *see* thiamine *on page 862*

thiamine (THYE a min)

Medication Safety Issues
Sound-alike/look-alike issues:
Thiamine may be confused with Tenormin®, Thalomid®, Thorazine®
International issues:
Doxal® [Brazil] may be confused with Doxil® which is a brand name for doxorubicin in the U.S.

Doxal® [Brazil]: Brand name for doxycycline in Austria; brand name for pyridoxine/thiamine combination in Brazil; brand name for doxepin in Finland

Synonyms aneurine hydrochloride; thiamin; thiamine hydrochloride; thiaminium chloride hydrochloride; vitamin B_1

Canadian Brand Names Betaxin®

Therapeutic Category Vitamin, Water Soluble

Use Treatment of thiamine deficiency including beriberi, Wernicke encephalopathy, Korsakoff syndrome, neuritis associated with pregnancy, or in alcoholic patients; dietary supplement

General Dosage Range
I.M., I.V.:
Children: 10-25 mg/dose daily (thiamine deficiency)

Adults: 5-30 mg/dose 3 times/day (thiamine deficiency) **or** 50-250 mg/day (Wernicke encephalopathy)
Oral:
Infants: 0.2-0.3 mg/day (adequate intake)

Children: 0.5-1.4 mg/day (recommended daily intake) **or** 5-50 mg/day (thiamine deficiency)

Adults: 1.1-1.4 mg/day (recommended daily intake) **or** 5-30 mg/day in 1-3 divided doses (thiamine deficiency)

Dosage Forms
Injection, solution: 100 mg/mL (2 mL)

Tablet, oral: 50 mg, 100 mg, 250 mg, 500 mg

thiamine hydrochloride *see* thiamine *on page 862*

thiaminium chloride hydrochloride *see* thiamine *on page 862*

thioguanine (thye oh GWAH neen)

Medication Safety Issues
Sound-alike/look-alike issues:
Thioguanine may be confused with thiotepa
High alert medication:
This medication is in a class the Institute for Safe Medication Practices (ISMP) includes among its list of drug classes which have a heightened risk of causing significant patient harm when used in error.
Other safety concerns:
6-thioguanine and 6-TG are error-prone abbreviations (associated with sixfold overdoses of thioguanine)
International issues:
Lanvis [Canada and multiple international markets] may be confused with Lantus brand name for insulin glargine [U.S., Canada, and multiple international markets]

Synonyms 2-amino-6-mercaptopurine; 6-TG (error-prone abbreviation); 6-thioguanine (error-prone abbreviation); TG; tioguanine

U.S. Brand Names Tabloid®

Canadian Brand Names Lanvis®

Therapeutic Category Antineoplastic Agent

Use Treatment of acute myelogenous (nonlymphocytic) leukemia (AML)

Dosage Forms
Tablet, oral:
Tabloid®: 40 mg

6-thioguanine (error-prone abbreviation) *see* thioguanine *on page 862*

Thiola® *see* tiopronin *on page 871*

thiopental (thye oh PEN tal)

Medication Safety Issues
High alert medication:
The Institute for Safe Medication Practices (ISMP) includes this medication among its list of drugs which have a heightened risk of causing significant patient harm when used in error.

Synonyms thiopental sodium

U.S. Brand Names Pentothal® [DSC]

Canadian Brand Names Pentothal®

Therapeutic Category Barbiturate

Controlled Substance C-III

Use Induction of anesthesia; control of convulsive states; treatment of elevated intracranial pressure

General Dosage Range Dosage adjustment recommended in patients with renal impairment
I.V.:
Infants <1 year: Anesthesia induction: 5-8 mg/kg
Children 1-12 years: Anesthesia induction: 5-6 mg/kg; Maintenance: 1 mg/kg as needed **or** 1.5-5 mg/kg/dose, repeat as needed
Children >12 years: Maintenance: 1 mg/kg as needed **or** 1.5-5 mg/kg/dose, repeat as needed
Adults: Anesthesia induction: 3-5 mg/kg; Maintenance: 25-100 mg as needed **or** 1.5-5 mg/kg/dose, repeat as needed **or** 75-250 mg/dose, repeat as needed

Dosage Forms
Injection, powder for reconstitution:
Pentothal®: 400 mg, 500 mg, 1 g

thiopental sodium *see* thiopental *on page 863*

thiophosphoramide *see* thiotepa *on page 864*

Thioplex *see* thiotepa *on page 864*

thioridazine (thye oh RID a zeen)

Medication Safety Issues
Sound-alike/look-alike issues:
Thioridazine may be confused with thiothixene, Thorazine®
Mellaril may be confused with Elavil®, Mebaral®
BEERS Criteria medication:
This drug may be inappropriate for use in geriatric patients (high severity risk).

Synonyms thioridazine hydrochloride

Therapeutic Category Phenothiazine Derivative

Use Management of schizophrenic patients who fail to respond adequately to treatment with other antipsychotic drugs, either because of insufficient effectiveness or the inability to achieve an effective dose due to intolerable adverse effects from those medications

General Dosage Range Oral:
Children >2-12 years: 0.5-3 mg/kg/day in 2-3 divided doses **or** 10-25 mg 2-3 times/day (maximum: 3 mg/kg/day)
Children >12 years and Adults: Initial: 50-100 mg 3 times/day; Maintenance: 150-800 mg/day in 2-4 divided doses (maximum: 800 mg/day) **or** Initial: 25 mg 3 times/day; Maintenance: 20-200 mg/day
Elderly: Initial: 10-25 mg 1-2 times/day; Maintenance: 10-400 mg/day in 1-2 divided doses (maximum: 400 mg/day)

Dosage Forms
Tablet, oral: 10 mg, 25 mg, 50 mg, 100 mg

thioridazine hydrochloride *see* thioridazine *on page 863*

thiosulfuric acid disodium salt *see* sodium thiosulfate *on page 824*

thiotepa (thye oh TEP a)

Medication Safety Issues
Sound-alike/look-alike issues:
Thiotepa may be confused with thioguanine
High alert medication:
This medication is in a class the Institute for Safe Medication Practices (ISMP) includes among its list of drugs which have a heightened risk of causing significant patient harm when used in error.
Administration issues:
Intrathecal medication safety: The American Society of Clinical Oncology (ASCO)/Oncology Nursing Society (ONS) chemotherapy administration safety standards (Jacobson, 2009) encourage the following safety measures for intrathecal chemotherapy:
• Intrathecal medication should not be prepared during the preparation of any other agents
• After preparation, store in an isolated location or container clearly marked with a label identifying as "intrathecal" use only
• Delivery to the patient should only be with other medications intended for administration into the central nervous system

Synonyms TESPA; thiophosphoramide; Thioplex; triethylenethiophosphoramide; TSPA

Therapeutic Category Antineoplastic Agent

Use Treatment of superficial papillary bladder cancer; palliative treatment of adenocarcinoma of breast or ovary; controlling intracavitary effusions caused by metastatic tumors

General Dosage Range Dosage adjustment recommended in patients who develop toxicities
I.V.: *Adults:* 0.3-0.4 mg/kg every 1-4 weeks
Intracavitary: *Adults:* 0.6-0.8 mg/kg
Intravesical: *Adults:* 60 mg retained for 2 hours once weekly for 4 weeks

Dosage Forms
Injection, powder for reconstitution: 15 mg

thiothixene (thye oh THIKS een)

Medication Safety Issues
Sound-alike/look-alike issues:
Thiothixene may be confused with FLUoxetine, thioridazine
Navane® may be confused with Norvasc®, Nubain®

Synonyms tiotixene

U.S. Brand Names Navane®

Canadian Brand Names Navane®

Therapeutic Category Thioxanthene Derivative

Use Management of schizophrenia

General Dosage Range Oral: *Adults:* Initial: 6-10 mg/day in 2-3 divided doses; Maintenance: 20-60 mg/day in 2-3 divided doses (maximum: 60 mg/day)

Dosage Forms
Capsule, oral: 1 mg, 2 mg, 5 mg, 10 mg
Navane®: 2 mg, 10 mg, 20 mg

thonzonium, neomycin, colistin, and hydrocortisone *see* neomycin, colistin, hydrocortisone, and thonzonium *on page 617*

Thorazine *see* chlorpromazine *on page 203*

Thorets [OTC] *see* benzocaine *on page 121*

Thrive™ [OTC] *see* nicotine *on page 625*

Thrombate III® *see* antithrombin III *on page 83*

Thrombi-Gel® *see* thrombin (topical) *on page 865*

Thrombin-JMI® *see* thrombin (topical) *on page 865*

Thrombin-JMI® Epistaxis Kit *see* thrombin (topical) *on page 865*

Thrombin-JMI® Pump Spray Kit *see* thrombin (topical) *on page 865*

Thrombin-JMI® Syringe Spray Kit *see* thrombin (topical) *on page 865*

thrombin (topical) (THROM bin, TOP i kal)

Medication Safety Issues
Administration issues:
For topical use only. Do not administer intravenously or intra-arterially.

To reduce the risk of intravascular administration, the Institute for Safe Medication Practices (ISMP) has the following recommendations:
- Prepare, label, and dispense topical thrombin from the pharmacy department (including doses used in the operating room).
- Do not leave vial or syringe at bedside.
- Add auxiliary label to all labels and syringes stating "For topical use only - do not inject".
- When appropriate, use solutions which can be applied with an absorbable gelatin sponge or use a dry form on oozing surfaces.
- When appropriate, use spray kits to help differentiate between parenteral products.

U.S. Brand Names Evithrom®; Recothrom®; Thrombi-Gel®; Thrombi-Pad®; Thrombin-JMI®; Thrombin-JMI® Epistaxis Kit; Thrombin-JMI® Pump Spray Kit; Thrombin-JMI® Syringe Spray Kit

Therapeutic Category Hemostatic Agent

Use Hemostasis whenever minor bleeding from capillaries and small venules is accessible

Thrombi-Gel®; Thrombi-Pad®: Temporary control as trauma dressing for moderate-to-severe bleeding wounds; control of surface bleeding from vascular access sites and percutaneous catheter/tubes

General Dosage Range Topical: *Children and Adults:* Dose based on severity of bleeding

Dosage Forms
Pad, topical [preservative free]:
Thrombi-Pad® 3x3: ≥200 units
Powder for reconstitution, topical:
Thrombin-JMI®: 5000 int. units, 20,000 int. units
Thrombin-JMI® Epistaxis kit: 5000 int. units
Thrombin-JMI® Pump Spray Kit: 20,000 int. units
Thrombin-JMI® Syringe Spray Kit: 5000 int. units; 20,000 int. units
Powder for reconstitution, topical [preservative free]:
Recothrom®: 5000 int. units; 20,000 int. units
Solution, topical:
Evithrom®: 800-1200 int. units/mL (2 mL, 5 mL, 20 mL)
Sponge, topical [preservative free]:
Thrombi-Gel® 10: ≥1000 units (10s)
Thrombi-Gel® 40: ≥1000 units (5s)
Thrombi-Gel® 100: ≥2000 units (5s)

Thrombi-Pad® *see* thrombin (topical) *on page 865*
thymocyte stimulating factor *see* aldesleukin *on page 47*
Thymoglobulin® *see* antithymocyte globulin (rabbit) *on page 84*
Thyrogen® *see* thyrotropin alpha *on page 866*

thyroid, desiccated (THYE roid DES i kay tid)

Medication Safety Issues
BEERS Criteria medication:
This drug may be inappropriate for use in geriatric patients (high severity risk).

Synonyms desiccated thyroid; levothyroxine and liothyronine; tetraiodothyronine and triiodothyronine; thyroid extract; thyroid USP

U.S. Brand Names Armour® Thyroid; Nature-Throid™; Westhroid™

Therapeutic Category Thyroid Product

Use Replacement or supplemental therapy in hypothyroidism; pituitary TSH suppressants (thyroid nodules, thyroiditis, multinodular goiter, thyroid cancer)

General Dosage Range Oral:
Children 0-6 months: 15-30 mg/day **or** 4.8-6 mg/kg/day
Children 6-12 months: 30-45 mg/day **or** 3.6-4.8 mg/kg/day
Children 1-5 years: 45-60 mg/day **or** 3-3.6 mg/kg/day
Children 6-12 years: 60-90 mg/day **or** 2.4-3 mg/kg/day
Children >12 years: >90 mg/day **or** 1.2-1.8 mg/kg/day

Adults: Initial: 15-30 mg/day; Maintenance: 60-120 mg/day

Dosage Forms
Tablet, oral:
Armour® Thyroid: 15 mg, 30 mg, 60 mg, 90 mg, 120 mg, 180 mg, 240 mg, 300 mg
Nature-Throid™: 16.25 mg, 32.5 mg, 65 mg, 130 mg, 195 mg
Westhroid™: 32.5 mg, 65 mg, 130 mg

thyroid extract *see* thyroid, desiccated *on page 865*

thyroid USP *see* thyroid, desiccated *on page 865*

Thyrolar® *see* liotrix *on page 530*

ThyroSafe™ *see* potassium iodide *on page 726*

Thyroshield™ [OTC] *see* potassium iodide *on page 726*

thyrotropin alpha (thye roe TROH pin AL fa)

Medication Safety Issues
Sound-alike/look-alike issues:
Thyrogen® may be confused with Thyrolar®

Synonyms human thyroid stimulating hormone; recombinant human thyrotropin; Rh-TSH; thyrotropin alpha; TSH

U.S. Brand Names Thyrogen®

Canadian Brand Names Thyrogen®

Therapeutic Category Diagnostic Agent

Use As an adjunctive diagnostic tool for serum thyroglobulin (Tg) testing; adjunctive treatment for radioiodine ablation of thyroid tissue remnants after total or near-total thyroidectomy in patients with well-differentiated thyroid cancer without evidence of metastatic disease

Potential clinical uses include: Patients with an undetectable Tg on thyroid hormone suppressive therapy to exclude the diagnosis of residual or recurrent thyroid cancer, patients requiring serum Tg testing and radioiodine imaging who are unwilling to undergo thyroid hormone withdrawal testing and whose treating physician believes that use of a less sensitive test is justified, patients who are either unable to mount an adequate endogenous TSH response to thyroid hormone withdrawal or in whom withdrawal is medically contraindicated, and patients without evidence of metastatic disease to ablate thyroid remnants (in combination with radioiodine [I^{131}]) following near-total thyroidectomy.

General Dosage Range I.M.: *Children >16 years and Adults:* 0.9 mg, followed 24 hours later by a second 0.9 mg dose

Dosage Forms
Injection, powder for reconstitution:
Thyrogen®: 1.1 mg

thyrotropin alpha *see* thyrotropin alpha *on page 866*

tiacumicin B *see* fidaxomicin (systemic) *on page 377*

tiagabine (tye AG a been)

Medication Safety Issues
Sound-alike/look-alike issues:
TiaGABine may be confused with tiZANidine

Synonyms tiagabine hydrochloride

Tall-Man tia**GAB**ine

U.S. Brand Names Gabitril®

Canadian Brand Names Gabitril®

Therapeutic Category Anticonvulsant

Use Adjunctive therapy in adults and children ≥12 years of age in the treatment of partial seizures

General Dosage Range Dosage adjustment recommended in patients on concomitant therapy
Oral:
Children 12-18 years: Initial: 4 mg once daily; Maintenance: 8-32 mg/day in 2-4 divided doses
Adults: Initial: 4 mg once daily; Maintenance: 8-56 mg/day in 2-4 divided doses

Dosage Forms
Tablet, oral:
Gabitril®: 2 mg, 4 mg, 12 mg, 16 mg

tiagabine hydrochloride *see* tiagabine *on page 866*

Tiamol® (Can) *see* fluocinonide *on page* 385

tiaprofenic acid *(Canada only)* (tye ah PRO fen ik AS id)

Canadian Brand Names Apo-Tiaprofenic®; Dom-Tiaprofenic; Nu-Tiaprofenic; PMS-Tiaprofenic; Teva-Tiaprofenic Acid

Therapeutic Category Nonsteroidal Antiinflammatory Drug (NSAID)

Use Relief of signs and symptoms of rheumatoid arthritis and osteoarthritis (degenerative joint disease)

General Dosage Range Oral: *Adults:* Immediate release: 600 mg/day in 2-3 divided doses (maximum: 600 mg/day); Sustained release: 600 mg once daily

Product Availability Not available in U.S.

Dosage Forms - Canada
Capsule, sustained release, oral: 300 mg
Tablet, oral: 200 mg, 300 mg

Tiazac® *see* diltiazem *on page* 286
Tiazac® XC (Can) *see* diltiazem *on page* 286

ticagrelor (tye KA grel or)

Synonyms AZD6140

U.S. Brand Names Brilinta™

Canadian Brand Names Brilinta™

Therapeutic Category Antiplatelet Agent; Antiplatelet Agent, Cyclopentyltriazolopyrimidine

Use Used in conjunction with aspirin for secondary prevention of thrombotic events in patients with unstable angina, non-ST-elevation myocardial infarction (NSTEMI), or ST-elevation myocardial infarction (STEMI) managed medically or with percutaneous coronary intervention (PCI) and/or coronary artery bypass graft (CABG)

General Dosage Range Oral: *Adults:* Loading dose: 180 mg; Maintenance: 90 mg twice daily

Dosage Forms
Tablet, oral:
Brilinta™: 90 mg
Dosage Forms - Canada
Tablet, oral:
Brilinta®: 90 mg

ticarcillin and clavulanate potassium (tye kar SIL in & klav yoo LAN ate poe TASS ee um)

Synonyms ticarcillin and clavulanic acid

U.S. Brand Names Timentin®

Canadian Brand Names Timentin®

Therapeutic Category Penicillin

Use Treatment of lower respiratory tract, urinary tract, skin and skin structures, bone and joint, gynecologic (endometritis) and intraabdominal (peritonitis) infections, and septicemia caused by susceptible organisms. Clavulanate expands activity of ticarcillin to include beta-lactamase producing strains of *S. aureus, H. influenzae, Bacteroides* species, and some other gram-negative bacilli

General Dosage Range Dosage adjustment recommended in patients with hepatic or renal impairment
I.V.:
Children and Adults <60 kg: 200-300 mg of ticarcillin component/kg/day in divided doses every 4-6 hours
Children ≥60 kg and Adults: 3.1 g (ticarcillin 3 g plus clavulanic acid 0.1 g) every 4-6 hours (maximum: 24 g of ticarcillin component/day)

Dosage Forms
Infusion [premixed, frozen]:
Timentin®: Ticarcillin 3 g and clavulanic acid 0.1 g (100 mL)
Injection, powder for reconstitution:
Timentin®: Ticarcillin 3 g and clavulanic acid 0.1 g (3.1 g, 31 g)

ticarcillin and clavulanic acid *see* ticarcillin and clavulanate potassium *on page* 867
TICE® BCG *see* BCG *on page* 115

ticlopidine (tye KLOE pi deen)

Medication Safety Issues
BEERS Criteria medication:
This drug may be inappropriate for use in geriatric patients (high severity risk).
Synonyms ticlopidine hydrochloride
Canadian Brand Names Apo-Ticlopidine®; Dom-Ticlopidine; Gen-Ticlopidine; Mylan-Ticlopidine; Novo-Ticlopidine; Nu-Ticlopidine; PMS-Ticlopidine; Sandoz-Ticlopidine; Teva-Ticlopidine
Therapeutic Category Antiplatelet Agent
Use Platelet aggregation inhibitor that reduces the risk of thrombotic stroke in patients who have had a stroke or stroke precursors. **Note:** Due to its association with life-threatening hematologic disorders, ticlopidine should be reserved for patients who are intolerant to aspirin, or who have failed aspirin therapy. Adjunctive therapy (with aspirin) following successful coronary stent implantation to reduce the incidence of subacute stent thrombosis.
General Dosage Range Oral: *Adults:* 250 mg twice daily
Dosage Forms
Tablet, oral: 250 mg

ticlopidine hydrochloride *see* ticlopidine *on page 868*
TIG *see* tetanus immune globulin (human) *on page 855*
Tigan® *see* trimethobenzamide *on page 891*

tigecycline (tye ge SYE kleen)

Synonyms GAR-936
U.S. Brand Names Tygacil®
Canadian Brand Names Tygacil®
Therapeutic Category Antibiotic, Glycylcycline
Use Treatment of complicated skin and skin structure infections caused by susceptible organisms, including methicillin-resistant *Staphylococcus aureus* and vancomycin-sensitive *Enterococcus faecalis*; complicated intraabdominal infections (cIAI); community-acquired pneumonia
General Dosage Range Dosage adjustment recommended in patients with hepatic impairment
I.V.: *Adults:* Initial: 100 mg as a single dose; Maintenance: 50 mg every 12 hours
Dosage Forms
Injection, powder for reconstitution:
Tygacil®: 50 mg

Tikosyn® *see* dofetilide *on page 303*
Tilia™ Fe *see* ethinyl estradiol and norethindrone *on page 355*

tiludronate (tye LOO droe nate)

Synonyms tiludronate disodium
U.S. Brand Names Skelid®
Therapeutic Category Bisphosphonate Derivative
Use Treatment of Paget disease of the bone (osteitis deformans) in patients who have a level of serum alkaline phosphatase (SAP) at least twice the upper limit of normal, or who are symptomatic, or who are at risk for future complications of their disease
General Dosage Range Oral: *Adults:* 400 mg once daily
Dosage Forms
Tablet, oral:
Skelid®: 200 mg

tiludronate disodium *see* tiludronate *on page 868*
Tim-AK (Can) *see* timolol (ophthalmic) *on page 869*
Time-C® [OTC] *see* ascorbic acid *on page 96*
Timentin® *see* ticarcillin and clavulanate potassium *on page 867*

timolol (systemic) (TIM oh lol)

Medication Safety Issues
Sound-alike/look-alike issues:
Timolol may be confused with atenolol, Tylenol®

Synonyms timolol maleate
Canadian Brand Names Apo-Timol®; Nu-Timolol; Teva-Timolol
Therapeutic Category Beta-Adrenergic Blocker, Nonselective
Use Treatment of hypertension and angina; to reduce mortality following myocardial infarction; prophylaxis of migraine
General Dosage Range Oral: *Adults:* Initial: 10 mg twice daily; Maintenance: 20-60 mg/day in 2 divided doses (maximum: 60 mg/day)
Dosage Forms
Tablet, oral: 5 mg, 10 mg, 20 mg

timolol (ophthalmic) (TIM oh lol)
Medication Safety Issues
Sound-alike/look-alike issues:
Timolol may be confused with atenolol, Tylenol®
Timoptic® may be confused with Betoptic® S, Talacen, Viroptic®
Other safety concerns:
Bottle cap color change: Timoptic®: Both the 0.25% and 0.5% strengths are now packaged in bottles with yellow caps; previously, the color of the cap on the product corresponded to different strengths.
International issues:
Betimol [U.S., Finland] may be confused with Betanol brand name for metipranolol [Monaco]
Synonyms timolol hemihydrate; timolol maleate
U.S. Brand Names Betimol®; Istalol®; Timolol GFS; Timoptic-XE®; Timoptic®; Timoptic® in OcuDose®
Canadian Brand Names Apo-Timop®; Dom-Timolol; Mylan-Timolol; Novo-Timol; PMS-Timolol; Sandoz-Timolol; Tim-AK; Timolol Maleate-EX; Timoptic-XE®; Timoptic®
Therapeutic Category Beta-Adrenergic Blocker, Nonselective; Ophthalmic Agent, Antiglaucoma
Use Treatment of elevated intraocular pressure such as glaucoma or ocular hypertension
General Dosage Range Ophthalmic:
Gel-forming solution: *Children and Adults:* Instill 1 drop (0.25% or 0.5%) once daily
Solution: *Children and Adults:* Initial: Instill 1 drop (0.25%) twice daily; Maintenance: Instill 1 drop (0.25% or 0.5%) 1-2 times daily (maximum: 2 drops/day [0.5%])
Dosage Forms
Gel forming solution, ophthalmic: 0.25% (5 mL); 0.5% (5 mL)
Timolol GFS: 0.25% (5 mL); 0.5% (5 mL)
Timoptic-XE®: 0.25% (5 mL); 0.5% (5 mL)
Solution, ophthalmic: 0.25% (5 mL, 10 mL, 15 mL); 0.5% (5 mL, 10 mL, 15 mL)
Betimol®: 0.25% (5 mL); 0.5% (5 mL, 10 mL, 15 mL)
Istalol®: 0.5% (2.5 mL, 5 mL)
Timoptic®: 0.25% (5 mL); 0.5% (5 mL, 10 mL)
Solution, ophthalmic [preservative free]:
Timoptic® in OcuDose®: 0.25% (0.2 mL); 0.5% (0.2 mL)

Tinamed® Corn and Callus Remover [OTC] *see* salicylic acid *on page 795*
Tinamed® Wart Remover [OTC] *see* salicylic acid *on page 795*
tincture of opium *see* opium tincture *on page 653*
Tindamax® *see* tinidazole *on page 870*
Ting® Cream [OTC] *see* tolnaftate *on page 876*
Ting® Spray Liquid [OTC] *see* tolnaftate *on page 876*
Ting® Spray Powder [OTC] *see* miconazole (topical) *on page 585*

tinidazole (tye NI da zole)

U.S. Brand Names Tindamax®
Therapeutic Category Amebicide; Antibiotic, Miscellaneous; Antiprotozoal, Nitroimidazole
Use Treatment of trichomoniasis caused by *T. vaginalis*; treatment of giardiasis caused by *G. duodenalis* (*G. lamblia*); treatment of intestinal amebiasis and amebic liver abscess caused by *E. histolytica*; treatment of bacterial vaginosis caused by *Bacteroides* spp, *Gardnerella vaginalis*, and *Prevotella* spp in nonpregnant females
General Dosage Range Oral:
Children >3 years: 50 mg/kg/day (maximum: 2 g/day)
Adults: 1-2 g/day
Dosage Forms
Tablet, oral:
Tindamax®: 250 mg, 500 mg

tinzaparin (tin ZA pa rin)

Medication Safety Issues
High alert medication:
The Institute for Safe Medication Practices (ISMP) includes this medication among its list of drug classes which have a heightened risk of causing significant patient harm when used in error.
2009 National Patient Safety Goals:
The Joint Commission (TJC) requires healthcare organizations that provide anticoagulant therapy to have a process in place to reduce the risk of anticoagulant-associated patient harm. Patients receiving anticoagulants should receive individualized care through a defined process that includes standardized ordering, dispensing, administration, monitoring and education. This does not apply to routine short-term use of anticoagulants for prevention of venous thromboembolism when the expectation is that the patient's laboratory values will remain within or close to normal values (NPSG.03.05.01).
Synonyms tinzaparin sodium
U.S. Brand Names Innohep® [DSC]
Canadian Brand Names Innohep®
Therapeutic Category Anticoagulant (Other)
Use Treatment of acute symptomatic deep vein thrombosis, with or without pulmonary embolism, in conjunction with warfarin sodium
General Dosage Range SubQ: *Adults:* 175 anti-Xa int. units/kg of body weight once daily

tinzaparin sodium *see* tinzaparin *on page 870*

tioconazole (tye oh KONE a zole)

Medication Safety Issues
Sound-alike/look-alike issues:
Tioconazole may be confused with terconazole
U.S. Brand Names 1-Day™ [OTC]; Vagistat®-1 [OTC]
Therapeutic Category Antifungal Agent
Use Local treatment of vulvovaginal candidiasis
General Dosage Range Intravaginal: *Adults:* Insert 1 applicatorful prior to bedtime, as a single dose
Dosage Forms
Ointment, vaginal:
1-Day™ [OTC]: 6.5% (4.6 g)
Vagistat®-1 [OTC]: 6.5% (4.6 g)

tioguanine *see* thioguanine *on page 862*

tiopronin (tye oh PROE nin)

U.S. Brand Names Thiola®

Therapeutic Category Urinary Tract Product

Use Prevention of kidney stone (cystine) formation in patients with severe homozygous cystinuria who have urinary cystine >500 mg/day who are resistant to treatment with high fluid intake, alkali and diet modification, or who have had adverse reactions to penicillamine

General Dosage Range Oral:

Children ≥9 years: Initial: 15 mg/kg/day in 3 divided doses

Adults: Initial: 800 mg/day in 3 divided doses; average dose: 1000 mg/day

Dosage Forms

Tablet, oral:

Thiola®: 100 mg

tiotixene *see* thiothixene *on page 864*

tiotropium (ty oh TRO pee um)

Medication Safety Issues

Sound-alike/look-alike issues:

Spiriva® may be confused with Inspra™, Serevent®

Tiotropium may be confused with ipratropium

Administration issues:

Spiriva® capsules for inhalation are for administration via HandiHaler® device and are **not** for oral use

Synonyms tiotropium bromide monohydrate

U.S. Brand Names Spiriva® HandiHaler®

Canadian Brand Names Spiriva®

Therapeutic Category Anticholinergic Agent

Use Maintenance treatment of bronchospasm associated with COPD (including bronchitis and emphysema); reduction of COPD exacerbations

General Dosage Range Inhalation: *Adults:* Contents of 1 capsule (18 mcg) once daily

Dosage Forms

Powder, for oral inhalation:

Spiriva® HandiHaler®: 18 mcg/capsule (5s, 30s, 90s)

tiotropium bromide monohydrate *see* tiotropium *on page 871*

tipranavir (tip RA na veer)

Synonyms PNU-140690E; TPV

U.S. Brand Names Aptivus®

Canadian Brand Names Aptivus®

Therapeutic Category Antiretroviral Agent, Protease Inhibitor

Use Treatment of HIV-1 infections in combination with ritonavir and other antiretroviral agents; limited to highly treatment-experienced or multiprotease inhibitor-resistant patients.

General Dosage Range Dosage adjustment recommended in patients on concomitant therapy

Oral:

Children ≥2 years: 12-14 mg/kg or 290-375 mg/m^2 (maximum: 500 mg/dose) twice daily

Adults: 500 mg twice daily

Dosage Forms

Capsule, soft gelatin, oral:

Aptivus®: 250 mg

Solution, oral:

Aptivus®: 100 mg/mL (95 mL)

tirofiban (tye roe FYE ban)

Medication Safety Issues

Sound-alike/look-alike issues:

Aggrastat® may be confused with Aggrenox®, argatroban

High alert medication:

The Institute for Safe Medication Practices (ISMP) includes this medication among its list of drugs which have a heightened risk of causing significant patient harm when used in error.

◀ **Synonyms** MK383; tirofiban hydrochloride
U.S. Brand Names Aggrastat®
Canadian Brand Names Aggrastat®
Therapeutic Category Antiplatelet Agent
Use Treatment of acute coronary syndrome (ie, unstable angina/non-ST-elevation myocardial infarction [UA/NSTEMI]) in combination with heparin
General Dosage Range Dosage adjustment recommended in patients with renal impairment
I.V.: *Adults:* Initial: 0.4 mcg/kg/minute for 30 minutes; Maintenance infusion: 0.1 mcg/kg/minute
Dosage Forms
Infusion, premixed in NS [preservative free]:
Aggrastat®: 50 mcg/mL (250 mL)

tirofiban hydrochloride *see* tirofiban *on page 871*
Tirosint® *see* levothyroxine *on page 522*
Tisseel *see* fibrin sealant *on page 376*
Tisseel VH S/D *see* fibrin sealant *on page 376*
Titralac™ [OTC] *see* calcium carbonate *on page 161*
Titralac® Plus [OTC] *see* calcium carbonate and simethicone *on page 162*
Ti-U-Lac® H (Can) *see* urea and hydrocortisone *on page 901*

tizanidine (tye ZAN i deen)

Medication Safety Issues
Sound-alike/look-alike issues:
TiZANidine may be confused with tiaGABine
Zanaflex® may be confused with Xiaflex™
Other safety concerns:
Zanaflex® capsules and Zanaflex® tablets (or generic tizanidine tablets) are not interchangeable
Synonyms Sirdalud®
Tall-Man tiZANidine
U.S. Brand Names Zanaflex Capsules®; Zanaflex®
Canadian Brand Names Apo-Tizanidine®; Gen-Tizanidine; Mylan-Tizanidine; Zanaflex®
Therapeutic Category Alpha$_2$-Adrenergic Agonist Agent
Use Skeletal muscle relaxant used for treatment of muscle spasticity
General Dosage Range Oral: *Adults:* Initial: 2-4 mg 3 times/day; Maintenance: 6-36 mg/day in 3 divided doses (maximum: 36 mg/day)
Dosage Forms
Capsule, oral:
Zanaflex Capsules®: 2 mg, 4 mg, 6 mg
Tablet, oral: 2 mg, 4 mg
Zanaflex®: 4 mg

TMC-114 *see* darunavir *on page 254*
TMC125 *see* etravirine *on page 362*
TMC278 *see* rilpivirine *on page 781*
TMP *see* trimethoprim *on page 892*
TMP-SMX *see* sulfamethoxazole and trimethoprim *on page 836*
TMP-SMZ *see* sulfamethoxazole and trimethoprim *on page 836*
TMX-67 *see* febuxostat *on page 368*
TMZ *see* temozolomide *on page 849*
T. N. Dickinson's® Hazelets® [OTC] *see* witch hazel *on page 923*
T. N. Dickinson's® Witch Hazel® Astringent [OTC] *see* witch hazel *on page 923*
T. N. Dickinson's® Witch Hazel® Hemorrhoidal [OTC] *see* witch hazel *on page 923*
TNKase® *see* tenecteplase *on page 850*
TOBI® *see* tobramycin (systemic, oral inhalation) *on page 873*
TOBI® Podhaler® (Can) *see* tobramycin (systemic, oral inhalation) *on page 873*
TobraDex® *see* tobramycin and dexamethasone *on page 874*
Tobradex® (Can) *see* tobramycin and dexamethasone *on page 874*

TobraDex® ST *see tobramycin and dexamethasone on page 874*

tobramycin (systemic, oral inhalation) (toe bra MYE sin)

Medication Safety Issues

Sound-alike/look-alike issues:

Tobramycin may be confused with Trobicin®, vancomycin

Nebcin® may be confused with Inapsine®, Naprosyn®, Nubain®

High alert medication:

The Institute for Safe Medication Practices (ISMP) includes this medication (intrathecal administration) among its list of drug classes which have a heightened risk of causing significant patient harm when used in error.

Synonyms tobramycin sulfate

U.S. Brand Names TOBI®

Canadian Brand Names TOBI®; TOBI® Podhaler®; Tobramycin Injection, USP

Therapeutic Category Antibiotic, Aminoglycoside

Use Treatment of documented or suspected infections caused by susceptible gram-negative bacilli, including *Pseudomonas aeruginosa*. Tobramycin solution for inhalation and powder for inhalation (Canadian availability; not available in the U.S.) are indicated for the management of cystic fibrosis patients (>6 years of age) with *Pseudomonas aeruginosa*.

General Dosage Range Dosage adjustment recommended for the I.M. and I.V. routes in patients with renal impairment

I.M.:

Infants and Children <5 years: 2.5 mg/kg every 8 hours

Children ≥5 years: 2-3.3 mg/kg every 6-8 hours

Adults: 1-2.5 mg/kg every 8-12 hours (1 mg/kg used for synergy) **or** 4-7 mg/kg/day as a single daily dose

Elderly: 1.5-5 mg/kg/day in 1-2 divided doses

I.V.:

Infants and Children <5 years: 2.5 mg/kg every 8 hours

Children ≥5 years: 2-3.3 mg/kg every 6-8 hours

Adults: 1-2.5 mg/kg every 8-12 hours (1 mg/kg/dose used for synergy) **or** 4-7 mg/kg/day as a single daily dose

Elderly: 1.5-5 mg/kg/day in 1-2 divided doses **or** 5-7 mg/kg given every 24, 36, or 48 hours based on Cl_{cr}

Inhalation: *Children ≥6 years and Adults:* 300 mg every 12 hours [TOBI®]

Dosage Forms

Infusion, premixed in NS: 80 mg (100 mL)

Injection, powder for reconstitution: 1.2 g

Injection, solution: 10 mg/mL (2 mL, 8 mL); 40 mg/mL (2 mL, 30 mL, 50 mL)

Solution, for nebulization [preservative free]:

TOBI®: 300 mg/5 mL (56s)

Dosage Forms - Canada

Powder, for oral inhalation [capsule]:

TOBI® Podhaler®: 28 mg/capsule (224s)

tobramycin (ophthalmic) (toe bra MYE sin)

Medication Safety Issues

Sound-alike/look-alike issues:

Tobramycin may be confused with Trobicin®, vancomycin

AKTob® may be confused with AK-Trol®

Tobrex® may be confused with TobraDex®

Synonyms tobramycin sulfate

U.S. Brand Names AK-Tob™; Tobrex®

Canadian Brand Names PMS-Tobramycin; Sandoz-Tobramycin; Tobrex®

Therapeutic Category Antibiotic, Aminoglycoside; Antibiotic, Ophthalmic

Use Treatment of superficial ophthalmic infections caused by susceptible bacteria

General Dosage Range Ophthalmic: *Children ≥2 months and Adults:* Ointment: Apply 2-3 times/day; for severe infections, apply every 3-4 hours; Solution: Instill 1-2 drops every 2-4 hours

Dosage Forms
Ointment, ophthalmic:
Tobrex®: 0.3% (3.5 g)
Solution, ophthalmic: 0.3% (5 mL)
AK-Tob™: 0.3% (5 mL)
Tobrex®: 0.3% (5 mL)

tobramycin and dexamethasone (toe bra MYE sin & deks a METH a sone)

Medication Safety Issues
Sound-alike/look-alike issues:
TobraDex® may be confused with Tobrex®
Synonyms dexamethasone and tobramycin
U.S. Brand Names TobraDex®; TobraDex® ST
Canadian Brand Names Tobradex®
Therapeutic Category Antibiotic/Corticosteroid, Ophthalmic
Use Treatment of external ocular infection caused by susceptible gram-negative bacteria and steroid responsive inflammatory conditions of the palpebral and bulbar conjunctiva, cornea, and anterior segment of the globe
General Dosage Range Ophthalmic: *Children ≥2 years and Adults:* Ointment: Apply ~1/2" ribbon up to 3-4 times/day; Suspension: Instill 1-2 drops every every 4-6 hours, may increase to 1-2 drops every 2 hours for 24-48 hours
Dosage Forms
Ointment, ophthalmic:
TobraDex®: Tobramycin 0.3% and dexamethasone 0.1% (3.5 g)
Suspension, ophthalmic: Tobramycin 0.3% and dexamethasone 0.1% (2.5 mL, 5 mL, 10 mL)
TobraDex®: Tobramycin 0.3% and dexamethasone 0.1% (2.5 mL, 5 mL, 10 mL)
TobraDex® ST: Tobramycin 0.3% and dexamethasone 0.05% (5 mL)

tobramycin and loteprednol etabonate see loteprednol and tobramycin *on page 539*
Tobramycin Injection, USP (Can) see tobramycin (systemic, oral inhalation) *on page 873*
tobramycin sulfate see tobramycin (ophthalmic) *on page 873*
tobramycin sulfate see tobramycin (systemic, oral inhalation) *on page 873*
Tobrex® see tobramycin (ophthalmic) *on page 873*

tocilizumab (toe si LIZ oo mab)

Synonyms atlizumab; MRA; R-1569; RoActemra®
U.S. Brand Names Actemra®
Canadian Brand Names Actemra®
Therapeutic Category Antirheumatic, Disease Modifying; Interleukin-6 Receptor Antagonist
Use Treatment of moderately- to severely-active rheumatoid arthritis in adult patients who have had an inadequate response to one or more TNF antagonists (as monotherapy or in combination with nonbiological disease-modifying antirheumatic drugs [DMARDs]); treatment of active systemic juvenile idiopathic arthritis (SJIA) (as monotherapy or in combination with methotrexate)
General Dosage Range Dosage adjustment recommended in patients who develop toxicities
I.V.:
Children ≥2 years and <30 kg: 12 mg/kg every 2 weeks
Children ≥2 years and ≥30 kg: 8 mg/kg every 2 weeks
Adults: 4-8 mg/kg every 4 weeks (maximum: 800 mg per infusion)
Dosage Forms
Injection, solution [preservative free]:
Actemra®: 20 mg/mL (4 mL, 10 mL, 20 mL)

Today® [OTC] see nonoxynol 9 *on page 632*
Tofranil® see imipramine *on page 467*
Tofranil-PM® see imipramine *on page 467*

tolazamide (tole AZ a mide)

Medication Safety Issues
Sound-alike/look-alike issues:
   TOLAZamide may be confused with tolazoline, TOLBUTamide
   Tolinase® may be confused with Orinase®
High alert medication:
   The Institute for Safe Medication Practices (ISMP) includes this medication among its list of drugs which have a heightened risk of causing significant patient harm when used in error.

Tall-Man TOLAZamide

Canadian Brand Names Tolinase®

Therapeutic Category Antidiabetic Agent, Oral

Use Adjunct to diet for the management of mild-to-moderately severe, stable, type 2 diabetes mellitus (noninsulin-dependent, NIDDM)

General Dosage Range Oral: *Adults:* Initial: 100-250 mg/day with first main meal of day; Maintenance: 100-1000 mg/day in 1-2 (doses >500 mg) divided doses (maximum: 1 g/day)

Dosage Forms
Tablet, oral: 250 mg, 500 mg

tolbutamide (tole BYOO ta mide)

Medication Safety Issues
Sound-alike/look-alike issues:
   TOLBUTamide may be confused with terbutaline, TOLAZamide
   Orinase® may be confused with Orabase®, Ornex®, Tolinase®
High alert medication:
   The Institute for Safe Medication Practices (ISMP) includes this medication among its list of drugs which have a heightened risk of causing significant patient harm when used in error.

Synonyms Orinase; tolbutamide sodium

Tall-Man TOLBUTamide

Canadian Brand Names Apo-Tolbutamide®

Therapeutic Category Antidiabetic Agent, Oral

Use Adjunct to diet for the management of type 2 diabetes mellitus (noninsulin-dependent, NIDDM)

General Dosage Range Oral:
   Adults: Initial: 1-2 g/day as a single dose or divided doses; Maintenance: 0.25-3 g/day as a single dose or divided doses
   Elderly: Initial: 0.25 g 1-3 times/day; Maintenance: 0.5-2 g/day in 1-3 divided doses (maximum: 3 g/day)

Dosage Forms
Tablet, oral: 500 mg

tolbutamide sodium *see* tolbutamide *on page 875*

tolcapone (TOLE ka pone)

U.S. Brand Names Tasmar®

Therapeutic Category Anti-Parkinson Agent

Use Adjunct to levodopa and carbidopa for the treatment of signs and symptoms of idiopathic Parkinson disease in patients with motor fluctuations not responsive to other therapies

General Dosage Range Oral: *Adults:* Initial: 100 mg 3 times/day; Maintenance: 100-200 mg 3 times/day

Dosage Forms
Tablet, oral:
   Tasmar®: 100 mg

Tolectin *see* tolmetin *on page 875*

Tolinase® (Can) *see* tolazamide *on page 875*

tolmetin (TOLE met in)

Synonyms Tolectin; tolmetin sodium

Therapeutic Category Analgesic, Nonnarcotic; Nonsteroidal Antiinflammatory Drug (NSAID)

Use Treatment of rheumatoid arthritis and osteoarthritis, juvenile idiopathic arthritis (JIA)

◀ **General Dosage Range Oral:**
Children ≥2 years: Initial: 20 mg/kg/day in 3-4 divided doses; Maintenance: 15-30 mg/kg/day in 3-4 divided doses (maximum: 30 mg/kg/day)
Adults: Initial: 400 mg 3 times/day; Maintenance: 600-1800 mg/day in 3 divided doses (maximum: 1.8 g/day)
Dosage Forms
Capsule, oral: 400 mg
Tablet, oral: 200 mg, 600 mg

tolmetin sodium *see* tolmetin *on page 875*

tolnaftate (tole NAF tate)

Medication Safety Issues
Sound-alike/look-alike issues:
Tolnaftate may be confused with Tornalate®
Tinactin® may be confused with Talacen

U.S. Brand Names Blis-To-Sol® [OTC]; Mycocide® NS [OTC]; Podactin Powder [OTC]; Tinactin® Antifungal Deodorant [OTC]; Tinactin® Antifungal Jock Itch [OTC]; Tinactin® Antifungal [OTC]; Tinaderm [OTC]; Ting® Cream [OTC]; Ting® Spray Liquid [OTC]

Canadian Brand Names Pitrex

Therapeutic Category Antifungal Agent

Use Treatment of tinea pedis, tinea cruris, tinea corporis

General Dosage Range Topical: *Children ≥2 years and Adults:* Apply to affected areas 2 times/day

Dosage Forms
Aerosol, topical:
Tinactin® Antifungal [OTC]: 1% (133 g, 150 g)
Tinactin® Antifungal Deodorant [OTC]: 1% (133 g)
Tinactin® Antifungal Jock Itch [OTC]: 1% (133 g)
Ting® Spray Liquid [OTC]: 1% (128 g)
Cream, topical: 1% (15 g, 30 g, 114 g)
Tinactin® Antifungal [OTC]: 1% (15 g, 30 g)
Tinactin® Antifungal Jock Itch [OTC]: 1% (15 g)
Ting® Cream [OTC]: 1% (15 g)
Liquid, topical:
Blis-To-Sol® [OTC]: 1% (30 mL, 55 mL)
Tinactin® Antifungal [OTC]: 1% (59 mL)
Powder, topical: 1% (45 g)
Podactin Powder [OTC]: 1% (60 g)
Tinactin® Antifungal [OTC]: 1% (108 g)
Solution, topical:
Mycocide® NS [OTC]: 1% (30 mL)
Tinaderm [OTC]: 1% (10 mL)

Toloxin® (Can) *see* digoxin *on page 283*

tolterodine (tole TER oh deen)

Medication Safety Issues
Sound-alike/look-alike issues:
Tolterodine may be confused with fesoterodine
Detrol® may be confused with Ditropan

Synonyms tolterodine tartrate

U.S. Brand Names Detrol®; Detrol® LA

Canadian Brand Names Detrol®; Detrol® LA; Unidet®

Therapeutic Category Anticholinergic Agent

Use Treatment of patients with an overactive bladder with symptoms of urinary frequency, urgency, or urge incontinence

General Dosage Range Dosage adjustment recommended in patients with hepatic or renal impairment and on concomitant therapy
Oral: *Adults:* Extended release: 2-4 mg once daily; Immediate release: 1-2 mg twice daily

---

Dosage Forms
Capsule, extended release, oral:
Detrol® LA: 2 mg, 4 mg
Tablet, oral:
Detrol®: 1 mg, 2 mg

tolterodine tartrate *see tolterodine on page 876*

tolvaptan (tol VAP tan)
Synonyms OPC-41061
U.S. Brand Names Samsca™
Therapeutic Category Vasopressin Antagonist
Use Treatment of clinically significant hypervolemic or euvolemic hyponatremia (associated with heart failure, cirrhosis or SIADH) with either a serum sodium <125 mEq/L or less marked hyponatremia that is symptomatic and resistant to fluid restriction
General Dosage Range Oral: *Adults:* 15-60 mg once daily
Dosage Forms
Tablet, oral:
Samsca™: 15 mg, 30 mg

tomoxetine *see atomoxetine on page 101*
Tomudex® (Can) *see raltitrexed (Canada only) on page 765*
Topactin (Can) *see fluocinonide on page 385*
Topamax® *see topiramate on page 877*
TopCare® Junior Strength [OTC] *see ibuprofen on page 460*
TopCare® Pain Relief PM [OTC] *see acetaminophen and diphenhydramine on page 27*
Topicaine® [OTC] *see lidocaine (topical) on page 524*
Topicort® *see desoximetasone on page 263*
Topicort® LP *see desoximetasone on page 263*
Topilene® (Can) *see betamethasone on page 129*

topiramate (toe PYRE a mate)
Medication Safety Issues
Sound-alike/look-alike issues:
Topamax® may be confused with Sporanox®, Tegretol®, Tegretol®-XR, Toprol-XL®
U.S. Brand Names Topamax®
Canadian Brand Names Apo-Topiramate®; CO Topiramate; Dom-Topiramate; Mint-Topiramate; Mylan-Topiramate; Novo-Topiramate; PHL-Topiramate; PMS-Topiramate; PRO-Topiramate; ratio-Topiramate; Sandoz-Topiramate; Topamax®; ZYM-Topiramate
Therapeutic Category Anticonvulsant
Use Monotherapy or adjunctive therapy for partial onset seizures and primary generalized tonic-clonic seizures; adjunctive treatment of seizures associated with Lennox-Gastaut syndrome; prophylaxis of migraine headache
General Dosage Range Dosage adjustment recommended in patients with renal impairment
Oral:
Children 2-9 years: Initial: 25 mg once daily **or** 1-3 mg/kg/day; Maintenance: 150-400 mg/day in 2 divided doses **or** 5-9 mg/kg/day in 2 divided doses
Children 10-16 years: Initial: 25 mg once or twice daily **or** 1-3 mg/kg/day; Maintenance: 5-9 mg/kg/day in 2 divided doses **or** 25-200 mg twice daily
Children ≥17 years: Initial: 25 mg once or twice daily; Maintenance: 100-200 mg twice daily
Adults: Initial: 25-50 mg/day in 1-2 divided doses; Maintenance: 50-200 mg twice daily
Dosage Forms
Capsule, sprinkle, oral: 15 mg, 25 mg
Topamax®: 15 mg, 25 mg
Tablet, oral: 25 mg, 50 mg, 100 mg, 200 mg
Topamax®: 25 mg, 50 mg, 100 mg, 200 mg

Topisone® (Can) *see betamethasone on page 129*
Toposar® *see etoposide on page 361*

topotecan (toe poe TEE kan)

Medication Safety Issues
Sound-alike/look-alike issues:
Hycamtin® may be confused with Hycomine®, Mycamine®
Topotecan may be confused with irinotecan
High alert medication:
This medication is in a class the Institute for Safe Medication Practices (ISMP) includes among its list of drug classes which have a heightened risk of causing significant patient harm when used in error.

Synonyms hycamptamine; SKF 104864; SKF 104864-A; topotecan hydrochloride

U.S. Brand Names Hycamtin®

Canadian Brand Names Hycamtin®; Topotecan For Injection

Therapeutic Category Antineoplastic Agent

Use Treatment of metastatic ovarian cancer, relapsed or refractory small cell lung cancer, recurrent or resistant (stage IVB) cervical cancer (in combination with cisplatin)

General Dosage Range Dosage adjustment recommended in patients with renal impairment or who develop toxicities
Oral: *Adults:* 2.3 mg/m^2/day for 5 days; repeated every 21 days
I.V.: *Adults:* IVPB: 1.5 mg/m^2/day for 5 days; repeated every 21 days **or** 0.75 mg/m^2/day for 3 days; repeated every 21 days

Dosage Forms
Capsule, oral:
Hycamtin®: 0.25 mg, 1 mg
Injection, powder for reconstitution: 4 mg
Hycamtin®: 4 mg
Injection, solution: 1 mg/mL (4 mL)

Topotecan For Injection (Can) *see* topotecan *on page 878*

topotecan hydrochloride *see* topotecan *on page 878*

Toprol-XL® *see* metoprolol *on page 581*

Topsyn® (Can) *see* fluocinonide *on page 385*

Toradol *see* ketorolac (systemic) *on page 501*

Toradol® (Can) *see* ketorolac (systemic) *on page 501*

Toradol® IM (Can) *see* ketorolac (systemic) *on page 501*

toremifene (tore EM i feen)

Synonyms FC1157a; toremifene citrate

U.S. Brand Names Fareston®

Canadian Brand Names Fareston®

Therapeutic Category Antineoplastic Agent

Use Treatment of metastatic breast cancer in postmenopausal women with estrogen receptor positive or estrogen receptor status unknown

General Dosage Range Oral: *Adults:* 60 mg once daily

Dosage Forms
Tablet, oral:
Fareston®: 60 mg

toremifene citrate *see* toremifene *on page 878*

Torisel® *see* temsirolimus *on page 849*

torsemide (TORE se mide)

Medication Safety Issues
Sound-alike/look-alike issues:
Torsemide may be confused with furosemide
Demadex® may be confused with Denorex®

U.S. Brand Names Demadex®

Therapeutic Category Diuretic, Loop

Use Management of edema associated with heart failure and hepatic or renal disease (including chronic renal failure); treatment of hypertension

General Dosage Range
  I.V.: *Adults:* 10-200 mg once daily
  Oral: *Adults:* 5-200 mg once daily (maximum: 200 mg/day)
Dosage Forms
  Injection, solution: 10 mg/mL (2 mL, 5 mL)
  Tablet, oral: 5 mg, 10 mg, 20 mg, 100 mg
    Demadex®: 5 mg, 10 mg, 20 mg, 100 mg

tositumomab I-131 *see tositumomab and iodine I 131 tositumomab on page 879*

tositumomab and iodine I 131 tositumomab
(toe si TYOO mo mab & EYE oh dyne eye one THUR tee one toe si TYOO mo mab)
Medication Safety Issues
  High alert medication:
    The Institute for Safe Medication Practices (ISMP) includes this medication among its list of drug classes which have a heightened risk of causing significant patient harm when used in error.
Synonyms 131 I anti-B1 antibody; 131 I-anti-B1 monoclonal antibody; anti-CD20-murine monoclonal antibody I-131; iodine I 131 tositumomab and tositumomab; tositumomab I-131
U.S. Brand Names Bexxar®
Therapeutic Category Antineoplastic Agent, Monoclonal Antibody; Radiopharmaceutical
Use Treatment of relapsed or refractory CD20 positive, low-grade, follicular, or transformed non-Hodgkin lymphoma (NHL)
General Dosage Range Dosage adjustment recommended in patients who develop toxicities
  I.V.:
    Tositumomab: *Adults:* Step 1: 450 mg; Step 2: 450 mg
    Iodine I-131 tositumomab (given after tositumomab): *Adults:* Step 1: I-131 5 mCi and tositumomab 35 mg; Step 2: I-131 (calculated to deliver 65-75 cGy total body irradiation) and tositumomab 35 mg
Dosage Forms
  Kit [dosimetric package]:
    Bexxar®: Tositumomab 225 mg/16.1 mL [2 vials], tositumomab 35 mg/2.5 mL [1 vial], and iodine I 131 tositumomab 0.1 mg/mL and 0.61mCi/mL (20 mL) [1 vial]
  Kit [therapeutic package]:
    Bexxar®: Tositumomab 225 mg/16.1 mL [2 vials], tositumomab 35 mg/2.5 mL [1 vial], and iodine I 131 tositumomab 1.1 mg/mL and 5.6 mCi/mL (20 mL) [1 or 2 vials]

total parenteral nutrition (TOE tal par EN ter al noo TRISH un)
Medication Safety Issues
  High alert medication:
    The Institute for Safe Medication Practices (ISMP) includes this medication among its list of drugs which have a heightened risk of causing significant patient harm when used in error.
Synonyms hyperal; hyperalimentation; parenteral nutrition; PN; TPN
Therapeutic Category Caloric Agent; Intravenous Nutritional Therapy
Use Infusion of nutrient solutions into the bloodstream to support nutritional needs during a time when patient is unable to absorb nutrients via the gastrointestinal tract, cannot take adequate nutrition orally or enterally, or have had (or are expected to have) inadequate oral intake for 7-14 days.
General Dosage Range I.V.: Dosage varies greatly depending on indication
Dosage Forms TPN is usually compounded from optimal combinations of macronutrients (water, protein, dextrose, and lipids) and micronutrients (electrolytes, trace elements, and vitamins) to meet the specific nutritional requirements of a patient. Individual hospitals may have designated standard TPN formulas. There are a few commercially-available amino acids with electrolytes solutions; however, these products may not meet an individual's specific nutrition requirements.

Totect® *see dexrazoxane on page 267*
Toviaz™ *see fesoterodine on page 374*
tPA *see alteplase on page 58*
TPN *see total parenteral nutrition on page 879*
TPV *see tipranavir on page 871*
tRA *see tretinoin (systemic) on page 885*
4 Trace Elements *see trace metals on page 880*
Trace Elements 4 Pediatric *see trace metals on page 880*

trace metals (trase MET als)

Synonyms chromium; copper; iodine; manganese; molybdenum; neonatal trace metals; selenium; zinc

U.S. Brand Names 4 Trace Elements; Multitrace®-4; Multitrace®-4 Concentrate; Multitrace®-4 Neonatal; Multitrace®-4 Pediatric; Multitrace®-5; Multitrace®-5 Concentrate; Trace Elements 4 Pediatric

Therapeutic Category Trace Element

Use Prevention and correction of trace metal deficiencies

General Dosage Range I.V.: *Infants, Children, and Adults:* Dosage varies greatly depending on indication

Dosage Forms

Injection, solution [combination products]:

Multitrace®-4: Chromium 4 mcg, copper 0.4 mg, manganese 0.1 mg, and zinc 1 mg per 1 mL (10 mL)

Multitrace®-4 Concentrate: Chromium 10 mcg, copper 1 mg, manganese 0.5 mg, and zinc 5 mg per 1 mL (1 mL, 10 mL)

Multitrace®-4 Neonatal: Chromium 0.85 mcg, copper 0.1 mg, manganese 0.025 mg, and zinc 1.5 mg per 1 mL (2 mL)

Multitrace®-5: Chromium 4 mcg, copper 0.4 mg, manganese 0.1 mg, selenium 20 mcg, and zinc 1 mg per 1 mL (10 mL)

Multitrace®-5 Concentrate: Chromium 10 mcg, copper 1 mg, manganese 0.5 mg, selenium 60 mcg, and zinc 5 mg per 1 mL (1 mL, 10 mL)

Trace Elements 4 Pediatric: Chromium 1 mcg, copper 0.1 mg, manganese 0.03 mg, and zinc 0.5 mg per 1 mL (10 mL)

Injection, solution [combination products, preservative free]:

4 Trace Elements: Chromium 2 mcg, copper 0.2 mg, manganese 0.16 mg, and zinc 0.8 mg per 1 mL (5 mL, 50 mL)

Multitrace®-4 Pediatric: Chromium 1 mcg, copper 0.1 mg, manganese 0.025 mg, and zinc 1 mg per 1 mL (3 mL)

Tracleer® *see* bosentan *on page 139*

Tradjenta™ *see* linagliptin *on page 528*

trajenta *see* linagliptin *on page 528*

Trajenta™ (Can) *see* linagliptin *on page 528*

Tramacet (Can) *see* acetaminophen and tramadol *on page 29*

tramadol (TRA ma dole)

Medication Safety Issues

Sound-alike/look-alike issues:

TraMADol may be confused with tapentadol, Toradol®, Trandate®, traZODone, Voltaren®

Ultram® may be confused with Ultane®, Ultracet®, Voltaren®

International issues:

Theradol [Netherlands] may be confused with Foradil brand name for formoterol [U.S., Canada, and multiple international markets], Terazol brand name for terconazole [U.S. and Canada], and Toradol brand name for ketorolac [Canada and multiple international markets]

Trexol [Mexico] may be confused with Trexall brand name for methotrexate [U.S.]; Truxal brand name for chlorprothixene [multiple international markets]

Synonyms tramadol hydrochloride

Tall-Man traMADol

U.S. Brand Names ConZip™; Rybix™ ODT; Ryzolt™; Ultram®; Ultram® ER

Canadian Brand Names Ralivia™ ER; Tridural™; Zytram® XL

Therapeutic Category Analgesic, Nonnarcotic

Use Relief of moderate to moderately-severe pain

Extended release formulations are indicated for patients requiring around-the-clock management of moderate to moderately-severe pain for an extended period of time

General Dosage Range Dosage adjustment recommended in patients with hepatic or renal impairment

Oral:

Immediate release:

Children ≥17 years: 50-100 mg every 4-6 hours (maximum: 400 mg/day)

Adults: 50-100 mg every 4-6 hours (maximum: 400 mg/day)

Elderly >75 years: Maximum: 300 mg/day

Extended release: *Adults:* 100-300 once daily (maximum: 300 mg/day)

Dosage Forms
 Capsule, variable release, oral:
  ConZip™: 100 mg [25 mg (immediate release) and 75 mg (extended release)]
  ConZip™: 200 mg [50 mg (immediate release) and 150 mg (extended release)]
  ConZip™: 300 mg [50 mg (immediate release) and 250 mg (extended release)]
 Tablet, oral: 50 mg
  Ultram®: 50 mg
 Tablet, extended release, oral: 100 mg, 200 mg, 300 mg
  Ryzolt™: 100 mg, 200 mg, 300 mg
  Ultram® ER: 100 mg, 200 mg, 300 mg
 Tablet, orally disintegrating, oral:
  Rybix™ ODT: 50 mg
Dosage Forms - Canada
 Tablet, extended release:
  Ralivia™ ER, Tridural™: 100 mg, 200 mg, 300 mg
  Zytram® XL: 75 mg, 100 mg, 150 mg, 200 mg, 300 mg, 400 mg

tramadol hydrochloride *see* tramadol *on page 880*
tramadol hydrochloride and acetaminophen *see* acetaminophen and tramadol *on page 29*
Trandate® *see* labetalol *on page 504*

trandolapril (tran DOE la pril)

U.S. Brand Names Mavik®
Canadian Brand Names Mavik®
Therapeutic Category Angiotensin-Converting Enzyme (ACE) Inhibitor
Use Treatment of hypertension alone or in combination with other antihypertensive agents; treatment of heart failure (HF) or left ventricular (LV) dysfunction after myocardial infarction (MI)
General Dosage Range Dosage adjustment recommended in patients with hepatic or renal impairment
 Oral: *Adults:* Initial: 1-2 mg once daily; Maintenance: 1-4 mg once daily
Dosage Forms
 Tablet, oral: 1 mg, 2 mg, 4 mg
  Mavik®: 1 mg, 2 mg, 4 mg

trandolapril and verapamil (tran DOE la pril & ver AP a mil)

Synonyms verapamil and trandolapril
U.S. Brand Names Tarka®
Canadian Brand Names Tarka®
Therapeutic Category Antihypertensive Agent, Combination
Use Treatment of hypertension; however, not indicated for initial treatment of hypertension
General Dosage Range Dosage adjustment recommended in patients with hepatic or renal impairment
 Oral: *Adults:* Trandolapril 1-4 mg and verapamil 180-240 mg once daily
Dosage Forms
 Tablet, variable release: Trandolapril 2 mg [immediate release] and verapamil 180 mg [sustained release]; Trandolapril 2 mg [immediate release] and verapamil 240 mg [sustained release]; Trandolapril 4 mg [immediate release] and verapamil 240 mg [sustained release]
 Tarka®:
  1/240: Trandolapril 1 mg [immediate release] and verapamil 240 mg [sustained release]
  2/180: Trandolapril 2 mg [immediate release] and verapamil 180 mg [sustained release]
  2/240: Trandolapril 2 mg [immediate release] and verapamil 240 mg [sustained release]
  4/240: Trandolapril 4 mg [immediate release] and verapamil 240 mg [sustained release]

tranexamic acid (tran eks AM ik AS id)

Medication Safety Issues
 Sound-alike/look-alike issues:
  Cyklokapron® may be confused with cycloSPORINE
U.S. Brand Names Cyklokapron®; Lysteda™
Canadian Brand Names Cyklokapron®; Tranexamic Acid Injection BP
Therapeutic Category Antihemophilic Agent

◀ **Use**
Solution for injection: Short-term use (2-8 days) in hemophilia patients to reduce or prevent hemorrhage and reduce need for replacement therapy during and following tooth extraction
Tablet: Treatment of cyclic heavy menstrual bleeding
General Dosage Range Dosage adjustment recommended in patients with renal impairment
I.V.: *Children and Adults:* Initial: 10 mg/kg as a single dose; Maintenance: 10 mg/kg/dose 3-4 times/day
Oral: *Adults:* 1300 mg 3 times daily (3900 mg/day)
Dosage Forms
Injection, solution:
Cyklokapron®: 100 mg/mL (10 mL)
Tablet, oral:
Lysteda™: 650 mg

Tranexamic Acid Injection BP (Can) *see* tranexamic acid *on page 881*
transamine sulphate *see* tranylcypromine *on page 882*
Transderm-V® (Can) *see* scopolamine (systemic) *on page 804*
Transderm-Nitro® (Can) *see* nitroglycerin *on page 629*
Transderm Scōp® *see* scopolamine (systemic) *on page 804*
Trans-Plantar® (Can) *see* salicylic acid *on page 795*
trans-**retinoic acid** *see* tretinoin (systemic) *on page 885*
trans-**retinoic acid** *see* tretinoin (topical) *on page 885*
Trans-Ver-Sal® [OTC] *see* salicylic acid *on page 795*
Trans-Ver-Sal® (Can) *see* salicylic acid *on page 795*
trans **vitamin A acid** *see* tretinoin (systemic) *on page 885*
Tranxene® T-Tab® *see* clorazepate *on page 225*

tranylcypromine (tran il SIP roe meen)

Synonyms transamine sulphate; tranylcypromine sulfate
U.S. Brand Names Parnate®
Canadian Brand Names Parnate®
Therapeutic Category Antidepressant, Monoamine Oxidase Inhibitor
Use Treatment of major depressive episode without melancholia
General Dosage Range Oral: *Adults:* 10-30 mg twice daily (maximum: 60 mg/day)
Dosage Forms
Tablet, oral: 10 mg
Parnate®: 10 mg

tranylcypromine sulfate *see* tranylcypromine *on page 882*

trastuzumab (tras TU zoo mab)

Medication Safety Issues
High alert medication:
This medication is in a class the Institute for Safe Medication Practices (ISMP) includes among its list of drug classes which have a heightened risk of causing significant patient harm when used in error.
Synonyms anti-c-erB-2; anti-ERB-2; MOAB HER2; rhuMAb HER2
U.S. Brand Names Herceptin®
Canadian Brand Names Herceptin®
Therapeutic Category Antineoplastic Agent
Use Treatment (adjuvant) of HER-2 overexpressing breast cancer; treatment of HER-2 overexpressing metastatic breast cancer; treatment of HER-2 overexpressing metastatic gastric or gastroesophageal junction adenocarcinoma (in patients who have not received prior treatment)
General Dosage Range Dosage adjustment recommended in patients who develop toxicities
I.V.: *Adults:* Loading dose: 4 mg/kg; Maintenance: 2 mg/kg once weekly **or** Loading dose: 8 mg/kg; Maintenance: 6 mg/kg every 3 weeks
Dosage Forms
Injection, powder for reconstitution:
Herceptin®: 440 mg

Trasylol® (Can) *see* aprotinin *on page 91*

Trav-L-Tabs® [OTC] *see* meclizine *on page 552*
Travasol® *see* amino acid injection *on page 65*
Travatan® [DSC] *see* travoprost *on page 883*
Travatan® (Can) *see* travoprost *on page 883*
Travatan Z® *see* travoprost *on page 883*

traveler's diarrhea and cholera vaccine *(Canada only)*
(TRAV uh lerz dahy uh REE uh & KOL er uh vak SEEN)

Synonyms *Vibrio cholera* and enterotoxigenic *Escherichia coli* vaccine; cholera and traveler's diarrhea vaccine; cholera vaccine; enterotoxigenic *Escherichia coli* and *Vibrio cholera* vaccine; oral cholera vaccine; traveller's diarrhea vaccine and cholera

Canadian Brand Names Dukoral®

Therapeutic Category Vaccine

Use Protection against traveler's diarrhea and/or cholera in adults and children ≥2 years of age who will be visiting areas where there is a risk of contracting traveler's diarrhea caused by enterotoxigenic *E. coli* (ETEC) or cholera caused by *V. cholerae* O1 (classical and El Tor biotypes; Inaba and Ogawa serotypes)

General Dosage Range Oral:
Children 2-6 years: Cholera: Primary immunization: 3 doses given at intervals of ≥1 week
Children ≥2 years: ETEC: Primary immunization: 2 doses given at intervals of ≥1 week
Children >6 years: Cholera: Primary immunization: 2 doses given at intervals of ≥1 week
Adults: Cholera: Primary immunization: 2 doses given at intervals of ≥1 week; ETEC: Primary immunization: 2 doses given at intervals of ≥1 week

Product Availability Not available in U.S.

Dosage Forms - Canada
Suspension [vial]:
Dukoral®: 2.5×10^{10} of each of the following *Vibrio cholerae* O1 strains: Inaba classic (heat inactivated), Inaba El Tor (formalin inactivated), Ogawa classic (heat inactivated), Ogawa classic (formalin inactivated), and 1 mg recombinant cholera toxin B subunit (rCTB) (3 mL)

traveller's diarrhea vaccine and cholera *see* traveler's diarrhea and cholera vaccine *(Canada only)* *on page 883*

travoprost (TRA voe prost)
Medication Safety Issues
Sound-alike/look-alike issues:
Travatan® may be confused with Xalatan®
U.S. Brand Names Travatan Z®; Travatan® [DSC]
Canadian Brand Names Travatan Z®; Travatan®
Therapeutic Category Prostaglandin, Ophthalmic
Use Reduction of elevated intraocular pressure in patients with open-angle glaucoma or ocular hypertension who are intolerant of the other IOP-lowering medications or insufficiently responsive (failed to achieve target IOP determined after multiple measurements over time) to another IOP-lowering medication
General Dosage Range Ophthalmic: *Adults:* Instill 1 drop into affected eye(s) once daily
Dosage Forms
Solution, ophthalmic:
Travatan Z®: 0.004% (2.5 mL, 5 mL)

travoprost and timolol *(Canada only)* (TRA voe prost & TIM oh lol)
Medication Safety Issues
Sound-alike/look-alike issues:
DuoTrav™ may be confused with DuoNeb®
Synonyms timolol maleate and travoprost
Canadian Brand Names DuoTrav™
Therapeutic Category Beta Blocker, Nonselective; Ophthalmic Agent, Antiglaucoma; Prostaglandin, Ophthalmic
Use Reduction of intraocular pressure (IOP) in patients with open-angle glaucoma or ocular hypertension who are insufficiently responsive to topical beta-blockers, prostaglandin analogues, or other IOP-reducing agents and in whom combination therapy is appropriate

◀ **General Dosage Range Ophthalmic:** *Adults:* Instill 1 drop into affected eye(s) once daily

Product Availability Not available in U.S.

Dosage Forms - Canada
Solution, ophthalmic:
DuoTrav™: Travoprost 0.004% and timolol 0.5%: (2.5 mL, 5 mL)

trazodone (TRAZ oh done)

Medication Safety Issues
Sound-alike/look-alike issues:
Desyrel may be confused with Demerol®, Delsym®, Zestril®
TraZODone may be confused with traMADol, ziprasidone
International issues:
Desyrel [Canada, Turkey] may be confused with Deseril brand name for methysergide [Australia, Belgium, Great Britain, Netherlands]

Synonyms Desyrel; trazodone hydrochloride

Tall-Man traZODone

U.S. Brand Names Oleptro™

Canadian Brand Names Apo-Trazodone D®; Apo-Trazodone®; Dom-Trazodone; Mylan-Trazodone; Novo-Trazodone; Nu-Trazodone; Nu-Trazodone D; Oleptro™; PHL-Trazodone; PMS-Trazodone; ratio-Trazodone; Teva-Trazodone; Trazorel®; ZYM-Trazodone

Therapeutic Category Antidepressant, Triazolopyridine

Use Treatment of major depressive disorder

General Dosage Range Oral:
Adults: Immediate release: Initial: 150 mg/day in 3 divided doses; Maintenance: 150-600 mg/day in 3 divided doses; Extended-release: Initial: 150 mg once daily; Maximum dose: 375 mg/day
Elderly: Immediate release: Initial: 25-50 mg at bedtime; Maintenance: 25-150 mg/day at bedtime

Dosage Forms
Tablet, oral: 50 mg, 100 mg, 150 mg, 300 mg
Tablet, extended release, oral:
Oleptro™: 150 mg, 300 mg

trazodone hydrochloride *see trazodone on page 884*

Trazorel® (Can) *see trazodone on page 884*

Treanda® *see bendamustine on page 119*

Trecator® *see ethionamide on page 358*

Trelstar® *see triptorelin on page 894*

TRENtal® *see pentoxifylline on page 689*

Trental® (Can) *see pentoxifylline on page 689*

treprostinil (tre PROST in il)

Synonyms treprostinil sodium

U.S. Brand Names Remodulin®; Tyvaso™

Canadian Brand Names Remodulin®

Therapeutic Category Vasodilator

Use
Injection: Treatment of pulmonary arterial hypertension (PAH) (WHO Group I) in patients with NYHA Class II-IV symptoms to decrease exercise-associated symptoms; to diminish clinical deterioration when transitioning from epoprostenol (I.V.)

Inhalation: Treatment of pulmonary arterial hypertension (PAH) (WHO Group I) in patients with NYHA Class III symptoms to improve exercise ability. **Note:** Nearly all controlled clinical trial experience has been with concomitant bosentan or sildenafil.

General Dosage Range Dosage adjustment recommended for the I.V. infusion and SubQ routes in patients with hepatic impairment
Inhalation: *Adults:* Initial: 18 mcg (or 3 inhalations) every 4 hours 4 times/day; Maintenance: Maximum dose: 54 mcg (or 9 inhalations) 4 times/day
I.V. Infusion, SubQ: *Adults:* Initial: 0.625-1.25 ng/kg/minute; Maintenance: 1.25-40 ng/kg/minute

Dosage Forms
 Injection, solution:
  Remodulin®: 1 mg/mL (20 mL); 2.5 mg/mL (20 mL); 5 mg/mL (20 mL); 10 mg/mL (20 mL)
 Solution, for oral inhalation:
  Tyvaso™: 0.6 mg/mL (2.9 mL)

treprostinil sodium *see* treprostinil *on page 884*

Tretin-X™ *see* tretinoin (topical) *on page 885*

tretinoin and clindamycin *see* clindamycin and tretinoin *on page 219*

tretinoin and mequinol *see* mequinol and tretinoin *on page 563*

tretinoin, fluocinolone acetonide, and hydroquinone *see* fluocinolone, hydroquinone, and tretinoin *on page 385*

tretinoin (systemic) (TRET i noyn)

Synonyms *trans* vitamin A acid; *trans*-retinoic acid; all-*trans* retinoic acid; all-*trans* vitamin A acid; ATRA; Ro 5488; tRA; tretinoinum; Vesanoid

Canadian Brand Names Vesanoid®

Therapeutic Category Antineoplastic Agent

Use Induction of remission in patients with acute promyelocytic leukemia (APL), French American British (FAB) classification M3 (including the M3 variant) characterized by t(15;17) translocation and/or PML/RARα gene presence

General Dosage Range Dosage adjustment recommended in patients who develop toxicities
 Oral: *Children and Adults:* Induction: 45 mg/m²/day in 2 divided doses (maximum duration of treatment: 90 days)

Dosage Forms
 Capsule, oral: 10 mg

tretinoin (topical) (TRET i noyn)

Medication Safety Issues
 Sound-alike/look-alike issues:
  Tretinoin may be confused with ISOtretinoin, Tenormin®, triamcinolone, trientine
 International issues:
  Renova [U.S., Canada] may be confused with Remov brand name for nimesulide [Italy]

Synonyms *trans*-retinoic acid; retinoic acid; vitamin A acid

U.S. Brand Names Atralin™; Avita®; Refissa™; Renova®; Retin-A Micro®; Retin-A®; Tretin-X™

Canadian Brand Names Rejuva-A®; Renova®; Retin-A Micro®; Retin-A®; Retinova®; Stieva-A

Therapeutic Category Retinoic Acid Derivative

Use Treatment of acne vulgaris; photodamaged skin; palliation of fine wrinkles, mottled hyperpigmentation, and tactile roughness of facial skin as part of a comprehensive skin care and sun avoidance program

General Dosage Range Topical: *Children >12 years and Adults:* Apply once daily **or** every other day

Dosage Forms
 Cream, topical: 0.025% (20 g, 45 g); 0.05% (20 g, 45 g); 0.1% (20 g, 45 g)
  Avita®: 0.025% (20 g, 45 g)
  Refissa™: 0.05% (40 g)
  Renova®: 0.02% (40 g, 44 g, 60 g)
  Retin-A®: 0.025% (20 g, 45 g); 0.05% (20 g, 45 g); 0.1% (20 g, 45 g)
  Tretin-X™: 0.025% (35 g); 0.0375% (35 g); 0.05% (35 g); 0.1% (35 g)
 Gel, topical: 0.01% (15 g, 45 g); 0.025% (15 g, 45 g)
  Atralin™: 0.05% (45 g)
  Avita®: 0.025% (20 g, 45 g)
  Retin-A Micro®: 0.04% (20 g, 45 g, 50 g); 0.1% (20 g, 45 g, 50 g)
  Retin-A®: 0.01% (15 g, 45 g); 0.025% (15 g, 45 g)
  Tretin-X™: 0.01% (35 g); 0.025% (35 g)

tretinoinum *see* tretinoin (systemic) *on page 885*

Trexall™ *see* methotrexate *on page 571*

Treximet™ *see* sumatriptan and naproxen *on page 839*

Trezix™ *see* acetaminophen, caffeine, and dihydrocodeine *on page 30*

triaconazole *see* terconazole *on page 853*

Triaderm (Can) *see* triamcinolone (topical) *on page 887*

Triall™ [DSC] *see* chlorpheniramine, phenylephrine, and methscopolamine *on page 200*

triamcinolone (systemic) (trye am SIN oh lone)

Medication Safety Issues

Sound-alike/look-alike issues:

Kenalog® may be confused with Ketalar®

Other safety concerns:

TAC (occasional abbreviation for triamcinolone) is an error-prone abbreviation (mistaken as tetracaine-adrenaline-cocaine)

Synonyms triamcinolone acetonide, parenteral; triamcinolone hexacetonide

U.S. Brand Names Aristospan®; Kenalog®-10; Kenalog®-40

Canadian Brand Names Aristospan®

Therapeutic Category Corticosteroid, Inhalant (Oral); Corticosteroid, Systemic

Use

Intraarticular (soft tissue): Acute gouty arthritis, acute/subacute bursitis, acute tenosynovitis, epicondylitis, rheumatoid arthritis, synovitis of osteoarthritis

Intralesional: Alopecia areata, discoid lupus erythematosus, keloids, granuloma annulare lesions (localized hypertrophic, infiltrated, or inflammatory), lichen planus plaques, lichen simplex chronicus plaques, psoriatic plaques, necrobiosis lipoidica diabeticorum, cystic tumors of aponeurosis or tendon (ganglia)

Oral inhalation: Control of bronchial asthma and related bronchospastic conditions

Systemic: Adrenocortical insufficiency, dermatologic diseases, endocrine disorders, gastrointestinal diseases, hematologic and neoplastic disorders, nervous system disorders, nephrotic syndrome, rheumatic disorders, allergic states, respiratory diseases, systemic lupus erythematosus (SLE), and other diseases requiring antiinflammatory or immunosuppressive effects

General Dosage Range

I.M.:

Children 6-12 years: Acetonide: Initial: 40 mg; Range: 2.5-100 mg/day

Children >12 years: Acetonide: Initial: 60 mg; Range: 2.5-100 mg/day

Adults: Acetonide: Initial: 60 mg; Range: 2.5-100 mg/day, may repeat with 20-100 mg when symptoms recur; Multiple sclerosis: 160 mg/day for 1 week, then 64 mg every other day

Intraarticular: *Adults:* Acetonide: 2.5-80 mg; Hexacetonide: 2-20 mg

Intradermal: *Adults:* Acetonide: 1 mg/site

Intralesional: *Adults:* Acetonide: 1-30 mg (usually 1 mg/injection site); Hexacetonide: Up to 0.5 mg/sq inch

Intrasynovial: *Adults:* Acetonide: 5-40 mg

Tendon Sheath: *Adults:* Acetonide: 2.5-10 mg

Dosage Forms

Injection, suspension:

Aristospan®: 5 mg/mL (5 mL); 20 mg/mL (1 mL, 5 mL)

Kenalog®-10: 10 mg/mL (5 mL)

Kenalog®-40: 40 mg/mL (1 mL, 5 mL, 10 mL)

triamcinolone (nasal) (trye am SIN oh lone)

Medication Safety Issues

Sound-alike/look-alike issues:

Nasacort® may be confused with NasalCrom®

Other safety concerns:

TAC (occasional abbreviation for triamcinolone) is an error-prone abbreviation (mistaken as tetracaine-adrenaline-cocaine)

Synonyms triamcinolone acetonide

U.S. Brand Names Nasacort® AQ

Canadian Brand Names Nasacort® AQ; Trinasal®

Therapeutic Category Corticosteroid, Nasal

Use Management of seasonal and perennial allergic rhinitis

General Dosage Range Inhalation:
Nasal inhaler:
Children 6-11 years: 220 mcg/day as 2 sprays in each nostril once daily
Children ≥12 years and Adults: 220-440 mcg/day as 2-4 sprays in each nostril 1-4 times/day
Nasal spray:
Children 2-5 years: 110 mcg/day as 1 spray in each nostril once daily (maximum: 110 mcg/day)
Children 6-11 years: Initial: 110 mcg/day as 1 spray in each nostril once daily; Maintenance: 110-220 mcg/day as 1-2 sprays in each nostril
Children ≥12 years and Adults: 110-220 mcg/day as 1-2 sprays in each nostril once daily
Dosage Forms
Suspension, intranasal: 55 mcg/inhalation (16.5 g)
Nasacort® AQ: 55 mcg/inhalation (16.5 g)

triamcinolone (ophthalmic) (trye am SIN oh lone)

Medication Safety Issues
Other safety concerns:
TAC (occasional abbreviation for triamcinolone) is an error-prone abbreviation (mistaken as tetracaine-adrenaline-cocaine)
Synonyms triamcinolone acetonide
U.S. Brand Names Triesence™
Therapeutic Category Corticosteroid, Ophthalmic
Use
Intavitreal: Treatment of sympathetic ophthalmia, temporal arteritis, uveitis, ocular inflammatory conditions unresponsive to topical corticosteroids
Triesence™: Visualization during vitrectomy
General Dosage Range Intravitreal: *Children and Adults:* Ocular disease: 4 mg as needed; visualization during vitrectomy: 1-4 mg
Dosage Forms
Injection, suspension, ophthalmic:
Triesence™: 40 mg/mL (1 mL)

triamcinolone (topical) (trye am SIN oh lone)

Medication Safety Issues
Sound-alike/look-alike issues:
Kenalog® may be confused with Ketalar®
Other safety concerns:
TAC (occasional abbreviation for triamcinolone) is an error-prone abbreviation (mistaken as tetracaine-adrenaline-cocaine)
U.S. Brand Names Kenalog®; Oralone®; Pediaderm™ TA; Trianex™; Triderm®; Zytopic™
Canadian Brand Names Kenalog®; Oracort; Triaderm
Therapeutic Category Corticosteroid, Topical
Use
Oral topical: Adjunctive treatment and temporary relief of symptoms associated with oral inflammatory lesions and ulcerative lesions resulting from trauma
Topical: Inflammatory dermatoses responsive to steroids
General Dosage Range Topical: *Adults:* Cream, ointment: Apply thin film to affected areas 2-4 times/day; Oral: Press a small dab (about 1/4") to the lesion until a thin film develops; Spray: Apply to affected area 3-4 times/day
Dosage Forms
Aerosol, topical:
Kenalog®: 0.2 mg/2-second spray (63 g)
Cream, topical: 0.025% (15 g, 80 g, 454 g); 0.1% (15 g, 30 g, 80 g, 454 g, 2240 g, 2270 g); 0.5% (15 g)
Pediaderm™ TA: 0.1% (30 g)
Triderm®: 0.1% (30 g, 85 g)
Zytopic™: 0.1% (85 g)
Lotion, topical: 0.025% (60 mL); 0.1% (60 mL)
Ointment, topical: 0.025% (15 g, 80 g, 454 g); 0.05% (430 g); 0.1% (15 g, 80 g, 454 g); 0.5% (15 g)
Trianex™: 0.05% (17 g, 85 g)
Paste, oral topical: 0.1% (5 g)
Oralone®: 0.1% (5 g)

triamcinolone acetonide *see* triamcinolone (nasal) *on page 886*

triamcinolone acetonide *see* triamcinolone (ophthalmic) *on page 887*

triamcinolone acetonide, parenteral *see* triamcinolone (systemic) *on page 886*

triamcinolone and nystatin *see* nystatin and triamcinolone *on page 642*

triamcinolone hexacetonide *see* triamcinolone (systemic) *on page 886*

Triaminic® Children's Chest & Nasal Congestion [OTC] *see* guaifenesin and phenylephrine *on page 428*

Triaminic® Children's Cough Long Acting [OTC] *see* dextromethorphan *on page 270*

Triaminic™ Children's Fever Reducer Pain Reliever [OTC] *see* acetaminophen *on page 23*

Triaminic® Children's Night Time Cold & Cough [OTC] *see* diphenhydramine and phenylephrine *on page 292*

Triaminic® Children's Softchews® Cough & Runny Nose [OTC] *see* dextromethorphan and chlorpheniramine *on page 271*

Triaminic® Children's Thin Strips® Night Time Cold & Cough [OTC] *see* diphenhydramine and phenylephrine *on page 292*

Triaminic® Cold & Allergy (Can) *see* chlorpheniramine and pseudoephedrine *on page 199*

Triaminic® Cold and Allergy [OTC] *see* chlorpheniramine and phenylephrine *on page 198*

Triaminic® Day Time Cold & Cough [OTC] *see* dextromethorphan and phenylephrine *on page 271*

Triaminic Thin Strips® Children's Cold with Stuffy Nose [OTC] *see* phenylephrine (systemic) *on page 696*

Triaminic Thin Strips® Children's Cough & Runny Nose [OTC] *see* diphenhydramine (systemic) *on page 290*

Triaminic Thin Strips® Children's Long Acting Cough [OTC] *see* dextromethorphan *on page 270*

Triaminic Thin Strips® Children's Day Time Cold & Cough [OTC] *see* dextromethorphan and phenylephrine *on page 271*

triamterene (trye AM ter een)

Medication Safety Issues
  Sound-alike/look-alike issues:
    Triamterene may be confused with trimipramine
    Dyrenium® may be confused with Pyridium®
U.S. Brand Names Dyrenium®
Therapeutic Category Diuretic, Potassium Sparing
Use Alone or in combination with other diuretics in treatment of edema and hypertension; decreases potassium excretion caused by kaliuretic diuretics
General Dosage Range Oral: *Adults:* 50-300 mg/day in 1-2 divided doses (maximum: 300 mg/day)
Dosage Forms
  Capsule, oral:
    Dyrenium®: 50 mg, 100 mg

triamterene and hydrochlorothiazide *see* hydrochlorothiazide and triamterene *on page 446*

Trianex™ *see* triamcinolone (topical) *on page 887*

Triatec-8 (Can) *see* acetaminophen and codeine *on page 26*

Triatec-8 Strong (Can) *see* acetaminophen and codeine *on page 26*

Triatec-30 (Can) *see* acetaminophen and codeine *on page 26*

Triaz® *see* benzoyl peroxide *on page 124*

triazolam (trye AY zoe lam)

Medication Safety Issues
  Sound-alike/look-alike issues:
    Triazolam may be confused with alPRAZolam
    Halcion® may be confused with halcinonide, Haldol®
  BEERS Criteria medication:
    This drug may be inappropriate for use in geriatric patients (high severity risk).
U.S. Brand Names Halcion®
Canadian Brand Names Apo-Triazo®; Gen-Triazolam; Halcion®; Mylan-Triazolam
Therapeutic Category Benzodiazepine

Controlled Substance C-IV

Use Short-term treatment of insomnia

General Dosage Range Dosage adjustment recommended in patients with hepatic impairment
Oral:
  Adults: 0.125-0.25 mg at bedtime (maximum: 0.5 mg/day)
  Elderly: Initial: 0.125 mg at bedtime (maximum: 0.25 mg/day)

Dosage Forms
  Tablet, oral: 0.125 mg, 0.25 mg
  Halcion®: 0.25 mg

Tri-B® [OTC] *see* folic acid, cyanocobalamin, and pyridoxine *on page 396*

tribavirin *see* ribavirin *on page 777*

Tribenzor™ *see* olmesartan, amlodipine, and hydrochlorothiazide *on page 646*

Tri Biozene [OTC] *see* bacitracin, neomycin, polymyxin B, and pramoxine *on page 112*

Tri-Buffered Aspirin [OTC] *see* aspirin *on page 98*

tricalcium phosphate *see* calcium phosphate (tribasic) *on page 165*

Tricardio B *see* folic acid, cyanocobalamin, and pyridoxine *on page 396*

TriCare® Prenatal *see* vitamins (multiple/prenatal) *on page 920*

TriCare® Prenatal DHA One® *see* vitamins (multiple/prenatal) *on page 920*

Tri-Chlor® *see* trichloroacetic acid *on page 889*

trichloroacetaldehyde monohydrate *see* chloral hydrate *on page 193*

trichloroacetic acid (trye klor oh a SEE tik AS id)

U.S. Brand Names Tri-Chlor®

Therapeutic Category Keratolytic Agent

Use Chemical used in compounding agents for the treatment of warts, skin resurfacing (chemical peels)

Dosage Forms
  Liquid, topical:
    Tri-Chlor®: 80% (15 mL)

Trichophyton skin test (trye koe FYE ton skin test)

Therapeutic Category Diagnostic Agent

Use Skin test in diagnosis of Type I hypersensitivity to *Trichophyton* fungus

General Dosage Range Intradermal: *Children and Adults:* 0.1 mL

Dosage Forms
  Injection, solution: 1:200 (2 mL)

Tricitrates *see* citric acid, sodium citrate, and potassium citrate *on page 214*

TriCor® *see* fenofibrate *on page 369*

tricosal *see* choline magnesium trisalicylate *on page 205*

Tri-Cyclen® (Can) *see* ethinyl estradiol and norgestimate *on page 357*

Tri-Cyclen® Lo (Can) *see* ethinyl estradiol and norgestimate *on page 357*

Triderm® *see* triamcinolone (topical) *on page 887*

Tridil *see* nitroglycerin *on page 629*

Tridural™ (Can) *see* tramadol *on page 880*

trien *see* trientine *on page 889*

trientine (TRYE en teen)

Medication Safety Issues
  Sound-alike/look-alike issues:
    Trientine may be confused with Trental®, tretinoin

Synonyms 2,2,2-tetramine; trien; trientine hydrochloride; triethylene tetramine dihydrochloride

U.S. Brand Names Syprine®

Canadian Brand Names Syprine®

Therapeutic Category Chelating Agent

Use Treatment of Wilson disease in patients intolerant to penicillamine

◄ **General Dosage Range Oral:**
Children <12 years: 20 mg/kg **or** 500-750 mg/day in 2-4 divided doses (maximum: 1.5 g/day)
Children ≥12 years and Adults: 750-1500 mg/day in 2-4 divided doses (maximum: 2 g/day)

Dosage Forms
Capsule, oral:
Syprine®: 250 mg

trientine hydrochloride *see trientine on page 889*
Triesence™ *see triamcinolone (ophthalmic) on page 887*
triethanolamine salicylate *see trolamine on page 894*
triethylene tetramine dihydrochloride *see trientine on page 889*
triethylenethiophosphoramide *see thiotepa on page 864*

trifluoperazine (trye floo oh PER a zeen)

Medication Safety Issues
Sound-alike/look-alike issues:
Trifluoperazine may be confused with triflupromazine, trihexyphenidyl
Stelazine® may be confused with selegiline
International issues:
Eskazine [Spain] may be confused with Ecazide, a brand name for captopril/hydrochlorothiazide [France, Spain]

Synonyms trifluoperazine hydrochloride
Canadian Brand Names Apo-Trifluoperazine®; Novo-Trifluzine; PMS-Trifluoperazine; Terfluzine
Therapeutic Category Phenothiazine Derivative
Use Treatment of schizophrenia; short-term treatment of generalized nonpsychotic anxiety
General Dosage Range Oral:
Children 6-12 years: Initial: 1 mg 1-2 times/day; Maintenance: 1-15 mg/day in 1-2 divided doses (maximum: 15 mg/day)
Adults: Inpatient: Initial: 2-5 mg twice daily; Maintenance: 15-40 mg/day in 2 divided doses (maximum: 40 mg/day); Outpatient: Initial: 1-3 mg twice daily (maximum: 40 mg/day)
Dosage Forms
Tablet, oral: 1 mg, 2 mg, 5 mg, 10 mg

trifluoperazine hydrochloride *see trifluoperazine on page 890*
trifluorothymidine *see trifluridine on page 890*

trifluridine (trye FLURE i deen)

Medication Safety Issues
Sound-alike/look-alike issues:
Viroptic® may be confused with Timoptic®
Synonyms F_3T; trifluorothymidine
U.S. Brand Names Viroptic®
Canadian Brand Names Sandoz-Trifluridine; Viroptic®
Therapeutic Category Antiviral Agent
Use Treatment of primary keratoconjunctivitis and recurrent epithelial keratitis caused by herpes simplex virus types I and II
General Dosage Range Ophthalmic: *Adults:* Initial: Instill 1 drop into affected eye(s) every 2 hours while awake (maximum: 9 drops/day); After re-epithelialization of corneal ulcer: 1 drop every 4 hours (maximum: 21 days of treatment)
Dosage Forms
Solution, ophthalmic: 1% (7.5 mL)
Viroptic®: 1% (7.5 mL)

Triglide® *see fenofibrate on page 369*
triglycerides, medium chain *see medium chain triglycerides on page 553*
Trihexyphen (Can) *see trihexyphenidyl on page 891*

trihexyphenidyl (trye heks ee FEN i dil)
Medication Safety Issues
Sound-alike/look-alike issues:
Trihexyphenidyl may be confused with trifluoperazine
Synonyms Artane; benzhexol hydrochloride; trihexyphenidyl hydrochloride
Canadian Brand Names PMS-Trihexyphenidyl; Trihexyphen; Trihexyphenidyl
Therapeutic Category Anti-Parkinson Agent; Anticholinergic Agent
Use Adjunctive treatment of Parkinson disease; treatment of drug-induced extrapyramidal symptoms
General Dosage Range Oral: *Adults:* Initial: 1 mg/day; Maintenance: 3-15 mg/day in 3-4 divided doses
Dosage Forms
Elixir, oral: 2 mg/5 mL (473 mL)
Tablet, oral: 2 mg, 5 mg

Trihexyphenidyl (Can) *see* trihexyphenidyl *on page 891*

trihexyphenidyl hydrochloride *see* trihexyphenidyl *on page 891*

TriHIBit® [DSC] *see* diphtheria, tetanus toxoids, and acellular pertussis vaccine and *Haemophilus influenzae* b conjugate vaccine *on page 297*

Tri-Legest™ Fe *see* ethinyl estradiol and norethindrone *on page 355*

Trileptal® *see* oxcarbazepine *on page 660*

TriLipix® *see* fenofibric acid *on page 369*

Trilisate *see* choline magnesium trisalicylate *on page 205*

Tri-Luma® *see* fluocinolone, hydroquinone, and tretinoin *on page 385*

TriLyte® *see* polyethylene glycol-electrolyte solution *on page 718*

trimebutine *(Canada only)* (trye me BYOO teen)
Synonyms trimebutine maleate
Canadian Brand Names Modulon®
Therapeutic Category Antispasmodic Agent, Gastrointestinal
Use Treatment and relief of symptoms associated with irritable bowel syndrome (IBS) (spastic colon). In postoperative paralytic ileus in order to accelerate the resumption of the intestinal transit following abdominal surgery.
General Dosage Range Oral: *Children ≥12 years and Adults:* 200 mg 3 times/day
Product Availability Not available in U.S.
Dosage Forms - Canada Tablet, oral: 100 mg, 200 mg

trimebutine maleate *see* trimebutine *(Canada only) on page 891*

trimethobenzamide (trye meth oh BEN za mide)
Medication Safety Issues
Sound-alike/look-alike issues:
Tigan® may be confused with Tiazac®, Ticar®, Ticlid®
Trimethobenzamide may be confused with metoclopramide, trimethoprim
BEERS Criteria medication:
This drug may be inappropriate for use in geriatric patients (high severity risk).
Synonyms trimethobenzamide hydrochloride
U.S. Brand Names Tigan®
Canadian Brand Names Tigan®
Therapeutic Category Anticholinergic Agent; Antiemetic
Use Treatment of postoperative nausea and vomiting; treatment of nausea associated with gastroenteritis
General Dosage Range
I.M.: *Adults:* 200 mg 3-4 times/day **or** 200 mg as a single dose, repeat 1 hour later
Oral: *Children >40 kg and Adults:* 300 mg 3-4 times/day
Dosage Forms
Capsule, oral: 300 mg
Tigan®: 300 mg
Injection, solution:
Tigan®: 100 mg/mL (20 mL)

◀ **Injection, solution** [preservative free]:
Tigan®: 100 mg/mL (2 mL)

trimethobenzamide hydrochloride *see* trimethobenzamide *on page 891*

trimethoprim (trye METH oh prim)
Medication Safety Issues
Sound-alike/look-alike issues:
Trimethoprim may be confused with trimethaphan
Synonyms TMP
U.S. Brand Names Primsol®
Canadian Brand Names Apo-Trimethoprim®
Therapeutic Category Antibiotic, Miscellaneous
Use Treatment of urinary tract infections due to susceptible strains of *E. coli, P. mirabilis, K. pneumoniae, Enterobacter* spp and coagulase-negative *Staphylococcus* including *S. saprophyticus*; acute otitis media due to susceptible strains of *S. pneumoniae* and *H. influenzae* in children
General Dosage Range Dosage adjustment recommended in patients with renal impairment
Oral:
Children ≥2 months: 4-12 mg/kg/day in divided doses every 12 hours
Adults: 100 mg once daily **or** 100 mg every 12 hours **or** 200 mg every 24 hours; up to 15mg/kg/day
Dosage Forms
Solution, oral:
Primsol®: 50 mg (base)/5 mL (473 mL)
Tablet, oral: 100 mg

trimethoprim and polymyxin B (trye METH oh prim & pol i MIKS in bee)
Synonyms polymyxin B and trimethoprim
U.S. Brand Names Polytrim®
Canadian Brand Names PMS-Polytrimethoprim; Polytrim™
Therapeutic Category Antibiotic, Ophthalmic
Use Treatment of surface ocular bacterial conjunctivitis and blepharoconjunctivitis
General Dosage Range Ophthalmic: *Children ≥2 months and Adults:* Instill 1 drop in affected eye(s) every 3 hours (maximum: 6 doses per day) for 7-10 days
Dosage Forms
Solution, ophthalmic: Trimethoprim 1 mg and polymyxin B 10,000 units per 1 mL (10 mL)
Polytrim®: Trimethoprim 1 mg and polymyxin B 10,000 units per 1 mL (10 mL)

trimethoprim and sulfamethoxazole *see* sulfamethoxazole and trimethoprim *on page 836*

trimipramine (trye MI pra meen)
Medication Safety Issues
Sound-alike/look-alike issues:
Trimipramine may be confused with triamterene, trimeprazine
Synonyms trimipramine maleate
U.S. Brand Names Surmontil®
Canadian Brand Names Apo-Trimip®; Nu-Trimipramine; Rhotrimine®; Surmontil®
Therapeutic Category Antidepressant, Tricyclic (Tertiary Amine)
Use Treatment of depression
General Dosage Range
Oral:
Adolescents: Initial: 50 mg/day (maximum: 100 mg/day)
Adults: 50-200 mg at bedtime (maximum: 200 mg/day [outpatient] or 300 mg/day [inpatient])
Elderly: 50-100 mg at bedtime (maximum: 100 mg/day)
Dosage Forms
Capsule, oral:
Surmontil®: 25 mg, 50 mg, 100 mg

trimipramine maleate *see* trimipramine *on page 892*
Trinasal® (Can) *see* triamcinolone (nasal) *on page 886*
TriNessa® *see* ethinyl estradiol and norgestimate *on page 357*

Trinipatch® (Can) *see* nitroglycerin *on page 629*
Tri-Norinyl® *see* ethinyl estradiol and norethindrone *on page 355*
Triostat® *see* liothyronine *on page 529*
Tripedia® [DSC] *see* diphtheria, tetanus toxoids, and acellular pertussis vaccine *on page 296*
Triphasil® (Can) *see* ethinyl estradiol and levonorgestrel *on page 353*
triple antibiotic *see* bacitracin, neomycin, and polymyxin B *on page 111*
triple sulfa *see* sulfabenzamide, sulfacetamide, and sulfathiazole *on page 834*
Triplex™ AD [DSC] *see* chlorpheniramine, pyrilamine, and phenylephrine *on page 202*
Tripohist™ D *see* triprolidine and pseudoephedrine *on page 893*

triprolidine and pseudoephedrine (trye PROE li deen & soo doe e FED rin)

Medication Safety Issues
Sound-alike/look-alike issues:
Aprodine® may be confused with Aphrodyne®
Synonyms pseudoephedrine and triprolidine
U.S. Brand Names Allerfrim [OTC]; Aprodine [OTC]; Genac™ [OTC] [DSC]; Pediatex® TD; Silafed [OTC]; Tripohist™ D
Canadian Brand Names Actifed®
Therapeutic Category Antihistamine/Decongestant Combination
Use Temporary relief of nasal congestion, decongest sinus openings, running nose, sneezing, itching of nose or throat and itchy, watery eyes due to common cold, hay fever, or other upper respiratory allergies
General Dosage Range Oral: *Children ≥6 years and Adults:* Dosage varies greatly depending on product
Dosage Forms
Liquid, oral:
Pediatex® TD: Triprolidine 0.938 mg and pseudoephedrine 10 mg per 1 mL
Tripohist™ D: Triprolidine 1.25 mg and pseudoephedrine 45 mg per 5 mL
Syrup, oral:
Allerfrim [OTC], Aprodine [OTC], Silafed [OTC]: Triprolidine 1.25 mg and pseudoephedrine 30 mg per 5 mL
Tablet, oral:
Allerfrim [OTC], Aprodine [OTC]: Triprolidine 2.5 mg and pseudoephedrine 60 mg

triprolidine, codeine, and pseudoephedrine *see* triprolidine, pseudoephedrine, and codeine *(Canada only) on page 893*

triprolidine, pseudoephedrine, and codeine (Canada only)
(trye PROE li deen, soo doe e FED rin, & KOE deen)
Medication Safety Issues
Sound-alike/look-alike issues:
Triacin-C® may be confused with triacetin
Synonyms codeine, pseudoephedrine, and triprolidine; codeine, triprolidine, and pseudoephedrine; Cotridin; pseudoephedrine, codeine, and triprolidine; pseudoephedrine, triprolidine, and codeine; triprolidine, codeine, and pseudoephedrine
Canadian Brand Names CoActifed®; Covan®; ratio-Cotridin
Therapeutic Category Antihistamine/Decongestant/Antitussive
Controlled Substance CDSA-I
Use Symptomatic relief of upper respiratory symptoms and cough
General Dosage Range Oral:
Children 2-6 years: 2.5 mL 4 times/day
Children 7-12 years: 5 mL 4 times/day **or** 1/2 tablet 4 times/day
Children >12 years and Adults: 10 mL 4 times/day **or** 1 tablet 4 times/day
Product Availability Not available in U.S.
Dosage Forms - Canada
Syrup, oral:
CoActifed®, ratio-Cotridin: Triprolidine 2 mg, pseudoephedrine 30 mg, and codeine 10 mg per 5 mL
CoVan®: Triprolidine 2 mg, pseudoephedrine 30 mg, and codeine 10 mg per 5 mL (500 mL)
Tablet, oral:
CoActifed®: Triprolidine 4 mg, pseudoephedrine 60 mg, and codeine 20 mg (50s)

TripTone® [OTC] see dimenhydrinate *on page 288*

triptorelin (trip toe REL in)

Synonyms AY-25650; CL-118,532; D-Trp(6)-LHRH; detryptoreline; triptorelin pamoate; tryptoreline
U.S. Brand Names Trelstar®
Canadian Brand Names Trelstar®
Therapeutic Category Luteinizing Hormone-Releasing Hormone Analog
Use Palliative treatment of advanced prostate cancer
General Dosage Range I.M.: *Adults:* 3.75 mg once every 4 weeks **or** 11.25 mg once every 12 weeks **or** 22.5 mg once every 24 weeks
Dosage Forms
  Injection, powder for reconstitution:
    Trelstar®: 3.75 mg, 11.25 mg, 22.5 mg

triptorelin pamoate see triptorelin *on page 894*
Triquilar® (Can) see ethinyl estradiol and levonorgestrel *on page 353*
tris buffer see tromethamine *on page 895*
Trisenox® see arsenic trioxide *on page 94*
tris(hydroxymethyl)aminomethane see tromethamine *on page 895*
trisodium calcium diethylenetriaminepentaacetate (Ca-DTPA) see diethylene triamine penta-acetic acid *on page 281*
Tri-Sprintec® see ethinyl estradiol and norgestimate *on page 357*
Trivagizole-3® (Can) see clotrimazole (topical) *on page 226*
trivalent inactivated influenza vaccine (TIV) see influenza virus vaccine (inactivated) *on page 473*
Tri-Vi-Sol® [OTC] see vitamins (multiple/pediatric) *on page 920*
Tri-Vi-Sol® With Iron [OTC] see vitamins (multiple/pediatric) *on page 920*
Trivora® see ethinyl estradiol and levonorgestrel *on page 353*
Trizivir® see abacavir, lamivudine, and zidovudine *on page 20*
Trocaine® [OTC] see benzocaine *on page 121*
Trocal® [OTC] see dextromethorphan *on page 270*

trolamine (TROLE a meen)

Medication Safety Issues
  Sound-alike/look-alike issues:
    Myoflex® may be confused with Mycelex®
  International issues:
    Biafine: Brand name for trolamine [multiple international markets], but also the brand name for sodium alginate [Portugal] and a topical emulsion [U.S.]
Synonyms TEAS; triethanolamine salicylate; trolamine salicylate
U.S. Brand Names Aspercreme® [OTC]; Flex-Power [OTC]; Mobisyl® [OTC]; Myoflex® [OTC]; Sportscreme® [OTC]
Canadian Brand Names Antiphlogistine Rub A-535 No Odour; Myoflex®
Therapeutic Category Analgesic, Topical
Use Relief of pain of muscular aches, rheumatism, neuralgia, sprains, arthritis on intact skin
General Dosage Range Topical: *Children ≥12 years and Adults:* Apply to affected area as needed up to 3-4 times/day
Dosage Forms
  Cream, topical:
    Aspercreme® [OTC]: 10% (35 g, 85 g, 142 g)
    Flex-Power [OTC]: 10% (57 g, 113 g)
    Mobisyl® [OTC]: 10% (100 g, 227 g)
    Myoflex® [OTC]: 10% (57 g, 113 g)
    Sportscreme® [OTC]: 10% (35 g, 85 g)
  Lotion, topical:
    Aspercreme® [OTC]: 10% (180 mL)

trolamine salicylate see trolamine *on page 894*
Trombovar® (Can) see sodium tetradecyl *on page 824*

tromethamine (troe METH a meen)

Medication Safety Issues
 Sound-alike/look-alike issues:
  Tromethamine may be confused with TrophAmine®

Synonyms tris buffer; tris(hydroxymethyl)aminomethane

U.S. Brand Names THAM®

Therapeutic Category Alkalinizing Agent

Use Correction of metabolic acidosis associated with cardiac bypass surgery or cardiac arrest; to correct excess acidity of stored blood that is preserved with acid citrate dextrose (ACD); indicated in infants needing alkalinization after receiving maximum sodium bicarbonate (8-10 mEq/kg/24 hours)

General Dosage Range
 I.V.:
  Infants: Initial: Approximately 1 mL/kg for each pH unit below 7.4; additional doses determined by changes in PaO_2, pH, and pCO_2
  Adults: 3.6-10.8 g (111-333 mL) **or** 9 mL/kg (maximum: 500 mg/kg) **or** 15-77 mL added to each 500 mL of blood
 Intraventricular: *Adults:* 3.6-10.8 g (111-333 mL) **or** 9 mL/kg (maximum: 500 mg/kg) **or** 15-77 mL added to each 500 mL of blood

Dosage Forms
 Injection, solution:
  THAM®: 18 g (500 mL)

Tronolane® Cream [OTC] *see* pramoxine *on page 730*

Tronolane® Suppository [OTC] *see* phenylephrine (topical) *on page 698*

Tropazone™ *see* emollients *on page 325*

TrophAmine® *see* amino acid injection *on page 65*

Tropicacyl® *see* tropicamide *on page 895*

tropicamide (troe PIK a mide)

Synonyms bistropamide

U.S. Brand Names Mydral™ [DSC]; Mydriacyl®; Tropicacyl®

Canadian Brand Names Diotrope®; Mydriacyl®

Therapeutic Category Anticholinergic Agent

Use Short-acting mydriatic used in diagnostic procedures; as well as preoperatively and postoperatively; treatment of some cases of acute iritis, iridocyclitis, and keratitis

General Dosage Range Ophthalmic: *Children and Adults:* 0.5%: Instill 1-2 drops 15-20 minutes before exam, may repeat; 1%: Instill 1-2 drops, may repeat in 5 minutes

Dosage Forms
 Solution, ophthalmic: 0.5% (15 mL); 1% (2 mL, 3 mL, 15 mL)
  Mydriacyl®: 1% (3 mL, 15 mL)
  Tropicacyl®: 0.5% (15 mL); 1% (15 mL)

tropicamide and hydroxyamphetamine *see* hydroxyamphetamine and tropicamide *on page 454*

Trosec (Can) *see* trospium *on page 895*

trospium (TROSE pee um)

Synonyms trospium chloride

U.S. Brand Names Sanctura®; Sanctura® XR

Canadian Brand Names Sanctura® XR; Trosec

Therapeutic Category Anticholinergic Agent

Use Treatment of overactive bladder with symptoms of urgency, incontinence, and urinary frequency

General Dosage Range Dosage adjustment recommended in patients with renal impairment
 Oral:
  Adults: Immediate release formulation: 20 mg twice daily; Extended release formulation: 60 mg once daily
  Elderly ≥75 years: Immediate release formulation: Initial: 20 mg at bedtime

◀ **Dosage Forms**
Capsule, extended release, oral:
Sanctura® XR: 60 mg
Tablet, oral: 20 mg
Sanctura®: 20 mg

trospium chloride *see* trospium *on page 895*
Trusopt® *see* dorzolamide *on page 307*
Truvada® *see* emtricitabine and tenofovir *on page 326*

trypsin, balsam Peru, and castor oil (TRIP sin, BAL sam pe RUE, & KAS tor oyl)

Medication Safety Issues
Sound-alike/look-alike issues:
Granulex® may be confused with Regranex®
Synonyms balsam Peru, castor oil, and trypsin; castor oil, trypsin, and balsam Peru
U.S. Brand Names Granulex®; Optase™; TBC; Vasolex™; Xenaderm®
Therapeutic Category Protectant, Topical
Use Treatment of decubitus ulcers, varicose ulcers, debridement of eschar, dehiscent wounds and sunburn; promote wound healing; reduce odor from necrotic wounds
General Dosage Range Topical: *Adults:* Apply a minimum of twice daily or as often as necessary
Dosage Forms
Aerosol, topical:
Granulex®: Trypsin 0.12 mg, balsam Peru 87 mg, and castor oil 788 mg per gram (60 g, 120 g)
TBC: Trypsin 0.1 mg, balsam Peru 72.5 mg, and castor oil 650 mg per 0.82 mL (60 g, 120 g)
Gel, topical:
Optase™: Trypsin 0.12 mg, balsam Peru 87 mg, and castor oil 788 mg per gram (95 g)
Ointment, topical:
Vasolex™: Trypsin 90 USP units, balsam Peru 87 mg, and castor oil 788 mg per gram (5 g, 30 g, 60 g)
Xenaderm®: Trypsin 90 USP units, balsam Peru 87 mg, and castor oil 788 mg per gram (30 g, 60 g)

tryptoreline *see* triptorelin *on page 894*
TSH *see* thyrotropin alpha *on page 866*
TSPA *see* thiotepa *on page 864*
TST *see* tuberculin tests *on page 896*
TT *see* tetanus toxoid (adsorbed) *on page 855*
tuberculin purified protein derivative *see* tuberculin tests *on page 896*
tuberculin skin test *see* tuberculin tests *on page 896*

tuberculin tests (too BER kyoo lin tests)

Medication Safety Issues
Sound-alike/look-alike issues:
Aplisol® may be confused with Anusol®, A.P.L.®, Aplitest®, Atropisol®
Administration issues:
Tuberculin products may be confused with tetanus toxoid products, poliovirus vaccine (inactivated), and influenza virus vaccine. Medication errors have occurred when tuberculin skin tests (PPD) have been inadvertently administered instead of tetanus toxoid products and influenza virus vaccine. These products are refrigerated and often stored in close proximity to each other.
Synonyms mantoux; PPD; TB skin test; TST; tuberculin purified protein derivative; tuberculin skin test
U.S. Brand Names Aplisol®; Tubersol®
Therapeutic Category Diagnostic Agent
Use Skin test in diagnosis of tuberculosis
General Dosage Range Intradermal: *Children and Adults:* 0.1 mL
Dosage Forms
Injection, solution:
Aplisol®: 5 TU/0.1 mL (1 mL, 5 mL)
Tubersol®: 5 TU/0.1 mL (1 mL, 5 mL)

Tubersol® *see* tuberculin tests *on page 896*
Tucks® Anti-Itch [OTC] *see* witch hazel *on page 923*
Tucks® Hemorrhoidal [OTC] *see* pramoxine *on page 730*

Tucks® Take Alongs® [OTC] *see* witch hazel *on page 923*

Tums® [OTC] *see* calcium carbonate *on page 161*

Tums® Dual Action [OTC] *see* famotidine, calcium carbonate, and magnesium hydroxide *on page 367*

Tums® E-X [OTC] *see* calcium carbonate *on page 161*

Tums® Extra Strength Sugar Free [OTC] *see* calcium carbonate *on page 161*

Tums® Quickpak [OTC] *see* calcium carbonate *on page 161*

Tums® Smoothies™ [OTC] *see* calcium carbonate *on page 161*

Tums® Ultra [OTC] *see* calcium carbonate *on page 161*

Tusscough DHC™ *see* dihydrocodeine, chlorpheniramine, and phenylephrine *on page 285*

Tussi-12® *see* carbetapentane and chlorpheniramine *on page 172*

Tussi-12® D [DSC] *see* carbetapentane, phenylephrine, and pyrilamine *on page 173*

Tussi-12® DS [DSC] *see* carbetapentane, phenylephrine, and pyrilamine *on page 173*

Tussi-12 S™ *see* carbetapentane and chlorpheniramine *on page 172*

Tussi-Bid® *see* guaifenesin and dextromethorphan *on page 427*

TussiCaps® *see* hydrocodone and chlorpheniramine *on page 448*

Tussigon® *see* hydrocodone and homatropine *on page 448*

Tussionex® *see* hydrocodone and chlorpheniramine *on page 448*

Tussizone-12 RF™ *see* carbetapentane and chlorpheniramine *on page 172*

Tusso-C™ *see* guaifenesin and codeine *on page 426*

Tusso™-DMR [DSC] *see* guaifenesin, dextromethorphan, and phenylephrine *on page 429*

T-Vites [OTC] *see* vitamins (multiple/oral) *on page 919*

TVP-1012 *see* rasagiline *on page 769*

Twelve Resin-K [OTC] *see* cyanocobalamin *on page 241*

Twilite® [OTC] *see* diphenhydramine (systemic) *on page 290*

Twinject® *see* epinephrine (systemic, oral inhalation) *on page 331*

Twinrix® *see* hepatitis A and hepatitis B recombinant vaccine *on page 437*

Twinrix® Junior (Can) *see* hepatitis A and hepatitis B recombinant vaccine *on page 437*

Twynsta® *see* telmisartan and amlodipine *on page 848*

Ty21a vaccine *see* typhoid vaccine *on page 898*

Tygacil® *see* tigecycline *on page 868*

Tykerb® *see* lapatinib *on page 512*

Tylenol® [OTC] *see* acetaminophen *on page 23*

Tylenol® (Can) *see* acetaminophen *on page 23*

Tylenol #2 *see* acetaminophen and codeine *on page 26*

Tylenol #3 *see* acetaminophen and codeine *on page 26*

Tylenol® 8 Hour [OTC] *see* acetaminophen *on page 23*

Tylenol® Allergy Multi-Symptom Nighttime [OTC] *see* acetaminophen, diphenhydramine, and phenylephrine *on page 33*

Tylenol® Arthritis Pain Extended Relief [OTC] *see* acetaminophen *on page 23*

Tylenol® Children's [OTC] *see* acetaminophen *on page 23*

Tylenol® Children's Meltaways [OTC] *see* acetaminophen *on page 23*

Tylenol® Children's Plus Cold and Allergy [OTC] *see* acetaminophen, diphenhydramine, and phenylephrine *on page 33*

Tylenol Codeine *see* acetaminophen and codeine *on page 26*

Tylenol® Cold Head Congestion Daytime [OTC] *see* acetaminophen, dextromethorphan, and phenylephrine *on page 32*

Tylenol® Cold Multi-Symptom Daytime [OTC] *see* acetaminophen, dextromethorphan, and phenylephrine *on page 32*

Tylenol® Cough & Sore Throat Nighttime [OTC] *see* acetaminophen, dextromethorphan, and doxylamine *on page 32*

Tylenol® Decongestant (Can) *see* acetaminophen and pseudoephedrine *on page 29*

Tylenol Elixir with Codeine (Can) *see* acetaminophen and codeine *on page 26*

Tylenol® Extra Strength [OTC] *see* acetaminophen *on page 23*

Tylenol® Infant's Concentrated [OTC] *see* acetaminophen *on page* 23
Tylenol® Jr. Meltaways [OTC] *see* acetaminophen *on page* 23
Tylenol No. 1 (Can) *see* acetaminophen and codeine *on page* 26
Tylenol No. 1 Forte (Can) *see* acetaminophen and codeine *on page* 26
Tylenol No. 2 with Codeine (Can) *see* acetaminophen and codeine *on page* 26
Tylenol No. 3 with Codeine (Can) *see* acetaminophen and codeine *on page* 26
Tylenol No. 4 with Codeine (Can) *see* acetaminophen and codeine *on page* 26
Tylenol® PM [OTC] *see* acetaminophen and diphenhydramine *on page* 27
Tylenol® Severe Allergy [OTC] *see* acetaminophen and diphenhydramine *on page* 27
Tylenol® Sinus (Can) *see* acetaminophen and pseudoephedrine *on page* 29
Tylenol® Sinus Congestion & Pain Daytime [OTC] *see* acetaminophen and phenylephrine *on page* 28
Tylenol® with Codeine No. 3 *see* acetaminophen and codeine *on page* 26
Tylenol® with Codeine No. 4 *see* acetaminophen and codeine *on page* 26
Tylenol® Women's Menstrual Relief [OTC] *see* acetaminophen and pamabrom *on page* 27
Tylox® *see* oxycodone and acetaminophen *on page* 662
type 4 and type 7 adenovirus vaccine *see* adenovirus (types 4, 7) vaccine *on page* 42
Typherix® (Can) *see* typhoid vaccine *on page* 898
Typhim Vi® *see* typhoid vaccine *on page* 898

typhoid vaccine (TYE foid vak SEEN)

Synonyms Ty21a vaccine; typhoid vaccine live oral Ty21a; Vi vaccine
U.S. Brand Names Typhim Vi®; Vivotif®
Canadian Brand Names Typherix®; Typhim Vi®; Vivotif®
Therapeutic Category Vaccine, Inactivated Bacteria
Use Active immunization against typhoid fever caused by *Salmonella typhi*
Not for routine vaccination. In the United States and Canada, use should be limited to:
  - Travelers to areas with a prolonged risk of exposure to *S. typhi*
  - Persons with intimate exposure to a *S. typhi* carrier
  - Laboratory technicians with exposure to *S. typhi*
  - Travelers with achlorhydria or hypochlorhydria (Canadian recommendation)
General Dosage Range
  I.M.: *Children ≥2 years and Adults:* 0.5 mL given at least 2 weeks prior to expected exposure; may repeat every 2 years
  Oral: *Children ≥6 years and Adults:* 1 capsule on alternate days for a total of 4 doses; may repeat full course every 5 years
Dosage Forms
  Capsule, enteric coated:
    Vivotif®: Viable *S. typhi* Ty21a 2-6.8 x 10^9 colony-forming units and nonviable *S. typhi* Ty21a 5-50 x 10^9 bacterial cells [contains lactose 100-180 mg/capsule and sucrose 26-130 mg/capsule]
  Injection, solution:
    Typhim Vi®: Purified Vi capsular polysaccharide 25 mcg/0.5 mL (0.5 mL, 10 mL) [derived from *S. typhi* Ty2 strain]
Dosage Forms - Canada
  Injection, solution:
    Typherix®: Vi capsular polysaccharide 25 mcg/0.5 mL (0.5 mL) [derived from *S. typhi* Ty2 strain]

typhoid vaccine live oral Ty21a *see* typhoid vaccine *on page* 898
Tysabri® *see* natalizumab *on page* 614
Tyvaso™ *see* treprostinil *on page* 884
Tyzeka® *see* telbivudine *on page* 847
Tyzine® *see* tetrahydrozoline (nasal) *on page* 857
Tyzine® Pediatric *see* tetrahydrozoline (nasal) *on page* 857
506U78 *see* nelarabine *on page* 616
U-90152S *see* delavirdine *on page* 257
UCB-P071 *see* cetirizine *on page* 189
U-Cort® *see* hydrocortisone (topical) *on page* 450

UK-88,525 *see* darifenacin *on page 253*
UK-427,857 *see* maraviroc *on page 549*
UK92480 *see* sildenafil *on page 811*
UK109496 *see* voriconazole *on page 921*
U-Kera E™ [DSC] *see* urea *on page 900*
Ulcerease® [OTC] *see* phenol *on page 694*
Ulcidine (Can) *see* famotidine *on page 366*
Ulesfia® *see* benzyl alcohol *on page 126*

ulipristal (ue li PRIS tal)

Medication Safety Issues
  Sound-alike/look-alike issues:
    Ulipristal may be confused with ursodiol
Synonyms ulipristal acetate
U.S. Brand Names ella®
Therapeutic Category Contraceptive; Progestin
Use Emergency contraception following unprotected intercourse or possible contraceptive failure
General Dosage Range Oral: *Adults:* 1 tablet (30 mg) as a single dose
Dosage Forms
  Tablet, oral:
    ella®: 30 mg

ulipristal acetate *see* ulipristal *on page 899*
Uloric® *see* febuxostat *on page 368*
Ultane® *see* sevoflurane *on page 810*
Ultiva® *see* remifentanil *on page 773*
Ultracaine® DS (Can) *see* articaine and epinephrine *on page 95*
Ultracaine® DS Forte (Can) *see* articaine and epinephrine *on page 95*
Ultracet® *see* acetaminophen and tramadol *on page 29*
Ultra Freeda A-Free [OTC] *see* vitamins (multiple/oral) *on page 919*
Ultra Freeda Iron-Free [OTC] *see* vitamins (multiple/oral) *on page 919*
Ultra Freeda With Iron [OTC] *see* vitamins (multiple/oral) *on page 919*
Ultram® *see* tramadol *on page 880*
Ultram® ER *see* tramadol *on page 880*
Ultra Mide 25® [OTC] *see* urea *on page 900*
UltraMide 25™ (Can) *see* urea *on page 900*
Ultramop™ (Can) *see* methoxsalen (systemic) *on page 572*
Ultraprin [OTC] *see* ibuprofen *on page 460*
Ultraquin™ (Can) *see* hydroquinone *on page 453*
Ultra-R® *see* barium *on page 114*
Ultrase® (Can) *see* pancrelipase *on page 670*
Ultrase® MT (Can) *see* pancrelipase *on page 670*
Ultra Tears® [OTC] *see* artificial tears *on page 96*
Ultravate® *see* halobetasol *on page 433*
Ultravist® *see* iopromide *on page 486*
Umecta® *see* urea *on page 900*
Umecta® Nail Film *see* urea *on page 900*
Umecta PD™ *see* urea *on page 900*
Unasyn® *see* ampicillin and sulbactam *on page 77*
Unburn® [OTC] *see* lidocaine (topical) *on page 524*

undecylenic acid and derivatives (un de sil EN ik AS id & dah RIV ah tivs)

Synonyms zinc undecylenate
U.S. Brand Names Fungi-Nail® [OTC]
Therapeutic Category Antifungal Agent

◄ **Use** Treatment of athlete's foot (tinea pedis); ringworm (except nails and scalp)

General Dosage Range Topical: *Children ≥2 years and Adults:* Apply twice daily to affected area

Dosage Forms

Solution, topical:

Fungi-Nail® [OTC]: Undecylenic acid 25% (29.57 mL)

Unidet® (Can) *see* tolterodine *on page 876*

Unipen® (Can) *see* nafcillin *on page 609*

Uniphyl (Can) *see* theophylline *on page 860*

Uniretic® *see* moexipril and hydrochlorothiazide *on page 595*

Unisom®-2 (Can) *see* doxylamine *on page 313*

Unisom® SleepGels® Maximum Strength [OTC] *see* diphenhydramine (systemic) *on page 290*

Unisom® SleepMelts™ [OTC] *see* diphenhydramine (systemic) *on page 290*

Unithroid® *see* levothyroxine *on page 522*

Univasc® *see* moexipril *on page 594*

Unna boot *see* zinc gelatin *on page 930*

Unna paste *see* zinc gelatin *on page 930*

Uramaxin® *see* urea *on page 900*

Uramaxin® GT *see* urea *on page 900*

Urasal® (Can) *see* methenamine *on page 569*

urate oxidase *see* rasburicase *on page 769*

urate oxidase, pegylated *see* pegloticase *on page 682*

urea (yoor EE a)

Synonyms carbamide

U.S. Brand Names Aqua Care® [OTC]; Aquaphilic® with Carbamide [OTC]; BP 50%; Carmol® 10 [OTC]; Carmol® 20 [OTC]; Carmol® 40; Carmol® Deep Cleansing [OTC]; DPM™ [OTC]; Gordon's® Urea [OTC]; Gormel® Ten [OTC]; Gormel® [OTC]; Hydro 35™; Hydro 40™; Kerafoam®; Kerafoam® 42; Keralac™; Keralac™ Nailstik; Keratol 40™ [DSC]; Kerol™; Kerol™ AD; Kerol™ Redi-Cloths; Kerol™ ZX; Lanaphilic® with Urea [OTC]; Nutraplus® [OTC]; Quinnostik; Rea Lo® 30 [OTC]; Rea Lo® 40; Remeven™; RevitaDERM® 40; U-Kera E™ [DSC]; Ultra Mide 25® [OTC]; Umecta PD™; Umecta®; Umecta® Nail Film; Uramaxin®; Uramaxin® GT; Ureacin-10® [OTC]; Ureacin-20® [OTC]; X-Viate™

Canadian Brand Names UltraMide 25™; Uremol®; Urisec®

Therapeutic Category Diuretic, Osmotic; Topical Skin Product

Use Keratolytic agent to soften nails or skin; OTC: Moisturizer for dry, rough skin

General Dosage Range Topical: *Adults:* Apply 1-3 times/day

Dosage Forms

Aerosol, topical:

Hydro 35™: 35% (150 g)

Hydro 40™: 40% (150 g)

Kerafoam® 42: 42% (60 g, 100 g)

Kerafoam®: 30% (60 g, 100 g)

Umecta®: 40% (113.4 g)

Uramaxin®: 20% (100 g)

Cloth, topical:

Kerol™ Redi-Cloths: 42% (30s)

Cream, topical: 40% (28 g, 30 g, 85 g, 199 g, 210 g)

Aqua Care® [OTC]: 10% (71 g)

Carmol® 20 [OTC]: 20% (90 g)

Carmol® 40: 40% (28 g, 85 g, 199 g)

DPM™ [OTC]: 20% (118 g)

Gordon's® Urea [OTC]: 40% (30 g)

Gormel® [OTC]: 20% (75 g, 120 g, 454 g, 2270 g)

Keralac™: 50% (142 g, 255 g)

Nutraplus® [OTC]: 10% (90 g, 454 g)

Rea Lo® 30 [OTC]: 30% (60 g, 240 g)

Rea Lo® 40: 40% (60 g, 240 g)

Remeven™: 50% (142 g, 255 g)

RevitaDERM® 40: 40% (112 g)

Uramaxin®: 45% (255 g)
Ureacin-20® [OTC]: 20% (113 g)
X-Viate™: 40% (29 g, 85 g, 199 g)
Emulsion, topical: 50% (300 g)
BP 50%: 50% (300 g)
Kerol™: 50% (284 g)
Kerol™ AD: 45% (240 mL)
Umecta PD™: 40% (198.5 g)
Umecta®: 40% (114 g, 227 g)
Gel, topical: 40% (15 mL); 50% (18 mL)
Carmol® 40: 40% (15 mL)
Keralac™: 50% (18 mL)
Uramaxin®: 45% (28 mL)
Uramaxin® GT: 45% (20 mL)
X-Viate™: 40% (15 mL)
Lotion, topical: 35% (207 mL, 325 mL); 40% (237 mL, 240 mL)
Aqua Care® [OTC]: 10% (240 mL)
Carmol® 10 [OTC]: 10% (180 mL)
Carmol® 40: 40% (237 mL)
Gormel® Ten [OTC]: 20% (240 mL)
Keralac™: 35% (207 mL, 325 mL)
Nutraplus® [OTC]: 10% (240 mL, 480 mL)
Ultra Mide 25® [OTC]: 25% (236 mL, 240 mL)
Uramaxin®: 45% (480 mL)
Ureacin-10® [OTC]: 10% (237 mL)
X-Viate™: 40% (237 mL)
Ointment, topical: 50% (45 g)
Aquaphilic® with Carbamide [OTC]: 10% (180 g, 454 g); 20% (454 g)
Keralac™: 50% (45 g)
Lanaphilic® with Urea [OTC]: 10% (454 g); 20% (454 g)
Shampoo, topical:
Carmol® Deep Cleansing [OTC]: 10% (240 mL)
Solution, topical: 50% (2.4 mL, 12 mL)
Keralac™ Nailstik: 50% (2.4 mL)
Kerol™ ZX: 50% (12 mL)
Quinnostik: 50% (2.4 mL)
Suspension, topical: 40% (18 mL); 50% (284 g)
Kerol™: 50% (284 g)
Umecta PD™: 40% (255.1 g)
Umecta®: 40% (283 g)
Umecta® Nail Film: 40% (3 mL, 18 mL)

urea and hydrocortisone (yoor EE a & hye droe KOR ti sone)

Synonyms hydrocortisone and urea
U.S. Brand Names Carmol-HC®
Canadian Brand Names Ti-U-Lac® H; Uremol® HC
Therapeutic Category Corticosteroid, Topical
Use Inflammation of corticosteroid-responsive dermatoses
General Dosage Range Topical: *Children and Adults:* Apply thin film and rub in well 2-4 times/day
Dosage Forms
  Cream:
    Carmol-HC®: Urea 10% and hydrocortisone 1% (30 g)

Ureacin-10® [OTC] see urea on page 900
Ureacin-20® [OTC] see urea on page 900
urea peroxide see carbamide peroxide on page 172
Urecholine® see bethanechol on page 131
Uremol® (Can) see urea on page 900
Uremol® HC (Can) see urea and hydrocortisone on page 901
Urex see methenamine on page 569

Urisec® (Can) *see* urea *on page 900*
Urispas® (Can) *see* flavoxate *on page 379*
Urocit®-K *see* potassium citrate *on page 725*

urofollitropin (yoor oh fol li TROE pin)

Synonyms follicle-stimulating hormone, human; FSH; hFSH
U.S. Brand Names Bravelle®
Canadian Brand Names Bravelle®; Fertinorm® H.P.
Therapeutic Category Gonadotropin; Ovulation Stimulator
Use Ovulation induction in patients who previously received pituitary suppression; development of multiple follicles with Assisted Reproductive Technologies (ART)
General Dosage Range
I.M.: *Adults (females):* Initial: 150 int. units once daily for 5 days; Maintenance: Up to 450 int. units/day (maximum: 12 days therapy)
SubQ: *Adults (females):* Initial: 150-225 int. units once daily for 5 days; Maintenance: Up to 450 int. units/day (maximum: 12 days therapy)
Dosage Forms
Injection, powder for reconstitution:
Bravelle®: 75 int. units

Uro-Mag® [OTC] *see* magnesium oxide *on page 546*
Uromax® (Can) *see* oxybutynin *on page 661*
Uroxatral® *see* alfuzosin *on page 50*
Urso® (Can) *see* ursodiol *on page 902*
Urso 250® *see* ursodiol *on page 902*
ursodeoxycholic acid *see* ursodiol *on page 902*

ursodiol (ur soe DYE ol)

Medication Safety Issues
Sound-alike/look-alike issues:
Ursodiol may be confused with ulipristal
Synonyms ursodeoxycholic acid
U.S. Brand Names Actigall®; Urso 250®; Urso Forte®
Canadian Brand Names Dom-Ursodiol C; PHL-Ursodiol C; PMS-Ursodiol C; Urso®; Urso® DS
Therapeutic Category Gallstone Dissolution Agent
Use
Actigall®: Gallbladder stone dissolution; prevention of gallstones in obese patients experiencing rapid weight loss
Urso®, Urso Forte®: Primary biliary cirrhosis
General Dosage Range Oral: *Adults:* 8-15 mg/kg/day in 2-4 divided doses **or** 300 mg twice daily
Dosage Forms
Capsule, oral: 300 mg
Actigall®: 300 mg
Tablet, oral: 250 mg, 500 mg
Urso 250®: 250 mg
Urso Forte®: 500 mg

Urso® DS (Can) *see* ursodiol *on page 902*
Urso Forte® *see* ursodiol *on page 902*

ustekinumab (yoo stek in YOO mab)

Medication Safety Issues
Sound-alike/look-alike issues:
Stelara™ may be confused with Aldara®
Ustekinumab may be confused with infliximab, rituximab
Synonyms CNTO 1275
U.S. Brand Names Stelara™
Canadian Brand Names Stelara™

Therapeutic Category Antipsoriatic Agent; Interleukin-12 Inhibitor; Interleukin-23 Inhibitor; Monoclonal Antibody
Use Treatment of moderate-to-severe plaque psoriasis
General Dosage Range Oral: *Adults:* ≤100 kg: 45 mg at 0- and 4 weeks, and then every 12 weeks; >100 kg: 45 mg or 90 mg at 0- and 4 weeks, and then every 12 weeks
Dosage Forms
  Injection, solution [preservative free]:
    Stelara™: 45 mg/0.5 mL (0.5 mL); 90 mg/mL (1 mL)

UTI Relief® [OTC] *see* phenazopyridine *on page* 692
Utradol™ (Can) *see* etodolac *on page* 360
Uvadex® *see* methoxsalen (systemic) *on page* 572

vaccinia immune globulin (intravenous)
(vax IN ee a i MYUN GLOB yoo lin IN tra VEE nus)
Synonyms VIGIV
U.S. Brand Names CNJ-016®
Therapeutic Category Immune Globulin
Use Treatment of infectious complications of smallpox (vaccinia virus) vaccination, such as eczema vaccinatum, progressive vaccinia, and severe generalized vaccinia; treatment of vaccinia infections in individuals with concurrent skin conditions or accidental virus exposure to eyes (except vaccinia keratitis), mouth, or other areas where viral infection would pose significant risk

CDC guidelines for use:
  Use is recommended for:
    - Inadvertent inoculation (considering severity, toxicity of affected person, and pain)
    - Eczema vaccinatum
    - Generalized vaccinia (severe form or if underlying illness is present)
    - Progressive vaccinia
  Use may be considered for:
    - Severe ocular complications except isolated keratitis
  Use is not recommended for:
    - Inadvertent inoculation that is not severe
    - Mild or limited generalized vaccinia
    - Nonspecific rashes, erythema multiforme, or Stevens-Johnson syndrome
    - Postvaccinial encephalitis or encephalomyelitis
General Dosage Range I.V.: *Adults:* Initial: 6000 units/kg; may repeat 6000-9000 units/kg if needed (maximum: 24,000 units/kg)
Dosage Forms Injection, solution [preservative free; solvent-detergent treated]:
  CNJ-016®: ≥50,000 units/15 mL (15 mL)

vaccinia vaccine *see* smallpox vaccine *on page* 817
Vagifem® *see* estradiol (topical) *on page* 344
Vagifem® 10 (Can) *see* estradiol (topical) *on page* 344
Vagi-Gard® [OTC] *see* povidone-iodine (topical) *on page* 727
Vagistat®-1 [OTC] *see* tioconazole *on page* 870

valacyclovir (val ay SYE kloe veer)
Medication Safety Issues
  Sound-alike/look-alike issues:
    Valtrex® may be confused with Keflex®, Valcyte®, Zovirax®
    ValACYclovir may be confused with acyclovir, valGANciclovir, vancomycin
Synonyms valacyclovir hydrochloride
Tall-Man valACYclovir
U.S. Brand Names Valtrex®
Canadian Brand Names Apo-Valacyclovir®; Mylan-Valacyclovir; PHL-Valacyclovir; PMS-Valacyclovir; PRO-Valacyclovir; Riva-Valacyclovir; Valtrex®
Therapeutic Category Antiviral Agent

◄ **Use** Treatment of herpes zoster (shingles) in immunocompetent patients; treatment of first-episode and recurrent genital herpes; suppression of recurrent genital herpes and reduction of heterosexual transmission of genital herpes in immunocompetent patients; suppression of genital herpes in HIV-infected individuals; treatment of herpes labialis (cold sores); chickenpox in immunocompetent children

General Dosage Range Dosage adjustment recommended in patients with renal impairment

Oral:

Children 2 to <12 years: 20 mg/kg/dose 3 times/day (maximum: 1 g 3 times/day)

Children ≥12 to <18 years: 2 g every 12 hours for 1 day **or** 20 mg/kg/dose 3 times/day (maximum: 1 g 3 times/day)

Adults: 500 mg to 1 g 1-3 times/day **or** 2 g every 12 hours for 1 day

Dosage Forms

Caplet, oral: 500 mg, 1 g

Valtrex®: 500 mg, 1 g

Tablet, oral: 500 mg, 1 g

valacyclovir hydrochloride *see valacyclovir on page 903*

Valcyte® *see valganciclovir on page 904*

23-valent pneumococcal polysaccharide vaccine *see pneumococcal polysaccharide vaccine (polyvalent) on page 715*

valganciclovir (val gan SYE kloh veer)

Medication Safety Issues

Sound-alike/look-alike issues:

Valcyte® may be confused with Valium®, Valtrex®

ValGANciclovir may be confused with valACYclovir

Synonyms valganciclovir hydrochloride

Tall-Man valGANciclovir

U.S. Brand Names Valcyte®

Canadian Brand Names Valcyte®

Therapeutic Category Antiviral Agent

Use Treatment of cytomegalovirus (CMV) retinitis in patients with acquired immunodeficiency syndrome (AIDS); prevention of CMV disease in high-risk patients (donor CMV positive/recipient CMV negative) undergoing kidney, heart, or kidney/pancreas transplantation

General Dosage Range Dosage adjustment recommended in patients with renal impairment

Oral:

Children 4 months to 16 years: Dose (mg) = 7 x body surface area x creatinine clearance once daily

Children >16 years and Adults: 900 mg 1-2 times/day

Dosage Forms

Powder for solution, oral:

Valcyte®: 50 mg/mL (100 mL)

Tablet, oral:

Valcyte®: 450 mg

valganciclovir hydrochloride *see valganciclovir on page 904*

Valisone® Scalp Lotion (Can) *see betamethasone on page 129*

Valium® *see diazepam on page 276*

Valorin [OTC] *see acetaminophen on page 23*

Valorin Extra [OTC] *see acetaminophen on page 23*

valproate semisodium *see divalproex on page 300*

valproate semisodium *see valproic acid on page 904*

valproate sodium *see valproic acid on page 904*

valproic acid (val PROE ik AS id)

Medication Safety Issues

Sound-alike/look-alike issues:

Depakene® may be confused with Depakote®

Valproate sodium may be confused with vecuronium

Synonyms 2-propylpentanoic acid; 2-propylvaleric acid; dipropylacetic acid; DPA; valproate semisodium; valproate sodium

U.S. Brand Names Depacon®; Depakene®; Stavzor™

Canadian Brand Names Apo-Valproic®; Depakene®; Epival® I.V.; Mylan-Valproic; PHL-Valproic Acid; PHL-Valproic Acid E.C.; PMS-Valproic Acid; PMS-Valproic Acid E.C.; ratio-Valproic; ratio-Valproic ECC; Rhoxal-valproic; Sandoz-Valproic

Therapeutic Category Anticonvulsant, Miscellaneous; Antimanic Agent; Histone Deacetylase Inhibitor

Use Monotherapy and adjunctive therapy in the treatment of patients with complex partial seizures; monotherapy and adjunctive therapy of simple and complex absence seizures; adjunctive therapy in patients with multiple seizure types that include absence seizures

Stavzor™: Mania associated with bipolar disorder; migraine prophylaxis

General Dosage Range Dosage adjustment recommended in patients with hepatic impairment

I.V.:
Children: Initial: 15 mg/kg/day; Maximum: 60 mg/kg/day
Children ≥10 years and Adults: Initial: 10-15 mg/kg/day; Maximum: 60 mg/kg/day

Oral:
Children: Initial: 15 mg/kg/day; Maximum: 60 mg/kg/day
Children ≥10 years and Adults: Seizures: Initial: 10-15 mg/kg/day; Maximum: 60 mg/kg/day
Children ≥12 years and Adults: Stavzor™: Initial: 250 mg twice daily; Maintenance: Up to 1000 mg/day
Adults: Mania (Stavzor™): Initial: 750 mg/day in divided doses; Maximum recommended dose: 60 mg/kg/day

Dosage Forms
Capsule, softgel, oral: 250 mg
Depakene®: 250 mg
Capsule, softgel, delayed release, oral:
Stavzor™: 125 mg, 250 mg, 500 mg
Injection, solution [preservative free]: 100 mg/mL (5 mL)
Depacon®: 100 mg/mL (5 mL)
Solution, oral: 250 mg/5 mL (473 mL, 480 mL)
Syrup, oral: 250 mg/5 mL (5 mL, 10 mL, 473 mL, 480 mL)
Depakene®: 250 mg/5 mL (473 mL)

valproic acid derivative *see* divalproex *on page 300*

valrubicin (val ROO bi sin)

Medication Safety Issues
Sound-alike/look-alike issues:
Valrubicin may be confused with DAUNOrubicin, DOXOrubicin, epirubicin, IDArubicin
Valstar® may be confused with valsartan
High alert medication:
The Institute for Safe Medication Practices (ISMP) includes this medication among its list of drug classes which have a heightened risk of causing significant patient harm when used in error.

Synonyms *N*-trifluoroacetyladriamycin-14-valerate; AD32

U.S. Brand Names Valstar®

Canadian Brand Names Valtaxin®

Therapeutic Category Antineoplastic Agent, Anthracycline

Use Intravesical therapy of BCG-refractory bladder carcinoma *in situ*

General Dosage Range Dosage adjustment recommended in patients who develop toxicities
Intravesical: *Adults:* 800 mg once weekly for 6 weeks

Dosage Forms
Injection, solution [preservative free]:
Valstar®: 40 mg/mL (5 mL)

valsartan (val SAR tan)

Medication Safety Issues
Sound-alike/look-alike issues:
Valsartan may be confused with losartan, Valstar™, Valturna®
Diovan® may be confused with Darvon®, Dioval®, Zyban®
International issues:
Diovan [U.S., Canada, and multiple international markets] may be confused with Dianben, a brand name for metformin [Spain]

U.S. Brand Names Diovan®

▶

◀ **Canadian Brand Names** CO Valsartan; Diovan®; Ran-Valsartan; Sandoz-Valsartan; Teva-Valsartan

Therapeutic Category Angiotensin II Receptor Antagonist

Use Alone or in combination with other antihypertensive agents in the treatment of essential hypertension; reduction of cardiovascular mortality in patients with left ventricular dysfunction postmyocardial infarction; treatment of heart failure (NYHA Class II-IV)

General Dosage Range Oral:

Children 6-16 years: Initial: 1.3 mg/kg once daily (maximum: 40 mg/day); Maintenance: Up to ≤2.7 mg/kg; 160 mg

Adults: Initial: 20-40 mg twice daily **or** 80-160 mg once daily; Maintenance: 80-160 mg twice daily (maximum: 320 mg/day)

Dosage Forms

Tablet, oral:

Diovan®: 40 mg, 80 mg, 160 mg, 320 mg

valsartan and aliskiren *see* aliskiren and valsartan *on page 53*

valsartan and amlodipine *see* amlodipine and valsartan *on page 71*

valsartan and hydrochlorothiazide (val SAR tan & hye droe klor oh THYE a zide)

Medication Safety Issues

Sound-alike/look-alike issues:

Diovan® may be confused with Darvon®, Dioval®, Zyban®

Synonyms hydrochlorothiazide and valsartan

U.S. Brand Names Diovan HCT®

Canadian Brand Names Diovan HCT®; Sandoz Valsartan HCT; Teva-Valsartan HCTZ; Valsartan-HCTZ

Therapeutic Category Antihypertensive Agent, Combination

Use Treatment of hypertension

General Dosage Range Oral: *Adults:* Valsartan 80-160 mg and hydrochlorothiazide 12.5-25 mg once daily (maximum: 25 mg/day [hydrochlorothiazide]; 320 mg/day [valsartan])

Dosage Forms

Tablet:

Diovan HCT®: 80 mg/12.5 mg: Valsartan 80 mg and hydrochlorothiazide 12.5 mg; 160 mg/12.5 mg: Valsartan 160 mg and hydrochlorothiazide 12.5 mg; 160 mg/25 mg: Valsartan 160 mg and hydrochlorothiazide 25 mg; 320 mg/12.5 mg: Valsartan 320 mg and hydrochlorothiazide 12.5 mg; 320 mg/25 mg: Valsartan 320 mg and hydrochlorothiazide 25 mg

Valsartan-HCTZ (Can) *see* valsartan and hydrochlorothiazide *on page 906*

valsartan, hydrochlorothiazide, and amlodipine *see* amlodipine, valsartan, and hydrochlorothiazide *on page 71*

Valstar® *see* valrubicin *on page 905*

Valtaxin® (Can) *see* valrubicin *on page 905*

Valtrex® *see* valacyclovir *on page 903*

Valturna® *see* aliskiren and valsartan *on page 53*

Val-Vanco (Can) *see* vancomycin *on page 906*

Vancenase *see* beclomethasone (oral inhalation) *on page 117*

Vanceril® AEM (Can) *see* beclomethasone (oral inhalation) *on page 117*

Vancocin® *see* vancomycin *on page 906*

vancomycin (van koe MYE sin)

Medication Safety Issues

Sound-alike/look-alike issues:

I.V. vancomycin may be confused with Invanz®

Vancomycin may be confused with clindamycin, gentamicin, tobramycin, valACYclovir, vecuronium, Vibramycin®

High alert medication:

The Institute for Safe Medication Practices (ISMP) includes this medication (intrathecal administration) among its list of drug classes which have a heightened risk of causing significant patient harm when used in error.

Synonyms vancomycin hydrochloride

U.S. Brand Names Vancocin®

Canadian Brand Names PMS-Vancomycin; Sterile Vancomycin Hydrochloride, USP; Val-Vanco; Vancocin®; Vancomycin Hydrochloride for Injection, USP

Therapeutic Category Antibiotic, Miscellaneous

Use Treatment of patients with infections caused by staphylococcal species and streptococcal species; used orally for staphylococcal enterocolitis or for antibiotic-associated pseudomembranous colitis produced by *C. difficile*

General Dosage Range Dosage adjustment recommended in patients with renal impairment

I.V.:
  Infants >1 month: 40-60 mg/kg/day in divided doses every 6 hours
  Children: 40-60 mg/kg/day in divided doses every 6 hours **or** 20 mg/kg as a single dose
  Adults: 30-60 mg/kg/day in divided doses every 6-12 hours **or** 500-750 mg every 6 hours **or** 1 g as a single dose

Intracatheter, intraventricular: *Children and Adults:* 2-5 mg/mL instilled into catheter port with a volume sufficient to fill the catheter (2-5 mL)

Intrathecal: *Children and Adults:* 5-20 mg/day

Oral:
  Children: 40 mg/kg/day in 3-4 divided doses (maximum: 2000 mg/day)
  Adults: 500-2000 mg/day in 3-4 divided doses (maximum: 2000 mg/day)

Dosage Forms
  Capsule, oral: Vancocin®: 125 mg, 250 mg
  Infusion, premixed iso-osmotic dextrose solution: 500 mg (100 mL); 750 mg (150 mL); 1 g (200 mL)
  Injection, powder for reconstitution: 500 mg, 750 mg, 1 g, 5 g, 10 g

vancomycin hydrochloride *see* vancomycin *on page 906*

Vancomycin Hydrochloride for Injection, USP (Can) *see* vancomycin *on page 906*

Vandazole® *see* metronidazole (topical) *on page 583*

vandetanib (van DET a nib)

Medication Safety Issues
  Sound-alike/look-alike issues:
    Vandetanib may be confused with dasatinib, erlotinib, gefitinib, imatinib, lapatinib, nilotinib, pazopanib, SORAfenib, SUNItinib, vemurafenib
  High alert medication:
    This medication is in a class the Institute for Safe Medication Practices (ISMP) includes among its list of drug classes which have a heightened risk of causing significant patient harm when used in error.

Synonyms AZD6474; Zactima; ZD6474; Zictifa

U.S. Brand Names Caprelsa®

Therapeutic Category Antineoplastic Agent, Tyrosine Kinase Inhibitor; Epidermal Growth Factor Receptor (EGFR) Inhibitor; Vascular Endothelial Growth Factor (VEGF) Inhibitor

Use Treatment of metastatic or unresectable locally advanced medullary thyroid cancer (symptomatic or progressive)

General Dosage Range Note: Do not initiate treatment unless QTcF <450 msec. Avoid concomitant use of QT-prolonging agents and strong CYP3A4 inducers. To reduce the risk of QT prolongation, maintain serum calcium and magnesium within normal limits and maintain serum potassium ≥4 mEq/L.

Medullary thyroid cancer, locally advanced or metastatic: Oral: 300 mg once daily, continue treatment until no longer clinically benefiting or until unacceptable toxicity

Dosage Forms
  Tablet, oral: 100 mg, 300 mg
  Caprelsa®: 100 mg, 300 mg

Vaniqa® *see* eflornithine *on page 322*

Vanos® *see* fluocinonide *on page 385*

Vanoxide-HC® *see* benzoyl peroxide and hydrocortisone *on page 125*

Vanquish® Extra Strength Pain Reliever [OTC] *see* acetaminophen, aspirin, and caffeine *on page 29*

Vantin *see* cefpodoxime *on page 183*

Vaprisol® *see* conivaptan *on page 234*

VAQTA® *see* hepatitis A vaccine *on page 437*

VAR *see* varicella virus vaccine *on page 908*

vardenafil (var DEN a fil)

Medication Safety Issues
Sound-alike/look-alike issues:
Vardenafil may be confused with sildenafil, tadalafil
Levitra® may be confused with Kaletra®, Lexiva®
Synonyms Staxyn™; vardenafil hydrochloride
U.S. Brand Names Levitra®; Staxyn™
Canadian Brand Names Levitra®
Therapeutic Category Phosphodiesterase (Type 5) Enzyme Inhibitor
Use Treatment of erectile dysfunction (ED)
General Dosage Range Dosage adjustment recommended in patients with hepatic impairment or on concomitant therapy
Oral:
Adults: Film-coated tablet (Levitra®): 2.5-20 mg as a single dose (maximum: 1 dose/day); Oral disintegrating tablet (Staxyn™): 10 mg as a single dose (maximum: 10 mg/day)
Elderly ≥65 years: 2.5-5 mg as a single dose (maximum: 1 dose/day)
Dosage Forms
Tablet, oral:
Levitra®: 2.5 mg, 5 mg, 10 mg, 20 mg
Tablet, orally disintegrating, oral:
Staxyn™: 10 mg

vardenafil hydrochloride see vardenafil on page 908

varenicline (var e NI kleen)

Synonyms varenicline tartrate
U.S. Brand Names Chantix®
Canadian Brand Names Champix®
Therapeutic Category Partial Nicotine Agonist
Use Treatment to aid in smoking cessation
General Dosage Range Dosage adjustment recommended in patients with renal impairment or who develop toxicities
Oral: *Adults:* Days 1-3: 0.5 mg once daily; Days 4-7: 0.5 mg twice daily; Maintenance (≥Day 8): 1 mg twice daily
Dosage Forms
Combination package, oral:
Chantix®: Tablet: 0.5 mg (11s) [white tablets] and Tablet: 1 mg (42s) [light blue tablets]
Tablet, oral:
Chantix®: 0.5 mg, 1 mg

varenicline tartrate see varenicline on page 908
Varibar® Honey see barium on page 114
Varibar® Nectar see barium on page 114
Varibar® Pudding see barium on page 114
Varibar® Thin Honey see barium on page 114
Varibar® Thin Liquid see barium on page 114
varicella, measles, mumps, and rubella vaccine see measles, mumps, rubella, and varicella virus vaccine on page 551

varicella virus vaccine (var i SEL a VYE rus vak SEEN)

Medication Safety Issues
Sound-alike/look-alike issues:
Varicella virus vaccine has been given in error (instead of the indicated varicella immune globulin) to pregnant women exposed to varicella.
Other safety concerns:
Both varicella vaccine and zoster vaccine are live, attenuated strains of varicella-zoster virus. Their indications, dosing, and composition are distinct. Varicella is indicated in children to prevent chickenpox, while zoster vaccine is indicated in older individuals to prevent reactivation of the virus

which causes shingles. Zoster vaccine is **not** a substitute for varicella vaccine and should not be used in children.

Synonyms chickenpox vaccine; VAR; varicella-zoster virus (VZV) vaccine (varicella); VZV vaccine (varicella)

U.S. Brand Names Varivax®

Canadian Brand Names Varilrix®; Varivax® III

Therapeutic Category Vaccine, Live Virus

Use Immunization against varicella in children ≥12 months of age and adults

The ACIP recommends vaccination for all children, adolescents, and adults who do not have evidence of immunity. Vaccination is especially important for:
- Persons with close contact to those at high risk for severe disease
- Persons living or working in environments where transmission is likely (teachers, child-care workers, residents and staff of institutional settings)
- Persons in environments where transmission has been reported
- Nonpregnant women of childbearing age
- Adolescents and adults in households with children
- International travelers

Postexposure prophylaxis: Vaccination within 3 days (possibly 5 days) after exposure to rash is effective in preventing illness or modifying severity of disease

General Dosage Range SubQ:
Children 12 months to 12 years: 0.5 mL as a single dose; may repeat in ≥3 months
Children ≥13 years and Adults: 2 doses of 0.5 mL separated by 4-8 weeks

Dosage Forms
Injection, powder for reconstitution [preservative free]:
Varivax®: 1350 PFU

Dosage Forms - Canada
Injection, powder for reconstitution [preservative free]:
Varivax® III: 1350 plaque-forming units (PFU)
Injection, powder for reconstitution:
Valrilix®: $10^{3.3}$ plaque-forming units (PFU)

varicella-zoster immune globulin (human)
(var i SEL a- ZOS ter i MYUN GLOB yoo lin HYU man)

Medication Safety Issues
Sound-alike/look-alike issues:
Varicella virus vaccine has been given in error (instead of the indicated varicella immune globulin) to pregnant women exposed to varicella.

Synonyms VZIG

Canadian Brand Names VariZIG™

Therapeutic Category Immune Globulin

Use In pregnant women, for the prevention or reduction in severity of maternal infection within 4 days of exposure to the varicella zoster virus.

General Dosage Range I.M., I.V.: *Adults:* 125 int. units/10 kg (minimum dose: 125 int. units; maximum dose: 625 int. units)

Dosage Forms - Canada
Injection, powder for reconstitution [preservative free]:
VariZIG™: 125 int. units [package with diluent] [

varicella-zoster virus (VZV) vaccine (varicella) *see* varicella virus vaccine *on page* 908

varicella-zoster (VZV) vaccine (zoster) *see* zoster vaccine *on page* 935

Varilrix® (Can) *see* varicella virus vaccine *on page* 908

Varivax® *see* varicella virus vaccine *on page* 908

Varivax® III (Can) *see* varicella virus vaccine *on page* 908

VariZIG™ (Can) *see* varicella-zoster immune globulin (human) *on page* 909

Vaseretic® *see* enalapril and hydrochlorothiazide *on page* 327

Vasocon® (Can) *see* naphazoline (ophthalmic) *on page* 611

Vasodilan *see* isoxsuprine *on page* 496

Vasolex™ *see* trypsin, balsam Peru, and castor oil *on page* 896

vasopressin (vay soe PRES in)

Medication Safety Issues

Administration issues:

Use care when prescribing and/or administering vasopressin solutions. Close attention should be given to concentration of solution, route of administration, dose, and rate of administration (units/minute, units/kg/minute, units/kg/hour).

Synonyms 8-arginine vasopressin; ADH; antidiuretic hormone; AVP

U.S. Brand Names Pitressin®

Canadian Brand Names Pressyn®; Pressyn® AR

Therapeutic Category Hormone, Posterior Pituitary

Use Treatment of central diabetes insipidus; differential diagnosis of diabetes insipidus

General Dosage Range I.M., SubQ:
Children: 2.5-10 units 2-4 times/day as needed
Adults: 5-10 units 2-4 times/day as needed

Dosage Forms

Injection, solution: 20 units/mL (0.5 mL, 1 mL, 10 mL)
Pitressin®: 20 units/mL (1 mL)

Vasotec® *see* enalapril *on page 326*
Vasotec® I.V. (Can) *see* enalapril *on page 326*
Vaxigrip® (Can) *see* influenza virus vaccine (inactivated) *on page 473*
VCF® [OTC] *see* nonoxynol 9 *on page 632*
Vectibix® *see* panitumumab *on page 672*
Vectical™ *see* calcitriol *on page 159*

vecuronium (vek ue ROE nee um)

Medication Safety Issues

Sound-alike/look-alike issues:

Vecuronium may be confused with valproate sodium, vancomycin

Norcuron® may be confused with Narcan®

High alert medication:

The Institute for Safe Medication Practices (ISMP) includes this medication among its list of drugs which have a heightened risk of causing significant patient harm when used in error.

Other safety concerns:

United States Pharmacopeia (USP) 2006: The Interdisciplinary Safe Medication Use Expert Committee of the USP has recommended the following:

- Hospitals, clinics, and other practice sites should institute special safeguards in the storage, labeling, and use of these agents and should include these safeguards in staff orientation and competency training.

- Healthcare professionals should be on high alert (especially vigilant) whenever a neuromuscular-blocking agent (NMBA) is stocked, ordered, prepared, or administered.

Synonyms ORG NC 45

Canadian Brand Names Norcuron®

Therapeutic Category Skeletal Muscle Relaxant

Use To facilitate endotracheal intubation and to relax skeletal muscles during surgery; to facilitate mechanical ventilation in ICU patients; does not relieve pain or produce sedation

General Dosage Range Dosage adjustment recommended in patients with hepatic impairment
I.V.: *Children ≥1 year and Adults:* Initial: 0.04-0.1 mg/kg; Maintenance: 0.01-0.015 mg/kg every 12-15 minutes **or** 0.8-1.2 mcg/kg/minute as a continuous infusion

Dosage Forms

Injection, powder for reconstitution: 10 mg, 20 mg

velaglucerase alfa (vel a GLOO ser ase AL fa)

Synonyms gene-activated human acid-beta-glucosidase; glcCerase

U.S. Brand Names VPRIV™

Canadian Brand Names VPRIV™

Therapeutic Category Enzyme

Use Long-term enzyme replacement therapy for patients with type 1 Gaucher disease

General Dosage Range I.V.: *Children ≥4 years and Adults:* 15-60 units/kg every other week
Dosage Forms
  Injection, powder for reconstitution:
    VPRIV™: 400 units

Velcade® *see bortezomib on page 139*
Veletri® *see epoprostenol on page 334*
Velivet™ *see ethinyl estradiol and desogestrel on page 351*
Veltin™ *see clindamycin and tretinoin on page 219*

vemurafenib (vem ue RAF e nib)

Medication Safety Issues
  Sound-alike/look-alike issues:
    Vemurafenib may be confused with sorafenib, vandetanib
  High alert medication:
    This medication is in a class the Institute for Safe Medication Practices (ISMP) includes among its list of drug classes which have a heightened risk of causing significant patient harm when used in error.
Synonyms BRAF(V600E) kinase inhibitor RO5185426; PLX4032; RG7024; RO5185426
U.S. Brand Names Zelboraf™
Therapeutic Category Antineoplastic Agent, BRAF Kinase Inhibitor
Use Treatment of unresectable or metastatic melanoma in patients with a BRAF^{V600E} mutation (as detected by an FDA-approved test)

Note: Not recommended in patients with wild-type BRAF melanoma
General Dosage Range Dosage adjustment recommended in patients who develop toxicities.
  Oral: *Adults:* 960 mg twice daily
Dosage Forms
  Tablet, oral:
    Zelboraf™: 240 mg

venlafaxine (ven la FAX een)

Medication Safety Issues
  Sound-alike/look-alike issues:
    Effexor® may be confused with Effexor XR®
U.S. Brand Names Effexor XR®; Effexor®
Canadian Brand Names CO Venlafaxine XR; Effexor XR®; Mylan-Venlafaxine XR; PMS-Venlafaxine XR; ratio-Venlafaxine XR; Riva-Venlafaxine XR; Sandoz-Venlafaxine XR; Teva-Venlafaxine XR; Venlafaxine XR
Therapeutic Category Antidepressant, Phenethylamine
Use Treatment of major depressive disorder, generalized anxiety disorder (GAD), social anxiety disorder (social phobia), panic disorder
General Dosage Range Dosage adjustment recommended in patients with hepatic or renal impairment
  Oral:
    Extended release: *Adults:* Initial: 37.5-75 mg/day once daily; Maintenance: 75-225 mg/day once daily (recommended maximum: 225 mg/day)
    Immediate release: *Adults:* Initial: 75 mg/day in 2-3 divided doses; Maintenance: 75-375 mg/day in 2-3 divided doses (recommended maximum: 375 mg/day)
Dosage Forms
  Capsule, extended release, oral: 37.5 mg, 75 mg, 150 mg
    Effexor XR®: 37.5 mg, 75 mg, 150 mg
  Tablet, oral: 25 mg, 37.5 mg, 50 mg, 75 mg, 100 mg
    Effexor®: 50 mg
  Tablet, extended release, oral: 37.5 mg, 75 mg, 150 mg, 225 mg

Venlafaxine XR (Can) *see venlafaxine on page 911*
Venofer® *see iron sucrose on page 492*
Ventavis® *see iloprost on page 465*
Ventolin® (Can) *see albuterol on page 45*
Ventolin® Diskus (Can) *see albuterol on page 45*
Ventolin® HFA *see albuterol on page 45*

Ventolin® I.V. Infusion (Can) *see* albuterol *on page 45*
Ventolin® Nebules P.F. (Can) *see* albuterol *on page 45*
VePesid *see* etoposide *on page 361*
Veracolate® [OTC] *see* bisacodyl *on page 134*
Veramyst® *see* fluticasone (nasal) *on page 393*

verapamil (ver AP a mil)

Medication Safety Issues
Sound-alike/look-alike issues:
Calan® may be confused with Colace®, diltiazem
Covera-HS® may be confused with Provera®
Isoptin® may be confused with Isopto® Tears
Verelan® may be confused with Virilon®, Voltaren®
High alert medication:
The Institute for Safe Medication Practices (ISMP) includes this medication (I.V. formulation) among its list of drug classes which have a heightened risk of causing significant patient harm when used in error.
Administration issues:
Significant differences exist between oral and I.V. dosing. Use caution when converting from one route of administration to another.
International issues:
Dilacor [Brazil] may be confused with Dilacor XR brand name for diltiazem [U.S.]

Synonyms iproveratril hydrochloride; verapamil hydrochloride

U.S. Brand Names Calan®; Calan® SR; Covera-HS®; Isoptin® SR; Verelan®; Verelan® PM

Canadian Brand Names Apo-Verap®; Apo-Verap® SR; Covera-HS®; Covera®; Dom-Verapamil SR; Isoptin® SR; Mylan-Verapamil; Mylan-Verapamil SR; Novo-Veramil; Novo-Veramil SR; Nu-Verap; Nu-Verap SR; PHL-Verapamil SR; PMS-Verapamil SR; PRO-Verapamil SR; Riva-Verapamil SR; Verapamil Hydrochloride Injection, USP; Verapamil SR; Verelan SRC

Therapeutic Category Antiarrhythmic Agent, Class IV; Calcium Channel Blocker

Use
Oral: Treatment of hypertension; angina pectoris (vasospastic, chronic stable, unstable) (Calan®, Covera-HS®); supraventricular tachyarrhythmia (PSVT, atrial fibrillation/flutter [rate control])
I.V.: Supraventricular tachyarrhythmia (PSVT, atrial fibrillation/flutter [rate control])

General Dosage Range
I.V.:
Children 1-15 years: 0.1-0.3 mg/kg/dose (maximum: 5 mg/dose); may repeat dose (maximum for second dose: 10 mg)
Adults: Initial dose: 2.5-5 mg; Second dose: 5-10 mg (maximum: 20-30 mg total dose)
Oral:
Extended release:
Adults: 180-480 mg once daily
Elderly: Initial: 100-180 mg once daily
Immediate release: *Adults:* Initial: 80-120 mg 3 times/day; Maintenance: 80-480 mg/day in 2-4 divided doses (maximum: 480 mg/day)
Sustained release:
Adults: 120-480 mg/day in 1-2 divided doses (maximum: 480 mg/day)
Elderly: Initial: 120 mg/day once daily; Maintenance: 120-360 mg/day in 1-2 divided doses

Dosage Forms
Caplet, sustained release, oral:
Calan® SR: 120 mg, 180 mg, 240 mg
Capsule, extended release, oral: 120 mg, 180 mg, 240 mg
Capsule, extended release, controlled onset, oral: 100 mg, 200 mg, 300 mg
Verelan® PM: 100 mg, 200 mg, 300 mg
Capsule, sustained release, oral: 120 mg, 180 mg, 240 mg, 360 mg
Verelan®: 120 mg, 180 mg, 240 mg, 360 mg
Injection, solution: 2.5 mg/mL (2 mL, 4 mL)
Tablet, oral: 40 mg, 80 mg, 120 mg
Calan®: 80 mg, 120 mg
Tablet, extended release, oral: 120 mg, 180 mg, 240 mg
Tablet, extended release, controlled onset, oral:
Covera-HS®: 180 mg, 240 mg

Tablet, sustained release, oral: 240 mg
  Isoptin® SR: 120 mg, 180 mg, 240 mg

verapamil and trandolapril *see* trandolapril and verapamil *on page 881*
verapamil hydrochloride *see* verapamil *on page 912*
Verapamil Hydrochloride Injection, USP (Can) *see* verapamil *on page 912*
Verapamil SR (Can) *see* verapamil *on page 912*
Verdeso® *see* desonide *on page 263*
Veregen™ *see* sinecatechins *on page 814*
Verelan® *see* verapamil *on page 912*
Verelan® PM *see* verapamil *on page 912*
Verelan SRC (Can) *see* verapamil *on page 912*
Veripred™ 20 *see* prednisolone (systemic) *on page 734*
Vermox *see* mebendazole *on page 552*
Vermox® (Can) *see* mebendazole *on page 552*
Versed *see* midazolam *on page 587*
Versel® (Can) *see* selenium sulfide *on page 807*
Versiclear™ *see* sodium thiosulfate *on page 824*

verteporfin (ver te POR fin)
U.S. Brand Names Visudyne®
Canadian Brand Names Visudyne®
Therapeutic Category Ophthalmic Agent
Use Treatment of predominantly classic subfoveal choroidal neovascularization due to macular degeneration, presumed ocular histoplasmosis, or pathologic myopia
General Dosage Range I.V.: *Adults:* 6 mg/m² body surface area
Dosage Forms
  Injection, powder for reconstitution:
    Visudyne®: 15 mg

Vesanoid *see* tretinoin (systemic) *on page 885*
Vesanoid® (Can) *see* tretinoin (systemic) *on page 885*
VESIcare® *see* solifenacin *on page 825*
Vexol® *see* rimexolone *on page 782*
VFEND® *see* voriconazole *on page 921*
Viactiv® [OTC] *see* vitamins (multiple/oral) *on page 919*
Viactiv® Calcium Flavor Glides™ [OTC] *see* vitamins (multiple/oral) *on page 919*
Viactiv® Flavor Glides [OTC] *see* vitamins (multiple/oral) *on page 919*
Viactiv® for Teens [OTC] *see* vitamins (multiple/oral) *on page 919*
Viactiv® With Calcium [OTC] *see* vitamins (multiple/oral) *on page 919*
Viagra® *see* sildenafil *on page 811*
Vibativ™ *see* telavancin *on page 847*
Vibramycin® *see* doxycycline *on page 312*
Vibra-Tabs® (Can) *see* doxycycline *on page 312*
***Vibrio cholera* and enterotoxigenic *Escherichia coli* vaccine** *see* traveler's diarrhea and cholera vaccine *(Canada only) on page 883*
Vicks® 44® Cough Relief [OTC] *see* dextromethorphan *on page 270*
Vicks® 44E [OTC] *see* guaifenesin and dextromethorphan *on page 427*
Vicks® Casero™ Chest Congestion Relief [OTC] *see* guaifenesin *on page 425*
Vicks® DayQuil® Cold & Flu Multi-Symptom [OTC] *see* acetaminophen, dextromethorphan, and phenylephrine *on page 32*
Vicks® DayQuil® Cough [OTC] *see* dextromethorphan *on page 270*
Vicks® DayQuil® Mucus Control [OTC] *see* guaifenesin *on page 425*
Vicks® DayQuil® Mucus Control DM [OTC] *see* guaifenesin and dextromethorphan *on page 427*
Vicks® DayQuil® Sinus [OTC] *see* acetaminophen and phenylephrine *on page 28*
Vicks® Formula 44® Sore Throat [OTC] *see* phenol *on page 694*

Vicks® NyQuil® D Cold & Flu Multi-Symptom [OTC] *see* acetaminophen, dextromethorphan, doxylamine, and pseudoephedrine *on page 33*

Vicks® NyQuil® Cold & Flu Multi-Symptom [OTC] *see* acetaminophen, dextromethorphan, and doxylamine *on page 32*

Vicks® Pediatric Formula 44E [OTC] *see* guaifenesin and dextromethorphan *on page 427*

Vicks® Sinex® VapoSpray™ 4 Hour Decongestant [OTC] *see* phenylephrine (nasal) *on page 697*

Vicks® Sinex® VapoSpray 12-Hour *see* oxymetazoline (nasal) *on page 664*

Vicks® Sinex® VapoSpray 12-Hour UltraFine Mist [OTC] *see* oxymetazoline (nasal) *on page 664*

Vicks® Sinex® VapoSpray Moisturizing 12-Hour UltraFine Mist [OTC] *see* oxymetazoline (nasal) *on page 664*

Vicks® Vitamin C [OTC] *see* ascorbic acid *on page 96*

Vicodin® *see* hydrocodone and acetaminophen *on page 446*

Vicodin® ES *see* hydrocodone and acetaminophen *on page 446*

Vicodin® HP *see* hydrocodone and acetaminophen *on page 446*

Vicoprofen® *see* hydrocodone and ibuprofen *on page 448*

Victoza® *see* liraglutide *on page 531*

Victrelis™ *see* boceprevir *on page 138*

Vidaza® *see* azacitidine *on page 106*

Videx® *see* didanosine *on page 281*

Videx® EC *see* didanosine *on page 281*

vigabatrin (vye GA ba trin)

Medication Safety Issues
Sound-alike/look-alike issues:
Vigabatrin may be confused with Vibativ™

U.S. Brand Names Sabril®

Canadian Brand Names Sabril®

Therapeutic Category Anticonvulsant

Use Treatment of infantile spasms; refractory complex partial seizures not controlled by usual treatments

Canadian labeling: Additional uses (not in U.S. labeling): Active management of partial or secondary generalized seizures not controlled by usual treatments

General Dosage Range Dosage adjustment recommended in patients with renal impairment
Oral:
Infants: 50-150 mg/kg/day in 2 divided doses
Adults: 1-3 g/day in 2 divided doses

Dosage Forms
Powder for solution, oral:
Sabril®: 500 mg/packet (50s)
Tablet, oral:
Sabril®: 500 mg

Dosage Forms - Canada
Powder for suspension, oral [sachets]:
Sabril®: 0.5 g

Vigamox® *see* moxifloxacin (ophthalmic) *on page 601*

VIGIV *see* vaccinia immune globulin (intravenous) *on page 903*

Viibryd™ *see* vilazodone *on page 914*

vilazodone (vil AZ oh done)

Synonyms EMD 68843; SB659746-A; vilazodone hydrochloride

U.S. Brand Names Viibryd™

Therapeutic Category Antidepressant, Selective Serotonin Reuptake Inhibitor/5-HT$_{1A}$ Receptor Partial Agonist

Use Treatment of major depressive disorder

General Dosage Range Dosage adjustment recommended in patients on concomitant therapy
  Oral: *Adults:* 10-40 mg once daily
Dosage Forms
  Tablet, oral:
    Viibryd™: 10 mg, 20 mg, 40 mg

vilazodone hydrochloride *see vilazodone on page 914*

Vimovo™ *see naproxen and esomeprazole on page 613*

Vimpat® *see lacosamide on page 505*

Vinacal™ *see vitamins (multiple/prenatal) on page 920*

Vinate® Care *see vitamins (multiple/prenatal) on page 920*

vinblastine (vin BLAS teen)

Medication Safety Issues
  Sound-alike/look-alike issues:
    VinBLAStine may be confused with vinCRIStine, vinorelbine
  High alert medication:
    The Institute for Safe Medication Practices (ISMP) includes this medication among its list of drug classes which have a heightened risk of causing significant patient harm when used in error.
  Administration issues:
    Must be dispensed in overwrap which bears the statement **"Do not remove covering until the moment of injection. Fatal if given intrathecally. For I.V. use only."** Syringes should be labeled: **"Fatal if given intrathecally. For I.V. use only."**
Synonyms vinblastine sulfate; vincaleukoblastine; VLB
Tall-Man vin**BLAS**tine
Therapeutic Category Antineoplastic Agent
Use Treatment of Hodgkin and non-Hodgkin lymphoma; testicular cancer; breast cancer; mycosis fungoides; Kaposi sarcoma; histiocytosis (Letterer-Siwe disease); choriocarcinoma
General Dosage Range Dosage adjustment recommended in patients with hepatic impairment
  I.V.:
    Children: Initial dose: 3-6.5 mg/m^2 every 7 days as needed
    Adults: Initial: 3.7 mg/m^2; adjust dose every 7 days; Second dose: 5.5 mg/m^2; Third dose: 7.4 mg/m^2; Fourth dose: 9.25 mg/m^2; Fifth dose: 11.1 mg/m^2; Usual range: 5.5-7.4 mg/m^2 every 7 days; Maximum dose: 18.5 mg/m^2
Dosage Forms
  Injection, powder for reconstitution: 10 mg
  Injection, solution: 1 mg/mL (10 mL)

vinblastine sulfate *see vinblastine on page 915*

vincaleukoblastine *see vinblastine on page 915*

Vincasar PFS® *see vincristine on page 915*

vincristine (vin KRIS teen)

Medication Safety Issues
  Sound-alike/look-alike issues:
    VinCRIStine may be confused with vinBLAStine, vinorelbine
    Oncovin® may be confused with Ancobon®
  High alert medication:
    This medication is in a class the Institute for Safe Medication Practices (ISMP) includes among its list of drug classes which have a heightened risk of causing significant patient harm when used in error.
  Administration issues:
    For I.V. use only. Fatal if administered by other routes. To prevent fatal inadvertent intrathecal injection, it is recommended that vincristine doses be dispensed in a small minibag. Vincristine should **NOT** be prepared during the preparation of any intrathecal medications. After preparation, store vincristine in a location **away** from the separate storage location recommended for intrathecal medications. Vincristine should **NOT** be delivered to the patient at the same time with any medications intended for central nervous system administration.
Synonyms leurocristine sulfate; vincristine sulfate
Tall-Man vin**CRIS**tine
U.S. Brand Names Vincasar PFS®

◄ **Canadian Brand Names** Vincristine Sulfate Injection

Therapeutic Category Antineoplastic Agent

Use Treatment of acute lymphocytic leukemia (ALL), Hodgkin lymphoma, non-Hodgkin lymphomas, Wilms tumor, neuroblastoma, rhabdomyosarcoma

General Dosage Range Dosage adjustment recommended in patients with hepatic impairment

I.V.:
Children ≤10 kg: 0.05 mg/kg once weekly (maximum: 2 mg/dose)
Children >10 kg: 1.5-2 mg/m^2/dose (maximum: 2 mg/dose)
Adults: 1.4 mg/m^2/dose (maximum: 2 mg/dose)

Dosage Forms
Injection, solution [preservative free]: 1 mg/mL (1 mL, 2 mL)
Vincasar PFS®: 1 mg/mL (1 mL, 2 mL)

vincristine sulfate *see* vincristine *on page 915*

Vincristine Sulfate Injection. (Can) *see* vincristine *on page 915*

vinorelbine (vi NOR el been)

Medication Safety Issues
Sound-alike/look-alike issues:
Vinorelbine may be confused with vinBLAStine, vinCRIStine
High alert medication:
This medication is in a class the Institute for Safe Medication Practices (ISMP) includes among its list of drug classes which have a heightened risk of causing significant patient harm when used in error.
Administration issues:
Vinorelbine is intended **for I.V. use only**: Inadvertent intrathecal administration of other vinca alkaloids has resulted in death. Syringes containing vinorelbine should be labeled **"For I.V. use only. Fatal if given intrathecally."** Vinorelbine should **NOT** be prepared during the preparation of any intrathecal medications. After preparation, store vinorelbine in a location **away** from the separate storage location recommended for intrathecal medications.

Synonyms dihydroxydeoxynorvinkaleukoblastine; vinorelbine tartrate

U.S. Brand Names Navelbine®

Canadian Brand Names Navelbine®; Vinorelbine Injection, USP; Vinorelbine Tartrate for Injection

Therapeutic Category Antineoplastic Agent

Use Treatment of nonsmall cell lung cancer (NSCLC)

General Dosage Range Dosage adjustment recommended in patients with hepatic impairment or who develop toxicities
I.V.: *Adults:* 25-30 mg/m^2/dose every 7 days

Dosage Forms
Injection, solution [preservative free]: 10 mg/mL (1 mL, 5 mL)
Navelbine®: 10 mg/mL (1 mL, 5 mL)

Vinorelbine Injection, USP (Can) *see* vinorelbine *on page 916*

vinorelbine tartrate *see* vinorelbine *on page 916*

Vinorelbine Tartrate for Injection (Can) *see* vinorelbine *on page 916*

Viokase® (Can) *see* pancrelipase *on page 670*

viosterol *see* ergocalciferol *on page 336*

Viracept® *see* nelfinavir *on page 616*

Viramune® *see* nevirapine *on page 621*

Viramune® XR™ *see* nevirapine *on page 621*

Virazole® *see* ribavirin *on page 777*

Viread® *see* tenofovir *on page 851*

Viroptic® *see* trifluridine *on page 890*

Viscoat® *see* sodium chondroitin sulfate and sodium hyaluronate *on page 820*

Viscous Lidocaine *see* lidocaine (topical) *on page 524*

Visicol® *see* sodium phosphates *on page 823*

Visine-A® [OTC] *see* naphazoline and pheniramine *on page 611*

Visine® Advanced Allergy (Can) *see* naphazoline and pheniramine *on page 611*

Visine® Advanced Relief [OTC] *see* tetrahydrozoline (ophthalmic) *on page 858*

Visine® L.R.® [OTC] *see* oxymetazoline (ophthalmic) *on page 665*
Visine® Original [OTC] *see* tetrahydrozoline (ophthalmic) *on page 858*
Visipaque™ *see* iodixanol *on page 484*
Viskazide® (Can) *see* pindolol and hydrochlorothiazide *(Canada only) on page 705*
Visken® (Can) *see* pindolol *on page 705*
Vistaril® *see* hydroxyzine *on page 456*
Vistide® *see* cidofovir *on page 208*
Visudyne® *see* verteporfin *on page 913*
Vita-C® [OTC] *see* ascorbic acid *on page 96*
Vitafol® *see* vitamins (multiple/oral) *on page 919*
Vitafol®-OB [OTC] *see* vitamins (multiple/prenatal) *on page 920*
Vitafol®-OB+DHA [OTC] *see* vitamins (multiple/prenatal) *on page 920*
Vitafol®-PN *see* vitamins (multiple/prenatal) *on page 920*
Vitalets [OTC] *see* vitamins (multiple/pediatric) *on page 920*
vitamin C *see* ascorbic acid *on page 96*
vitamin D₃ and alendronate *see* alendronate and cholecalciferol *on page 49*
vitamin D and calcium carbonate *see* calcium and vitamin D *on page 160*

vitamin A (VYE ta min aye)

Medication Safety Issues
  Sound-alike/look-alike issues:
    Aquasol® may be confused with Anusol®
Synonyms oleovitamin A
U.S. Brand Names A-25 [OTC]; A-Natural [OTC]; A-Natural-25 [OTC]; Aquasol A®
Therapeutic Category Vitamin, Fat Soluble
Use Treatment and prevention of vitamin A deficiency; parenteral (I.M.) route is indicated when oral administration is not feasible or when absorption is insufficient (malabsorption syndrome)
General Dosage Range I.M., Oral: *Children and Adults:* Dosage varies greatly depending on indication
Dosage Forms
  Capsule, oral:
    A-25 [OTC]: 25,000 units
  Capsule, softgel, oral: 10,000 units
    A-Natural [OTC]: 10,000 units
    A-Natural-25 [OTC]: 25,000 units
  Injection, solution:
    Aquasol A®: 50,000 units/mL (2 mL)
  Tablet, oral: 10,000 units, 15,000 units

vitamin A acid *see* tretinoin (topical) *on page 885*

vitamin A and vitamin D (VYE ta min aye & VYE ta min dee)

Synonyms cod liver oil
U.S. Brand Names A and D® Original [OTC]; Baza® Clear [OTC]; Sween Cream® [OTC]
Therapeutic Category Protectant, Topical
Use Temporary relief of discomfort due to chapped skin, diaper rash, minor burns, abrasions, as well as irritations associated with ostomy skin care
General Dosage Range Topical: *Children and Adults:* Apply locally as needed
Dosage Forms
  Capsule, softgel: Vitamin A 1250 int. units and vitamin D 135 int. units; vitamin A 1250 int. units and vitamin D 130 int. units; vitamin A 5,000 int. units and vitamin D 400 int. units; vitamin A 10,000 int. units and vitamin D 400 int. units; vitamin A 10,000 int. units and vitamin D 5000 int. units; vitamin A 25,000 int. units and vitamin D 1000 int. units
  Cream:
    Sween Cream® [OTC]: 2 g, 57 g, 85 g, 142 g, 184 g, 339 g
  Ointment: 0.9 g, 5 g, 60 g, 120 g, 454 g
    A and D® Original [OTC]: 45 g, 120 g, 454 g
    Baza® Clear [OTC]: 50 g, 150 g, 240 g
  Tablet: Vitamin A 10,000 int. units and vitamin D 400 int. units

vitamin B₁ *see* thiamine *on page 862*
vitamin B₂ *see* riboflavin *on page 778*
vitamin B₃ *see* niacin *on page 622*
vitamin B₃ *see* niacinamide *on page 623*
vitamin B₅ *see* pantothenic acid *on page 673*
vitamin B₆ *see* pyridoxine *on page 758*
vitamin B₁₂ *see* cyanocobalamin *on page 241*

vitamin B complex combinations (VYE ta min bee KOM pleks kom bi NAY shuns)

Medication Safety Issues
Sound-alike/look-alike issues:
Nephrocaps® may be confused with Nephro-Calci®
Renal Caps may be confused with Renagel®, Renvela®
Surbex® may be confused with Sebex®, Suprax®, Surfak®

Synonyms B complex combinations; B vitamin combinations

Therapeutic Category Vitamin, Water Soluble

Use Supplement for use in the wasting syndrome in chronic renal failure, uremia, impaired metabolic functions of the kidney, dialysis; labeled for OTC use as a dietary supplement

General Dosage Range
Oral: *Adults:* Dosage varies greatly depending on product

Dosage Forms Content varies depending on product used. For more detailed information on ingredients in these and other multivitamins, please refer to package labeling.

vitamin D2 *see* ergocalciferol *on page 336*
Vitamin D3 [OTC] *see* cholecalciferol *on page 204*

vitamin E (VYE ta min ee)

Medication Safety Issues
Sound-alike/look-alike issues:
Aquasol E® may be confused with Anusol®

Synonyms *d*-alpha tocopherol; *dl*-alpha tocopherol

U.S. Brand Names Alph-E [OTC]; Alph-E-Mixed [OTC]; Aqua Gem-E™ [OTC]; Aquasol E® [OTC]; d-Alpha Gems™ [OTC]; E-Gems® Elite [OTC]; E-Gems® Plus [OTC]; E-Gems® [OTC]; E-Gem® Lip Care [OTC]; E-Gem® [OTC]; Ester-E™ [OTC]; Gamma E-Gems® [OTC]; Gamma-E PLUS [OTC]; High Gamma Vitamin E Complete™ [OTC]; Key-E® Kaps [OTC]; Key-E® Powder [OTC]; Key-E® [OTC]

Therapeutic Category Vitamin, Fat Soluble; Vitamin, Topical

Use Dietary supplement

General Dosage Range
Oral:
Children: 1 unit/kg/day **or** 100-750 units/day
Adults: 30-1600 units/day **or** 1000 units twice daily
Topical: *Adults:* Apply a thin layer over affected area

Dosage Forms
Capsule, oral: 1000 int. units
Key-E® Kaps [OTC]: 200 int. units, 400 int. units
Capsule, liquid, oral: 400 int. units
Capsule, softgel, oral: 100 int. units, 200 int. units, 400 int. units, 600 int. units, 1000 int. units, 200 units, 1000 units
Alph-E [OTC]: 200 int. units, 400 int. units, 1000 int. units
Alph-E-Mixed [OTC]: 200 int. units, 400 int. units, 1000 int. units
Aqua Gem-E™ [OTC]: 200 int. units, 400 int. units
d-Alpha Gems™ [OTC]: 400 int. units
E-Gems® [OTC]: 30 int. units, 100 int. units, 200 int. units, 400 int. units, 600 int. units, 800 int. units, 1000 int. units, 1200 int. units
E-Gems® Elite [OTC]: 400 int. units
E-Gems® Plus [OTC]: 200 int. units, 400 int. units, 800 int. units
Ester-E™ [OTC]: 400 int. units

Gamma E-Gems® [OTC]: 90 int. units
Gamma-E PLUS [OTC]: 200 int. units
High Gamma Vitamin E Complete™ [OTC]: 200 int. units
Cream, topical: 1000 int. units/120 g (120 g); 100 int. units/g (57 g, 60 g); 30,000 int. units/57 g (57 g)
Key-E® [OTC]: 30 int. units/g (57 g, 120 g, 600 g)
Lip balm, topical:
E-Gem® Lip Care [OTC]: 1000 int. units/tube
Liquid, oral/topical: 1150 int. units/1.25 mL (30 mL, 60 mL, 120 mL)
Oil, oral/topical: 100 int. units/0.25 mL (74 mL)
E-Gem® [OTC]: 10 int. units/drop (15 mL, 60 mL)
Oil, topical:
Alph-E [OTC]: 28,000 int. units/30 mL (30 mL)
Ointment, topical:
Key-E® [OTC]: 30 int. units/g (57 g, 113 g, 500 g)
Powder, oral:
Key-E® Powder [OTC]: (15 g, 75 g, 1000 g)
Solution, oral: 15 int. units/0.3 mL (30 mL)
Aquasol E® [OTC]: 15 int. units/0.3 mL (12 mL, 30 mL)
Suppository, rectal/vaginal:
Key-E® [OTC]: 30 int. units (12s, 24s)
Tablet, oral: 100 int. units, 200 int. units, 400 int. units, 500 int. units
Key-E® [OTC]: 200 int. units, 400 int. units

vitamin G *see* riboflavin *on page* 778
vitamin K₁ *see* phytonadione *on page* 703

vitamins (multiple/injectable) (VYE ta mins, MUL ti pul/in JEK ti bal)

U.S. Brand Names Infuvite® Adult; Infuvite® Pediatric; M.V.I. Adult™; M.V.I.®-12; M.V.I® Pediatric
Therapeutic Category Vitamin
Use Nutritional supplement in patients receiving parenteral nutrition or requiring intravenous administration
General Dosage Range I.V.:
Children ≥3 kg to 11 years: 5 mL/day
Children >11 years and Adults: 10 mL/day
Dosage Forms Content varies depending on product used. For more detailed information on ingredients in these and other multivitamins, please refer to package labeling.

vitamins (multiple/oral) (VYE ta mins, MUL ti pul/OR al)

Medication Safety Issues
Sound-alike/look-alike issues:
Theragran® may be confused with Phenergan®
Viactiv® may be confused with Vibativ™

Synonyms multiple vitamins; therapeutic multivitamins; vitamins, multiple (oral); vitamins, multiple (therapeutic); vitamins, multiple with iron
U.S. Brand Names Androvite® [OTC]; CalciFolic-D™; Centamin [OTC]; Centrum Cardio® [OTC]; Centrum Performance® [OTC]; Centrum® Silver® Ultra Men's [OTC]; Centrum® Silver® Ultra Women's [OTC]; Centrum® Silver® [OTC]; Centrum® Ultra Men's [OTC]; Centrum® Ultra Women's [OTC]; Centrum® [OTC]; Diatx®Zn; Drinkables® Fruits and Vegetables [OTC]; Drinkables® MultiVitamins [OTC]; Encora®; Foltrin®; Freedavite [OTC]; Geri-Freeda [OTC]; Geriation [OTC]; Geritol Complete® [OTC]; Geritol Extend® [OTC]; Geritol® Tonic [OTC]; Glutofac®-MX; Glutofac®-ZX; Gynovite® Plus [OTC]; Hemocyte Plus®; Hi-Kovite [OTC]; Iberet®-500 [OTC] [DSC]; Monocaps [OTC]; Myadec® [OTC]; Nutrimin-Plus [OTC]; Ocuvite® Adult 50+ [OTC]; Ocuvite® Extra® [OTC]; Ocuvite® Lutein [OTC]; Ocuvite® [OTC]; One A Day® Cholesterol Plus [OTC]; One A Day® Energy [OTC]; One A Day® Essential [OTC]; One A Day® Maximum [OTC]; One A Day® Men's 50+ Advantage [OTC]; One A Day® Men's Health Formula [OTC]; One A Day® Teen Advantage for Her [OTC]; One A Day® Teen Advantage for Him [OTC]; One A Day® Weight Smart® Advanced [OTC]; One A Day® Women's 50+ Advantage [OTC]; One A Day® Women's Active Mind & Body [OTC]; One A Day® Women's [OTC]; Optivite® P.M.T. [OTC]; PreserVision® AREDS [OTC]; PreserVision® Lutein [OTC]; Quintabs [OTC]; Quintabs-M Iron-Free [OTC]; Quintabs-M [OTC]; Renax®; Renax® 5.5; Replace Without Iron [OTC]; Replace [OTC]; Repliva 21/7®; SourceCF®; Strovite®; Strovite® Advance; Strovite® Forte; Strovite® Plus; T-Vites [OTC]; Ultra Freeda A-Free [OTC]; Ultra Freeda Iron-Free [OTC]; Ultra Freeda With Iron [OTC]; Viactiv®

◀ Calcium Flavor Glides™ [OTC]; Viactiv® Flavor Glides [OTC]; Viactiv® for Teens [OTC]; Viactiv® With Calcium [OTC]; Viactiv® [OTC]; Vitafol®; Xtramins [OTC]; Yelets [OTC]

Therapeutic Category Vitamin

Use Prevention/treatment of vitamin and mineral deficiencies; labeled for OTC use as a dietary supplement

General Dosage Range Oral: *Adults:* 1 tablet/capsule **or** 5-15 mL once daily

Dosage Forms Content varies depending on product used. For more detailed information on ingredients in these and other multivitamins, please refer to package labeling.

vitamins, multiple (oral) *see* vitamins (multiple/oral) *on page 919*

vitamins (multiple/pediatric) (VYE ta mins, MUL ti pul/pe de AT rik)

Synonyms children's vitamins; multivitamins/fluoride

U.S. Brand Names ADEKs® [OTC]; AquADEKs™ [OTC]; Centrum Kids® [OTC]; Flintstones™ Complete [OTC]; Flintstones™ Gummies [OTC]; Flintstones™ Plus Bone Building Support Gummies [OTC]; Flintstones™ Plus Bone Building Support [OTC]; Flintstones™ Plus Immunity Support Gummies [OTC]; Flintstones™ Plus Immunity Support [OTC]; Flintstones™ Plus Iron [OTC]; Flintstones™ Sour Gummies [OTC]; My First Flintstones™ [OTC]; MyKidz Iron FL™; MyKidz Iron™ [OTC]; One A Day® Kids Jolly Rancher™ Gummies [OTC]; One A Day® Kids Jolly Rancher™ Sour Gummies [OTC]; One A Day® Kids Scooby-Doo!™ Complete [OTC]; One A Day® Kids Scooby-Doo!™ Gummies [OTC]; Poly-Vi-Sol® With Iron [OTC]; Poly-Vi-Sol® [OTC]; SourceCF® [OTC]; Tri-Vi-Sol® With Iron [OTC]; Tri-Vi-Sol® [OTC]; Vitalets [OTC]

Therapeutic Category Vitamin

Use Prevention/treatment of vitamin deficiency; products containing fluoride are used to prevent dental caries; labeled for OTC use as a dietary supplement

General Dosage Range Oral: *Children:* Daily dose varies greatly depending on product

Dosage Forms Content varies depending on product used. For more detailed information on ingredients in these and other multivitamins, please refer to package labeling.

vitamins (multiple/prenatal) (VYE ta mins, MUL ti pul/pree NAY tal)

Medication Safety Issues

Sound-alike/look-alike issues:

PreCare® may be confused with Precose®

Synonyms prenatal vitamins

U.S. Brand Names A-Free Prenatal [OTC]; CitraNatal® Harmony™; CitraNatal™ 90 DHA; CitraNatal™ Assure; CitraNatal™ B-Calm; CitraNatal™ DHA; CitraNatal™ Rx; Concept DHA™; Concept OB™; Duet®; Duet® Balanced DHA^ec; Femecal OB; Folcaps™ Care One; Foltabs™ Prenatal; Foltabs™ Prenatal Plus DHA; Gesticare®; Gesticare® DHA; KPN Prenatal [OTC]; Mini-Prenatal [OTC]; Multi-Nate 30; NataChew® [OTC]; NataFort® [OTC]; Néevo®; Néevo® DHA; One A Day® Women's Prenatal [OTC]; OptiNate®; Paire OB™ Plus DHA; PreCare®; PreferaOB®; PreferaOB® + DHA; PreferaOB® One™; Prenatabs FA; Prenatal One Daily [OTC]; Prenatal Rx 1; Prenatal With Beta Carotene [OTC]; Prenate DHA™; Prenate Elite®; Prenate Essential™; PreNexa® Premier; PrimaCare® One; Select-OB™; Stuart Prenatal® [OTC]; Tandem® DHA; Tandem® OB; TriCare® Prenatal; TriCare® Prenatal DHA One®; Vinacal™; Vinate® Care; Vitafol®-OB [OTC]; Vitafol®-OB+DHA [OTC]; Vitafol®-PN; VitaPhil + DHA

Therapeutic Category Vitamin

Use Nutritional supplement for use prior to conception, during pregnancy, and postnatal (in lactating and nonlactating women)

General Dosage Range Oral: *Adults:* 1 tablet/capsule once daily **or** 4 teaspoonfuls/day once daily or in divided doses

Dosage Forms Content varies depending on product used. For more detailed information on ingredients in these and other multivitamins, please refer to package labeling.

vitamins, multiple (therapeutic) *see* vitamins (multiple/oral) *on page 919*

vitamins, multiple with iron *see* vitamins (multiple/oral) *on page 919*

VitaPhil + DHA *see* vitamins (multiple/prenatal) *on page 920*

Vita-Respa® *see* folic acid, cyanocobalamin, and pyridoxine *on page 396*

Vitrase® *see* hyaluronidase *on page 443*

Vitrasert® *see* ganciclovir (ophthalmic) *on page 410*

Vivacaine™ *see* bupivacaine and epinephrine *on page 148*

Vi vaccine *see* typhoid vaccine *on page 898*
Vivactil® *see* protriptyline *on page 751*
Viva-Drops® [OTC] *see* artificial tears *on page 96*
Vivaglobin® [DSC] *see* immune globulin *on page 468*
Vivaglobin® (Can) *see* immune globulin *on page 468*
Vivarin® [OTC] *see* caffeine *on page 157*
Vivelle-Dot® *see* estradiol (systemic) *on page 343*
Vivitrol® *see* naltrexone *on page 610*
Vivotif® *see* typhoid vaccine *on page 898*
VLB *see* vinblastine *on page 915*
VM-26 *see* teniposide *on page 850*
Volibris® (Can) *see* ambrisentan *on page 62*
Voltaren *see* diclofenac (systemic) *on page 277*
Voltaren® (Can) *see* diclofenac (systemic) *on page 277*
Voltaren® Emulgel™ (Can) *see* diclofenac (topical) *on page 279*
Voltaren® Gel *see* diclofenac (topical) *on page 279*
Voltaren Ophtha® (Can) *see* diclofenac (ophthalmic) *on page 278*
Voltaren Ophthalmic® *see* diclofenac (ophthalmic) *on page 278*
Voltaren Rapide® (Can) *see* diclofenac (systemic) *on page 277*
Voltaren SR® (Can) *see* diclofenac (systemic) *on page 277*
Voltaren®-XR *see* diclofenac (systemic) *on page 277*
VoLumen® *see* barium *on page 114*
Voluven® *see* tetrastarch *on page 858*
von willebrand factor/factor VIII complex *see* antihemophilic factor/von Willebrand factor complex (human) *on page 82*

voriconazole (vor i KOE na zole)

Synonyms UK109496
U.S. Brand Names VFEND®
Canadian Brand Names VFEND®
Therapeutic Category Antifungal Agent
Use Treatment of invasive aspergillosis; treatment of esophageal candidiasis; treatment of candidemia (in nonneutropenic patients); treatment of disseminated *Candida* infections of the skin and viscera; treatment of serious fungal infections caused by *Scedosporium apiospermum* and *Fusarium* spp (including *Fusarium solani*) in patients intolerant of, or refractory to, other therapy
General Dosage Range Dosage adjustment recommended in patients with hepatic impairment
  I.V.: *Children ≥12 years and Adults:* Initial: 6 mg/kg every 12 hours for 2 doses; Maintenance: 3-4 mg/kg every 12 hours
  Oral: *Children ≥12 years and Adults:* 100-300 mg every 12 hours
Dosage Forms
  Injection, powder for reconstitution:
    VFEND®: 200 mg
  Powder for suspension, oral:
    VFEND®: 40 mg/mL (70 mL)
  Tablet, oral: 50 mg, 200 mg
    VFEND®: 50 mg, 200 mg

vorinostat (vor IN oh stat)

Medication Safety Issues
  Sound-alike/look-alike issues:
    Vorinostat may be confused with Votrient™
  High alert medication:
    The Institute for Safe Medication Practices (ISMP) includes this medication among its list of drug classes which have a heightened risk of causing significant patient harm when used in error.
Synonyms SAHA; suberoylanilide hydroxamic acid
U.S. Brand Names Zolinza®
Canadian Brand Names Zolinza®

◄ **Therapeutic Category** Antineoplastic Agent, Histone Deacetylase Inhibitor
Use Treatment of progressive, persistent, or recurrent cutaneous T-cell lymphoma (CTCL)
General Dosage Range Dosage adjustment recommended in patients who develop toxicities
 Oral: *Adults:* 400 mg once daily
Dosage Forms
 Capsule, oral:
 Zolinza®: 100 mg

VoSoL® *see* acetic acid *on page 35*

VoSol® HC *see* acetic acid, propylene glycol diacetate, and hydrocortisone *on page 35*

VoSpire ER® *see* albuterol *on page 45*

Votrient™ *see* pazopanib *on page 676*

VP-16 *see* etoposide *on page 361*

VP-16-213 *see* etoposide *on page 361*

VPRIV™ *see* velaglucerase alfa *on page 910*

VRT111950 *see* telaprevir *on page 846*

VSL #3® [OTC] *see* Lactobacillus *on page 506*

VSL #3®-DS *see* Lactobacillus *on page 506*

Vumon® *see* teniposide *on page 850*

Vusion® *see* miconazole and zinc oxide *on page 586*

V.V.S.® *see* sulfabenzamide, sulfacetamide, and sulfathiazole *on page 834*

VWF/FVIII concentrate *see* antihemophilic factor/von Willebrand factor complex (human) *on page 82*

VWF:RCo *see* antihemophilic factor/von Willebrand factor complex (human) *on page 82*

vWF:RCof *see* antihemophilic factor/von Willebrand factor complex (human) *on page 82*

VX-950 *see* telaprevir *on page 846*

Vyloma™ (Can) *see* imiquimod *on page 467*

Vytorin® *see* ezetimibe and simvastatin *on page 364*

Vyvanse® *see* lisdexamfetamine *on page 531*

Vyvanse™ (Can) *see* lisdexamfetamine *on page 531*

VZIG *see* varicella-zoster immune globulin (human) *on page 909*

VZV vaccine (varicella) *see* varicella virus vaccine *on page 908*

VZV vaccine (zoster) *see* zoster vaccine *on page 935*

warfarin (WAR far in)

Medication Safety Issues
 Sound-alike/look-alike issues:
 Coumadin® may be confused with Avandia®, Cardura®, Compazine®, Kemadrin®
 Jantoven® may be confused with Janumet®, Januvia®
 High alert medication:
 The Institute for Safe Medication Practices (ISMP) includes this medication among its list of drugs which have a heightened risk of causing significant patient harm when used in error.
 2009 National Patient Safety Goals:
 The Joint Commission on Accreditation of Healthcare Organizations requires healthcare organizations that provide anticoagulant therapy to have a process in place to reduce the risk of anticoagulant-associated patient harm. Patients receiving anticoagulants should receive individualized care through a defined process that includes standardized ordering, dispensing, administration, monitoring and education. This does not apply to routine short-term use of anticoagulants for prevention of venous thromboembolism when the expectation is that the patient's laboratory values will remain within or close to normal values (NPSG.03.05.01).

Synonyms warfarin sodium

U.S. Brand Names Coumadin®; Jantoven®

Canadian Brand Names Apo-Warfarin®; Coumadin®; Mylan-Warfarin; Novo-Warfarin; Taro-Warfarin

Therapeutic Category Anticoagulant (Other)

Use Prophylaxis and treatment of thromboembolic disorders (eg, venous, pulmonary) and embolic complications arising from atrial fibrillation or cardiac valve replacement; adjunct to reduce risk of systemic embolism (eg, recurrent MI, stroke) after myocardial infarction

General Dosage Range
I.V.: *Adults:* 2-5 mg once daily
Oral:
  Adults: Initial: 2-5 mg daily for 2 days; Maintenance: 2-10 mg daily
  Elderly: Initial: ≤5 mg/day; Maintenance: 2-5 mg/day
Dosage Forms
Injection, powder for reconstitution:
  Coumadin®: 5 mg
Tablet, oral: 1 mg, 2 mg, 2.5 mg, 3 mg, 4 mg, 5 mg, 6 mg, 7.5 mg, 10 mg
  Coumadin®: 1 mg, 2 mg, 2.5 mg, 3 mg, 4 mg, 5 mg, 6 mg, 7.5 mg, 10 mg
  Jantoven®: 1 mg, 2 mg, 2.5 mg, 3 mg, 4 mg, 5 mg, 6 mg, 7.5 mg, 10 mg

warfarin sodium *see* warfarin *on page 922*
Wartec® (Can) *see* podofilox *on page 716*
Wart-Off® Maximum Strength [OTC] *see* salicylic acid *on page 795*
4-Way® 12 Hour [OTC] *see* oxymetazoline (nasal) *on page 664*
4 Way® Fast Acting [OTC] *see* phenylephrine (nasal) *on page 697*
4 Way® Menthol [OTC] *see* phenylephrine (nasal) *on page 697*
4-Way® Saline Moisturizing Mist [OTC] *see* sodium chloride *on page 818*
Welchol® *see* colesevelam *on page 231*
Wellbutrin® *see* bupropion *on page 150*
Wellbutrin XL® *see* bupropion *on page 150*
Wellbutrin® XL (Can) *see* bupropion *on page 150*
Wellbutrin SR® *see* bupropion *on page 150*
Wellbutrin® SR (Can) *see* bupropion *on page 150*
Westcort® *see* hydrocortisone (topical) *on page 450*
Westhroid™ *see* thyroid, desiccated *on page 865*

wheat dextrin (weet DEKS trin)

Synonyms dextrin; resistant dextrin; resistant maltodextrin
U.S. Brand Names Benefiber® Plus Calcium [OTC]; Benefiber® [OTC]
Therapeutic Category Fiber Supplement; Laxative, Bulk-Producing
Use OTC labeling: Dietary fiber supplement
General Dosage Range Oral: *Children and Adults:* Dosage varies greatly depending on product
Dosage Forms
Caplet, oral:
  Benefiber® [OTC]: 1.3 g
Powder, oral:
  Benefiber® [OTC]: (80 g, 155 g, 161 g, 245 g, 267 g, 350 g, 477 g, 529 g); 3.5 g/packet (8s, 16s, 28s)
  Benefiber® Plus Calcium [OTC]: (424 g)
Tablet, chewable, oral:
  Benefiber® [OTC]: 2.7 g
  Benefiber® Plus Calcium [OTC]: 2.7 g

Wilate® *see* antihemophilic factor/von Willebrand factor complex (human) *on page 82*
Winpred™ (Can) *see* prednisone *on page 735*
WinRho® SDF *see* Rh₀(D) immune globulin *on page 776*

witch hazel (witch HAY zel)

Synonyms hamamelis water
U.S. Brand Names Dickinson's® Witch Hazel Astringent Cleanser [OTC]; Dickinson's® Witch Hazel Cleansing Astringent [OTC]; Dickinson's® Witch Hazel [OTC]; Medi Pads [OTC]; Preparation H® Medicated Wipes [OTC]; T. N. Dickinson's® Hazelets® [OTC]; T. N. Dickinson's® Witch Hazel® Astringent [OTC]; T. N. Dickinson's® Witch Hazel® Hemorrhoidal [OTC]; Tucks® Anti-Itch [OTC]; Tucks® Take Alongs® [OTC]
Canadian Brand Names Preparation H® Cleansing Pads
Therapeutic Category Astringent

◀ **Use** After-stool wipe to remove most causes of local irritation; temporary management of vulvitis, pruritus ani and vulva; help relieve the discomfort of simple hemorrhoids, anorectal surgical wounds, and episiotomies

General Dosage Range Topical: *Children ≥12 years and Adults:* Apply to anorectal area as needed up to 6 times daily or after each bowel movement

Dosage Forms

Liquid, topical:
Dickinson's® Witch Hazel Astringent Cleanser [OTC]: 99.5% (3785 mL)
Dickinson's® Witch Hazel Cleansing Astringent [OTC]: 99.5% (59 mL, 237 mL, 473 mL)
T. N. Dickinson's® Witch Hazel® Astringent [OTC]: 100% (59 mL, 237 mL, 473 mL)

Pad, topical:
Dickinson's® Witch Hazel [OTC]: 99% (60s)
Dickinson's® Witch Hazel Cleansing Astringent [OTC]: 99% (20s)
Medi Pads [OTC]: 50% (100s)
Preparation H® Medicated Wipes [OTC]: 50% (8s, 48s, 96s)
T. N. Dickinson's® Hazelets® [OTC]: 100% (50s, 60s)
T. N. Dickinson's® Witch Hazel® Hemorrhoidal [OTC]: 50% (100s)
Tucks® Anti-Itch [OTC]: 50% (40s, 100s)

Towelette, topical:
Tucks® Take Alongs® [OTC]: 50% (12s)

Wound Wash Saline™ [OTC] *see* sodium chloride *on page* 818
WR-2721 *see* amifostine *on page* 63
WR-139007 *see* dacarbazine *on page* 248
WR-139013 *see* chlorambucil *on page* 193
WR-139021 *see* carmustine *on page* 177
Wycillin [DSC] *see* penicillin G procaine *on page* 685
Wycillin® (Can) *see* penicillin G procaine *on page* 685
Wytensin® (Can) *see* guanabenz *on page* 430
Xalacom™ (Can) *see* latanoprost and timolol *(Canada only) on page* 513
Xalatan® *see* latanoprost *on page* 513
Xamiol® (Can) *see* calcipotriene and betamethasone *on page* 158
Xanax® *see* alprazolam *on page* 56
Xanax TS™ (Can) *see* alprazolam *on page* 56
Xanax XR® *see* alprazolam *on page* 56
Xarelto® *see* rivaroxaban *on page* 786
Xatral (Can) *see* alfuzosin *on page* 50
Xeloda® *see* capecitabine *on page* 168
Xenaderm® *see* trypsin, balsam Peru, and castor oil *on page* 896
Xenazine® *see* tetrabenazine *on page* 856
Xenical® *see* orlistat *on page* 655
Xeomin® *see* incobotulinumtoxinA *on page* 470
Xerac™ AC *see* aluminum chloride hexahydrate *on page* 59
Xerclear *see* acyclovir and hydrocortisone *on page* 39
Xerese™ *see* acyclovir and hydrocortisone *on page* 39
Xgeva™ *see* denosumab *on page* 259
Xiaflex™ *see* collagenase (systemic) *on page* 232
Xibrom® [DSC] *see* bromfenac *on page* 142
Xifaxan® *see* rifaximin *on page* 780
Xigris® *see* drotrecogin alfa *on page* 315
xilep *see* rufinamide *on page* 793
Xodol® 5/300 *see* hydrocodone and acetaminophen *on page* 446
Xodol® 7.5/300 *see* hydrocodone and acetaminophen *on page* 446
Xodol® 10/300 *see* hydrocodone and acetaminophen *on page* 446
Xolair® *see* omalizumab *on page* 648
Xolegel® *see* ketoconazole (topical) *on page* 500
Xopenex® *see* levalbuterol *on page* 516

Xopenex HFA™ *see* levalbuterol *on page 516*
XP13512 *see* gabapentin enacarbil *on page 406*
Xpect™ [OTC] *see* guaifenesin *on page 425*
XRP6258 *see* cabazitaxel *on page 156*
X-Seb T® Pearl [OTC] *see* coal tar and salicylic acid *on page 228*
X-Seb T® Plus [OTC] *see* coal tar and salicylic acid *on page 228*
Xtramins [OTC] *see* vitamins (multiple/oral) *on page 919*
X-Viate™ *see* urea *on page 900*
Xylac (Can) *see* loxapine *on page 541*
Xylocaine® *see* lidocaine (systemic) *on page 523*
Xylocaine® *see* lidocaine (topical) *on page 524*
Xylocaine® Dental *see* lidocaine (systemic) *on page 523*
Xylocaine® MPF *see* lidocaine (systemic) *on page 523*
Xylocaine® MPF With Epinephrine *see* lidocaine and epinephrine *on page 525*
Xylocaine Viscous *see* lidocaine (topical) *on page 524*
Xylocaine® With Epinephrine *see* lidocaine and epinephrine *on page 525*
Xylocard® (Can) *see* lidocaine (systemic) *on page 523*
Xyntha® *see* antihemophilic factor (recombinant) *on page 81*
Xyntha® Solofuse™ *see* antihemophilic factor (recombinant) *on page 81*
Xyrem® *see* sodium oxybate *on page 822*
Xyzal® *see* levocetirizine *on page 519*
Y-90 ibritumomab *see* ibritumomab *on page 460*
Y-90 zevalin *see* ibritumomab *on page 460*
Yasmin® *see* ethinyl estradiol and drospirenone *on page 352*
Yaz® *see* ethinyl estradiol and drospirenone *on page 352*
Yelets [OTC] *see* vitamins (multiple/oral) *on page 919*

yellow fever vaccine (YEL oh FEE ver vak SEEN)

U.S. Brand Names YF-VAX®
Canadian Brand Names YF-VAX®
Therapeutic Category Vaccine, Live Virus
Use Induction of active immunity against yellow fever virus, primarily among persons traveling or living in areas where yellow fever infection exists and laboratory workers who may be exposed to the virus; vaccination may also be required for some international travelers

The Advisory Committee on Immunization Practices (ACIP) recommends vaccination for:
• Persons traveling to or living in areas at risk for yellow fever transmission
• Persons traveling to countries which require vaccination for international travel
• Laboratory personnel who may be exposed to the yellow fever virus or concentrated preparations of the vaccine

Although the vaccine is approved for use in children ≥9 months of age, the CDC recommends use in children as young as 6 months under unusual circumstances (eg, travel to an area where exposure is unavoidable). Children <6 months of age should **never** receive the vaccine.
General Dosage Range SubQ: *Children ≥9 months and Adults:* Initial: 0.5 mL as a single dose
Dosage Forms
  Injection, powder for reconstitution [17D-204 strain]:
    YF-VAX®: ≥4.74 Log_{10} plaque-forming units (PFU) per 0.5 mL dose

Yervoy™ *see* ipilimumab *on page 488*
YF-VAX® *see* yellow fever vaccine *on page 925*
YM087 *see* conivaptan *on page 234*
YM905 *see* solifenacin *on page 825*
YM-08310 *see* amifostine *on page 63*
Yodoxin® *see* iodoquinol *on page 484*
Z4942 *see* ifosfamide *on page 464*
Zactima *see* vandetanib *on page 907*

Zaditor® [OTC] *see* ketotifen (ophthalmic) *on page 503*
Zaditor® (Can) *see* ketotifen (ophthalmic) *on page 503*

zafirlukast (za FIR loo kast)

Medication Safety Issues
  Sound-alike/look-alike issues:
    Accolate® may be confused with Accupril®, Accutane®, Aclovate®
Synonyms ICI-204,219
U.S. Brand Names Accolate®
Canadian Brand Names Accolate®
Therapeutic Category Leukotriene Receptor Antagonist
Use Prophylaxis and chronic treatment of asthma in adults and children ≥5 years of age
General Dosage Range Oral:
  Children 5-11 years: 10 mg twice daily
  Children ≥12 years and Adults: 20 mg twice daily
Dosage Forms
  Tablet, oral: 10 mg, 20 mg
    Accolate®: 10 mg, 20 mg

zaleplon (ZAL e plon)

Medication Safety Issues
  Sound-alike/look-alike issues:
    Sonata® may be confused with Soriatane®
    Zaleplon may be confused with Zelapar®, Zemplar®, zolpidem, ZyPREXA® Zydis®
U.S. Brand Names Sonata®
Therapeutic Category Hypnotic, Nonbenzodiazepine (Pyrazolopyrimidine)
Controlled Substance C-IV
Use Short-term (7-10 days) treatment of insomnia (has been demonstrated to be effective for up to 5 weeks in controlled trial)
General Dosage Range Dosage adjustment recommended in patients with hepatic impairment
  Oral:
    Adults: 5-20 mg at bedtime
    Elderly: 5 mg at bedtime (maximum: 10 mg/day)
Dosage Forms
  Capsule, oral: 5 mg, 10 mg
    Sonata®: 5 mg, 10 mg

Zamicet™ *see* hydrocodone and acetaminophen *on page 446*
Zanaflex® *see* tizanidine *on page 872*
Zanaflex Capsules® *see* tizanidine *on page 872*

zanamivir (za NA mi veer)

Medication Safety Issues
  Sound-alike/look-alike issues:
    Relenza® may be confused with Albenza®, Aplenzin™
U.S. Brand Names Relenza®
Canadian Brand Names Relenza®
Therapeutic Category Antiviral Agent, Inhalation Therapy
Use Treatment of uncomplicated acute illness due to influenza virus A and B in patients who have been symptomatic for no more than 2 days; prophylaxis against influenza virus A and B

The Advisory Committee on Immunization Practices (ACIP) recommends that **treatment** be considered for the following:
  • Persons with severe, complicated or progressive illness
  • Hospitalized persons

- Persons at higher risk for influenza complications:
  - Children <2 years of age (highest risk in children <6 months of age)
  - Adults ≥65 years of age
  - Persons with chronic disorders of the pulmonary (including asthma) or cardiovascular systems (except hypertension)
  - Persons with chronic metabolic diseases (including diabetes mellitus), hepatic disease, renal dysfunction, hematologic disorders (including sickle cell disease), or immunosuppression (including immunosuppression caused by medications or HIV)
  - Persons with neurologic/neuromuscular conditions (including conditions such as spinal cord injuries, seizure disorders, cerebral palsy, stroke, mental retardation, moderate to severe developmental delay, or muscular dystrophy) which may compromise respiratory function, the handling of respiratory secretions, or that can increase the risk of aspiration
  - Pregnant or postpartum women (≤2 weeks after delivery)
  - Persons <19 years of age on long-term aspirin therapy
  - American Indians and Alaskan Natives
  - Persons who are morbidly obese (BMI ≥40)
  - Residents of nursing homes or other chronic care facilities
- Use may also be considered for previously healthy, nonhigh-risk outpatients with confirmed or suspected influenza based on clinical judgment when treatment can be started within 48 hours of illness onset.

The ACIP recommends that **prophylaxis** be considered for the following:
- Postexposure prophylaxis may be considered for family or close contacts of suspected or confirmed cases, who are at higher risk of influenza complications, and who have not been vaccinated against the circulating strain at the time of the exposure.
- Postexposure prophylaxis may be considered for unvaccinated healthcare workers who had occupational exposure without protective equipment.
- Preexposure prophylaxis should only be used for persons at very high risk of influenza complications who cannot be otherwise protected at times of high risk for exposure.
- Prophylaxis should also be administered to all eligible residents of institutions that house patients at high risk when needed to control outbreaks.

General Dosage Range Oral inhalation:
Children ≥5 years: Prophylaxis: 10 mg once daily
Children ≥7 years: Treatment: 10 mg twice daily
Adolescents and Adults: Prophylaxis: 10 mg once to twice daily; Treatment: 10 mg twice daily

Dosage Forms
Powder, for oral inhalation:
Relenza®: 5 mg/blister (20s)

Zanosar® see streptozocin *on page 831*

Zantac® see ranitidine *on page 767*

Zantac 75® [OTC] see ranitidine *on page 767*

Zantac 75® (Can) see ranitidine *on page 767*

Zantac 150® [OTC] see ranitidine *on page 767*

Zantac® EFFERdose® see ranitidine *on page 767*

Zantac Maximum Strength Non-Prescription (Can) see ranitidine *on page 767*

Zapzyt® [OTC] see benzoyl peroxide *on page 124*

Zapzyt® Acne Wash [OTC] see salicylic acid *on page 795*

Zapzyt® Pore Treatment [OTC] see salicylic acid *on page 795*

Zarah® see ethinyl estradiol and drospirenone *on page 352*

Zarontin® see ethosuximide *on page 358*

Zaroxolyn® see metolazone *on page 581*

Zavesca® see miglustat *on page 589*

Zazole™ [DSC] see terconazole *on page 853*

Z-chlopenthixol see zuclopenthixol *(Canada only) on page 935*

ZD1033 see anastrozole *on page 79*

ZD1694 see raltitrexed *(Canada only) on page 765*

ZD1839 see gefitinib *on page 412*

ZD6474 see vandetanib *on page 907*

ZD9238 see fulvestrant *on page 404*

ZDV *see* zidovudine *on page* 929

ZDV, abacavir, and lamivudine *see* abacavir, lamivudine, and zidovudine *on page* 20

ZDX *see* goserelin *on page* 424

Zeasorb®-AF [OTC] *see* miconazole (topical) *on page* 585

Zebeta® *see* bisoprolol *on page* 136

Zebutal® *see* butalbital, acetaminophen, and caffeine *on page* 152

Zegerid® *see* omeprazole and sodium bicarbonate *on page* 650

Zegerid OTC™ [OTC] *see* omeprazole and sodium bicarbonate *on page* 650

Zelapar® *see* selegiline *on page* 806

Zelboraf™ *see* vemurafenib *on page* 911

Zeldox *see* ziprasidone *on page* 931

Zeldox® (Can) *see* ziprasidone *on page* 931

Zelnorm® *see* tegaserod *on page* 846

Zelnorm® [DSC] (Can) *see* tegaserod *on page* 846

Zemaira® *see* alpha$_1$-proteinase inhibitor *on page* 55

Zemplar® *see* paricalcitol *on page* 675

Zemuron® *see* rocuronium *on page* 788

Zenapax® [DSC] *see* daclizumab *on page* 249

Zenapax® (Can) *see* daclizumab *on page* 249

Zenchent™ *see* ethinyl estradiol and norethindrone *on page* 355

Zenhale™ (Can) *see* mometasone and formoterol *on page* 596

Zenpep™ *see* pancrelipase *on page* 670

Zeosa™ *see* ethinyl estradiol and norethindrone *on page* 355

Zerit® *see* stavudine *on page* 830

ZerLor™ [DSC] *see* acetaminophen, caffeine, and dihydrocodeine *on page* 30

Zestoretic® *see* lisinopril and hydrochlorothiazide *on page* 532

Zestril® *see* lisinopril *on page* 531

Zetar® [OTC] *see* coal tar *on page* 227

Zetia® *see* ezetimibe *on page* 364

Zevalin® *see* ibritumomab *on page* 460

Zgesic *see* acetaminophen and phenyltoloxamine *on page* 28

Ziac® *see* bisoprolol and hydrochlorothiazide *on page* 136

Ziagen® *see* abacavir *on page* 20

Ziana™ *see* clindamycin and tretinoin *on page* 219

ziconotide (zi KOE no tide)

Medication Safety Issues
High alert medication:
The Institute for Safe Medication Practices (ISMP) includes this medication among its list of drugs which have a heightened risk of causing significant patient harm when used in error.

U.S. Brand Names Prialt®

Therapeutic Category Analgesic, Nonnarcotic; Calcium Channel Blocker, N-Type

Use Management of severe chronic pain in patients requiring intrathecal (I.T.) therapy and who are intolerant or refractory to other therapies

General Dosage Range Dosage adjustment recommended in patients who develop toxicities
I.T.: *Adults:* Initial dose: ≤2.4 mcg/day (0.1 mcg/hour); Maintenance range: 2.4-19.2 mcg/day (0.1-0.8 mcg/hour) (maximum: 19.2 mcg/day [0.8 mcg/hour])

Dosage Forms
Injection, solution [preservative free]:
Prialt®: 25 mcg/mL (20 mL); 100 mcg/mL (1 mL, 5 mL)

Zictifa *see* vandetanib *on page* 907

zidovudine (zye DOE vyoo deen)

Medication Safety Issues
Sound-alike/look-alike issues:
Azidothymidine may be confused with azaTHIOprine, aztreonam
Retrovir® may be confused with acyclovir, ritonavir
Other safety concerns:
AZT is an error-prone abbreviation (mistaken as azathioprine, aztreonam)

Synonyms azidothymidine; AZT (error-prone abbreviation); compound S; ZDV

U.S. Brand Names Retrovir®

Canadian Brand Names Apo-Zidovudine®; AZT™; Novo-AZT; Retrovir®; Retrovir® (AZT™)

Therapeutic Category Antiviral Agent

Use Treatment of HIV infection in combination with at least two other antiretroviral agents; prevention of maternal/fetal HIV transmission as monotherapy

General Dosage Range Dosage adjustment recommended in patients with renal impairment or who develop toxicities

I.V.:
Infants <30 weeks gestation at birth: 1.5 mg/kg/dose every 12 hours; at 4 weeks of age advance to 1.5 mg/kg/dose every 8 hours
Infants ≥30 weeks and <35 weeks gestation at birth: 2 mg/kg/dose every 12 hours; at 2 weeks of age, advance to 1.5 mg/kg/dose every 8 hours
Infants (full term): 1.5 mg/kg/dose every 6 hours
Children 6 weeks to <12 years: 120 mg/m^2/dose every 6 hours **or** 20 mg/m^2/hour as a continuous infusion
Children ≥12 years and Adults: 1 mg/kg/dose every 4 hours around-the-clock **or** 2 mg/kg bolus followed by 1 mg/kg/hour continuous infusion

Oral:
Infants <30 weeks gestation at birth: 2 mg/kg/dose every 12 hours; at 4 weeks of age advance to 2 mg/kg/dose every 8 hours
Infants ≥30 weeks and <35 weeks gestation at birth: 2 mg/kg/dose every 12 hours; at 2 weeks of age, advance to 2 mg/kg/dose every 8 hours
Infants (full term): 2 mg/kg/dose every 6 hours
Children 4 weeks to <18 years: 240 mg/m^2 every 12 hours (maximum 300 mg every 12 hours) **or** 160 mg/m^2/dose every 8 hours (maximum: 200 mg every 8 hours)
4 to <9 kg: 12 mg/kg/dose twice daily **or** 8 mg/kg/dose 3 times/day
≥9 to <30 kg: 9 mg/kg/dose twice daily **or** 6 mg/kg/dose 3 times/day
≥30 kg and Adults: 300 mg twice daily **or** 200 mg 3 times/day

Dosage Forms
Capsule, oral: 100 mg
Retrovir®: 100 mg
Injection, solution [preservative free]:
Retrovir®: 10 mg/mL (20 mL)
Syrup, oral: 50 mg/5 mL (240 mL)
Retrovir®: 50 mg/5 mL (240 mL)
Tablet, oral: 300 mg
Retrovir®: 300 mg

zileuton (zye LOO ton)

U.S. Brand Names Zyflo CR®; Zyflo®

Therapeutic Category 5-Lipoxygenase Inhibitor

Use Prophylaxis and chronic treatment of asthma

General Dosage Range Oral:
Extended release: *Children ≥12 years and Adults:* 1200 mg twice daily
Immediate release: *Children ≥12 years and Adults:* 600 mg 4 times/day
Dosage Forms
Tablet, oral:
Zyflo®: 600 mg [scored]
Tablet, extended release, oral:
Zyflo CR®: 600 mg

Zinacef® *see* cefuroxime *on page 185*
zinc *see* trace metals *on page 880*
Zinc 15 [OTC] *see* zinc sulfate *on page 931*

zinc acetate (zink AS e tate)
U.S. Brand Names Galzin®
Therapeutic Category Trace Element
Use Maintenance treatment of Wilson disease following initial chelation therapy
General Dosage Range Oral:
Children ≥10 years and Adults (pregnant females): 75-150 mg/day in 3 divided doses
Adults (males and nonpregnant females): 150 mg/day in 3 divided doses
Dosage Forms
Capsule, oral:
Galzin®: Elemental zinc 25 mg, Elemental zinc 50 mg

Zincate® *see* zinc sulfate *on page 931*

zinc chloride (zink KLOR ide)
Therapeutic Category Trace Element
Use Cofactor for replacement therapy to different enzymes; helps maintain normal growth rates, normal skin hydration, and senses of taste and smell
General Dosage Range I.V.:
Premature infants <1500 g up to 3 kg: 300 mcg/kg/day
Infants (full term) and Children ≤5 years: 100 mcg/kg/day to I.V. fluid
Adults: 2-6 mg/day, up to 12.2 mg/L TPN **or** 17.1 mg/kg of stool or ileostomy output
Dosage Forms
Injection, solution [preservative free]: 1 mg/mL (10 mL)

zinc diethylenetriaminepentaacetate (Zn-DTPA) *see* diethylene triamine penta-acetic acid *on page 281*
Zincfrin® (Can) *see* phenylephrine and zinc sulfate *(Canada only) on page 698*

zinc gelatin (zink JEL ah tin)
Synonyms dome paste bandage; Unna boot; Unna paste; zinc gelatin boot
U.S. Brand Names Gelucast®
Therapeutic Category Protectant, Topical
Use As a protectant and to support varicosities and similar lesions of the lower limbs
General Dosage Range Topical: *Adults:* Apply externally as an occlusive boot
Dosage Forms
Bandage: 3" x 10 yards; 4" x 10 yards
Gelucast®: 3" x 10 yards; 4" x 10 yards

zinc gelatin boot *see* zinc gelatin *on page 930*
Zincofax® (Can) *see* zinc oxide *on page 930*
Zincon® [OTC] *see* pyrithione zinc *on page 759*

zinc oxide (zink OKS ide)
Synonyms base ointment; lassar's zinc paste
U.S. Brand Names Ammens® Original Medicated [OTC]; Ammens® Shower Fresh [OTC]; Balmex® [OTC]; Boudreaux's® Butt Paste [OTC]; Critic-Aid Skin Care® [OTC]; Desitin® Creamy [OTC]; Desitin® [OTC]

Canadian Brand Names Zincofax®

Therapeutic Category Topical Skin Product

Use Protective coating for mild skin irritations and abrasions; soothing and protective ointment to promote healing of chapped skin, diaper rash

General Dosage Range Topical: *Children and Adults:* Apply as required to affected areas several times daily

Dosage Forms

Cream, topical:
  Balmex® [OTC]: 11.3% (60 g, 120 g, 480 g)
Cream, topical [stick]:
  Balmex® [OTC]: 11.3% (56 g)
Ointment, topical: 20% (30 g, 60 g, 454 g); 40% (120 g)
  Desitin® [OTC]: 40% (30 g, 60 g, 90 g, 120 g, 270 g, 480 g)
  Desitin® Creamy [OTC]: 10% (60 g, 120 g)
Paste, topical:
  Boudreaux's® Butt Paste [OTC]: 16% (30 g, 60 g, 120 g, 480 g)
  Critic-Aid Skin Care® [OTC]: 20% (71 g, 170 g)
Powder, topical:
  Ammens® Original Medicated [OTC], Ammens® Shower Fresh [OTC]: 9.1% (312 g)

zinc oxide and miconazole nitrate *see* miconazole and zinc oxide *on page 586*

zinc sulfate (zink SUL fate)

Medication Safety Issues
  Sound-alike/look-alike issues:
    ZnSO₄ is an error-prone abbreviation (mistaken as morphine sulfate)

Synonyms ZnSO₄ (error-prone abbreviation)

U.S. Brand Names Orazinc® 110 [OTC]; Orazinc® 220 [OTC]; Zinc 15 [OTC]; Zincate®

Canadian Brand Names Anuzinc; Rivasol

Therapeutic Category Electrolyte Supplement, Oral

Use Zinc supplement (oral and parenteral); may improve wound healing in those who are deficient

General Dosage Range

I.V.:
  Premature infants (<1500 g up to 3 kg): 300 mcg/kg/day
  Infants (full term) and Children ≤5 years: 100 mcg/kg/day
  Adults: 2.5-6 mg/day **or** 12.2 mg/L of TPN **or** 17.1 mg/kg of stool or ileostomy output
Oral:
  Children: 0.5-1 mg elemental zinc/kg/day divided in 1-3 doses
  Adults: 110-220 mg (25-50 mg elemental zinc) 3 times/day

Dosage Forms

Capsule, oral: 220 mg
  Orazinc® 220 [OTC]: 220 mg
  Zincate®: 220 mg
Injection, solution [preservative free]: Elemental zinc 1 mg/mL (10 mL); Elemental zinc 5 mg/mL (5 mL)
Tablet, oral: 220 mg
  Orazinc® 110 [OTC]: 110 mg
  Zinc 15 [OTC]: 66 mg

zinc sulfate and phenylephrine *see* phenylephrine and zinc sulfate *(Canada only) on page 698*
zinc undecylenate *see* undecylenic acid and derivatives *on page 899*
Zinecard® *see* dexrazoxane *on page 267*

ziprasidone (zi PRAS i done)

Medication Safety Issues
  Sound-alike/look-alike issues:
    Ziprasidone may be confused with TraZODone

Synonyms Zeldox; ziprasidone hydrochloride; ziprasidone mesylate

U.S. Brand Names Geodon®

Canadian Brand Names Zeldox®

Therapeutic Category Antipsychotic Agent

Use Treatment of schizophrenia; treatment of acute manic or mixed episodes associated with bipolar disorder with or without psychosis; maintenance treatment of bipolar disorder as an adjunct to lithium or valproate; acute agitation in patients with schizophrenia

General Dosage Range
I.M.: *Adults:* 10 mg every 2 hours **or** 20 mg every 4 hours (maximum: 40 mg/day)
Oral: *Adults:* Initial: 20-40 mg twice daily; Maintenance: 20-80 mg twice daily (maximum: 200 mg/day)

Dosage Forms
Capsule, oral:
Geodon®: 20 mg, 40 mg, 60 mg, 80 mg
Injection, powder for reconstitution:
Geodon®: 20 mg

ziprasidone hydrochloride *see* ziprasidone *on page 931*
ziprasidone mesylate *see* ziprasidone *on page 931*
Zipsor™ *see* diclofenac (systemic) *on page 277*
Zirgan® *see* ganciclovir (ophthalmic) *on page 410*
Zithranol®-RR *see* anthralin *on page 80*
Zithromax® *see* azithromycin (systemic) *on page 108*
Zithromax® TRI-PAK™ *see* azithromycin (systemic) *on page 108*
Zithromax® Z-PAK® *see* azithromycin (systemic) *on page 108*
Zmax® *see* azithromycin (systemic) *on page 108*
Zn-DTPA *see* diethylene triamine penta-acetic acid *on page 281*
ZNP® [OTC] *see* pyrithione zinc *on page 759*
ZnSO₄ (error-prone abbreviation) *see* zinc sulfate *on page 931*
Zocor® *see* simvastatin *on page 813*
ZoDerm® *see* benzoyl peroxide *on page 124*
ZoDerm® Hydrating Wash™ *see* benzoyl peroxide *on page 124*
ZoDerm® Redi-Pads™ *see* benzoyl peroxide *on page 124*
Zofran® *see* ondansetron *on page 651*
Zofran® ODT *see* ondansetron *on page 651*
zol 446 *see* zoledronic acid *on page 932*
Zoladex® *see* goserelin *on page 424*
Zoladex® LA (Can) *see* goserelin *on page 424*
zoledronate *see* zoledronic acid *on page 932*

zoledronic acid (zoe le DRON ik AS id)

Medication Safety Issues
Sound-alike/look-alike issues:
Zometa® may be confused with Zofran®, Zoladex®
Other safety concerns:
Duplicate therapy issues: Reclast® and Aclasta® contain zoledronic acid, which is the same ingredient contained in Zometa®; patients receiving Zometa® should not be treated with Reclast® or Aclasta®

Synonyms CGP-42446; zol 446; zoledronate
U.S. Brand Names Reclast®; Zometa®
Canadian Brand Names Aclasta®; Zometa®
Therapeutic Category Bisphosphonate Derivative
Use
Oncology-related uses: Treatment of hypercalcemia of malignancy (albumin-corrected serum calcium >12 mg/dL); treatment of multiple myeloma; treatment of bone metastases of solid tumors
Nononcology uses: Treatment of Paget disease of bone; treatment of osteoporosis in postmenopausal women (to reduce the incidence of fractures or to reduce the incidence of new clinical fractures in patients with low-trauma hip fracture); prevention of osteoporosis in postmenopausal women, treatment of osteoporosis in men (to increase bone mass); treatment and prevention of glucocorticoid-induced osteoporosis (in patients initiating or continuing prednisone ≥7.5 mg/day [or equivalent] and expected to remain on glucocorticoids for at least 12 months)

General Dosage Range
I.V.:
Children: Dosage not established
Adults:
Zometa®: 4 mg as a single dose [hypercalcemia of malignancy] or 4 mg every 3-4 weeks [multiple myeloma or metastatic bone lesions]
Reclast®: 5 mg [Paget disease] or 5 mg once a year or every 2 years [osteoporosis]
Dosage Forms
Infusion, premixed:
Reclast®: 5 mg (100 mL)
Zometa®: 4 mg (100 mL)
Injection, solution:
Zometa®: 4 mg/5 mL (5 mL)
Dosage Forms - Canada
Infusion, solution [premixed]:
Aclasta®: 5 mg (100 mL)

Zolinza® *see* vorinostat *on page 921*

zolmitriptan (zohl mi TRIP tan)
Medication Safety Issues
Sound-alike/look-alike issues:
ZOLMitriptan may be confused with SUMAtriptan
Synonyms 311C90
Tall-Man ZOLMitriptan
U.S. Brand Names Zomig-ZMT®; Zomig®
Canadian Brand Names Mylan-Zolmitriptan; PMS-Zolmitriptan; PMS-Zolmitriptan ODT; Sandoz-Zolmitriptan; Sandoz-Zolmitriptan ODT; Teva-Zolmitriptan; Teva-Zolmitriptan OD; Zomig®; Zomig® Nasal Spray; Zomig® Rapimelt
Therapeutic Category Antimigraine Agent; Serotonin Agonist
Use Acute treatment of migraine with or without aura
General Dosage Range Dosage adjustment recommended in patients with hepatic impairment
Nasal inhalation: *Adults:* 1 spray (5 mg) at the onset of migraine headache; may repeat in 2 hours if no relief (maximum: 10 mg/24 hours)
Oral: *Adults:* 1.25-2.5 mg at the onset of migraine headache; may repeat in 2 hours if no relief (maximum: 10 mg/24 hours)
Dosage Forms
Solution, intranasal:
Zomig®: 5 mg/0.1 mL (0.1 mL)
Tablet, oral:
Zomig®: 2.5 mg, 5 mg
Tablet, orally disintegrating, oral:
Zomig-ZMT®: 2.5 mg, 5 mg

Zoloft® *see* sertraline *on page 809*

zolpidem (zole PI dem)
Medication Safety Issues
Sound-alike/look-alike issues:
Ambien® may be confused with Abilify®, Ativan®, Ambi 10®
Zolpidem may be confused with lorazepam, zaleplon
International issues:
Ambien® may be confused with Ambyen which is a brand name for amiodarone in Great Britain
Synonyms zolpidem tartrate
U.S. Brand Names Ambien CR®; Ambien®; Edluar™; Zolpimist®
Therapeutic Category Hypnotic, Nonbarbiturate
Controlled Substance C-IV
Use
Ambien®, Edluar™, Zolpimist®: Short-term treatment of insomnia (with difficulty of sleep onset)
Ambien CR®: Treatment of insomnia (with difficulty of sleep onset and/or sleep maintenance)

◀ **General Dosage Range** Dosage adjustment recommended in patients with hepatic impairment.
Oral:
Immediate release tablet, spray, sublingual tablet:
Adults: 10 mg immediately before bedtime
Elderly: 5 mg immediately before bedtime
Extended release tablet:
Adults: 12.5 mg immediately before bedtime
Elderly: 6.25 mg immediately before bedtime
Dosage Forms
Solution, oral:
Zolpimist®: 5 mg/actuation (8.2 g)
Tablet, oral: 5 mg, 10 mg
Ambien®: 5 mg, 10 mg
Tablet, sublingual:
Edluar™: 5 mg, 10 mg
Tablet, extended release, oral: 6.25 mg, 12.5 mg
Ambien CR®: 6.25 mg, 12.5 mg

zolpidem tartrate *see* zolpidem *on page 933*
Zolpimist® *see* zolpidem *on page 933*
Zolvit™ *see* hydrocodone and acetaminophen *on page 446*
Zometa® *see* zoledronic acid *on page 932*
Zomig® *see* zolmitriptan *on page 933*
Zomig® Nasal Spray (Can) *see* zolmitriptan *on page 933*
Zomig® Rapimelt (Can) *see* zolmitriptan *on page 933*
Zomig-ZMT® *see* zolmitriptan *on page 933*
Zonalon® *see* doxepin (topical) *on page 309*
Zonatuss™ *see* benzonatate *on page 124*
Zonegran® *see* zonisamide *on page 934*

zonisamide (zoe NIS a mide)
Medication Safety Issues
Sound-alike/look-alike issues:
Zonegran® may be confused with SINEquan®
Zonisamide may be confused with lacosamide
U.S. Brand Names Zonegran®
Therapeutic Category Anticonvulsant, Sulfonamide
Use Adjunct treatment of partial seizures in children >16 years of age and adults with epilepsy
General Dosage Range Oral: *Children >16 years and Adults:* Initial: 100 mg/day; Maintenance: 100-600 mg/day (maximum: 600 mg/day)
Dosage Forms
Capsule, oral: 25 mg, 50 mg, 100 mg
Zonegran®: 25 mg, 100 mg

zopiclone *(Canada only)* (ZOE pi clone)
Canadian Brand Names Apo-Zopiclone®; CO Zopiclone; Dom-Zopiclone; Imovane®; Mylan-Zopiclone; Novo-Zopiclone; Nu-Zopiclone; PHL-Zopiclone; PMS-Zopiclone; PRO-Zopiclone; RAN™-Zopiclone; ratio-Zopiclone; Rhovane®; Riva-Zopiclone; Sandoz-Zopiclone
Therapeutic Category Hypnotic
Use Short-term and symptomatic relief of insomnia
General Dosage Range Dosage adjustment recommended in patients with hepatic and renal impairment, elderly and debilitated patients, and patients with chronic respiratory insufficiency.
Oral:
Adults: 3.75-7.5 mg once daily at bedtime
Elderly: Initial: 3.75 mg once daily at bedtime
Product Availability Not available in U.S.
Dosage Forms - Canada
Tablet, oral: 5 mg, 7.5 mg

Zorbtive® *see* somatropin *on page 826*
Zorcaine™ *see* articaine and epinephrine *on page 95*
Zortress® *see* everolimus *on page 362*
ZOS *see* zoster vaccine *on page 935*
Zostavax® *see* zoster vaccine *on page 935*

zoster vaccine (ZOS ter vak SEEN)

Medication Safety Issues
  Administration issues:
    Both varicella vaccine and zoster vaccine are live, attenuated strains of varicella-zoster virus. Their indications, dosing, and composition are distinct. Varicella vaccine is indicated for the prevention of chickenpox, while zoster vaccine is indicated in older individuals to prevent reactivation of the virus which causes shingles. Zoster vaccine is **not** a substitute for varicella vaccine and should not be used in children.

Synonyms shingles vaccine; varicella-zoster (VZV) vaccine (zoster); VZV vaccine (zoster); ZOS
U.S. Brand Names Zostavax®
Canadian Brand Names Zostavax®
Therapeutic Category Vaccine
Use Prevention of herpes zoster (shingles) in patients ≥50 years of age
  The Advisory Committee on Immunization Practices (ACIP) recommends routine vaccination of all patients ≥60 years of age, including:
  • Patients who report a previous episode of zoster.
  • Patients with chronic medical conditions (eg, chronic renal failure, diabetes mellitus, rheumatoid arthritis, chronic pulmonary disease) unless those conditions are contraindications.
  • Residents of nursing homes and other long-term care facilities ≥60 years of age, without contraindications.
General Dosage Range SubQ: *Adults ≥50 years:* 0.65 mL as a single dose
Dosage Forms
  Injection, powder for reconstitution [preservative free]:
    Zostavax®: 19,400 PFU

Zostrix® [OTC] *see* capsaicin *on page 169*
Zostrix® (Can) *see* capsaicin *on page 169*
Zostrix® Diabetic Foot Pain [OTC] *see* capsaicin *on page 169*
Zostrix®-HP [OTC] *see* capsaicin *on page 169*
Zostrix® H.P. (Can) *see* capsaicin *on page 169*
Zosyn® *see* piperacillin and tazobactam sodium *on page 707*
Zovia® *see* ethinyl estradiol and ethynodiol diacetate *on page 353*
Zovirax® *see* acyclovir (systemic) *on page 39*
Zovirax® *see* acyclovir (topical) *on page 39*
Z-Pak *see* azithromycin (systemic) *on page 108*
zuclopenthixol acetate *see* zuclopenthixol *(Canada only) on page 935*

zuclopenthixol *(Canada only)* (zoo kloe pen THIX ol)

Synonyms Z-chlopenthixol; zuclopenthixol acetate; zuclopenthixol decanoate; zuclopenthixol dihydrochloride
Canadian Brand Names Clopixol-Acuphase®; Clopixol®; Clopixol® Depot
Therapeutic Category Antipsychotic Agent
Use Management of schizophrenia; acetate injection is intended for short-term acute treatment; decanoate injection is for long-term management; hydrochloride tablets may be used in either the initial or maintenance phase
General Dosage Range
  I.M.: *Adults:* Acetate: Initial: 50-150 mg, may repeat in 2-3 days (maximum: 4 doses or 400 mg during treatment course; maximum treatment course: 2 weeks); Decanoate: Initial: 100-400 mg every 2 weeks (usual maintenance: 150-300 mg every 2-4 weeks)
  Oral: *Adults:* Initial: 10-50 mg/day in 2-3 divided doses; usual dosage range for acute therapy: 20-60 mg/day (maximum: 100 mg/day); usual maintenance dose: 20-40 mg/day
Product Availability Not available in U.S.

◀ **Dosage Forms - Canada**
Injection:
Clopixol Acuphase®: 50 mg/mL [zuclopenthixol 42.5 mg/mL] (1 mL, 2 mL)
Clopixol® Depot: 200 mg/mL [zuclopenthixol 144.4 mg/mL] (10 mL)
Tablet, oral:
Clopixol®: 10 mg, 25 mg, 40 mg

zuclopenthixol decanoate *see* zuclopenthixol *(Canada only) on page 935*
zuclopenthixol dihydrochloride *see* zuclopenthixol *(Canada only) on page 935*
Zuplenz® *see* ondansetron *on page 651*
Zutripro™ *see* hydrocodone, chlorpheniramine, and pseudoephedrine *on page 449*
Zyban® *see* bupropion *on page 150*
Zyclara® *see* imiquimod *on page 467*
Zydone® *see* hydrocodone and acetaminophen *on page 446*
Zyflo® *see* zileuton *on page 929*
Zyflo CR® *see* zileuton *on page 929*
Zylet® *see* loteprednol and tobramycin *on page 539*
Zyloprim® *see* allopurinol *on page 54*
ZYM-Amlodipine (Can) *see* amlodipine *on page 69*
Zymar® [DSC] *see* gatifloxacin *on page 411*
Zymar® (Can) *see* gatifloxacin *on page 411*
Zymaxid™ *see* gatifloxacin *on page 411*
ZYM-Bisoprolol (Can) *see* bisoprolol *on page 136*
ZYM-Carvedilol (Can) *see* carvedilol *on page 178*
ZYM-Cholestyramine-Light (Can) *see* cholestyramine resin *on page 205*
ZYM-Cholestyramine-Regular (Can) *see* cholestyramine resin *on page 205*
ZYM-Clonazepam (Can) *see* clonazepam *on page 222*
ZYM-Fluconazole (Can) *see* fluconazole *on page 381*
ZYM-Fluoxetine (Can) *see* fluoxetine *on page 389*
ZYM-Mirtazapine (Can) *see* mirtazapine *on page 592*
ZYM-Ondansetron (Can) *see* ondansetron *on page 651*
ZYM-Pioglitazone (Can) *see* pioglitazone *on page 706*
ZYM-Pravastatin (Can) *see* pravastatin *on page 732*
ZYM-Simvastatin (Can) *see* simvastatin *on page 813*
ZYM-Sotalol (Can) *see* sotalol *on page 828*
ZYM-Topiramate (Can) *see* topiramate *on page 877*
ZYM-Trazodone (Can) *see* trazodone *on page 884*
Zypram™ *see* pramoxine and hydrocortisone *on page 731*
ZyPREXA® *see* olanzapine *on page 645*
Zyprexa® (Can) *see* olanzapine *on page 645*
ZyPREXA® IntraMuscular *see* olanzapine *on page 645*
Zyprexa® Intramuscular (Can) *see* olanzapine *on page 645*
ZyPREXA® Relprevv™ *see* olanzapine *on page 645*
ZyPREXA® Zydis® *see* olanzapine *on page 645*
Zyprexa® Zydis® (Can) *see* olanzapine *on page 645*
ZyrTEC-D® Allergy & Congestion [OTC] *see* cetirizine and pseudoephedrine *on page 189*
ZyrTEC® Allergy [OTC] *see* cetirizine *on page 189*
ZyrTEC® Children's Allergy [OTC] *see* cetirizine *on page 189*
ZyrTEC® Children's Hives Relief [OTC] *see* cetirizine *on page 189*
ZyrTEC® Itchy Eye [OTC] *see* ketotifen (ophthalmic) *on page 503*
Zytiga™ *see* abiraterone acetate *on page 21*
Zytopic™ *see* triamcinolone (topical) *on page 887*
Zytram® XL (Can) *see* tramadol *on page 880*
Zyvox® *see* linezolid *on page 529*
Zyvoxam® (Can) *see* linezolid *on page 529*

CHEMOTHERAPY REGIMENS

5 + 2 (Cytarabine-Daunorubicin) (AML Induction)

Use Leukemia, acute myeloid

Regimen
Cytarabine: I.V.: 100 mg/m^2/day continuous infusion days 1 to 5
[total dose/cycle = 500 mg/m^2]
Daunorubicin: I.V.: 45 mg/m^2/day I.V. bolus days 1 and 2
[total dose/cycle = 90 mg/m^2]
May administer a second induction cycle if needed

5 + 2 (Cytarabine-Daunorubicin) (AML Postremission)

Use Leukemia, acute myeloid

Regimen
Cytarabine: I.V.: 100 mg/m^2/day continuous infusion days 1 to 5
[total dose/cycle = 500 mg/m^2]
Daunorubicin: I.V.: 45 mg/m^2/day I.V. bolus days 1 and 2
[total dose/cycle = 90 mg/m^2]
Administer 2 courses

5 + 2 + 5 (Cytarabine-Daunorubicin-Etoposide) (AML Consolidation)

Use Leukemia, acute myeloid

Regimen
Cytarabine: I.V.: 100 mg/m^2/day continuous infusion days 1 to 5
[total dose/cycle = 500 mg/m^2]
Daunorubicin: I.V.: 50 mg/m^2/day I.V. bolus days 1 and 2
[total dose/cycle = 100 mg/m^2]
Etoposide: I.V.: 75 mg/m^2/day over 1 hour days 1 to 5
[total dose/cycle = 375 mg/m^2]
Administer 2 courses

5 + 2 (Cytarabine-Idarubicin) (AML Consolidation)

Use Leukemia, acute myeloid

Regimen
Cytarabine: I.V.: 100 mg/m^2/day continuous infusion days 1 to 5
[total dose/cycle = 500 mg/m^2]
Idarubicin: I.V.: 13 mg/m^2/day I.V. bolus days 1 and 2
[total dose/cycle = 26 mg/m^2]
Administer 2 courses

5 + 2 (Cytarabine-Mitoxantrone) (AML Consolidation)

Use Leukemia, acute myeloid

Regimen
Cytarabine: I.V.: 100 mg/m^2/day continuous infusion days 1 to 5
[total dose/cycle = 500 mg/m^2]
Mitoxantrone: I.V.: 12 mg/m^2/day days 1 and 2
[total dose/cycle = 24 mg/m^2]
Administered every 28 days for a total of 2 cycles

7 + 3 + 7 (Cytarabine-Daunorubicin-Etoposide) (AML Induction)

Use Leukemia, acute myeloid

Regimen
Cytarabine: I.V.: 100 mg/m^2/day continuous infusion days 1 to 7
[total dose/cycle = 700 mg/m^2]
Daunorubicin: I.V.: 50 mg/m^2/day days 1, 2, and 3
[total dose/cycle = 150 mg/m^2]
Etoposide: I.V.: 75 mg/m^2/day over 1 hour days 1 to 7
[total dose/cycle = 525 mg/m^2]
Up to 3 induction cycles may be given based on individual response

7 + 3 (Cytarabine-Daunorubicin) (AML Induction)

Use Leukemia, acute myeloid

Regimen NOTE: Multiple variations are listed.

Variation 1:
 Cytarabine: I.V.: 100 mg/m^2/day continuous infusion days 1 to 7
  [total dose/cycle = 700 mg/m^2]
 Daunorubicin: I.V.: 45 mg/m^2/day I.V. bolus days 1, 2, and 3
  [total dose/cycle = 135 mg/m^2]
 May administer a second induction cycle if needed

Variation 2 (≥60 years of age):
 Cytarabine: I.V.: 100 mg/m^2/day continuous infusion days 1 to 7
  [total dose/cycle = 700 mg/m^2]
 Daunorubicin: I.V.: 30 mg/m^2/day days 1, 2, and 3
  [total dose/cycle = 90 mg/m^2]
 May administer a second induction cycle if needed (at a reduced dose of daunorubicin [45 mg/m^2])

Variation 3 (between 17 and 60 years of age):
 Cytarabine: I.V.: 100 mg/m^2/day continuous infusion days 1 to 7
  [total dose/cycle = 700 mg/m^2]
 Daunorubicin: I.V.: 90 mg/m^2/day I.V. bolus days 1, 2, and 3
  [total dose/cycle = 270 mg/m^2]
 May administer a second induction cycle if needed

Variation 4 (<60 years of age):
 Cytarabine: I.V.: 200 mg/m^2/day continuous infusion days 1 to 7
  [total dose/cycle = 1400 mg/m^2]
 Daunorubicin: I.V.: 45 mg/m^2/day I.V. bolus days 1, 2, and 3
  [total dose/cycle = 135 mg/m^2]
 May administer a second induction cycle if needed

7 + 3 (Cytarabine-Idarubicin) (AML Induction)

Use Leukemia, acute myeloid

Regimen NOTE: Multiple variations are listed.

Variation 1:
 Cytarabine: I.V.: 100 mg/m^2/day continuous infusion days 1 to 7
  [total dose/cycle = 700 mg/m^2]
 Idarubicin: I.V.: 12 mg/m^2/day slow I.V. infusion days 1, 2, and 3
  [total dose/cycle = 36 mg/m^2]
 May administer a second induction cycle if needed

Variation 2:
 Cytarabine: I.V.: 100 mg/m^2/day continuous infusion days 1 to 7
  [total dose/cycle = 700 mg/m^2]
 Idarubicin: I.V.: 13 mg/m^2/day slow I.V. infusion days 1, 2, and 3
  [total dose/cycle = 39 mg/m^2]
 May administer a second induction cycle if needed

7 + 3 (Cytarabine-Mitoxantrone) (AML Induction)

Use Leukemia, acute myeloid

Regimen

Induction:
 Cytarabine: I.V.: 100 mg/m^2/day continuous infusion days 1 to 7
  [total dose/cycle = 700 mg/m^2]
 Mitoxantrone: I.V.: 12 mg/m^2/day days 1, 2, and 3
  [total dose/cycle = 36 mg/m^2]

Reinduction if needed:
 Cytarabine: I.V.: 100 mg/m^2/day continuous infusion days 1 to 5
  [total dose/cycle = 500 mg/m^2]
 Mitoxantrone: I.V.: 12 mg/m^2/day days 1 and 2
  [total dose/cycle = 24 mg/m^2]

AAV (DD)

Use Wilms tumor

Regimen
Dactinomycin: I.V.: 15 mcg/kg/day days 1 to 5 of weeks 0, 13, 26, 39, 52, and 65
[total dose/cycle = 450 mcg/kg]
Doxorubicin: I.V.: 20 mg/m^2/day days 1, 2, and 3 of weeks 6, 19, 32, 45, and 58
[total dose/cycle = 300 mg/m^2]
Vincristine: I.V.: 1.5 mg/m^2 day 1 of weeks 0-10, 13, 14, 26, 27, 39, 40, 52, 53, 65, and 66
[total dose/cycle = 31.5 mg/m^2]

Abiraterone-Prednisone (Prostate Cancer)

Use Prostate cancer

Regimen
Abiraterone acetate: Oral: 1000 mg once a day
Prednisone: Oral: 5 mg twice a day

ABVD

Use Lymphoma, Hodgkin disease

Regimen
Doxorubicin: I.V.: 25 mg/m^2/day days 1 and 15
[total dose/cycle = 50 mg/m^2]
Bleomycin: I.V.: 10 units/m^2/day days 1 and 15
[total dose/cycle = 20 units/m^2]
Vinblastine: I.V.: 6 mg/m^2/day days 1 and 15
[total dose/cycle = 12 mg/m^2]
Dacarbazine: I.V.: 375 mg/m^2/day days 1 and 15
[total dose/cycle = 750 mg/m^2]
Repeat cycle every 28 days for 6-8 cycles

AC

Use Breast cancer

Regimen NOTE: Multiple variations are listed.
Variation 1: AC (conventional):
Doxorubicin: I.V.: 60 mg/m^2 day 1
[total dose/cycle = 60 mg/m^2]
Cyclophosphamide: I.V.: 600 mg/m^2 day 1
[total dose/cycle = 600 mg/m^2]
Repeat cycle every 21 days
Variation 2:
Cyclophosphamide: Oral: 200 mg/m^2/day days 3 to 6
[total dose/cycle = 800 mg/m^2]
Doxorubicin: I.V.: 40 mg/m^2 day 1
[total dose/cycle = 40 mg/m^2]
Repeat cycle every 3 weeks for 3 cycles, then every 4 weeks

AC/Paclitaxel (Sequential)

Use Breast cancer

Regimen
Variation 1: AC + Paclitaxel (conventional):
Doxorubicin: I.V.: 60 mg/m^2 day 1
[total dose/cycle = 60 mg/m^2]
Cyclophosphamide: I.V.: 600 mg/m^2 day 1
[total dose/cycle = 600 mg/m^2]
Repeat cycle every 21 days for 4 cycles
followed by
Paclitaxel: I.V.: 175 mg/m^2 day 1
[total dose/cycle = 175 mg/m^2]
Repeat cycle every 21 days for 4 cycles

Variation 2: AC + Paclitaxel (dose dense):
Doxorubicin: I.V.: 60 mg/m^2 day 1
[total dose/cycle = 60 mg/m^2]
Cyclophosphamide: I.V.: 600 mg/m^2 day 1
[total dose/cycle = 600 mg/m^2]
Filgrastim: SubQ: 5 mcg/kg/day days 3 to 10
[total dose/cycle = 40 mcg/kg]
Repeat cycle every 14 days for 4 cycles
followed by
Paclitaxel: I.V.: 175 mg/m^2 day 1
[total dose/cycle = 175 mg/m^2]
Filgrastim: SubQ: 5 mcg/kg/day days 3 to 10
[total dose/cycle = 40 mcg/kg]
Repeat cycle every 14 days for 4 cycles

AC-Paclitaxel-Trastuzumab

Use Breast cancer
Regimen NOTE: Multiple variations are listed.
Variation 1:
Doxorubicin: I.V.: 60 mg/m^2 day 1
[total dose/cycle = 60 mg/m^2]
Cyclophosphamide: I.V.: 600 mg/m^2 day 1
[total dose/cycle = 600 mg/m^2]
Repeat cycle every 21 days for 4 cycles
followed by
Paclitaxel: I.V.: 175 mg/m^2 day 1
[total dose/cycle = 175 mg/m^2]
Trastuzumab: I.V.: 4 mg/kg (loading dose) day 1 (cycle 1 only)
[total dose/cycle = 4 mg/kg]
  followed by I.V.: 2 mg/kg/day days 8 and 15 (cycle 1)
    [total dose/cycle = 4 mg/kg]
    then I.V.: 2 mg/kg/day days 1, 8, and 15 (cycles 2, 3, and 4)
      [total dose/cycle = 6 mg/kg]
Repeat cycle every 21 days for 4 cycles
followed by
Trastuzumab: I.V.: 2 mg/kg weekly for 40 weeks
Variation 2:
Doxorubicin: I.V.: 60 mg/m^2 day 1
[total dose/cycle = 60 mg/m^2]
Cyclophosphamide: I.V.: 600 mg/m^2 day 1
[total dose/cycle = 600 mg/m^2]
Repeat cycle every 21 days for 4 cycles
followed by
Paclitaxel: I.V.: 80 mg/m^2 day 1 week 13
[total dose/cycle = 80 mg/m^2]
Trastuzumab: I.V.: 4 mg/kg (loading dose) day 1 week 13 only
[total dose/cycle = 4 mg/kg]
followed by
Paclitaxel: I.V.: 80 mg/m^2 weekly
[total dose/cycle = 80 mg/m^2]
Trastuzumab: I.V.: 2 mg/kg /weekly
[total dose/cycle = 2 mg/kg]
Repeat cycle every week for 11 cycles
followed by
Trastuzumab: I.V.: 2 mg/kg/weekly for 40 weeks

AD

Use Soft tissue sarcoma

Regimen

NOTE: Multiple variations are listed.

Variation 1 (metastatic):

Doxorubicin: I.V.: 15 mg/m^2/day continuous infusion days 1 to 4

[total dose/cycle = 60 mg/m^2]

Dacarbazine: I.V.: 187.5 mg/m^2/day continuous infusion days 1 to 4

[total dose/cycle = 750 mg/m^2]

Repeat cycle every 21 days; maximum lifetime doxorubicin dose of 450 mg/m^2

Variation 2 (metastatic):

Doxorubicin: I.V.: 60 mg/m^2 I.V. bolus day 1

[total dose/cycle = 60 mg/m^2]

Dacarbazine: I.V.: 750 mg/m^2/day I.V. bolus day 1

[total dose/cycle = 750 mg/m^2]

Repeat cycle every 21 days; maximum lifetime doxorubicin dose of 450 mg/m^2

Variation 3 (metastatic):

Doxorubicin: I.V.: 15 mg/m^2/day continuous infusion days 1 to 4

[total dose/cycle = 60 mg/m^2]

Dacarbazine: I.V.: 250 mg/m^2/day continuous infusion days 1 to 4

[total dose/cycle = 1000 mg/m^2]

Repeat cycle every 21 days

Variation 4 (metastatic):

Doxorubicin: I.V.: 60 mg/m^2 day 1

[total dose/cycle = 60 mg/m^2]

Dacarbazine: I.V.: 250 mg/m^2/day days 1 to 5

[total dose/cycle = 1250 mg/m^2]

Repeat cycle every 21 days until disease progression; when maximum lifetime doxorubicin dose received, continue with single agent dacarbazine

AI

Use Soft tissue sarcoma

Regimen NOTE: Multiple variations are listed.

Variation 1:

Doxorubicin: I.V.: 25 mg/m^2/day continuous infusion days 1, 2, and 3

[total dose/cycle = 75 mg/m^2]

Ifosfamide: I.V.: 2 g/m^2/day days 1 to 5

[total dose/cycle = 10 g/m^2]

Mesna: I.V.: 400 mg/m^2 day 1

followed by I.V.: 1200 mg/m^2/day continuous infusion days 1 to 5

[total dose/cycle = 6400 mg/m^2]

Repeat cycle every 3 weeks

Variation 2:

Doxorubicin: I.V.: 30 mg/m^2/day continuous infusion days 1, 2, and 3

[total dose/cycle = 90 mg/m^2]

Ifosfamide: I.V.: 2.5 g/m^2/day days 1 to 4

[total dose/cycle = 10 g/m^2]

Mesna: I.V.: 500 mg/m^2 day 1

followed by I.V.: 1500 mg/m^2/day continuous infusion days 1 to 4

[total dose/cycle = 6500 mg/m^2]

Filgrastim: SubQ: 5 mcg/kg/day days 5 through ANC recovery

Repeat cycle every 3 weeks

AP

Use Endometrial cancer

Regimen

Doxorubicin: I.V.: 60 mg/m^2 day 1

[total dose/cycle = 60 mg/m^2]

Cisplatin: I.V.: 60 mg/m^2 day 1

[total dose/cycle = 60 mg/m^2]

Repeat cycle every 21-28 days

AVD

Use Wilms tumor

Regimen
Dactinomycin: I.V.: 15 mcg/kg/day days 1 to 5 of weeks 0, 13, 26, 39, 52, and 65
[total dose/cycle = 450 mcg/kg]
Doxorubicin: I.V.: 60 mg/m^2 day 1 of weeks 6, 19, 32, 45, and 58
[total dose/cycle = 300 mg/m^2]
Vincristine: I.V.: 1.5 mg/m^2 day 1 of weeks 1 to 8, 13, 14, 26, 27, 39, 40, 52, 53, 65, and 66
[total dose/cycle = 27 mg/m^2]

AV (EE)

Use Wilms tumor

Regimen
Dactinomycin: I.V.: 15 mcg/kg/day days 1 to 5 of weeks 0, 5, 13, and 26
[total dose/cycle = 300 mcg/kg]
Vincristine: I.V.: 1.5 mg/m^2/dose day 1 of weeks 1 to 10, and days 1 and 5 of weeks 13 and 26
[total dose/cycle = 21 mg/m^2]

AV (K)

Use Wilms tumor

Regimen
Dactinomycin: I.V.: 15 mcg/kg/day days 1 to 5 of weeks 0, 5, 13, 22, 31, 40, 49, and 58
[total dose/cycle = 600 mcg/kg]
Vincristine: I.V.: 1.5 mg/m^2/dose day 1 of weeks 0-10, 15-20, 24-29, 33-38, 42-47, 51-56, and 60-65
[total dose/cycle = 70.5 mg/m^2]

AV (L)

Use Wilms tumor

Regimen
Dactinomycin: I.V.: 15 mcg/kg/day days 1 to 5 of weeks 0 and 5
[total dose/cycle = 150 mcg/kg]
Vincristine: I.V.: 1.5 mg/m^2 day 1 of weeks 0-10
[total dose/cycle = 16.5 mg/m^2]

AV (Wilms Tumor)

Use Wilms tumor

Regimen
Dactinomycin: I.V.: 15 mcg/kg/day days 1 to 5 of weeks 0, 13, 26, 39, 52, and 65
[total dose/cycle = 450 mcg/kg]
Vincristine: I.V.: 1.5 mg/m^2/dose day 1 of weeks 1 to 8, 13, 14, 26, 27, 39, 40, 52, 53, 65, and 66
[total dose/cycle = 27 mg/m^2]

Azacitidine (AML Regimen)

Use Leukemia, acute myeloid

Regimen
Azacitidine: SubQ: 75 mg/m^2/day days 1 to 7
[total dose/cycle = 525 mg/m^2]
Repeat cycle every 28 days (for a minimum of 6 cycles [Fenaux, 2010]) as long as tolerated and maintaining response

BEACOPP-14 (Hodgkin Lymphoma)

Use Lymphoma, Hodgkin disease

Regimen
Bleomycin: I.V.: 10 units/m^2 day 8
[total dose/cycle = 10 units/m^2]
Etoposide: I.V.: 100 mg/m^2/day days 1, 2, and 3
[total dose/cycle = 300 mg/m^2]
Doxorubicin: I.V.: 25 mg/m^2 day 1
[total dose/cycle = 25 mg/m^2]

◀ Cyclophosphamide: I.V.: 650 mg/m^2 day 1
[total dose/cycle = 650 mg/m^2]
Vincristine: I.V.: 1.4 mg/m^2 (maximum dose: 2 mg) day 8
[total dose/cycle = 1.4 mg/m^2; maximum: 2 mg]
Procarbazine: Oral: 100 mg/m^2/day days 1 to 7
[total dose/cycle = 700 mg/m^2]
Prednisone: Oral: 80 mg/m^2/day days 1 to 7
[total dose/cycle = 560 mg/m^2]
Filgrastim: SubQ: 300 or 480 mcg/day days 8 to13
Repeat cycle every 14 days for a total of 8 cycles

BEACOPP Escalated (Hodgkin Lymphoma)

Use Lymphoma, Hodgkin disease
Regimen NOTE: Multiple variations are listed.
Variation 1:
Bleomycin: I.V.: 10 units/m^2 day 8
[total dose/cycle = 10 units/m^2]
Etoposide: I.V.: 200 mg/m^2/day days 1, 2, and 3
[total dose/cycle = 600 mg/m^2]
Doxorubicin: I.V.: 35 mg/m^2 day 1
[total dose/cycle = 35 mg/m^2]
Cyclophosphamide: I.V.: 1200 mg/m^2 day 1
[total dose/cycle = 1200 mg/m^2]
Vincristine: I.V.: 1.4 mg/m^2 (maximum dose: 2 mg) day 8
[total dose/cycle = 1.4 mg/m^2: maximum: 2 mg]
Procarbazine: Oral: 100 mg/m^2/day days 1 to 7
[total dose/cycle = 700 mg/m^2]
Prednisone: Oral: 40 mg/m^2/day days 1 to 14
[total dose/cycle = 560 mg/m^2]
Filgrastim: SubQ: 300 or 480 mcg/day day 8 until leukocyte recovery (3 days at >1000/mm^3)
Repeat cycle every 21 days for a total of 8 cycles
Variation 2:
Bleomycin: I.V.: 10 units/m^2 day 8
[total dose/cycle = 10 units/m^2]
Etoposide: I.V.: 200 mg/m^2/day days 1, 2, and 3
[total dose/cycle = 600 mg/m^2]
Doxorubicin: I.V.: 35 mg/m^2 day 1
[total dose/cycle = 35 mg/m^2]
Cyclophosphamide: I.V.: 1250 mg/m^2 day 1
[total dose/cycle = 1250 mg/m^2]
Vincristine: I.V.: 1.4 mg/m^2 (maximum dose: 2 mg) day 8
[total dose/cycle = 1.4 mg/m^2; maximum: 2 mg]
Procarbazine: Oral: 100 mg/m^2/day days 1 to 7
total dose/cycle = 700 mg/m^2]
Prednisone: Oral: 40 mg/m^2/day days 1 to 14
[total dose/cycle = 560 mg/m^2]
Filgrastim: SubQ: Daily (dose not specified) beginning day 8 until leukocyte recovery
Repeat cycle every 21 days for a total of 8 cycles
Variation 3:
Bleomycin: I.V.: 10 units/m^2 day 8
[total dose/cycle = 10 units/m^2]
Etoposide: I.V.: 200 mg/m^2/day days 1, 2, and 3
[total dose/cycle = 600 mg/m^2]
Doxorubicin: I.V.: 35 mg/m^2 day 1
[total dose/cycle = 35 mg/m^2]
Cyclophosphamide: I.V.: 1250 mg/m^2 day 1
[total dose/cycle = 1250 mg/m^2]
Mesna: I.V.: 250 mg/m^2 day 1
[total dose/cycle = 250 mg/m^2]
Mesna: Oral: 500 mg/m^2/dose at hour 2 and hour 5 day 1
[total dose/cycle = 1000 mg/m^2]

Vincristine: I.V.: 1.4 mg/m^2 (maximum dose: 2 mg) day 8
  [total dose/cycle = 1.4 mg/m^2; maximum: 2 mg]
Procarbazine: Oral: 100 mg/m^2/day days 1 to 7
  [total dose/cycle = 700 mg/m^2]
Prednisone: Oral: 40 mg/m^2/day days 1 to 7
  [total dose/cycle = 280 mg/m^2]
Filgrastim: SubQ: (dose not specified)
Repeat cycle every 21 days for a total of 6 cycles
Variation 4:
Bleomycin: I.V.: 10 units/m^2 day 8
  [total dose/cycle = 10 units/m^2]
Etoposide: I.V.: 200 mg/m^2/day days 1, 2, and 3
  [total dose/cycle = 600 mg/m^2]
Doxorubicin: I.V.: 35 mg/m^2 day 1
  [total dose/cycle = 35 mg/m^2]
Cyclophosphamide: I.V.: 1250 mg/m^2 day 1
  [total dose/cycle = 1250 mg/m^2]
Mesna: I.V.: 250 mg/m^2/dose at hours 0, 4, and 8 day 1
  [total dose/cycle = 750 mg/m^2]
Vincristine: I.V.: 1.4 mg/m^2 (maximum dose: 2 mg) day 8
  [total dose/cycle = 1.4 mg/m^2; maximum: 2 mg]
Procarbazine: Oral: 100 mg/m^2/day days 1 to 7
  [total dose/cycle = 700 mg/m^2]
Prednisone: Oral: 40 mg/m^2/day days 1 to 14
  [total dose/cycle = 560 mg/m^2]
Filgrastim: SubQ: 300 or 480 mcg/day day 8 until leukocyte recovery (3 days at >1000/mm^3)
Repeat cycle every 21 days for a total of 8 cycles
Variation 5 (studied in children):
Bleomycin: I.V.: 10 units/m^2 day 8
  [total dose/cycle = 10 units/m^2]
Etoposide: I.V.: 200 mg/m^2/day days 1, 2, and 3
  [total dose/cycle = 600 mg/m^2]
Doxorubicin: I.V.: 35 mg/m^2 day 1
  [total dose/cycle = 35 mg/m^2]
Cyclophosphamide: I.V.: 1200 mg/m^2 day 1
  [total dose/cycle = 1200 mg/m^2]
Vincristine: I.V.: 2 mg/m^2 (maximum dose: 2 mg) day 8
  [total dose/cycle = 2 mg/m^2; maximum: 2 mg]
Procarbazine: Oral: 100 mg/m^2/day days 1 to 7
  [total dose/cycle = 700 mg/m^2]
Prednisone: Oral: 40 mg/m^2/day days 1 to 14
  [total dose/cycle = 560 mg/m^2]
Repeat cycle every 21 days for 4 cycles (may repeat with 4 more cycles if "slow early responder")

BEACOPP Standard (Hodgkin Lymphoma)

Use Lymphoma, Hodgkin disease
Regimen NOTE: Multiple variations are listed.
Variation 1:
Bleomycin: I.V.: 10 units/m^2 day 8
  [total dose/cycle = 10 units/m^2]
Etoposide: I.V.: 100 mg/m^2/day days 1, 2, and 3
  [total dose/cycle = 300 mg/m^2]
Doxorubicin: I.V.: 25 mg/m^2 day 1
  [total dose/cycle = 25 mg/m^2]
Cyclophosphamide: I.V.: 650 mg/m^2 day 1
  [total dose/cycle = 650 mg/m^2]
Vincristine: I.V.: 1.4 mg/m^2 (maximum dose: 2 mg) day 8
  [total dose/cycle = 1.4 mg/m^2; maximum: 2 mg]
Procarbazine: Oral: 100 mg/m^2/day days 1 to 7
  [total dose/cycle = 700 mg/m^2]
Prednisone: Oral: 40 mg/m^2/day days 1 to 14
  [total dose/cycle = 560 mg/m^2]
Repeat cycle every 21 days for a total of 8 cycles

◀ Variation 2:

Bleomycin: I.V.: 10 units/m^2 day 8
[total dose/cycle = 10 units/m^2]

Etoposide: I.V.: 100 mg/m^2/day days 1, 2, and 3
[total dose/cycle = 300 mg/m^2]

Doxorubicin: I.V.: 25 mg/m^2 day 1
[total dose/cycle = 25 mg/m^2]

Cyclophosphamide: I.V.: 650 mg/m^2 day 1
[total dose/cycle = 650 mg/m^2]

Vincristine: I.V.: 1.4 mg/m^2 (maximum dose: 2 mg) day 8
[total dose/cycle = 1.4 mg/m^2; maximum: 2 mg]

Procarbazine: Oral: 100 mg/m^2/day days 1 to 7
[total dose/cycle = 700 mg/m^2]

Prednisone: Oral: 40 mg/m^2/day days 1 to 7
[total dose/cycle = 280 mg/m^2]

Repeat cycle every 21 days for a total of 6 cycles

Variation 3:

Bleomycin: I.V.: 10 units/m^2 day 8
[total dose/cycle = 10 units/m^2]

Etoposide: Oral: 50 mg/m^2/day days 3 to 12
[total dose/cycle = 500 mg/m^2]

Doxorubicin: I.V.: 40 mg/m^2 day 1
[total dose/cycle = 40 mg/m^2]

Cyclophosphamide: I.V.: 650 mg/m^2 day 1
[total dose/cycle = 650 mg/m^2]

Vincristine: I.V.: 1.4 mg/m^2 (maximum dose: 2 mg) day 8
[total dose/cycle = 1.4 mg/m^2; maximum: 2 mg]

Procarbazine: Oral: 100 mg/m^2/day days 1 to 7
[total dose/cycle = 700 mg/m^2]

Prednisone: Oral: 40 mg/m^2/day days 1 to 14
[total dose/cycle = 560 mg/m^2]

Repeat cycle every 21 days for a total of 8 cycles

Variation 4:

Bleomycin: I.V.: 10 units/m^2 day 8
[total dose/cycle = 10 units/m^2]

Etoposide: I.V.: 100 mg/m^2/day days 1, 2, and 3
[total dose/cycle = 300 mg/m^2]

Doxorubicin: I.V.: 25 mg/m^2 day 1
[total dose/cycle = 25 mg/m^2]

Cyclophosphamide: I.V.: 650 mg/m^2 day 1
[total dose/cycle = 650 mg/m^2]

Vincristine: I.V.: 2 mg day 8
[total dose/cycle = 2 mg]

Procarbazine: Oral: 100 mg/m^2/day days 1 to 7
[total dose/cycle = 700 mg/m^2]

Prednisone: Oral: 40 mg/m^2/day days 1 to 7
[total dose/cycle = 280 mg/m^2]

Repeat cycle every 21 days for a total of 8 cycles

Bendamustine-Rituximab

Use Lymphoma, non-Hodgkin (mantle cell or low-grade NHL)

Regimen NOTE: Multiple variations are listed.

Variation 1:

Pretreatment:

Rituximab: I.V.: 375 mg/m^2 1 week before the start of cycle 1
[total dose/pretreatment = 375 mg/m^2]

Cycles:
   Rituximab: I.V.: 375 mg/m^2 day 1
   [total dose/cycle = 375 mg/m^2]
   Bendamustine: I.V.: 90 mg/m^2 days 2 and 3
   [total dose/cycle = 180 mg/m^2]
   Repeat cycle every 4 weeks for up to 4 cycles
Post-Treatment:
   Rituximab: I.V.: 375 mg/m^2 4 weeks after the last cycle
   [total dose/post-treatment = 375 mg/m^2]
Variation 2:
   Pretreatment:
   Rituximab: I.V.: 375 mg/m^2 1 week before the start of cycle 1
   [total dose/pretreatment = 375 mg/m^2]
   Cycles:
   Rituximab: I.V.: 375 mg/m^2 day 1
   [total dose/cycle = 375 mg/m^2]
   Bendamustine: I.V.: 90 mg/m^2 days 2 and 3
   [total dose/cycle = 180 mg/m^2]
   Repeat cycle every 4 weeks for 4-6 cycles
Post-Treatment:
   Rituximab: I.V.: 375 mg/m^2 4 weeks after the last cycle
   [total dose/post-treatment = 375 mg/m^2]

BEP (Ovarian Cancer)

Use Ovarian cancer

Regimen
Bleomycin: I.V.: 20 units/m^2 (maximum dose: 30 units) day 1
   [total dose/cycle = 20 units/m^2]
Etoposide: I.V.: 75 mg/m^2/day days 1 to 5
   [total dose/cycle = 375 mg/m^2]
   or I.V.: 75 mg/m^2/day days 1 to 4 (if received prior radiation therapy)
   [total dose/cycle = 300 mg/m^2]
Cisplatin: I.V.: 20 mg/m^2/day days 1 to 5
   [total dose/cycle = 100 mg/m^2]
Repeat cycle every 3 weeks for 4 cycles

BEP (Ovarian Cancer, Testicular Cancer)

Use Ovarian cancer; Testicular cancer

Regimen
Bleomycin: I.V.: 30 units/day days 2, 9, and 16
   [total dose/cycle = 90 units]
Etoposide: I.V.: 100 mg/m^2/day days 1 to 5
   [total dose/cycle = 500 mg/m^2]
   or I.V.: 120 mg/m^2/day days 1, 2, and 3
   [total dose/cycle = 360 mg/m^2]
Cisplatin: I.V.: 20 mg/m^2/day days 1 to 5
   [total dose/cycle = 100 mg/m^2]
Repeat cycle every 21 days

BEP (Testicular Cancer)

Use Testicular cancer

Regimen NOTE: Multiple variations are listed.
Variation 1:
   Bleomycin: I.V.: 30 units/day days 1, 8, and 15
   [total dose/cycle = 90 units]
   Etoposide: I.V.: 100 mg/m^2/day days 1 to 5
   [total dose/cycle = 500 mg/m^2]
   Cisplatin: I.V.: 20 mg/m^2/day days 1 to 5
   [total dose/cycle = 100 mg/m^2]
   Repeat cycle every 21 days for 3-4 cycles

Variation 2:
Bleomycin: I.V.: 30 units/day days 2, 9, and 16
[total dose/cycle = 90 units]
Etoposide: I.V.: 100 mg/m^2/day days 1 to 5
[total dose/cycle = 500 mg/m^2]
Cisplatin: I.V.: 20 mg/m^2/day days 1 to 5
[total dose/cycle = 100 mg/m^2]
Repeat cycle every 21 days
Variation 3:
Bleomycin: I.V.: 30 units once weekly
[total dose/cycle = 90 units]
Etoposide: I.V.: 120 mg/m^2/day days 1, 3, and 5
[total dose/cycle = 360 mg/m^2]
Cisplatin: I.V.: 20 mg/m^2/day days 1 to 5
[total dose/cycle = 100 mg/m^2]
Repeat cycle every 21 days
Variation 4:
Bleomycin: I.V.: 30 units/day days 1, 8, and 15
[total dose/cycle = 90 units]
Etoposide: I.V.: 165 mg/m^2/day days 1, 2, and 3
[total dose/cycle = 495 mg/m^2]
Cisplatin: I.V.: 50 mg/m^2/day days 1 and 2
[total dose/cycle = 100 mg/m^2]
Repeat cycle every 21 days

Bevacizumab-Capecitabine (Breast Cancer)

Use Breast cancer

Regimen NOTE: Multiple variations are listed.
Variation 1:
Capecitabine: Oral: 1250 mg/m^2 twice daily days 1 to 14
[total dose/cycle = 35,000 mg/m^2]
Bevacizumab: I.V.: 15 mg/kg day 1
[total dose/cycle = 15 mg/kg]
Repeat cycle every 21 days for up to 35 cycles
Variation 2:
Capecitabine: Oral: 2000 mg/m^2/day days 1 to 14
[total dose/cycle = 28,000 mg/m^2]
Bevacizumab: I.V.: 15 mg/kg day 1
[total dose/cycle = 15 mg/kg]
Repeat cycle every 21 days

Bevacizumab-Cisplatin-Gemcitabine (NSCLC)

Use Lung cancer, nonsmall cell

Regimen
Bevacizumab: I.V.: 7.5 or 15 mg/kg/dose day 1
[total dose/cycle = 7.5 or 15 mg/kg]
Cisplatin: I.V.: 80 mg/m^2/dose day 1
[total dose/cycle = 80 mg/m^2]
Gemcitabine: I.V.: 1250 mg/m^2/dose days 1 and 8
[total dose/cycle = 2500 mg/m^2]
Repeat cycle every 21 days for up to 6 cycles (bevacizumab monotherapy may be continued thereafter until disease progression)

Bevacizumab-Fluorouracil-Leucovorin

Use Colorectal cancer

Regimen
Bevacizumab: I.V.: 5 mg/kg/day days 1, 15, 29, and 43
[total dose/cycle = 20 mg/kg]
Leucovorin: I.V.: 500 mg/m^2/day days 1, 8, 15, 22, 29, and 36
[total dose/cycle = 3000 mg/m^2]

Fluorouracil: I.V.: 500 mg/m^2/day days 1, 8, 15, 22, 29, and 36
[total dose/cycle = 3000 mg/m^2]
Repeat cycle every 56 days

Bevacizumab-Interferon Alfa (RCC)

Use Renal cell cancer
Regimen NOTE: Multiple variations are listed.
Variation 1:
Interferon Alfa-2a: SubQ: 9 million units 3 times/week
[total dose/cycle = 54 million units]
Bevacizumab: I.V.: 10 mg/kg day 1
[total dose/cycle = 10 mg/kg]
Repeat cycle every 14 days for up to 1 year or until disease progression
Variation 2:
Interferon Alfa-2b: SubQ: 9 million units 3 times/week
[total dose/cycle = 108 million units]
Bevacizumab: I.V.: 10 mg/kg day 1 and 15
[total dose/cycle = 20 mg/kg]
Repeat cycle every 28 days until disease progression or unacceptable toxicity

Bevacizumab-Irinotecan (Glioblastoma)

Use Brain tumors
Regimen Note: Patients receiving concurrent antiepileptic enzyme-inducing drugs received an increased
dose of irinotecan (340 mg/m^2/dose).
Bevacizumab: I.V.: 10 mg/kg day 1
[total dose/cycle = 10 mg/kg]
Irinotecan: I.V.: 125 mg/m^2 day 1
[total dose/cycle = 125 mg/m^2]
Repeat cycle every 14 days

Bevacizumab-Oxaliplatin-Fluorouracil-Leucovorin

Use Colorectal cancer
Regimen
Bevacizumab: I.V.: 10 mg/kg day 1
[total dose/cycle = 10 mg/kg]
Oxaliplatin: I.V.: 85 mg/m^2 day 1
[total dose/cycle = 85 mg/m^2]
Leucovorin: I.V.: 200 mg/m^2/day days 1 and 2
[total dose/cycle = 400 mg/m^2]
Fluorouracil: I.V. bolus: 400 mg/m^2/day days 1 and 2
followed by I.V.: 600 mg/m^2 continuous infusion over 22 hours days 1 and 2
[total dose/cycle = 2000 mg/m^2]
Repeat cycle every 14 days

Bicalutamide-Goserelin

Use Prostate cancer
Regimen
Bicalutamide: Oral: 50 mg/day
[total dose/cycle = 1400 mg]
Goserelin acetate: SubQ: 3.6 mg day 1
[total dose/cycle = 3.6 mg]
Repeat cycle every 28 days

Bicalutamide-Leuprolide

Use Prostate cancer
Regimen
Bicalutamide: Oral: 50 mg/day
[total dose/cycle = 1400 mg]
Leuprolide depot: I.M.: 7.5 mg day 1
[total dose/cycle = 7.5 mg]
Repeat cycle every 28 days

BOLD

Use Melanoma

Regimen

Dacarbazine: I.V.: 200 mg/m^2/day days 1 to 5
[total dose/cycle = 1000 mg/m^2]
Vincristine: I.V.: 1 mg/m^2/day days 1 and 4
[total dose/cycle = 2 mg/m^2]
Bleomycin: I.V.: 15 units/day days 2 and 5
[total dose/cycle = 30 units]
Lomustine: Oral: 80 mg day 1
[total dose/cycle = 80 mg]
Repeat cycle every 4 weeks

BOLD + Interferon

Use Melanoma

Regimen NOTE: Multiple variations are listed.

Variation 1:
Bleomycin: I.V.: 15 units/day days 2 and 5
[total dose/cycle = 30 units]
Vincristine: I.V.: 1 mg/m^2/day days 1 and 4
[total dose/cycle = 2 mg/m^2]
Lomustine: Oral: 80 mg day 1
[total dose/cycle = 80 mg]
Dacarbazine: I.V.: 200 mg/m^2/day days 1 to 5
[total dose/cycle = 1000 mg/m^2]
Interferon Alfa-2b: SubQ: 3 million units/day days 8 to 49 (cycles 1 and 2)
[total dose through day 49 = 126 million units]
followed by SubQ: 6 million units 3 times/week (beginning day 50 and subsequent cycles)
[total dose/cycle = 72 million units]
Repeat cycle every 4 weeks

Variation 2:
Bleomycin: I.V.: 30 units day 1
[total dose/cycle = 30 units]
Vincristine: I.V.: 2 mg day 1
[total dose/cycle = 2 mg]
Lomustine: Oral: 80 mg day 1
[total dose/cycle = 80 mg]
Dacarbazine: I.V.: 700 mg/m^2 day 1
[total dose/cycle = 700 mg/m^2]
Interferon Alfa-2b: SubQ: 3 million units 3 times/week
[total dose/cycle = 36 million units]
Repeat cycle every 4 weeks

Variation 3:
Bleomycin: I.V.: 15 units/day days 2 and 5
[total dose/cycle = 30 units]
Vincristine: I.V.: 1-2 mg/day days 1 and 4
[total dose/cycle = 2-4 mg]
Lomustine: Oral: 80 mg day 1
[total dose/cycle = 80 mg]
Dacarbazine: I.V.: 200 mg/m^2/day days 1 to 5
[total dose/cycle = 1000 mg/m^2]
Interferon Alfa-2b: SubQ: 6 million units 3 times/week, for 6 doses, starting day 8
[total dose/cycle = 36 million units]
Repeat cycle every 4 weeks

Variation 4:
Bleomycin: I.V.: 15 units/day days 2 and 5
[total dose/cycle = 30 units]
Vincristine: I.V.: 1 mg/m^2/day (maximum dose: 2 mg) days 1 and 4
[total dose/cycle = 2 mg/m^2]
Lomustine: Oral: 80 mg day 1
[total dose/cycle = 80 mg]

Dacarbazine: I.V.: 200 mg/m^2/day days 1 to 5
[total dose/cycle = 1000 mg/m^2]
Interferon Alfa-2b: SubQ: 3 million units/day days 8, 10, 12, 15, 17, and 19
[total dose/cycle = 18 million units]
Repeat cycle every 4 weeks

BOLD (Melanoma)

Use Melanoma

Regimen NOTE: Multiple variations are listed.
Variation 1:
Bleomycin: SubQ: 7.5 units/day days 1 and 4 (cycle 1 only)
followed by SubQ: 15 units/day days 1 and 4 (subsequent cycles)
[total dose/cycle = 45 units; maximum total dose (all cycles): 400 units]
Vincristine: I.V.: 1 mg/m^2/day days 1 and 5
[total dose/cycle = 2 mg/m^2]
Lomustine: Oral: 80 mg/m^2 (maximum dose: 150 mg) day 1
[total dose/cycle = 80 mg/m^2]
Dacarbazine: I.V.: 200 mg/m^2/day (maximum dose: 400 mg) days 1 to 5
[total dose/cycle = 1000 mg/m^2; maximum: 2000 mg]
Repeat cycle every 4-6 weeks
Variation 2:
Bleomycin: I.V.: 15 units/day days 1 and 4
[total dose/cycle = 30 units]
Vincristine: I.V.: 1 mg/m^2/day days 1 and 5
[total dose/cycle = 2 mg/m^2]
Lomustine: Oral: 80 mg/m^2 (maximum dose: 150 mg) day 1
[total dose/cycle = 80 mg/m^2]
Dacarbazine: I.V.: 200 mg/m^2/day days 1 to 5
[total dose/cycle = 1000 mg/m^2]
Repeat cycle every 4 weeks
Variation 3:
Bleomycin: I.V.: 15 units/day days 1 and 4
[total dose/cycle = 30 units]
Vincristine: I.V.: 1 mg/m^2 day 1
[total dose/cycle = 1 mg/m^2]
Lomustine: Oral: 80 mg/m^2 day 3 (odd numbered cycles)
[total dose/cycle = 80 mg/m^2; every other cycle]
Dacarbazine: I.V.: 200 mg/m^2/day days 1 to 5
[total dose/cycle = 1000 mg/m^2]
Repeat cycle every 4 weeks

Bortezomib-Dexamethasone (Amyloidosis)

Use Systemic light chain amyloidosis
Regimen
Bortezomib: I.V.: 1.3 mg/m^2/dose days 1, 4, 8, and 11
[total dose/cycle = 5.2 mg/m^2]
Dexamethasone: Oral: 40 mg/day days 1 to 4
[total dose/cycle = 160 mg]
Repeat cycle every 21 days

Bortezomib-Dexamethasone (Multiple Myeloma)

Use Multiple myeloma
Regimen NOTE: Multiple variations are listed.
Variation 1:
Cycles 1 and 2:
Bortezomib: I.V.: 1.3 mg/m^2/day days 1, 4, 8, and 11
[total dose/cycle = 5.2 mg/m^2]
Dexamethasone: Oral: 40 mg/day days 1 to 4 and days 9 to 12
[total dose/cycle = 320 mg]
Treatment cycle is 21 days

Cycles 3 and 4:
Bortezomib: I.V.: 1.3 mg/m^2/day days 1, 4, 8, and 11
[total dose/cycle = 5.2 mg/m^2]
Dexamethasone: Oral: 40 mg/day days 1 to 4
[total dose/cycle = 160 mg]
Treatment cycle is 21 days
Variation 2:
Cycles 1 and 2:
Bortezomib: I.V.: 1.3 mg/m^2/day days 1, 4, 8, and 11
[total dose/cycle = 5.2 mg/m^2]
Treatment cycle is 21 days
Cycles 3 through 6 (begin dexamethasone after cycle 2 if partial response not achieved or after cycle 4 if complete response not achieved):
Bortezomib: I.V.: 1.3 mg/m^2/day days 1, 4, 8, and 11
[total dose/cycle = 5.2 mg/m^2]
Dexamethasone: Oral: 40 mg/day days 1 and 2
[total dose/cycle = 80 mg]
Treatment cycle is 21 days (for up to a total of 6 cycles)

Bortezomib-Dexamethasone-Rituximab (Waldenstrom Macroglobulinemia)

Use Waldenstrom Macroglobulinemia
Regimen
Bortezomib: I.V.: 1.3 mg/m^2 days 1, 4, 8, and 11
[total dose/cycle = 5.2 mg/m^2]
Dexamethasone: I.V.: 40 mg days 1, 4, 8, and 11
[total dose/cycle = 160 mg]
Rituximab: I.V.: 375 mg/m^2 day 11
[total dose/cycle = 375 mg/m^2]
Repeat cycle every 21 days for 4 cycles, followed by a 12 week interruption, then repeat cycle every 12 weeks for 4 cycles

Bortezomib-Doxorubicin-Dexamethasone

Use Multiple myeloma
Regimen NOTE: Multiple variations are listed.
Variation 1:
Cycle 1:
Bortezomib: I.V.: 1.3 mg/m^2/day days 1, 4, 8, and 11
[total dose/cycle = 5.2 mg/m^2]
Dexamethasone: Oral: 40 mg/day days 1 to 4, 8 to 11, and 15 to 18
[total dose/cycle = 480 mg]
Doxorubicin: I.V.: 4.5 or 9 mg/m^2/day days 1 to 4
[total dose/cycle = 18 or 36 mg/m^2]
Treatment cycle is 21 days
Cycles 2-4:
Bortezomib: I.V.: 1.3 mg/m^2/day days 1, 4, 8, and 11
[total dose/cycle = 5.2 mg/m^2]
Dexamethasone: Oral: 40 mg/day days 1 to 4
[total dose/cycle = 160 mg]
Doxorubicin: I.V.: 4.5 or 9 mg/m^2/day days 1 to 4
[total dose/cycle = 18 or 36 mg/m^2]
Treatment cycle is 21 days
Variation 2:
Cycle 1:
Bortezomib: I.V.: 1 mg/m^2/day days 1, 4, 8, and 11
[total dose/cycle = 4 mg/m^2]
Dexamethasone: Oral: 40 mg/day days 1 to 4, 8 to 11, and 15 to 18
[total dose/cycle = 480 mg]
Doxorubicin: I.V.: 9 mg/m^2/day days 1 to 4
[total dose/cycle = 36 mg/m^2]
Treatment cycle is 21 days

Cycles 2-4:
  Bortezomib: I.V.: 1 mg/m^2/day days 1, 4, 8, and 11
    [total dose/cycle = 4 mg/m^2]
  Dexamethasone: Oral: 40 mg/day days 1 to 4
    [total dose/cycle = 160 mg]
  Doxorubicin: I.V.: 9 mg/m^2/day days 1 to 4
    [total dose/cycle = 36 mg/m^2]
  Treatment cycle is 21 days
Variation 3:
  Bortezomib: I.V.: 1.3 mg/m^2/day days 1, 4, 8, and 11
    [total dose/cycle = 5.2 mg/m^2]
  Dexamethasone: Oral: 40 mg/day days 1 to 4
    [total dose/cycle = 160 mg]
  Doxorubicin: I.V.: 20 mg/m^2/day days 1 and 4
    [total dose/cycle = 40 mg/m^2]
  Repeat cycle every 28 days for up to 6 cycles

Bortezomib-Doxorubicin (Liposomal)

Use Multiple myeloma

Regimen
  Bortezomib: I.V.: 1.3 mg/m^2/day days 1, 4, 8, and 11
    [total dose/cycle = 5.2 mg/m^2]
  Doxorubicin (liposomal): I.V.: 30 mg/m^2 day 4
    [total dose/cycle = 30 mg/m^2]
  Repeat cycle every 21 days for up to 8 cycles

Bortezomib-Doxorubicin (Liposomal)-Dexamethasone

Use Multiple myeloma

Regimen
  Bortezomib: I.V.: 1.3 mg/m^2/day days 1, 4, 8, and 11
    [total dose/cycle = 5.2 mg/m^2]
  Doxorubicin (Liposomal): I.V.: 30 mg/m^2 day 1
    [total dose/cycle = 30 mg/m^2]
  Dexamethasone: Oral: 40 mg/day days 1 to 4
    [total dose/cycle = 160 mg]
  Repeat cycle every 28 days for up to 6 cycles

Bortezomib-Melphalan-Prednisone-Thalidomide

Use Multiple myeloma

Regimen
  Bortezomib: I.V.: 1-1.3 mg/m^2/day days 1, 4, 15, and 22
    [total dose/cycle = 4-5.2 mg/m^2]
  Melphalan: Oral: 6 mg/m^2/day days 1 to 5
    [total dose/cycle = 30 mg/m^2]
  Prednisone: Oral: 60 mg/m^2/day days 1 to 5
    [total dose/cycle = 300 mg/m^2]
  Thalidomide: Oral: 50 mg/day days 1 to 35
    [total dose/cycle = 1750 mg]
  Repeat cycle every 35 days for 6 cycles

Bortezomib-Rituximab (Waldenstrom Macroglobulinemia)

Use Waldenstrom Macroglobulinemia

Regimen
  Bortezomib: I.V.: 1.6 mg/m^2/day days 1, 8, and 15 (cycles 1 to 6)
    [total dose/cycle = 4.8 mg/m^2]
  Rituximab: I.V.: 375 mg/m^2/day days 1, 8, 15, and 22 (cycles 1 and 4 only)
    [total dose/cycle (cycles 1 and 4 only) = 1500 mg/m^2]
  Repeat cycle every 28 days for a total of 6 cycles; bortezomib administered for all 6 cycles and rituximab administered cycles 1 and 4 only

Bortezomib (Waldenstrom Macroglobulinemia)

Use Waldenstrom Macroglobulinemia

Regimen
Bortezomib: I.V.: 1.3 mg/m^2/day days 1, 4, 8, and 11
[total dose/cycle = 5.2 mg/m^2]
Repeat cycle every 21 days until disease progression or until 2 cycles after a complete response

Cabazitaxel-Prednisone (Prostate Cancer)

Use Prostate cancer

Regimen
Cabazitaxel: I.V.: 25 mg/m^2/dose day 1
[total dose/cycle = 25 mg/m^2]
Prednisone: Oral: 10 mg once daily
[total dose/cycle = 210 mg]
Repeat cycle every 21 days

CAF

Use Breast cancer

Regimen NOTE: Multiple variations are listed.
Variation 1:
Cyclophosphamide: Oral: 100 mg/m^2/day days 1 to 14
[total dose/cycle = 1400 mg/m^2]
Doxorubicin: I.V.: 30 mg/m^2/day days 1 and 8
[total dose/cycle = 60 mg/m^2]
Fluorouracil: I.V.: 500 mg/m^2/day days 1 and 8
[total dose/cycle = 1000 mg/m^2]
Repeat cycle every 28 days
Variation 2:
Cyclophosphamide: Oral: 100 mg/m^2/day days 1 to 14
[total dose/cycle = 1400 mg/m^2]
Doxorubicin: I.V.: 25 mg/m^2/day days 1 and 8
[total dose/cycle = 50 mg/m^2]
Fluorouracil: I.V.: 500 mg/m^2/day days 1 and 8
[total dose/cycle = 1000 mg/m^2]
Repeat cycle every 28 days

CAP

Use Bladder cancer

Regimen
Cyclophosphamide: I.V.: 400 mg/m^2 day 1
[total dose = 400 mg/m^2]
Doxorubicin: I.V.: 40 mg/m^2 day 1
[total dose = 40 mg/m^2]
Cisplatin: I.V.: 60 mg/m^2 day 1
[total dose = 60 mg/m^2]
Repeat cycle every 21 days

Capecitabine + Docetaxel (Breast Cancer)

Use Breast cancer

Regimen NOTE: Multiple variations are listed.
Variation 1:
Capecitabine: Oral: 1250 mg/m^2 twice daily days 1 to 14
[total dose/cycle = 35,000 mg/m^2]
Docetaxel: I.V.: 75 mg/m^2 day 1
[total dose/cycle = 75 mg/m^2]
Repeat cycle every 3 weeks

Variation 2:

Capecitabine: Oral: 1000 mg/m^2 twice daily days 2 to 15
[total dose/cycle = 28,000 mg/m^2]
Docetaxel: I.V.: 75 mg/m^2 day 1
[total dose/cycle = 75 mg/m^2]
Repeat cycle every 3 weeks

Variation 3:

Capecitabine: Oral: 937.5 mg/m^2 twice daily days 2 to 15
[total dose/cycle = 26,250 mg/m^2]
Docetaxel: I.V.: 60 mg/m^2 day 1
[total dose/cycle = 60 mg/m^2]
Repeat cycle every 3 weeks

Capecitabine-Docetaxel (Gastric Cancer)

Use Gastric cancer

Regimen NOTE: Multiple variations are listed.

Variation 1:

Capecitabine: Oral: 1000 mg/m^2 twice daily days 1 to 14
[total dose/cycle = 28,000 mg/m^2]
Docetaxel: I.V.: 75 mg/m^2 day 1
[total dose/cycle = 75 mg/m^2]
Repeat cycle every 3 weeks for up to 9 cycles or until disease progression or unacceptable toxicity

Variation 2:

Capecitabine: Oral: 1000 mg/m^2 twice daily days 1 to 14
[total dose/cycle = 28,000 mg/m^2]
Docetaxel: I.V.: 36 mg/m^2 days 1 and 8
[total dose/cycle = 72 mg/m^2]
Repeat cycle every 3 weeks until disease progression or unacceptable toxicity

Variation 3:

Capecitabine: Oral: 825 mg/m^2 twice daily days 1 to 14
[total dose/cycle = 23,100 mg/m^2]
Docetaxel: I.V.: 75 mg/m^2 day 1
[total dose/cycle = 75 mg/m^2]
Repeat cycle every 3 weeks until disease progression

Variation 4:

Capecitabine: Oral: 1250 mg/m^2 twice daily days 1 to 14
[total dose/cycle = 35,000 mg/m^2]
Docetaxel: I.V.: 75 mg/m^2 day 1
[total dose/cycle = 75 mg/m^2]
Repeat cycle every 3 weeks until disease progression for up to a maximum of 6 cycles

Capecitabine-Docetaxel (NSCLC)

Use Lung cancer, nonsmall cell

Regimen NOTE: Multiple variations are listed.

Variation 1:

Capecitabine: Oral: 1000 mg/m^2 twice daily days 1 to 14
[total dose/cycle = 28,000 mg/m^2]
Docetaxel: I.V.: 36 mg/m^2 days 1 and 8
[total dose/cycle = 72 mg/m^2]
Repeat cycle every 3 weeks

Variation 2:

Capecitabine: Oral: 625 mg/m^2 twice daily days 5 to 18
[total dose/cycle = 17,500 mg/m^2]
Docetaxel: I.V.: 36 mg/m^2 days 1, 8, and 15
[total dose/cycle = 108 mg/m^2]
Repeat cycle every 4 weeks

Capecitabine + Lapatinib (Breast Cancer)

Use Breast cancer

Regimen
Capecitabine: Oral: 1000 mg/m^2 twice daily days 1 to 14
[total dose/cycle = 28,000 mg/m^2]
Lapatinib: Oral: 1250 mg/day days 1 to 21
[total dose/cycle = 26,250 mg]
Repeat cycle every 3 weeks

Capecitabine-Trastuzumab

Use Breast cancer

Regimen NOTE: Multiple variations are listed.
Variation 1:
Cycle 1:
Capecitabine: Oral: 1250 mg/m^2 twice daily days 1 to 14
[total dose/cycle 1 = 35,000 mg/m^2]
Trastuzumab: I.V.: 4 mg/kg (loading dose) day 1 cycle 1
followed by I.V.: 2 mg/kg/day days 8 and 15 cycle 1
[total dose/cycle 1 = 8 mg/kg]
Treatment cycle is 21 days
Subsequent cycles:
Capecitabine: Oral: 1250 mg/m^2 twice daily days 1 to 14
[total dose/cycle = 35,000 mg/m^2]
Trastuzumab: I.V.: 2 mg/kg/day days 1, 8, and 15
[total dose/cycle = 6 mg/kg]
Repeat cycle every 21 days
Variation 2:
Cycle 1:
Capecitabine: Oral: 1250 mg/m^2 twice daily days 1 to 14
[total dose/cycle 1 = 35,000 mg/m^2]
Trastuzumab: I.V.: 8 mg/kg (loading dose) day 1 cycle 1
[total dose/cycle 1 = 8 mg/kg]
Treatment cycle is 21 days
Subsequent cycles:
Capecitabine: Oral: 1250 mg/m^2 twice daily days 1 to 14
[total dose/cycle = 35,000 mg/m^2]
Trastuzumab: I.V.: 6 mg/kg day 1
[total dose/cycle = 6 mg/kg]
Repeat cycle every 21 days

CAPOX (Biliary Cancer)

Use Biliary adenocarcinoma

Regimen
Capecitabine: Oral: 1000 mg/m^2/dose twice daily days 1 to 14
[total dose/cycle = 28,000 mg/m^2]
Oxaliplatin: I.V.: 130 mg/m^2 over 2 hours day 1
[total dose/cycle = 130 mg/m^2]
Repeat cycle every 3 weeks

CAPOX (Colorectal Cancer)

Use Colorectal cancer

Regimen Note: Multiple variations are listed.
Variation 1:
Oxaliplatin: I.V.: 130 mg/m^2 day 1
[total dose/cycle = 130 mg/m^2]
Capecitabine: Oral: 2500 mg/m^2/day days 1 to 14
[total dose/cycle = 35,000 mg/m^2]
Repeat cycle every 21 days

Variation 2:
  Oxaliplatin: I.V.: 85 mg/m^2 day 1
  [total dose/cycle = 85 mg/m^2]
  Capecitabine: Oral: 3500 mg/m^2/day days 1 to 7
  [total dose/cycle = 24,500 mg/m^2]
  Repeat cycle every 14 days
Variation 3:
  Oxaliplatin: I.V.: 50-80 mg/m^2/day days 1, 8, 22, and 29
  [total dose/cycle = 200-320 mg/m^2]
  Capecitabine: Oral: 1650 mg/m^2/day days 1 to 14 and 22 to 35
  [total dose/cycle = 46,200 mg/m^2]
Variation 4:
  Oxaliplatin: I.V.: 70 mg/m^2/day days 1 and 8
  [total dose/cycle = 140 mg/m^2]
  Capecitabine: Oral: 2000 mg/m^2/day days 1 to 14
  [total dose/cycle = 28,000 mg/m^2]
  Repeat cycle every 21 days
Variation 5:
  Oxaliplatin: I.V.: 120 mg/m^2 day 1
  [total dose/cycle = 120 mg/m^2]
  Capecitabine: Oral: 2500 mg/m^2/day days 1 to 14
  [total dose/cycle = 35,000 mg/m^2]
  Repeat cycle every 21 days
Variation 6:
  Oxaliplatin: I.V.: 85 mg/m^2 day 1
  [total dose/cycle = 85 mg/m^2]
  Capecitabine: Oral: 2500 mg/m^2/day days 1 to 7
  [total dose/cycle = 17,500 mg/m^2]
  or Capecitabine: Oral: 3000 mg/m^2/day days 1 to 7
  [total dose/cycle = 21,000 mg/m^2]
  or Capecitabine: Oral: 3500 mg/m^2/day days 1 to 7
  [total dose/cycle = 24,500 mg/m^2]
  or Capecitabine: Oral: 4000 mg/m^2/day days 1 to 7
  [total dose/cycle = 28,000 mg/m^2]
  Repeat cycle every 14 days
Variation 7:
  Oxaliplatin: I.V.: 130 mg/m^2 day 1
  [total dose/cycle = 130 mg/m^2]
  Capecitabine: Oral: 1000 mg/m^2 twice daily days 1 (beginning with evening dose) to 15 (ending with morning dose)
  [total dose/cycle = 28,000 mg/m^2]
  Repeat cycle every 21 days

CAPOX (Pancreatic Cancer)

Use Pancreatic cancer
Regimen NOTE: Multiple variations are listed.
  Variation 1 (patients ≤65 years of age or ECOG PS <2):
  Capecitabine: Oral: 1000 mg/m^2/dose twice daily days 1 to 14
  [total dose/cycle = 28,000 mg/m^2]
  Oxaliplatin: I.V.: 130 mg/m^2/dose over 2 hours day 1
  [total dose/cycle = 130 mg/m^2]
  Repeat cycle every 21 days until disease progression or unacceptable toxicity
  Variation 2 (patients >65 years of age or ECOG PS of 2):
  Capecitabine: Oral: 750 mg/m^2/dose twice daily days 1 to 14
  [total dose/cycle = 21,000 mg/m^2]
  Oxaliplatin: I.V.: 110 mg/m^2/dose over 2 hours day 1
  [total dose/cycle = 110 mg/m^2]
  Repeat cycle every 21 days until disease progression or unacceptable toxicity

Carboplatin-Cetuximab (Head and Neck Cancer)

Use Head and neck cancer

Regimen
Cycle 1:
Cetuximab: I.V.: 400 mg/m^2 (loading dose) day 1 (week 1, cycle 1 only)
[total loading dose = 400 mg/m^2]
followed by I.V.: 250 mg/m^2/day days 8 and 15
[total dose/cycle 1 = 900 mg/m^2]
Carboplatin: I.V.: AUC 5 day 1
[total dose/cycle = AUC = 5]
Treatment cycle is 3 weeks
Subsequent cycles:
Cetuximab: I.V.: 250 mg/m^2/day days 1, 8, and 15
[total dose/cycle = 750 mg/m^2]
Carboplatin: I.V.: AUC 5 day 1
[total dose/cycle = AUC = 5]
Repeat cycle every 3 weeks until disease progression or unacceptable toxicity for up to a maximum of 8 cycles

CE (Retinoblastoma)

Use Retinoblastoma

Regimen
Etoposide: I.V.: 100 mg/m^2/day over 1 hour days 1 to 5
[total dose/cycle = 500 mg/m^2]
Carboplatin: I.V.: 160 mg/m^2/day over 1 hour days 1 to 5
[total dose/cycle = 800 mg/m^2]
Repeat cycle in 21 to 28 days for a total of 2 cycles

Carboplatin-Irinotecan (Small Cell Lung Cancer)

Use Lung cancer, small cell

Regimen NOTE: Multiple variations are listed.
Variation 1:
Carboplatin: I.V.: Target AUC 5 (Calvert formula) day 1
[total dose/cycle = AUC = 5]
Irinotecan: I.V.: 175 mg/m^2/dose day 1
[total dose/cycle = 175 mg/m^2]
Repeat cycle every 21 days for a total of 4 cycles
Variation 2:
Carboplatin: I.V.: Target AUC 5 (Calvert formula) day 1
[total dose/cycle = AUC = 5]
Irinotecan: I.V.: 50 mg/m^2/dose days 1, 8, and 15
[total dose/cycle = 150 mg/m^2]
Repeat cycle every 28 days

Carboplatin-Paclitaxel (Cervical Cancer)

Use Cervical cancer

Regimen NOTE: Multiple variations are listed.
Variation 1:
Paclitaxel: I.V.: 175 mg/m^2 over 3 hours day 1 (reduce to 155 mg/m^2 over 3 hours day 1 if prior pelvic irradiation)
[total dose/cycle = 175 (or 155) mg/m^2]
Carboplatin: I.V.: AUC 5 or 6 day 1
[total dose/cycle = AUC = 5 or 6]
Repeat cycle every 28 days for up to a total of 6-9 cycles
Variation 2:
Paclitaxel: I.V.: 175 mg/m^2 over 3 hours day 1
[total dose/cycle = 175 mg/m^2]
Carboplatin: I.V.: AUC 5 day 1
[total dose/cycle = AUC = 5]
Repeat cycle every 21 days for 6-9 cycles

Carboplatin-Paclitaxel (Ovarian Cancer)

Use Ovarian cancer

Regimen NOTE: Multiple variations are listed.

Variation 1:

Carboplatin: I.V.: AUC 7.5 day 1

[total dose/cycle = AUC = 7.5]

Paclitaxel: I.V.: 175 mg/m^2 over 3 hours day 1

[total dose/cycle = 175 mg/m^2]

Repeat cycle every 3 weeks for a total for 6 cycles

Variation 2:

Carboplatin: I.V.: AUC 5-6 day 1

[total dose/cycle = AUC = 5-6]

Paclitaxel: I.V.: 175 mg/m^2 over 3 hours day 1

[total dose/cycle = 175 mg/m^2]

Repeat cycle every 3 weeks for a total of 6-8 cycles

Variation 3:

Carboplatin: I.V.: AUC 5 day 1

[total dose/cycle = AUC = 5]

Paclitaxel: I.V.: 175 mg/m^2 over 3 hours day 1

[total dose/cycle = 175 mg/m^2]

Repeat cycle every 3 weeks for 6 cycles

Variation 4:

Carboplatin: I.V.: AUC 6 (maximum dose: 880 mg) day 1

[total dose/cycle = AUC = 6; maximum dose: 880 mg]

Paclitaxel: I.V.: 185 mg/m^2 (maximum dose: 400 mg) over 3 hours day 1

[total dose/cycle = 185 mg/m^2; maximum dose: 400 mg]

Repeat cycle every 3 weeks

Variation 5:

Carboplatin: I.V.: AUC 7.5 day 1

[total dose/cycle = AUC = 7.5]

Paclitaxel: I.V.: 175 mg/m^2 over 3 hours day 1

[total dose/cycle = 175 mg/m^2]

Repeat cycle every 3 weeks for 3-6 cycles

Carboplatin-Paclitaxel (Unknown Primary)

Use Unknown primary (adenocarcinoma)

Regimen

Carboplatin: I.V.: Target AUC 6 day 1

[total dose/cycle = AUC = 6]

followed by

Paclitaxel: I.V.: 200 mg/m^2 infused over 3 hours day 1

[total dose/cycle = 200 mg/m^2]

Filgrastim: SubQ: 300 mcg/day days 5 to 12

[total dose/cycle = 2400 mcg]

Repeat cycle every 21 days for a total of 6 or 8 cycles

Carbo-Tax (NSCLC)

Use Lung cancer, nonsmall cell

Regimen

Paclitaxel: I.V.: 135-215 mg/m^2 infused over 24 hours day 1

[total dose/cycle = 135-215 mg/m^2]

or I.V.: 175 mg/m^2 infused over 3 hours day 1

[total dose/cycle = 175 mg/m^2]

followed by

Carboplatin: I.V.: Target AUC 7.5

[total dose/cycle = AUC = 7.5]

Repeat cycle every 21 days

CaT (NSCLC)

Use Lung cancer, nonsmall cell

Regimen NOTE: Multiple variations are listed.

Variation 1:

Paclitaxel: I.V.: 175 mg/m^2 day 1

[total dose/cycle = 175 mg/m^2]

or I.V.: 135 mg/m^2 continuous infusion day 1

[total dose/cycle = 135 mg/m^2]

Carboplatin: I.V.: AUC 7.5 day 1 or 2

[total dose/cycle = AUC = 7.5]

Repeat cycle every 21 days

Variation 2:

Paclitaxel: I.V.: 225 mg/m^2 day 1

[total dose/cycle = 225 mg/m^2]

Carboplatin: I.V.: AUC 6 day 1

[total dose/cycle = AUC = 6]

Repeat cycle every 21 days

CAVE

Use Lung cancer, small cell

Regimen

Cyclophosphamide: I.V.: 750 mg/m^2 day 1

[total dose/cycle = 750 mg/m^2]

Doxorubicin: I.V.: 50 mg/m^2 day 1

[total dose/cycle = 50 mg/m^2]

Vincristine: I.V.: 1.4 mg/m^2 (maximum dose: 2 mg) day 1

[total dose/cycle = 1.4 mg/m^2]

Etoposide: I.V.: 60-100 mg/m^2/day days 1, 2, and 3

[total dose/cycle = 180-300 mg/m^2]

Repeat cycle every 21 days

CAV-P/VP

Use Neuroblastoma

Regimen

Course 1, 2, 4, and 6:

Cyclophosphamide: I.V.: 70 mg/kg/day days 1 and 2

[total dose/cycle = 140 mg/kg]

Doxorubicin: I.V.: 25 mg/m^2/day continuous infusion days 1, 2, and 3

[total dose/cycle = 75 mg/m^2]

Vincristine: I.V.: 0.033 mg/kg/day continuous infusion days 1, 2, and 3

[total dose/cycle = 0.099 mg/kg]

Vincristine: I.V.: 1.5 mg/m^2 day 9

[total dose/cycle = 1.5 mg/m^2]

Course 3, 5, and 7:

Etoposide: I.V.: 200 mg/m^2/day days 1, 2, and 3

[total dose/cycle = 600 mg/m^2]

Cisplatin: I.V.: 50 mg/m^2/day days 1 to 4

[total dose/cycle = 200 mg/m^2]

CC

Use Ovarian cancer

Regimen

Carboplatin: I.V.: Target AUC 5-7.5 day 1

[total dose/cycle = AUC = 5-7.5]

Cyclophosphamide: I.V.: 600 mg/m^2 day 1

[total dose/cycle = 600 mg/m^2]

Repeat cycle every 28 days

CCDT (Melanoma)

Use Melanoma

Regimen
Dacarbazine: I.V.: 220 mg/m^2/day days 1, 2, and 3, every 21 to 28 days
  [total dose/cycle = 660 mg/m^2]
Carmustine: I.V.: 150 mg/m^2 day 1, every 42 to 56 days
  [total dose/cycle = 150 mg/m^2]
Cisplatin: I.V.: 25 mg/m^2/day days 1, 2, and 3, every 21 to 28 days
  [total dose/cycle = 75 mg/m^2]
Tamoxifen: Oral: 20 mg/day (use of tamoxifen is optional)

CDDP/VP-16

Use Brain tumors

Regimen
Cisplatin: I.V.: 90 mg/m^2 day 1
  [total dose/cycle = 90 mg/m^2]
Etoposide: I.V.: 150 mg/m^2/day days 3 and 4
  [total dose/cycle = 300 mg/m^2]
Repeat cycle every 21 days

CE-CAdO

Use Neuroblastoma

Regimen
Carboplatin: I.V.: 160 mg/m^2/day days 1 to 5
  [total dose/cycle = 800 mg/m^2]
Etoposide: I.V.: 100 mg/m^2/day days 1 to 5
  [total dose/cycle = 500 mg/m^2]
or
Carboplatin: I.V.: 200 mg/m^2/day days 1, 2, and 3
  [total dose/cycle = 600 mg/m^2]
Etoposide: I.V.: 150 mg/m^2/day days 1, 2, and 3
  [total dose/cycle = 450 mg/m^2]
and
Cyclophosphamide: I.V.: 300 mg/m^2/day days 1 to 5
  [total dose/cycle = 1500 mg/m^2]
Doxorubicin: I.V.: 60 mg/m^2 day 5
  [total dose/cycle = 60 mg/m^2]
Vincristine: I.V.: 1.5 mg/m^2/day days 1 and 5
  [total dose/cycle = 3 mg/m^2]
Repeat cycle every 21 days

CEF

Use Breast cancer

Regimen
Cyclophosphamide: Oral: 75 mg/m^2/day days 1 to 14
  [total dose/cycle = 1050 mg/m^2]
Epirubicin: I.V.: 60 mg/m^2/day days 1 and 8
  [total dose/cycle = 120 mg/m^2]
Fluorouracil: I.V.: 500 mg/m^2/day days 1 and 8
  [total dose/cycle = 1000 mg/m^2]
Repeat cycle every 28 days

CE (Neuroblastoma)

Use Neuroblastoma

Regimen
Carboplatin: I.V.: 500 mg/m^2/day days 1 and 2
  [total dose/cycle = 1000 mg/m^2]
Etoposide: I.V.: 100 mg/m^2/day days 1, 2, and 3
  [total dose/cycle = 300 mg/m^2]
Repeat cycle every 21-28 days

CEPP(B)

Use Lymphoma, non-Hodgkin

Regimen
Cyclophosphamide: I.V.: 600-650 mg/m^2/day days 1 and 8
 [total dose/cycle = 1200-1300 mg/m^2]
Etoposide: I.V.: 70-85 mg/m^2/day days 1, 2, and 3
 [total dose/cycle = 210-255 mg/m^2]
Procarbazine: Oral: 60 mg/m^2/day days 1 to 10
 [total dose/cycle = 600 mg/m^2]
Prednisone: Oral: 60 mg/m^2/day days 1 to 10
 [total dose/cycle = 600 mg/m^2]
Bleomycin: I.V.: 15 units/m^2/day days 1 and 15 (Bleomycin is sometimes omitted)
 [total dose/cycle = 30 units/m^2]
Repeat cycle every 28 days

Cetuximab (Biweekly)-Irinotecan

Use Colorectal cancer

Regimen
Cycle 1:
 Cetuximab: I.V.: 500 mg/m^2 over 120 minutes day 1 (cycle 1 only)
 [total dose/cycle = 500 mg/m^2]
 Irinotecan: I.V.: 180 mg/m^2 day 1
 [total dose/cycle = 180 mg/m^2]
Subsequent cycles:
 Cetuximab: I.V.: 500 mg/m^2 over 60 minutes day 1
 [total dose/cycle = 500 mg/m^2]
 Irinotecan: I.V.: 180 mg/m^2 day 1
 [total dose/cycle = 180 mg/m^2]
Repeat cycle every 14 days

Cetuximab-Carboplatin-Fluorouracil (Head and Neck Cancer)

Use Head and neck cancer

Regimen
Cycle 1:
 Cetuximab: I.V.: 400 mg/m^2 (loading dose) day 1 (week 1, cycle 1 only)
 [total loading dose = 400 mg/m^2]
 followed by I.V.: 250 mg/m^2/day days 8 and 15
 [total dose/cycle 1 = 900 mg/m^2]
 Carboplatin: I.V.: AUC 5 day 1
 [total dose/cycle = AUC = 5]
 Fluorouracil: I.V.: 1000 mg/m^2/day continuous infusion days 1 to 4
 [total dose/cycle = 4000 mg/m^2]
 Treatment cycle is 3 weeks
Subsequent cycles:
 Cetuximab: I.V.: 250 mg/m^2/day days 1, 8, and 15
 [total dose/cycle = 750 mg/m^2]
 Carboplatin: I.V.: AUC 5 day 1
 [total dose/cycle = AUC = 5]
 Fluorouracil: I.V.: 1000 mg/m^2/day continuous infusion days 1 to 4
 [total dose/cycle = 4000 mg/m^2]
 Repeat cycle every 3 weeks for a total of up to 6 cycles (cetuximab monotherapy may be continued thereafter until disease progression or unacceptable toxicity)

Cetuximab-Cisplatin-Fluorouracil (Head and Neck Cancer)

Use Head and neck cancer

Regimen

Cycle 1:

Cetuximab: I.V.: 400 mg/m^2 (loading dose) day 1 (week 1, cycle 1 only)
[total loading dose = 400 mg/m^2]
  followed by I.V.: 250 mg/m^2/day days 8 and 15
    [total dose/cycle 1 = 900 mg/m^2]
Cisplatin: I.V.: 100 mg/m^2 day 1
[total dose/cycle = 100 mg/m^2]
Fluorouracil: I.V.: 1000 mg/m^2/day continuous infusion days 1 to 4
[total dose/cycle = 4000 mg/m^2]
Treatment cycle is 3 weeks

Subsequent cycles:

Cetuximab: I.V.: 250 mg/m^2/day days 1, 8, and 15
[total dose/cycle = 750 mg/m^2]
Cisplatin: I.V.: 100 mg/m^2 day 1
[total dose/cycle = 100 mg/m^2]
Fluorouracil: I.V.: 1000 mg/m^2/day continuous infusion days 1 to 4
[total dose/cycle = 4000 mg/m^2]
Repeat cycle every 3 weeks for a total of up to 6 cycles (cetuximab monotherapy may be continued thereafter until disease progression or unacceptable toxicity)

Cetuximab-Cisplatin-Vinorelbine

Use Lung cancer, nonsmall cell

Regimen

Cycle 1:

Cetuximab: I.V.: 400 mg/m^2 (loading dose) day 1 (week 1, cycle 1 only)
[total loading dose = 400 mg/m^2]
  followed by I.V.: 250 mg/m^2/dose days 8 and 15
    [total dose/cycle 1 = 900 mg/m^2]
Cisplatin: I.V.: 80 mg/m^2/dose day 1
[total dose/cycle = 80 mg/m^2]
Vinorelbine: I.V.: 25 mg/m^2/dose days 1 and 8
[total dose/cycle = 50 mg/m^2]
Treatment cycle is 3 weeks

Subsequent cycles:

Cetuximab: I.V.: 250 mg/m^2/day days 1, 8, and 15
[total dose/cycle = 750 mg/m^2]
Cisplatin: I.V.: 80 mg/m^2 day 1
[total dose/cycle = 80 mg/m^2]
Vinorelbine: I.V.: 25 mg/m^2/dose days 1 and 8
[total dose/cycle = 50 mg/m^2]
Repeat cycle every 3 weeks

Cetuximab-FOLFOX4

Use Colorectal cancer

Regimen

Cycle 1:

Cetuximab: I.V.: 400 mg/m^2 (loading dose) day 1 (week 1, cycle 1 only)
  followed by I.V.: 250 mg/m^2/day day 8
    [total dose/cycle 1 = 650 mg/m^2]
Oxaliplatin: I.V.: 85 mg/m^2 (over 2 hours) day 1
[total dose/cycle = 85 mg/m^2]
Leucovorin: I.V.: 200 mg/m^2/day (over 2 hours) days 1 and 2
[total dose/cycle = 400 mg/m^2]
Fluorouracil: I.V. bolus: 400 mg/m^2/day days 1 and 2
  followed by I.V.: 600 mg/m^2 continuous infusion (over 22 hours) days 1 and 2
    [total dose/cycle = 2000 mg/m^2]
Note: Bolus fluorouracil and continuous infusion are both given on each day.
Treatment cycle is 14 days

◄ Subsequent cycles:
Cetuximab: I.V.: 250 mg/m^2/day days 1 and 8
[total dose/cycle = 500 mg/m^2]
Oxaliplatin: I.V.: 85 mg/m^2 day 1
[total dose/cycle = 85 mg/m^2]
Leucovorin: I.V.: 200 mg/m^2/day (over 2 hours) days 1 and 2
[total dose/cycle = 400 mg/m^2]
Fluorouracil: I.V. bolus: 400 mg/m^2/day days 1 and 2
followed by I.V.: 600 mg/m^2 continuous infusion (over 22 hours) days 1 and 2
[total dose/cycle = 2000 mg/m^2]
Note: Bolus fluorouracil and continuous infusion are both given on each day.
Repeat cycle every 14 days

Cetuximab-Irinotecan

Use Colorectal cancer
Regimen NOTE: Multiple variations are listed.
Variation 1:
Cycle 1:
Cetuximab: I.V.: 400 mg/m^2 (loading dose) day 1 (week 1, cycle 1 only)
[total loading dose = 400 mg/m^2]
followed by I.V.: 250 mg/m^2/day days 8, 15, 22, 29, and 36
[total dose/cycle 1 = 1650 mg/m^2]
Irinotecan: I.V.: 125 mg/m^2/day days 1, 8, 15, and 22
[total dose/cycle = 500 mg/m^2]
Subsequent cycles:
Cetuximab: I.V.: 250 mg/m^2/day days 1, 8, 15, 22, 29, and 36
[total dose/cycle = 1500 mg/m^2]
Irinotecan: I.V.: 125 mg/m^2/day days 1, 8, 15, and 22
[total dose/cycle = 500 mg/m^2]
Repeat cycle every 42 days
Variation 2:
Cycle 1:
Cetuximab: I.V.: 400 mg/m^2 (loading dose) day 1 (week 1, cycle 1 only)
[total loading dose = 400 mg/m^2]
followed by I.V.: 250 mg/m^2 day 8
[total dose/cycle 1 = 650 mg/m^2]
Irinotecan: I.V.: 180 mg/m^2 day 1
[total dose/cycle = 180 mg/m^2]
Subsequent cycles:
Cetuximab: I.V.: 250 mg/m^2/day days 1 and 8
[total dose/cycle = 500 mg/m^2]
Irinotecan: I.V.: 180 mg/m^2 day 1
[total dose/cycle = 180 mg/m^2]
Repeat cycle every 14 days
Variation 3:
Cycle 1:
Cetuximab: I.V.: 400 mg/m^2 (loading dose) day 1 (week 1, cycle 1 only)
[total loading dose = 400 mg/m^2]
followed by I.V.: 250 mg/m^2/day days 8 and 15 (cycle 1)
[total dose/cycle 1 = 900 mg/m^2]
Irinotecan: I.V.: 350 mg/m^2 day 1
[total dose/cycle = 350 mg/m^2]
Subsequent cycles:
Cetuximab: I.V.: 250 mg/m^2/day days 1, 8, and 15
[total dose/cycle = 750 mg/m^2]
Irinotecan: I.V.: 350 mg/m^2 day 1
[total dose/cycle = 350 mg/m^2]
Repeat cycle every 21 days

CEV

Use Rhabdomyosarcoma

Regimen
Carboplatin: I.V.: 500 mg/m^2 day 1
[total dose/cycle = 500 mg/m^2]
Epirubicin: I.V.: 150 mg/m^2 day 1
[total dose/cycle = 150 mg/m^2]
Vincristine: I.V.: 1.5 mg/m^2/day days 1 and 7
[total dose/cycle = 3 mg/m^2]
Repeat cycle every 21 days

CHAMOCA (Modified Bagshawe Regimen)

Use Gestational trophoblastic tumor

Regimen NOTE: Multiple variations are listed.
Variation 1:
Hydroxyurea: Oral: 500 mg every 6 hours, for 4 doses, day 1 (start at 6 AM)
[total dose/cycle = 2000 mg]
Dactinomycin: I.V.: 0.2 mg/day days 1, 2, and 3 (give at 7 PM)
followed by I.V.: 0.5 mg/day days 4 and 5 (give at 7 PM)
[total dose/cycle = 1.6 mg]
Cyclophosphamide: I.V.: 500 mg/m^2/day days 3 and 8 (give at 7 PM)
[total dose/cycle = 1000 mg/m^2]
Vincristine: I.V.: 1 mg/m^2 (maximum dose: 2 mg) day 2 (give at 7 AM)
[total dose/cycle = 1 mg/m^2; maximum: 2 mg]
Methotrexate: I.V. bolus: 100 mg/m^2 day 2 (give at 7 PM)
followed by I.V.: 200 mg/m^2 continuous infusion over 12 hours day 2
[total dose/cycle = 300 mg/m^2]
Leucovorin: I.M.: 14 mg every 6 hours, for 6 doses, days 3, 4, and 5 (begin at 7 PM on day 3; start 24 hours after the start of methotrexate)
[total dose/cycle = 84 mg]
Doxorubicin: I.V.: 30 mg/m^2 day 8 (give at 7 PM)
[total dose/cycle = 30 mg/m^2]
Repeat cycle every 18 days or as toxicity permits (cycle may be repeated 10 days after last treatment)
Variation 2:
Hydroxyurea: Oral: 500 mg every 12 hours, for 4 doses, days 1 and 2 (usually started in early morning)
[total dose/cycle = 2000 mg]
Dactinomycin: I.V.: 10 mcg/kg/day days 5, 6, and 7
[total dose/cycle = 30 mcg/kg]
Vincristine: I.V.: 1 mg/m^2 day 3
[total dose/cycle = 1 mg/m^2]
Methotrexate: I.V. bolus: 100 mg/m^2 day 3
followed by I.V.: 200 mg/m^2 continuous infusion over 12 hours day 3
[total dose/cycle = 300 mg/m^2]
Leucovorin: I.M.: 10 mg/m^2 every 12 hours, for 4 doses, days 4 and 5 (start 24 hours after the start of methotrexate)
[total dose/cycle = 40 mg/m^2]
Cyclophosphamide: I.V.: 600 mg/m^2 day 5
[total dose/cycle = 600 mg/m^2]
Doxorubicin: I.V.: 30 mg/m^2 day 10
[total dose/cycle = 30 mg/m^2]
Repeat cycle every 3 weeks
Variation 3:
Hydroxyurea: Oral: 500 mg every 12 hours, for 4 doses, days 1 and 2 (usually started in early morning)
[total dose/cycle = 2000 mg/m^2]
Vincristine: I.V.: 1 mg/m^2 day 3
[total dose/cycle = 1 mg/m^2]
Methotrexate: I.V. bolus: 100 mg/m^2 day 3
followed by I.V.: 200 mg/m^2 continuous infusion over 12 hours day 3
[total dose/cycle = 300 mg/m^2]
Leucovorin: I.M.: 14 mg every 6 hours, for 6 doses, days 4, 5, and 6 (start 24 hours after start of methotrexate)
[total dose/cycle = 84 mg]

◄ Dactinomycin: I.V.: 0.2 mg/day days 2, 3, and 4
　followed by I.V.: 0.5 mg/day days 5 and 6
　[total dose/cycle = 1.6 mg]
Cyclophosphamide: I.V.: 500 mg/m^2 day 4
　[total dose/cycle = 500 mg/m^2]
Doxorubicin: I.V.: 30 mg/m^2 day 9
　[total dose/cycle = 30 mg/m^2]
Melphalan: I.V.: 6 mg/m^2 day 9
　[total dose/cycle = 6 mg/m^2]
Repeat cycle approximately every 3 weeks
Variation 4:
Hydroxyurea: Oral: 500 mg 4 times/day, for 4 doses, day 1
　[total dose/cycle = 2000 mg/m^2]
Vincristine: I.V.: 1 mg/m^2 day 2
　[total dose/cycle = 1 mg/m^2]
Methotrexate: I.V. bolus: 100 mg/m^2 day 2
　followed by I.V.: 200 mg/m^2 continuous infusion over 12 hours day 2
　[total dose/cycle = 300 mg/m^2]
Leucovorin: I.M.: 14 mg every 6 hours, for 6 doses, days 3, 4, and 5 (start 24 hours after the start of methotrexate)
　[total dose/cycle = 84 mg]
Dactinomycin: I.V.: 0.2 mg days 1, 2, and 3
　followed by I.V.: 0.5 mg days 4 and 5
　[total dose/cycle = 1.6 mg]
Cyclophosphamide: I.V.: 500 mg/m^2 day 3
　[total dose/cycle = 500 mg/m^2]
Cyclophosphamide: I.V.: 300 mg/m^2 on day 8
　[total dose/cycle = 300 mg/m^2]
Doxorubicin: I.V.: 30 mg/m^2 day 8
　[total dose/cycle = 30 mg/m^2]
Repeat cycle approximately every 3 weeks

CHAMOMA (Bagshawe Regimen)

Use Gestational trophoblastic tumor

Regimen

Hydroxyurea: Oral: 500 mg every 12 hours, for 4 doses, days 1 and 2
　[total dose/cycle = 2000 mg]
Vincristine: I.V.: 1 mg/m^2 day 3
　[total dose/cycle = 1 mg/m^2]
Methotrexate: I.V. bolus: 100 mg/m^2 day 3
　followed by I.V.: 200 mg/m^2 continuous infusion over 12 hours day 3
　[total dose/cycle = 300 mg/m^2]
Leucovorin: I.M.: 12 mg/m^2 every 12 hours, for 4 doses, days 4 and 5 (start 12 hours after the end of methotrexate infusion)
　[total dose/cycle = 48 mg/m^2]
Dactinomycin: I.V.: 10 mcg/kg/day days 5, 6, and 7
　[total dose/cycle = 30 mcg/kg]
Cyclophosphamide: I.V.: 600 mg/m^2 day 5
　[total dose/cycle = 600 mg/m^2]
Doxorubicin: I.V.: 30 mg/m^2 day 10
　[total dose/cycle = 30 mg/m^2]
Melphalan: I.V.: 6 mg/m^2 day 10
　[total dose/cycle = 6 mg/m^2]
Repeat cycle approximately every 3 weeks

Chlorambucil-VPP (Hodgkin Lymphoma)

Use Lymphoma, Hodgkin disease

Regimen

Chlorambucil: Oral: 6 mg/m^2/day (maximum dose: 10 mg) days 1 to 14
　[total dose/cycle = 84 mg/m^2]
Vinblastine: I.V.: 6 mg/m^2/day (maximum dose: 10 mg) days 1 and 8
　[total dose/cycle = 12 mg/m^2]

Procarbazine: Oral: 100 mg/m²/day (maximum dose: 150 mg) days 1 to 14
  [total dose/cycle = 1400 mg/m²]
Prednisone: Oral: 40-50 mg/day days 1 to 14
  [total dose/cycle = 560-700 mg]
Repeat cycle every 28 days

CHL + PRED

Use Leukemia, chronic lymphocytic
Regimen
  Chlorambucil: Oral: 0.4 mg/kg/day for 1 day every other week; increase initial dose of 0.4 mg/kg by 0.1 mg/kg every 2 weeks until toxicity or disease control is achieved
  Prednisone: Oral: 100 mg/day for 2 days every other week

CHOP

Use Lymphoma, non-Hodgkin
Regimen NOTE: Multiple variations are listed.
  Variation 1:
  Cyclophosphamide: I.V.: 750 mg/m² day 1
    [total dose/cycle = 750 mg/m²]
  Doxorubicin: I.V.: 50 mg/m² day 1
    [total dose/cycle = 50 mg/m²]
  Vincristine: I.V.: 1.4 mg/m² (maximum dose: 2 mg) day 1
    [total dose/cycle = 1.4 mg/m²; maximum: 2 mg]
  Prednisone: Oral: 100 mg/day days 1 to 5
    [total dose/cycle = 500 mg]
  Repeat cycle every 21 days for 6 to 8 cycles
  Variation 2 (dose intensity/dose-dense):
  Cyclophosphamide: I.V.: 1600 mg/m² day 1
    [total dose/cycle = 1600 mg/m²]
  Doxorubicin: I.V.: 65 mg/m² day 1
    [total dose/cycle = 65 mg/m²]
  Vincristine: I.V.: 1.4 mg/m² day 1
    [total dose/cycle = 1.4 mg/m²]
  Prednisone: Oral: 100 mg/day days 1 to 5
    [total dose/cycle = 500 mg]
  Filgrastim: SubQ: 5 mcg/kg days 2 to 11 or until ANC >10,000/mm³
  Repeat cycle every 14 days for 6 cycles
  Variation 3 (dose-dense):
  Cyclophosphamide: I.V.: 750 mg/m² day 1
    [total dose/cycle = 750 mg/m²]
  Doxorubicin: I.V.: 50 mg/m² day 1
    [total dose/cycle = 50 mg/m²]
  Vincristine: I.V.: 2 mg day 1
    [total dose/cycle = 2 mg]
  Prednisone: Oral: 100 mg/day days 1 to 5
    [total dose/cycle = 500 mg]
  Filgrastim: SubQ: 300 mcg/day (<75 kg patient) or 480 mcg/day (≥75 kg patient) days 4 to 13
  Repeat cycle every 14 days for 6 cycles
  Variation 4 (localized disease; chemotherapy plus radiotherapy):
  Cyclophosphamide: I.V.: 750 mg/m² day 1
    [total dose/cycle = 750 mg/m²]
  Doxorubicin: I.V.: 50 mg/m² day 1
    [total dose/cycle = 50 mg/m²]
  Vincristine: I.V.: 1.4 mg/m² (maximum dose: 2 mg) day 1
    [total dose/cycle = 1.4 mg/m²; maximum: 2 mg]
  Prednisone: Oral: 100 mg/day days 1 to 5
    [total dose/cycle = 500 mg]
  Repeat cycle every 21 days for 3 cycles followed by radiation therapy
  Variation 5 (HIV-associated NHL):
  Cyclophosphamide: I.V.: 750 mg/m² day 1
    [total dose/cycle = 750 mg/m²]

◄ Doxorubicin: I.V.: 50 mg/m^2 day 1
  [total dose/cycle = 50 mg/m^2]
Vincristine: I.V.: 1.4 mg/m^2 (maximum dose: 2 mg) day 1
  [total dose/cycle = 1.4 mg/m^2; maximum: 2 mg]
Prednisone: Oral: 100 mg/day days 1 to 5
  [total dose/cycle = 500 mg]
Filgrastim: SubQ: 300 mcg/day (<70 kg patient) or 480 mcg/day (>70 kg patient) days 4 to 13
Repeat cycle every 21 days; minimum of 4 cycles or 2 cycles beyond complete remission

CI (Neuroblastoma)

Use Neuroblastoma
Regimen
Ifosfamide: I.V.: 1500 mg/m^2/day days 1, 2, and 3
  [total dose/cycle = 4500 mg/m^2]
Mesna: I.V.: 500 mg/m^2 every 3 hours, for 3 doses each day, days 1, 2, and 3
  [total dose/cycle = 4500 mg/m^2]
Carboplatin: I.V.: 400 mg/m^2 day 4
  [total dose/cycle = 400 mg/m^2]
Repeat cycle every 21-28 days

CISCA

Use Bladder cancer
Regimen
Cyclophosphamide: I.V.: 650 mg/m^2 day 1
  [total dose = 650 mg/m^2]
Doxorubicin: I.V.: 50 mg/m^2 day 1
  [total dose = 50 mg/m^2]
Cisplatin: I.V.: 100 mg/m^2 day 2
  [total dose = 100 mg/m^2]
Repeat cycle every 21-28 days

Cisplatin-Capecitabine (Esophageal Cancer)

Use Esophageal cancer
Regimen
Cisplatin: I.V.: 80 mg/m^2 over 2 hours day 1
  [total dose/cycle = 80 mg/m^2]
Capecitabine: Oral: 1000 mg/m^2/dose twice daily, days 1 to 14
  [total dose/cycle = 28,000 mg/m^2]
Repeat cycle every 3 weeks until disease progression or unacceptable toxicity

Cisplatin-Capecitabine (Gastric Cancer)

Use Gastric cancer
Regimen
Cisplatin: I.V.: 80 mg/m^2 over 2 hours day 1
  [total dose/cycle = 80 mg/m^2]
Capecitabine: Oral: 1000 mg/m^2/dose twice daily, days 1 to 14
  [total dose/cycle = 28,000 mg/m^2]
Repeat cycle every 3 weeks until disease progression or unacceptable toxicity

Cisplatin-Cetuximab (Head and Neck Cancer)

Use Head and neck cancer
Regimen NOTE: Multiple variations are listed.
Variation 1:
Cycle 1:
Cetuximab: I.V.: 400 mg/m^2 (loading dose) day 1 (week 1, cycle 1 only)
  [total loading dose = 400 mg/m^2]
  followed by I.V.: 250 mg/m^2/day days 8, 15, and 22
    [total dose/cycle 1 = 1150 mg/m^2]
Cisplatin: I.V.: 100 mg/m^2 day 1
  [total dose/cycle = 100 mg/m^2]
Treatment cycle is 4 weeks

Subsequent cycles:
　Cetuximab: I.V.: 250 mg/m^2/day days 1, 8, 15, and 22
　　[total dose/cycle = 1000 mg/m^2]
　Cisplatin: I.V.: 100 mg/m^2 day 1
　　[total dose/cycle = 100 mg/m^2]
　Repeat cycle every 4 weeks
Variation 2:
　Cycle 1:
　Cetuximab: I.V.: 400 mg/m^2 (loading dose) day 1 (week 1, cycle 1 only)
　　[total loading dose = 400 mg/m^2]
　　followed by I.V.: 250 mg/m^2/day days 8 and 15
　　　[total dose/cycle 1 = 900 mg/m^2]
　Cisplatin: I.V.: 75-100 mg/m^2 day 1
　　[total dose/cycle = 75-100 mg/m^2]
　Treatment cycle is 3 weeks
　Subsequent cycles:
　Cetuximab: I.V.: 250 mg/m^2/day days 1, 8, and 15
　　[total dose/cycle = 750 mg/m^2]
　Cisplatin: I.V.: 75-100 mg/m^2 day 1
　　[total dose/cycle = 75-100 mg/m^2]
　Repeat cycle every 3 weeks

Cisplatin-Cytarabine-Dexamethasone (NHL Regimen)

Use Lymphoma, non-Hodgkin
Regimen NOTE: Multiple variations are listed.
Variation 1:
　Dexamethasone: I.V. or Oral: 40 mg/day days 1 to 4
　　[total dose/cycle = 160 mg]
　Cisplatin: I.V.: 100 mg/m^2 over 24 hours day 1
　　[total dose/cycle = 100 mg/m^2]
　Cytarabine: I.V.: 2000 mg/m^2 every 12 hours for 2 doses day 2 (begins at the end of the cisplatin infusion)
　　[total dose/cycle = 4000 mg/m^2]
　Repeat cycle every 3-4 weeks for 6-10 cycles
Variation 2 (patients >70 years of age):
　Dexamethasone: I.V. or Oral: 40 mg/day days 1 to 4
　　[total dose/cycle = 160 mg]
　Cisplatin: I.V.: 100 mg/m^2 over 24 hours day 1
　　[total dose/cycle = 100 mg/m^2]
　Cytarabine: I.V.: 1000 mg/m^2 every 12 hours for 2 doses day 2 (begins at the end of the cisplatin infusion)
　　[total dose/cycle = 2000 mg/m^2]
　Repeat cycle every 3-4 weeks for 6-10 cycles

Cisplatin-Dacarbazine-Interferon Alfa-2b-Aldesleukin

Use Melanoma
Regimen
Cisplatin: I.V.: 25 mg/m^2/day days 1, 2, and 3
　[total dose/cycle = 75 mg/m^2]
Dacarbazine: 250 mg/m^2/day days 1, 2, and 3
　[total dose/cycle = 750 mg/m^2]
Interferon Alfa-2b: SubQ: 5 million units/m^2/day days 6, 8, 10, 13, and 15
　[total dose/cycle = 25 million units/m^2]
Aldesleukin: I.V.: 18 million units/m^2/day days 6 to 10, 13, 14, and 15
　[total dose/cycle = 144 million units/m^2]
Repeat cycle every 28 days

Cisplatin-Etoposide (NSCLC)

Use Lung cancer, nonsmall cell
Regimen NOTE: Multiple variations are listed.

Variation 1:
Cisplatin: I.V.: 80 mg/m^2 day 1
[total dose/cycle = 80 mg/m^2]
Etoposide: I.V.: 100 mg/m^2/day days 1, 2, and 3
[total dose/cycle = 300 mg/m^2]
Repeat cycle every 21 days for a total of 4 cycles
Variation 2:
Cisplatin: I.V.: 100 mg/m^2 day 1
[total dose/cycle = 100 mg/m^2]
Etoposide: I.V.: 100 mg/m^2/day days 1, 2, and 3
[total dose/cycle = 300 mg/m^2]
Repeat cycle every 28 days for a total of 3 cycles
Variation 3:
Cisplatin: I.V.: 100 mg/m^2 day 1
[total dose/cycle = 100 mg/m^2]
Etoposide: I.V.: 100 mg/m^2/day days 1, 2, and 3
[total dose/cycle = 300 mg/m^2]
Repeat cycle every 28 days for a total of 4 cycles
Variation 4:
Cisplatin: I.V.: 120 mg/m^2/day days 1, 29, and 71
[total dose/treatment = 360 mg/m^2]
Etoposide: I.V.: 100 mg/m^2/day days 1, 2, 3, 29, 30, 31, 71, 72, and 73
[total dose/treatment = 900 mg/m^2]
Variation 5:
Cisplatin: I.V.: 75 mg/m^2 day 1
[total dose/cycle = 75 mg/m^2]
Etoposide: I.V.: 100 mg/m^2/day days 1, 2, and 3
[total dose/cycle = 300 mg/m^2]
Repeat cycle every 21 days for up to 10 cycles

Cisplatin-Fluorouracil (Bladder Cancer)

Use Bladder cancer

Regimen In combination with radiation therapy
Note: Begin infusion(s) 2 hours before radiation therapy on days 1, 3, 15, and 17:
Cisplatin: I.V.: 15 mg/m^2/day over 2 hours days 1, 2, 3, 15, 16, and 17
[total dose/cycle = 90 mg/m^2]
Fluorouracil: I.V.: 400 mg/m^2/day over 2 hours days 1, 2, 3, 15, 16, and 17
[total dose/cycle = 2400 mg/m^2]

Cisplatin-Fluorouracil (Cervical Cancer)

Use Cervical cancer

Regimen NOTE: Multiple variations are listed.
Variation 1 (with concurrent radiation therapy):
Cisplatin: I.V.: 75 mg/m^2 day 1
[total dose/cycle = 75 mg/m^2]
Fluorouracil: I.V.: 1000 mg/m^2/day continuous infusion days 1 to 4 (96 hours)
[total dose/cycle = 4000 mg/m^2]
Repeat cycle every 21 days for a total 3 cycles
Variation 2 (with concurrent radiation therapy):
Cisplatin: I.V.: 50 mg/m^2 day 1 starting 4 hours before radiotherapy
[total dose/cycle = 50 mg/m^2]
Fluorouracil: I.V.: 1000 mg/m^2/day continuous infusion days 2 to 5 (96 hours)
[total dose/cycle = 4000 mg/m^2]
Repeat cycle every 28 days for a total of 2 cycles
Variation 3 (cycles 1 and 2 are with concurrent radiation therapy):
Cisplatin: I.V.: 70 mg/m^2 day 1
[total dose/cycle = 70 mg/m^2]
Fluorouracil: I.V.: 1000 mg/m^2/day continuous infusion days 1 to 4 (96 hours)
[total dose/cycle = 4000 mg/m^2]
Repeat cycle every 21 days for a total of 4 cycles

Cisplatin-Fluorouracil (Esophageal Cancer)

Use Esophageal cancer

Regimen NOTE: Multiple variations are listed.

Variation 1:

Cisplatin: I.V.: 100 mg/m^2/dose day 1

[total dose/cycle = 100 mg/m^2]

Fluorouracil: I.V.: 1000 mg/m^2/day continuous infusion days 1 to 5

[total dose/cycle = 5000 mg/m^2]

Repeat cycle every 28 days until disease progression or unacceptable toxicity.

Variation 2:

Cycles 1 to 3 (prior to surgery):

Cisplatin: I.V.: 100 mg/m^2/dose day 1

[total dose/cycle = 100 mg/m^2]

Fluorouracil: I.V.: 1000 mg/m^2/day continuous infusion days 1 to 5

[total dose/cycle = 5000 mg/m^2]

Treatment cycles 1-3 are 28 days each

Cycles 4 and 5 (postoperative):

Cisplatin: I.V.: 75 mg/m^2/dose day 1

[total dose/cycle = 75 mg/m^2]

Fluorouracil: I.V.: 1000 mg/m^2/day continuous infusion days 1 to 5

[total dose/cycle = 5000 mg/m^2]

Treatment cycles 4 and 5 are 28 days each

Variation 3 (in combination with radiation therapy):

Cycle 1:

Cisplatin: I.V.: 75 mg/m^2/dose day 1

[total dose/cycle = 75 mg/m^2]

Fluorouracil: I.V.: 1000 mg/m^2/day continuous infusion days 1 to 4

[total dose/cycle = 4000 mg/m^2]

Treatment cycle is 28 days

Cycles 2 to 4:

Cisplatin: I.V.: 75 mg/m^2/dose day 1

[total dose/cycle = 75 mg/m^2]

Fluorouracil: I.V.: 1000 mg/m^2/day continuous infusion days 1 to 4

[total dose/cycle = 4000 mg/m^2]

Repeat cycle every 21 days for 3 more cycles (total of 4 cycles)

Variation 4 (in combination with radiation therapy):

Cisplatin: I.V.: 100 mg/m^2/dose day 1

[total dose/cycle = 100 mg/m^2]

Fluorouracil: I.V.: 1000 mg/m^2/day continuous infusion days 1 to 4

[total dose/cycle = 4000 mg/m^2]

Repeat cycle every 28 days for total of 2 cycles

Variation 5 (in combination with radiation therapy):

Cisplatin: I.V.: 75 mg/m^2/dose day 1

[total dose/cycle = 75 mg/m^2]

Fluorouracil: I.V.: 1000 mg/m^2/day continuous infusion days 1 to 4

[total dose/cycle = 4000 mg/m^2]

Repeat cycle every 28 days for 4 cycles

Variation 6 (in combination with radiation therapy):

Cycles 1 and 2:

Cisplatin: I.V.: 75 mg/m^2/dose day 1

[total dose/cycle = 75 mg/m^2]

Fluorouracil: I.V.: 1000 mg/m^2/day continuous infusion days 1 to 4

[total dose/cycle = 4000 mg/m^2]

Treatment cycles 1 and 2 are 28 days each; cycle 2 is followed by a 2-week rest

Cycles 3 and 4 (begin cycle 3 at week 11):

Cisplatin: I.V.: 75 mg/m^2/dose day 1

[total dose/cycle = 75 mg/m^2]

Fluorouracil: I.V.: 1000 mg/m^2/day continuous infusion days 1 to 4

[total dose/cycle = 4000 mg/m^2]

Treatment cycles 3 and 4 are 28 days each

Variation 7 (in combination with radiation therapy):
Cycles 1 to 4:
Cisplatin: I.V.: 15 mg/m^2/day days 1 to 5
[total dose/cycle = 75 mg/m^2]
Fluorouracil: I.V.: 800 mg/m^2/day continuous infusion days 1 to 5
[total dose/cycle = 4000 mg/m^2]
Repeat cycles 1-4 every 21 days; cycle 4 is followed by a 1-week rest
Cycles 5 (begin cycle 5 at week 14):
Cisplatin: I.V.: 15 mg/m^2/day days 1 to 5
[total dose/cycle = 75 mg/m^2]
Fluorouracil: I.V.: 800 mg/m^2/day continuous infusion days 1 to 5
[total dose/cycle = 4000 mg/m^2]
Variation 8:
Cisplatin: I.V.: 80 mg/m^2/dose day 1
[total dose/cycle = 80 mg/m^2]
Fluorouracil: I.V.: 800 mg/m^2/day continuous infusion days 1 to 5
[total dose/cycle = 4000 mg/m^2]
Repeat cycle every 21 days until disease progression or unacceptable toxicity.

Cisplatin-Fluorouracil (Gastric Cancer)

Use Gastric cancer

Regimen NOTE: Multiple variations are listed.
Variation 1:
Cisplatin: I.V.: 100 mg/m^2 day 1
[total dose/cycle = 100 mg/m^2]
Fluorouracil: I.V.: 1000 mg/m^2/day continuous infusion days 1 to 5
[total dose/cycle = 5000 mg/m^2]
Repeat cycle every 4 weeks until disease progression or unacceptable toxicity
Variation 2:
Cisplatin: I.V.: 80 mg/m^2 over 2 hours day 1
[total dose/cycle = 80 mg/m^2]
Fluorouracil: I.V.: 800 mg/m^2/day continuous infusion days 1 to 5
[total dose/cycle = 4000 mg/m^2]
Repeat cycle every 21 days until disease progression or unacceptable toxicity
Variation 3:
Fluorouracil: I.V.: 1000 mg/m^2/day continuous infusion days 1 to 5
[total dose/cycle = 5000 mg/m^2]
Cisplatin: I.V.: 100 mg/m^2 day 2
[total dose/cycle = 100 mg/m^2]
Repeat cycle every 4 weeks

Cisplatin-Fluorouracil (Head and Neck Cancer)

Use Head and neck cancer

Regimen NOTE: Multiple variations are listed.
Variation 1:
Cisplatin: I.V.: 100 mg/m^2 day 1
[total dose/cycle = 100 mg/m^2]
Fluorouracil: I.V.: 1000 mg/m^2/day continuous infusion days 1 to 4
[total dose/cycle = 4000 mg/m^2]
Repeat cycle every 3 weeks
Variation 2:
Cisplatin: I.V.: 100 mg/m^2 day 1
[total dose/cycle = 100 mg/m^2]
Fluorouracil: I.V.: 1000 mg/m^2/day continuous infusion days 1 to 4
[total dose/cycle = 4000 mg/m^2]
Repeat cycle every 3 or 4 weeks
Variation 3:
Cisplatin: I.V.: 100 mg/m^2 day 1
[total dose/cycle = 100 mg/m^2]
Fluorouracil: I.V.: 1000 mg/m^2/day continuous infusion days 1 to 5
[total dose/cycle = 5000 mg/m^2]
Repeat cycle every 3 or 4 weeks

Variation 4:
  Cisplatin: I.V.: 60 mg/m^2 day 1
  [total dose/cycle = 60 mg/m^2]
  Fluorouracil: I.V.: 800 mg/m^2/day continuous infusion days 1 to 5
  [total dose/cycle = 4000 mg/m^2]
  Repeat cycle every 14 days
Variation 5:
  Cisplatin: I.V.: 20 mg/m^2/day days 1 to 5
  [total dose/cycle = 100 mg/m^2]
  Fluorouracil: I.V.: 200 mg/m^2/day days 1 to 5
  [total dose/cycle = 1000 mg/m^2]
  Repeat cycle every 3 weeks
Variation 6:
  Cisplatin: I.V.: 80 mg/m^2 continuous infusion day 1
  [total dose/cycle = 80 mg/m^2]
  Fluorouracil: I.V.: 800 mg/m^2/day continuous infusion days 2 to 6
  [total dose/cycle = 4000 mg/m^2]
  Repeat cycle every 3 weeks
Variation 7:
  Cisplatin: I.V.: 75 mg/m^2 day 1
  [total dose/cycle = 75 mg/m^2]
  Fluorouracil: I.V.: 1000 mg/m^2/day continuous infusion days 1 to 4
  [total dose/cycle = 4000 mg/m^2]
  Repeat cycle every 4 weeks
Variation 8:
  Cisplatin: I.V.: 120 mg/m^2 day 1
  [total dose/cycle = 120 mg/m^2]
  Fluorouracil: I.V.: 1000 mg/m^2/day continuous infusion days 1 to 5
  [total dose/cycle = 5000 mg/m^2]
  Repeat cycle every 3 weeks
Variation 9:
  Cisplatin: I.V.: 25 mg/m^2/day continuous infusion days 1 to 4
  [total dose/cycle = 100 mg/m^2]
  Fluorouracil: I.V.: 1000 mg/m^2/day days 1 to 4
  [total dose/cycle = 4000 mg/m^2]
  Repeat cycle every 3 weeks
Variation 10:
  Fluorouracil: I.V.: 350 mg/m^2/day continuous infusion days 1 to 5
  [total dose/cycle = 1750 mg/m^2]
  Cisplatin: I.V.: 50 mg/m^2 day 6
  [total dose/cycle = 50 mg/m^2]
  Repeat cycle every 3 weeks
Variation 11:
  Cisplatin: I.V.: 5 mg/m^2/day continuous infusion days 1 to 14
  [total dose/cycle = 70 mg/m^2]
  Fluorouracil: I.V.: 200 mg/m^2/day continuous infusion days 1 to 14
  [total dose/cycle = 2800 mg/m^2]
  With concurrent radiation therapy, cycle does not repeat
Variation 12 (administer during the final 2 weeks of radiation therapy; weeks 6 and 7):
  Cisplatin: I.V.: 10 mg/m^2/day days 1 to 5 beginning week 6
  [total dose/week = 50 mg/m^2]
  Fluorouracil: I.V.: 400 mg/m^2/day continuous infusion days 1 to 5 beginning week 6
  [total dose/week = 2000 mg/m^2]
  Repeat cycle one time in week 7

Variation 13:
  Cisplatin: I.V.: 100 mg/m^2/day day 1 (concurrent with radiation therapy)
    [total dose/cycle = 100 mg/m^2]
  Repeat cycle every 3 weeks for a total of 3 cycles
  Followed by (postradiation chemotherapy; begin 4 weeks after radiotherapy or the last cisplatin dose):
  Cisplatin: I.V.: 80 mg/m^2 day 1
    [total dose/cycle = 80 mg/m^2]
  Fluorouracil: I.V.: 1000 mg/m^2/day continuous infusion days 1 to 4
    [total dose/cycle = 4000 mg/m^2]
  Repeat cycle every 4 weeks for a total of 3 cycles

Cisplatin-Gemcitabine (Cervical Cancer)

Use Cervical cancer
Regimen NOTE: Multiple variations are listed.
  Variation 1:
    Gemcitabine: I.V.: 1250 mg/m^2/day days 1 and 8
      [total dose/cycle = 2500 mg/m^2]
    Cisplatin: I.V.: 50 mg/m^2 day 1
      [total dose/cycle = 50 mg/m^2]
    Repeat cycle every 21 days for up to a total of 6 cycles
  Variation 2:
    Gemcitabine: I.V.: 1000 mg/m^2/day days 1 and 8
      [total dose/cycle = 2000 mg/m^2]
    Cisplatin: I.V.: 50 mg/m^2 day 1
      [total dose/cycle = 50 mg/m^2]
    Repeat cycle every 21 days for up to a total of 6 cycles; responders may continue beyond 6 cycles

Cisplatin-Irinotecan (NSCLC)

Use Lung cancer, nonsmall cell
Regimen
  Cisplatin: I.V.: 80 mg/m^2 day 1
    [total dose/cycle = 80 mg/m^2]
  Irinotecan: I.V.: 60 mg/m^2/dose days 1, 8, and 15
    [total dose/cycle = 180 mg/m^2]
  Repeat cycle every 28 days for at least 3 more cycles or until disease progression or unacceptable toxicity·

Cisplatin-Irinotecan (Small Cell Lung Cancer)

Use Lung cancer, small cell
Regimen NOTE: Multiple variations are listed.
  Variation 1:
    Cisplatin: I.V.: 60 mg/m^2 day 1
      [total dose/cycle = 60 mg/m^2]
    Irinotecan: I.V.: 60 mg/m^2/dose days 1, 8, and 15
      [total dose/cycle = 180 mg/m^2]
    Repeat cycle every 28 days for 4 cycles
  Variation 2:
    Cisplatin: I.V.: 30 mg/m^2 days 1 and 8
      [total dose/cycle = 60 mg/m^2]
    Irinotecan: I.V.: 65 mg/m^2/dose days 1 and 8
      [total dose/cycle = 130 mg/m^2]
    Repeat cycle every 21 days for at least 4 cycles

Cisplatin-Paclitaxel (Cervical Cancer)

Use Cervical cancer
Regimen
  Paclitaxel: I.V.: 135 mg/m^2 continuous infusion over 24 hours day 1
    [total dose/cycle = 135 mg/m^2]
  Cisplatin: I.V.: 50 mg/m^2 day 2
    [total dose/cycle = 50 mg/m^2]
  Repeat cycle every 21 days for up to a total of 6 cycles; responders may continue beyond 6 cycles

Cisplatin-Paclitaxel (Head and Neck Cancer)

Use Head and neck cancer

Regimen NOTE: Multiple variations are listed.
Variation 1 (with concurrent radiation therapy):
Paclitaxel: I.V.: 30 mg/m^2 day 1
[total dose/week = 30 mg/m^2]
Cisplatin: I.V.: 20 mg/m^2 day 2
[total dose/week = 20 mg/m^2]
Repeat every week for a total of 7 weeks
Variation 2:
Paclitaxel: I.V.: 175 mg/m^2 dose over 3 hours day 1
[total dose/cycle = 175 mg/m^2]
Cisplatin: I.V.: 75 mg/m^2/dose day 1
[total dose/cycle = 75 mg/m^2]
Repeat cycle every 3 weeks

Cisplatin-Paclitaxel (Intraperitoneal Regimen)

Use Ovarian cancer

Regimen Note: I.P. therapies administered in 2 liters warmed saline
Paclitaxel: I.V.: 135 mg/m^2 continuous infusion (over 24 hours) day 1
[total dose/cycle = 135 mg/m^2]
Cisplatin: I.P.: 100 mg/m^2 day 2
[total dose/cycle = 100 mg/m^2]
Paclitaxel: I.P.: 60 mg/m^2 day 8
[total dose/cycle = 60 mg/m^2]
Repeat cycle every 21 days for 6 cycles

Cisplatin-Paclitaxel (Ovarian Cancer)

Use Ovarian cancer

Regimen NOTE: Multiple variations are listed.
Variation 1:
Paclitaxel: I.V.: 135 mg/m^2 continuous infusion over 24 hours day 1
[total dose/cycle = 135 mg/m^2]
Cisplatin: I.V.: 75 mg/m^2 day 2
[total dose/cycle = 75 mg/m^2]
Repeat cycle every 21 days for a total of 6 cycles
Variation 2:
Paclitaxel: I.V.: 175 mg/m^2 over 3 hours day 1
[total dose/cycle = 175 mg/m^2]
Cisplatin: I.V.: 75 mg/m^2 day 1
[total dose/cycle = 75 mg/m^2]
Repeat cycle every 21 days for a total of at least 6 cycles
Variation 3:
Paclitaxel: I.V.: 185 mg/m^2 (maximum dose: 400 mg) over 3 hours day 1
[total dose/cycle = 185 mg/m^2; maximum: 400 mg]
Cisplatin: I.V.: 75 mg/m^2 (maximum dose: 165 mg) day 1
[total dose/cycle = 75 mg/m^2; maximum: 165 mg]
Repeat cycle every 21 days

Cisplatin-Pemetrexed (Mesothelioma)

Use Malignant pleural mesothelioma

Regimen
Pemetrexed: I.V.: 500 mg/m^2 infused over 10 minutes day 1
[total dose/cycle = 500 mg/m^2]
Cisplatin: I.V.: 75 mg/m^2 infused over 2 hours day 1 (start 30 minutes after pemetrexed)
[total dose/cycle = 75 mg/m^2]
Repeat cycle every 21 days

Cisplatin-Topotecan (Cervical Cancer)

Use Cervical cancer

◀ **Regimen** NOTE: Multiple variations are listed.
Variation 1 (Body surface area capped at 2 m^2 maximum):
Topotecan: I.V.: 0.75 mg/m^2/day days 1, 2, and 3
[total dose/cycle = 2.25 mg/m^2]
Cisplatin: I.V.: 50 mg/m^2 day 1 only
[total dose/cycle = 50 mg/m^2]
Repeat cycle every 21 days for up to a total of 6 cycles; responders may continue beyond 6 cycles
Variation 2:
Topotecan: I.V.: 0.75 mg/m^2/day days 1, 2, and 3
[total dose/cycle = 2.25 mg/m^2]
Cisplatin: I.V.: 50 mg/m^2 day 1 only
[total dose/cycle = 50 mg/m^2]
Repeat cycle every 21 days for up to a total of 6 cycles; responders may continue beyond 6 cycles

Cisplatin-Vinblastine-Dacarbazine (Melanoma)

Use Melanoma

Regimen NOTE: Multiple variations are listed.
Variation 1:
Cisplatin: I.V.: 20 mg/m^2/day days 2 to 5
[total dose/cycle = 80 mg/m^2]
Vinblastine: I.V.: 1.6 mg/m^2/day days 1 to 5
[total dose/cycle = 8 mg/m^2]
Dacarbazine: I.V.: 800 mg/m^2 day 1
[total dose/cycle = 800 mg/m^2]
Repeat cycle every 21 days
Variation 2:
Cisplatin: I.V.: 20 mg/m^2/day days 1 to 4
[total dose/cycle = 80 mg/m^2]
Vinblastine: I.V.: 2 mg/m^2/day days 1 to 4
[total dose/cycle = 8 mg/m^2]
Dacarbazine: I.V.: 800 mg/m^2 day 1
[total dose/cycle = 800 mg/m^2]
Repeat cycle every 21 days

Cisplatin-Vinblastine (NSCLC)

Use Lung cancer, nonsmall cell

Regimen NOTE: Multiple variations are listed.
Variation 1:
Cisplatin: I.V.: 80 mg/m^2/day days 1, 22, 43, and 64
[total dose/treatment = 320 mg/m^2]
Vinblastine: I.V.: 4 mg/m^2/day days 1, 8, 15, 22, 29, 43, and 57
[total dose/treatment = 28 mg/m^2]
Variation 2:
Cisplatin: I.V.: 100 mg/m^2/day days 1, 29, and 57
[total dose/treatment = 300 mg/m^2]
Vinblastine: I.V.: 4 mg/m^2/day days 1, 8, 15, 22, 29, 43, and 57
[total dose/treatment = 28 mg/m^2]
Variation 3:
Cisplatin: I.V.: 100 mg/m^2/day days 1, 29, 57, and 85
[total dose/treatment = 400 mg/m^2]
Vinblastine: I.V.: 4 mg/m^2/day days 1, 8, 15, 22, 29, 43, 57, 71, and 85
[total dose/treatment = 36 mg/m^2]
Variation 4:
Cisplatin: I.V.: 120 mg/m^2/day days 1, 29, and 71
[total dose/treatment = 360 mg/m^2]
Vinblastine: I.V.: 4 mg/m^2/day days 1, 8, 15, 22, 29, 43, 57, and 71
[total dose/treatment = 32 mg/m^2]

Cisplatin-Vinorelbine (Cervical Cancer)

Use Cervical cancer

Regimen NOTE: Multiple variations are listed.

Variation 1:
  Cisplatin: I.V.: 50 mg/m^2 day 1
    [total dose/cycle = 50 mg/m^2]
  Vinorelbine: I.V.: 30 mg/m^2/day days 1 and 8
    [total dose/cycle = 60 mg/m^2]
  Repeat cycle every 21 days for up to a total of 6 cycles; responders may continue beyond 6 cycles
Variation 2:
  Cisplatin: I.V.: 80 mg/m^2 day 1
    [total dose/cycle = 80 mg/m^2]
  Vinorelbine: I.V.: 25 mg/m^2/day days 1 and 8
    [total dose/cycle = 50 mg/m^2]
  Repeat cycle every 21 days for a total of 3-6 cycles

CLAG (AML Induction)

Use Leukemia, acute myeloid

Regimen
  Cladribine: I.V.: 5 mg/m^2/day over 2 hours days 1 to 5
    [total dose/cycle = 25 mg/m^2]
  Cytarabine: I.V.: 2 g/m^2/day over 4 hours days 1 to 5 (begin 2 hours after cladribine)
    [total dose/cycle = 10 g/m^2]
  Filgrastim: SubQ: 300 mcg daily days 0 to 5 (start 24 hours prior to chemotherapy; for a total of 6 days)
    [total dose/cycle = 1800 mcg]
  May administer a second induction cycle if needed

CLAG-M (AML Induction)

Use Leukemia, acute myeloid

Regimen
  Cladribine: I.V.: 5 mg/m^2/day over 2 hour days 1 to 5
    [total dose/cycle = 25 mg/m^2]
  Cytarabine: I.V.: 2 g/m^2/day over 4 hours days 1 to 5 (begin 2 hours after cladribine)
    [total dose/cycle = 10 g/m^2]
  Mitoxantrone: I.V.: 10 mg/m^2/day days 1 to 3
    [total dose/cycle = 30 mg/m^2]
  Filgrastim: SubQ: 300 mcg daily days 0 to 5 (start 24 hours prior to chemotherapy; for a total of 6 days)
    [total dose/cycle = 1800 mcg]
  May administer a second induction cycle if needed

Clofarabine (AML Consolidation)

Use Leukemia, acute myeloid

Regimen
  Clofarabine: I.V.: 20 mg/m^2/day over 1 hour days 1 to 5
    [total dose/cycle = 100 mg/m^2]
  Up to a maximum total of 6 cycles (including induction/reinduction) may be administered

Clofarabine (AML Induction)

Use Leukemia, acute myeloid

Regimen
  Induction:
  Clofarabine: I.V.: 30 mg/m^2/day over 1 hour days 1 to 5
    [total dose/cycle = 150 mg/m^2]
  Reinduction (if needed) after day 28 of induction:
  Clofarabine: I.V.: 20 mg/m^2/day over 1 hour days 1 to 5
    [total dose/cycle = 100 mg/m^2]

Clofarabine-Cytarabine (AML Consolidation)

Use Leukemia, acute myeloid

Regimen
  Clofarabine: I.V.: 30 mg/m^2/day infusion over 1 hour on days 1, 2, and 3
    [total dose/cycle = 90 mg/m^2]
  Cytarabine: SubQ: 20 mg/m^2/day days 1 to 7 (4 hours after clofarabine on days 1, 2, and 3)
    [total dose/cycle = 140 mg/m^2]
  Repeat cycle every 4 to 7 weeks; up to a total of 12 consolidation cycles may be administered

Clofarabine-Cytarabine (AML Induction)

Use Leukemia, acute myeloid

Regimen
Clofarabine: I.V.: 30 mg/m^2/day infusion over 1 hour on days 1 to 5
[total dose/cycle = 150 mg/m^2]
Cytarabine: SubQ: 20 mg/m^2/day days 1 to 14 (4 hours after clofarabine on days 1 to 5)
[total dose/cycle = 280 mg/m^2]
A second induction cycle may be administered if needed

CMF

Use Breast cancer

Regimen NOTE: Multiple variations are listed.
Variation 1:
Methotrexate: I.V.: 40 mg/m^2/day days 1 and 8
[total dose/cycle = 80 mg/m^2]
Fluorouracil: I.V.: 600 mg/m^2/day days 1 and 8
[total dose/cycle = 1200 mg/m^2]
Cyclophosphamide: Oral: 100 mg/m^2/day days 1 to 14
[total dose/cycle = 1400 mg/m^2]
Repeat cycle every 28 days
Variation 2 (>60 years of age):
Methotrexate: I.V.: 30 mg/m^2/day days 1 and 8
[total dose/cycle = 60 mg/m^2]
Fluorouracil: I.V.: 400 mg/m^2/day days 1 and 8
[total dose/cycle = 800 mg/m^2]
Cyclophosphamide: Oral: 100 mg/m^2/day days 1 to 14
[total dose/cycle = 1400 mg/m^2]
Repeat cycle every 28 days

CMF-IV

Use Breast cancer

Regimen
Cyclophosphamide: I.V.: 600 mg/m^2 day 1
[total dose/cycle = 600 mg/m^2]
Methotrexate: I.V.: 40 mg/m^2 day 1
[total dose/cycle = 40 mg/m^2]
Fluorouracil: I.V.: 600 mg/m^2 day 1
[total dose/cycle = 600 mg/m^2]
Repeat cycle every 21 or 28 days

CMV

Use Bladder cancer

Regimen
Cisplatin: I.V.: 100 mg/m^2 infused over 4 hours (start at least 12 hours after methotrexate) day 2
[total dose = 100 mg/m^2]
Methotrexate: I.V.: 30 mg/m^2/day days 1 and 8
[total dose = 60 mg/m^2]
Vinblastine: I.V.: 4 mg/m^2/day days 1 and 8
[total dose = 8 mg/m^2]
Repeat cycle every 21 days

CNOP

Use Lymphoma, non-Hodgkin

Regimen
Cyclophosphamide: I.V.: 750 mg/m^2 day 1
[total dose/cycle = 750 mg/m^2]
Mitoxantrone: I.V.: 10 mg/m^2 day 1
[total dose/cycle = 10 mg/m^2]

Vincristine: I.V.: 1.4 mg/m^2 day 1
  [total dose/cycle = 1.4 mg/m^2]
Prednisone: Oral: 50 mg/m^2/day days 1 to 5
  [total dose/cycle = 250 mg/m^2]
Repeat cycle every 21 days

CODOX-M

Use Lymphoma, non-Hodgkin

Regimen
Variation 1:
  Cyclophosphamide: I.V.: 800 mg/m^2 day 1
    followed by I.V.: 200 mg/m^2/day days 2 to 5
      [total dose/cycle = 1600 mg/m^2]
  Vincristine: I.V.: 1.5 mg/m^2/dose (no maximum dose) days 1 and 8
    [total dose/cycle = 3 mg/m^2]
  Doxorubicin: I.V.: 40 mg/m^2/dose day 1
    [total dose/cycle = 40 mg/m^2]
  Methotrexate: I.V.: 1200 mg/m^2 (loading dose) over 1 hour
    followed by I.V.: 240 mg/m^2/hour for 23 hours day 10
      [total dose/cycle = 6720 mg/m^2]
  Leucovorin: I.V.: 192 mg/m^2/dose day 11 (begin 36 hours after the start of methotrexate infusion)
    followed by I.V.: 12 mg/m^2/dose every 6 hours until methotrexate level <5 x 10^{-8}M
  Cytarabine: I.T.: 70 mg/dose (adjust to age-appropriate dose if <3 years of age) day 1
    [total dose/cycle = 70 mg]
  Methotrexate: I.T.: 12 mg/dose (adjust to age-appropriate dose if <3 years of age) day 3
    [total dose/cycle = 12 mg]
  Repeat cycle when ANC >1000/m^3 for a total of three cycles
Variation 2:
  Cyclophosphamide: I.V.: 800 mg/m^2/dose day 1
    followed by I.V.: 200 mg/m^2/dose days 2 to 5
      [total dose/cycle = 1600 mg/m^2]
  Vincristine: I.V.: 1.5 mg/m^2/dose (maximum dose: 2 mg) days 1 and 8
    [total dose/cycle = 3 mg/m^2; maximum: 4 mg/cycle]
  Doxorubicin: I.V.: 40 mg/m^2/dose day 1
    [total dose/cycle = 40 mg/m^2]
  Methotrexate: I.V.: 1200 mg/m^2 (loading dose) over 1 hour
    followed by I.V.: 240 mg/m^2/hour for 23 hours day 10
      [total dose/cycle = 6720 mg/m^2]
  Leucovorin: I.V.: 192 mg/m^2/dose day 11 (begin 36 hours after the start of methotrexate infusion)
    followed by I.V.: 12 mg/m^2/dose every 6 hours until methotrexate level <5 x 10^{-8}M
  Cytarabine: I.T.: 70 mg/dose days 1 and 3
    [total dose/cycle = 140 mg]
  Methotrexate: I.T.: 12 mg/dose day 15
    [total dose/cycle = 12 mg]
  Leucovorin: Oral: 15 mg/dose day 16 (24 hours after I.T. methotrexate)
  Filgrastim: 5 mcg/kg/day beginning day 13, continue until ANC >1000/mm^3
  Repeat cycle when ANC >1000/mm^3 for a total of three cycles
Variation 3:
  Cyclophosphamide: I.V.: 800 mg/m^2/dose days 1 and 2
    [total dose/cycle = 1600 mg/m^2]
  Vincristine: I.V.: 1.4 mg/m^2/dose (maximum dose: 2 mg) days 1 and 10
    [total dose/cycle = 2.8 mg/m^2; maximum: 4 mg/cycle]
  Doxorubicin: I.V.: 50 mg/m^2/dose day 1
    [total dose/cycle = 50 mg/m^2]
  Methotrexate: I.V.: 3 g/m^2 day 10
    [total dose/cycle = 3 g/m^2]
  Leucovorin: I.V.: 200 mg/m^2/dose day 11
    followed by Oral, I.V.: 15 mg/m^2/dose every 6 hours until methotrexate level <0.1 Mmol/L
  Cytarabine: I.T.: 50 mg/dose day 1
    [total dose/cycle = 50 mg]
  Hydrocortisone: I.T.: 50 mg/dose day 1
    [total dose/cycle = 50 mg]

◄ Methotrexate: I.T.: 12 mg/dose day 1
 [total dose/cycle = 12 mg]
 Filgrastim: SubQ: Dose not specified; days 3 to 8 and day 12 until ANC >1000/mm^3
 Repeat cycle when ANC >1000/mm^3 for a total of three cycles

CODOX-M/IVAC

Use Lymphoma, non-Hodgkin (Burkitt)

Regimen NOTE: Multiple variations are listed.

 Variation 1:

CODOX-M (Cycles 1 and 3; cycles begin when ANC >1000/mm^3)
 Cyclophosphamide: I.V.: 800 mg/m^2/dose day 1
  followed by I.V.: 200 mg/m^2/dose days 2 to 5
   [total dose/cycle = 1600 mg/m^2]
 Vincristine: I.V.: 1.5 mg/m^2/dose (no maximum dose) days 1 and 8 (cycle 1) and days 1, 8, and 15 (cycle 3)
   [total dose/cycle = 3-4.5 mg/m^2]
 Doxorubicin: I.V.: 40 mg/m^2/dose day 1
   [total dose/cycle = 40 mg/m^2]
 Methotrexate: I.V.: 1200 mg/m^2 (loading dose) over 1 hour
  followed by I.V.: 240 mg/m^2/hour for 23 hours day 10
   [total dose/cycle = 6720 mg/m^2]
 Leucovorin: I.V.: 192 mg/m^2/dose day 11 (begin 36 hours after the start of methotrexate infusion)
  followed by I.V.: 12 mg/m^2/dose every 6 hours until methotrexate level <5 x 10^{-8}M
 Cytarabine: I.T.: 70 mg/dose (adjust to age-appropriate dose if <3 years of age) days 1 and 3
   [total dose/cycle = 140 mg]
 Methotrexate: I.T.: 12 mg/dose (adjust to age-appropriate dose if <3 years of age) day 15
   [total dose/cycle = 12 mg]
 Sargramostim: SubQ: 7.5 mcg/kg/day beginning day 13, continue until ANC >1000/mm^3
 Note: If CNS disease present, administer additional I.T. treatment in cycle 1: Cytarabine 70 mg/dose (adjust to age-appropriate dose if <3 years of age) on day 5 and methotrexate 12 mg/dose (adjust to age-appropriate dose if <3 years of age) on day 17

IVAC (Cycles 2 and 4; cycles begin when ANC >1000/mm^3)
 Ifosfamide: I.V.: 1500 mg/m^2/dose days 1 to 5
   [total dose/cycle = 7500 mg/m^2]
 Mesna: I.V.: 360 mg/m^2/dose every 3 hours days 1 to 5
 Etoposide: I.V.: 60 mg/m^2/dose days 1 to 5
   [total dose/cycle = 300 mg/m^2]
 Cytarabine: I.V.: 2 g/m^2/dose every 12 hours, for 4 doses, days 1 and 2
   [total dose/cycle = 8 g/m^2]
 Methotrexate: I.T.: 12 mg/dose day 5
   [total dose/cycle = 12 mg]
 Sargramostim: SubQ: 7.5 mcg/kg/day beginning day 7, continue until ANC >1000/mm^3
 Note: If CNS disease present, administer additional I.T. treatment in cycle 2: Cytarabine 70 mg/dose (adjust to age-appropriate dose if <3 years of age) on days 7 and 9

 Variation 2:

CODOX-M (Cycles 1 and 3; cycles begin when ANC >1000/mm^3)
 Cyclophosphamide: I.V.: 800 mg/m^2/dose day 1
  followed by I.V.: 200 mg/m^2/dose days 2 to 5
   [total dose/cycle = 1600 mg/m^2]
 Vincristine: I.V.: 1.5 mg/m^2/dose (maximum: dose 2 mg) days 1 and 8
   [total dose/cycle = 3 mg/m^2; maximum: 4 mg/cycle]
 Doxorubicin: I.V.: 40 mg/m^2/dose day 1
   [total dose/cycle = 40 mg/m^2]
 Methotrexate: I.V.: 300 mg/m^2 (100 mg/m^2 if >65 years of age) (loading dose) over 1 hour
  followed by I.V.: 2700 mg/m^2 (900 mg/m^2 if >65 years of age) over 23 hours day 10
   [total dose/cycle = 3000 mg/m^2 (1000 mg/m^2 if >65 years of age)]
 Leucovorin: I.V.: 15 mg/m^2/dose every 3 hours beginning day 11 (begin 36 hours after the start of methotrexate infusion) for 5 doses
  followed by I.V.: 15 mg/m^2/dose every 6 hours until methotrexate level <5 x 10^{-8}M
 Cytarabine: I.T.: 70 mg/dose days 1 and 3
   [total dose/cycle = 140 mg]

Methotrexate: I.T.: 12 mg/dose day 15
  [total dose/cycle = 12 mg]
Leucovorin: Oral: 15 mg/dose day 16 (24 hours after I.T. methotrexate)
Filgrastim: SubQ: 5 mcg/kg/day beginning day 13, continue until ANC >1000/mm^3
Note: If CNS disease present, administer additional I.T. treatment: Cytarabine 70 mg/dose on day 5 and methotrexate 12 mg/dose (with leucovorin rescue) on day 17
IVAC (Cycles 2 and 4; cycles begin when ANC >1000/mm^3)
Ifosfamide: I.V.: 1500 mg/m^2/dose (1000 mg/m^2/dose if >65 years of age) days 1 to 5
  [total dose/cycle = 7500 mg/m^2 (5000 mg/m^2 if >65 years of age)]
Mesna: I.V.: 300 mg/m^2/dose (200 mg/m^2/dose if >65 years of age) mixed with each ifosfamide dose
  followed by I.V.: 300 mg/m^2/dose (200 mg/m^2/dose if >65 years of age) every 4 hours for 2 doses/ day days 1 to 5
  [total dose/cycle = 4500 mg/m^2 (3000 mg/m^2/dose if >65 years of age)]
Etoposide: I.V.: 60 mg/m^2/dose days 1 to 5
  [total dose/cycle = 300 mg/m^2]
Cytarabine: I.V.: 2 g/m^2/dose (1 g/m^2/dose if >65 years of age) every 12 hours, for 4 doses, days 1 and 2
  [total dose/cycle = 8 g/m^2 (4 g/m^2 if >65 years of age)]
Methotrexate: I.T.: 12 mg day 5
  [total dose/cycle = 12 mg]
Leucovorin: Oral: 15 mg/dose day 6 (24 hours after I.T. methotrexate)
Filgrastim: SubQ: 5 mcg/kg/day beginning day 7, continue until ANC >1000/mm^3
Note: If CNS disease present, administer additional I.T. treatment: Cytarabine 70 mg/dose on days 7 and 9
Variation 3:
CODOX-M (Cycles 1 and 3; cycles begin when ANC >1000/mm^3)
Cyclophosphamide: I.V.: 800 mg/m^2/dose day 1
  followed by I.V.: 200 mg/m^2/dose days 2 to 5
  [total dose/cycle = 1600 mg/m^2]
Vincristine: I.V.: 1.5 mg/m^2/dose (maximum dose: 2 mg) days 1 and 8
  [total dose/cycle = 3 mg/m^2; maximum: 4 mg/cycle]
Doxorubicin: I.V.: 40 mg/m^2/dose day 1
  [total dose/cycle = 40 mg/m^2]
Methotrexate: I.V.: 1200 mg/m^2 (loading dose) over 1 hour
  followed by I.V.: 240 mg/m^2/hour for 23 hours day 10
  [total dose/cycle = 6720 mg/m^2]
Leucovorin: I.V.: 192 mg/m^2/dose day 11 (begin 36 hours after the start of methotrexate infusion)
  followed by I.V.: 12 mg/m^2/dose every 6 hours until methotrexate level <5 x 10^{-8}M
Cytarabine: I.T.: 70 mg/dose days 1 and 3
  [total dose/cycle = 140 mg]
Methotrexate: I.T.: 12 mg/dose day 15
  [total dose/cycle = 12 mg]
Leucovorin: Oral: 15 mg/dose day 16 (24 hours after I.T. methotrexate)
Filgrastim: SubQ: 5 mcg/kg/day beginning day 13, continue until ANC >1000/mm^3
Note: If CNS disease present, administer additional I.T. treatment in cycle 1: Cytarabine 70 mg/dose (15 mg if via Ommaya reservoir) on day 5 and methotrexate 12.5 mg/dose (2 mg if via Ommaya reservoir) on day 17
IVAC (Cycles 2 and 4; cycles begin when ANC >1000/mm^3)
Ifosfamide: I.V.: 1500 mg/m^2/dose days 1 to 5
  [total dose/cycle = 7500 mg/m^2]
Mesna: I.V.: 360 mg/m^2/dose mixed with each ifosfamide dose
  followed by I.V.: 360 mg/m^2/dose every 3 hours for 7 doses/day days 1 to 5
  [total dose/cycle = 14,400 mg/m^2]
Etoposide: I.V.: 60 mg/m^2/dose days 1 to 5
  [total dose/cycle = 300 mg/m^2]
Cytarabine: I.V.: 2 g/m^2/dose every 12 hours, for 4 doses, days 1 and 2
  [total dose/cycle = 8 g/m^2]
Methotrexate: I.T.: 12 mg/dose day 5
  [total dose/cycle = 12 mg]
Leucovorin: Oral: 15 mg/dose day 6 (24 hours after I.T. methotrexate)
Filgrastim: SubQ: 5 mcg/kg/day beginning day 7, continue until ANC >1000/mm^3

◄ **Note:** If CNS disease present, administer additional I.T. treatment in cycle 2: Cytarabine 70 mg/dose (15 mg if via Ommaya reservoir) on days 7 and 9

Variation 4:

CODOX-M (Cycles 1 and 3; cycles begin when ANC >1000/mm^3)

Cyclophosphamide: I.V.: 800 mg/m^2/dose days 1 and 2
[total dose/cycle = 1600 mg/m^2]
Vincristine: I.V.: 1.4 mg/m^2/dose (maximum dose: 2 mg) days 1 and 10
[total dose/cycle = 2.8 mg/m^2; maximum: 4 mg/cycle]
Doxorubicin: I.V.: 50 mg/m^2/dose day 1
[total dose/cycle = 50 mg/m^2]
Methotrexate: I.V.: 3 g/m^2 day 10
[total dose/cycle = 3 g/m^2]
Leucovorin: I.V.: 200 mg/m^2/dose day 11
followed by Oral, I.V.: 15 mg/m^2/dose every 6 hours until methotrexate level <0.1 Mmol/L
Cytarabine: I.T.: 50 mg/dose days 1 and 3
[total dose/cycle = 100 mg]
Hydrocortisone: I.T.: 50 mg/dose days 1 and 3
[total dose/cycle = 100 mg]
Methotrexate: I.T.: 12 mg/dose day 1
[total dose/cycle = 12 mg]
Filgrastim: SubQ: Dose not specified, days 3 to 8 and day 12 until ANC >1000 mm^3
Note: If CNS disease present, administer additional I.T. treatment in cycle 1: Cytarabine 50 mg/dose on day 5 and methotrexate 12 mg/dose on day 10

IVAC (Cycles 2 and 4; cycles begin when ANC >1000/mm^3)

Ifosfamide: I.V.: 1500 mg/m^2/dose days 1 to 5
[total dose/cycle = 7500 mg/m^2]
Mesna: I.V.: 1500 mg/m^2/day (in divided doses) days 1 to 5
[total dose/cycle = 7500 mg/m^2]
Etoposide: I.V.: 60 mg/m^2/dose days 1 to 5
[total dose/cycle = 300 mg/m^2]
Cytarabine: I.V.: 2 g/m^2/dose every 12 hours, for 4 doses, days 1 and 2
[total dose/cycle = 8 g/m^2]
Methotrexate: I.T.: 12 mg/dose day 5
[total dose/cycle = 12 mg]
Hydrocortisone: I.T.: 50 mg/dose day 5
[total dose/cycle = 50 mg]
Filgrastim: SubQ: Dose not specified, daily beginning day 6 until ANC >1000 mm^3
Note: If CNS disease present, administer additional I.T. treatment in cycle 2: Cytarabine 50 mg/dose on days 3 and 5

COMLA

Use Lymphoma, non-Hodgkin

Regimen

Cyclophosphamide: I.V.: 1500 mg/m^2 day 1
[total dose/cycle = 1500 mg/m^2]
Vincristine: I.V.: 1.4 mg/m^2/day (maximum dose: 2 mg) days 1, 8, and 15
[total dose/cycle = 4.2 mg/m^2]
Methotrexate: I.V.: 120 mg/m^2/day days 22, 29, 36, 43, 50, 57, 64, and 71
[total dose/cycle = 960 mg/m^2]
Leucovorin: Oral: 25 mg/m^2 every 6 hours for 4 doses (beginning 24 hours after each methotrexate dose)
[total dose/cycle = 800 mg/m^2]
Cytarabine: I.V.: 300 mg/m^2/day days 22, 29, 36, 43, 50, 57, 64, and 71
[total dose/cycle = 2400 mg/m^2]
Repeat cycle every 85 days

COP-BLAM

Use Lymphoma, non-Hodgkin

Regimen

Cyclophosphamide: I.V.: 400 mg/m^2 day 1
[total dose/cycle = 400 mg/m^2]
Vincristine: I.V.: 1 mg/m^2 day 1
[total dose/cycle = 1 mg/m^2]

Prednisone: Oral: 40 mg/m^2/day days 1 to 10
  [total dose/cycle = 400 mg/m^2]
Bleomycin: I.V.: 15 mg day 14
  [total dose/cycle = 15 mg]
Doxorubicin: I.V.: 40 mg/m^2 day 1
  [total dose/cycle = 40 mg/m^2]
Procarbazine: Oral: 100 mg/m^2/day days 1 to 10
  [total dose/cycle = 1000 mg/m^2]

COPE

Use Brain tumors
Regimen
  Cycle A:
  Vincristine: I.V.: 0.065 mg/kg/day (maximum dose: 1.5 mg) days 1 and 8
    [total dose/cycle = 0.13 mg/kg]
  Cyclophosphamide: I.V.: 65 mg/kg day 1
    [total dose/cycle = 65 mg/kg]
  Cycle B:
  Cisplatin: I.V.: 4 mg/kg day 1
    [total dose/cycle = 4 mg/kg]
  Etoposide: I.V.: 6.5 mg/kg/day days 3 and 4
    [total dose/cycle = 13 mg/kg]
  Repeat cycle every 28 days in the following sequence: AABAAB

COPP

Use Lymphoma, non-Hodgkin
Regimen
  Cyclophosphamide: I.V.: 450-650 mg/m^2/day days 1 and 8
    [total dose/cycle = 900-1300 mg/m^2]
  Vincristine: I.V.: 1.4-2 mg/m^2/day (maximum dose: 2 mg) days 1 and 8
    [total dose/cycle = 2.8-4 mg/m^2]
  Procarbazine: Oral: 100 mg/m^2/day days 1 to 14
    [total dose/cycle = 1400 mg/m^2]
  Prednisone: Oral: 40 mg/m^2/day days 1 to 14
    [total dose/cycle = 560 mg/m^2]
  Repeat cycle every 3-4 weeks

CP (Leukemia)

Use Leukemia, chronic lymphocytic
Regimen
  Chlorambucil: Oral: 30 mg/m^2 day 1
    [total dose/cycle = 30 mg/m^2]
  Prednisone: Oral: 80 mg/day days 1 to 5
    [total dose/cycle = 400 mg]
  Repeat cycle every 14 days

CP (Ovarian Cancer)

Use Ovarian cancer
Regimen
  Cyclophosphamide: I.V.: 750 mg/m^2 day 1
    [total dose/cycle = 750 mg/m^2]
  Cisplatin: I.V.: 75 mg/m^2 day 1
    [total dose/cycle = 75 mg/m^2]
  Repeat cycle every 21 days

CVD-Interleukin-Interferon (Melanoma)

Use Melanoma
Regimen NOTE: Multiple variations are listed.
  Variation 1:
  Cisplatin: I.V.: 20 mg/m^2/day days 1 to 4 and 22 to 25
    [total dose/cycle = 160 mg/m^2]

Vinblastine: I.V.: 1.5 mg/m^2/day days 1 to 4 and 22 to 25
[total dose/cycle = 12 mg/m^2]
Dacarbazine: I.V.: 800 mg/m^2/day days 1 and 22
[total dose/cycle = 1600 mg/m^2]
Aldesleukin: I.V.: 9 million units/m^2/day continuous infusion days 5 to 8, 17 to 20, and 26 to 29
[total dose/cycle = 108 million units/m^2]
Interferon alfa-2b: SubQ: 5 million units/m^2/day days 5 to 9, 17 to 21, and 26 to 30
[total dose/cycle = 75 million units/m^2]
Repeat every 42 days (maximum of five 21-day cycles for cytokine [interleukin and interferon] component)
Variation 2:
Cisplatin: I.V.: 20 mg/m^2/day days 1 to 4
[total dose/cycle = 80 mg/m^2]
Vinblastine: I.V.: 1.6 mg/m^2/day days 1 to 4
[total dose/cycle = 6.4 mg/m^2]
Dacarbazine: I.V.: 800 mg/m^2 day 1
[total dose/cycle = 800 mg/m^2]
Aldesleukin: I.V.: 9 million units/m^2/day continuous infusion days 1 to 4
[total dose/cycle = 36 million units/m^2]
Interferon alfa-2a: SubQ: 5 million units/m^2/day days 1 to 5, 7, 9, 11, and 13
[total dose/cycle = 45 million units/m^2]
Repeat cycle every 21 days for a total of 6 cycles
Variation 3:
Cisplatin: I.V.: 20 mg/m^2/day days 1 to 4
[total dose/cycle = 80 mg/m^2]
Vinblastine: I.V.: 1.2 mg/m^2/day days 1 to 4
[total dose/cycle = 4.8 mg/m^2]
Dacarbazine: I.V.: 800 mg/m^2 day 1
[total dose/cycle = 800 mg/m^2]
Aldesleukin: I.V.: 9 million units/m^2/day continuous infusion days 1 to 4
[total dose/cycle = 36 million units/m^2]
Interferon alfa-2b: SubQ: 5 million units/m^2/day days 1 to 5, 8, 10, and 12
[total dose/cycle = 40 million units/m^2]
Repeat cycle every 21 days (maximum: 4 cycles)

CVP (Leukemia)

Use Leukemia, chronic lymphocytic
Regimen NOTE: Multiple variations are listed.
Variation 1:
Cyclophosphamide: Oral: 300 or 400 mg/m^2/day days 1 to 5
[total dose/cycle = 1500 or 2000 mg/m^2]
Vincristine: I.V.: 1.4 mg/m^2 (maximum dose: 2 mg) day 1
[total dose/cycle = 1.4 mg/m^2]
Prednisone: Oral: 100 mg/m^2/day days 1 to 5
[total dose/cycle = 500 mg/m^2]
Repeat cycle every 21 days
Variation 2:
Cyclophosphamide: I.V.: 800 mg/m^2 day 1
[total dose/cycle = 800 mg/m^2]
Vincristine: I.V.: 1.4 mg/m^2 (maximum dose: 2 mg) day 1
[total dose/cycle = 1.4 mg/m^2]
Prednisone: Oral: 100 mg/m^2/day days 1 to 5
[total dose/cycle = 500 mg/m^2]
Repeat cycle every 21 days

CVP (Lymphoma, non-Hodgkin)

Use Lymphoma, non-Hodgkin
Regimen NOTE: Multiple variations are listed.
Variation 1:
Cyclophosphamide: I.V.: 750 mg/m^2 day 1
[total dose/cycle = 750 mg/m^2]

Vincristine: I.V.: 1.2 mg/m^2 day 1
  [total dose/cycle = 1.2 mg/m^2]
Prednisone: Oral: 40 mg/m^2/day days 1 to 5
  [total dose/cycle = 200 mg/m^2]
Repeat cycle every 21 days for up to 10 cycles
Variation 2:
  Cyclophosphamide: I.V.: 750 mg/m^2 day 1
  [total dose/cycle = 750 mg/m^2]
  Vincristine: I.V.: 1.2 mg/m^2 day 1 (maximum dose: 2 mg)
  [total dose/cycle = 1.2 mg/m^2 (maximum: 2 mg)]
  Prednisone: Oral: 40 mg/m^2/day days 1 to 5
  [total dose/cycle = 200 mg/m^2]
Repeat cycle every 28 days for up to 8 cycles
Variation 3:
  Cyclophosphamide: I.V.: 750 mg/m^2 day 1
  [total dose/cycle = 750 mg/m^2]
  Vincristine: I.V.: 1.4 mg/m^2 day 1 (maximum dose: 2 mg)
  [total dose/cycle = 1.4 mg/m^2 (maximum: 2 mg)]
  Prednisone: Oral: 40 mg/m^2/day days 1 to 5
  [total dose/cycle = 200 mg/m^2]
Repeat cycle every 21 days for up to 8 cycles
Variation 4:
  Cyclophosphamide: Oral: 400 mg/m^2/day days 1 to 5
  [total dose/cycle = 2000 mg/m^2]
  Vincristine: I.V.: 1.4 mg/m^2 day 1 (maximum dose: 2 mg)
  [total dose/cycle = 1.4 mg/m^2 (maximum: 2 mg)]
  Prednisone: Oral: 100 mg/m^2/day days 1 to 5
  [total dose/cycle = 500 mg/m^2]
Repeat cycle every 21 days

Cyclophosphamide-Fludarabine-Alemtuzumab-Rituximab (CLL)

Use Leukemia, chronic lymphocytic
Regimen
Variation 1:
  Cyclophosphamide: I.V.: 200 mg/m^2/day days 3, 4, and 5
  [total dose/cycle = 600 mg/m^2]
  Fludarabine: I.V.: 20 mg/m^2/day days 3, 4, and 5
  [total dose/cycle = 60 mg/m^2]
  Rituximab: I.V.: 375-500 mg/m^2/dose day 2
  [total dose/cycle = 375-500 mg/m^2]
  Alemtuzumab: I.V.: 30 mg/dose days 1, 3, and 5
  [total dose/cycle = 90 mg]
Repeat cycle every 28 days for up to a total of 6 cycles
Variation 2:
  Cyclophosphamide: I.V.: 200 mg/m^2/day days 3, 4, and 5
  [total dose/cycle = 600 mg/m^2]
  Fludarabine: I.V.: 20 mg/m^2/day days 3, 4, and 5
  [total dose/cycle = 60 mg/m^2]
  Rituximab: I.V.: 375-500 mg/m^2/dose day 2
  [total dose/cycle = 375-500 mg/m^2]
  Alemtuzumab: I.V.: 30 mg/dose days 1, 3, and 5
  [total dose/cycle = 90 mg]
  Pegfilgrastim: SubQ: 6 mg with each cycle
Repeat cycle every 28 days for a total of 6 cycles
Variation 3:
  Cyclophosphamide: I.V.: 250 mg/m^2/day days 3, 4, and 5
  [total dose/cycle = 750 mg/m^2]
  Fludarabine: I.V.: 25 mg/m^2/day days 3, 4, and 5
  [total dose/cycle = 75 mg/m^2]
  Rituximab: I.V.: 375-500 mg/m^2/dose day 2
  [total dose/cycle = 375-500 mg/m^2]

Alemtuzumab: I.V.: 30 mg/dose days 1, 3, and 5
[total dose/cycle = 90 mg]
Repeat cycle every 28 days for a total of 6 cycles

Cytarabine (High Dose)-Daunorubicin (AML Induction)

Use Leukemia, acute myeloid

Regimen
Cytarabine: I.V.: 2 g/m^2/day over 1 hour every 12 hours days 1 to 6 (12 total doses)
[total dose/cycle = 24 g/m^2]
Daunorubicin: I.V.: 45 mg/m^2/day I.V. bolus days 7 to 9
[total dose/cycle = 135 mg/m^2]

Cytarabine (High Dose)-Daunorubicin-Etoposide (AML Induction)

Use Leukemia, acute myeloid

Regimen
Daunorubicin: I.V.: 50 mg/m^2/day days 1, 2, and 3
[total dose/cycle = 150 mg/m^2]
Cytarabine: I.V.: 3 g/m^2/dose over 3 hours every 12 hours days 1, 3, 5, and 7 (8 total doses)
[total dose/cycle = 24 g/m^2]
Etoposide: I.V.: 75 mg/m^2/day days 1 to 7
[total dose/cycle = 525 mg/m^2]
Up to 3 induction cycles may be given based on individual response

Cytarabine (High-Dose Single-Agent AML Induction Regimen)

Use Leukemia, acute myeloid

Regimen NOTE: Multiple variations are listed.
Variation 1 (ages 14 to 50 years):
Cytarabine: I.V.: 3 g/m^2 over 2 hours every 12 hours days 1 to 6 (total of 12 doses)
[total dose/cycle = 36 g/m^2]
May administer a second induction cycle if needed
Variation 2 (ages >50 years):
Cytarabine: I.V.: 2 g/m^2 over 2 hours every 12 hours days 1 to 6 (total of 12 doses)
[total dose/cycle = 24 g/m^2]
May administer a second induction cycle if needed

Cytarabine (SubQ Single-Agent AML Induction Regimen)

Use Leukemia, acute myeloid

Regimen NOTE: Multiple variations are listed.
Variation 1 (>50 years of age):
Cytarabine: SubQ: 20 mg/m^2/day days 1 to 14
[total dose/cycle = 280 mg/m^2]
Repeat cycle every 28 days for at least 4 cycles
Variation 2 (>65 years of age):
Cytarabine: SubQ: 10 mg/m^2/day every 12 hours days 1 to 21
[total dose/cycle = 420 mg/m^2]
After 15 days, a second induction course may be administered if needed

CYVADIC

Use Sarcoma

Regimen
Cyclophosphamide: I.V.: 500 mg/m^2 day 1
[total dose/cycle = 500 mg/m^2]
Vincristine: I.V.: 1.4 mg/m^2/day days 1 and 5
[total dose/cycle = 2.8 mg/m^2]
Doxorubicin: I.V.: 50 mg/m^2 day 1
[total dose/cycle = 50 mg/m^2]
Dacarbazine: I.V.: 250 mg/m^2/day days 1 to 5
[total dose/cycle = 1250 mg/m^2]
Repeat cycle every 21 days

Dacarbazine-Carboplatin-Aldesleukin-Interferon
Use Melanoma
Regimen
Dacarbazine: I.V.: 750 mg/m²/day days 1 and 22
  [total dose/cycle = 1500 mg/m²]
Carboplatin: I.V.: 400 mg/m²/day days 1 and 22
  [total dose/cycle = 800 mg/m²]
Aldesleukin: SubQ: 4,800,000 units every 8 hours days 36 and 57
  [total dose/cycle = 28,800,000 units]
   then 4,800,000 units every 12 hours days 37 and 58
   [total dose/cycle = 19,200,000 units]
     then 4,800,000 units/day days 38 to 40, 43 to 47, 50 to 54, 59 to 61, 65 to 68, 71 to 75
      [total dose/cycle = 120,000,000 units]
Interferon alpha-2a: SubQ: 6,000,000 units days 38, 40, 43, 45, 47, 50, 52, 54, 59, 61, 64, 66, 68, 71, 73, and 75
  [total dose/cycle = 96,000,000 units]
Repeat cycle every 78 days for 3 cycles

Dartmouth Regimen
Use Melanoma
Regimen NOTE: Multiple variations are listed.
Variation 1:
 Cisplatin: I.V.: 25 mg/m²/day days 1, 2, and 3
  [total dose/cycle = 75 mg/m²]
 Dacarbazine: I.V.: 220 mg/m²/day days 1, 2, and 3
  [total dose/cycle = 660 mg/m²]
 Carmustine: I.V.: 150 mg/m² day 1 (every other cycle)
  [total dose/cycle = 150 mg/m²; every other cycle]
 Tamoxifen: Oral: 10 mg twice daily (begin 1 week before chemotherapy)
  [total dose/cycle = 420 mg]
 Repeat cycle every 21 days
Variation 2:
 Carmustine: I.V.: 150 mg/m² day 1
  [total dose/cycle = 150 mg/m²]
 Cisplatin: I.V.: 25 mg/m²/day days 1, 2, 3, 22, 23, and 24
  [total dose/cycle = 150 mg/m²]
 Dacarbazine: I.V.: 220 mg/m²/day days 1, 2, 3, 22, 23, and 24
  [total dose/cycle = 1320 mg/m²]
 Tamoxifen: Oral: 10 mg twice daily days 1 to 42
  [total dose/cycle = 840 mg]
 Repeat cycle every 42 days
Variation 3:
 Carmustine: I.V.: 150 mg/m² day 1
  [total dose/cycle = 150 mg/m²]
 Cisplatin: I.V.: 25 mg/m²/day days 1, 2, 3, 22, 23, and 24
  [total dose/cycle = 150 mg/m²]
 Dacarbazine: I.V.: 220 mg/m²/day days 1, 2, 3, 22, 23, and 24
  [total dose/cycle = 1320 mg/m²]
 Tamoxifen: Oral: 160 mg/day days -6 to 0 (cycle 1 only)
  [total dose/cycle = 1120 mg]
   followed by Oral: 40 mg/day days 1 to 42
    [total dose/cycle = 1680 mg]
 Repeat cycle every 42 days
Variation 4:
 Carmustine: I.V.: 150 mg/m² day 1
  [total dose/cycle = 150 mg/m²]
 Cisplatin: I.V.: 25 mg/m²/day days 1, 2, 3, 29, 30, and 31
  [total dose/cycle = 150 mg/m²]
 Dacarbazine: I.V.: 220 mg/m²/day days 1, 2, 3, 29, 30, and 31
  [total dose/cycle = 1320 mg/m²]

◀

Tamoxifen: Oral: 10-20 mg twice daily days 1 to 56
[total dose/cycle = 1120-2240 mg]
Repeat cycle every 56 days
Variation 5:
Cisplatin: I.V.: 25 mg/m^2/day days 1, 2, and 3
[total dose/cycle = 75 mg/m^2]
Dacarbazine: I.V.: 220 mg/m^2/day days 1, 2, and 3
[total dose/cycle = 660 mg/m^2]
Carmustine: I.V.: 100 mg/m^2 day 1 (give in cycles 1, 3, and 6 **only**)
[total dose/cycles 1, 3, and 6 = 100 mg/m^2]
Tamoxifen: Oral: 160 mg loading dose immediately before cycle 1
[total dose/loading dose + cycle 1 = 580 mg]
followed by Oral: 20 mg daily days 1 to 21
[total dose/subsequent cycles = 420 mg]
Repeat cycle every 21 days
Note: Tamoxifen is continued until 3 weeks after last cycle.

Decitabine (AML Regimen)

Use Leukemia, acute myeloid
Regimen
Decitabine: I.V.: 20 mg/m^2/day over 1 hour days 1 to 5
[total dose/cycle = 100 mg/m^2]
Repeat cycle every 28 days

Decitabine (MDS Low Dose Regimen)

Use Myelodysplastic syndrome
Regimen NOTE: Multiple variations are listed.
Variation 1:
Decitabine: I.V.: 20 mg/m^2/day over 1 hour days 1 to 5
[total dose/cycle = 100 mg/m^2]
Repeat cycle every 28 days
Variation 2:
Decitabine: I.V.: 15 mg/m^2/dose over 3 hours every 8 hours days 1 to 3 (total of 45 mg/m^2/day)
[total dose/cycle = 135 mg/m^2]
Repeat cycle every 6 weeks

DHAP (Hodgkin)

Use Lymphoma, Hodgkin
Regimen
Salvage treatment:
Dexamethasone: I.V.: 40 mg/day days 1 to 4
[total dose/cycle = 160 mg]
Cisplatin: I.V.: 100 mg/m^2 continuous infusion for 24 hours day 1
[total dose/cycle = 100 mg/m^2]
Cytarabine: I.V.: 2000 mg/m^2 over 3 hours every 12 hours day 2 (total of 2 doses)
[total dose/cycle = 4000 mg/m^2]
Filgrastim: SubQ: 5 mcg/kg/day beginning 24 hours after last dose of cytarabine, continue until leukocytes ≥2500/mm^3 for 3 days
Administer 2 cycles

Docetaxel-Bevacizumab

Use Breast cancer
Regimen NOTE: Multiple variations are listed.
Variation 1:
Docetaxel: I.V.: 100 mg/m^2 day 1
[total dose/cycle = 100 mg/m^2]
Bevacizumab: I.V.: 7.5 mg/kg day 1
[total dose/cycle = 7.5 mg/kg]
Repeat cycle every 21 days (administer docetaxel for up to 9 cycles, bevacizumab until disease progression or unacceptable toxicity)

Variation 2:
Docetaxel: I.V.: 100 mg/m^2 day 1
[total dose/cycle = 100 mg/m^2]
Bevacizumab: I.V.: 15 mg/kg day 1
[total dose/cycle = 15 mg/kg]
Repeat cycle every 21 days (administer docetaxel for up to 9 cycles, bevacizumab until disease progression or unacceptable toxicity)

Docetaxel-Carboplatin (Ovarian Cancer)

Use Ovarian cancer

Regimen NOTE: Multiple variations are listed.
Variation 1:
Docetaxel: I.V.: 60 mg/m^2 day 1
[total dose/cycle = 60 mg/m^2]
Carboplatin: I.V.: Target AUC 6
[total dose/cycle = AUC = 6]
Repeat cycle every 21 days for 6 cycles
Variation 2:
Docetaxel: I.V.: 75 mg/m^2 day 1
[total dose/cycle = 75 mg/m^2]
Carboplatin: I.V.: AUC 5 day 1
[total dose/cycle = AUC = 5]
Repeat cycle every 21 days for 6 cycles

Docetaxel-Carboplatin (Unknown Primary)

Use Unknown primary (adenocarcinoma)

Regimen
Docetaxel: I.V.: 65 mg/m^2 infused over 1 hour day 1
[total dose/cycle = 65 mg/m^2]
followed by
Carboplatin: I.V.: Target AUC 6 day 1
[total dose/cycle = AUC = 6]
Repeat cycle every 21 days for up to a total of 8 cycles

Docetaxel-Cisplatin

Use Lung cancer, nonsmall cell

Regimen
Docetaxel: I.V.: 75 mg/m^2 day 1
[total dose/cycle = 75 mg/m^2]
Cisplatin: I.V.: 75 mg/m^2 day 1
[total dose/cycle = 75 mg/m^2]
Repeat cycle every 21 days

Docetaxel-Cisplatin-Fluorouracil (Gastric/Esophageal Cancer)

Use Esophageal cancer; Gastric cancer

Regimen NOTE: Multiple variations are listed.
Variation 1:
Docetaxel: I.V.: 75 mg/m^2 day 1
[total dose/cycle = 75 mg/m^2]
Cisplatin: I.V.: 75 mg/m^2 day 1
[total dose/cycle = 75 mg/m^2]
Fluorouracil: I.V.: 750 mg/m^2/day continuous infusion days 1 to 5
[total dose/cycle = 3750 mg/m^2]
Repeat cycle every 21 days until disease progression or unacceptable toxicity

Variation 2:
Docetaxel: I.V.: 75 mg/m^2 day 1
[total dose/cycle = 75 mg/m^2]
Cisplatin: I.V.: 75 mg/m^2 over 4 hours day 1
[total dose/cycle = 75 mg/m^2]
Fluorouracil: I.V.: 300 mg/m^2/day continuous infusion days 1 to 14
[total dose/cycle = 4200 mg/m^2]
Repeat cycle every 21 days until disease progression or unacceptable toxicity for up to a maximum of 8 cycles

Docetaxel-Cisplatin-Fluorouracil (Head and Neck Cancer)

Use Head and neck cancer
Regimen NOTE: Multiple variations are listed.
Variation 1:
Docetaxel: I.V.: 75 mg/m^2 day 1
[total dose/cycle = 75 mg/m^2]
Cisplatin: I.V.: 75 mg/m^2 day 1
[total dose/cycle = 75 mg/m^2]
Fluorouracil: I.V.: 750 mg/m^2/day continuous infusion days 1 to 5
[total dose/cycle = 3750 mg/m^2]
Repeat cycle every 21 days for 4 cycles
Variation 2:
Docetaxel: I.V.: 75 mg/m^2 day 1
[total dose/cycle = 75 mg/m^2]
Cisplatin: I.V.: 75-100 mg/m^2 day 1
[total dose/cycle = 75-100 mg/m^2]
Fluorouracil: I.V.: 1000 mg/m^2/day continuous infusion days 1 to 4
[total dose/cycle = 4000 mg/m^2]
Repeat cycle every 21 days for total of 3 cycles

Docetaxel-Cisplatin-Fluorouracil (Unknown Primary)

Use Unknown primary (squamous cell)
Regimen
Docetaxel: I.V.: 75 mg/m^2 day 1
[total dose/cycle = 75 mg/m^2]
Cisplatin: I.V.: 75 mg/m^2 day 1
[total dose/cycle = 75 mg/m^2]
Fluorouracil: I.V.: 750 mg/m^2/day continuous infusion days 1 to 5
[total dose/cycle = 3750 mg/m^2]
Repeat cycle every 21 days for a total of 3 cycles

Docetaxel-Cisplatin (Unknown Primary)

Use Unknown primary (adenocarcinoma)
Regimen
Docetaxel: I.V.: 75 mg/m^2 infused over 1 hour day 1
[total dose/cycle = 75 mg/m^2]
followed by
Cisplatin: I.V.: 75 mg/m^2 infused over 1 hour day 1
[total dose/cycle = 75 mg/m^2]
Repeat cycle every 21 days for up to a total of 8 cycles

Docetaxel-Cyclophosphamide (TC)

Use Breast cancer
Regimen
Docetaxel: I.V.: 75 mg/m^2 day 1
[total dose/cycle = 75 mg/m^2]
Cyclophosphamide: I.V.: 600 mg/m^2 day 1
[total dose/cycle = 600 mg/m^2]
Repeat cycle every 21 days for 4 cycles

Docetaxel-Doxorubicin (Breast Cancer)

Use Breast cancer

Regimen
Doxorubicin: I.V.: 50 mg/m^2 day 1
  [total dose/cycle = 50 mg/m^2]
Docetaxel: I.V.: 75 mg/m^2 day 1
  [total dose/cycle = 75 mg/m^2]
Repeat cycle every 3 weeks for up to 8 cycles

Docetaxel-FEC

Use Breast cancer

Regimen
Cycles 1, 2, and 3:
Docetaxel: I.V.: 80-100 mg/m^2 day 1
  [total dose/cycle = 80-100 mg/m^2]
Repeat cycle every 21 days for 3 cycles
Cycles 4, 5, and 6 (FEC):
Fluorouracil: I.V.: 600 mg/m^2 day 1
  [total dose/cycle = 600 mg/m^2]
Epirubicin: I.V.: 60 mg/m^2 day 1
  [total dose/cycle = 60 mg/m^2]
Cyclophosphamide: I.V.: 600 mg/m^2 day 1
  [total dose/cycle = 600 mg/m^2]
Repeat FEC cycle every 21 days for total of 3 cycles

Docetaxel-Oxaliplatin-Fluorouracil (Esophageal Cancer)

Use Esophageal cancer

Regimen
Docetaxel: I.V.: 50 mg/m^2 day 1
  [total dose/cycle = 50 mg/m^2]
Oxaliplatin: I.V.: 85 mg/m^2 day 1
  [total dose/cycle = 85 mg/m^2]
Fluorouracil: I.V.: 2400 mg/m^2 continuous infusion over 46 hours starting day 1
  [total dose/cycle = 2400 mg/m^2]
Repeat cycle every 14 days.

Docetaxel-Oxaliplatin-Leucovorin-Fluorouracil (Esophageal Cancer)

Use Esophageal cancer

Regimen
Docetaxel: I.V.: 50 mg/m^2 day 1
  [total dose/cycle = 50 mg/m^2]
Oxaliplatin: I.V.: 85 mg/m^2 day 1
  [total dose/cycle = 85 mg/m^2]
Leucovorin: I.V.: 200 mg/m^2 day 1
  [total dose/cycle = 200 mg/m^2]
Fluorouracil: I.V.: 2600 mg/m^2/day continuous infusion over 24 hours day 1
  [total dose/cycle = 2600 mg/m^2]
Repeat cycle every 14 days until disease progression or unacceptable toxicity for up to a total of 8 cycles.

Docetaxel-Oxaliplatin (Ovarian Cancer)

Use Ovarian cancer

Regimen
Docetaxel: I.V.: 75 mg/m^2/dose over 60 minutes day 1
  [total dose/cycle = 75 mg/m^2]
Oxaliplatin: I.V.: 100 mg/m^2/dose over 2 hours day 1
  [total dose/cycle = 100 mg/m^2]
Repeat cycle every 21 days

Docetaxel-Prednisone

Use Prostate cancer

◀ **Regimen**
Docetaxel: I.V.: 75 mg/m^2 day 1
[total dose/cycle = 75 mg/m^2]
Prednisone: Oral: 5 mg twice daily
[total dose/cycle = 210 mg]
Repeat cycle every 21 days for up to 10 cycles

Docetaxel-Trastuzumab

Use Breast cancer
Regimen
Cycle 1:
Docetaxel: I.V.: 100 mg/m^2 day 1
[total dose/cycle 1 = 100 mg/m^2]
Trastuzumab: I.V.: 4 mg/kg (loading dose) day 1 cycle 1
followed by I.V.: 2 mg/kg/day days 8 and 15 cycle 1
[total dose/cycle 1 = 8 mg/kg]
Treatment cycle is 21 days
Subsequent cycles:
Docetaxel: I.V.: 100 mg/m^2 day 1
[total dose/cycle = 100 mg/m^2]
Trastuzumab: I.V.: 2 mg/kg/day days 1, 8, and 15
[total dose/cycle = 6 mg/kg]
Repeat cycle every 21 days for a total of at least 6 cycles (continue weekly trastuzumab until disease progression)

Docetaxel-Trastuzumab-Carboplatin

Use Breast cancer
Regimen
Cycle 1:
Trastuzumab: I.V.: 4 mg/kg (loading dose) day 1 cycle 1
followed by I.V.: 2 mg/kg/day days 8 and 15 cycle 1
[total dose/cycle 1 = 8 mg/kg]
Docetaxel: I.V.: 75 mg/m^2 day 2
[total dose/cycle 1 = 75 mg/m^2]
Carboplatin: I.V.: AUC 6 day 2
[total dose/cycle 1 = AUC = 6]
Treatment cycle is 21 days
Subsequent cycles:
Trastuzumab: I.V.: 2 mg/kg/day days 1, 8, and 15
[total dose/cycle = 6 mg/kg]
Docetaxel: I.V.: 75 mg/m^2 day 1
[total dose/cycle = 75 mg/m^2]
Carboplatin: I.V.: AUC 6 day 1
[total dose/cycle = AUC = 6]
Repeat cycle every 21 days for a total of ~6 cycles (continue weekly trastuzumab for 1 year after chemotherapy, or until disease progression or unacceptable toxicity)

Docetaxel-Trastuzumab-Cisplatin

Use Breast cancer
Regimen
Cycle 1:
Trastuzumab: I.V.: 4 mg/kg (loading dose) day 1 cycle 1
followed by I.V.: 2 mg/kg/day days 8 and 15 cycle 1
[total dose/cycle 1 = 8 mg/kg]
Docetaxel: I.V.: 75 mg/m^2 day 2
[total dose/cycle 1 = 75 mg/m^2]
Cisplatin: I.V.: 75 mg/m^2 day 2
[total dose/cycle 1 = 75 mg/m^2]
Treatment cycle is 21 days

Subsequent cycles:
  Trastuzumab: I.V.: 2 mg/kg/day days 1, 8, and 15
    [total dose/cycle = 6 mg/kg]
  Docetaxel: I.V.: 75 mg/m^2 day 1
    [total dose/cycle = 75 mg/m^2]
  Cisplatin: I.V.: 75 mg/m^2 day 1
    [total dose/cycle = 75 mg/m^2]
  Repeat cycle every 21 days for a total of ~6 cycles (continue weekly trastuzumab for 1 year after chemotherapy, or until disease progression or unacceptable toxicity)

Docetaxel-Trastuzumab-FEC

Use Breast cancer

Regimen
  Cycle 1:
  Trastuzumab: I.V.: 4 mg/kg (loading dose) day 1 cycle 1
    followed by I.V.: 2 mg/kg/day days 8 and 15 cycle 1
      [total dose/cycle 1 = 8 mg/kg]
  Docetaxel: I.V.: 80-100 mg/m^2 day 1
    [total dose/cycle 1 = 80-100 mg/m^2]
  Treatment cycle is 21 days
  Cycles 2 and 3:
  Trastuzumab: I.V.: 2 mg/kg/day days 1, 8, and 15
    [total dose/cycle = 6 mg/kg]
  Docetaxel: I.V.: 80-100 mg/m^2 day 1
    [total dose/cycle = 80-100 mg/m^2]
  Treatment cycle is 21 days
  Cycles 4, 5, and 6 (FEC):
  Fluorouracil: I.V.: 600 mg/m^2 day 1
    [total dose/cycle = 600 mg/m^2]
  Epirubicin: I.V.: 60 mg/m^2 day 1
    [total dose/cycle = 60 mg/m^2]
  Cyclophosphamide: I.V.: 600 mg/m^2 day 1
    [total dose/cycle = 600 mg/m^2]
  Repeat FEC cycle every 21 days for total of 3 cycles

Docetaxel (Weekly Regimen)

Use Prostate cancer

Regimen
  Docetaxel: I.V.: 40 mg/m^2 days 1, 8, and 15
    [total dose/cycle = 120 mg/m^2]
  Repeat cycle every 4 weeks

Docetaxel (Weekly)-Trastuzumab

Use Breast cancer

Regimen
  Cycle 1:
  Docetaxel: I.V.: 35 mg/m^2/day days 1, 8, and 15
    [total dose/cycle 1 = 105 mg/m^2]
  Trastuzumab: I.V.: 4 mg/kg (loading dose) day 0 cycle 1
    followed by I.V.: 2 mg/kg/day days 8 and 15 cycle 1
      [total dose/cycle 1 = 8 mg/kg]
  Treatment cycle is 28 days
  Subsequent cycles:
  Docetaxel: I.V.: 35 mg/m^2/day days 1, 8, and 15
    [total dose/cycle = 105 mg/m^2]
  Trastuzumab: I.V.: 2 mg/kg/day days 1, 8, and 15
    [total dose/cycle = 6 mg/kg]
  Repeat cycle every 28 days

Dox-CMF (Sequential)

Use Breast cancer

◀ **Regimen**
Doxorubicin: I.V.: 75 mg/m^2 day 1
[total dose/cycle = 75 mg/m^2]
Repeat cycle every 21 days for 4 cycles
followed by (after completing Cycle 4)
Cyclophosphamide: I.V.: 600 mg/m^2 day 1
[total dose/cycle = 600 mg/m^2]
Methotrexate: I.V.: 40 mg/m^2 day 1
[total dose/cycle = 40 mg/m^2]
Fluorouracil: I.V.: 600 mg/m^2 day 1
[total dose/cycle = 600 mg/m^2]
Repeat cycle every 21 days for 8 cycles

Doxorubicin + Ketoconazole

Use Prostate cancer
Regimen
Doxorubicin: I.V.: 20 mg/m^2 continuous infusion day 1
[total dose/cycle = 20 mg/m^2]
Ketoconazole: Oral: 400 mg 3 times/day days 1 to 7
[total dose/cycle = 8400 mg]
Repeat cycle every 7 days

Doxorubicin + Ketoconazole/Estramustine + Vinblastine

Use Prostate cancer
Regimen
Doxorubicin: I.V.: 20 mg/m^2/day days 1, 15, and 29
[total dose/cycle = 60 mg/m^2]
Ketoconazole: Oral: 400 mg 3 times/day days 1 to 7, 15 to 21, and 29 to 35
[total dose/cycle = 25,200 mg]
Estramustine: Oral: 140 mg 3 times/day days 8 to 14, 22 to 28, and 36 to 42
[total dose/cycle = 8820 mg]
Vinblastine: I.V.: 5 mg/m^2/day days 8, 22, and 36
[total dose/cycle = 15 mg/m^2]
Repeat cycle every 8 weeks

Doxorubicin (Liposomal)-Docetaxel (Breast Cancer)

Use Breast cancer
Regimen
Doxorubicin (liposomal): I.V.: 30 mg/m^2 over 1 hour day 1
[total dose/cycle = 30 mg/m^2]
Docetaxel: I.V.: 60 mg/m^2 over 1 hour day 1
[total dose/cycle = 60 mg/m^2]
Repeat cycle every 3 weeks until disease progression or unacceptable toxicity

Doxorubicin (Liposomal)-Vincristine-Dexamethasone

Use Multiple myeloma
Regimen NOTE: Multiple variations are listed.
Variation 1:
Doxorubicin, liposomal: I.V.: 40 mg/m^2 day 1
[total dose/cycle = 40 mg/m^2]
Vincristine: I.V.: 2 mg day 1
[total dose/cycle = 2 mg]
Dexamethasone: Oral or I.V.: 40 mg/day days 1 to 4
[total dose/cycle = 160 mg]
Repeat cycle every 4 weeks
Variation 2:
Doxorubicin, liposomal: I.V.: 40 mg/m^2 day 1
[total dose/cycle = 40 mg/m^2]
Vincristine: I.V.: 1.4 mg/m^2 (maximum dose: 2 mg) day 1
[total dose/cycle = 1.4 mg/m^2; maximum: 2 mg]

Dexamethasone: Oral: 40 mg/day days 1 to 4
[total dose/cycle = 160 mg]
Repeat cycle every 4 weeks

DTPACE

Use Multiple myeloma

Regimen
Dexamethasone: Oral: 40 mg/day days 1 to 4
[total dose/cycle = 160 mg]
Thalidomide: Oral: 400 mg/day
[total dose/cycle = 11,200 - 16,800 mg]
Cisplatin: I.V.: 10 mg/m^2/day continuous infusion days 1 to 4
[total dose/cycle = 40 mg/m^2]
Doxorubicin: I.V.: 10 mg/m^2/day continuous infusion days 1 to 4
[total dose/cycle = 40 mg/m^2]
Cyclophosphamide: I.V.: 400 mg/m^2 continuous infusion days 1 to 4
[total dose/cycle = 1600 mg/m^2]
Etoposide: I.V.: 40 mg/m^2 continuous infusion days 1 to 4
[total dose/cycle = 160 mg/m^2]
Repeat cycle every 4-6 weeks

DVP

Use Leukemia, acute lymphocytic

Regimen Induction:
Daunorubicin: I.V.: 25 mg/m^2/day days 1, 8, and 15
[total dose/cycle = 75 mg/m^2]
Vincristine: I.V.: 1.5 mg/m^2/day (maximum dose: 2 mg) days 1, 8, 15, and 22
[total dose/cycle = 6 mg/m^2]
Prednisone: Oral: 60 mg/m^2/day days 1 to 28 then taper over next 14 days
[total dose/cycle = 1680 mg/m^2 + taper over next 14 days]
Administer single cycle; used in conjunction with intrathecal chemotherapy

EC (NSCLC)

Use Lung cancer, nonsmall cell

Regimen
Etoposide: I.V.: 120 mg/m^2/day days 1, 2, and 3
[total dose/cycle = 360 mg/m^2]
Carboplatin: I.V.: AUC 6 day 1
[total dose/cycle = AUC = 6]
Repeat cycle every 21-28 days

EC (Small Cell Lung Cancer)

Use Lung cancer, small cell

Regimen NOTE: Multiple variations are listed.
Variation 1:
Etoposide: I.V.: 100-120 mg/m^2/day days 1, 2, and 3
[total dose/cycle = 300-360 mg/m^2]
Carboplatin: I.V.: 325-400 mg/m^2 day 1
[total dose/cycle = 325-400 mg/m^2]
Repeat cycle every 28 days
Variation 2:
Etoposide: I.V.: 120 mg/m^2/day days 1, 2, and 3
[total dose/cycle = 360 mg/m^2]
Carboplatin: I.V.: AUC 6 day 1
[total dose/cycle = AUC = 6]
Repeat cycle every 21-28 days

EE

Use Wilms tumor

Regimen

Dactinomycin: I.V.: 15 mcg/kg/day days 1 to 5 of weeks 0, 5, 13, and 24
[total dose/cycle = 300 mcg/kg]
Vincristine: I.V.: 1.5 mg/m^2 day 1 of weeks 1-10, 13, 14, 24, and 25
[total dose/cycle = 21 mg/m^2]

EE-4A

Use Wilms tumor

Regimen

Dactinomycin: I.V.: 45 mcg/kg day 1 of weeks 0, 3, 6, 9, 12, 15, and 18
[total dose/cycle = 315 mcg/kg]
Vincristine: I.V.: 2 mg/m^2 day 1 of weeks 1-10, 12, 15, and 18
[total dose/cycle = 26 mg/m^2]

EMA/CO

Use Gestational trophoblastic tumor

Regimen NOTE: Multiple variations are listed.

Variation 1:

Etoposide: I.V.: 100 mg/m^2/day days 1 and 2
[total dose/cycle = 200 mg/m^2]
Methotrexate: I.V.: 300 mg/m^2 continuous infusion over 12 hours day 1
[total dose/cycle = 300 mg/m^2]
Dactinomycin: I.V. push: 0.5 mg/day days 1 and 2
[total dose/cycle = 1 mg]
Leucovorin: Oral, I.M.: 15 mg twice daily for 2 days (start 24 hours after the start of methotrexate) days 2 and 3
[total dose/cycle = 60 mg]
Alternate weekly with:
Cyclophosphamide: I.V.: 600 mg/m^2 day 1
[total dose/cycle = 600 mg/m^2]
Vincristine: I.V. push: 0.8 mg/m^2 (maximum dose: 2 mg) day 1
[total dose/cycle = 0.8 mg/m^2]
Repeat cycle every 2 weeks

Variation 2:

Dactinomycin: I.V.: 0.5 mg/day days 1 and 2
[total dose/cycle = 1 mg]
Etoposide: I.V.: 100 mg/m^2/day days 1 and 2
[total dose/cycle = 200 mg/m^2]
Methotrexate: I.V. bolus: 100 mg/m^2 then 200 mg/m^2 continuous infusion over 12 hours day 1
[total dose/cycle = 300 mg/m^2]
Leucovorin: Oral, I.M.: 15 mg every 12 hours for 4 doses (start 24 hours after methotrexate) days 2 and 3
[total dose/cycle = 60 mg]
Vincristine: I.V.: 1 mg/m^2 day 8
[total dose/cycle = 1 mg/m^2]
Cyclophosphamide: I.V.: 600 mg/m^2 day 8
[total dose/cycle = 600 mg/m^2]
Repeat cycle every 2 weeks

Variation 3:

Dactinomycin: I.V.: 0.5 mg/day days 1 and 2
[total dose/cycle = 1 mg]
Etoposide: I.V.: 100 mg/m^2/day days 1 and 2
[total dose/cycle = 200 mg/m^2]
Methotrexate: I.V.: 300 mg/m^2 continuous infusion over 12 hours day 1
[total dose/cycle = 300 mg/m^2]
Leucovorin: Oral, I.M.: 15 mg every 12 hours for 4 doses (start 24 hours after start of methotrexate) days 2 and 3
[total dose/cycle = 60 mg]

Vincristine: I.V.: 1 mg/m^2 day 8
  [total dose/cycle = 1 mg/m^2]
Cyclophosphamide: I.V.: 600 mg/m^2 day 8
  [total dose/cycle = 600 mg/m^2]
Repeat cycle every 2 weeks
Variation 4:
  Dactinomycin: I.V.: 0.35 mg/m^2/day days 1 and 2
  [total dose/cycle = 0.7 mg/m^2]
  Etoposide: I.V.: 100 mg/m^2/day days 1 and 2
  [total dose/cycle = 200 mg/m^2]
  Methotrexate: I.V. bolus: 100 mg/m^2 then 200 mg/m^2 continuous infusion over 12 hours day 1
  [total dose/cycle = 300 mg/m^2]
  Leucovorin: Oral, I.M.: 15 mg every 12 hours for 4 doses (start 24 hours after start of methotrexate) days
  2 and 3
  [total dose/cycle = 60 mg]
  Vincristine: I.V.: 1 mg/m^2 day 8
  [total dose/cycle = 1 mg/m^2]
  Cyclophosphamide: I.V.: 600 mg/m^2 day 8
  [total dose/cycle = 600 mg/m^2]
Repeat cycle every 2 weeks
Variation 5 (patients with brain metastases):
  Dactinomycin: I.V.: 0.5 mg/day days 1 and 2
  [total dose/cycle = 1 mg]
  Etoposide:I.V.: 100 mg/m^2/day days 1 and 2
  [total dose/cycle = 200 mg/m^2]
  Methotrexate: I.V.: 1 g/m^2 continuous infusion over 12 hours day 1
  [total dose/cycle = 1 g/m^2]
  Leucovorin: I.M.: 20 mg/m^2 every 6 hours for 12 doses (start 24 hours after start of methotrexate) days
  2, 3, and 4
  [total dose/cycle = 240 mg/m^2]
  Vincristine: I.V.: 1 mg/m^2 day 8
  [total dose/cycle = 1 mg/m^2]
  Cyclophosphamide: I.V.: 600 mg/m^2 day 8
  [total dose/cycle = 600 mg/m^2]
Repeat cycle every 2 weeks
Variation 6 (patients with brain metastases):
  Dactinomycin: I.V.: 0.5 mg/day days 1 and 2
  [total dose/cycle = 1 mg]
  Etoposide: I.V.: 100 mg/m^2/day days 1 and 2
  [total dose/cycle = 200 mg/m^2]
  Methotrexate: I.V.: 1 g/m^2 continuous infusion over 12 hours day 1
  [total dose/cycle = 1 g/m^2]
  Leucovorin: Oral, I.M.: 30 mg/m^2 every 12 hours for 6 doses (start 32 hours after start of methotrexate)
  days 2, 3, and 4
  [total dose/cycle = 180 mg/m^2]
  Vincristine: I.V.: 1 mg/m^2 day 8
  [total dose/cycle = 1 mg/m^2]
  Cyclophosphamide: I.V.: 600 mg/m^2 day 8
  [total dose/cycle = 600 mg/m^2]
Repeat cycle every 2 weeks
Variation 7:
  Dactinomycin: I.V.: 0.5 mg/day days 1 and 2
  [total dose/cycle = 1 mg]
  Etoposide: I.V.: 100 mg/m^2/day days 1 and 2
  [total dose/cycle = 200 mg/m^2]
  Methotrexate: I.V.: 1 g/m^2 continuous infusion over 24 hours day 1
  [total dose/cycle = 1 g/m^2]
  Leucovorin: Oral, I.M.: 15 mg every 8 hours for 9 doses (start 32 hours after start of methotrexate) days
  2, 3, and 4
  [total dose/cycle = 135 mg/m^2]

Vincristine: I.V.: 1 mg/m^2 day 8
[total dose/cycle = 1 mg/m^2]
Cyclophosphamide: I.V.: 600 mg/m^2 day 8
[total dose/cycle = 600 mg/m^2]
Repeat cycle every 2 weeks
Variation 8 (patients with lung metastases):
Dactinomycin: I.V.: 0.5 mg/day days 1 and 2
[total dose/cycle = 1 mg]
Etoposide: I.V.: 100 mg/m^2/day days 1 and 2
[total dose/cycle = 200 mg/m^2]
Methotrexate: I.V. bolus: 100 mg/m^2 then 200 mg/m^2 continuous infusion over 12 hours day 1
[total dose/cycle = 300 mg/m^2]
Leucovorin: Oral, I.M.: 15 mg every 12 hours for 4 doses (start 24 hours after start of methotrexate) days 2 and 3
[total dose/cycle = 60 mg]
Vincristine: I.V.: 1 mg/m^2 day 8
[total dose/cycle = 1 mg/m^2]
Cyclophosphamide: I.V.: 600 mg/m^2 day 8
[total dose/cycle = 600 mg/m^2]
Methotrexate: I.T.: 10 mg day 1 (every other cycle)
[total dose/cycle = 10 mg, every other cycle]
Repeat cycle every 2 weeks
Variation 9 (patients with lung metastases):
Dactinomycin: I.V.: 0.5 mg/day days 1 and 2
[total dose/cycle = 1 mg]
Etoposide: I.V.: 100 mg/m^2/day days 1 and 2
[total dose/cycle = 200 mg/m^2]
Methotrexate: I.V. bolus: 100 mg/m^2 then 200 mg/m^2 continuous infusion over 12 hours day 1
[total dose/cycle = 300 mg/m^2]
Leucovorin: Oral, I.M.: 15 mg every 12 hours for 4 doses (start 24 hours after start of methotrexate) days 2 and 3
[total dose/cycle = 60 mg]
Vincristine: I.V.: 1 mg/m^2 day 8
[total dose/cycle = 1 mg/m^2]
Cyclophosphamide: I.V.: 600 mg/m^2 day 8
[total dose/cycle = 600 mg/m^2]
Methotrexate: I.T.: 12.5 mg day 8
[total dose/cycle = 12.5 mg]
Repeat cycle every 2 weeks

EP (Small Cell Lung Cancer)

Use Lung cancer, small cell
Regimen NOTE: Multiple variations are listed below.
Variation 1:
Etoposide: I.V.: 100 mg/m^2/day days 1, 2, and 3
[total dose/cycle = 300 mg/m^2]
Cisplatin: I.V.: 100 mg/m^2 day 1
[total dose/cycle = 100 mg/m^2]
Repeat cycle every 21 days
Variation 2:
Etoposide: I.V.: 80 mg/m^2/day days 1, 2, and 3
[total dose/cycle = 240 mg/m^2]
Cisplatin: I.V.: 80 mg/m^2 day 1
[total dose/cycle = 80 mg/m^2]
Repeat cycle every 21-28 days

EP/EMA

Use Gestational trophoblastic tumor
Regimen NOTE: Multiple variations are listed.
Variation 1:
Etoposide: I.V.: 150 mg/m^2 day 1
[total dose/cycle = 150 mg/m^2]

Cisplatin: I.V.: 25 mg/m^2 infused over 4 hours for 3 consecutive doses, day 1
[total dose/cycle = 75 mg/m^2]
Alternate weekly with:
Etoposide: I.V.: 100 mg/m^2 day 1
[total dose/cycle = 100 mg/m^2]
Methotrexate: I.V.: 300 mg/m^2 infused over 12 hours day 1
[total dose/cycle = 300 mg/m^2]
Dactinomycin: I.V. push: 0.5 mg day 1
[total dose/cycle = 0.5 mg]
Leucovorin: Oral, I.M.: 15 mg twice daily for 2 days (start 24 hours after the start of methotrexate) days 2 and 3
[total dose/cycle = 60 mg]
Variation 2:
Dactinomycin: I.V.: 0.5 mg/day days 1 and 2
[total dose/cycle = 1 mg]
Etoposide: I.V.: 100 mg/m^2/day days 1 and 2
[total dose/cycle = 200 mg/m^2]
Methotrexate: I.V.: 300 mg/m^2 continuous infusion over 12 hours day 1
[total dose/cycle = 300 mg/m^2]
Leucovorin: Oral, I.M.: 15 mg every 12 hours for 4 doses (start 24 hours after start of methotrexate) days 2 and 3
[total dose/cycle = 60 mg]
Etoposide: I.V.: 150 mg/m^2 day 8
[total dose/cycle = 150 mg/m^2]
Cisplatin: I.V.: 75 mg/m^2 day 8
[total dose/cycle = 75 mg/m^2]
Repeat cycle every 2 weeks

Epirubicin-Cisplatin-Capecitabine (Esophageal Cancer)

Use Esophageal cancer

Regimen
Epirubicin: I.V.: 50 mg/m^2 day 1
[total dose/cycle = 50 mg/m^2]
Cisplatin: I.V.: 60 mg/m^2 day 1
[total dose/cycle = 60 mg/m^2]
Capecitabine: Oral: 625 mg/m^2 twice daily days 1 to 21
[total dose/cycle = 26,250 mg/m^2]
Repeat cycle every 21 days for up to 8 cycles

Epirubicin-Cisplatin-Fluorouracil (Gastric/Esophageal Cancer)

Use Esophageal cancer; Gastric cancer

Regimen NOTE: Multiple variations are listed.
Variation 1:
Epirubicin: I.V.: 50 mg/m^2 day 1
[total dose/cycle = 50 mg/m^2]
Cisplatin: I.V.: 60 mg/m^2 day 1
[total dose/cycle = 60 mg/m^2]
Fluorouracil: I.V.: 200 mg/m^2/day continuous infusion days 1 to 21
[total dose/cycle = 4200 mg/m^2]
Repeat cycle every 3 weeks for up to a maximum of 8 cycles
Variation 2:
Epirubicin: I.V.: 50 mg/m^2 day 1
[total dose/cycle = 50 mg/m^2]
Cisplatin: I.V.: 60 mg/m^2 day 1
[total dose/cycle = 60 mg/m^2]
Fluorouracil: I.V.: 200 mg/m^2/day continuous infusion days 1 to 21
[total dose/cycle = 4200 mg/m^2]
Repeat cycle every 3 weeks for up to 6 cycles (3 cycles before surgery and 3 cycles postoperatively)

Epirubicin-Oxaliplatin-Capecitabine

Use Esophageal cancer; Gastric cancer

◀ **Regimen**
Epirubicin: I.V.: 50 mg/m^2 day 1
[total dose/cycle = 50 mg/m^2]
Oxaliplatin: I.V.: 130 mg/m^2 day 1
[total dose/cycle = 130 mg/m^2]
Capecitabine: Oral: 625 mg/m^2 twice daily days 1 to 21
[total dose/cycle = 26,250 mg/m^2]
Repeat cycle every 21 days for up to 8 cycles

Epirubicin-Oxaliplatin-Fluorouracil (Esophageal Cancer)

Use Esophageal cancer

Regimen
Epirubicin: I.V.: 50 mg/m^2 day 1
[total dose/cycle = 50 mg/m^2]
Oxaliplatin: I.V.: 130 mg/m^2 day 1
[total dose/cycle = 130 mg/m^2]
Fluorouracil: I.V.: 200 mg/m^2/day continuous infusion days 1 to 21
[total dose/cycle = 4200 mg/m^2]
Repeat cycle every 21 days for up to 8 cycles

EP (NSCLC)

Use Lung cancer, nonsmall cell

Regimen
Etoposide: I.V.: 80-120 mg/m^2/day days 1, 2, and 3
[total dose/cycle = 240-360 mg/m^2]
Cisplatin: I.V.: 80-100 mg/m^2 day 1
[total dose/cycle = 80-100 mg/m^2]
Repeat cycle every 21-28 days

EPOCH Dose-Adjusted (AIDS-Related Lymphoma)

Use Lymphoma, AIDS-related

Regimen
Etoposide: I.V.: 50 mg/m^2/day continuous infusion days 1 to 4
[total dose/cycle = 200 mg/m^2]
Vincristine: I.V.: 0.4 mg/m^2/day continuous infusion days 1 to 4
[total dose/cycle = 1.6 mg/m^2]
Doxorubicin: I.V.: 10 mg/m^2/day continuous infusion days 1 to 4
[total dose/cycle = 40 mg/m^2]
Cyclophosphamide: I.V.: 375 mg/m^2 day 5 for CD4+ cells ≥100/mm^3 **or** 187 mg/m^2 day 5 for CD4+ cells <100/mm^3
[total dose/cycle = 187-375 mg/m^2]
Prednisone: Oral: 60 mg/m^2/day days 1 to 5
[total dose/cycle = 300 mg/m^2]
Filgrastim: SubQ: 5 mcg/kg/day beginning day 6; continue until ANC >5000/mm^3 (past nadir)
Repeat cycle every 21 days for 6 cycles with cyclophosphamide dose adjusted based on previous cycle nadir according to the following schedule:
Nadir ANC >500/mm^3: Increase cyclophosphamide dose by 187 mg/m^2 above previous cycle dose (maximum dose: 750 mg/m^2)
Nadir ANC <500/mm^3 or platelet <25,000/mm^3: Decrease cyclophosphamide dose by 187 mg/m^2 below previous cycle dose

EPOCH Dose-Adjusted (NHL)

Use Lymphoma, non-Hodgkin

Regimen
Etoposide: I.V.: 50 mg/m^2/day continuous infusion days 1 to 4
[total dose/cycle = 200 mg/m^2]
Vincristine: I.V.: 0.4 mg/m^2/day continuous infusion days 1 to 4
[total dose/cycle = 1.6 mg/m^2]
Doxorubicin: I.V.: 10 mg/m^2/day continuous infusion days 1 to 4
[total dose/cycle = 40 mg/m^2]

Cyclophosphamide: I.V.: 750 mg/m^2 day 5
[total dose/cycle = 750 mg/m^2]
Prednisone: Oral: 60 mg/m^2 twice daily days 1 to 5
total dose/cycle = 600 mg/m^2]
Filgrastim: SubQ: 5 mcg/kg/day beginning day 6; continue until ANC >5000/mm^3
Repeat cycle every 21 days with etoposide, doxorubicin, and cyclophosphamide dose adjustments (based on CBC 2 times/week) according to the following schedule:
Nadir ANC ≥500/mm^3: 20% increase (above previous cycle) for etoposide, doxorubicin, and cyclophosphamide
Nadir ANC <500/mm^3 (on 1 or 2 measurements): Same doses as previous cycle
Nadir ANC <500/mm^3 (on ≥3 measurements) or nadir platelet <25,000/mm^3 (on 1 measurement): 20% decrease below previous cycle for etoposide, doxorubicin, and cyclophosphamide (dosing adjustments below starting dose levels only apply to cyclophosphamide)

EPOCH (Dose-Adjusted)-Rituximab (NHL)

Use Lymphoma, non-Hodgkin

Regimen NOTE: Multiple variations are listed.
Variation 1:
Rituximab: I.V.: 375 mg/m^2 day 1
[total dose/cycle = 375 mg/m^2]
Etoposide: I.V.: 50 mg/m^2/day continuous infusion days 1 to 4
[total dose/cycle = 200 mg/m^2]
Vincristine: I.V.: 0.4 mg/m^2/day continuous infusion days 1 to 4
[total dose/cycle = 1.6 mg/m^2]
Doxorubicin: I.V.: 10 mg/m^2/day continuous infusion days 1 to 4
[total dose/cycle = 40 mg/m^2]
Cyclophosphamide: I.V.: 750 mg/m^2 day 5
[total dose/cycle = 750 mg/m^2]
Prednisone: Oral: 60 mg/m^2 twice daily days 1 to 5
[total dose/cycle = 600 mg/m^2]
Filgrastim: SubQ: 5 mcg/kg/day beginning day 6; continue until ANC >5000/mm^3
Repeat cycle every 21 days (for at least 2 cycles beyond best response; minimum of 6 cycles) with etoposide, doxorubicin, and cyclophosphamide dose adjustments (based on CBC 2 times/week) according to the following schedule:
Nadir ANC ≥500/mm^3: 20% increase (above previous cycle) for etoposide, doxorubicin, and cyclophosphamide
Nadir ANC <500/mm^3 (on 1 or 2 measurements): Same doses as previous cycle
Nadir ANC <500/mm^3 (on ≥3 measurements): 20% decrease below previous cycle for etoposide, doxorubicin, and cyclophosphamide (dosing adjustments below starting dose levels only apply to cyclophosphamide)
Variation 2:
Rituximab: I.V.: 375 mg/m^2 day 1
[total dose/cycle = 375 mg/m^2]
Etoposide: I.V.: 50 mg/m^2/day continuous infusion days 1 to 4
[total dose/cycle = 200 mg/m^2]
Vincristine: I.V.: 0.4 mg/m^2/day continuous infusion days 1 to 4
[total dose/cycle = 1.6 mg/m^2]
Doxorubicin: I.V.: 10 mg/m^2/day continuous infusion days 1 to 4
[total dose/cycle = 40 mg/m^2]
Cyclophosphamide: I.V.: 750 mg/m^2 day 5
[total dose/cycle = 750 mg/m^2]
Prednisone: Oral: 60 mg/m^2/day days 1 to 5
[total dose/cycle = 300 mg/m^2]
Filgrastim: SubQ: 5 mcg/kg/day beginning day 6; continue until ANC >500/mm^3
Repeat cycle every 21 days (for 6-8 cycles); refer to variation 1 for dose adjustments

EPOCH (NHL)

Use Lymphoma, non-Hodgkin

Regimen NOTE: Multiple variations are listed.
Variation 1:
Etoposide: I.V.: 50 mg/m^2/day continuous infusion days 1 to 4
[total dose/cycle = 200 mg/m^2]

◄ Vincristine: I.V.: 0.4 mg/m^2/day continuous infusion days 1 to 4
 [total dose/cycle = 1.6 mg/m^2]
Doxorubicin: I.V.: 10 mg/m^2/day continuous infusion days 1 to 4
 [total dose/cycle = 40 mg/m^2]
Cyclophosphamide: I.V.: 750 mg/m^2 day 5
 [total dose/cycle = 750 mg/m^2]
Prednisone: Oral: 60 mg/m^2/day days 1 to 5
 [total dose/cycle = 300 mg/m^2]
Repeat cycle (with cyclophosphamide dose adjustments if needed based on ANC) every 21 days (best response seen in a median of 4 cycles)
Variation 2:
Etoposide: I.V.: 50 mg/m^2/day continuous infusion days 1 to 4
 [total dose/cycle = 200 mg/m^2]
Vincristine: I.V.: 0.4 mg/m^2/day continuous infusion days 1 to 4
 [total dose/cycle = 1.6 mg/m^2]
Doxorubicin: I.V.: 10 mg/m^2/day continuous infusion days 1 to 4
 [total dose/cycle = 40 mg/m^2]
Cyclophosphamide: I.V.: 750 mg/m^2 day 6
 [total dose/cycle = 750 mg/m^2]
Prednisone: Oral: 60 mg/m^2/day days 1 to 6
 [total dose/cycle = 360 mg/m^2]
Repeat cycle (with cyclophosphamide dose adjustments if needed based on ANC) every 21 days (best response seen in a median of 4 cycles)

EPOCH-Rituximab (NHL)

Use Lymphoma, non-Hodgkin
Regimen
Rituximab: I.V.: 375 mg/m^2 day 1
 [total dose/cycle = 375 mg/m^2]
Etoposide: I.V.: 65 mg/m^2/day continuous infusion days 2, 3, and 4
 [total dose/cycle = 195 mg/m^2]
Vincristine: I.V.: 0.5 mg/m^2/day continuous infusion days 2, 3, and 4
 [total dose/cycle = 1.5 mg/m^2]
Doxorubicin: I.V.: 15 mg/m^2/day continuous infusion days 2, 3, and 4
 [total dose/cycle = 45 mg/m^2]
Cyclophosphamide: I.V.: 750 mg/m^2 day 5
 [total dose/cycle = 750 mg/m^2]
Prednisone: Oral: 60 mg/m^2/day days 1 to 14
 [total dose/cycle = 840 mg/m^2]
Repeat cycle every 21 days for 4-6 cycles

EP/PE

Use Lung cancer, nonsmall cell
Regimen
Etoposide: I.V.: 120 mg/m^2/day days 1, 2, and 3
 [total dose/cycle = 360 mg/m^2]
Cisplatin: I.V.: 60-120 mg/m^2 day 1
 [total dose/cycle = 60-120 mg/m^2]
Repeat cycle every 21-28 days

EP (Testicular Cancer)

Use Testicular cancer
Regimen NOTE: Multiple variations are listed.
Variation 1:
Etoposide: I.V.: 100 mg/m^2/day days 1 to 5
 [total dose/cycle = 500 mg/m^2]
Cisplatin: I.V.: 20 mg/m^2/day days 1 to 5
 [total dose/cycle = 100 mg/m^2]
Repeat cycle every 21 days

Variation 2:
  Etoposide: I.V.: 120 mg/m^2/day days 1, 2, and 3
    [total dose/cycle = 360 mg/m^2]
  Cisplatin: I.V.: 20 mg/m^2/day days 1 to 5
    [total dose/cycle = 100 mg/m^2]
  Repeat cycle every 3 or 4 weeks
Variation 3:
  Etoposide: I.V.: 120 mg/m^2/day days 1, 3, and 5
    [total dose/cycle = 360 mg/m^2]
  Cisplatin: I.V.: 20 mg/m^2/day days 1 to 5
    [total dose/cycle = 100 mg/m^2]
  Repeat cycle every 3 weeks

ESHAP

Use Lymphoma, non-Hodgkin

Regimen NOTE: Multiple variations are listed.
  Variation 1:
    Etoposide: I.V.: 40 mg/m^2/day days 1 to 4
      [total dose/cycle = 160 mg/m^2]
    Methylprednisolone: I.V.: 250-500 mg/day days 1 to 5
      [total dose/cycle = 1250-2500 mg]
    Cytarabine: I.V.: 2000 mg/m^2 day 5
      [total dose/cycle = 2000 mg/m^2]
    Cisplatin: I.V.: 25 mg/m^2/day continuous infusion days 1 to 4
      [total dose/cycle = 100 mg/m^2]
    Repeat cycle every 21-28 days
  Variation 2:
    Etoposide: I.V.: 40 mg/m^2/day days 1 to 4
      [total dose/cycle = 160 mg/m^2]
    Methylprednisolone: I.V.: 500 mg/day days 1 to 5
      [total dose/cycle = 2500 mg]
    Cytarabine: I.V.: 2000 mg/m^2 day 5
      [total dose/cycle = 2000 mg/m^2]
    Cisplatin: I.V.: 25 mg/m^2/day continuous infusion days 1 to 4
      [total dose/cycle = 100 mg/m^2]
    Repeat cycle every 21-28 days
  Variation 3:
    Etoposide: I.V.: 60 mg/m^2/day days 1 to 4
      [total dose/cycle = 240 mg/m^2]
    Methylprednisolone: I.V.: 500 mg/day days 1 to 4
      [total dose/cycle = 2000 mg]
    Cytarabine: I.V.: 2000 mg/m^2 day 5
      [total dose/cycle = 2000 mg/m^2]
    Cisplatin: I.V.: 25 mg/m^2/day continuous infusion days 1 to 4
      [total dose/cycle = 100 mg/m^2]
    Repeat cycle every 21 days

ESHAP (Hodgkin)

Use Lymphoma, Hodgkin

Regimen
  Etoposide: I.V.: 40 mg/m^2 /day days 1 to 4
    [total dose/cycle = 160 mg/m^2]
  Methylprednisolone: I.V.: 500 mg/day days 1 to 4
    [total dose/cycle = 2000 mg]
  Cisplatin: I.V.: 25 mg/m^2/day days 1 to 4
    [total dose/cycle = 100 mg/m^2]
  Cytarabine: I.V.: 2000 mg/m^2 day 5
    [total dose/cycle = 2000 mg/m^2]
  Filgrastim: SubQ: 5 mcg/kg/day days 6 to 18
  Repeat cycle every 21 to 28 days for 3 cycles (if transplant candidate) or 6 cycles (nontransplant candidate)

Estramustine + Docetaxel

Use Prostate cancer

Regimen NOTE: Multiple variations are listed.

Variation 1:
Docetaxel: I.V.: 20-80 mg/m^2 day 2
[total dose/cycle = 20-80 mg/m^2]
Estramustine: Oral: 280 mg 3 times/day days 1 to 5
[total dose/cycle = 4200 mg]
Repeat cycle every 21 days

Variation 2:
Docetaxel: I.V.: 20-80 mg/m^2 day 2
[total dose/cycle = 20-80 mg/m^2]
Estramustine: Oral: 14 mg/kg/day days 1 to 21
[total dose/cycle = 294 mg/kg]
Repeat cycle every 21 days

Variation 3:
Docetaxel: I.V.: 35 mg/m^2/day days 2 and 9
[total dose/cycle = 70 mg/m^2]
Estramustine: Oral: 420 mg 3 times/day for 4 doses, then 280 mg 3 times/day for 5 doses days 1, 2, 3, 8, 9, and 10
[total dose/cycle = 6160 mg]
Repeat cycle every 21 days

Variation 4:
Docetaxel: I.V.: 60 mg/m^2 day 2 cycle 1
[total dose/cycle = 60 mg/m^2]
followed by I.V.: 60-70 mg/m^2 day 2 (subsequent cycles)
[total dose/cycle = 60-70 mg/m^2]
Estramustine: Oral: 280 mg 3 times/day days 1 to 5
[total dose/cycle = 4200 mg]
Repeat cycle every 21 days for up to 12 cycles

Estramustine + Docetaxel + Calcitriol

Use Prostate cancer

Regimen

Cycle 1:
Calcitriol: Oral: 60 mcg (in divided doses) day 1
[total dose/cycle = 60 mcg]
Estramustine: Oral: 280 mg 3 times/day days 1 to 5
[total dose/cycle = 4200 mg]
Docetaxel: I.V.: 60 mg/m^2 day 2
[total dose/cycle = 60 mg/m^2]
Treatment cycle is 21 days

Subsequent cycles:
Calcitriol: Oral: 60 mcg (in divided doses) day 1
[total dose/cycle = 60 mcg]
Estramustine: Oral: 280 mg 3 times/day days 1 to 5
[total dose/cycle = 4200 mg]
Docetaxel: I.V.: 70 mg/m^2 day 2
[total dose/cycle = 70 mg/m^2]
Repeat cycle every 21 days for up to 12 cycles

Estramustine + Docetaxel + Carboplatin

Use Prostate cancer

Regimen

Docetaxel: I.V.: 70 mg/m^2 day 2
[total dose/cycle = 70 mg/m^2]
Estramustine: Oral: 280 mg 3 times/day days 1 to 5
[total dose/cycle = 4200 mg]
Carboplatin: I.V.: Target AUC 5 day 2
[total dose/cycle = AUC = 5]
Repeat cycle every 3 weeks

Estramustine + Docetaxel + Hydrocortisone

Use Prostate cancer

Regimen
Docetaxel: I.V.: 70 mg/m^2 day 2
  [total dose/cycle = 70 mg/m^2]
Estramustine: Oral: 10 mg/kg/day days 1 to 5
  [total dose/cycle = 50 mg/kg]
Hydrocortisone: Oral: 40 mg daily
  [total dose/cycle = 840 mg]
Repeat cycle every 3 weeks

Estramustine + Docetaxel + Prednisone

Use Prostate cancer

Regimen
Estramustine: Oral: 280 mg 3 times/day days 1 to 5 and days 7 to 11
  [total dose/cycle = 8400 mg]
Docetaxel: I.V.: 70 mg/m^2 day 2
  [total dose/cycle = 70 mg/m^2]
Prednisone: Oral: 10 mg daily
  [total dose/cycle = 210 mg]
Repeat cycle every 21 days for up to 6 cycles

Estramustine + Etoposide

Use Prostate cancer

Regimen NOTE: Multiple variations are listed.
Variation 1:
  Estramustine: Oral: 15 mg/kg/day days 1 to 21
    [total dose/cycle = 315 mg/kg]
  Etoposide: Oral: 50 mg/m^2/day days 1 to 21
    [total dose/cycle = 1050 mg/m^2]
  Repeat cycle every 4 weeks
Variation 2:
  Estramustine: Oral: 10 mg/kg/day days 1 to 21
    [total dose/cycle = 210 mg/kg]
  Etoposide: Oral: 50 mg/m^2/day days 1 to 21
    [total dose/cycle = 1050 mg/m^2]
  Repeat cycle every 4 weeks
Variation 3:
  Estramustine: Oral: 140 mg 3 times/day days 1 to 21
    [total dose/cycle = 8820 mg]
  Etoposide: Oral: 50 mg/m^2/day days 1 to 21
    [total dose/cycle = 1050 mg/m^2]
  Repeat cycle every 4 weeks

Estramustine-Paclitaxel

Use Prostate cancer

Regimen NOTE: Multiple variations are listed.
Variation 1:
  Paclitaxel: I.V.: 30-35 mg/m^2/day continuous infusion (given in 2-3 divided doses daily) either days 1 to 4 or days 2 to 5
    [total dose/cycle = 120-140 mg/m^2]
  Estramustine: Oral: 600 mg/m^2/day days 1 to 21
    [total dose/cycle = 12,600 mg/m^2]
  Repeat cycle every 21 days
Variation 2:
  Paclitaxel: I.V. 60-107 mg/m^2 infused over 3 hours weekly for 6 weeks
    [total dose/cycle = 360-642 mg/m^2]
  Estramustine: Oral: 280 mg twice daily 3 days/week for 6 weeks
    [total dose/cycle = 3360 mg]
  Repeat cycle every 8 weeks

◄ Variation 3:
  Paclitaxel: I.V. 150 mg/m^2/day days 2, 9, and 16
    [total dose/cycle = 450 mg/m^2]
  Estramustine: Oral: 280 mg 3 times/day days 1, 2, 3, 8, 9, 10, 15, 16, and 17
    [total dose/week = 7560 mg/m^2]
  Repeat cycle every 4 weeks
Variation 4:
  Paclitaxel: I.V.: 100 mg/m^2/day days 2, 9, and 16
    [total dose/cycle = 300 mg/m^2]
  Estramustine: Oral: 280 mg 3 times/day days 1, 2, 3, 8, 9, 10, 15, 16, and 17
    [total dose/cycle = 7560 mg]
  Repeat cycle every 4 weeks

Estramustine-Vinblastine

Use Prostate cancer

Regimen NOTE: Multiple variations are listed.
Variation 1:
  Estramustine: Oral: 10 mg/kg/day days 1 to 42
    [total dose/cycle = 420 mg/kg]
  Vinblastine: I.V.: 4 mg/m^2/day days 1, 8, 15, 22, 29, and 36
    [total dose/cycle = 24 mg/m^2]
  Repeat cycle every 8 weeks
Variation 2:
  Estramustine: Oral: 600 mg/m^2/day days 1 to 42
    [total dose/cycle = 25,200 mg/m^2]
  Vinblastine: I.V.: 4 mg/m^2/day days 1, 8, 15, 22, 29, and 36
    [total dose/cycle = 24 mg/m^2]
  Repeat cycle every 8 weeks

Estramustine + Vinorelbine

Use Prostate cancer

Regimen NOTE: Multiple variations are listed.
Variation 1:
  Estramustine: Oral: 140 mg 3 times/day days 1 to 14
    [total dose/cycle = 5880 mg]
  Vinorelbine: I.V.: 25 mg/m^2/day days 1 and 8
    [total dose/cycle = 50 mg/m^2]
  Repeat cycle every 21 days
Variation 2:
  Estramustine: Oral: 280 mg 3 times/day days 1, 2, and 3
    [total dose/cycle = 2520 mg/m^2]
  Vinorelbine: I.V.: 15 or 20 mg/m^2 day 2
    [total dose/cycle = 15 or 20 mg/m^2]
  Repeat cycle weekly for 8 weeks, then every other week

Etoposide-Carboplatin (Ovarian Cancer)

Use Ovarian cancer

Regimen
  Etoposide: I.V.: 120 mg/m^2/day days 1, 2, and 3
    [total dose/cycle = 360 mg/m^2]
  Carboplatin: I.V.: 400 mg/m^2 day 1
    [total dose/cycle = 400 mg/m^2]
  Repeat cycle every 28 days for a total of 3 cycles

FAC

Use Breast cancer

Regimen NOTE: Multiple variations are listed below.
Variation 1:
  Fluorouracil: I.V.: 500 mg/m^2/day days 1 and 8
    [total dose/cycle = 1000 mg/m^2]
    or 500 mg/m^2 day 1
      [total dose/cycle = 500 mg/m^2]

Doxorubicin: I.V.: 50 mg/m^2 day 1
  [total dose/cycle = 50 mg/m^2]
Cyclophosphamide: I.V.: 500 mg/m^2 day 1
  [total dose/cycle = 500 mg/m^2]
Repeat cycle every 21-28 days
Variation 2:
Fluorouracil: I.V.: 200 mg/m^2/day days 1, 2, and 3
  [total dose/cycle = 600 mg/m^2]
Doxorubicin: I.V.: 40 mg/m^2 day 1
  [total dose/cycle = 40 mg/m^2]
Cyclophosphamide: I.V.: 400 mg/m^2 day 1
  [total dose/cycle = 400 mg/m^2]
Repeat cycle every 28 days
Variation 3:
Fluorouracil: I.V.: 400 mg/m^2/day days 1 and 8
  [total dose/cycle = 800 mg/m^2]
Doxorubicin: I.V.: 40 mg/m^2 day 1
  [total dose/cycle = 40 mg/m^2]
Cyclophosphamide: I.V.: 400 mg/m^2 day 1
  [total dose/cycle = 400 mg/m^2]
Repeat cycle every 28 days
Variation 4:
Fluorouracil: I.V.: 600 mg/m^2/day days 1 and 8
  [total dose/cycle = 1200 mg/m^2]
Doxorubicin: I.V.: 60 mg/m^2 day 1
  [total dose/cycle = 60 mg/m^2]
Cyclophosphamide: I.V.: 600 mg/m^2 day 1
  [total dose/cycle = 600 mg/m^2]
Repeat cycle every 28 days
Variation 5:
Fluorouracil: I.V.: 300 mg/m^2/day days 1 and 8
  [total dose/cycle = 600 mg/m^2]
Doxorubicin: I.V.: 30 mg/m^2 day 1
  [total dose/cycle = 30 mg/m^2]
Cyclophosphamide: I.V.: 300 mg/m^2 day 1
  [total dose/cycle = 300 mg/m^2]
Repeat cycle every 28 days

FEC

Use Breast cancer
Regimen
Fluorouracil: I.V.: 500 mg/m^2 day 1
  [total dose/cycle = 500 mg/m^2]
Cyclophosphamide: I.V.: 500 mg/m^2 day 1
  [total dose/cycle = 500 mg/m^2]
Epirubicin: I.V.: 100 mg/m^2 day 1
  [total dose/cycle = 100 mg/m^2]
Repeat cycle every 21 days

FL

Use Prostate cancer
Regimen NOTE: Multiple variations are listed.
Variation 1:
Flutamide: Oral: 250 mg every 8 hours
  [total dose/cycle = 21,000 mg]
Leuprolide acetate: SubQ: 1 mg/day
  [total dose/cycle = 28 mg]
Repeat cycle every 28 days
Variation 2:
Flutamide: Oral: 250 mg every 8 hours
  [total dose/cycle = 67,500 mg]

Leuprolide acetate depot: I.M.: 22.5 mg day 1
[total dose/cycle = 22.5 mg]
Repeat cycle every 3 months

FLAG (AML Induction)

Use Leukemia, acute myeloid

Regimen NOTE: Multiple variations are listed below.
Variation 1:
Fludarabine: I.V.: 30 mg/m^2/day over 30 minutes days 1 to 5
[total dose/cycle = 150 mg/m^2]
Cytarabine: I.V.: 2 g/m^2/day over 4 hours days 1 to 5 (begin 4 hours after fludarabine infusion)
[total dose/cycle = 10 g/m^2]
Filgrastim: SubQ: 300 mcg 12 hours prior to start of fludarabine then 300 mcg/day days 2 through 5
[total dose/cycle = 1500 mcg]
followed by Filgrastim: SubQ: 300 mcg/day beginning one week after the end of treatment and
continuing until complete neutrophil recovery
Variation 2:
Fludarabine: I.V.: 30 mg/m^2/day over 30 minutes days 1 to 5
[total dose/cycle = 150 mg/m^2]
Cytarabine: I.V.: 2 g/m^2/day over 4 hours days 1 to 5 (begin 3.5 hours after end of fludarabine infusion)
[total dose/cycle = 10 g/m^2]
Filgrastim: SubQ: 5 mcg/kg/day beginning 24 hours prior to start of fludarabine and continuing until ANC
>500 mm^3
May repeat cycle one time for partial remission
Variation 3:
Fludarabine: I.V.: 30 mg/m^2/day over 30 minutes days 1 to 5
[total dose/cycle = 150 mg/m^2]
Cytarabine: I.V.: 2 g/m^2/day over 2 hours days 1 to 5 (begin 4 hours after the start of fludarabine
infusion)
[total dose/cycle = 10 g/m^2]
Filgrastim: SubQ or I.V.: 300 mcg/day beginning the day prior to start of chemotherapy and continuing
during chemotherapy and until ANC >1000 mm^3
May receive a second cycle
Variation 4:
Fludarabine: I.V.: 25 mg/m^2/day over 30 minutes days 1 to 5
[total dose/cycle = 125 mg/m^2]
Cytarabine: I.V.: 2 g/m^2/day over 4 hours days 1 to 5 (begin 4 hours after start of fludarabine infusion)
[total dose/cycle = 10 g/m^2]
Filgrastim: SubQ: 5 mcg/kg/day beginning 24 hours prior to start of cytarabine and continuing until ANC
>500 mm^3
May repeat cycle in patients with complete remission and partial remission

FLAG-IDA

Use Leukemia, acute myeloid

Regimen NOTE: Multiple variations are listed.
Variation 1:
Fludarabine: I.V.: 30 mg/m^2/day over 30 minutes days 1 to 5
[total dose/cycle = 150 mg/m^2]
Cytarabine: I.V.: 2 g/m^2/day over 4 hours days 1 to 5 (begin 4 hours after the start of fludarabine)
[total dose/cycle = 10 g/m^2]
Idarubicin: I.V.: 10 mg/m^2/day days 1, 2, and 3
[total dose/cycle = 30 mg/m^2]
Filgrastim: SubQ: 5 mcg/kg from day 6 until ANC >500/mm^3
Variation 2:
Fludarabine: I.V.: 30 mg/m^2/day over 30 minutes days 1 to 5
[total dose/cycle = 150 mg/m^2]
Cytarabine: I.V.: 2 g/m^2/day over 2 hours days 1 to 5 (begin 4 hours after the start of fludarabine
infusion)
[total dose/cycle = 10 g/m^2]
Idarubicin: I.V.: 8 mg/m^2/day over 30 minutes days 1, 2, and 3
[total dose/cycle = 24 mg/m^2]

Filgrastim: SubQ or I.V.: 300 mcg/day beginning the day prior to start of chemotherapy and continuing during chemotherapy and until ANC >1000/mm^3

May receive up to 2 cycles

Variation 3:

Fludarabine: I.V.: 30 mg/m^2/day over 30 minutes days 1 to 4
[total dose/cycle = 120 mg/m^2]

Cytarabine: I.V.: 2 g/m^2/day over 4 hours days 1 to 4 (begin 4 hours after fludarabine treatment)
[total dose/cycle = 8 g/m^2]

Idarubicin: I.V.: 10 mg/m^2/day days 1, 2, and 3
[total dose/cycle = 30 mg/m^2]

Filgrastim: Sub Q: see article for dose and frequency

FLOX (Nordic FLOX)

Use Colorectal cancer

Regimen

Oxaliplatin: I.V.: 85 mg/m^2 day 1
[total dose/cycle = 85 mg/m^2]

Fluorouracil: I.V.: 500 mg/m^2/day days 1 and 2
[total dose/cycle = 1000 mg/m^2]

Leucovorin: I.V.: 60 mg/m^2/day days 1 and 2
[total dose/cycle = 120 mg/m^2]

Repeat cycle every 2 weeks

Fludarabine-Alemtuzumab (CLL)

Use Leukemia, chronic lymphocytic

Regimen

Prior to Cycle 1 (days -14 to -1):

Alemtuzumab dose escalation (on consecutive days): I.V.: 3 mg/dose/day (repeat until tolerated); when tolerated, increase to 10 mg/dose/day (repeat until tolerated); when tolerated, increase to 30 mg/dose

Cycle 1 (begin when alemtuzumab successfully escalated to 30 mg, but no more than 14 days from dose escalation protocol):

Alemtuzumab: I.V.: 30 mg/dose over 2 hours days 1, 2, and 3
[total dose/cycle = 90 mg]

Fludarabine: I.V.: 30 mg/m^2/day over 15-30 minutes days 1, 2, and 3 (begin with alemtuzumab at full dose)
[total dose/cycle = 90 mg/m^2]

Repeat cycle in 28 days

Cycles 2-4:

Alemtuzumab: I.V.: 30 mg/dose (over 4 hours day 1; over 2 hours days 2 and 3) days 1, 2, and 3
[total dose/cycle = 90 mg]

Fludarabine: I.V.: 30 mg/m^2/day over 15-30 minutes days 1, 2, and 3
[total dose/cycle = 90 mg/m^2]

Repeat cycle every 28 days; may administer an additional 2 cycles (cycles 5 and 6) if respond (and tolerate)

Fludarabine-Cyclophosphamide (CLL)

Use Leukemia, chronic lymphocytic

Regimen NOTE: Multiple variations are listed.

Variation 1:

Fludarabine: I.V.: 25 mg/m^2/day days 1, 2, and 3
[total dose/cycle = 75 mg/m^2]

Cyclophosphamide: I.V.: 250 mg/m^2/day days 1, 2, and 3
[total dose/cycle = 750 mg/m^2]

Repeat cycle every 4 weeks for up to 6 cycles

Variation 2:

Fludarabine: I.V.: 30 mg/m^2/day days 1, 2, and 3
[total dose/cycle = 90 mg/m^2]

Cyclophosphamide: I.V.: 250 mg/m^2/day days 1, 2, and 3
[total dose/cycle = 750 mg/m^2]

Repeat cycle every 4 weeks for up to 6 cycles

◀ Variation 3:
  Cyclophosphamide: I.V.: 600 mg/m^2 day 1
  [total dose/cycle = 600 mg/m^2]
  Fludarabine: I.V.: 20 mg/m^2/day days 1 to 5
  [total dose/cycle = 100 mg/m^2]
  Repeat cycle every 4 weeks for up to 6 cycles
Variation 4:
  Fludarabine: I.V.: 30 mg/m^2/day days 1, 2, and 3
  [total dose/cycle = 90 mg/m^2]
  Cyclophosphamide: I.V.: 300 mg/m^2/day days 1, 2, and 3
  [total dose/cycle = 900 mg/m^2]
  Repeat cycle every 4 weeks for up to 6 cycles
Variation 5:
  Fludarabine: I.V.: 30 mg/m^2/day days 1, 2, and 3
  [total dose/cycle = 90 mg/m^2]
  Cyclophosphamide: I.V.: 300 mg/m^2/day days 1, 2, and 3
  [total dose/cycle = 900 mg/m^2]
  Repeat cycle every 4-6 weeks for up to 6 cycles

Fludarabine-Cyclophosphamide-Mitoxantrone-Rituximab

Use Lymphoma, non-Hodgkin

Regimen NOTE: Multiple variations are listed.
  Consider pretherapy cytoreduction with cyclophosphamide 200 mg/m^2/day for 3-5 days for patients with high tumor burden and/or lymphocytes >20,000/mm^3
Variation 1:
  Rituximab: I.V.: 375 mg/m^2/dose day 1
  [total dose/cycle = 375 mg/m^2]
  Fludarabine: I.V.: 25 mg/m^2/day days 2, 3, and 4
  [total dose/cycle = 75 mg/m^2]
  Cyclophosphamide: I.V.: 200 mg/m^2/day days 2, 3, and 4
  [total dose/cycle = 600 mg/m^2]
  Mitoxantrone: I.V.: 8 mg/m^2/dose day 2
  [total dose/cycle = 8 mg/m^2]
  Repeat cycle every 28 days for total of 4 cycles
Variation 2 (with maintenance rituximab):
  Rituximab: I.V.: 375 mg/m^2/dose day 1
  [total dose/cycle = 375 mg/m^2]
  Fludarabine: I.V.: 25 mg/m^2/day days 2, 3, and 4
  [total dose/cycle = 75 mg/m^2]
  Cyclophosphamide: I.V.: 200 mg/m^2/day days 2, 3, and 4
  [total dose/cycle = 600 mg/m^2]
  Mitoxantrone: I.V.: 8 mg/m^2/dose day 2
  [total dose/cycle = 8 mg/m^2]
  Repeat cycle every 28 days for total of 4 cycles
  followed by:
    Maintenance rituximab (begin 3 months after completion of cycle 4):
    Rituximab: I.V.: 375 mg/m^2/dose day 1, 8, 15, and 22
    [total dose/cycle = 1500 mg/m^2]
    Repeat maintenance cycle (once) in 6 months

Fludarabine-Cyclophosphamide (NHL-Mantle Cell)

Use Lymphoma, non-Hodgkin (mantle cell)

Regimen NOTE: Multiple variations are listed.
  Variation 1:
  Fludarabine: I.V.: 20 mg/m^2/day days 1 to 5
  [total dose/cycle = 100 mg/m^2]
  Cyclophosphamide: I.V.: 800 mg/m^2/dose day 1
  [total dose/cycle = 800 mg/m^2]
  Repeat cycle every 3-4 weeks for up to a total of 5 cycles
  Variation 2:
  Fludarabine: I.V.: 20 mg/m^2/day days 1 to 5
  [total dose/cycle = 100 mg/m^2]

Cyclophosphamide: I.V.: 1000 mg/m^2/dose day 1
 [total dose/cycle = 1000 mg/m^2]
Repeat cycle every 3-4 weeks for up to a total of 5 cycles
Variation 3:
 Fludarabine: I.V.: 25 mg/m^2/day days 1 to 4
 [total dose/cycle = 100 mg/m^2]
 Cyclophosphamide: I.V.: 1000 mg/m^2/dose day 1
 [total dose/cycle = 1000 mg/m^2]
 Repeat cycle every 3-4 weeks for up to a total of 5 cycles

Fludarabine-Cyclophosphamide-Rituximab (CLL)

Use Leukemia, chronic lymphocytic

Regimen
Cycle 1:
 Rituximab: I.V.: 375 mg/m^2 day 1
 [total dose/cycle = 375 mg/m^2]
 Fludarabine: I.V.: 25 mg/m^2/day days 2, 3, and 4
 [total dose/cycle = 75 mg/m^2]
 Cyclophosphamide: I.V.: 250 mg/m^2/day days 2, 3, and 4
 [total dose/cycle = 750 mg/m^2]
 Treatment cycle is 4 weeks
Cycles 2-6:
 Rituximab: I.V.: 500 mg/m^2 day 1
 [total dose/cycle = 500 mg/m^2]
 Fludarabine: I.V.: 25 mg/m^2/day days 1, 2, and 3
 [total dose/cycle = 75 mg/m^2]
 Cyclophosphamide: I.V.: 250 mg/m^2/day days 1, 2, and 3
 [total dose/cycle = 750 mg/m^2]
 Repeat cycle every 4 weeks

Fludarabine-Cyclophosphamide-Rituximab (NHL-Follicular)

Use Lymphoma, non-Hodgkin (Follicular lymphoma)

Regimen
Cycle 1:
 Rituximab: I.V.: 375 mg/m^2 day 15
 [total dose/cycle = 375 mg/m^2]
 Fludarabine: I.V.: 25 mg/m^2/day days 1, 2, and 3
 [total dose/cycle = 75 mg/m^2]
 Cyclophosphamide: I.V.: 300 mg/m^2/day days 1, 2, and 3
 [total dose/cycle = 900 mg/m^2]
 Treatment cycle is 3 weeks
Cycles 2-4:
 Rituximab: I.V.: 375 mg/m^2 day 1
 [total dose/cycle = 375 mg/m^2]
 Fludarabine: I.V.: 25 mg/m^2/day days 1, 2, and 3
 [total dose/cycle = 75 mg/m^2]
 Cyclophosphamide: I.V.: 300 mg/m^2/day days 1, 2, and 3
 [total dose/cycle = 900 mg/m^2]
 Each treatment cycle is 3 weeks

Fludarabine-Mitoxantrone

Use Lymphoma, non-Hodgkin

Regimen
Fludarabine: I.V.: 25 mg/m^2/day days 1, 2, and 3
 [total dose/cycle = 75 mg/m^2]
Mitoxantrone: I.V.: 10 mg/m^2/dose day 1
 [total dose/cycle = 10 mg/m^2]
Repeat cycle every 21 days for total of 6 cycles

Fludarabine-Mitoxantrone-Dexamethasone (NHL)

Use Lymphoma, non-Hodgkin

◄ **Regimen**
Fludarabine: I.V.: 25 mg/m^2/day days 1, 2, and 3
[total dose/cycle = 75 mg/m^2]
Mitoxantrone: I.V.: 10 mg/m^2/dose day 1
[total dose/cycle = 10 mg/m^2]
Dexamethasone: I.V. or Oral: 20 mg/day days 1 to 5
[total dose/cycle = 100 mg]
Repeat cycle every 28 days for up to a total of 8 cycles

Fludarabine-Mitoxantrone-Dexamethasone-Rituximab

Use Lymphoma, non-Hodgkin
Regimen
Cycle 1:
Rituximab: I.V.: 375 mg/m^2/day days 1 and 8
[total dose/cycle = 750 mg/m^2]
Fludarabine: I.V.: 25 mg/m^2/day days 1, 2, and 3
[total dose/cycle = 75 mg/m^2]
Mitoxantrone: I.V.: 10 mg/m^2/dose day 1
[total dose/cycle = 10 mg/m^2]
Dexamethasone: I.V. or Oral: 20 mg/m^2/day days 1 to 5
[total dose/cycle = 100 mg/m^2]
Treatment cycle is 28 days
Cycles 2-5:
Rituximab: I.V.: 375 mg/m^2 day 1
[total dose/cycle = 375 mg/m^2]
Fludarabine: I.V.: 25 mg/m^2/day days 2, 3, and 4
[total dose/cycle = 75 mg/m^2]
Mitoxantrone: I.V.: 10 mg/m^2/dose day 2
[total dose/cycle = 10 mg/m^2]
Dexamethasone: I.V. or Oral: 20 mg/m^2/day days 1 to 5
[total dose/cycle = 100 mg/m^2]
Repeat cycle every 28 days
Cycles 6-8:
Fludarabine: I.V.: 25 mg/m^2/day days 1, 2, and 3
[total dose/cycle = 75 mg/m^2]
Mitoxantrone: I.V.: 10 mg/m^2/dose day 1
[total dose/cycle = 10 mg/m^2]
Dexamethasone: I.V. or Oral: 20 mg/m^2/day days 1 to 5
[total dose/cycle = 100 mg/m^2]
Repeat cycle every 28 days
followed by:
Interferon maintenance:
Interferon alfa-2b: SubQ: 3 million units/m^2 days 1 to 14
[total dose/cycle = 42 million units/m^2]
Dexamethasone: Oral: 8 mg/day days 1, 2, and 3
[total dose/cycle = 24 mg]
Repeat cycle every month for 1 year

Fludarabine-Mitoxantrone-Rituximab

Use Lymphoma, non-Hodgkin
Regimen
Fludarabine: I.V.: 25 mg/m^2/day days 1, 2, and 3
[total dose/cycle = 75 mg/m^2]
Mitoxantrone: I.V.: 10 mg/m^2/dose day 1
[total dose/cycle = 10 mg/m^2]
Repeat cycle every 21 days for total of 6 cycles
followed by:
Sequential rituximab (after completion of cycle 6):
Rituximab: I.V.: 375 mg/m^2/dose weekly for 4 doses
[total dose/4 weeks = 1500 mg/m^2]

Fludarabine-Rituximab (CLL)

Use Leukemia, chronic lymphocytic

Regimen
Rituximab: I.V.: 375 mg/m²/day days 1 and 4 (cycle 1); day 1 (cycles 2 to 6)
Fludarabine: I.V.: 25 mg/m²/day days 1 to 5
Repeat cycle every 4 weeks

Fludarabine-Rituximab (NHL-Follicular)

Use Lymphoma, non-Hodgkin (follicular lymphoma)

Regimen
Week 1:
Rituximab: I.V.: 375 mg/m²/dose for 2 doses 4 days apart
[total dose/week = 750 mg/m²]
Week 2:
Fludarabine: I.V.: 25 mg/m²/day days 1 to 5
[total dose/week = 125 mg/m²]
Week 5:
Rituximab: I.V.: 375 mg/m²/dose day 5
[total dose/week = 375 mg/m²]
Week 6:
Fludarabine: I.V.: 25 mg/m²/day days 1 to 5
[total dose/week = 125 mg/m²]
Week 10:
Fludarabine: I.V.: 25 mg/m²/day days 1 to 5
[total dose/week = 125 mg/m²]
Week 13:
Rituximab: I.V.: 375 mg/m²/dose day 5
[total dose/week = 375 mg/m²]
Week 14:
Fludarabine: I.V.: 25 mg/m²/day days 1 to 5
[total dose/week = 125 mg/m²]
Week 18:
Fludarabine: I.V.: 25 mg/m²/day days 1 to 5
[total dose/week = 125 mg/m²]
Week 21:
Rituximab: I.V.: 375 mg/m²/dose day 5
[total dose/week = 375 mg/m²]
Week 22:
Fludarabine: I.V.: 25 mg/m²/day days 1 to 5
[total dose/week = 125 mg/m²]
Week 26:
Rituximab: I.V.: 375 mg/m²/dose for 2 doses 4 days apart
[total dose/week = 750 mg/m²]

Fluorouracil-Carboplatin (Head and Neck Cancer)

Use Head and neck cancer

Regimen NOTE: Multiple variations are listed.
Variation 1:
Fluorouracil: I.V.: 600 mg/m²/day continuous infusion days 1 to 4
[total dose/cycle = 2400 mg/m²]
Carboplatin: I.V.: 70 mg/m²/day days 1 to 4
[total dose/cycle = 280 mg/m²]
Repeat cycle every 3 weeks for 3 cycles
Variation 2:
Fluorouracil: I.V.: 1000 mg/m²/day continuous infusion days 1 to 4
[total dose/cycle = 4000 mg/m²]
Carboplatin: I.V.: 300 mg/m²/dose day 1 (may escalate to 360 mg/m²/dose in future cycles for grade 0
or 1 hematologic toxicity)
[total dose/cycle = 300-360 mg/m²]
Repeat cycle every 28 weeks

◄ Variation 3:
Carboplatin: I.V.: 400 mg/m^2 day 1
[total dose/cycle = 400 mg/m^2]
Fluorouracil: I.V.: 1000 mg/m^2/day continuous infusion days 1 to 4
[total dose/cycle = 4000 mg/m^2]
Repeat cycle every 28 days for a total of 2 or 3 cycles

Fluorouracil-Hydroxyurea (Head and Neck Cancer)

Use Head and neck cancer

Regimen NOTE: Administered with concurrent radiation therapy
Fluorouracil: I.V.: 800 mg/m^2/day continuous infusion days 1 to 5
[total dose/cycle = 4000 mg/m^2]
Hydroxyurea: Oral: 1000 mg/dose every 12 hours for 11 doses beginning day 1
[total dose/cycle = 11,000 mg]
Repeat cycle every other week for a total therapy duration of 13 weeks

Fluorouracil-Leucovorin

Use Colorectal cancer

Regimen NOTE: Multiple variations are listed.
Variation 1 (Mayo Regimen):
Fluorouracil: I.V.: 370-425 mg/m^2/day days 1 to 5
[total dose/cycle = 1850-2125 mg/m^2]
Leucovorin: I.V.: 20 mg/m^2/day days 1 to 5
[total dose/cycle = 100 mg/m^2]
Repeat cycle at 4 weeks, 8 weeks, and every 5 weeks thereafter
Variation 2:
Fluorouracil: I.V.: 400 mg/m^2/day days 1 to 5
[total dose/cycle = 2000 mg/m^2]
Leucovorin: I.V.: 20 mg/m^2/day days 1 to 5
[total dose/cycle = 100 mg/m^2]
Repeat cycle every 28 days
Variation 3:
Fluorouracil: I.V.: 500 mg/m^2 day 1
[total dose/cycle = 500 mg/m^2]
Leucovorin: I.V.: 20 mg/m^2 (2-hour infusion) day 1
[total dose/cycle = 20 mg/m^2]
Repeat cycle weekly
Variation 4:
Fluorouracil: I.V.: 600 mg/m^2 weekly for 6 weeks
[total dose/cycle = 3600 mg/m^2]
Leucovorin: I.V.: 500 mg/m^2 (3-hour infusion) weekly for 6 weeks
[total dose/cycle = 3000 mg/m^2]
Repeat cycle every 8 weeks
Variation 5:
Fluorouracil: I.V.: 600 mg/m^2 weekly for 6 weeks
[total dose/cycle = 3600 mg/m^2]
Leucovorin: I.V.: 500 mg/m^2 (2-hour infusion) weekly for 6 weeks
[total dose/cycle = 3000 mg/m^2]
Repeat cycle every 8 weeks
Variation 6:
Fluorouracil: I.V.: 600 mg/m^2 weekly
[total dose/cycle = 600 mg/m^2]
Leucovorin: I.V.: 500 mg/m^2 (2-hour infusion) weekly
[total dose/cycle = 500 mg/m^2]
Repeat cycle weekly
Variation 7:
Fluorouracil: I.V.: 2600 mg/m^2 continuous infusion over 24 hours day 1
[total dose/cycle = 2600 mg/m^2]
Leucovorin: I.V.: 500 mg/m^2 continuous infusion over 24 hours day 1
[total dose/cycle = 500 mg/m^2]
Repeat cycle weekly

Variation 8:
  Fluorouracil: I.V.: 2600 mg/m^2 continuous infusion over 24 hours day 1
    [total dose/cycle = 2600 mg/m^2]
  Leucovorin: I.V.: 300 mg/m^2 (maximum dose: 500 mg) continuous infusion over 24 hours day 1
    [total dose/cycle = 300 mg/m^2; maximum: 500 mg]
  Repeat cycle weekly
Variation 9:
  Fluorouracil: I.V.: 2600 mg/m^2 continuous infusion over 24 hours once weekly for 6 weeks
    [total dose/cycle = 15,600 mg/m^2]
  Leucovorin: I.V.: 500 mg/m^2 over 2 hours once weekly for 6 weeks
    [total dose/cycle = 3000 mg/m^2]
  Repeat cycle every 8 weeks
Variation 10:
  Fluorouracil: I.V.: 2300 mg/m^2 continuous infusion over 24 hours day 1
    [total dose/cycle = 2300 mg/m^2]
  Leucovorin: I.V.: 50 mg/m^2 continuous infusion over 24 hours day 1
    [total dose/cycle = 50 mg/m^2]
  Repeat cycle weekly
Variation 11:
  Fluorouracil: I.V.: 200 mg/m^2/day continuous infusion days 1 to 14
    [total dose/cycle = 2800 mg/m^2]
  Leucovorin: I.V.: 5 mg/m^2/day continuous infusion days 1 to 14
    [total dose/cycle = 70 mg/m^2]
  Repeat cycle every 28 days
Variation 12:
  Cycle 1:
    Fluorouracil: I.V.: 200 mg/m^2/day continuous infusion for 4 weeks
      [total dose/cycle = 5600 mg/m^2]
    Leucovorin: I.V.: 20 mg/m^2/day days 1, 8, 15, 22
      [total dose/cycle = 80 mg/m^2]
    Treatment cycle is 6 weeks
  Subsequent cycles (starting week 7):
    Fluorouracil: 200 mg/m^2 continuous infusion days 1 to 21
      [total dose/cycle = 4200 mg/m^2]
    Leucovorin: I.V.: 20 mg/m^2/day days 1, 8, and 15
      [total dose/cycle = 60 mg/m^2]
    Repeat cycle every 4 weeks

Fluorouracil-Leucovorin-Irinotecan (Saltz Regimen)

Use Colorectal cancer

Regimen
  Fluorouracil: I.V.: 500 mg/m^2/day days 1, 8, 15, and 22
    [total dose/cycle = 2000 mg/m^2]
  Leucovorin: I.V.: 20 mg/m^2/day days 1, 8, 15, and 22
    [total dose/cycle = 80 mg/m^2]
  Irinotecan: I.V.: 125 mg/m^2/day days 1, 8, 15, and 22
    [total dose/cycle = 500 mg/m^2]
  Repeat cycle every 42 days

Fluorouracil-Leucovorin-Oxaliplatin (Esophageal Cancer)

Use Esophageal Cancer

Regimen NOTE: Multiple variations are listed.
  Variation 1:
    Oxaliplatin: I.V.: 85 mg/m^2/dose over 2 hours day 1
      [total dose/cycle = 85 mg/m^2]
    Leucovorin: I.V.: 200 mg/m^2/dose over 2 hours day 1
      [total dose/cycle = 200 mg/m^2]
    Fluorouracil: I.V.: 2600 mg/m^2/dose continuous infusion over 24 hours day 1
      [total dose/cycle = 2600 mg/m^2]
    Repeat cycle every 2 weeks until disease progression or unacceptable toxicity.

◀ Variation 2:
Oxaliplatin: I.V.: 85 mg/m^2/dose over 2 hours day 1
[total dose/cycle = 85 mg/m^2]
Leucovorin: I.V.: 500 mg/m^2/day over 2 hours days 1 and 2
[total dose/cycle = 1000 mg/m^2]
Fluorouracil: I.V. bolus: 400 mg/m^2/day days 1 and 2
followed by I.V.: 600 mg/m^2/day continuous infusion over 22 hours days 1 and 2
[total dose/cycle = 2000 mg/m^2]
Repeat cycle every 2 weeks for 4 cycles (if achieve stable disease or response, continue until disease progression or unacceptable toxicity).
Variation 3:
Oxaliplatin: I.V.: 85 mg/m^2/dose day 1
[total dose/cycle = 85 mg/m^2]
Leucovorin: I.V.: 200 mg/m^2/day over 2 hours days 1 and 2
[total dose/cycle = 400 mg/m^2]
Fluorouracil: I.V. bolus: 400 mg/m^2/day days 1 and 2
followed by I.V.: 600 mg/m^2/day continuous infusion over 22 hours days 1 and 2
[total dose/cycle = 2000 mg/m^2]
Repeat cycle every 2 weeks for 6 cycles (3 cycles with radiation therapy and 3 cycles after completion of radiation therapy).

Fluorouracil-Leucovorin-Oxaliplatin (Gastric Cancer)

Use Gastric cancer
Regimen NOTE: Multiple variations are listed below.
Variation 1:
Oxaliplatin: I.V.: 85 mg/m^2/dose over 2 hours day 1
[total dose/cycle = 85 mg/m^2]
Leucovorin: I.V.: 200 mg/m^2/dose over 2 hours day 1
[total dose/cycle = 200 mg/m^2]
Fluorouracil: I.V.: 2600 mg/m^2/dose continuous infusion over 24 hours day 1
[total dose/cycle = 2600 mg/m^2]
Repeat cycle every 2 weeks until disease progression or unacceptable toxicity
Variation 2:
Oxaliplatin: I.V.: 100 mg/m^2/dose over 2 hours day 1
[total dose/cycle = 100 mg/m^2]
Leucovorin: I.V.: 400 mg/m^2/dose over 2 hours day 1
[total dose/cycle = 400 mg/m^2]
Fluorouracil: I.V. bolus: 400 mg/m^2/dose over 10 minutes day 1
followed by I.V.: 3000 mg/m^2 continuous infusion over 46 hours beginning day 1
[total dose/cycle = 3400 mg/m^2]
Repeat cycle every 2 weeks until disease progression or unacceptable toxicity for at least 6 cycles
Variation 3:
Oxaliplatin: I.V.: 85 mg/m^2/dose over 2 hours day 1
[total dose/cycle = 85 mg/m^2]
Leucovorin: I.V.: 500 mg/m^2/dose over 2 hours day 1
[total dose/cycle = 500 mg/m^2]
Fluorouracil: I.V.: 2600 mg/m^2/dose continuous infusion over 24 hours day 1
[total dose/cycle = 2600 mg/m^2]
Repeat cycle every 2 weeks until disease progression or unacceptable toxicity

Fluorouracil-Mitomycin (Anal Cancer)

Use Anal cancer
Regimen NOTE: Multiple variations are listed below.
Variation 1 (in combination with radiotherapy):
Fluorouracil: I.V.: 1000 mg/m^2/day continuous infusion days 1 to 4 and days 29 to 32
[total dose/cycle = 8000 mg/m^2]
Mitomycin: I.V.: 10 mg/m^2/day (maximum dose: 20 mg) days 1 and 29
[total dose/cycle = 20 mg/m^2; maximum: 40 mg]
Variation 2 (in combination with radiotherapy):
Fluorouracil: I.V.: 1000 mg/m^2/day continuous infusion days 1 to 4
[total dose/cycle = 4000 mg/m^2]

Mitomycin: I.V.: 10 mg/m^2/dose (maximum dose: 20 mg) day 1
  [total dose/cycle = 10 mg/m^2; maximum: 20 mg]
  Repeat cycle in 28 days (total of 2 cycles)

FOLFIRI (Colorectal Cancer)

Use Colorectal cancer

Regimen NOTE: Multiple variations are listed below.
 Variation 1:
 Cycles 1 and 2:
  Irinotecan: I.V.: 180 mg/m^2 over 90 minutes day 1
   [total dose/cycle = 180 mg/m^2]
  Leucovorin: I.V.: 400 mg/m^2 over 2 hours day 1
   [total dose/cycle = 400 mg/m^2]
  Fluorouracil: I.V. bolus: 400 mg/m^2 day 1
   followed by I.V.: 2400 mg/m^2 continuous infusion (over 46 hours) beginning day 1
    [total fluorouracil dose/cycle = 2800 mg/m^2]
  Repeat cycle in 14 days
 Subsequent cycles:
  Irinotecan: I.V.: 180 mg/m^2 over 90 minutes day 1
   [total dose/cycle = 180 mg/m^2]
  Leucovorin: I.V.: 400 mg/m^2 over 2 hours day 1
   [total dose/cycle = 400 mg/m^2]
  Fluorouracil: I.V. bolus: 400 mg/m^2 day 1
   followed by I.V.: 3000 mg/m^2 continuous infusion (over 46 hours) beginning day 1
    [total fluorouracil dose/cycle = 3400 mg/m^2]
  Repeat cycle every 14 days until disease progression or unacceptable toxicity
 Variation 2:
  Irinotecan: I.V.: 180 mg/m^2 over 90 minutes day 1
   [total dose/cycle = 180 mg/m^2]
  Leucovorin: I.V.: 200 mg/m^2/day over 2 hours days 1 and 2
   [total dose/cycle = 400 mg/m^2]
  Fluorouracil: I.V. bolus: 400 mg/m^2/day days 1 and 2
   followed by I.V.: 600 mg/m^2/day continuous infusion (over 22 hours each day) on days 1 and 2
    [total fluorouracil dose/cycle = 2000 mg/m^2]
  Repeat cycle every 14 days until disease progression or unacceptable toxicity
 Variation 3:
  Irinotecan: I.V.: 180 mg/m^2 over 1 hour day 1
   [total dose/cycle = 180 mg/m^2]
  Leucovorin: I.V.: 100 mg/m^2/day over 2 hours days 1 and 2
   [total dose/cycle = 200 mg/m^2]
  Fluorouracil: I.V. bolus: 400 mg/m^2/day days 1 and 2
   followed by I.V.: 600 mg/m^2/day continuous infusion (over 22 hours each day) on days 1 and 2
    [total fluorouracil dose/cycle = 2000 mg/m^2]
  Repeat cycle every 14 days for up to 12 cycles or until disease progression or unacceptable toxicity
 Variation 4:
  Irinotecan: I.V.: 180 mg/m^2 over 90 minutes day 1
   [total dose/cycle = 180 mg/m^2]
  Leucovorin: I.V.: 400 mg/m^2 over 2 hours day 1
   [total dose/cycle = 400 mg/m^2]
  Fluorouracil: I.V. bolus: 400 mg/m^2 day 1
   followed by I.V.: 2400 mg/m^2 continuous infusion (over 46 hours) beginning day 1
    [total fluorouracil dose/cycle = 2800 mg/m^2]
  Repeat cycle every 14 days until disease progression or unacceptable toxicity

FOLFIRINOX (Pancreatic Cancer)

Use Pancreatic cancer

Regimen
 Oxaliplatin: I.V.: 85 mg/m^2/dose over 2 hours day 1
  [total dose/cycle = 85 mg/m^2]
 Irinotecan: I.V.: 180 mg/m^2/dose over 90 minutes day 1
  [total dose/cycle = 180 mg/m^2]

Leucovorin: I.V.: 400 mg/m^2/dose over 2 hours day 1
  [total dose/cycle = 400 mg/m^2]
Fluorouracil: I.V. bolus: 400 mg/m^2/dose day 1
  followed by I.V.: 2400 mg/m^2 continuous infusion over 46 hours beginning day 1
  [total dose/cycle = 2800 mg/m^2]
  Note: Bolus fluorouracil and continuous infusion are both given on day 1.
  Repeat cycle every 14 days for 12 cycles or until disease progression or unacceptable toxicity

FOLFOX 1

Use Colorectal cancer
Regimen
Oxaliplatin: I.V.: 130 mg/m^2 day 1 (every other cycle)
  [total dose/cycle = 130 mg/m^2]
Leucovorin: I.V.: 500 mg/m^2/day days 1 and 2
  [total dose/cycle = 1000 mg/m^2]
Fluorouracil: I.V.: 1.5-2 g/m^2/day continuous infusion days 1 and 2
  [total dose/cycle = 3-4 g/m^2]
Repeat cycle every 14 days

FOLFOX 2

Use Colorectal cancer
Regimen
Oxaliplatin: I.V.: 100 mg/m^2 day 1
  [total dose/cycle = 100 mg/m^2]
Leucovorin: I.V.: 500 mg/m^2/day days 1 and 2
  [total dose/cycle = 1000 mg/m^2]
Fluorouracil: I.V.: 1.5-2 g/m^2/day continuous infusion days 1 and 2
  [total dose/cycle = 3-4 g/m^2]
Repeat cycle every 14 days

FOLFOX 3

Use Colorectal cancer
Regimen
Oxaliplatin: I.V.: 85 mg/m^2 day 1
  [total dose/cycle = 85 mg/m^2]
Leucovorin: I.V.: 500 mg/m^2/day days 1 and 2
  [total dose/cycle = 1000 mg/m^2]
Fluorouracil: I.V.: 1.5-2 g/m^2/day continuous infusion days 1 and 2
  [total dose/cycle = 3-4 g/m^2]
Repeat cycle every 14 days

FOLFOX 4

Use Colorectal cancer
Regimen
Oxaliplatin: I.V.: 85 mg/m^2 day 1
  [total dose/cycle = 85 mg/m^2]
Leucovorin: I.V.: 200 mg/m^2/day days 1 and 2
  [total dose/cycle = 400 mg/m^2]
Fluorouracil: I.V. bolus: 400 mg/m^2/day days 1 and 2
  [total dose/cycle = 800 mg/m^2]
  followed by I.V.: 600 mg/m^2 continuous infusion (over 22 hours) days 1 and 2
  [total dose/cycle = 1200 mg/m^2]
  Note: Bolus fluorouracil and continuous infusion are both given on each day.
  Repeat cycle every 14 days

FOLFOX 6

Use Colorectal cancer
Regimen
Oxaliplatin: I.V.: 100 mg/m^2 day 1
  [total dose/cycle = 100 mg/m^2]

Leucovorin: I.V.: 400 mg/m^2 day 1
[total dose/cycle = 400 mg/m^2]
Fluorouracil: I.V. bolus: 400 mg/m^2 day 1
[total dose/cycle = 400 mg/m^2]
   followed by I.V.: 2.4-3 g/m^2 continuous infusion (46 hours) extending over days 1 and 2
   [total dose/cycle = 2.4-3 g/m^2]
Repeat cycle every 14 days

FOLFOX 7

Use Colorectal cancer
Regimen
Oxaliplatin: I.V.: 130 mg/m^2 day 1
[total dose/cycle = 130 mg/m^2]
Leucovorin: I.V.: 400 mg/m^2 day 1
[total dose/cycle = 400 mg/m^2]
Fluorouracil: I.V. bolus: 400 mg/m^2 day 1
[total dose/cycle = 400 mg/m^2]
   followed by I.V.: 2.4 g/m^2 continuous infusion (46 hours) extending over days 1 and 2
   [total dose/cycle = 2.4 g/m^2]
Repeat cycle every 14 days

FOLFOXIRI (Colorectal)

Use Colorectal cancer
Regimen
Irinotecan: I.V.: 165 mg/m^2 over 1 hour day 1
[total dose/cycle = 165 mg/m^2]
Oxaliplatin: I.V.: 85 mg/m^2 over 2 hours day 1
[total dose/cycle = 85 mg/m^2]
Leucovorin: I.V.: 200 mg/m^2 over 2 hours day 1
[total dose/cycle = 200 mg/m^2]
Fluorouracil: I.V.: 3200 mg/m^2 continuous infusion over 48 hours beginning day 1
[total dose/cycle = 3200 mg/m^2]
Repeat cycle every 14 days for a maximum of 12 cycles

FU-LV-CPT-11

Use Colorectal cancer
Regimen NOTE: Multiple variations are listed below.
Variation 1:
Irinotecan: I.V.: 350 mg/m^2 day 1
[total dose/cycle = 350 mg/m^2]
Leucovorin: I.V.: 20 mg/m^2/day days 22 to 26
[total dose/cycle = 100 mg/m^2]
Fluorouracil: I.V.: 425 mg/m^2/day days 22 to 26
[total dose/cycle = 2125 mg/m^2]
Repeat cycle every 6 weeks
Variation 2:
Irinotecan: I.V.: 80 mg/m^2 day 1
[total dose/cycle = 80 mg/m^2]
Fluorouracil: I.V.: 2300 mg/m^2 continuous infusion day 1
[total dose/cycle = 2300 mg/m^2]
Leucovorin: I.V.: 500 mg/m^2 day 1
[total dose/cycle = 500 mg/m^2]
Repeat cycle weekly
or
Irinotecan: I.V.: 180 mg/m^2 day 1
[total dose/cycle = 180 mg/m^2]
Leucovorin: I.V.: 200 mg/m^2/day days 1 and 2
[total dose/cycle = 400 mg/m^2]

Fluorouracil: I.V.: 400 mg/m^2/day days 1 and 2
  [total dose/cycle = 800 mg/m^2]
  followed by I.V.: 600 mg/m^2/day continuous infusion days 1 and 2
    [total dose/cycle = 1200 mg/m^2]
Repeat cycle every 2 weeks
Variation 3:
Irinotecan: I.V.: 175 mg/m^2 day 1
  [total dose/cycle = 175 mg/m^2]
Leucovorin: I.V.: 250 mg/m^2 day 2
  [total dose/cycle = 250 mg/m^2]
Fluorouracil: I.V.: 950 mg/m^2 day 2
  [total dose/cycle = 950 mg/m^2]
or
Irinotecan: I.V.: 200 mg/m^2 day 1
  [total dose/cycle = 200 mg/m^2]
Leucovorin: I.V.: 250 mg/m^2 day 2
  [total dose/cycle = 250 mg/m^2]
Fluorouracil: I.V.: 850 mg/m^2 day 2
  [total dose/cycle = 850 mg/m^2]
Repeat cycle every other week

FZ

Use Prostate cancer
Regimen NOTE: Multiple variations are listed below.
Variation 1:
Flutamide: Oral: 250 mg every 8 hours
  [total dose/cycle = 21,000 mg]
Goserelin acetate: SubQ: 3.6 mg day 1
  [total dose/cycle = 3.6 mg]
Repeat cycle every 28 days
Variation 2:
Flutamide: Oral: 250 mg every 8 hours
  [total dose/cycle = 67,500 mg]
Goserelin acetate: SubQ: 10.8 mg day 1
  [total dose/cycle = 10.8 mg]
Repeat cycle every 3 months

Gemcitabine-Capecitabine (Biliary Cancer)

Use Biliary adenocarcinoma
Regimen
Gemcitabine: I.V.: 1000 mg/m^2/day over 30 minutes days 1 and 8
  [total dose/cycle = 2000 mg/m^2]
Capecitabine: Oral: 650 mg/m^2 twice daily days 1 to 14
  [total dose/cycle = 18,200 mg/m^2]
Repeat cycle every 21 days until disease progression or unacceptable toxicity

Gemcitabine-Capecitabine (Pancreatic Cancer)

Use Pancreatic cancer
Regimen NOTE: Multiple variations are listed below.
Variation 1:
Gemcitabine: I.V.: 1000 mg/m^2/day over 30 minutes days 1 and 8
  [total dose/cycle = 2000 mg/m^2]
Capecitabine: Oral: 650 mg/m^2/dose twice daily days 1 to 14
  [total dose/cycle = 18,200 mg/m^2]
Repeat cycle every 21 days until disease progression (maximum duration: 24 weeks)
Variation 2:
Gemcitabine: I.V.: 1000 mg/m^2/day over 30 minutes days 1, 8, and 15
  [total dose/cycle = 3000 mg/m^2]
Capecitabine: Oral: 830 mg/m^2/dose twice daily days 1 to 21
  [total dose/cycle = 34,860 mg/m^2]
Repeat cycle every 28 days until disease progression or unacceptable toxicity

Gemcitabine-Capecitabine (RCC)

Use Renal cell cancer

Regimen NOTE: Multiple variations are listed.

Variation 1:

Gemcitabine: I.V.: 1000 mg/m^2/day days 1, 8, and 15

[total dose/cycle = 3000 mg/m^2]

Capecitabine: Oral: 830 mg/m^2/dose twice daily on days 1 to 21

[total dose/cycle = 34,860 mg/m^2]

Repeat cycle every 28 days

Variation 2 (for patients with Cl$_{cr}$ 30-50 mL/minute):

Gemcitabine: I.V.: 1000 mg/m^2/day days 1, 8, and 15

[total dose/cycle = 3000 mg/m^2]

Capecitabine: Oral: 622 mg/m^2/dose twice daily on days 1 to 21

[total dose/cycle = 26,124 mg/m^2]

Repeat cycle every 28 days

Variation 3:

Gemcitabine: I.V.: 1200 mg/m^2/day days 1 and 8

[total dose/cycle = 2400 mg/m^2]

Capecitabine: Oral: 1300 mg/m^2/dose twice daily on days 1 to 14

[total dose/cycle = 36,400 mg/m^2]

Repeat cycle every 21 days for up to 6 cycles

Gemcitabine-Carboplatin (Bladder Cancer)

Use Bladder cancer

Regimen

Gemcitabine: I.V.: 1000 mg/m^2/day days 1 and 8

[total dose/cycle = 2000 mg/m^2]

Carboplatin: I.V.: AUC 5 day 1

[total dose/cycle = AUC = 5]

Repeat cycle every 21 days for up to 6 cycles

Gemcitabine-Carboplatin (NSCLC)

Use Lung cancer, nonsmall cell

Regimen NOTE: Multiple variations are listed.

Variation 1:

Gemcitabine: I.V.: 1000 mg/m^2/dose days 1, 8, and 15

[total dose/cycle = 3000 mg/m^2]

Carboplatin: I.V.: AUC 5 day 1

[total dose/cycle = AUC = 5]

Repeat cycle every 28 days for up to 4 cycles

Variation 2:

Gemcitabine: I.V.: 1000 or 1100 mg/m^2/day days 1 and 8

[total dose/cycle = 2000 or 2200 mg/m^2]

Carboplatin: I.V.: AUC 5 day 8

[total dose/cycle = AUC = 5]

Repeat cycle every 28 days

Gemcitabine-Carboplatin (Ovarian Cancer)

Use Ovarian cancer

Regimen

Gemcitabine: I.V.: 1000 mg/m^2/day days 1 and 8

[total dose/cycle = 2000 mg/m^2]

Carboplatin: I.V.: AUC 4 day 1

[total dose/cycle = AUC = 4]

Repeat cycle every 21 days for 6-10 cycles

Gemcitabine-Cisplatin (Biliary Cancer)

Use Biliary adenocarcinoma

Regimen NOTE: Multiple variations are listed.

Variation 1:
Gemcitabine: I.V.: 1250 mg/m^2/dose days 1 and 8
[total dose/cycle = 2500 mg/m^2]
Cisplatin: I.V.: 75 mg/m^2/dose day 1
[total dose/cycle = 75 mg/m^2]
Repeat cycle every 3 weeks
Variation 2:
Gemcitabine: I.V.: 1000 mg/m^2/dose days 1 and 8
[total dose/cycle = 2000 mg/m^2]
Cisplatin: I.V.: 70 mg/m^2/dose day 1
[total dose/cycle = 70 mg/m^2]
Repeat cycle every 3 weeks (maximum: 6 cycles)

Gemcitabine-Cisplatin (Bladder Cancer)

Use Bladder cancer
Regimen
Gemcitabine: I.V.: 1000 mg/m^2/day days 1, 8, and 15
[total dose/cycle = 3000 mg/m^2]
Cisplatin: I.V.: 70 mg/m^2 day 2
[total dose/cycle = 70 mg/m^2]
Repeat cycle every 28 days for 6 cycles

Gemcitabine-Cisplatin (Mesothelioma)

Use Malignant pleural mesothelioma
Regimen NOTE: Multiple variations are listed.
Variation 1:
Cisplatin: I.V.: 100 mg/m^2 infused over 1 hour day 1
[total dose/cycle = 100 mg/m^2]
Gemcitabine: I.V.: 1000 mg/m^2/dose over 30 minutes days 1, 8, and 15
[total dose/cycle = 3000 mg/m^2]
Repeat cycle every 28 days for up to a total of 6 cycles
Variation 2:
Gemcitabine: I.V.: 1250 mg/m^2/dose over 30 minutes days 1 and 8
[total dose/cycle = 2500 mg/m^2]
Cisplatin: I.V.: 80 mg/m^2 infused over 3 hours day 1
[total dose/cycle = 80 mg/m^2]
Repeat cycle every 21 days for up to a total of 6 cycles

Gemcitabine-Cisplatin (NSCLC)

Use Lung cancer, nonsmall cell
Regimen NOTE: Multiple variations are listed.
Variation 1:
Gemcitabine: I.V.: 1000 mg/m^2/day days 1, 8, and 15
[total dose/cycle = 3000 mg/m^2]
Cisplatin: I.V.: 100 mg/m^2 day 1
[total dose/cycle = 100 mg/m^2]
Repeat cycle every 28 days
Variation 2:
Gemcitabine: I.V.: 1250 mg/m^2/day days 1 and 8
[total dose/cycle = 2500 mg/m^2]
Cisplatin: I.V.: 100 mg/m^2 day 1
[total dose/cycle = 100 mg/m^2]
Repeat cycle every 21 days
Variation 3:
Gemcitabine: I.V.: 1000 mg/m^2/day days 1 and 8
[total dose/cycle = 2000 mg/m^2]
Cisplatin: I.V.: 80 mg/m^2 day 1
[total dose/cycle = 80 mg/m^2]
Repeat cycle every 21 days

Variation 4:
  Gemcitabine: I.V.: 1250 mg/m^2/day days 1 and 8
    [total dose/cycle = 2500 mg/m^2]
  Cisplatin: I.V.: 75 mg/m^2 day 1
    [total dose/cycle = 75 mg/m^2]
  Repeat cycle every 21 days for up to 6 cycles
Variation 5:
  Gemcitabine: I.V.: 1000 mg/m^2/day days 1, 8, and 15
    [total dose/cycle = 3000 mg/m^2]
  Cisplatin: I.V.: 100 mg/m^2 day 15
    [total dose/cycle = 100 mg/m^2]
  Repeat cycle every 28 days
Variation 6:
  Gemcitabine: I.V.: 1000 mg/m^2/day days 1, 8, and 15
    [total dose/cycle = 3000 mg/m^2]
  Cisplatin: I.V.: 100 mg/m^2 day 2
    [total dose/cycle = 100 mg/m^2]
  Repeat cycle every 28 days for 5 cycles
Variation 7:
  Gemcitabine: I.V.: 1200 mg/m^2/day days 1, 8, and 15
    [total dose/cycle = 3600 mg/m^2]
  Cisplatin: I.V.: 100 mg/m^2 day 15
    [total dose/cycle = 100 mg/m^2]
  Repeat cycle every 28 days for up to 6 cycles
Variation 8 (patients ≥70 years of age):
  Gemcitabine: I.V.: 1000 mg/m^2/day days 1 and 8
    [total dose/cycle = 2000 mg/m^2]
  Cisplatin: I.V.: 60 mg/m^2 day 1
    [total dose/cycle = 60 mg/m^2]
  Repeat cycle every 21 days for up to 6 cycles

Gemcitabine-Cisplatin (Pancreatic Cancer)

Use Pancreatic cancer
Regimen
  Cisplatin: I.V.: 50 mg/m^2 infused over 1 hour days 1 and 15
    [total dose/cycle = 100 mg/m^2]
  Gemcitabine: I.V.: 1000 mg/m^2/dose over 30 minutes days 1 and 15
    [total dose/cycle = 2000 mg/m^2]
  Repeat cycle every 28 days

Gemcitabine-Cisplatin (Unknown Primary)

Use Unknown primary (adenocarcinoma)
Regimen
  Gemcitabine: I.V.: 1250 mg/m^2/day days 1 and 8
    [total dose/cycle = 2500 mg/m^2]
  Cisplatin: I.V.: 100 mg/m^2 infused over 1 hour day 1
    [total dose/cycle = 100 mg/m^2]
  Repeat cycle every 21 days

Gemcitabine-Docetaxel (Sarcoma)

Use Osteosarcoma; Soft tissue sarcoma
Regimen
  Gemcitabine: I.V.: 675 mg/m^2/day days 1 and 8
    [total dose/cycle = 1350 mg/m^2]
  Docetaxel: I.V.: 100 mg/m^2 day 8
    [total dose/cycle = 100 mg/m^2]
  Repeat cycle every 21 days

Gemcitabine-Docetaxel (Unknown Primary)

Use Unknown primary (adenocarcinoma)

Regimen
Gemcitabine: I.V.: 1000 mg/m^2/day days 1 and 8
[total dose/cycle = 2000 mg/m^2]
Docetaxel: I.V.: 75 mg/m^2 infused over 1 hour day 8
[total dose/cycle = 75 mg/m^2]
Repeat cycle every 21 days for up to a total of 6 cycles

Gemcitabine-Erlotinib (Pancreatic Cancer)

Use Pancreatic cancer
Regimen
Cycle 1:
Gemcitabine: I.V.: 1000 mg/m^2/day days 1, 8, 15, 22, 29, 36, and 43 (cycle 1 only)
[total dose/cycle 1 = 7000 mg/m^2]
Erlotinib: Oral: 100 mg once daily days 1 to 56
[total dose/cycle 1 = 5600 mg]
Treatment cycle is 56 days
Subsequent cycles:
Gemcitabine: I.V.: 1000 mg/m^2/day days 1, 8, and 15
[total dose/cycle = 3000 mg/m^2]
Erlotinib: Oral: 100 mg once daily days 1 to 28
[total dose/cycle = 2800 mg]
Repeat cycle every 28 days

Gemcitabine-Fluorouracil (RCC)

Use Renal cell cancer
Regimen
Gemcitabine: I.V.: 600 mg/m^2/day days 1, 8, and 15
[total dose/cycle = 1800 mg/m^2]
Fluorouracil: I.V.: 150 mg/m^2/day continuous infusion days 1 to 21
[total dose/cycle = 3150 mg/m^2]
Repeat cycle every 28 days for at least 2 cycles

Gemcitabine-Oxaliplatin (Pancreatic Cancer)

Use Pancreatic cancer
Regimen
Gemcitabine: I.V.: 1000 mg/m^2/day (infused at 10 mg/m^2/minute) day 1
[total dose/cycle = 1000 mg/m^2]
Oxaliplatin: I.V.: 100 mg/m^2/day (over 2 hours) day 2
[total dose/cycle = 100 mg/m^2]
Repeat cycle every 14 days

Gemcitabine-Oxaliplatin-Rituximab (NHL)

Use Lymphoma, non-Hodgkin
Regimen
Oxaliplatin: I.V.: 100 mg/m^2/dose day 1
[total dose/cycle = 100 mg/m^2]
Gemcitabine: I.V.: 1000 mg/m^2/dose day 1
[total dose/cycle = 1000 mg/m^2]
Rituximab: I.V.: 375 mg/m^2/dose day 1
[total dose/cycle = 375 mg/m^2]
Repeat cycle every 3 weeks (for a total of 6-8 cycles)

Gemcitabine-Paclitaxel (Breast Cancer)

Use Breast cancer
Regimen
Paclitaxel: I.V.: 175 mg/m^2 (infused over 3 hours) day 1
[total dose/cycle = 175 mg/m^2]
Gemcitabine: I.V.: 1250 mg/m^2/day days 1 and 8
[total dose/cycle = 2500 mg/m^2]
Repeat cycle every 21 days until disease progression or unacceptable toxicity

Gemcitabine-Paclitaxel (Ovarian Cancer)

Use Ovarian cancer

Regimen
Paclitaxel: I.V.: 110 mg/m^2/dose over 1 hour days 1, 8, and 15
[total dose/cycle = 330 mg/m^2]
Gemcitabine: I.V.: 1000 mg/m^2/dose days 1, 8, and 15
[total dose/cycle = 3000 mg/m^2]
Repeat cycle every 4 weeks for a maximum of 6 cycles

Gemcitabine-Vinorelbine (NSCLC)

Use Lung cancer, nonsmall cell

Regimen NOTE: Multiple variations are listed.
Variation 1:
Gemcitabine: I.V.: 1200 mg/m^2/day days 1 and 8
[total dose/cycle = 2400 mg/m^2]
Vinorelbine: I.V.: 30 mg/m^2/day days 1 and 8
[total dose/cycle = 60 mg/m^2]
Repeat cycle every 21 days for 6 cycles
Variation 2:
Gemcitabine: I.V.: 1000 mg/m^2/day days 1, 8, and 15
[total dose/cycle = 3000 mg/m^2]
Vinorelbine: I.V.: 20 mg/m^2/day days 1, 8, and 15
[total dose/cycle = 60 mg/m^2]
Repeat cycle every 28 days for a maximum of 6 cycles
Variation 3:
Gemcitabine: I.V.: 800 mg/m^2/day days 1, 8, and 15
[total dose/cycle = 2400 mg/m^2]
Vinorelbine: I.V.: 20 mg/m^2/day days 1, 8, and 15
[total dose/cycle = 60 mg/m^2]
Repeat cycle every 28 days for up to 6 cycles

Gemcitabine-Vinorelbine (Sarcoma)

Use Soft tissue sarcoma

Regimen NOTE: Multiple variations are listed.
Variation 1:
Vinorelbine: I.V.: 25 mg/m^2/dose over 10 minutes days 1 and 8
[total dose/cycle = 50 mg/m^2]
Gemcitabine: I.V.: 800 mg/m^2/dose over 90 minutes days 1 and 8
[total dose/cycle = 1600 mg/m^2]
Repeat cycle every 21 days until disease progression or unacceptable toxicity
Variation 2 (modification for toxicity):
Vinorelbine: I.V.: 25 mg/m^2/dose over 10 minutes days 1 and 15
[total dose/cycle = 50 mg/m^2]
Gemcitabine: I.V.: 800 mg/m^2/dose over 90 minutes days 1 and 15
[total dose/cycle = 1600 mg/m^2]
Repeat cycle every 28 days until disease progression or unacceptable toxicity

GEMOX (Biliary Cancer)

Use Biliary adenocarcinoma

Regimen
Gemcitabine: I.V.: 1000 mg/m^2 day 1
[total dose/cycle = 1000 mg/m^2]
Oxaliplatin: I.V.: 100 mg/m^2 day 2
[total dose/cycle = 100 mg/m^2]
Repeat cycle every 2 weeks

GEMOX (Testicular Cancer)

Use Testicular cancer

Regimen NOTE: Multiple variations are listed.

◄ Variation 1:
  Gemcitabine: I.V.: 1000 mg/m^2/dose over 30 minutes days 1 and 8
    [total dose/cycle = 2000 mg/m^2]
  Oxaliplatin: I.V.: 130 mg/m^2/dose over 2 hours day 1
    [total dose/cycle = 130 mg/m^2]
  Repeat cycle every 21 days for a total of at least 2 cycles (maximum: 6 cycles)
Variation 2:
  Gemcitabine: I.V.: 1250 mg/m^2/dose over 30 minutes days 1 and 8
    [total dose/cycle = 2500 mg/m^2]
  Oxaliplatin: I.V.: 130 mg/m^2/dose over 2 hours day 1
    [total dose/cycle = 130 mg/m^2]
  Repeat cycle every 21 days

Gemcitabine-Vinorelbine-Doxorubicin (Liposomal)

Use Lymphoma, Hodgkin disease

Regimen NOTE: Multiple variations are listed.
 Variation 1 (for transplant-naive patients):
  Vinorelbine: I.V.: 20 mg/m^2/day over 6-10 minutes days 1 and 8
    [total dose/cycle = 40 mg/m^2]
  Gemcitabine: I.V.: 1000 mg/m^2/day over 30 minutes days 1 and 8
    [total dose/cycle = 2000 mg/m^2]
  Doxorubicin liposomal: I.V.: 15 mg/m^2/day over 30-60 minutes days 1 and 8
    [total dose/cycle = 30 mg/m^2]
  Repeat cycle every 21 days for a total of 2 to 6 cycles
 Variation 2 (for patients with prior transplant):
  Vinorelbine: I.V.: 15 mg/m^2/day over 6-10 minutes days 1 and 8
    [total dose/cycle = 30 mg/m^2]
  Gemcitabine: I.V.: 800 mg/m^2/day over 30 minutes days 1 and 8
    [total dose/cycle = 1600 mg/m^2]
  Doxorubicin liposomal: I.V.: 10 mg/m^2/day over 30-60 minutes days 1 and 8
    [total dose/cycle = 20 mg/m^2]
  Repeat cycle every 21 days for a total of 2 to 6 cycles

HDMTX

Use Osteosarcoma

Regimen
 Methotrexate: I.V.: 12 g/m^2/week for 2-12 weeks
   [total dose/cycle = 24-144 g/m^2]
 Leucovorin calcium rescue: Oral, I.V.: 15 mg/m^2 every 6 hours (beginning 30 hours after the beginning of
  the 4-hour methotrexate infusion) for 10 doses; **serum methotrexate levels must be monitored**
   [total dose/cycle = 150 mg/m^2]

HIPE-IVAD

Use Neuroblastoma

Regimen
 Cisplatin: I.V.: 40 mg/m^2/day days 1 to 5
   [total dose/cycle = 200 mg/m^2]
 Etoposide: I.V.: 100 mg/m^2/day days 1 to 5
   [total dose/cycle = 500 mg/m^2]
 Ifosfamide: I.V.: 3 g/m^2/day days 21 to 23
   [total dose/cycle = 9 g/m^2]
 Mesna: I.V.: 3 g/m^2/day continuous infusion days 21, 22, and 23
   [total dose/cycle = 9 g/m^2]
 Vincristine: I.V.: 1.5 mg/m^2 day 21
   [total dose/cycle = 1.5 mg/m^2]
 Doxorubicin: I.V.: 60 mg/m^2 day 23
   [total dose/cycle = 60 mg/m^2]
 Repeat cycle every 28 days

Hyper-CVAD + Imatinib

Use Leukemia, acute lymphocytic

Regimen
Cycle A: (Cycles 1, 3, 5, and 7)
  Imatinib: Oral: 400 mg/day days 1 to 14
    [total dose/cycle = 5600 mg]
  Cyclophosphamide: I.V.: 300 mg/m^2 every 12 hours, for 6 doses, days 1, 2, and 3
    [total dose/cycle = 1800 mg/m^2]
  Mesna: I.V. 600 mg/m^2/day continuous infusion days 1, 2, and 3
    [total dose/cycle = 1800 mg/m^2]
  Vincristine: I.V.: 2 mg/day days 4 and 11
    [total dose/cycle = 4 mg]
  Doxorubicin: I.V.: 50 mg/m^2/day continuous infusion day 4
    [total dose/cycle = 50 mg/m^2]
  Dexamethasone: Oral, I.V.: 40 mg/day days 1 to 4 and 11 to 14
    [total dose/cycle = 320 mg]
Cycle B: (Cycles 2, 4, 6, and 8)
  Imatinib: Oral: 400 mg/day days 1 to 14
    [total dose/cycle = 5600 mg]
  Methotrexate: I.V.: 1 g/m^2/day continuous infusion day 1
    [total dose/cycle = 1 g/m^2]
  Leucovorin: I.V.: 50 mg then 15 mg every 6 hours, for 8 doses (start 12 hours after the end of the methotrexate infusion)
    [total dose/cycle = 170 mg]
  Cytarabine: I.V.: 3 g/m^2 every 12 hours for 4 doses, days 2 and 3
    [total dose/cycle = 12 g/m^2]
Repeat every 6 weeks in the following sequence: ABABABAB
CNS Prophylaxis
  Methotrexate: I.T.: 12 mg/day day 2
    [total dose/cycle = 12 mg/day]
  or 6 mg into Ommaya day 2
    [total dose/cycle = 6 mg/day]
  Cytarabine: I.T.: 100 mg/day day 7 or 8
    [total dose/cycle = 100 mg/day]
  Repeat cycle every 3 weeks for 3 or 4 cycles
Maintenance (POMP)
  Imatinib: Oral: 600 mg/day
    [total dose/cycle = 18,000 mg]
  Vincristine: I.V.: 2 mg/day day 1
    [total dose/cycle = 2 mg]
  Prednisone: Oral: 200 mg/day days 1 to 5
    [total dose/cycle = 1000 mg/m^2]
  Repeat cycle every month (except months 6 and 13) for 13 months
Intensification
  Imatinib: Oral: 400 mg/day days 1 to 14
    [total dose/cycle = 5600 mg]
  Cyclophosphamide: I.V.: 300 mg/m^2 every 12 hours, for 6 doses, days 1, 2, and 3
    [total dose/cycle = 1800 mg/m^2]
  Mesna: I.V.: 600 mg/m^2/day continuous infusion days 1, 2, and 3
    [total dose/cycle = 1800 mg/m^2]
  Vincristine: I.V.: 2 mg/day days 4 and 11
    [total dose/cycle = 4 mg]
  Doxorubicin: 50 mg/m^2/day continuous infusion day 4
    [total dose/cycle = 50 mg/m^2]
  Dexamethasone: I.V. or Oral: 40 mg/day days 1 to 4 and 11 to 14
    [total dose/cycle = 320 mg]
  Cycle is given in months 6 and 13 during maintenance

Hyper-CVAD (Leukemia, Acute Lymphocytic)
Use Leukemia, acute lymphocytic
Regimen NOTE: Multiple variations are listed.
  Variation 1:
  Cycle A: (Cycles 1, 3, 5, and 7)
    Cyclophosphamide: I.V.: 300 mg/m^2 every 12 hours, for 6 doses, days 1, 2, and 3
      [total dose/cycle = 1800 mg/m^2]

Mesna: I.V.: 1200 mg/m^2/day continuous infusion days 1, 2, and 3
  [total dose/cycle = 3600 mg/m^2]
Vincristine: I.V.: 2 mg/day days 4 and 11
  [total dose/cycle = 4 mg]
Doxorubicin: I.V.: 50 mg/m^2 day 4
  [total dose/cycle = 50 mg/m^2]
Dexamethasone: (route not specified): 40 mg/day days 1 to 4 and 11 to 14
  [total dose/cycle = 320 mg]
Cycle B: (Cycles 2, 4, 6, and 8)
Methotrexate: I.V.: 1 g/m^2 continuous infusion day 1
  [total dose/cycle = 1g/m^2]
Leucovorin: (route not specified): 15 mg every 6 hours, for 8 doses (start 12 hours after end of
  methotrexate infusion)
  [total dose/cycle = 120 mg]
Cytarabine: I.V.: 3 g/m^2 every 12 hours, for 4 doses, days 2 and 3
  [total dose/cycle = 12 g/m^2]
Methylprednisolone: I.V.: 50 mg twice daily, for 6 doses, days 1, 2, and 3
  [total dose/cycle = 300 mg/m^2]
Repeat every 6 weeks in the following sequence: ABABABAB
CNS Prophylaxis
Methotrexate: I.T.: 12 mg/day day 2
  [total dose/cycle = 12 mg]
or 6 mg/day into Ommaya day 2
  [total dose/cycle = 6 mg]
Cytarabine: I.T: 100 mg day 8
  [total dose/cycle = 100 mg]
Repeat cycle every 3 weeks
Maintenance (POMP)
Mercaptopurine: Oral: 50 mg 3 times/day
  [total dose/cycle = 4200-4650 mg]
Vincristine: I.V.: 2 mg day 1
  [total dose/cycle = 2 mg]
Methotrexate: Oral: 20 mg/m^2/day days 1, 8, 15, and 22
  [total dose/cycle = 80 mg/m^2]
Prednisone: Oral: 200 mg/day days 1 to 5
  [total dose/cycle = 1000 mg/m^2]
or
Mercaptopurine: I.V.: 1 g/m^2/day days 1 to 5
  [total dose/cycle = 5 g/m^2]
Vincristine: I.V.: 2 mg day 1
  [total dose/cycle = 2 mg]
Methotrexate: I.V.: 10 mg/m^2/day days 1 to 5
  [total dose/cycle = 50 mg/m^2]
Prednisone: Oral: 200 mg/day days 1 to 5
  [total dose/cycle = 1000 mg/m^2]
Repeat cycles every month for 2 years
Variation 2:
Cycle A: (Cycles 1, 3, 5, and 7)
Cyclophosphamide: I.V.: 300 mg/m^2 every 12 hours, for 6 doses, days 1, 2, and 3
  [total dose/cycle = 1800 mg/m^2]
Mesna: I.V.: 600 mg/m^2/day continuous infusion days 1, 2, and 3
  [total dose/cycle = 1800 mg/m^2]
Vincristine: I.V.: 2 mg/day days 4 and 11
  [total dose/cycle = 4 mg]
Doxorubicin: I.V.: 50 mg/m^2 day 4
  [total dose/cycle = 50 mg/m^2]
Dexamethasone: Oral, I.V.: 40 mg/day days 1 to 4 and 11 to 14
  [total dose/cycle = 320 mg]
Cycle B: (Cycles 2, 4, 6, and 8)
Methotrexate: I.V.: 1 g/m^2 continuous infusion day 1
  [total dose/cycle = 1 g/m^2]

Leucovorin: I.V.: 50 mg (start 12 hours after end of methotrexate infusion)
  followed by I.V.: 15 mg every 6 hours, for 8 doses
    [total dose/cycle = 170 mg]
Cytarabine: I.V.: 3 g/m^2 every 12 hours, for 4 doses, days 2 and 3
  [total dose/cycle = 12 g/m^2]
Repeat every 6 weeks in the following sequence: ABABABAB
CNS Prophylaxis
Methotrexate: I.T.: 12 mg day 2
  [total dose/cycle = 12 mg]
  or 6 mg into Ommaya day 2
  [total dose/cycle = 6 mg]
Cytarabine: I.T.: 100 mg day 7
  [total dose/cycle = 100 mg]
Repeat cycle every 3 weeks
Variation 3:
 Cycle A: (Cycles 1, 3, 5, and 7)
  Cyclophosphamide: I.V.: 300 mg/m^2 every 12 hours, for 6 doses, days 1, 2, and 3
    [total dose/cycle = 1800 mg/m^2]
  Mesna: I.V.: 600 mg/m^2/day continuous infusion days 1, 2, and 3
    [total dose/cycle = 1800 mg/m^2]
  Vincristine: I.V.: 2 mg/day days 4 and 11
    [total dose/cycle = 4 mg]
  Doxorubicin: I.V.: 50 mg/m^2 continuous infusion day 4
    [total dose/cycle = 50 mg/m^2]
  Dexamethasone: Oral, I.V.: 40 mg/day days 1 to 4 and 11 to 14
    [total dose/cycle = 320 mg]
 Cycle B: (Cycles 2, 4, 6, and 8)
  Methotrexate: I.V.: 200 mg/m^2 day 1
    followed by I.V.: 800 mg/m^2 continuous infusion day 1
    [total dose/cycle = 1 g/m^2]
  Leucovorin: I.V.: 50 mg (start 12 hours after end of methotrexate infusion)
    followed by I.V.: 15 mg every 6 hours, for 8 doses
    [total dose/cycle = 170 mg]
  Cytarabine: I.V.: 3 g/m^2 every 12 hours, for 4 doses, days 2 and 3
    [total dose/cycle = 12 g/m^2]
  Repeat every 6 weeks in the following sequence: ABABABAB
CNS Prophylaxis
Methotrexate: I.T.: 12 mg day 2
  [total dose/cycle = 12 mg]
  or 6 mg into Ommaya day 2
  [total dose/cycle = 6 mg]
Cytarabine: I.T.: 100 mg day 7 **or** 8
  [total dose/cycle = 100 mg]
Repeat cycles every 3 weeks for 6 or 8 cycles
Maintenance (POMP)
Mercaptopurine: Oral: 50 mg 3 times/day
  [total dose/cycle = 4200-4650 mg]
Vincristine: I.V.: 2 mg day 1
  [total dose/cycle = 2 mg]
Methotrexate: Oral, I V: 20 mg/m^2/ day days 1, 8, 15, and 22
  [total dose/cycle = 80 mg/m^2]
Prednisone: Oral: 200 mg/day days 1 to 5
  [total dose/cycle = 1000 mg/m^2]
or
Mercaptopurine: I.V.: 1 g/m^2/day days 1 to 5
  [total dose/cycle = 5 g/m^2]
Vincristine: I.V.: 2 mg day 1
  [total dose/cycle = 2 mg]
Methotrexate: I.V.: 10 mg/m^2/day days 1 to 5
  [total dose/cycle = 50 mg/m^2]
Prednisone: Oral: 200 mg/day days 1 to 5
  [total dose/cycle = 1000 mg]
Repeat cycles every month (except months 7 and 11 or 9 and 12) for 2 years

Intensification

Etoposide: I.V.: 100 mg/m^2/day days 1 to 5
[total dose/cycle = 500 mg/m^2]
Pegaspargase: I.V.: 2500 units/m^2 day 1
[total dose/cycle = 2500 units/m^2]
Given during months 9 and 12 of maintenance
or
Methotrexate: I.V.: 100 mg/m^2/day days 1, 8, 15, and 22
[total dose/cycle = 400 mg/m^2]
Asparaginase: I.V.: 20,000 units/day days 2, 9, 16, and 23
[total dose/cycle = 80,000 units]
Given during months 7 and 11 of maintenance

Variation 4:

Cycle A: (Cycles 1, 3, 5, and 7)

Cyclophosphamide: I.V.: 300 mg/m^2 every 12 hours, for 6 doses, days 1, 2, and 3
[total dose/cycle = 1800 mg/m^2]
Mesna: I.V.: 600 mg/m^2/day continuous infusion days 1, 2, and 3
[total dose/cycle = 1800 mg/m^2]
Vincristine: I.V.: 2 mg/day days 4 and 11
[total dose/cycle = 4 mg]
Doxorubicin: I.V.: 50 mg/m^{2}day 4
[total dose/cycle = 50 mg/m^2]
Dexamethasone: (route not specified): 40 mg/day days 1 to 4 and 11 to 14
[total dose/cycle = 320 mg]

Cycle B: (Cycles 2, 4, 6, and 8)

Methotrexate: I.V.: 200 mg/m^2 day 1
followed by I.V.: 800 mg/m^2 continuous infusion day 1
[total dose/cycle = 1 g/m^2]
Leucovorin: (route not specified): 15 mg every 6 hours, for 8 doses (start 24 hours after end of methotrexate infusion)
[total dose/cycle = 120 mg]
Cytarabine: I.V.: 3 g/m^2 every 12 hours, for 4 doses, days 2 and 3
[total dose/cycle = 12 g/m^2]
Repeat every 6 weeks in the following sequence: ABABABAB

CNS Prophylaxis

Methotrexate: I.T.: 12 mg day 2
[total dose/cycle = 12 mg]
Cytarabine: I.T.: 100 mg day 8
[total dose/cycle = 100 mg]
Repeat cycle every 3 weeks for 4 or 8 cycles

Maintenance (POMP)

Mercaptopurine: Oral: 50 mg 3 times/day
[total dose/cycle = 4200-4650 mg]
Vincristine: I.V.: 2 mg day 1
[total dose/cycle = 2 mg]
Methotrexate: Oral: 20 mg/m^2/day days 1, 8, 15, and 22
[total dose/cycle = 80 mg/m^2]
Prednisone: Oral: 200 mg/day days 1 to 5
[total dose/cycle = 1000 mg/m^2]
or
Mercaptopurine: I.V.: 1 g/m^2/day days 1 to 5
[total dose/cycle = 5 g/m^2]
Vincristine: I.V.: 2 mg day 1
[total dose/cycle = 2 mg]
Methotrexate: I.V.: 10 mg/m^2/day days 1 to 5
[total dose/cycle = 50 mg/m^2]
Prednisone: Oral: 200 mg/day days 1 to 5
[total dose/cycle = 1000 mg/m^2]
or
Interferon alfa: SubQ: 5 million units/m^2 daily
[total dose/cycle = 140-155 million units/m^2]

Cytarabine: SubQ: 10 mg daily
  [total dose/cycle = 280-310 mg]
Repeat cycles every month for 2 years
Variation 5:
 Cycle A: (Cycles 1, 4, 6, and 8)
  Cyclophosphamide: I.V.: 300 mg/m^2 every 12 hours, for 6 doses, days 1, 2, and 3
   [total dose/cycle = 1800 mg/m^2]
  Mesna: I.V.: 600 mg/m^2/day continuous infusion days 1, 2, and 3
   [total dose/cycle = 1800 mg/m^2]
  Vincristine: I.V.: 2 mg/day days 4 and 11
   [total dose/cycle = 4 mg]
  Doxorubicin: I.V.: 50 mg/m^2 continuous infusion day 4
   [total dose/cycle = 50 mg/m^2]
  Dexamethasone: Oral, I.V.: 40 mg/day days 1 to 4 and 11 to 14
   [total dose/cycle = 320 mg]
 Cycle B: (Cycles 3, 5, 7, and 9)
  Methotrexate: I.V.: 200 mg/m^2 day 1
   followed by I.V.: 800 mg/m^2 continuous infusion day 1
   [total dose/cycle = 1 g/m^2]
  Leucovorin: I.V.: 50 mg (start 12 hours after end of methotrexate infusion)
   followed by I.V.: 15 mg every 6 hours, for 8 doses
   [total dose/cycle = 170 mg]
  Cytarabine: I.V.: 3 g/m^2 every 12 hours, for 4 doses, days 2 and 3
   [total dose/cycle = 12 g/m^2]
 Cycle C: Liposomal Daunorubicin/Cytarabine (Cycle 2):
  Daunorubicin, liposomal: I.V.: 150 mg/m^2/day days 1 and 2
   [total dose/cycle = 300 mg/m^2]
  Cytarabine: I.V.: 1.5 g/m^2/day continuous infusion days 1 and 2
   [total dose/cycle = 3 g/m^2]
  Prednisone: Oral: 200 mg/day days 1 to 5
   [total dose/cycle = 1000 mg]
  Administer in the following sequence: ACBABABA (Cycle C does not repeat)
CNS Prophylaxis
  Methotrexate: I.T.: 12 mg day 2
   [total dose/cycle = 12 mg]
  or 6 mg into Ommaya day 2
   [total dose/cycle = 6 mg]
  Cytarabine: I.T.: 100 mg day 7 **or** 8
   [total dose/cycle = 100 mg]
  Repeat cycle every 3 weeks for 6 or 8 cycles
Maintenance (POMP)
  Mercaptopurine: I.V.: 1 g/m^2/day days 1 to 5
   [total dose/cycle = 5 g/m^2]
  Vincristine: I.V.: 2 mg day 1
   [total dose/cycle = 2 mg]
  Methotrexate: I.V.: 10 mg/m^2/day days 1 to 5
   [total dose/cycle = 50 mg/m^2]
  Prednisone: Oral: 200 mg/day days 1 to 5
   [total dose/cycle = 1000 mg]
  Repeat cycles monthly, except months 6, 7, 18, and 19 for 3 years
Intensification
  Methotrexate: I.V.: 100 mg/m^2/day days 1, 8, 15, and 22
   [total dose/cycle = 400 mg/m^2]
  Asparaginase: I.V.: 20,000 units/day days 2, 9, 16, and 23
   [total dose/cycle = 80,000 units]
  Given during months 6 and 18 of maintenance
  Cyclophosphamide: I.V.: 300 mg/m^2 every 12 hours, for 6 doses, days 1, 2, and 3
   [total dose/cycle = 1800 mg/m^2]
  Mesna: I.V.: 600 mg/m^2/day continuous infusion days 1, 2, and 3
   [total dose/cycle = 1800 mg/m^2]
  Vincristine: I.V.: 2 mg/day days 4 and 11
   [total dose/cycle = 4 mg]

Doxorubicin: I.V.: 50 mg/m^2/day continuous infusion day 4
[total dose/cycle = 50 mg/m^2]
Dexamethasone: Oral, I.V.: 40 mg/day days 1 to 4 and 11 to 14
[total dose/cycle = 320 mg]
Given during months 7 and 19 of maintenance

Hyper-CVAD (Lymphoma, non-Hodgkin)

Use Lymphoma, non-Hodgkin
Regimen
Cycle A: (Cycles 1, 3, 5, and 7)
Cyclophosphamide: I.V.: 300 mg/m^2 every 12 hours, for 6 doses, days 1, 2, and 3
[total dose/cycle = 1800 mg/m^2]
Vincristine: I.V.: 2 mg/day days 4 and 11
[total dose/cycle = 4 mg]
Doxorubicin: I.V.: 25 mg/m^2/day continuous infusion days 4 and 5
[total dose/cycle = 50 mg/m^2]
Dexamethasone: Oral, I.V.: 40 mg/day days 1 to 4 and 11 to 14
[total dose/cycle = 320 mg]
Cycle B: (Cycles 2, 4, 6, and 8)
Methotrexate: I.V.: 200 mg/m^2 day 1
followed by I.V.: 800 mg/m^2 continuous infusion day 1
[total dose/cycle = 1 g/m^2]
Leucovorin: Oral: 50 mg
followed by Oral: 15 mg every 6 hours, for 8 doses (start 24 hours after end of methotrexate infusion)
[total dose/cycle = 170 mg]
Cytarabine: I.V.: 3 g/m^2 every 12 hours, for 4 doses, days 2 and 3
[total dose/cycle = 12 g/m^2]
Repeat every 6 weeks in the following sequence: ABABABAB

Hyper-CVAD (Multiple Myeloma)

Use Multiple myeloma
Regimen
Cyclophosphamide: I.V.: 300 mg/m^2 every 12 hours, for 6 doses, days 1, 2, and 3
[total dose/cycle = 1800 mg/m^2]
Mesna: I.V.: 600 mg/m^2/day continuous infusion days 1, 2, and 3
[total dose/cycle = 1800 mg/m^2]
Doxorubicin: I.V.: 25 mg/m^2/day continuous infusion days 4 and 5
[total dose/cycle = 50 mg/m^2]
Vincristine: I.V.: 1 mg/day continuous infusion days 4 and 5
followed by I.V.: 2 mg day 11
[total dose/cycle = 4 mg]
Dexamethasone: Oral, I.V.: 20 mg/m^2/day days 1 to 5 and 11 to 14
[total dose/cycle = 180 mg/m^2]
Repeat cycle once if ≥50% reduction in myeloma protein
Maintenance
Cyclophosphamide: Oral: 125 mg/m^2 every 12 hours, for 10 doses, days 1 to 5
[total dose/cycle = 1250 mg/m^2]
Dexamethasone: Oral: 20 mg/m^2/day days 1 to 5
[total dose/cycle = 100 mg/m^2]
Repeat maintenance cycle every 5 weeks

Hyper-CVAD + Rituximab

Use Lymphona, non-Hodgkin (mantle cell)
Regimen
Cycle A: (Cycles 1, 3, 5 [and 7, if needed])
Rituximab: I.V.: 375 mg/m^2 day 1
[total dose/cycle = 375 mg/m^2]
Cyclophosphamide: I.V.: 300 mg/m^2 every 12 hours, for 6 doses, days 2, 3, and 4
[total dose/cycle = 1800 mg/m^2]
Mesna: I.V.: 600 mg/m^2 continuous infusion days 2, 3, and 4
[total dose/cycle = 1800 mg/m^2]

Vincristine: I.V.: 1.4 mg/m^2 (maximum dose: 2 mg) days 5 and 12
  [total dose/cycle = 2.8 mg/m^2; maximum: 4 mg]
Doxorubicin: I.V.: 16.7 mg/m^2 continuous infusion days 5, 6, and 7
  [total dose/cycle = 50.1 mg/m^2]
Dexamethasone: Oral, I.V.: 40 mg/day days 2 to 5 and 12 to 15
  [total dose/cycle = 320 mg]
Cycle B: (Cycles 2, 4, 6 [and 8, if needed])
Rituximab: I.V.: 375 mg/m^2 day 1
  [total dose/cycle = 375 mg/m^2]
Methotrexate: I.V.: 200 mg/m^2 day 2
  followed by I.V.: 800 mg/m^2 continuous infusion day 2
  [total dose/cycle = 1000 mg/m^2]
Leucovorin: Oral: 50 mg (start 12 hours after the end of the methotrexate infusion)
  followed by Oral: 15 mg every 6 hours, for 8 doses
  [total dose/cycle = 170 mg]
Cytarabine: I.V.: 3 g/m^2 every 12 hours, for 4 doses, day 3 and 4
  [total dose/cycle = 12 g/m^2]
Repeat every 6 weeks in the following sequence: ABABABAB

ICE (Lymphoma, non-Hodgkin)

Use Lymphoma, non-Hodgkin
Regimen
Etoposide: I.V.: 100 mg/m^2/day days 1, 2, and 3
  [total dose/cycle = 300 mg/m^2]
Carboplatin: I.V.: AUC 5 (maximum dose: 800 mg) day 2
  [total dose/cycle = AUC = 5]
Ifosfamide: I.V.: 5000 mg/m^2 continuous infusion day 2
  [total dose/cycle = 5000 mg/m^2]
Mesna: I.V.: 5000 mg/m^2 continuous infusion day 2
  [total dose/cycle = 5000 mg/m^2]
Filgrastim: SubQ: 5 mcg/kg/day days 5-12 (cycles 1 and 2 only)
  [total dose/cycle = 40 mcg/kg]
  followed by SubQ: 10 mcg/kg/day day 5 through completion of leukaphoresis (cycle 3 only)
Repeat cycle every 2 weeks for 3 cycles

ICE (Sarcoma)

Use Osteosarcoma; Soft tissue sarcoma
Regimen
Ifosfamide: I.V.: 1500 mg/m^2/day days 1, 2, and 3
  [total dose/cycle = 4500 mg/m^2]
Carboplatin: I.V.: 300-635 mg/m^2 day 3
  [total dose/cycle = 300-635 mg/m^2]
Etoposide: I.V.: 100 mg/m^2/day days 1, 2, and 3
  [total dose/cycle = 300 mg/m^2]
Mesna: I.V.: 500 mg/m^2 prior to each ifosfamide, and every 3 hours for 2 more doses/day days 1, 2, and 3
  [total dose/cycle = 4500 mg/m^2]
Repeat cycle every 21-28 days

ICE-T

Use Breast cancer; Soft tissue sarcoma
Regimen
Ifosfamide: I.V.: 1250 mg/m^2/day days 1, 2, and 3
  [total dose/cycle = 3750 mg/m^2]
Carboplatin: I.V.: 300 mg/m^2 day 1
  [total dose/cycle = 300 mg/m^2]
Etoposide: I.V.: 80 mg/m^2/day days 1, 2, and 3
  [total dose/cycle = 240 mg/m^2]
Paclitaxel: I.V.: 175 mg/m^2 day 4
  [total dose/cycle = 175 mg/m^2]

◀ Mesna: I.V.: 250 mg prior to ifosfamide days 1, 2, and 3
   followed by: Oral: 500 mg at 4 and 8 hours after ifosfamide days 1, 2, and 3
   [total dose/cycle = I.V. 750 mg; Oral: 3000 mg]
or
Mesna: I.V.: 1250 mg/m^2/day over 6 hours, days 1, 2, and 3
[total dose/cycle = 3750 mg/m^2]
Repeat cycle every 28 days

IE

Use Soft tissue sarcoma
Regimen
Etoposide: I.V.: 100 mg/m^2/day days 1, 2, and 3
[total dose/cycle = 300 mg/m^2]
Ifosfamide: I.V.: 2500 mg/m^2/day days 1, 2, and 3
[total dose/cycle = 7500 mg/m^2]
Mesna: I.V.: 500 mg/m^2 prior to ifosfamide, after ifosfamide, and every 4 hours for 3 more doses (total of 5 doses/day) days 1, 2, and 3
[total dose/cycle = 7500 mg/m^2]
Repeat cycle every 28 days

IMVP-16

Use Lymphoma, non-Hodgkin
Regimen
Ifosfamide: I.V.: 4 g/m^2 continuous infusion over 24 hours day 1
[total dose/cycle = 4 g/m^2]
Mesna: I.V.: 800 mg/m^2 bolus prior to ifosfamide, then 4 g/m^2 continuous infusion over 12 hours concurrent with ifosfamide, then 2.4 g/m^2 continuous infusion over 12 hours after ifosfamide infusion day 1
[total dose/cycle = 7.2 g/m^2]
Methotrexate: I.V.: 30 mg/m^2/day days 3 and 10
[total dose/cycle = 60 mg/m^2]
Etoposide: I.V.: 100 mg/m^2/day days 1, 2, and 3
[total dose/cycle = 300 mg/m^2]
Repeat cycle every 21-28 days

Interferon Alfa-2b-Cytarabine (CML)

Use Chronic Myeloid Leukemia
Regimen
Interferon Alfa-2b: SubQ: 5 million units/m^2/dose days 1 to 30
[total dose/cycle = 150 million units/m^2]
Hydroxyurea: Oral: 50 mg/kg/day (use lower dose based on WBC counts) until complete hematologic remission
Cytarabine: SubQ: 20 mg/m^2/dose days 15 to 24
[total dose/cycle = 200 mg/m^2]
Repeat cycle every month until complete cytogenic remission or unacceptable toxicity

Interleukin 2-Interferon Alfa-2 (RCC)

Use Renal cell cancer
Regimen
Induction (2 cycles):
Aldesleukin: I.V.: 18 million units/m^2/day continuous infusion days 1 to 5 and days 12 to 16
[total dose/cycle = 180 million units/m^2]
Repeat aldesleukin induction cycle one time (total of 2 cycles) after a 3-week rest between cycles
Interferon Alfa-2: SubQ: 6 million units/dose 3 times weekly continuously (no rest break) during induction cycles
[total dose/week = 18 million units/week]
Maintenance (begin after a 3-week aldesleukin rest):
Aldesleukin: I.V.: 18 million units/m^2/day continuous infusion days 1 to 5
[total dose/cycle = 90 million units/m^2]
Repeat aldesleukin maintenance cycle 3 times (total of 4 maintenance cycles) after 3-week rest between cycles

Interferon Alfa-2: SubQ: 6 million units/dose 3 times weekly continuously (no rest break) during maintenance cycles
[total dose/week = 18 million units/week]

IPA

Use Hepatoblastoma

Regimen
Ifosfamide: I.V.: 500 mg/m^2 day 1
  [total dose/cycle = 500 mg/m^2]
  followed by I.V.: 1000 mg/m^2/day continuous infusion days 1 to 3
    [total dose/cycle = 3000 mg/m^2]
Cisplatin: I.V.: 20 mg/m^2/day days 4 to 8
  [total dose/cycle = 100 mg/m^2]
Doxorubicin: I.V.: 30 mg/m^2/day continuous infusion days 9 and 10
  [total dose/cycle = 60 mg/m^2]
Repeat cycle every 21 days

Irinotecan-Capecitabine (Esophageal Cancer)

Use Esophageal cancer

Regimen NOTE: Multiple variations are listed.
Variation 1:
  Irinotecan: I.V.: 250 mg/m^2/dose day 1
    [total dose/cycle = 250 mg/m^2]
  Capecitabine: Oral: 1000 mg/m^2/dose twice daily days 1 to 14
    [total dose/cycle = 28000 mg/m^2]
  Repeat cycle every 21 days until disease progression or unacceptable toxicity
Variation 2:
  Irinotecan: I.V.: 250 mg/m^2/dose day 1
    [total dose/cycle = 250 mg/m^2]
  Capecitabine: Oral: 1000 mg/m^2/dose twice daily days 1 to 14
    [total dose/cycle = 28000 mg/m^2]
  Repeat cycle every 21 days for up to 24 weeks

Irinotecan-Capecitabine (Gastric Cancer)

Use Gastric cancer

Regimen NOTE: Multiple variations are listed.
Variation 1:
  Irinotecan: I.V.: 250 mg/m^2/dose day 1
    [total dose/cycle = 250 mg/m^2]
  Capecitabine: Oral: 1000 mg/m^2/dose twice daily days 1 to 14
    [total dose/cycle = 28000 mg/m^2]
  Repeat cycle every 21 days until disease progression or unacceptable toxicity
Variation 2:
  Irinotecan: I.V.: 250 mg/m^2/dose day 1
    [total dose/cycle = 250 mg/m^2]
  Capecitabine: Oral: 1000 mg/m^2/dose twice daily days 1 to 14
    [total dose/cycle = 28000 mg/m^2]
  Repeat cycle every 21 days for up to 24 weeks

Irinotecan-Cisplatin (Esophageal Cancer)

Use Esophageal cancer

Regimen NOTE: Multiple variations are listed.
Variation 1:
  Cisplatin: I.V.: 30 mg/m^2/dose days 1, 8, 15, and 22
    [total dose/cycle = 120 mg/m^2]
  Irinotecan: I.V.: 65 mg/m^2/dose days 1, 8, 15, and 22
    [total dose/cycle = 260 mg/m^2]
  Repeat cycle every 6 weeks until disease progression.
Variation 2 (with concurrent radiation therapy):
  Cisplatin: I.V.: 30 mg/m^2/dose on day 1 and 8
    [total dose/cycle = 60 mg/m^2]

◄ Irinotecan: I.V.: 65 mg/m^2/dose day 1 and 8
　　[total dose/cycle = 130 mg/m^2]
　Treatment cycle is 21 days; cycle is not repeated.
　Variation 3:
　Cisplatin: I.V.: 30 mg/m^2/dose on days 1, 8, 22, and 29
　　[total dose/cycle = 120 mg/m^2]
　Irinotecan: I.V.: 50 mg/m^2/dose on days 1, 8, 22, and 29
　　[total dose/cycle = 200 mg/m^2]
　Administered (with concurrent radiation therapy) over one 5-week treatment cycle.
　Followed by: Postoperative therapy:
　Cisplatin: I.V.: 30 mg/m^2/dose on days 1 and 8
　　[total dose/cycle = 60 mg/m^2]
　Irinotecan: I.V.: 65 mg/m^2/dose on days 1 and 8
　　[total dose/cycle = 130 mg/m^2]
　Repeat postop cycle every 21 days for a total of 3 cycles.
　Variation 4:
　Cisplatin: I.V.: 30 mg/m^2/dose on day 1 and 8
　　[total dose/cycle = 60 mg/m^2]
　Irinotecan: I.V.: 65 mg/m^2/dose day 1 and 8
　　[total dose/cycle = 130 mg/m^2]
　Repeat cycle every 21 days.

Irinotecan-Cisplatin (Gastric Cancer)

Use Gastric cancer
Regimen
　Irinotecan: I.V.: 65 mg/m^2/dose over 90 minutes days 1, 8, 15, and 22
　　[total dose/cycle = 260 mg/m^2]
　Cisplatin: I.V.: 30 mg/m^2/dose over 1 hour days 1, 8, 15, and 22
　　[total dose/cycle = 120 mg/m^2]
　Repeat cycle every 6 weeks until disease progression or unacceptable toxicity

Irinotecan-Fluorouracil-Leucovorin (Esophageal Cancer)

Use Esophageal cancer
Regimen NOTE: Multiple variations are listed.
　Variation 1:
　Irinotecan: I.V.: 80 mg/m^2/dose days 1, 8, 15, 22, 29, and 36
　　[total dose/week = 480 mg/m^2]
　Fluorouracil: I.V.: 2000 mg/m^2/dose continuous infusion over 24 hours days 1, 8, 15, 22, 29, and 36
　　[total dose/cycle = 12,000 mg/m^2]
　Leucovorin: I.V.: 500 mg/m^2/dose continuous infusion over 24 hours days 1, 8, 15, 22, 29, and 36
　　[total dose/week = 3000 mg/m^2]
　Repeat cycle every 8 weeks until disease progression or unacceptable toxicity.
　Variation 2:
　Irinotecan: I.V.: 80 mg/m^2/dose day 1
　　[total dose/cycle = 80 mg/m^2]
　Leucovorin: I.V.: 500 mg/m^2/dose over 2 hours day 1
　　[total dose/cycle = 500 mg/m^2]
　Fluorouracil: I.V.: 2000 mg/m^2/dose continuous infusion over 22 hours day 1 (begin immediately after leucovorin)
　　[total dose/cycle = 2000 mg/m^2]
　Repeat every week for 6 weeks followed by a 1-week rest, continue until disease progression or unacceptable toxicity.

Irinotecan-Leucovorin-Fluorouracil (Gastric Cancer)

Use Gastric cancer
Regimen NOTE: Multiple variations are listed.
　Variation 1:
　Irinotecan: I.V.: 80 mg/m^2/dose day 1
　　[total dose/week = 80 mg/m^2]
　Leucovorin: I.V.: 500 mg/m^2/dose over 2 hours day 1
　　[total dose/week = 500 mg/m^2]

Fluorouracil: I.V.: 2000 mg/m^2/dose continuous infusion over 22 hours day 1
  [total dose/week = 2000 mg/m^2]
  Repeat cycle weekly for 6 weeks followed by a 1-week rest; repeat until disease progression or unacceptable toxicity
Variation 2:
  Irinotecan: I.V.: 180 mg/m^2/dose day 1
  [total dose/cycle = 180 mg/m^2]
  Leucovorin: I.V.: 200 mg/m^2/dose over 2 hours days 1 and 2
  [total dose/cycle = 400 mg/m^2]
  Fluorouracil: I.V. bolus: 400 mg/m^2 days 1 and 2
  followed by I.V.: 600 mg/m^2/dose continuous infusion over 22 hours days 1 and 2
    [total dose/cycle = 2000 mg/m^2]
  Repeat cycle every 14 days for at least 4 cycles or until disease progression or unacceptable toxicity

Irinotecan-Temozolomide (Ewing Sarcoma)

Use Ewing sarcoma
Regimen
  Irinotecan: I.V.: 20 mg/m^2/dose days 1 to 5 and days 8 to 12
  [total dose/cycle = 200 mg/m^2]
  Temozolomide: Oral: 100 mg/m^2/dose days 1 to 5
  [total dose/cycle = 500 mg/m^2]
  Repeat cycle every 21 days

Ixabepilone-Capecitabine

Use Breast cancer
Regimen
  Capecitabine: Oral: 1000 mg/m^2 twice daily days 1 to 14
  [total dose/cycle = 28,000 mg/m^2]
  Ixabepilone: I.V.: 40 mg/m^2 day 1
  [total dose/cycle = 40 mg/m^2]
  Repeat cycle every 3 weeks

Lapatinib-Letrozole (Breast Cancer)

Use Breast cancer
Regimen
  Lapatinib: Oral: 1500 mg/day days 1 to 28
  [total dose/cycle = 42,000 mg]
  Letrozole: Oral: 2.5 mg/day days 1 to 28
  [total dose/cycle = 70 mg]
  Repeat cycle every 28 days until disease progression

Lapatinib-Trastuzumab (Breast Cancer)

Use Breast cancer
Regimen
  Week 1:
    Trastuzumab: I.V.: 4 mg/kg (loading dose) day 1
    [total dose/week 1 = 4 mg/kg]
    Lapatinib: Oral: 1000 mg/day days 1 to 7
    [total dose/week = 7000 mg]
  Subsequent weeks:
    Trastuzumab: I.V.: 2 mg/kg day 1
    [total dose/week = 2 mg/kg]
    Lapatinib: Oral: 1000 mg/day days 1 to 7
    [total dose/week = 7000 mg]
  Repeat weekly

Larson Regimen (ALL)

Use Leukemia, acute lymphocytic
Regimen NOTE: Multiple variations are listed.

1037

◀ Variation 1 (CALGB 8811):
Induction, patients <60 years of age (4-week cycle):
Cyclophosphamide: I.V.: 1200 mg/m² day 1
[total dose/cycle = 1200 mg/m²]
Daunorubicin: I.V.: 45 mg/m²/dose days 1, 2, and 3
[total dose/cycle = 135 mg/m²]
Vincristine: I.V.: 2 mg/dose days 1, 8, 15, and 22
[total dose/cycle = 8 mg]
Prednisone: Oral: 60 mg/m²/dose days 1 to 21
[total dose/cycle = 1260 mg/m²]
Asparaginase: SubQ: 6000 units/m²/dose days 5, 8, 11, 15, 18, and 22
[total dose/cycle ≥ 36,000 units/m²]
Induction, patients ≥60 years of age (4-week cycle):
Cyclophosphamide: I.V.: 800 mg/m² day 1
[total dose/cycle = 800 mg/m²]
Daunorubicin: I.V.: 30 mg/m²/dose days 1, 2, and 3
[total dose/cycle = 90 mg/m²]
Vincristine: I.V.: 2 mg/dose days 1, 8, 15, and 22
[total dose/cycle = 8 mg]
Prednisone: Oral: 60 mg/m²/dose days 1 to 7
[total dose/cycle = 420 mg/m²]
Asparaginase: SubQ: 6000 units/m²/dose days 5, 8, 11, 15, 18, and 22
[total dose/cycle = 36,000 units/m²]
Early intensification (4-week cycle; repeat cycle once):
Methotrexate: I.T.: 15 mg/dose day 1
[total dose/cycle = 15 mg]
Cyclophosphamide: I.V.: 1000 mg/m² day 1
[total dose/cycle = 1000 mg/m²]
Mercaptopurine: Oral: 60 mg/m²/dose days 1 to 14
[total dose/cycle = 840 mg/m²]
Cytarabine: SubQ: 75 mg/m²/dose days 1 to 4 and 8 to 11
[total dose/cycle = 600 mg/m²]
Vincristine: I.V.: 2 mg/dose days 15 and 22
[total dose/cycle = 4 mg]
Asparaginase: SubQ: 6000 units/m²/dose days 15, 18, 22, and 25
[total dose/cycle = 24,000 units/m²]
CNS prophylaxis/interim maintenance (12 week duration; with cranial irradiation days 1 to 12):
Methotrexate: I.T.: 15 mg/dose days 1, 8, 15, 22, and 29
[total dose/cycle = 75 mg]
Mercaptopurine: Oral: 60 mg/m²/dose days 1 to 70
[total dose/cycle = 4200 mg/m²]
Methotrexate: Oral: 20 mg/m²/dose days 36, 43, 50, 57, and 64
[total dose/cycle = 100 mg/m²]
Late intensification (8-week cycle):
Doxorubicin: I.V.: 30 mg/m²/dose days 1, 8, and 15
[total dose/cycle = 90 mg/m²]
Vincristine: I.V.: 2 mg/dose days 1, 8, and 15
[total dose/cycle = 6 mg]
Dexamethasone: Oral: 10 mg/m²/dose days 1 to 14
[total dose/cycle = 140 mg/m²]
Cyclophosphamide: I.V.: 1000 mg/m² day 29
[total dose/cycle = 1000 mg/m²]
Thioguanine: Oral: 60 mg/m²/dose days 29 to 42
[total dose/cycle = 840 mg/m²]
Cytarabine: SubQ: 75 mg/m²/dose days 29 to 32 and 36 to 39
[total dose/cycle = 600 mg/m²]
Maintenance (continue until 24 months from diagnosis):
Vincristine: I.V. 2 mg/dose day 1 every 4 weeks
[total dose/4 weeks = 2 mg]
Prednisone: Oral: 60 mg/m²/dose days 1 to 5 every 4 weeks
[total dose/4 weeks = 300 mg/m²]

Methotrexate: Oral: 20 mg/m^2/dose days 1, 8, 15, and 22
[total dose/phase = 80 mg/m^2]
Mercaptopurine: Oral: 60 mg/m^2/dose days 1 to 28
[total dose/phase = 1680 mg/m^2]
Variation 2 (with G-CSF; CALGB 9111):
Induction, patients <60 years of age (4-week cycle):
Cyclophosphamide: I.V.: 1200 mg/m^2 day 1
[total dose/cycle = 1200 mg/m^2]
Daunorubicin: I.V.: 45 mg/m^2/dose days 1, 2, and 3
[total dose/cycle = 135 mg/m^2]
Vincristine: I.V.: 2 mg/dose days 1, 8, 15, and 22
[total dose/cycle = 8 mg]
Prednisone: Oral: 60 mg/m^2/dose days 1 to 21
[total dose/cycle = 1260 mg/m^2]
Asparaginase: SubQ, I.M.: 6000 units/m^2/dose days 5, 8, 11, 15, 18, and 22
[total dose/cycle = 36,000 units/m^2]
Filgrastim: SubQ: 5 mcg/kg/day starting day 4; continue for at least 7 days and until ANC ≥1000/mm^3
on two draws, 24 hours apart
Induction, patients ≥60 years of age (4-week cycle):
Cyclophosphamide: I.V.: 800 mg/m^2 day 1
[total dose/cycle = 800 mg/m^2]
Daunorubicin: I.V.: 30 mg/m^2/dose days 1, 2, and 3
[total dose/cycle = 90 mg/m^2]
Vincristine: I.V.: 2 mg/dose days 1, 8, 15, and 22
[total dose/cycle = 8 mg]
Prednisone: Oral: 60 mg/m^2/dose days 1 to 7
[total dose/cycle = 420 mg/m^2]
Asparaginase: SubQ, I.M.: 6000 units/m^2/dose days 5, 8, 11, 15, 18, and 22
[total dose/cycle = 36,000 units/m^2]
Filgrastim: SubQ: 5 mcg/kg/day starting day 4; continue for at least 7 days and until ANC ≥1000/mm^3
on two draws, 24 hours apart
Early intensification (4-week cycle; repeat cycle once):
Methotrexate: I.T.: 15 mg/dose day 1
[total dose/cycle = 15 mg]
Cyclophosphamide: I.V.: 1000 mg/m^2 day 1
[total dose/cycle = 1000 mg/m^2]
Mercaptopurine: Oral: 60 mg/m^2/dose days 1 to 14
[total dose/cycle = 840 mg/m^2]
Cytarabine: SubQ: 75 mg/m^2/dose days 1 to 4 and 8 to 11
[total dose/cycle = 600 mg/m^2]
Vincristine: I.V.: 2 mg/dose days 15 and 22
[total dose/cycle = 4 mg]
Asparaginase: SubQ, I.M.: 6000 units/m^2/dose days 15, 18, 22, and 25
[total dose/cycle = 24,000 units/m^2]
Filgrastim: SubQ: 5 mcg/kg/day starting day 2; continue at least 14 days and until ANC ≥5000/mm^3 on
two draws, 24 hours apart
CNS prophylaxis/interim maintenance (12-week duration; with cranial irradiation days 1 to 12):
Methotrexate: I.T.: 15 mg/dose days 1, 8, 15, 22, and 29
[total dose/cycle = 75 mg]
Mercaptopurine: Oral: 60 mg/m^2/dose days 1 to 70
[total dose/cycle = 4200 mg/m^2]
Methotrexate: Oral: 20 mg/m^2/dose days 36, 43, 50, 57, and 64
[total dose/cycle = 100 mg/m^2]
Late intensification (8-week cycle):
Doxorubicin: I.V.: 30 mg/m^2/dose days 1, 8, and 15
[total dose/cycle = 90 mg/m^2]
Vincristine: I.V.: 2 mg/dose days 1, 8, and 15
[total dose/cycle = 6 mg]
Dexamethasone: Oral: 10 mg/m^2/dose days 1 to 14
[total dose/cycle = 140 mg/m^2]
Cyclophosphamide: I.V.: 1000 mg/m^2 day 29
[total dose/cycle = 1000 mg/m^2]

◄

Thioguanine: Oral: 60 mg/m^2/dose days 29 to 42
  [total dose/cycle = 840 mg/m^2]
Cytarabine: SubQ: 75 mg/m^2/dose days 29 to 32 and 36 to 39
  [total dose/cycle = 600 mg/m^2]
Maintenance (continue until 24 months from diagnosis):
Vincristine: I.V.: 2 mg/dose day 1 every 4 weeks
  [total dose/4 weeks = 2 mg]
Prednisone: Oral: 60 mg/m^2/dose days 1 to 5 every 4 weeks
  [total dose/4 weeks = 300 mg/m^2]
Methotrexate: Oral: 20 mg/m^2/dose days 1, 8, 15, and 22
  [total dose/phase = 80 mg/m^2]
Mercaptopurine: Oral: 60 mg/m^2/dose days 1 to 28
  [total dose/phase = 1680 mg/m^2]

Lenalidomide-Dexamethasone

Use Multiple myeloma
Regimen
Lenalidomide: Oral: 25 mg/day days 1 to 21
  [total dose/cycle = 525 mg]
Dexamethasone: Oral: 40 mg/day days 1 to 4, 9 to 12, and 17 to 20 (cycles 1 to 4)
  [total dose/cycle = 480 mg]
Dexamethasone: Oral 40 mg/day days 1 to 4 (cycle 5 and beyond)
  [total dose/cycle = 160 mg]
Repeat cycle every 28 days

Lenalidomide-Dexamethasone (Low Dose)

Use Multiple myeloma
Regimen
Lenalidomide: Oral: 25 mg/day days 1 to 21
  [total dose/cycle = 525 mg]
Dexamethasone: Oral: 40 mg/day days 1, 8, 15, and 22
  [total dose/cycle = 160 mg]
Repeat cycle every 28 days

Linker Protocol (ALL)

Use Leukemia, acute lymphocytic
Regimen
Remission induction:
Daunorubicin: I.V.: 50 mg/m^2/day days 1, 2, and 3
  [total dose/cycle = 150 mg/m^2]
Vincristine: I.V.: 2 mg/day days 1, 8, 15, and 22
  [total dose/cycle = 8 mg]
Prednisone: Oral: 60 mg/m^2/day days 1 to 28
  [total dose/cycle = 1680 mg/m^2]
Asparaginase: I.M.: 6000 units/m^2/day days 17 to 28
  [total dose/cycle = 72,000 units/m^2]
If residual leukemia in bone marrow on day 14:
Daunorubicin: I.V.: 50 mg/m^2 day 15
  [total dose/cycle = 50 mg/m^2]
If residual leukemia in bone marrow on day 28:
Daunorubicin: I.V.: 50 mg/m^2/day days 29 and 30
  [total dose/cycle = 100 mg/m^2]
Vincristine: I.V.: 2 mg/day days 29 and 36
  [total dose/cycle = 4 mg]
Prednisone: Oral: 60 mg/m^2/day days 29 to 42
  [total dose/cycle = 840 mg/m^2]
Asparaginase: I.M.: 6000 units/m^2/day days 29 to 35
  [total dose/cycle = 42,000 units/m^2]

Consolidation therapy:
Treatment A (cycles 1, 3, 5, and 7)
  Daunorubicin: I.V.: 50 mg/m^2/day days 1 and 2
    [total dose/cycle = 100 mg/m^2]
  Vincristine: I.V.: 2 mg/day days 1 and 8
    [total dose/cycle = 4 mg]
  Prednisone: Oral: 60 mg/m^2/day days 1 to 14
    [total dose/cycle = 840 mg/m^2]
  Asparaginase: I.M.: 12,000 units/m^2/day days 2, 4, 7, 9, 11, and 14
    [total dose/cycle = 72,000 units/m^2]
Treatment B (cycles 2, 4, 6, and 8)
  Teniposide: I.V.: 165 mg/m^2/day days 1, 4, 8, and 11
    [total dose/cycle = 660 mg/m^2]
  Cytarabine: I.V.: 300 mg/m^2/day days 1, 4, 8, and 11
    [total dose/cycle = 1200 mg/m^2]
Treatment C (cycle 9)
  Methotrexate: I.V.: 690 mg/m^2 continuous infusion over 42 hours day 1
    [total dose/cycle = 690 mg/m^2]
  Leucovorin: I.V.: 15 mg/m^2 every 6 hours for 12 doses (start at end of methotrexate infusion)
    [total dose/cycle = 180 mg/m^2]
Administer remission induction regimen for one cycle only. Repeat consolidation cycle every 28 days.

MACOP-B

Use Lymphoma, non-Hodgkin
Regimen
  Methotrexate: I.V. bolus: 100 mg/m^2 weeks 2, 6, 10
    followed by I.V.: 300 mg/m^2 over 4 hours weeks 2, 6, and 10
    [total dose/cycle = 1200 mg/m^2]
  Doxorubicin: I.V.: 50 mg/m^2 weeks 1, 3, 5, 7, 9, and 11
    [total dose/cycle = 300 mg/m^2]
  Cyclophosphamide: I.V.: 350 mg/m^2 weeks 1, 3, 5, 7, 9, and 11
    [total dose/cycle = 2100 mg/m^2]
  Vincristine: I.V.: 1.4 mg/m^2 (maximum dose: 2 mg) weeks 2, 4, 6, 8, 10, and 12
    [total dose/cycle = 8.4 mg/m^2; maximum: 12 mg]
  Bleomycin: I.V.: 10 units/m^2 weeks 4, 8, and 12
    [total dose/cycle = 30 units/m^2]
  Prednisone: Oral: 75 mg/day for 12 weeks, then taper over 2 weeks
  Leucovorin calcium: Oral: 15 mg/m^2 every 6 hours, for 6 doses (beginning 24 hours after methotrexate) weeks 2, 6, and 10
    [total dose/cycle = 270 mg/m^2]
  Administer one cycle

MAID (Sarcoma)

Use Sarcoma
Regimen NOTE: Multiple variations are listed.
  Variation 1:
  Mesna: I.V.: 2000 mg/m^2/day continuous infusion days 1 to 4
    [total dose/cycle = 8000 mg/m^2]
  Doxorubicin: I.V.: 15 mg/m^2/day continuous infusion days 1 to 4
    [total dose/cycle = 60 mg/m^2]
  Ifosfamide: I.V.: 2000 mg/m^2/day continuous infusion days 1, 2, and 3
    [total dose/cycle = 6000 mg/m^2]
  Dacarbazine: I.V.: 250 mg/m^2/day continuous infusion days 1 to 4
    [total dose/cycle = 1000 mg/m^2]
  Repeat cycle every 21 days until disease progression or until maximum lifetime cumulative doxorubicin dose of 450 mg/m^2
  Variation 2:
  Mesna: I.V.: 2500 mg/m^2/day continuous infusion days 1 to 4
    [total dose/cycle = 10,000 mg/m^2]
  Doxorubicin: I.V.: 20 mg/m^2/day continuous infusion days 1, 2, and 3
    [total dose/cycle = 60 mg/m^2]

Ifosfamide: I.V.: 2500 mg/m^2/day continuous infusion days 1, 2, and 3
[total dose/cycle = 7500 mg/m^2]
Dacarbazine: I.V.: 300 mg/m^2/day continuous infusion days 1, 2, and 3
[total dose/cycle = 900 mg/m^2]
Repeat cycle every 21 days (delay 1 week for leukopenia or thrombocytopenia)
Variation 3 (if prior pelvic irradiation):
Mesna: I.V.: 2500 mg/m^2/day continuous infusion days 1 to 4
[total dose/cycle = 10,000 mg/m^2]
Doxorubicin: I.V.: 20 mg/m^2/day continuous infusion days 1, 2, and 3
[total dose/cycle = 60 mg/m^2]
Ifosfamide: I.V.: 1500 mg/m^2/day continuous infusion days 1, 2, and 3
[total dose/cycle = 4500 mg/m^2]
Dacarbazine: I.V.: 300 mg/m^2/day continuous infusion days 1, 2, and 3
[total dose/cycle = 900 mg/m^2]
Repeat cycle every 21 days (delay 1 week for leukopenia or thrombocytopenia)
Variation 4:
Mesna: I.V.: 2500 mg/m^2/day continuous infusion days 1 to 4
[total dose/cycle = 10,000 mg/m^2]
Doxorubicin: I.V.: 15 mg/m^2/day continuous infusion days 1 to 4
[total dose/cycle = 60 mg/m^2]
Ifosfamide: I.V.: 2000 mg/m^2/day continuous infusion days 1, 2, and 3
[total dose/cycle = 6000 mg/m^2]
Dacarbazine: I.V.: 250 mg/m^2/day continuous infusion days 1 to 4
[total dose/cycle = 1000 mg/m^2]
Repeat cycle every 21 days (or when adequate hematologic recovery)

m-BACOD

Use Lymphoma, non-Hodgkin

Regimen

Methotrexate: I.V.: 200 mg/m^2/day days 8 and 15
[total dose/cycle = 400 mg/m^2]
Leucovorin calcium: Oral: 10 mg/m^2 every 6 hours for 8 doses (beginning 24 hours after each methotrexate dose) days 9 and 16
[total dose/cycle = 160 mg/m^2]
Bleomycin: I.V.: 4 units/m^2 day 1
[total dose/cycle = 4 units/m^2]
Doxorubicin: I.V.: 45 mg/m^2 day 1
[total dose/cycle = 45 mg/m^2]
Cyclophosphamide: I.V.: 600 mg/m^2 day 1
[total dose/cycle = 600 mg/m^2]
Vincristine: I.V.: 1 mg/m^2 day 1
[total dose/cycle = 1 mg/m^2]
Dexamethasone: Oral: 6 mg/m^2/day days 1 to 5
[total dose/cycle = 30 mg/m^2]
Repeat cycle every 21 days

MEC (AML Induction)

Use Leukemia, acute myeloid

Regimen

Variation 1:
Mitoxantrone: I.V.: 12 mg/m^2/day over 30 minutes days 1, 2, and 3
[total dose/cycle = 36 mg/m^2]
Cytarabine: I.V.: 500 mg/m^2/day continuous infusion days 1, 2, and 3 and days 8, 9, and 10
[total dose/cycle = 3000 mg/m^2]
Etoposide: I.V.: 200 mg/m^2/day continuous infusion days 8, 9, and 10
[total dose/cycle = 600 mg/m^2]
May administer a second induction cycle if needed

Variation 2:
Etoposide: I.V.: 80 mg/m^2/day over 1 hour days 1 to 6
[total dose/cycle = 480 mg/m^2]
Cytarabine: I.V.: 1 g/m^2/day over 6 hours days 1 to 6
[total dose/cycle = 6 g/m^2]
Mitoxantrone: I.V.: 6 mg/m^2/day I.V. bolus days 1 to 6 (3 hours after the end of the cytarabine infusion)
[total dose/cycle = 36 mg/m^2]

Melphalan-Prednisone-Bortezomib (Multiple Myeloma)

Use Multiple myeloma

Regimen NOTE: Multiple variations are listed.
Variation 1:
Bortezomib: I.V.: 1.3 mg/m^2/day days 1, 4, 8, 11, 22, 25, 29, and 32
[total dose/cycle = 10.4 mg/m^2]
Melphalan: Oral: 9 mg/m^2/day days 1 to 4
[total dose/cycle = 36 mg/m^2]
Prednisone: Oral: 60 mg/m^2/day days 1 to 4
[total dose/cycle = 240 mg/m^2]
Repeat cycle every 42 days for 4 cycles
followed by
Bortezomib: I.V.: 1.3 mg/m^2/day days 1, 8, 22, and 29
[total dose/cycle = 5.2 mg/m^2]
Melphalan: Oral: 9 mg/m^2/day days 1 to 4
[total dose/cycle = 36 mg/m^2]
Prednisone: Oral: 60 mg/m^2/day days 1 to 4
[total dose/cycle = 240 mg/m^2]
Repeat cycle every 42 days for 5 cycles
Variation 2:
Bortezomib: I.V.: 1-1.3 mg/m^2/day days 1, 4, 8, 11, 22, 25, 29, and 32
[total dose/cycle = 8-10.4 mg/m^2]
Melphalan: Oral: 9 mg/m^2/day days 1 to 4
[total dose/cycle = 36 mg/m^2]
Prednisone: Oral: 60 mg/m^2/day days 1 to 4
[total dose/cycle = 240 mg/m^2]
Repeat cycle every 42 days for 4 cycles
followed by
Bortezomib: I.V.: 1-1.3 mg/m^2/day days 1, 8, 15, and 22
[total dose/cycle = 4-5.2 mg/m^2]
Melphalan: Oral: 9 mg/m^2/day days 1 to 4
[total dose/cycle = 36 mg/m^2]
Prednisone: Oral: 60 mg/m^2/day days 1 to 4
[total dose/cycle = 240 mg/m^2]
Repeat cycle every 35 days for 5 cycles

Melphalan-Prednisone (Multiple Myeloma)

Use Multiple myeloma

Regimen NOTE: Multiple variations are listed.
Variation 1:
Melphalan: Oral: 0.25 mg/kg/dose days 1 to 4
[total dose/cycle = 1 mg/kg]
Prednisone: Oral: 2 mg/kg/dose days 1 to 4
[total dose/cycle = 8 mg/kg]
Repeat cycle every 6 weeks for a total of 12 cycles
Variation 2:
Melphalan: Oral: 4 mg/m^2/dose days 1 to 7
[total dose/cycle = 28 mg/m^2]
Prednisone: Oral: 40 mg/m^2/dose days 1 to 7
[total dose/cycle = 280 mg/m^2]
Repeat cycle every 4 weeks for a total of 6 cycles

Variation 3:
  Melphalan: Oral: 9 mg/m^2/dose days 1 to 4
    [total dose/cycle = 36 mg/m^2]
  Prednisone: Oral: 60 mg/m^2/dose days 1 to 4
    [total dose/cycle = 240 mg/m^2]
  Repeat cycle every 6 weeks for a total of 9 cycles
Variation 4:
  Melphalan: Oral: 6 mg/m^2/dose days 1 to 7
    [total dose/cycle = 42 mg/m^2]
  Prednisone: Oral: 60 mg/m^2/dose days 1 to 7
    [total dose/cycle = 420 mg/m^2]
  Repeat cycle every 4 weeks for a total of 6 cycles
  Followed by (in responders):
    Interferon alfa: SubQ: 3 million units/dose 3 times/week until relapse
    Dexamethasone: Oral: 40 mg/dose days 1 to 4 every 2 months until relapse

Melphalan-Prednisone-Thalidomide (Multiple Myeloma)

Use Multiple myeloma
Regimen NOTE: Multiple variations are listed below.
Variation 1:
  Melphalan: Oral: 4 mg/m^2/day days 1 to 7
    [total dose/cycle = 28 mg/m^2]
  Prednisone: Oral: 40 mg/m^2/day days 1 to 7
    [total dose/cycle = 280 mg/m^2]
  Thalidomide: Oral: 100 mg/day days 1 to 28
    [total dose/cycle = 2800 mg]
  Repeat cycle every 28 days for 6 cycles
  followed by
  Thalidomide: Oral: 100 mg daily (as maintenance)
Variation 2:
  Melphalan: Oral: 0.25 mg/kg/dose days 1 to 4
    [total dose/cycle = 1 mg/kg]
  Prednisone: Oral: 2 mg/kg/dose days 1 to 4
    [total dose/cycle = 8 mg/kg]
  Thalidomide: Oral: 100-400 mg/day days 1 to 42
    [total dose/cycle = 4200-16,800 mg]
  Repeat cycle every 6 weeks for a total of 12 cycles (discontinue thalidomide on day 4 of the last cycle)

Methotrexate-Vinblastine (Desmoid Tumor)

Use Soft tissue sarcoma (desmoid tumor)
Regimen
  Methotrexate: I.V.: 30 mg/m^2 every 7-10 days
    [total dose/treatment = 30 mg/m^2]
  Vinblastine: I.V.: 6 mg/m^2 every 7-10 days
    [total dose/treatment = 6 mg/m^2]
  Continue treatment for 1 year (52 treatments)

MINE

Use Lymphoma, non-Hodgkin
Regimen
  Mesna: I.V.: 1.33 g/m^2/day concurrent with ifosfamide dose, then 500 mg orally (4 hours after each ifosfamide infusion) days 1, 2, and 3
    [total dose/cycle = 3.99 g/m^2/1500 mg]
  Ifosfamide: I.V.: 1.33 g/m^2/day days 1, 2, and 3
    [total dose/cycle = 3.99 g/m^2]
  Mitoxantrone: I.V.: 8 mg/m^2 day 1
    [total dose/cycle = 8 mg/m^2]
  Etoposide: I.V.: 65 mg/m^2/day days 1, 2, and 3
    [total dose/cycle = 195 mg/m^2]
  Repeat cycle every 28 days

MINE-ESHAP (Hodgkin)

Use Lymphoma, Hodgkin

Regimen

Refractory disease (alternate MINE regimen with ESHAP regimen for a total of 2 MINE cycles and 2 ESHAP cycles):

MINE Regimen:

Mesna: I.V.: 2250 mg/m^2/day days 1, 2, and 3
 [total dose/cycle = 6750 mg/m^2]
Ifosfamide: I.V.: 1500 mg/m^2/day days 1, 2, and 3
 [total dose/cycle = 4500 mg/m^2]
Mitoxantrone: I.V.: 10 mg/m^2 day 1
 [total dose/cycle = 10 mg/m^2]
Etoposide: I.V.: 80 mg/m^2/day days 1, 2, and 3
 [total dose/cycle = 240 mg/m^2]
Treatment cycle is 28 days

ESHAP Regimen:

Etoposide: I.V.: 40 mg/m^2/day days 1 to 4
 [total dose/cycle = 160 mg/m^2]
Methylprednisolone: I.V.: 250 mg/day days 1 to 4
 [total dose/cycle = 1000 mg]
Cisplatin: I.V.: 25 mg/m^2/day continuous infusion over 21 hours days 1 to 4
 [total dose/cycle = 100 mg/m^2]
Cytarabine: I.V.: 2000 mg/m^2 day 5
 [total dose/cycle = 2000 mg/m^2]
Treatment cycle is 28 days

MINE-ESHAP (NHL)

Use Lymphoma, non-Hodgkin

Regimen

Relapsed NHL (In patients achieving a complete remission, administer 6 cycles of MINE regimen, followed by 3 cycles of ESHAP regimen):

MINE regimen:

Mesna: I.V.: 1330 mg/m^2/day over 1 hour days 1, 2, and 3
 [total I.V. dose/cycle = 4000 mg/m^2]
 Followed by Mesna: Oral: 500 mg (4 hours after ifosfamide) days 1, 2, and 3
  [total oral dose/cycle = 1500 mg]
Ifosfamide: I.V.: 1330 mg/m^2/day over 1 hour days 1, 2, and 3
 [total dose/cycle = 4000 mg/m^2]
Mitoxantrone: I.V.: 8 mg/m^2 day 1
 [total dose/cycle = 8 mg/m^2]
Etoposide: I.V.: 65 mg/m^2/day over 1 hour days 1, 2, and 3
 [total dose/cycle = 195 mg/m^2]
Repeat MINE cycle every 21 days for 6 cycles, followed by 3 cycles of ESHAP

ESHAP Regimen:

Etoposide: I.V.: 60 mg/m^2/day over 1 hour days 1 to 4
 [total dose/cycle = 240 mg/m^2]
Methylprednisolone: I.V.: 500 mg/day days 1 to 4
 [total dose/cycle = 2000 mg]
Cisplatin: I.V.: 25 mg/m^2/day continuous infusion days 1 to 4
 [total dose/cycle = 100 mg/m^2]
Cytarabine: I.V.: 2000 mg/m^2 over 2 hours day 5
 [total dose/cycle = 2000 mg/m^2]
Repeat ESHAP cycle every 21 days for 3 cycles

mini-BEAM

Use Lymphoma, Hodgkin disease

Regimen

Carmustine: I.V.: 60 mg/m^2 over 30 minutes day 1
 [total dose/cycle = 60 mg/m^2]
Etoposide: I.V.: 75 mg/m^2/day over 30 minutes days 2 to 5
 [total dose/cycle = 300 mg/m^2]

Cytarabine: I.V.: 100 mg/m^2 every 12 hours days 2 to 5 (total of 8 doses)
[total dose/cycle = 800 mg/m^2]
Melphalan: I.V.: 30 mg/m^2 over 15 minutes day 6
[total dose/cycle = 30 mg/m^2]
Repeat cycle every 4 to 6 weeks

Mitoxantrone-Etoposide (AML Induction)

Use Leukemia, acute myeloid

Regimen
Mitoxantrone: I.V.: 10 mg/m^2/day over ≤15 minutes days 1 to 5
[total dose/cycle = 50 mg/m^2]
Etoposide: I.V.: 100 mg/m^2/day over 30 minutes days 1 to 5
[total dose/cycle = 500 mg/m^2]
May administer a second induction cycle if needed

Mitoxantrone + Hydrocortisone

Use Prostate cancer

Regimen
Mitoxantrone: I.V.: 14 mg/m^2 day 1
[total dose/cycle = 14 mg/m^2]
Hydrocortisone: Oral: 40 mg daily
[total dose/cycle = 840 mg]
Repeat cycle every 3 weeks

Mitoxantrone-Prednisone (Prostate Cancer)

Use Prostate cancer

Regimen NOTE: Multiple variations are listed.
Variation 1:
Mitoxantrone: I.V.: 12 mg/m^2 day 1
[total dose/cycle = 12 mg/m^2]
Prednisone: Oral: 5 mg twice daily
[total dose/cycle = 210 mg]
Repeat cycle every 21 days for up to a total of 10 cycles
Variation 2:
Cycle 1:
Mitoxantrone: I.V.: 12 mg/m^2 day 1
[total dose/cycle = 12 mg/m^2]
Prednisone: Oral: 5 mg twice daily
[total dose/cycle = 210 mg]
Treatment cycle is 21 days
Cycle 2 and beyond:
Mitoxantrone: I.V.: 12-14 mg/m^2 day 1 (increase to 14 mg/m^2 if no grade 3/4 adverse events)
[total dose/cycle = 12-14 mg/m^2]
Prednisone: Oral: 5 mg twice daily
[total dose/cycle = 210 mg]
Repeat cycle every 21 days for up to a maximum cumulative mitoxantrone dose of 144 mg/m^2
Variation 3:
Cycle 1:
Mitoxantrone: I.V.: 12 mg/m^2 day 1
[total dose/cycle = 12 mg/m^2]
Prednisone: Oral: 5 mg twice daily
[total dose/cycle = 210 mg]
Treatment cycle is 21 days
Cycles 2-8:
Mitoxantrone: I.V.: 12-14 mg/m^2 day 1 (increase to 14 mg/m^2 if granulocyte nadir is >1000/mm^3 and platelet nadir >50,000/ mm^3)
[total dose/cycle = 12-14 mg/m^2]
Prednisone: Oral: 5 mg twice daily
[total dose/cycle = 210 mg]
Treatment cycle is 21 days for up to a total of 8 cycles

MOPP/ABVD

Use Lymphoma, Hodgkin disease

Regimen NOTE: Multiple variations are listed.

Variation 1:

Mechlorethamine: I.V.: 6 mg/m^2/day days 1 and 8
[total dose/cycle = 12 mg/m^2]
Vincristine: I.V.: 1.4 mg/m^2/day (maximum dose: 2 mg) days 1 and 8
[total dose/cycle = 2.8 mg/m^2]
Procarbazine: I.V.: 100 mg/m^2/day days 1 to 14
[total dose/cycle = 1400 mg/m^2]
Prednisone: Oral: 40 mg/m^2/day days 1 to 14 (during cycles 1, 4, 7, and 10 only)
[total dose/cycle = 560 mg/m^2]
Doxorubicin: I.V.: 25 mg/m^2/day days 29 and 43
[total dose/cycle = 50 mg/m^2]
Bleomycin: I.V.: 10 units/m^2/day days 29 and 43
[total dose/cycle = 20 units/m^2]
Vinblastine: I.V.: 6 mg/m^2/day days 29 and 43
[total dose/cycle = 12 mg/m^2]
Dacarbazine: I.V.: 375 mg/m^2/day days 29 and 43
[total dose/cycle = 750 mg/m^2]
Repeat cycle every 56 days

Variation 2:

Mechlorethamine: I.V.: 6 mg/m^2/day days 1 and 8
[total dose/cycle = 12 mg/m^2]
Vincristine: I.V.: 1.4 mg/m^2/day (maximum dose: 2 mg) days 1 and 8
[total dose/cycle = 2.8 mg/m^2]
Procarbazine: I.V.: 100 mg/m^2/day days 1 to 14
[total dose/cycle = 1400 mg/m^2]
Prednisone: Oral: 40 mg/m^2/day days 1 to 14 (during cycles 1 and 7 only)
[total dose/cycle = 560 mg/m^2]
Doxorubicin: I.V.: 25 mg/m^2/day days 29 and 43
[total dose/cycle = 50 mg/m^2]
Bleomycin: I.V.: 10 units/m^2/day days 29 and 43
[total dose/cycle = 20 units/m^2]
Vinblastine: I.V.: 6 mg/m^2/day days 29 and 43
[total dose/cycle = 12 mg/m^2]
Dacarbazine: I.V.: 375 mg/m^2/day days 29 and 43
[total dose/cycle = 750 mg/m^2]
Repeat cycle every 56 days

Variation 3:

Mechlorethamine: I.V.: 6 mg/m^2/day days 1 and 8
[total dose/cycle = 12 mg/m^2]
Vincristine: I.V.: 1.4 mg/m^2/day (maximum dose: 2 mg) days 1 and 8
[total dose/cycle = 2.8 mg/m^2]
Procarbazine: I.V.: 100 mg/m^2/day days 1 to 14
[total dose/cycle = 1400 mg/m^2]
Prednisone: Oral: 40 mg/m^2/day days 1 to 14 (every cycle)
[total dose/cycle = 560 mg/m^2]
Doxorubicin: I.V.: 25 mg/m^2/day days 29 and 43
[total dose/cycle = 50 mg/m^2]
Bleomycin: I.V.: 10 units/m^2/day days 29 and 43
[total dose/cycle = 20 units/m^2]
Vinblastine: I.V.: 6 mg/m^2/day days 29 and 43
[total dose/cycle = 12 mg/m^2]
Dacarbazine: I.V.: 375 mg/m^2/day days 29 and 43
[total dose/cycle = 750 mg/m^2]
Repeat cycle every 56 days

◄ Variation 4:
  MOPP Regimen:
  Mechlorethamine: I.V.: 6 mg/m^2/day days 1 and 8
    [total dose/cycle = 12 mg/m^2]
  Vincristine: I.V.: 1.4 mg/m^2/day (maximum dose: 2 mg) days 1 and 8
    [total dose/cycle = 2.8 mg/m^2]
  Procarbazine: I.V.: 100 mg/m^2/day days 1 to 14
    [total dose/cycle = 1400 mg/m^2]
  Prednisone: Oral: 25 mg/m^2/day days 1 to 14
    [total dose/cycle = 350 mg/m^2]
  ABVD Regimen:
  Doxorubicin: I.V.: 25 mg/m^2/day days 1 and 15
    [total dose/cycle = 50 mg/m^2]
  Bleomycin: I.V.: 6 units/m^2/day days 1 and 15
    [total dose/cycle = 12 units/m^2]
  Vinblastine: I.V.: 6 mg/m^2/day days 1 and 15
    [total dose/cycle = 12 mg/m^2]
  Dacarbazine: I.V.: 250 mg/m^2/day days 1 and 15
    [total dose/cycle = 500 mg/m^2]
  Each regimen cycle is 28 days. Administer regimens in alternating fashion as follows: 2 cycles of MOPP alternating with 2 cycles of ABVD for a total of 8 cycles
Variation 5 (pediatrics):
  Mechlorethamine: I.V.: 6 mg/m^2/day days 1 and 8
    [total dose/cycle = 12 mg/m^2]
  Vincristine: I.V.: 1.4 mg/m^2/day days 1 and 8
    [total dose/cycle = 2.8 mg/m^2]
  Procarbazine: Oral: 100 mg/m^2/day days 1 to 14
    [total dose/cycle = 1400 mg/m^2]
  Prednisone: Oral: 40 mg/m^2/day days 1 to 14
    [total dose/cycle = 560 mg/m^2]
  Doxorubicin: I.V.: 25 mg/m^2/day days 29 and 42
    [total dose/cycle = 50 mg/m^2]
  Bleomycin: I.V.: 10 units/m^2/day days 29 and 42
    [total dose/cycle = 20 units/m^2]
  Vinblastine: I.V.: 6 mg/m^2/day days 29 and 42
    [total dose/cycle = 12 mg/m^2]
  Dacarbazine: I.V.: 150 mg/m^2/day days 29 to 33
    [total dose/cycle = 750 mg/m^2]
  Repeat cycle every 56 days for 4 cycles
Variation 6 (pediatrics):
  Mechlorethamine: I.V.: 6 mg/m^2/day days 1 and 8
    [total dose/cycle = 12 mg/m^2]
  Vincristine: I.V.: 1.4 mg/m^2/day days 1 and 8
    [total dose/cycle = 2.8 mg/m^2]
  Procarbazine: Oral: 100 mg/m^2/day days 1 to 14
    [total dose/cycle = 1400 mg/m^2]
  Prednisone: Oral: 40 mg/m^2/day days 1 to 14
    [total dose/cycle = 560 mg/m^2]
  Doxorubicin: I.V.: 25 mg/m^2/day days 29 and 42
    [total dose/cycle = 50 mg/m^2]
  Bleomycin: I.V.: 10 units/m^2/day days 29 and 42
    [total dose/cycle = 20 units/m^2]
  Vinblastine: I.V.: 6 mg/m^2/day days 29 and 42
    [total dose/cycle = 12 mg/m^2]
  Dacarbazine: I.V.: 375 mg/m^2/day days 29 and 43
    [total dose/cycle = 750 mg/m^2]
  Repeat cycle every 56 days for 4 cycles

MOPP/ABV Hybrid

Use Lymphoma, Hodgkin disease

Regimen
  Mechlorethamine: I.V.: 6 mg/m^2 day 1
    [total dose/cycle = 6 mg/m^2]
  Vincristine: I.V.: 1.4 mg/m^2 (maximum dose: 2 mg) day 1
    [total dose/cycle = 1.4 mg/m^2]
  Procarbazine: Oral: 100 mg/m^2/day days 1 to 7
    [total dose/cycle = 700 mg/m^2]
  Prednisone: Oral: 40 mg/m^2/day days 1 to 14
    [total dose/cycle = 560 mg/m^2]
  Doxorubicin: I.V.: 35 mg/m^2 day 8
    [total dose/cycle = 35 mg/m^2]
  Bleomycin: I.V.: 10 units/m^2 day 8
    [total dose/cycle = 10 units/m^2]
  Vinblastine: I.V.: 6 mg/m^2 day 8
    [total dose/cycle = 6 mg/m^2]
  Repeat cycle every 28 days

MOPP (Hodgkin Lymphoma)

Use Lymphoma, Hodgkin
Regimen NOTE: Multiple variations are listed.
  Variation 1:
    Mechlorethamine: I.V.: 6 mg/m^2/day days 1 and 8
      [total dose/cycle = 12 mg/m^2]
    Vincristine: I.V.: 1.4 mg/m^2/day days 1 and 8
      [total dose/cycle = 2.8 mg/m^2]
    Procarbazine: Oral: 100 mg/m^2/day days 1 to 14
      [total dose/cycle = 1400 mg/m^2]
    Prednisone: Oral: 40 mg/m^2/day days 1 to 14 (cycles 1 and 4)
      [total dose/cycle = 560 mg/m^2]
    Repeat cycle every 28 days for 6 cycles
  Variation 2:
    Mechlorethamine: I.V.: 6 mg/m^2/day days 1 and 8
      [total dose/cycle = 12 mg/m^2]
    Vincristine: I.V.: 1.4 mg/m^2/day (maximum dose: 2 mg) days 1 and 8
      [total dose/cycle = 2.8 mg/m^2; maximum dose/cycle: 4 mg]
    Procarbazine: Oral: 100 mg/m^2/day days 1 to 14
      [total dose/cycle = 1400 mg/m^2]
    Prednisone: Oral: 40 mg/m^2/day days 1 to 14 (cycles 1 and 4)
      [total dose/cycle = 560 mg/m^2]
    Repeat cycle every 28 days for 6-8 cycles

MOPP (Medulloblastoma)

Use Brain tumors
Regimen
  Mechlorethamine: I.V.: 3 mg/m^2/day days 1 and 8
    [total dose/cycle = 6 mg/m^2]
  Vincristine: I.V.: 1.4 mg/m^2/day (maximum dose: 2 mg) days 1 and 8
    [total dose/cycle = 2.8 mg/m^2]
  Prednisone: Oral: 40 mg/m^2/day days 1 to 10
    [total dose/cycle = 400 mg/m^2]
  Procarbazine: Oral: 50 mg day 1
    [total dose/cycle = 50 mg]
    followed by Oral: 100 mg day 2
      [total dose/cycle = 100 mg]
      followed by Oral: 100 mg/m^2/day days 3 to 10
        [total dose/cycle = 800 mg/m^2]
  Repeat cycle every 28 days

MTX/6-MP/VP (Maintenance)

Use Leukemia, acute lymphocytic

◀ **Regimen**
Methotrexate: Oral: 20 mg/m^2 weekly
[total dose/cycle = 80 mg/m^2]
Mercaptopurine: Oral: 75 mg/m^2/day
[total dose/cycle = 2250 mg/m^2]
Vincristine: I.V.: 1.5 mg/m^2 day 1
[total dose/cycle = 1.5 mg/m^2]
Prednisone: Oral: 40 mg/m^2/day days 1 to 5
[total dose/cycle = 200 mg/m^2]
Repeat monthly for 2-3 years

MTX-CDDPAdr

Use Osteosarcoma
Regimen
Cisplatin: I.V.: 75 mg/m^2 day 1 of cycles 1-7, then 120 mg/m^2 for cycles 8, 9, and 10
Doxorubicin: I.V.: 25 mg/m^2/day days 1, 2, and 3 of cycles 1 to 7
Methotrexate: I.V.: 12 g/m^2/day days 21 and 28
Leucovorin calcium rescue: I.V.: 20 mg/m^2 every 3 hours (beginning 16 hours after completion of methotrexate) for 8 doses, then orally every 6 hours for 8 doses

M-VAC (Bladder Cancer)

Use Bladder cancer
Regimen NOTE: Multiple variations are listed.
Variation 1:
Methotrexate: I.V.: 30 mg/m^2/day days 1, 15, and 22
[total dose/cycle = 90 mg/m^2]
Vinblastine: I.V.: 3 mg/m^2/day days 2, 15, and 22
[total dose/cycle = 9 mg/m^2]
Doxorubicin: I.V.: 30 mg/m^2 day 2
[total dose/cycle = 30 mg/m^2]
Cisplatin: I.V.: 70 mg/m^2 day 2
[total dose/cycle = 70 mg/m^2]
Repeat cycle every 4 weeks
Variation 2:
Methotrexate: I.V.: 40 or 50 mg/m^2/day days 1, 15, and 22
[total dose/cycle = 120 or 150 mg/m^2]
Vinblastine: I.V.: 4 or 5 mg/m^2/day days 2, 15, and 22
[total dose/cycle = 12 or 15 mg/m^2]
Doxorubicin: I.V.: 40 or 50 mg/m^2 day 2
[total dose/cycle = 40 or 50 mg/m^2]
Cisplatin: I.V.: 100 mg/m^2 day 2
[total dose/cycle = 100 mg/m^2]
Repeat cycle every 4 weeks
Variation 3:
Methotrexate: I.V.: 30 mg/m^2/day days 1, 15, and 22
[total dose/cycle = 90 mg/m^2]
Vinblastine: I.V.: 3 mg/m^2 day 2
[total dose/cycle = 3 mg/m^2]
Doxorubicin: I.V.: 30 mg/m^2 day 2
[total dose/cycle = 30 mg/m^2]
Cisplatin: I.V.: 70 mg/m^2 day 2
[total dose/cycle = 70 mg/m^2]
Repeat cycle every 4 weeks
Variation 4:
Methotrexate: I.V.: 60 mg/m^2 day 1
[total dose/cycle = 60 mg/m^2]
followed by I.V.: 30 mg/m^2 day 16
[total dose/cycle = 30 mg/m^2]
Vinblastine: I.V.: 4 mg/m^2/day days 2 and 16
[total dose/cycle = 8 mg/m^2]

Doxorubicin: I.V.: 60 mg/m^2 day 2
  [total dose/cycle = 60 mg/m^2]
Cisplatin: I.V.: 100 mg/m^2 day 2
  [total dose/cycle = 100 mg/m^2]
Repeat cycle every 23 days
Variation 5:
  Methotrexate: I.V.: 30 mg/m^2/day days 1, 16, and 23
    [total dose/cycle = 90 mg/m^2]
  Vinblastine: I.V.: 4 mg/m^2/day days 1, 16, and 23
    [total dose/cycle = 12 mg/m^2]
  Doxorubicin: I.V.: 60 mg/m^2 day 2
    [total dose/cycle = 60 mg/m^2]
  Cisplatin: I.V.: 100 mg/m^2 day 2
    [total dose/cycle = 100 mg/m^2]
  Repeat cycle every 23 days
Variation 6:
  Methotrexate: I.V.: 30 or 35 mg/m^2 day 1
    [total dose/cycle = 30 or 35 mg/m^2]
  Vinblastine: I.V.: 3 or 3.5 mg/m^2 day 2
    [total dose/cycle = 3 or 3.5 mg/m^2]
  Doxorubicin: I.V.: 30 or 35 mg/m^2 day 2
    [total dose/cycle = 30 or 35 mg/m^2]
  Cisplatin: I.V.: 70 or 80 mg/m^2 day 2
    [total dose/cycle = 70 or 80 mg/m^2]
  Repeat cycle every 2 weeks
Variation 7:
  Methotrexate: I.V.: 30 mg/m^2 day 1
    [total dose/cycle = 30 mg/m^2]
  Vinblastine: I.V.: 3 mg/m^2 day 2
    [total dose/cycle = 3 mg/m^2]
  Doxorubicin: I.V.: 30 mg/m^2 day 2
    [total dose/cycle = 30 mg/m^2]
  Cisplatin: I.V.: 70 mg/m^2 day 2
    [total dose/cycle = 70 mg/m^2]
  Repeat cycle every 14 days
Variation 8:
  Methotrexate: I.V.: 30 mg/m^2/day days 1, 15, and 22
    [total dose/cycle = 90 mg/m^2]
  Vinblastine: I.V.: 3 mg/m^2/day days 1, 15, and 22
    [total dose/cycle = 9 mg/m^2]
  Doxorubicin: I.V.: 45 mg/m^2 day 2
    [total dose/cycle = 45 mg/m^2]
  Cisplatin: I.V.: 70 mg/m^2 day 2
    [total dose/cycle = 70 mg/m^2]
  Repeat cycle every 4 weeks
Variation 9:
  Methotrexate: I.V.: 40 mg/m^2/day days 1 and 15
    [total dose/cycle = 80 mg/m^2]
  Vinblastine: I.V.: 4 mg/m^2/day days 1, 16, and 23
    [total dose/cycle = 12 mg/m^2]
  Doxorubicin: I.V.: 60 mg/m^2 day 2
    [total dose/cycle = 60 mg/m^2]
  Cisplatin: I.V.: 100 mg/m^2 day 2
    [total dose/cycle = 100 mg/m^2]
  Repeat cycle every 23 days
Variation 10:
  Methotrexate: I.V.: 30 mg/m^2/day days 1, 15, and 22
    [total dose/cycle = 90 mg/m^2]
  Vinblastine: I.V.: 3 mg/m^2/day days 1, 16, and 22
    [total dose/cycle = 9 mg/m^2]
  Doxorubicin: I.V.: 30 mg/m^2 day 1
    [total dose/cycle = 30 mg/m^2]

Cisplatin: I.V.: 70 mg/m^2 day 1
[total dose/cycle = 70 mg/m^2]
Repeat cycle every 4 weeks

Variation 11:
Methotrexate: I.V.: 30 mg/m^2/day days 1, 15, and 22
[total dose/cycle = 90 mg/m^2]
Vinblastine: I.V.: 3 mg/m^2/day days 2, 15, and 22
[total dose/cycle = 9 mg/m^2]
Doxorubicin: I.V.: 30 mg/m^2 day 2
[total dose/cycle = 30 mg/m^2]
Cisplatin: I.V.: 70 mg/m^2 day 2
[total dose/cycle = 70 mg/m^2]
Leucovorin: Oral: 15 mg every 6 hours for 4 doses days 2, 16, and 23
[total dose/cycle = 180 mg]
Repeat cycle every 4 weeks

Variation 12:
Methotrexate: I.V.: 30 mg/m^2/day days 1 and 15
[total dose/cycle = 60 mg/m^2]
Vinblastine: I.V.: 3 mg/m^2/day days 2 and 15
[total dose/cycle = 6 mg/m^2]
Doxorubicin: I.V.: 30 or 40 mg/m^2 day 3
[total dose/cycle = 30 or 40 mg/m^2]
Cisplatin: I.V.: 70 mg/m^2 day 2
[total dose/cycle = 70 mg/m^2]
Repeat cycle every 4 weeks

Variation 13:
Methotrexate: I.V.: 30 mg/m^2/day days 1 and 15
[total dose/cycle = 60 mg/m^2]
Vinblastine: I.V.: 3 mg/m^2/day days 2 and 15
[total dose/cycle = 6 mg/m^2]
Doxorubicin: I.V.: 30 or 40 mg/m^2 day 2
[total dose/cycle = 30 or 40 mg/m^2]
Cisplatin: I.V.: 70 mg/m^2 day 2
[total dose/cycle = 70 mg/m^2]
Repeat cycle every 4 weeks

M-VAC (Endometrial Cancer)

Use Endometrial cancer

Regimen
Methotrexate: I.V.: 30 mg/m^2/day days 1, 15, and 22
[total dose/cycle = 90 mg/m^2]
Vinblastine: I.V.: 3 mg/m^2/day days 2, 15, and 22
[total dose/cycle = 9 mg/m^2]
Doxorubicin: I.V.: 30 mg/m^2/day day 2
[total dose/cycle = 30 mg/m^2]
Cisplatin: I.V.: 70 mg/m^2/day day 2
[total dose/cycle = 70 mg/m^2]
Repeat cycle every 4 weeks

N6 Protocol

Use Neuroblastoma

Regimen
Course 1, 2, 4, and 6:
Cyclophosphamide: I.V.: 70 mg/kg/day days 1 and 2
[total dose/cycle = 140 mg/kg]
Doxorubicin: I.V.: 25 mg/m^2/day continuous infusion days 1, 2, and 3
[total dose/cycle = 75 mg/m^2]
Vincristine: I.V.: 0.033 mg/kg/day continuous infusion days 1, 2, and 3
[total dose/cycle = 0.099 mg/kg]
Vincristine: I.V.: 1.5 mg/m^2 day 9
[total dose/cycle = 1.5 mg/m^2]

Course 3, 5, and 7:
  Etoposide: I.V.: 200 mg/m^2/day days 1, 2, and 3
    [total dose/cycle = 600 mg/m^2]
  Cisplatin: I.V.: 50 mg/m^2/day days 1 to 4
    [total dose/cycle = 200 mg/m^2]

OFAR (CLL)

Use Leukemia, chronic lymphocytic
Regimen
  Cycle 1:
  Oxaliplatin: I.V.: 25 mg/m^2/dose day 1 to 4
    [total dose/cycle = 100 mg/m^2]
  Fludarabine: I.V.: 30 mg/m^2/dose days 2 and 3
    [total dose/cycle = 60 mg/m^2]
  Cytarabine: I.V.: 1000 mg/m^2/dose over 2 hours days 2 and 3
    [total dose/cycle = 2000 mg/m^2]
  Rituximab: I.V.: 375 mg/m^2 day 3
    [total dose/cycle = 375 mg/m^2]
  Treatment cycle is 4 weeks
  Cycles 2-6:
  Oxaliplatin: I.V.: 25 mg/m^2/dose day 1 to 4
    [total dose/cycle = 100 mg/m^2]
  Fludarabine: I.V.: 30 mg/m^2/dose days 2 and 3
    [total dose/cycle = 60 mg/m^2]
  Cytarabine: I.V.: 1000 mg/m^2/dose over 2 hours days 2 and 3
    [total dose/cycle = 2000 mg/m^2]
  Rituximab: I.V.: 375 mg/m^2 day 1
    [total dose/cycle = 375 mg/m^2]
  Repeat cycle every 4 weeks (maximum: 6 cycles)

Oxaliplatin-Cytarabine-Dexamethasone (NHL Regimen)

Use Lymphoma, non-Hodgkin
Regimen
  Dexamethasone: I.V. or Oral: 40 mg/day days 1 to 4
    [total dose/cycle = 160 mg]
  Oxaliplatin: I.V.: 130 mg/m^2 over 2 hours day 1
    [total dose/cycle = 130 mg/m^2]
  Cytarabine: I.V.: 2000 mg/m^2 over 3 hours every 12 hours for 2 doses day 2
    [total dose/cycle = 4000 mg/m^2]
  Repeat cycle every 3 weeks

Oxaliplatin-Fluorouracil (Esophageal Cancer)

Use Esophageal cancer
Regimen In combination with radiation therapy:
  Oxaliplatin: I.V.: 85 mg/m^2/day over 2 hours days 1, 15, and 29
    [total dose/cycle = 255 mg/m^2]
  Fluorouracil: I.V.: 180 mg/m^2/day continuous infusion days 8 to 42
    [total dose/cycle = 6300 mg/m^2]

PAC (CAP)

Use Ovarian cancer
Regimen
  Cisplatin: I.V.: 50 mg/m^2 day 1
    [total dose/cycle = 50 mg/m^2]
  Doxorubicin: I.V.: 50 mg/m^2 day 1
    [total dose/cycle = 50 mg/m^2]
  Cyclophosphamide: I.V.: 1000 mg/m^2 day 1
    [total dose/cycle = 1000 mg/m^2]
  Repeat cycle every 21 days for 8 cycles

PA-CI

Use Hepatoblastoma

Regimen NOTE: Multiple variations are listed.

Variation 1:

Cisplatin: I.V.: 90 mg/m^2 day 1

[total dose/cycle = 90 mg/m^2]

Doxorubicin: I.V.: 20 mg/m^2/day continuous infusion days 2 to 5

[total dose/cycle = 80 mg/m^2]

Repeat cycle every 21 days

Variation 2:

Cisplatin: I.V.: 20 mg/m^2/day days 1 to 4

[total dose/cycle = 80 mg/m^2]

Doxorubicin: I.V.: 100 mg/m^2 continuous infusion day 1

[total dose/cycle = 100 mg/m^2]

Repeat cycle every 21-28 days

Paclitaxel-Bevacizumab

Use Breast cancer

Regimen

Paclitaxel: I.V.: 90 mg/m^2/day days 1, 8, and 15

[total dose/cycle = 270 mg/m^2]

Bevacizumab: I.V.: 10 mg/kg/day days 1 and 15

[total dose/cycle = 20 mg/kg]

Repeat cycle every 28 days

Paclitaxel-Carboplatin-Bevacizumab

Use Lung cancer, nonsquamous, nonsmall cell

Regimen

Paclitaxel: I.V.: 200 mg/m^2 infused over 3 hours day 1

[total dose/cycle = 200 mg/m^2]

followed by

Carboplatin: I.V.: Target AUC 6 day 1

[total dose/cycle = AUC = 6]

followed by

Bevacizumab: I.V.: 15 mg/kg day 1

[total dose/cycle = 15 mg/kg]

Repeat cycle every 21 days for 6 cycles

Paclitaxel-Carboplatin (Bladder Cancer)

Use Bladder cancer

Regimen

Paclitaxel: I.V.: 200 mg/m^2 or 225 mg/m^2 day 1

[total dose/cycle = 200 or 225 mg/m^2]

Carboplatin: I.V.: AUC 5-6 day 1

[total dose/cycle = AUC = 5-6]

Repeat cycle every 21 days

Paclitaxel-Carboplatin (Esophageal Cancer)

Use Esophageal cancer

Regimen

Paclitaxel: I.V.: 50 mg/m^2/dose over 1 hour days 1, 8, 15, 22, and 29

[total dose/cycle = 250 mg/m^2]

Carboplatin: I.V.: AUC = 2 days 1, 8, 15, 22, and 29

[total dose/cycle = AUC = 10]

Administer with concurrent radiation therapy; cycle does not repeat.

Paclitaxel-Carboplatin-Etoposide (Unknown Primary)

Use Unknown primary, adenocarcinoma

Regimen
Paclitaxel: I.V.: 200 mg/m^2 infused over 1 hour day 1
[total dose/cycle = 200 mg/m^2]
followed by
Carboplatin: I.V.: Target AUC 6 day 1
[total dose/cycle = AUC = 6]
Etoposide: Oral: 50 mg/day days 1, 3, 5, 7, and 9
and Oral: 100 mg/day days 2, 4, 6, 8, and 10
[total dose/cycle = 750 mg]
Repeat cycle every 21 days for a total of 4-8 cycles

Paclitaxel-Carboplatin-Gemcitabine

Use Bladder cancer

Regimen
Paclitaxel: I.V.: 200 mg/m^2 day 1
[total dose/cycle = 200 mg/m^2]
Gemcitabine: I.V.: 1000 mg/m^2/day days 1 and 8
[total dose/cycle = 2000 mg/m^2]
Carboplatin: I.V.: AUC 5 day 1
[total dose/cycle = AUC = 5]
Repeat cycle every 21 days

Paclitaxel-Carboplatin-Gemcitabine (Unknown Primary)

Use Unknown primary (adenocarcinoma)

Regimen
Paclitaxel: I.V.: 200 mg/m^2 infused over 1 hour day 1
[total dose/cycle = 200 mg/m^2]
Carboplatin: I.V.: Target AUC 5 day 1
[total dose/cycle = AUC = 5]
Gemcitabine: I.V.: 1000 mg/m^2/dose days 1 and 8
[total dose/cycle = 2000 mg/m^2]
Repeat cycle every 21 days for a total of 4 cycles

Paclitaxel-Cetuximab

Use Head and neck cancer

Regimen
Week 1:
Paclitaxel: I.V.: 80 mg/m^2 day 1
[total dose/week 1 = 80 mg/m^2]
Cetuximab: I.V.: 400 mg/m^2 (loading dose) day 1 (week 1 only)
[total loading dose (week 1) = 400 mg/m^2]
Subsequent weeks:
Paclitaxel: I.V.: 80 mg/m^2 day 1
[total dose/week = 80 mg/m^2]
Cetuximab: I.V.: 250 mg/m^2 day 1
[total dose/week = 250 mg/m^2]

Paclitaxel-Cisplatin (Esophageal Cancer)

Use Esophageal cancer

Regimen NOTE: Multiple variations are listed.
Variation 1:
Paclitaxel: I.V.: 50 mg/m^2/dose over 1 hour days 1, 8, 15, 22, and 29
[total dose/cycle = 250 mg/m^2]

Cisplatin: I.V.: 30 mg/m^2/dose days 1, 8, 15, 22, and 29
  [total dose/cycle = 150 mg/m^2]
Administered (with concurrent radiation therapy) over one 5-week treatment cycle.
Followed by: Postoperative therapy:
Paclitaxel: I.V.: 175 mg/m^2/dose day 1
  [total dose/cycle = 175 mg/m^2]
Cisplatin: I.V.: 75 mg/m^2/dose day 1
  [total dose/cycle = 75 mg/m^2]
Repeat postop cycle every 21 days for a total of 3 cycles.
Variation 2:
Paclitaxel: I.V.: 60 mg/m^2/dose over 3 hours days 1, 8, 15, and 22
  [total dose/cycle = 240 mg/m^2]
Cisplatin: I.V.: 75 mg/m^2/dose over 2 hours day 1
  [total dose/cycle = 75 mg/m^2]
Filgrastim: SubQ: 5 mcg/kg/day starting day 23; continue until ANC >10,000/mm^3
Administer with concurrent radiation therapy; cycle does not repeat.
Variation 3:
Paclitaxel: I.V.: 90 mg/m^2/dose over 3 hours day 1
  [total dose/cycle = 90 mg/m^2]
Cisplatin: I.V.: 50 mg/m^2/dose over 1 hour day 1
  [total dose/cycle = 50 mg/m^2]
Repeat cycle every 14 days until disease progression or unacceptable toxicity.

Paclitaxel-Cisplatin-Fluorouracil (Esophageal Cancer)

Use Esophageal cancer
Regimen
Paclitaxel: I.V.: 175 mg/m^2 over 3 hours day 1
  [total dose/cycle = 175 mg/m^2]
Cisplatin: I.V.: 20 mg/m^2/day days 1 to 5 for cycles 1, 2, and 3
  [total dose/cycle = 100 mg/m^2]
  then 15 mg/m^2/day days 1 to 5
    [total dose/cycle = 75 mg/m^2]
Fluorouracil: I.V.: 750 mg/m^2/day continuous infusion days 1 to 5
  [total dose/cycle = 3750 mg/m^2]
Repeat cycle every 28 days

Paclitaxel-Cisplatin-Fluorouracil (Unknown Primary)

Use Unknown primary (squamous cell)
Regimen
Paclitaxel: I.V.: 175 mg/m^2 over 3 hours day 1
  [total dose/cycle = 175 mg/m^2]
Cisplatin: I.V.: 100 mg/m^2 day 2
  [total dose/cycle = 100 mg/m^2]
Fluorouracil: I.V.: 500 mg/m^2/day continuous infusion days 2 to 6
  [total dose/cycle = 2500 mg/m^2]
Repeat cycle every 21 days for a total of 3 cycles

Paclitaxel + Estramustine + Carboplatin

Use Prostate cancer
Regimen
Paclitaxel: I.V.: 100 mg/m^2 day 3 each week
  [total dose/cycle = 400 mg/m^2]
Estramustine: Oral: 10 mg/kg/day days 1 to 5 each week
  [total dose/cycle = 200 mg/kg]
Carboplatin: I.V.: Target AUC 6 day 3
  [total dose/cycle = AUC = 6]
Repeat cycle every 28 days

Paclitaxel + Estramustine + Etoposide

Use Prostate cancer

Regimen
Paclitaxel: I.V.: 135 mg/m^2 day 2
  [total dose/cycle = 135 mg/m^2]
Estramustine: Oral: 280 mg 3 times/day days 1 to 14
  [total dose/cycle = 11,760 mg]
Etoposide: Oral: 100 mg/day days 1 to 14
  [total dose/cycle = 1400 mg]
Repeat cycle every 21 days

Paclitaxel-Fluorouracil (Esophageal Cancer)

Use Esophageal cancer
Regimen
Paclitaxel: I.V.: 45 mg/m^2/dose over 3 hours day 1
  [total dose/cycle = 45 mg/m^2]
Fluorouracil: I.V.: 300 mg/m^2/day continuous infusion days 1 to 5
  [total dose/cycle = 1500 mg/m^2]
Repeat cycle weekly for 5 weeks; administer concurrent with radiation therapy; cycle does not repeat.

Paclitaxel-Gemcitabine

Use Bladder cancer
Regimen
Paclitaxel: I.V.: 200 mg/m^2 day 1
  [total dose/cycle = 200 mg/m^2]
Gemcitabine: I.V.: 1000 mg/m^2/day days 1, 8, and 15
  [total dose/cycle = 3000 mg/m^2]
Repeat cycle every 21 days for a maximum of 6 cycles

Paclitaxel-Ifosfamide-Cisplatin

Use Testicular cancer
Regimen
Paclitaxel: I.V.: 250 mg/m^2 continuous infusion day 1
  [total dose/cycle = 250 mg/m^2]
Ifosfamide: I.V.: 1500 mg/m^2/day days 2 to 5
  [total dose/cycle = 6000 mg/m^2]
Cisplatin: I.V.: 25 mg/m^2/day days 2 to 5
  [total dose/cycle = 100 mg/m^2]
Mesna: I.V.: 500 mg/m^2 prior to ifosfamide and every 4 hours for 2 doses, days 2 to 5
  [total dose/cycle = 6000 mg/m^2]
Repeat cycle every 21 days for 4 cycles

Paclitaxel-Vinorelbine

Use Breast cancer
Regimen NOTE: Multiple variations are listed.
Variation 1:
  Paclitaxel: I.V.: 135 mg/m^2 day 1
    [total dose/cycle = 135 mg/m^2]
  Vinorelbine: I.V.: 30 mg/m^2 day 1
    [total dose/cycle = 30 mg/m^2]
  Repeat cycle every 21 days
Variation 2:
  Paclitaxel: I.V.: 150 mg/m^2 day 1
    [total dose/cycle = 150 mg/m^2]
  Vinorelbine: I.V.: 25 mg/m^2 day 1
    [total dose/cycle = 25 mg/m^2]
  Repeat cycle every 21 days
Variation 3:
  Paclitaxel: I.V.: 135 mg/m^2 day 1
    [total dose/cycle = 135 mg/m^2]
  Vinorelbine: I.V.: 30 mg/m^2/day days 1 and 8
    [total dose/cycle = 60 mg/m^2]
  Repeat cycle every 28 days

PC (NSCLC)

Use Lung cancer, nonsmall cell

Regimen NOTE: Multiple variations are listed.

Variation 1:

Paclitaxel: I.V.: 175-225 mg/m^2 day 1

[total dose/cycle = 175-225 mg/m^2]

Carboplatin: I.V.: Target AUC 5-7 day 1

[total dose/cycle = AUC = 5-7]

Repeat cycle every 21 days for 2-8 cycles

Variation 2:

Paclitaxel: I.V.: 175 mg/m^2 day 1

[total dose/cycle = 175 mg/m^2]

Cisplatin: I.V.: 80 mg/m^2 day 1

[total dose/cycle = 80 mg/m^2]

Repeat cycle every 21 days

Variation 3:

Paclitaxel: I.V.: 135 mg/m^2 continuous infusion day 1

[total dose/cycle = 135 mg/m^2]

Carboplatin: I.V.: AUC 7.5 day 2

[total dose/cycle = AUC = 7.5]

Repeat cycle every 21 days

Variation 4:

Paclitaxel: I.V.: 135 mg/m^2 continuous infusion day 1

[total dose/cycle = 135 mg/m^2]

Cisplatin: I.V.: 75 mg/m^2 day 2

[total dose/cycle = 75 mg/m^2]

Repeat cycle every 21 days

PCR

Use Leukemia, chronic lymphocytic

Regimen NOTE: Multiple variations are listed.

Variation 1:

Cycle 1:

Cyclophosphamide: I.V.: 600 mg/m^2 day 1

[total dose/cycle = 600 mg/m^2]

Pentostatin: I.V.: 4 mg/m^2 day 1

[total dose/cycle = 4 mg/m^2]

Treatment cycle is 3 weeks

Cycles 2-6:

Cyclophosphamide: I.V.: 600 mg/m^2 day 1

[total dose/cycle = 600 mg/m^2]

Pentostatin: I.V.: 4 mg/m^2 day 1

[total dose/cycle = 4 mg/m^2]

Rituximab: I.V.: 375 mg/m^2 day 1

[total dose/cycle = 375 mg/m^2]

Repeat cycle every 3 weeks

Variation 2:

Cycle 1:

Pentostatin: I.V.: 2 mg/m^2 day 1

[total dose/cycle = 2 mg/m^2]

Cyclophosphamide: I.V.: 600 mg/m^2 day 1

[total dose/cycle = 600 mg/m^2]

Rituximab: I.V.: 100 mg/m^2 day 1 only

followed by I.V.: 375 mg/m^2/day days 3 and 5 only

[total dose/cycle 1 = 850 mg/m^2]

Treatment cycle is 3 weeks

Cycles 2-6:
  Pentostatin: I.V.: 2 mg/m^2 day 1
    [total dose/cycle = 2 mg/m^2]
  Cyclophosphamide: I.V.: 600 mg/m^2 day 1
    [total dose/cycle = 600 mg/m^2]
  Rituximab: I.V.: 375 mg/m^2 day 1
    [total dose/cycle = 375 mg/m^2]
  Repeat cycle every 3 weeks

PCV (Brain Tumor Regimen)

Use Brain tumors

Regimen NOTE: Multiple variations are listed.
Variation 1:
  Lomustine: Oral: 110 mg/m^2 day 1
    [total dose/cycle = 110 mg/m^2]
  Procarbazine: Oral: 60 mg/m^2/day days 8 to 21
    [total dose/cycle = 840 mg/m^2]
  Vincristine: I.V.: 1.4 mg/m^2/day (maximum dose: 2 mg) days 8 and 29
    [total dose/cycle = 2.8 mg/m^2; maximum: 4 mg]
  Repeat cycle every 6 weeks for a total of 6 cycles
Variation 2:
  Lomustine: Oral: 110 mg/m^2 day 1
    [total dose/cycle = 110 mg/m^2]
  Procarbazine: Oral: 60 mg/m^2/day days 8 to 21
    [total dose/cycle = 840 mg/m^2]
  Vincristine: I.V.: 1.4 mg/m^2/day (maximum dose: 2 mg) days 8 and 29
    [total dose/cycle = 2.8 mg/m^2; maximum: 4 mg]
  Repeat cycle every 6 weeks for a total of 7 cycles
Variation 3:
  Procarbazine: Oral: 75 mg/m^2/day days 8 to 21
    [total dose/cycle = 1050 mg/m^2]
  Lomustine: Oral: 130 mg/m^2 day 1
    [total dose/cycle = 130 mg/m^2]
  Vincristine: I.V.: 1.4 mg/m^2/day (no maximum) days 8 and 29
    [total dose/cycle = 2.8 mg/m^2; no maximum]
  Repeat cycle every 6 weeks for a total of 6 cycles
Variation 4:
  Procarbazine: Oral: 75 mg/m^2/day days 8 to 21
    [total dose/cycle = 1050 mg/m^2]
  Lomustine: Oral: 130 mg/m^2 day 1
    [total dose/cycle = 130 mg/m^2]
  Vincristine: I.V.: 1.4 mg/m^2/day (no maximum) days 8 and 29
    [total dose/cycle = 2.8 mg/m^2; no maximum]
  Repeat cycle every 6 weeks for up to a total of 4 cycles
Variation 5:
  Lomustine: Oral: 110 mg/m^2 day 1
    [total dose/cycle = 110 mg/m^2]
  Procarbazine: Oral: 60 mg/m^2/day days 8 to 21
    [total dose/cycle = 840 mg/m^2]
  Vincristine: I.V.: 1.4 mg/m^2/day days 8 and 29
    [total dose/cycle = 2.8 mg/m^2]
  Repeat cycle every 6-8 weeks for 1 year

Pemetrexed (Bladder Cancer Regimen)

Use Bladder cancer

Regimen
Pemetrexed: I.V.: 500 mg/m^2 infused over 10 minutes day 1
  [total dose/cycle = 500 mg/m^2]
Repeat cycle every 21 days

Pemetrexed-Carboplatin (Mesothelioma)

Use Malignant pleural mesothelioma

Regimen
Pemetrexed: I.V.: 500 mg/m^2 infused over 10 minutes day 1
[total dose/cycle = 500 mg/m^2]
Carboplatin: I.V.: AUC 5 infused over 30 minutes day 1 (start 30 minutes after pemetrexed)
[total dose/cycle = AUC = 5]
Repeat cycle every 21 days

Pemetrexed-Cisplatin (NSCLC)

Use Lung cancer, nonsmall cell

Regimen
Pemetrexed: I.V.: 500 mg/m^2/dose day 1
[total dose/cycle = 500 mg/m^2]
Cisplatin: I.V.: 75 mg/m^2/dose day 1
[total dose/cycle = 75 mg/m^2]
Repeat cycle every 21 days for up to 6 cycles

Pentostatin-Cyclophosphamide

Use Leukemia, chronic lymphocytic

Regimen
Cyclophosphamide: I.V.: 600 mg/m^2 day 1
[total dose/cycle = 600 mg/m^2]
Pentostatin: I.V.: 4 mg/m^2 day 1
[total dose/cycle = 4 mg/m^2]
Repeat cycle every 3 weeks for up to 6 cycles

POC

Use Brain tumors

Regimen
Prednisone: Oral: 40 mg/m^2/day days 1 to 14
[total dose/cycle = 560 mg/m^2]
Vincristine: I.V.: 1.5 mg/m^2/day (maximum dose: 2 mg) days 1, 8, and 15
[total dose/cycle = 4.5 mg/m^2]
Lomustine: Oral: 100 mg/m^2 day 1
[total dose/cycle = 100 mg/m^2]
Repeat cycle every 6 weeks

POG-8651

Use Osteosarcoma

Regimen
(Surgery at week 10)
Methotrexate: I.V.: 12 g/m^2 weeks 0, 1, 5, 6, 13, 14, 18, 19, 23, 24, 37, and 38
[total dose/cycle = 144 g/m^2]
Leucovorin: (route not specified): 15 mg every 6 hours for 10 doses, weeks 0, 1, 5, 6, 13, 14, 18, 19, 23, 24, 37, and 38
[total dose/cycle = 1800 mg]
Doxorubicin: I.V.: 37.5 mg/m^2/dose days 1 and 2 of weeks 2, 7, 25, and 28
followed by I.V.: 30 mg/m^2/dose days 1, 2, and 3 of week 20
[total dose/cycle = 390 mg/m^2]
Cisplatin: I.V.: 60 mg/m^2/day days 1 and 2, weeks 2, 7, 25, and 28
[total dose/cycle = 480 mg/m^2]
Cyclophosphamide: I.V.: 600 mg/m^2/day days 1, 2, and 3, weeks 15, 31, 34, 39, and 42
[total dose/cycle = 9000 mg/m^2]
Bleomycin: I.V.: 15 units/m^2/day days 1, 2, and 3, weeks 15, 31, 34, 39, and 42
[total dose/cycle = 225 units/m^2]

Dactinomycin: I.V.: 0.6 mg/m^2/day days 1, 2, and 3, weeks 15, 31, 34, 39, and 42
[total dose/cycle = 9 mg/m^2]
or
(Surgery at week 0)
Methotrexate: 12 g/m^2 weeks 3, 4, 8, 9, 13, 14, 18, 19, 23, 24, 37, and 38
[total dose/cycle = 144 g/m^2]
Leucovorin: (route not specified): 15 mg every 6 hours for 10 doses, weeks 3, 4, 8, 9, 13, 14, 18, 19, 23, 24, 37, and 38
[total dose/cycle = 1800 mg]
Doxorubicin: I.V.: 37.5 mg/m^2/day days 1 and 2, weeks 5, 10, 25, and 28 and 30 mg/m^2 days 1, 2, and 3, week 20
[total dose/cycle = 390 mg/m^2]
Cisplatin: I.V.: 60 mg/m^2/day days 1 and 2, weeks 5, 10, 25, and 28
[total dose/cycle = 480 mg/m^2]
Cyclophosphamide: I.V.: 600 mg/m^2/day days 1, 2, and 3, weeks 15, 31, 34, 39, and 42
[total dose/cycle = 9000 mg/m^2]
Bleomycin: I.V.: 15 units/m^2/day days 1, 2, and 3, weeks 15, 31, 34, 39, and 42
[total dose/cycle = 225 units/m^2]
Dactinomycin: I.V.: 0.6 mg/m^2/day days 1, 2, and 3, weeks 15, 31, 34, 39, and 42
[total dose/cycle = 9 mg/m^2]

POMP

Use Leukemia, acute lymphocytic
Regimen Maintenance:
Mercaptopurine: Oral: 50 mg 3 times/day
[total dose/cycle = 4200-4650 mg]
Methotrexate: Oral: 20 mg/m^2 once weekly
[total dose/cycle = 80 mg/m^2]
Vincristine: I.V.: 2 mg day 1
[total dose/cycle = 2 mg]
Prednisone: Oral: 200 mg/day days 1 to 5
[total dose/cycle = 1000 mg]
Repeat cycle monthly for 2 years

Pro-MACE-CytaBOM

Use Lymphoma, non-Hodgkin
Regimen
Prednisone: Oral: 60 mg/m^2/day days 1 to 14
[total dose/cycle = 840 mg/m^2]
Doxorubicin: I.V.: 25 mg/m^2 day 1
[total dose/cycle = 25 mg/m^2]
Cyclophosphamide: I.V.: 650 mg/m^2 day 1
[total dose/cycle = 650 mg/m^2]
Etoposide: I.V.: 120 mg/m^2 day 1
[total dose/cycle = 120 mg/m^2]
Cytarabine: I.V.: 300 mg/m^2 day 8
[total dose/cycle = 300 mg/m^2]
Bleomycin: I.V.: 5 units/m^2 day 8
[total dose/cycle = 5 units/m^2]
Vincristine: I.V.: 1.4 mg/m^2 (maximum dose: 2 mg) day 8
[total dose/cycle = 1.4 mg/m^2]
Methotrexate: I.V.: 120 mg/m^2 day 8
[total dose/cycle = 120 mg/m^2]
Leucovorin: Oral: 25 mg/m^2 every 6 hours for 4 doses (start 24 hours after methotrexate dose) day 9
[total dose/cycle = 100 mg/m^2]
Repeat cycle every 21 days

PVA (POG 8602)

Use Leukemia, acute lymphocytic

◄ **Regimen**
Induction:
Prednisone: Oral: 40 mg/m^2/day (maximum dose: 60 mg) given in 3 divided doses days 0 to 28
[total dose/cycle = 1160 mg/m^2]
Vincristine: I.V.: 1.5 mg/m^2/day (maximum dose: 2 mg) days 0, 7, 14, and 21
[total dose/cycle = 6 mg/m^2; maximum: 8 mg]
Asparaginase: I.M.: 6000 units/m^2 3 times per week for 2 weeks
[total dose/cycle = 36,000 units/m^2]
Intrathecal therapy (triple): Days 0 and 22
Leucovorin: Route and dose not specified: Single dose 24 hours after every intrathecal treatment days 1 and 23
Administer one cycle only
CNS consolidation:
Mercaptopurine: Oral: 75 mg/m^2/day days 29 to 43
[total dose/cycle = 1125 mg/m^2]
Intrathecal therapy (triple): Days 29 and 36
Leucovorin: Route and dose not specified: Single dose 24 hours after every intrathecal treatment days 30 and 37
Administer one cycle only
Intensification:
Regimen A:
Methotrexate: I.V.: 1000 mg/m^2 continuous infusion over 24 hours day 1
[total dose/cycle = 1000 mg/m^2]
Cytarabine: I.V.: 1000 mg/m^2 continuous infusion over 24 hours day 1 (start 12 hours after start of methotrexate)
[total dose/cycle = 1000 mg/m^2]
Leucovorin: I.M., I.V., or Oral: 30 mg/m^2 at 24 and 36 hours after the start of methotrexate
[total dose/cycle = 60 mg/m^2]
   followed by I.M., I.V., or Oral: 3 mg/m^2 at 48, 60, and 72 hours after the start of methotrexate
   [total dose/cycle = 9 mg/m^2]
Repeat cycle every 3 weeks for 6 cycles (administered weeks 7, 10, 13, 16, 19, and 22)
Intrathecal therapy (triple): Weeks 9, 12, 15, and 18
Leucovorin: Route and dose not specified: Single dose 24 hours after every intrathecal treatment weeks 9, 12, 15, and 18
or
Regimen B:
Methotrexate: I.V.: 1000 mg/m^2 continuous infusion over 24 hours day 1
[total dose/cycle = 1000 mg/m^2]
Cytarabine: I.V.: 1000 mg/m^2 continuous infusion over 24 hours day 1 (start 12 hours after methotrexate)
[total dose/cycle = 1000 mg/m^2]
Leucovorin: I.M., I.V., or Oral: 30 mg/m^2 at 24 and 36 hours after the start of methotrexate
[total dose/cycle = 60 mg/m^2]
   followed by I.M., I.V., or Oral: 3 mg/m^2 at 48, 60, and 72 hours after the start of methotrexate
   [total dose/cycle = 9 mg/m^2]
Repeat cycle every 12 weeks for 6 cycles (administer weeks 7, 19, 31, 43, 55, and 67)
Intrathecal therapy (triple): Weeks 9, 12, 15, and 18
Leucovorin: Route and dose not specified: Single dose 24 hours after every intrathecal treatment weeks 9, 12, 15, and 18
Maintenance:
Regimen A:
Methotrexate: I.M.: 20 mg/m^2 weekly, weeks 25 to 156
[total dose/cycle = 2640 mg/m^2]
Mercaptopurine: Oral: 75 mg/m^2 daily, weeks 25 to 156
[total dose/cycle = 69,300 mg/m^2]
Intrathecal therapy (triple): Every 8 weeks, weeks 26 through 105
Leucovorin: Route and dose not specified: Single dose 24 hours after every intrathecal treatment weeks 26 through 105
Prednisone: Oral: 40 mg/m^2/day (maximum dose: 60 mg) days 1 to 7 (given in 3 divided doses), weeks 8, 17, 25, 41, 57, 73, 89, and 105
[total dose/cycle = 2240 mg/m^2; maximum: 3360 mg]

Vincristine: I.V.: 1.5 mg/m^2/day (maximum dose: 2 mg) day 1, weeks 8, 9, 17, 18, 25, 26, 41, 42, 57, 58, 73, 74, 89, 90, 105, and 106
[total dose/cycle = 24 mg/m^2; maximum: 32 mg]
or
Regimen B:
Methotrexate: I.M.: 20 mg/m^2 weekly, weeks 22-28, 34-40, 46-52, and 58-64
[total dose/cycle = 560 mg/m^2]
Mercaptopurine: Oral: 75 mg/m^2 daily for 7 weeks, weeks 22-28, 34-40, 46-52, and 58-64
[total dose/cycle = 14700 mg/m^2]
followed by
Methotrexate: I.M.: 20 mg/m^2 weekly, weeks 70 to 156
[total dose/cycle = 1720 mg/m^2]
Mercaptopurine: Oral: 75 mg/m^2 daily, weeks 70 to 156
[total dose/cycle = 45,150 mg/m^2]
Intrathecal therapy (triple): Every 8 weeks, weeks 26 through 105
Leucovorin: Route and dose not specified: Single dose 24 hours after every intrathecal treatment weeks 26 through 105
Prednisone: Oral: 40 mg/m^2/day (maximum dose: 60 mg) days 1 to 7 (given in 3 divided doses), weeks 8, 17, 25, 41, 57, 73, 89, and 105
[total dose/cycle = 2240 mg/m^2]
Vincristine: I.V.: 1.5 mg/m^2/day (maximum dose: 2 mg) day 1, weeks 8, 9, 17, 18, 25, 26, 41, 42, 57, 58, 73, 74, 89, 90, 105, and 106
[total dose/cycle = 24 mg/m^2; maximum dose: 32 mg]

PVB

Use Testicular cancer
Regimen NOTE: Multiple variations are listed.
Variation 1:
Cisplatin: I.V.: 20 mg/m^2/day days 1 to 5
[total dose/cycle = 100 mg/m^2]
Vinblastine: I.V.: 0.2 mg/kg/day days 1 and 2
[total dose/cycle = 0.4 mg/kg]
Bleomycin: I.V.: 30 units/day days 2, 9, and 16
[total dose/cycle = 90 units]
Repeat cycle every 3 weeks
Variation 2:
Cisplatin: I.V.: 20 mg/m^2/day days 1 to 5
[total dose/cycle = 100 mg/m^2]
Vinblastine: I.V.: 0.15 mg/kg/day days 1 and 2
[total dose/cycle = 0.3 mg/kg]
Bleomycin: I.V.: 30 units/day days 2, 9, and 16
[total dose/cycle = 90 units]
Repeat cycle every 3 weeks
Variation 3:
Cisplatin: I.V.: 20 mg/m^2/day days 1 to 5
[total dose/cycle = 100 mg/m^2]
Vinblastine: I.V.: 6 mg/m^2/day days 1 and 2
[total dose/cycle = 12 mg/m^2]
Bleomycin: I.M.: 30 units/day days 2, 9, and 16
[total dose/cycle = 90 units]
Repeat cycle every 3 weeks

PVDA

Use Leukemia, acute lymphocytic
Regimen Induction:
Prednisone: Oral: 60 mg/m^2/day days 1 to 28
[total dose/cycle = 1680 mg/m^2]
Vincristine: I.V.: 1.5 mg/m^2/day days 1, 8, 15, and 22
[total dose/cycle = 6 mg/m^2]

◀ Daunorubicin: I.V.: 25 mg/m^2/day days 1, 8, 15, and 22
[total dose/cycle = 100 mg/m^2]
Asparaginase: I.M., SubQ, or I.V.: 5000 units/m^2/day days 1 to 14
[total dose/cycle = 70,000 units/m^2]
Administer one cycle only; used in conjunction with intrathecal chemotherapy

Raltitrexed-Cisplatin (Mesothelioma)

Use Malignant pleural mesothelioma

Regimen
Raltitrexed: I.V.: 3 mg/m^2 infused over 15 minutes day 1
[total dose/cycle = 3 mg/m^2]
Cisplatin: I.V.: 80 mg/m^2 infused over 1-2 hours day 1
[total dose/cycle = 80 mg/m^2]
Repeat cycle every 21 days until disease progression or unacceptable toxicity.

R-CVP

Use Lymphoma, non-Hodgkin

Regimen
Rituximab: I.V.: 375 mg/m^2 day 1
[total dose/cycle = 375 mg/m^2]
Cyclophosphamide: I.V.: 750 mg/m^2 day 1
[total dose/cycle = 750 mg/m^2]
Vincristine: I.V.: 1.4 mg/m^2 day 1
[total dose/cycle = 1.4 mg/m^2]
Prednisone: Oral: 40 mg/m^2/day days 1 to 5
[total dose/cycle = 200 mg/m^2]
Repeat cycle every 21 days

Regimen A1

Use Neuroblastoma

Regimen
Cyclophosphamide: I.V.: 1.2 g/m^2 day 1
[total dose/cycle = 1.2 g/m^2]
Vincristine: I.V.: 1.5 mg/m^2 day 1
[total dose/cycle = 1.5 mg/m^2]
Doxorubicin: I.V.: 40 mg/m^2 day 3
[total dose/cycle = 40 mg/m^2]
Cisplatin: I.V.: 90 mg/m^2 day 5
[total dose/cycle = 90 mg/m^2]
Repeat cycle every 28 days

Regimen A2

Use Neuroblastoma

Regimen
Cyclophosphamide: I.V.: 1.2 g/m^2 day 1
[total dose/cycle = 1.2 g/m^2]
Etoposide: I.V.: 100 mg/m^2/day days 1 to 5
[total dose/cycle = 500 mg/m^2]
Doxorubicin: I.V.: 40 mg/m^2 day 3
[total dose/cycle = 40 mg/m^2]
Cisplatin: I.V.: 90 mg/m^2 day 5
[total dose/cycle = 90 mg/m^2]
Repeat cycle every 28 days

RICE

Use Lymphoma, non-Hodgkin

Regimen
Rituximab: I.V.: 375 mg/m^2/day days -2 and 1 (cycle 1)
[total dose/cycle = 750 mg/m^2]
Rituximab: I.V.: 375 mg/m^2 day 1 (cycles 2 and 3)
[total dose/cycle = 375 mg/m^2]

Etoposide: I.V.: 100 mg/m^2/day days 3, 4, and 5
[total dose/cycle = 300 mg/m^2]
Carboplatin: I.V.: AUC = 5 (maximum dose: 800 mg) day 4
[total dose/cycle = AUC = 5]
Ifosfamide: I.V.: 5000 mg/m^2 continuous infusion day 4
[total dose/cycle = 5000 mg/m^2]
Mesna: I.V.: 5000 mg/m^2 continuous infusion day 4
[total dose/cycle = 5000 mg/m^2]
Filgrastim: SubQ: 5 mcg/kg/day days 7 to 14 (cycles 1 and 2)
[total dose/cycle = 40 mcg/kg]
Filgrastim: SubQ: 10 mcg/kg/day days 7 to 14 (cycle 3)
[total dose/cycle = 80 mcg/kg]
Repeat cycle every 2 weeks

Rituximab-CHOP (NHL)

Use Lymphoma, non-Hodgkin

Regimen NOTE: Multiple variations are listed.

Variation 1 (diffuse large B-cell lymphoma):
Rituximab: I.V.: 375 mg/m^2 day 1
[total dose/cycle = 375 mg/m^2]
Cyclophosphamide: I.V.: 750 mg/m^2 day 1
[total dose/cycle = 750 mg/m^2]
Doxorubicin: I.V.: 50 mg/m^2 day 1
[total dose/cycle = 50 mg/m^2]
Vincristine: I.V.: 1.4 mg/m^2 (maximum dose: 2 mg) day 1
[total dose/cycle = 1.4 mg/m^2; maximum: 2 mg]
Prednisone: Oral: 40 mg/m^2/day days 1 to 5
[total dose/cycle = 200 mg/m^2]
Repeat cycle every 21 days for a total of 8 cycles

Variation 2 (low-grade or follicular lymphoma):
Rituximab: I.V.: 375 mg/m^2 administer 7 and 2 days prior to the start of cycle 1 of CHOP, 2 days prior to the start of cycles 3 and 5 of CHOP, and after the 6th cycle of CHOP on days 134 and 141 (total of 6 doses of rituximab)
CHOP:
Cyclophosphamide: I.V.: 750 mg/m^2 day 1
[total dose/cycle = 750 mg/m^2]
Doxorubicin: I.V.: 50 mg/m^2 day 1
[total dose/cycle = 50 mg/m^2]
Vincristine: I.V.: 1.4 mg/m^2 (maximum dose: 2 mg) day 1
[total dose/cycle = 1.4 mg/m^2; maximum: 2 mg]
Prednisone: Oral: 100 mg/m^2/day days 1 to 5
[total dose/cycle = 500 mg/m^2]
Repeat each CHOP cycle every 21 days for a total of 6 CHOP cycles

Variation 3 (dose-dense R-CHOP in aggressive CD20-expressing B-cell lymphomas):
Pre-treatment (to improve performance status and diminish adverse effects to cycle 1):
Vincristine: I.V.: 1 mg 1 week before cycle 1
Prednisone: Oral: 100 mg/day for 7 days 1 week before cycle 1
Rituximab: I.V.: 375 mg/m^2 day 1
[total dose/cycle = 375 mg/m^2]
Cyclophosphamide: I.V.: 750 mg/m^2 day 1
[total dose/cycle = 750 mg/m^2]
Doxorubicin: I.V.: 50 mg/m^2 day 1
[total dose/cycle = 50 mg/m^2]
Vincristine: I.V.: 2 mg day 1
[total dose/cycle = 2 mg]
Prednisone: Oral: 100 mg/day days 1 to 5
[total dose/cycle = 500 mg]
Filgrastim (dose and route not specified): Daily beginning day 4 until leukocyte recovery
Repeat cycle every 14 days for a total of 6 cycles

Variation 4 (diffuse large B-cell lymphoma):

Rituximab: I.V.: 375 mg/m^2 days -7, 1, 22, and 43

[total dose/cycle = 1400 mg/m^2]

Cyclophosphamide: I.V.: 750 mg/m^2 days 3, 24, and 45

[total dose/cycle = 2250 mg/m^2]

Doxorubicin: I.V.: 50 mg/m^2 days 3, 24, and 45

[total dose/cycle = 150 mg/m^2]

Vincristine: I.V.: 1.4 mg/m^2 (maximum dose: 2 mg) days 3, 24, and 45

[total dose/cycle = 4.2 mg/m^2; maximum: 6 mg/cycle]

Prednisone: Oral: 100 mg/day for 5 days starting on days 3, 24, and 45

[total dose/cycle = 1500 mg]

Cycle does not repeat; followed by radiation therapy beginning on day 66

Variation 5 (diffuse large B-cell lymphoma):

Rituximab: I.V.: 375 mg/m^2 administer 7 and 3 days prior to the start of cycle 1 of CHOP, 2 days prior to the start of cycles 3 and 5 of CHOP, and 2 days before cycle 7 (if administered)

CHOP:

Cyclophosphamide: I.V.: 750 mg/m^2 day 1

[total dose/cycle = 750 mg/m^2]

Doxorubicin: I.V.: 50 mg/m^2 day 1

[total dose/cycle = 50 mg/m^2]

Vincristine: I.V.: 1.4 mg/m^2 (maximum dose: 2 mg) day 1

[total dose/cycle = 1.4 mg/m^2; maximum: 2 mg]

Prednisone: Oral: 100 mg/m^2/day days 1 to 5

[total dose/cycle = 500 mg/m^2]

Repeat each CHOP cycle every 21 days for a total of 6 CHOP cycles

Variation 6 (mantle cell lymphoma):

Rituximab: I.V.: 375 mg/m^2 day 0 (administer the day before CHOP)

[total dose/cycle = 375 mg/m^2]

Cyclophosphamide: I.V.: 750 mg/m^2 day 1

[total dose/cycle = 750 mg/m^2]

Doxorubicin: I.V.: 50 mg/m^2 day 1

[total dose/cycle = 50 mg/m^2]

Vincristine: I.V.: 1.4 mg/m^2 (maximum dose: 2 mg) day 1

[total dose/cycle = 1.4 mg/m^2; maximum: 2 mg]

Prednisone: Oral: 100 mg/m^2/day days 1 to 5

[total dose/cycle = 500 mg/m^2]

Repeat cycle every 21 days for a total of 6 cycles

Variation 7 (follicular lymphoma):

Rituximab: I.V.: 375 mg/m^2 day 0 (administer the day before CHOP)

[total dose/cycle = 375 mg/m^2]

Cyclophosphamide: I.V.: 750 mg/m^2 day 1

[total dose/cycle = 750 mg/m^2]

Doxorubicin: I.V.: 50 mg/m^2 day 1

[total dose/cycle = 50 mg/m^2]

Vincristine: I.V.: 1.4 mg/m^2 (maximum dose: 2 mg) day 1

[total dose/cycle = 1.4 mg/m^2; maximum: 2 mg]

Prednisone: Oral: 100 mg/m^2/day days 1 to 5

[total dose/cycle = 500 mg/m^2]

Repeat cycle every 21 days for a total of 6-8 cycles

Variation 8 (follicular lymphoma):
  Rituximab: I.V.: 375 mg/m^2 day 1
    [total dose/cycle = 375 mg/m^2]
  Cyclophosphamide: I.V.: 750 mg/m^2 day 1
    [total dose/cycle = 750 mg/m^2]
  Doxorubicin: I.V.: 50 mg/m^2 day 1
    [total dose/cycle = 50 mg/m^2]
  Vincristine: I.V.: 1.4 mg/m^2 (maximum dose: 2 mg) day 1
    [total dose/cycle = 1.4 mg/m^2; maximum: 2 mg]
  Prednisone: Oral: 100 mg/day days 1 to 5
    [total dose/cycle = 500 mg]
  Repeat cycle every 21 days for a total of 6 cycles
  followed by (maintenance rituximab):
    Rituximab: I.V.: 375 mg/m^2 day 1
      [total dose/cycle = 375 mg/m^2]
  Repeat every 3 months until relapse or for a maximum of 2 years

Stanford V Regimen

Use Lymphoma, Hodgkin disease

Regimen NOTE: Multiple variations are listed.
Variation 1:
  Mechlorethamine: I.V.: 6 mg/m^2/dose weeks 1, 5, and 9
    [total dose/cycle = 18 mg/m^2]
  Doxorubicin: I.V.: 25 mg/m^2/dose weeks 1, 3, 5, 7, 9, and 11
    [total dose/cycle = 150 mg/m^2]
  Vinblastine: I.V.: 6 mg/m^2/dose weeks 1, 3, 5, 7, 9, and 11
    [total dose/cycle = 36 mg/m^2]
  Vincristine: I.V.: 1.4 mg/m^2/dose (maximum dose: 2 mg) weeks 2, 4, 6, 8, 10, and 12
    [total dose/cycle = 8.4 mg/m^2; maximum: 12 mg]
  Bleomycin: I.V.: 5 units/m^2/dose weeks 2, 4, 6, 8, 10, and 12
    [total dose/cycle = 30 units/m^2]
  Etoposide: I.V.: 60 mg/m^2/day for 2 consecutive days, weeks 3, 7, and 11
    [total dose/cycle = 360 mg/m^2]
  Prednisone: Oral: 40 mg/m^2 every other day for 10 weeks
    [total dose prior to taper = 1400 mg/m^2]
    followed by tapering of prednisone dose during weeks 11 and 12
  Treatment cycle is 12 weeks
Variation 2:
  Mechlorethamine: I.V.: 6 mg/m^2/dose weeks 1 and 5
    [total dose/cycle = 12 mg/m^2]
  Doxorubicin: I.V.: 25 mg/m^2/dose weeks 1, 3, 5, and 7
    [total dose/cycle = 100 mg/m^2]
  Vinblastine: I.V.: 6 mg/m^2/dose weeks 1, 3, 5, and 7
    [total dose/cycle = 24 mg/m^2]
  Vincristine: I.V.: 1.4 mg/m^2/dose (maximum dose: 2 mg) weeks 2, 4, 6, and 8
    [total dose/cycle = 5.6 mg/m^2; maximum: 8 mg]
  Bleomycin: I.V.: 5 units/m^2/dose weeks 2, 4, 6, and 8
    [total dose/cycle = 20 units/m^2]
  Etoposide: I.V.: 60 mg/m^2/day days 15 and 16 and 43 and 44
    [total dose/cycle = 240 mg/m^2]
  Prednisone: Oral: 40 mg/m^2 days 1 to 36
    [total dose prior to taper = 1440 mg/m^2]
    followed by tapering of prednisone dose during weeks 7 and 8
  Treatment cycle is 8 weeks

TAC

Use Breast cancer

Regimen NOTE: Multiple variations are listed.
Variation 1:
  Docetaxel: I.V.: 75 mg/m^2 day 1
    [total dose/cycle = 75 mg/m^2]

Doxorubicin: I.V.: 50 mg/m^2 day 1
  [total dose/cycle = 50 mg/m^2]
Cyclophosphamide: I.V.: 500 mg/m^2 day 1
  [total dose/cycle = 500 mg/m^2]
Repeat cycle every 3 weeks
Variation 2:
Docetaxel: I.V.: 60 mg/m^2 day 1
  [total dose/cycle = 60 mg/m^2]
Doxorubicin: I.V.: 60 mg/m^2 day 1
  [total dose/cycle = 60 mg/m^2]
Cyclophosphamide: I.V.: 600 mg/m^2 day 1
  [total dose/cycle = 600 mg/m^2]
Repeat cycle every 3 weeks

Temozolomide-Rituximab (CNS Lymphoma)

Use Primary CNS lymphoma

Regimen NOTE: Multiple variations are listed.
Variation 1:
Combination therapy (cycles 1-4):
  Rituximab: I.V.: 375 mg/m^2/dose day 1
    [total dose/cycle = 375 mg/m^2]
  Temozolomide: Oral: 150 mg/m^2/day days 1 to 5
    [total dose/cycle = 750 mg/m^2]
  Repeat cycle every 28 days for a total of 4 cycles
followed by
Maintenance therapy:
  Temozolomide: Oral: 150 mg/m^2/day days 1 to 5
    [total dose/cycle = 750 mg/m^2]
  Repeat cycle every 28 days for a total of 8 cycles
Variation 2:
Combination therapy (cycles 1 and 2):
  Rituximab: I.V.: 750 mg/m^2/dose days 1, 8, 15, and 22
    [total dose/cycle = 3000 mg/m^2]
  Temozolomide: Oral: 150 mg/m^2/day days 1 to 7
    [total dose/cycle = 1050 mg/m^2]
  Repeat cycle every 28 days for a total of 2 cycles
followed by
Maintenance therapy:
  Temozolomide: Oral: 150 mg/m^2/day days 1 to 5
    [total dose/cycle = 750 mg/m^2]
  Repeat cycle every 28 days

Thalidomide-Dexamethasone

Use Multiple myeloma

Regimen NOTE: Multiple variations are listed.
Variation 1 (refractory):
Thalidomide: Oral: 100 mg/day days 1 to 28
  [total dose/cycle = 2800 mg]
Dexamethasone: Oral: 40 mg/day days 1 to 4
  [total dose/cycle = 160 mg]
Repeat cycle every 28 days
Variation 2 (refractory):
Thalidomide: Oral: 200 mg/day days 1 to 14 (cycle 1)
  followed by Oral: 400 mg/day days 15 to 28 (cycle 1)
  [total dose/cycle = 8400 mg]
Thalidomide: Oral: 400 mg/day days 1 to 28 (subsequent cycles)
  [total dose/cycle = 11,200 mg]
Dexamethasone: Oral: 20 mg/m^2/day days 1 to 4, 9 to 12, and 17 to 20 (cycle 1)
  [total dose/cycle = 240 mg/m^2]
  followed by Oral: 20 mg/m^2/day days 1 to 4 (subsequent cycles)
    [total dose/cycle = 80 mg/m^2]
Repeat cycle every 28 days

Variation 3 (newly diagnosed):
  Thalidomide: Oral: 200 mg/day days 1 to 28
    [total dose/cycle = 5600 mg]
  Dexamethasone: Oral: 40 mg/day days 1 to 4, 9 to 12, and 17 to 20
    [total dose/cycle = 480 mg]
  Repeat cycle every 28 days
Variation 4 (newly diagnosed):
  Thalidomide: Oral: 50 mg/day days 1 to 14
    followed by Oral: 100 mg/day days 15 to 28 (cycle 1)
      [total dose/cycle 1 = 2100 mg]
      followed by Oral: 200 mg/day days 1 to 28 (starting with cycle 2 and subsequent cycles)
        [total dose/cycle = 5600 mg]
  Dexamethasone: Oral: 40 mg/day days 1 to 4, 9 to 12, and 17 to 20 (cycles 1 to 4)
    [total dose/cycle 1 to 4 = 480 mg]
    followed by Oral: 40 mg/day days 1 to 4 (starting with cycle 5 and subsequent cycles)
      [total dose/cycle = 160 mg]
  Repeat cycle every 28 days until disease progression or unacceptable toxicity
Variation 5 (newly diagnosed):
  Thalidomide: Oral: 100 mg/day days 1 to 14
    followed by Oral: 200 mg/day days 15 to 28 (cycle 1)
      [total dose/cycle = 4200 mg]
      followed by Oral: 200 mg/day days 1 to 28 (starting with cycle 2 and subsequent cycles)
        [total dose/cycle = 5600 mg]
  Dexamethasone: Oral: 40 mg/day days 1 to 4, 9 to 12, and 17 to 20 (odd cycles)
    [total dose/cycle = 480 mg]
  Dexamethasone: Oral: 40 mg/day days 1 to 4 (even cycles)
    [total dose/cycle = 160 mg]
  Repeat cycle every 28 days for a total of 4 cycles
Variation 6 (newly diagnosed induction):
  Thalidomide: Oral: 50 mg/day; may escalate by 50 mg per week to a maximum dose of 400 mg/day
    [total dose/cycle = up to 14,000 mg]
  Dexamethasone: Oral: 40 mg/day days 1 to 4, 9 to 12, and 17 to 20
    [total dose/cycle = 480 mg]
  Repeat cycle every 35 days for a total of 3 cycles

Topotecan-Cyclophosphamide (Ewing Sarcoma)

Use Ewing sarcoma
Regimen
Cyclophosphamide: I.V.: 250 mg/m^2/dose days 1 to 5
  [total dose/cycle = 1250 mg/m^2]
Topotecan: I.V.: 0.75 mg/m^2/dose days 1 to 5
  [total dose/cycle = 3.75 mg/m^2]
Repeat cycle every 21 days

Topotecan (Oral)-Cisplatin

Use Lung cancer, small cell
Regimen
Topotecan: Oral: 1.7 mg/m^2/day days 1 to 5
  [total dose/cycle = 8.5 mg/m^2]
Cisplatin: I.V.: 60 mg/m^2 day 5 only
  [total dose/cycle = 60 mg/m^2]
Repeat cycle every 21 days for 4 cycles (or for 2 cycles beyond best response)

Topotecan Oral Regimen (Ovarian Cancer)

Use Ovarian cancer
Regimen
Topotecan: Oral: 2.3 mg/m^2/day days 1 to 5
  [total dose/cycle = 11.5 mg/m^2]
Repeat cycle every 21 days until disease progression or for at least 4 cycles after achieve stable disease

Topotecan Oral Regimen (SCLC)

Use Lung cancer, small cell

Regimen NOTE: Multiple variations are listed.

Variation 1:

Topotecan: Oral: 2.3 mg/m^2/day days 1 to 5

[total dose/cycle = 11.5 mg/m^2]

Repeat cycle every 21 days until disease progression or until 2 cycles after best response

Variation 2:

Topotecan: Oral: 2.3 mg/m^2/day days 1 to 5

[total dose/cycle = 11.5 mg/m^2]

Repeat cycle every 21 days for at least 4 treatment cycles

Topotecan (Weekly)

Use Lung cancer, small cell; Ovarian cancer

Regimen

Topotecan: I.V.: 4 mg/m^2/day days 1, 8, and 15

[total dose/cycle = 12 mg/m^2]

Repeat cycle every 28 days

Trabectedin-Doxorubicin (Liposomal) (Ovarian Cancer)

Use Ovarian cancer

Regimen

Doxorubicin (liposomal): I.V.: 30 mg/m^2 over 90 minutes day 1

[total dose/cycle = 30 mg/m^2]

Trabectedin: I.V.: 1.1 mg/m^2 over 3 hours (via central line) day 1

[total dose/cycle = 1.1 mg/m^2]

Repeat cycle every 3 weeks until disease progression or for 2 cycles beyond confirmed complete response.

Trastuzumab-Cisplatin-Capecitabine (Gastric Cancer)

Use Gastric cancer

Regimen

Cycle 1:

Capecitabine: Oral: 1000 mg/m^2/dose twice daily days 1 to 14

[total dose/cycle = 28,000 mg/m^2]

Cisplatin: I.V.: 80 mg/m^2/dose day 1

[total dose/cycle = 80 mg/m^2]

Trastuzumab: I.V.: 8 mg/kg/dose (loading dose) day 1

[total dose/cycle 1 = 8 mg/kg]

Treatment cycle is 21 days

Cycles 2-6:

Capecitabine: Oral: 1000 mg/m^2/dose twice daily days 1 to 14

[total dose/cycle = 28,000 mg/m^2]

Cisplatin: I.V.: 80 mg/m^2/dose day 1

[total dose/cycle = 80 mg/m^2]

Trastuzumab: I.V.: 6 mg/kg/dose day 1

[total dose/cycle = 6 mg/kg]

Treatment cycle is 21 days

Subsequent cycles:

Trastuzumab: I.V.: 6 mg/kg/dose day 1

[total dose/cycle = 6 mg/kg]

Repeat cycle every 3 weeks until disease progression or unacceptable toxicity

Trastuzumab-Cisplatin-Fluorouracil (Gastric Cancer)

Use Gastric cancer

Regimen

Cycle 1:

Fluorouracil: I.V.: 800 mg/m^2/day continuous infusion days 1 to 5

[total dose/cycle = 4000 mg/m^2]

Cisplatin: I.V.: 80 mg/m^2/dose day 1
  [total dose/cycle = 80 mg/m^2]
Trastuzumab: I.V.: 8 mg/kg/dose (loading dose) day 1
  [total dose/cycle 1 = 8 mg/kg]
Treatment cycle is 21 days
Cycles 2-6:
Fluorouracil: I.V.: 800 mg/m^2/day continuous infusion days 1 to 5
  [total dose/cycle = 4000 mg/m^2]
Cisplatin: I.V.: 80 mg/m^2/dose day 1
  [total dose/cycle = 80 mg/m^2]
Trastuzumab: I.V.: 6 mg/kg/dose day 1
  [total dose/cycle = 6 mg/kg]
Treatment cycle is 21 days
Subsequent cycles:
Trastuzumab: I.V.: 6 mg/kg/dose day 1
  [total dose/cycle = 6 mg/kg]
Repeat cycle every 3 weeks until disease progression or unacceptable toxicity

Trastuzumab-Paclitaxel

Use Breast cancer
Regimen NOTE: Multiple variations are listed.
Variation 1:
Cycle 1:
Paclitaxel: I.V.: 175 mg/m^2 day 1
  [total dose/cycle = 175 mg/m^2]
Trastuzumab: I.V.: 4 mg/kg (loading dose) day 1
  followed by I.V.: 2 mg/kg/day days 8 and 15
  [total dose/cycle 1 = 8 mg/kg]
Treatment cycle is 21 days
Subsequent cycles:
Paclitaxel: I.V.: 175 mg/m^2 day 1
  [total dose/cycle = 175 mg/m^2]
Trastuzumab: I.V.: 2 mg/kg/day days 1, 8, and 15
  [total dose/cycle = 6 mg/kg]
Repeat cycle every 21 days for a total of at least 6 cycles
Variation 2:
Cycle 1:
Trastuzumab: I.V.: 4 mg/kg (loading dose) day 1
  followed by I.V.: 2 mg/kg/day days 8 and 15
  [total dose/cycle 1 = 8 mg/kg]
Paclitaxel: I.V.: 175 mg/m^2 day 2
  [total dose/cycle = 175 mg/m^2]
Treatment cycle is 21 days
Subsequent cycles:
Trastuzumab: I.V.: 2 mg/kg/day days 1, 8, and 15
  [total dose/cycle = 6 mg/kg]
Paclitaxel: I.V.: 175 mg/m^2 day 2
  [total dose/cycle = 175 mg/m^2]
Repeat cycle every 21 days for a total of at least 6 cycles (continue weekly trastuzumab after chemotherapy until disease progression or unacceptable toxicity)

Trastuzumab-Paclitaxel-Carboplatin

Use Breast cancer
Regimen
Cycle 1:
Trastuzumab: I.V.: 4 mg/kg (loading dose) day 1
  followed by I.V.: 2 mg/kg/day days 8 and 15
  [total dose/cycle 1 = 8 mg/kg]
Paclitaxel: I.V.: 175 mg/m^2 day 2
  [total dose/cycle = 175 mg/m^2]
Carboplatin: I.V.: AUC 6 day 2
  [total dose/cycle = AUC = 6]
Treatment cycle is 21 days

◀

Subsequent cycles:
Trastuzumab: I.V.: 2 mg/kg/day days 1, 8, and 15
[total dose/cycle = 6 mg/kg]
Paclitaxel: I.V.: 175 mg/m² day 2
[total dose/cycle = 175 mg/m²]
Carboplatin: I.V.: AUC 6 day 2
[total dose/cycle = AUC = 6]
Repeat cycle every 21 days for a total of at least 6 cycles (continue weekly trastuzumab after chemotherapy until disease progression or unacceptable toxicity)

Trastuzumab-Paclitaxel (Weekly)

Use Breast cancer

Regimen NOTE: Multiple variations are listed.
Variation 1:
Week 1:
Trastuzumab: I.V.: 4 mg/kg (loading dose) day 1
[total dose/week 1 = 4 mg/kg]
Paclitaxel: I.V.: 90 mg/m² day 2
[total dose/week 1 = 90 mg/m²]
Subsequent weeks:
Paclitaxel: I.V.: 90 mg/m² day 1
[total dose/week = 90 mg/m²]
Trastuzumab: I.V.: 2 mg/kg day 1
[total dose/week = 2 mg/kg]
Repeat weekly
Variation 2:
Week 1:
Trastuzumab: I.V.: 4 mg/kg (loading dose) day 1
[total dose/week 1 = 4 mg/kg]
Paclitaxel: I.V.: 80 mg/m² day 1
[total dose/week 1 = 80 mg/m²]
Subsequent weeks:
Trastuzumab: I.V.: 2 mg/kg day 1
[total dose/week = 2 mg/kg]
Paclitaxel: I.V.: 80 mg/m² day 1
[total dose/week = 80 mg/m²]
Repeat weekly

Tretinoin-Arsenic Trioxide (APL)

Use Leukemia, acute promyelocytic

Regimen
Induction (continue until <5% blasts in marrow and no abnormal promyelocytes):
Tretinoin: Oral: 45 mg/m²/day (in 2 divided doses) day 1 up to day 85
[total induction dose = up to 3825 mg/m²]
Arsenic Trioxide: I.V.: 0.15 mg/kg/day over 1 hour beginning day 10 up to day 85
[total induction dose = up to 11.25 mg/kg]
Postremission therapy (beginning with complete remission):
Tretinoin: Oral: 45 mg/m²/day weeks 1, 2, 5, 6, 9, 10, 13, 14, 17, 18, 21, 22, 25, 26
[total postremission dose = 4410 mg/m²]
Arsenic Trioxide: I.V.: 0.15 mg/kg/day Monday through Friday weeks 1 to 4, 9 to 12, 17 to 20, and 25 to 28
[total postremission dose = 12 mg/kg]

Tretinoin-Daunorubicin (APL)

Use Leukemia, acute promyelocytic

Regimen
Induction:
Tretinoin: Oral: 45 mg/m²/day (in 2 divided doses) day 1 until hematologic complete remission
Daunorubicin: I.V.: 60 mg/m²/day days 1, 2, and 3
[total dose/cycle = 180 mg/m²]

Consolidation:
 Course 1:
  Daunorubicin: I.V.: 60 mg/m^2/day days 1, 2, and 3
   [total dose/cycle = 180 mg/m^2]
 Course 2:
  Daunorubicin: I.V.: 45 mg/m^2/day days 1, 2, and 3
   [total dose/cycle = 135 mg/m^2]
Maintenance:
 Mercaptopurine: Oral: 90 mg/m^2 daily
  [total dose/cycle = 8100 mg/m^2 (90 days)]
 Methotrexate: Oral: 15 mg/m^2 weekly
  [total dose/cycle = 180 mg/m^2]
 Tretinoin: Oral: 45 mg/m^2/day (in 2 divided doses) days 1 to 15
  [total dose/cycle = 675 mg/m^2]
 Repeat cycle every 3 months for 2 years

Tretinoin-Daunorubicin-Cytarabine (APL)

Use Leukemia, acute promyelocytic
Regimen NOTE: Multiple variations are listed.
 Variation 1 (patients ≤60 years of age and WBC <10,000/mm^3):
  Induction:
   Tretinoin: Oral: 45 mg/m^2/day (in 2 divided doses) day 1 until hematologic complete remission
   Daunorubicin: I.V.: 60 mg/m^2/day days 1, 2, and 3
    [total dose/cycle = 180 mg/m^2]
   Cytarabine: I.V.: 200 mg/m^2/day days 3 to 10
    [total dose/cycle = 1400 mg/m^2]
  Consolidation:
   Course 1:
    Daunorubicin: I.V.: 60 mg/m^2/day days 1, 2, and 3
     [total dose/cycle = 180 mg/m^2]
    Cytarabine: I.V.: 200 mg/m^2/day days 1 to 7
     [total dose/cycle = 1400 mg/m^2]
   Course 2:
    Daunorubicin: I.V.: 45 mg/m^2/day days 1, 2, and 3
     [total dose/cycle = 135 mg/m^2]
    Cytarabine: I.V.: 1000 mg/m^2/dose every 12 hours for 8 doses
     [total dose/cycle = 8000 mg/m^2]
  Maintenance:
   Mercaptopurine: Oral: 90 mg/m^2 daily
    [total dose/cycle = 8100 mg/m^2 (90 days)]
   Methotrexate: Oral: 15 mg/m^2 weekly
    [total dose/cycle = 180 mg/m^2]
   Tretinoin: Oral: 45 mg/m^2/day (in 2 divided doses) days 1 to 15
    [total dose/cycle = 675 mg/m^2]
   Repeat cycle every 3 months for 2 years
 Variation 2 (patients ≤60 years of age and WBC ≥10,000/mm^3):
  Induction:
   Tretinoin: Oral: 45 mg/m^2/day (in 2 divided doses) day 1 until hematologic complete remission
   Daunorubicin: I.V.: 60 mg/m^2/day days 1, 2, and 3
    [total dose/cycle = 180 mg/m^2]
   Cytarabine: I.V.: 200 mg/m^2/day days 3 to 10
    [total dose/cycle = 1400 mg/m^2]
  Consolidation:
   Course 1:
    Daunorubicin: I.V.: 60 mg/m^2/day days 1, 2, and 3
     [total dose/cycle = 180 mg/m^2]
    Cytarabine: I.V.: 200 mg/m^2/day days 1 to 7
     [total dose/cycle = 1400 mg/m^2]

Course 2:
Daunorubicin: I.V.: 45 mg/m^2/day days 1, 2, and 3
[total dose/cycle = 135 mg/m^2]
Cytarabine: I.V.: 2000 mg/m^2/dose every 12 hours for 10 doses
[total dose/cycle = 20,000 mg/m^2]
Intrathecal prophylaxis: Five intrathecal injections: First dose in between induction and consolidation and 2 doses during each consolidation phase:
Methotrexate (preservative free): I.T.: 15 mg
Cytarabine (preservative free): I.T.: 50 mg
Corticosteroids (preservative free): I.T.: Dose unspecified
Maintenance:
Mercaptopurine: Oral: 90 mg/m^2 daily
[total dose/cycle = 8100 mg/m^2 (90 days)]
Methotrexate: Oral: 15 mg/m^2 weekly
[total dose/cycle = 180 mg/m^2]
Tretinoin: Oral: 45 mg/m^2/day (in 2 divided doses) days 1 to 15
[total dose/cycle = 675 mg/m^2]
Repeat cycle every 3 months for 2 years
Variation 3 (patients >60 years of age and WBC >10,000/mm^3):
Induction:
Tretinoin: Oral: 45 mg/m^2/day (in 2 divided doses) day 1 until hematologic complete remission
Daunorubicin: I.V.: 60 mg/m^2/day days 1, 2, and 3
[total dose/cycle = 180 mg/m^2]
Cytarabine: I.V.: 200 mg/m^2/day days 3 to 10
[total dose/cycle = 1400 mg/m^2]
Consolidation:
Course 1:
Daunorubicin: I.V.: 60 mg/m^2/day days 1, 2, and 3
[total dose/cycle = 180 mg/m^2]
Cytarabine: I.V.: 200 mg/m^2/day days 1 to 7
[total dose/cycle = 1400 mg/m^2]
Course 2:
Daunorubicin: I.V.: 45 mg/m^2/day days 1, 2, and 3
[total dose/cycle = 135 mg/m^2]
Cytarabine: I.V.: 1000 mg/m^2/dose every 12 hours for 8 doses
[total dose/cycle = 8,000 mg/m^2]
Intrathecal prophylaxis: Five intrathecal injections: First dose in between induction and consolidation and 2 doses during each consolidation phase:
Methotrexate (preservative free): I.T.: 15 mg
Cytarabine (preservative free): I.T.: 50 mg
Corticosteroids (preservative free): I.T.: Dose unspecified
Maintenance:
Mercaptopurine: Oral: 90 mg/m^2 daily
[total dose/cycle = 8100 mg/m^2 (90 days)]
Methotrexate: Oral: 15 mg/m^2 weekly
[total dose/cycle = 180 mg/m^2]
Tretinoin: Oral: 45 mg/m^2/day (in 2 divided doses) days 1 to 15
[total dose/cycle = 675 mg/m^2]
Repeat cycle every 3 months for 2 years

Tretinoin-Idarubicin (APL)

Use Leukemia, acute promyelocytic
Regimen NOTE: Multiple variations are listed.
Variation 1:
Induction:
Tretinoin: Oral: 45 mg/m^2/day (in 2 divided doses) day 1 up to 90 days
[total dose/cycle = up to 4050 mg/m^2]
≤20 years: Oral: 25 mg/m^2/day (in 2 divided doses) day 1 up to 90 days
[total dose/cycle = up to 2250 mg/m^2]
Idarubicin: I.V.: 12 mg/m^2/day days 2, 4, 6, and 8 (omit day 8 for patients >70 years of age)
[total dose/cycle = 36-48 mg/m^2]

Consolidation (administer courses sequentially at 1-month intervals for 3 months):
Course 1:
  Idarubicin: I.V.: 5 mg/m^2/day days 1 to 4
   [total dose/cycle = 20 mg/m^2]
  or
  Idarubicin: I.V.: 7 mg/m^2/day days 1 to 4
   [total dose/cycle = 28 mg/m^2]
  Tretinoin: Oral: 45 mg/m^2/day (in 2 divided doses) days 1 to 15
   [total dose/cycle = 675 mg/m^2]
Course 2:
  Mitoxantrone: I.V.: 10 mg/m^2/day days 1 to 5
   [total dose/cycle = 50 mg/m^2]
  or
  Mitoxantrone: I.V.: 10 mg/m^2/day days 1 to 5
   [total dose/cycle = 50 mg/m^2]
  Tretinoin: Oral: 45 mg/m^2/day (in 2 divided doses) days 1 to 15
   [total dose/cycle = 675 mg/m^2]
Course 3:
  Idarubicin: I.V.: 12 mg/m^2 day 1
   [total dose/cycle = 12 mg/m^2]
  or
  Idarubicin: I.V.: 12 mg/m^2/day days 1 and 2
   [total dose/cycle = 24 mg/m^2]
  Tretinoin: Oral: 45 mg/m^2/day (in 2 divided doses) days 1 to 15
   [total dose/cycle = 675 mg/m^2]
Maintenance:
  Mercaptopurine: Oral: 50 mg/m^2 daily
   [total dose/cycle = 4500 mg/m^2 (90 days)]
  Methotrexate: I.M.: 15 mg/m^2 weekly
   [total dose/cycle = 180 mg/m^2]
  Tretinoin: Oral: 45 mg/m^2/day (in 2 divided doses) days 1 to 15
   [total dose/cycle = 675 mg/m^2]
  Repeat cycle every 3 months for 2 years
Variation 2:
Induction:
  Tretinoin: Oral: 45 mg/m^2/day (in 2 divided doses) day 1 up to 90 days
   [total dose/cycle = up to 4050 mg/m^2]
    <15 years: Oral: 25 mg/m^2/day (in 2 divided doses) day 1 up to 90 days
     [total dose/cycle = up to 2250 mg/m^2]
  Idarubicin: I.V.: 12 mg/m^2/day days 2, 4, 6, and 8
   [total dose/cycle = 48 mg/m^2]
Consolidation (administer courses sequentially at 1-month intervals for 3 months):
Course 1:
  Idarubicin: I.V.: 5 mg/m^2/day days 1 to 4
   [total dose/cycle = 20 mg/m^2]
Course 2:
  Mitoxantrone: I.V.: 10 mg/m^2/day days 1 to 5
   [total dose/cycle = 50 mg/m^2]
Course 3:
  Idarubicin: I.V.: 12 mg/m^2 day 1
   [total dose/cycle = 12 mg/m^2]
Maintenance:
  Mercaptopurine: Oral: 90 mg/m^2 daily
   [total dose/cycle = 8100 mg/m^2 (90 days)]
  Methotrexate: I.M.: 15 mg/m^2 weekly
   [total dose/cycle = 180 mg/m^2]
  Tretinoin: Oral: 45 mg/m^2/day (in 2 divided doses) days 1 to 15
   [total dose/cycle = 675 mg/m^2]
  Repeat cycle every 3 months for 2 years

◄ Variation 3 (patients ≥60 years of age):
Induction:
Tretinoin: Oral: 45 mg/m^2/day (in 2 divided doses) day 1 up to 90 days
  [total dose/cycle = up to 4050 mg/m^2]
Idarubicin: I.V.: 12 mg/m^2/day days 2, 4, 6, and 8 (omit day 8 for patients ≥70 years of age)
  [total dose/cycle = 36-48 mg/m^2]
Consolidation (administer courses sequentially at 1-month intervals for 3 months):
Course 1:
Idarubicin: I.V.: 5 mg/m^2/day days 1 to 4
  [total dose/cycle = 20 mg/m^2]
Tretinoin: Oral: 45 mg/m^2/day (in 2 divided doses) days 1 to 15 (if intermediate or high risk)
  [total dose/cycle = 675 mg/m^2]
Course 2:
Mitoxantrone: I.V.: 10 mg/m^2/day days 1 to 5
  [total dose/cycle = 50 mg/m^2]
Tretinoin: Oral: 45 mg/m^2/day (in 2 divided doses) days 1 to 15 (if intermediate or high risk)
  [total dose/cycle = 675 mg/m^2]
Course 3:
Idarubicin: I.V.: 12 mg/m^2 day 1
  [total dose/cycle = 12 mg/m^2]
Tretinoin: Oral: 45 mg/m^2/day (in 2 divided doses) days 1 to 15 (if intermediate or high risk)
  [total dose/cycle = 675 mg/m^2]
Maintenance:
Mercaptopurine: Oral: 50 mg/m^2 daily
  [total dose/cycle = 4500 mg/m^2 (90 days)]
Methotrexate: I.M.: 15 mg/m^2 weekly
  [total dose/cycle = 180 mg/m^2]
Tretinoin: Oral: 45 mg/m^2/day (in 2 divided doses) days 1 to 15
  [total dose/cycle = 675 mg/m^2]
Repeat cycle every 3 months for 2 years

VAC Alternating With IE (Ewing Sarcoma)

Use Ewing sarcoma
Regimen
Cycle A: (Odd numbered cycles)
Cyclophosphamide: I.V.: 1200 mg/m^2 day 1 (followed by mesna; dose not specified)
  [total dose/cycle = 1200 mg/m^2]
Vincristine: I.V.: 2 mg/m^2 (maximum dose: 2 mg) day 1
  [total dose/cycle = 2 mg/m^2; maximum: 2 mg]
Doxorubicin: I.V.: 75 mg/m^2 day 1, for 5 cycles (maximum cumulative dose: 375 mg/m^2)
  [total dose/cycle = 75 mg/m^2; maximum cumulative dose: 375 mg/m^2]
Dactinomycin: I.V.: 1.25 mg/m^2 day 1, begin cycle 11 (after reaching maximum cumulative doxorubicin dose)
  [total dose/cycle = 1.25 mg/m^2]
Cycle B: (Even numbered cycles)
Ifosfamide: I.V.: 1800 mg/m^2/day days 1 to 5 (given with mesna)
  [total dose/cycle = 9000 mg/m^2]
Etoposide: I.V.: 100 mg/m^2/day days 1 to 5
  [total dose/cycle = 500 mg/m^2]
Alternate Cycles A and B, administering a cycle every 3 weeks (alternating in the following sequence: ABABAB) for 17 cycles

VAC Pulse

Use Rhabdomyosarcoma
Regimen
Vincristine: I.V.: 2 mg/m^2/dose (maximum dose: 2 mg/dose) every 7 days, for 12 weeks
Dactinomycin: I.V.: 0.015 mg/kg/day (maximum dose: 0.5 mg/day) days 1 to 5, every 3 months for 5 courses
Cyclophosphamide: Oral, I.V.: 10 mg/kg/day for 7 days, repeat every 6 weeks

VAC (Rhabdomyosarcoma)

Use Rhabdomyosarcoma
Regimen
Induction (weeks 1 to 17):
Vincristine: I.V. push: 1.5 mg/m^2 (maximum dose: 2 mg) day 1 of weeks 1 to 13, then one dose at week 17
Dactinomycin: I.V. push: 0.015 mg/kg/day (maximum dose: 0.5 mg) days 1 to 5 of weeks 1, 4, 7, and 17
Cyclophosphamide: I.V.: 2.2 g/m^2 day 1 of weeks 1, 4, 7, 10, 13, and 17
Continuation (weeks 21 to 44):
Vincristine: I.V. push: 1.5 mg/m^2 (maximum dose: 2 mg) day 1 of weeks 21 to 26, 30 to 35, and 39 to 44
Dactinomycin: I.V. push: 0.015 mg/kg/day (maximum dose: 0.5 mg) days 1 to 5 of weeks 21, 24, 30, 33, 39, and 42
Cyclophosphamide: I.V.: 2.2 g/m^2 day 1 of weeks 21, 24, 30, 33, 39, and 42

VAD

Use Multiple myeloma
Regimen
Vincristine: I.V.: 0.4 mg/day continuous infusion days 1 to 4
[total dose/cycle = 1.6 mg]
Doxorubicin: I.V.: 9 mg/m^2/day continuous infusion days 1 to 4
[total dose/cycle = 36 mg/m^2]
Dexamethasone: Oral: 40 mg/day days 1 to 4, 9 to 12, and 17 to 20
[total dose/cycle = 480 mg]
Repeat cycle every 28-35 days

VAD/CVAD

Use Leukemia, acute lymphocytic
Regimen Induction cycle:
Vincristine: I.V.: 0.4 mg/day continuous infusion days 1 to 4 and 24 to 27
[total dose/cycle = 3.2 mg]
Doxorubicin: I.V.: 12 mg/m^2/day continuous infusion days 1 to 4 and 24 to 27
[total dose/cycle = 96 mg/m^2]
Dexamethasone: Oral: 40 mg/day days 1 to 4, 9 to 12, 17 to 20, 24 to 27, 32 to 35, and 40 to 43
[total dose/cycle = 960 mg]
Cyclophosphamide: I.V.: 1 g/m^2 day 24
[total dose/cycle = 1 g/m^2]
Administer one cycle only

VBMCP (Multiple Myeloma)

Use Multiple myeloma
Regimen NOTE: Multiple variations are listed.
Variation 1:
Vincristine: I.V.: 1.2 mg/m^2 day 1
[total dose/cycle = 1.2 mg/m^2]
Carmustine: I.V.: 20 mg/m^2 day 1
[total dose/cycle = 20 mg/m^2]
Melphalan: Oral: 8 mg/m^2/day days 1 to 4
[total dose/cycle = 32 mg/m^2]
Cyclophosphamide: I.V.: 400 mg/m^2 day 1
[total dose/cycle = 400 mg/m^2]
Prednisone: Oral: 40 mg/m^2/day days 1 to 7
[total dose/cycle = 280 mg/m^2]
Repeat cycle every 35 days for up to 2 years or until disease progression
Variation 2:
Vincristine: I.V.: 1.2 mg/m^2 (maximum dose: 2 mg) day 1
[total dose/cycle = 1.2 mg/m^2; maximum: 2 mg]
Carmustine: I.V.: 20 mg/m^2 day 1
[total dose/cycle = 20 mg/m^2]
Melphalan: Oral: 8 mg/m^2/day days 1 to 4
[total dose/cycle = 32 mg/m^2]

◀ Cyclophosphamide: I.V.: 400 mg/m^2 day 1
  [total dose/cycle = 400 mg/m^2]
Prednisone: Oral: 40 mg/m^2/day days 1 to 7 (all cycles)
  [total dose/cycle = 280 mg/m^2]
    followed by Oral: 20 mg/m^2/day days 8 to 14 (first 3 cycles only)
    [total dose/cycle = 140 mg/m^2]
Repeat cycle every 35 days

VBP

Use Testicular cancer
Regimen
Vinblastine: I.V.: 0.15 mg/kg/day days 1 and 2
  [total dose/cycle = 0.3 mg/kg]
Bleomycin: I.V.: 30 units/day days 2, 9, and 16
  [total dose/cycle = 90 units]
Cisplatin: I.V.: 20 mg/m^2/day days 1 to 5
  [total dose/cycle = 100 mg/m^2]
Repeat cycle every 21 days for 4 cycles

VCAP

Use Multiple myeloma
Regimen
Vincristine: I.V.: 1 mg/m^2 (maximum dose: 1.5 mg) day 1
  [total dose/cycle = 1 mg/m^2]
Cyclophosphamide: Oral: 125 mg/m^2/day days 1 to 4
  [total dose/cycle = 500 mg/m^2]
Doxorubicin: I.V.: 30 mg/m^2 day 1
  [total dose/cycle = 30 mg/m^2]
Prednisone: Oral: 60 mg/m^2/day days 1 to 4
  [total dose/cycle = 240 mg/m^2]
Repeat cycle every 21 days for 6-12 months

VDA-C (Wilms Tumor)

Use Wilms tumor
Regimen
Dactinomycin: I.V.: 15 mcg/kg/day days 1 to 5 of weeks 0, 13, 26, 39, 52, and 65
  [total dose/cycle = 450 mcg/kg]
Cyclophosphamide: I.V.: 10 mg/kg/day days 1, 2, and 3 of weeks 6, 13, 19, 26, 32, 39, 45, 52, 58, and 65
  [total dose/cycle = 300 mg/kg]
Doxorubicin: I.V.: 20 mg/m^2/day days 1, 2, and 3 of weeks 6, 19, 32, 45, and 58
  [total dose/cycle = 300 mg/m^2]
Vincristine: I.V.: 1.5 mg/m^2 day 1 of weeks 1-10, 13, 14, 19, 20, 26, 27, 32, 33, 39, 40, 45, 46, 52, 53, 58, 59, 65, and 66
  [total dose/cycle = 42 mg/m^2]

VIM-D (Hodgkin Lymphoma)

Use Lymphoma, Hodgkin disease
Regimen
Etoposide: I.V.: 100 mg/m^2 over 30 minutes day 1
  [total dose/cycle = 100 mg/m^2]
Ifosfamide: I.V.: 4 g/m^2 continuous infusion over 24 hours day 1
  [total dose/cycle = 4 g/m^2]
Mesna: I.V.: 1 g/m^2 I.V. bolus day 1
    followed by: Mesna: I.V.: 6 g/m^2 continuous infusion over 36 hours
    [total dose/cycle = 7 g/m^2]
Mitoxantrone: I.V.: 10 mg/m^2 I.V. bolus day 1
  [total dose/cycle = 10 mg/m^2]
Dexamethasone: Oral: 40 mg/day days 1 to 5
  [total dose/cycle = 200 mg]
Repeat cycle every 28 days; treat 3 cycles post remission

Vincristine-Dactinomycin-Cyclophosphamide (Ovarian Cancer)

Use Ovarian cancer (germ cell tumor)

Regimen NOTE: Multiple variations are listed.

Variation 1:

Vincristine: I.V.: 1.5 mg/m^2 (maximum dose: 2 mg) days 1, 8, 15, and 22 for 2-3 cycles
[total dose/cycle = 6 mg/m^2 (maximum: 8 mg)] for 2-3 cycles
Dactinomycin: I.V.: 300 mcg/m^2/day days 1 to 5
[total dose/cycle = 1500 mcg/m^2]
Cyclophosphamide: I.V.: 150 mg/m^2/day days 1 to 5
[total dose/cycle = 750 mg/m^2]
Repeat cycle every 4 weeks for at least 10 cycles; vincristine is only administered for 8-12 weeks

Variation 2:

Vincristine: I.V.: 1-1.5 mg/m^2 day 1
[total dose/cycle = 1-1.5 mg/m^2]
Dactinomycin: I.V.: 500 mcg/day days 1 to 5
[total dose/cycle = 2500 mcg]
Cyclophosphamide: I.V.: 5-7 mg/kg/day days 1 to 5
[total dose/cycle = 25-35 mg/kg]
Repeat cycle every 4 weeks for up to 12 cycles

Vinorelbine-Cisplatin

Use Lung cancer, nonsmall cell

Regimen NOTE: Multiple variations are listed.

Variation 1:

Cisplatin: I.V.: 50 mg/m^2/day days 1 and 8
[total dose/cycle = 100 mg/m^2]
Vinorelbine: I.V.: 25 mg/m^2/day days 1, 8, 15, and 22
[total dose/cycle = 100 mg/m^2]
Repeat cycle every 28 days for total of 4 cycles

Variation 2:

Vinorelbine: I.V.: 25 mg/m^2/day days 1, 8, 15, and 22
[total dose/cycle = 100 mg/m^2]
Cisplatin: I.V.: 100 mg/m^2 day 1
[total dose/cycle = 100 mg/m^2]
Repeat cycle every 28 days

Variation 3:

Vinorelbine: I.V.: 30 mg/m^2 weekly
Cisplatin: I.V.: 120 mg/m^2/day days 1 and 29, then once every 6 weeks

Variation 4:

Vinorelbine: I.V.: 30 mg/m^2/day days 1, 8, and 15
[total dose/cycle = 90 mg/m^2]
Cisplatin: I.V.: 80 mg/m^2 day 1
[total dose/cycle = 80 mg/m^2]
Repeat cycle every 21 days for total of 4 cycles
Note: Vinorelbine treatment is discontinued after day 1 of cycle 4

Variation 5:

Vinorelbine: I.V.: 30 mg/m^2/day days 1, 8, 15, and 22
[total dose/cycle = 120 mg/m^2]
Cisplatin: I.V.: 100 mg/m^2 day 1
[total dose/cycle = 100 mg/m^2]
Repeat cycle every 28 days for total of 3 or 4 cycles
Note: Vinorelbine treatment is discontinued after day 1 of last treatment cycle

Vinorelbine-FEC

Use Breast cancer

Regimen

Cycles 1 and 2:

Vinorelbine: I.V.: 25 mg/m^2/day days 1, 8, and 15
[total dose/cycle = 75 mg/m^2]
Treatment cycle is 21 days

◀

Cycle 3:
 Vinorelbine: I.V.: 25 mg/m^2/day days 1 and 8
  [total dose/cycle 3 = 50 mg/m^2]
 Treatment cycle is 21 days
Cycles 4, 5, and 6 (FEC):
 Fluorouracil: I.V.: 600 mg/m^2 day 1
  [total dose/cycle = 600 mg/m^2]
 Epirubicin: I.V.: 60 mg/m^2 day 1
  [total dose/cycle = 60 mg/m^2]
 Cyclophosphamide: I.V.: 600 mg/m^2 day 1
  [total dose/cycle = 600 mg/m^2]
 Repeat FEC cycle every 21 days for total of 3 cycles

Vinorelbine-Trastuzumab

Use Breast cancer

Regimen
Week 1:
 Trastuzumab: I.V.: 4 mg/kg (loading dose) day 1 week 1
  [total dose/week 1 = 4 mg/kg]
 Vinorelbine: I.V.: 25 mg/m^2 day 1
  [total dose/week 1 = 25 mg/m^2]
Subsequent weeks:
 Trastuzumab: I.V.: 2 mg/kg (loading dose) day 1
  [total dose/week = 2 mg/kg]
 Vinorelbine: I.V.: 25 mg/m^2 day 1
  [total dose/week = 25 mg/m^2]
 Repeat weekly

Vinorelbine-Trastuzumab-FEC

Use Breast cancer

Regimen
Cycle 1:
 Trastuzumab: I.V.: 4 mg/kg (loading dose) day 1 cycle 1
 followed by I.V.: 2 mg/kg/day days 8 and 15 cycle 1
  [total dose/cycle 1 = 8 mg/kg]
 Vinorelbine: I.V.: 25 mg/m^2/day days 1, 8, and 15
  [total dose/cycle 1 = 75 mg/m^2]
 Treatment cycle is 21 days
Cycle 2:
 Trastuzumab: I.V.: 2 mg/kg/day days 1, 8, and 15
  [total dose/cycle = 6 mg/kg]
 Vinorelbine: I.V.: 25 mg/m^2/day days 1, 8, and 15
  [total dose/cycle 2 = 75 mg/m^2]
 Treatment cycle is 21 days
Cycle 3:
 Trastuzumab: I.V.: 2 mg/kg/day days 1, 8, and 15
  [total dose/cycle = 6 mg/kg]
 Vinorelbine: I.V.: 25 mg/m^2/day days 1 and 8
  [total dose/cycle 3 = 50 mg/m^2]
 Treatment cycle is 21 days
Cycles 4, 5, and 6 (FEC):
 Fluorouracil: I.V.: 600 mg/m^2 day 1
  [total dose/cycle = 600 mg/m^2]
 Epirubicin: I.V.: 60 mg/m^2 day 1
  [total dose/cycle = 60 mg/m^2]
 Cyclophosphamide: I.V.: 600 mg/m^2 day 1
  [total dose/cycle = 600 mg/m^2]
 Repeat FEC cycle every 21 days for total of 3 cycles

VIP (Etoposide) (Testicular Cancer)

Use Testicular cancer

Regimen NOTE: Multiple variations are listed.
Variation 1:
  Etoposide: I.V.: 75 mg/m^2/day days 1 to 5
    [total dose/cycle = 375 mg/m^2]
  Ifosfamide: I.V.: 1200 mg/m^2/day days 1 to 5
    [total dose/cycle = 6000 mg/m^2]
  Cisplatin: I.V.: 20 mg/m^2/day days 1 to 5
    [total dose/cycle = 100 mg/m^2]
  Mesna: I.V.: 400 mg/m^2 day 1 only
    followed by I.V.: 1200 mg/m^2/day continuous infusion days 1 to 5
      [total dose/cycle = 6400 mg/m^2]
  Repeat cycle every 21 days for 4 cycles
Variation 2:
  Etoposide: I.V.: 100 mg/m^2/day days 1 to 5
    [total dose/cycle = 500 mg/m^2]
  Ifosfamide: I.V.: 1200 mg/m^2/day days 1 to 5
    [total dose/cycle = 6000 mg/m^2]
  Cisplatin: I.V.: 20 mg/m^2/day days 1 to 5
    [total dose/cycle = 100 mg/m^2]
  Mesna: I.V.: 200 mg/m^2 every 4 hours, for 3 doses each day, days 1, 2, and 3
    [total dose/cycle = 1800 mg/m^2]
  Repeat cycle every 21 days
Variation 3:
  Ifosfamide: I.V.: 2500 mg/m^2/day days 1 and 2
    [total dose/cycle = 5000 mg/m^2]
  Mesna: I.V.: 2400 mg/m^2/day days 1 and 2
    [total dose/cycle = 4800 mg/m^2]
  Etoposide: I.V.: 100 mg/m^2/day days 3, 4, and 5
    [total dose/cycle = 300 mg/m^2]
  Cisplatin: I.V.: 40 mg/m^2/day days 3, 4, and 5
    [total dose/cycle = 120 mg/m^2]
  Repeat cycle every 21 days
Variation 4:
  Etoposide: I.V.: 75 mg/m^2/day days 1 to 5
    [total dose/cycle = 375 mg/m^2]
  Ifosfamide: I.V.: 1200 mg/m^2/day days 1 to 5
    [total dose/cycle = 6000 mg/m^2]
  Cisplatin: I.V.: 20 mg/m^2/day days 1 to 5
    [total dose/cycle = 100 mg/m^2]
  Mesna: I.V.: 120 mg/m^2 day 1 only
    followed by I.V.: 1200 mg/m^2/day continuous infusion days 1 to 5
      [total dose/cycle = 6120 mg/m^2]
  Repeat cycle every 21 days for 4 cycles

VIP (Small Cell Lung Cancer)

Use Lung cancer, small cell
Regimen
  Etoposide: I.V.: 75 mg/m^2/day days 1 to 4
    [total dose/cycle = 300 mg/m^2]
  Ifosfamide: I.V.: 1200 mg/m^2/day days 1 to 4
    [total dose/cycle = 4800 mg/m^2]
  Cisplatin: I.V.: 20 mg/m^2/day days 1 to 4
    [total dose/cycle = 80 mg/m^2]
  Mesna: I.V.: 300 mg/m^2 day 1 only
    followed by I.V.: 1200 mg/m^2/day continuous infusion days 1 to 4
      [total dose/cycle = 5100 mg/m^2]
  Repeat cycle every 21 days

VIP (Vinblastine) (Testicular Cancer)

Use Testicular cancer

◀ **Regimen** NOTE: Multiple variations are listed.
  Variation 1:
    Vinblastine: I.V.: 0.11 mg/kg/day days 1 and 2
      [total dose/cycle = 0.22 mg/kg]
    Ifosfamide: I.V.: 1200 mg/m^2/day days 1 to 5
      [total dose/cycle = 6000 mg/m^2]
    Cisplatin: I.V.: 20 mg/m^2/day days 1 to 5
      [total dose/cycle = 100 mg/m^2]
    Mesna: I.V.: 400 mg/m^2 day 1
    followed by I.V.: 1200 mg/m^2/day continuous infusion days 1 to 5
      [total dose/cycle = 6400 mg/m^2]
    Repeat cycle every 21 days for 4 cycles
  Variation 2:
    Vinblastine: I.V.: 6 mg/m^2/day days 1 and 2
      [total dose/cycle = 12 mg/m^2]
    Ifosfamide: I.V.: 1500 mg/m^2/day days 1 to 5
      [total dose/cycle = 7500 mg/m^2]
    Cisplatin: I.V.: 20 mg/m^2/day days 1 to 5
      [total dose/cycle = 100 mg/m^2]
    Mesna: I.V.: 300 mg/m^2 3 times/day days 1 to 5
      [total dose/cycle = 4500 mg/m^2]
    Repeat cycle every 21 days for 4 cycles

VP (Small Cell Lung Cancer)

Use Lung cancer, small cell

Regimen
  Etoposide: I.V.: 100 mg/m^2/day days 1 to 4
    [total dose/cycle = 400 mg/m^2]
  Cisplatin: I.V.: 20 mg/m^2/day days 1 to 4
    [total dose/cycle = 80 mg/m^2]
  Repeat cycle every 21 days

CHEMOTHERAPY REGIMEN INDEX

◀ **GASTROINTESTINAL**

Pancreatic Cancer

GENITOURINARY

Bladder Cancer

Prostate Cancer

Renal Cell Cancer

Testicular Cancer

APPENDIX TABLE OF CONTENTS

Visit the**Point** http://thepoint.lww.com/QL2012 for exclusive access to:

Apothecary/Metric Conversions

Pounds/Kilograms Conversion

Temperature Conversion

Pharmaceutical Manufacturers and Distributors

Multivitamin Products

Refer to the inside front cover of this book for your online access code.

ABBREVIATIONS & SYMBOLS COMMONLY USED IN MEDICAL ORDERS

Abbreviations Which May Be Used in This Reference

Abbreviation	Meaning
5-HT	5-hydroxytryptamine
AAP	American Academy of Pediatrics
ABG	arterial blood gases
ABW	adjusted body weight
AACT	American Academy of Clinical Toxicology
ACC	American College of Cardiology
ACE	angiotensin converting enzyme
ACLS	advanced cardiac life support
ACOG	American College of Obstetricians and Gynecologists
ACTH	adrenocorticotrophic hormone
ADH	alcohol dehydrogenase
ADHD	attention-deficit/hyperactivity disorder
ADLs	activities of daily living
AED	antiepileptic drug
AHA	American Heart Association
AIDS	acquired immune deficiency syndrome
AIMS	Abnormal Involuntary Movement Scale
ALS	amyotrophic lateral sclerosis
ALT	alanine aminotransferase
AMA	American Medical Association
ANC	absolute neutrophil count
aPTT	activated partial thromboplastin
ARB	angiotensin receptor blocker
ARDS	acute respiratory distress syndrome
AST	aspartate aminotransferase
AUC	area under the curve
BDI	Beck Depression Inventory
BEC	blood ethanol concentration
BLS	basic life support
BMI	body mass index
BMT	bone marrow transplant
BP	blood pressure
BPH	benign prostatic hyperplasia
BPRS	Brief Psychiatric Rating Scale
BSA	body surface area
BUN	blood urea nitrogen
CABG	coronary artery bypass graft
CAD	coronary artery disease
CAN	Canadian
CAPD	continuous ambulatory peritoneal dialysis
CAS	chemical abstract service
CBC	complete blood count
CBT	cognitive behavioral therapy
Cl_{cr}	creatinine clearance

Abbreviations Which May Be Used in This Reference (continued)

Abbreviation	Meaning
CDC	Centers for Disease Control and Prevention
CF	cystic fibrosis
CGI	Clinical Global Impression
CHD	coronary heart disease
CHF	congestive heart failure; chronic heart failure
CIE	chemotherapy-induced emesis
C-II	schedule two controlled substance
C-III	schedule three controlled substance
C-IV	schedule four controlled substance
C-V	schedule five controlled substance
CIV	continuous I.V. infusion
C_{max}	maximum plasma concentration
C_{min}	minimum plasma concentration
CMV	cytomegalovirus
CNS	central nervous system or coagulase negative staphylococcus
COLD	chronic obstructive lung disease
COPD	chronic obstructive pulmonary disease
COX	cyclooxygenase
CPK	creatine phosphokinase
CRF	chronic renal failure
CRP	C-reactive protein
CRRT	continuous renal replacement therapy
CSF	cerebrospinal fluid
CSII	continuous subcutaneous insulin infusion
CT	computed tomography
CVA	cerebrovascular accident
CVVH	continuous venovenous hemofiltration
CVVHD	continuous venovenous hemodialysis
CVVHDF	continuous venovenous hemodiafiltration
CYP	cytochrome
D_5W	dextrose 5% in water
DBP	diastolic blood pressure
DEHP	di(3-ethylhexyl)phthalate
DIC	disseminated intravascular coagulation
DM	diabetes mellitus
DMARD	disease modifying antirheumatic drug
DSC	discontinued
DSM-IV	Diagnostic and Statistical Manual
DVT	deep vein thrombosis
EBV	Epstein-Barr virus
ECG	electrocardiogram
ECMO	extracorporeal membrane oxygenation
ECT	electroconvulsive therapy
ED	emergency department
EEG	electroencephalogram
EF	ejection fraction
EG	ethylene glycol
EGA	estimated gestational age
EIA	enzyme immunoassay

Abbreviation	Meaning
ELISA	enzyme-linked immunosorbent assay
EPS	extrapyramidal side effects
ESR	erythrocyte sedimentation rate
ESRD	end stage renal disease
EtOH	alcohol
FDA	Food and Drug Administration
FTT	failure to thrive
GABA	gamma-aminobutyric acid
GAD	generalized anxiety disorder
GERD	gastroesophageal reflux disease
GFR	glomerular filtration rate
GGT	gamma-glutamyltransferase
GI	gastrointestinal
GU	genitourinary
GVHD	graft versus host disease
HAM-A	Hamilton Anxiety Scale
HAM-D	Hamilton Depression Scale
HDL	high density lipoprotein
HF	heart failure
HFSA	Heart Failure Society of America
HIV	human immunodeficiency virus
HMG-CoA	3-hydroxy-3-methylglutaryl-coenzyme A
HOCM	hypertrophic obstructive cardiomyopathy
HPA	hypothalamic-pituitary-adrenal
HSV	herpes simplex virus
HTN	hypertension
HUS	hemolytic uremic syndrome
IBD	inflammatory bowel disease
IBS	irritable bowel syndrome
IBW	ideal body weight
ICD	implantable cardioverter defibrillator
ICH	intracranial hemorrhage
ICP	intracranial pressure
IDDM	insulin dependent diabetes mellitus
IDSA	Infectious Diseases Society of America
IHSS	idiopathic hypertrophic subaortic stenosis
I.M.	intramuscular
INR	international normalized ration
Int. unit	international unit
IOP	intraocular pressure
IUGR	intrauterine growth retardation
I.V.	intravenous
JIA	juvenile idiopathic arthritis
JNC	Joint National Committee
KIU	kallikrein inhibitor unit
LAMM	L-α-acetyl methadol
LDH	lactate dehydrogenase
LDL	low density lipoprotein
LFT	liver function test

Abbreviations Which May Be Used in This Reference *(continued)*

Abbreviation	Meaning
LGA	large for gestational age
LR	lactated ringers
LVEF	left ventricular ejection fraction
LVH	left ventricular hypertrophy
MADRS	Montgomery Asbery Depression Rating Scale
MAOIs	monamine oxidase inhibitors
MDD	major depressive disorder
MDRD	modification of diet in renal disease
MDRSP	multidrug resistant *streptococcus pneumoniae*
mEq	milliequivalent
mg	milligram
MI	myocardial infarction
mL	milliliter
mm	millimeter
mM	millimolar
mm Hg	millimeters of mercury
MMSE	mini mental status examination
M/P	milk to plasma ratio
MPS I	mucopolysaccharidosis I
MRHD	maximum recommended human dose
MRI	magnetic resonance imaging
MUGA	multiple gated acquisition scan
NAS	neonatal abstinence syndrome
NF	National Formulary
NFD	Nephrogenic fibrosing dermopathy
ng	nanogram
NIDDM	Noninsulin dependent diabetes mellitus
NKA	no known allergies
NKDA	No known drug allergies
NMDA	n-methyl-d-aspartic acid
NMS	neuroleptic malignant syndrome
NNRTI	nonnucleoside reverse transcriptase inhibitor
NRTI	nucleoside reverse transcriptase inhibitor
NS	normal saline
NSAID	nonsteroidal antiinflammatory drug
NSF	nephrogenic systemic fibrosis
NSTEMI	Non-ST-elevation myocardial infarction
OA	osteoarthritis
OCD	obsessive-compulsive disorder
OHSS	ovarian hyperstimulation syndrome
OTC	over-the-counter
PAT	paroxysmal atrial tachycardia
PD	Parkinson disease; peritoneal dialysis
PDA	patent ductus arteriosus
PDE-5	phosphodiesterase-5
PE	pulmonary embolus
PEG tube	percutaneous endoscopic gastrostomy tube
PHN	post-herpetic neuralgia
PID	pelvic inflammatory disease

Abbreviations Which May Be Used in This Reference *(continued)*

Abbreviation	Meaning
PMDD	premenstrual dysphoric disorder
PONV	postoperative nausea and vomiting
PPN	peripheral parenteral nutrition
PROM	premature rupture of membranes
PSVT	paroxysmal supraventricular tachycardia
PT	prothrombin time
PTSD	post-traumatic stress disorder
PTT	partial thromboplastin time
PUD	peptic ulcer disease
PVD	peripheral vascular disease
QT_c	corrected QT interval
QT_c-F	corrected QT interval by Fredricia formula
RA	rheumatoid arthritis
REM	rapid eye movement
RPLS	reversible posterior leukoencephalopathy syndrome
SA	sinoatrial
SAD	seasonal affective disorder
SAH	subarachnoid hemorrhage
SBE	subacute bacterial endocarditis
SBP	systolic blood pressure
S_{Cr}	serum creatinine
SERM	selective estrogen receptor modulator
SGA	small for gestational age
SGOT	serum glutamic oxaloacetic aminotransferase
SGPT	serum glutamic pyruvate transaminase
SI	International System of Units or Systeme international d'Unites
SIADH	syndrome of inappropriate antidiuretic hormone secretion
SLE	systemic lupus erythematosus
SNRI	serotonin norepinephrine reuptake inhibitor
SSKI	saturated solution of potassium iodide
SSRIs	selective serotonin reuptake inhibitors
STD	sexually transmitted disease
STEM I	ST-elevation myocardial infarction
SubQ	subcutaneous
supp	suppository
SVT	supraventricular tachycardia
SWFI	sterile water for injection
syr	syrup
$T_{1/2}$	half-life
tab	tablet
TB	tuberculosis
TC	total cholesterol
TCA	tricyclic antidepressant
TD	tardive dyskinesia
TG	triglyceride
TIA	transient ischemic attack
TMA	thrombotic microangiopathy
T_{max}	time to maximum observed concentration, plasma
TNF	Tumor necrosis factor

Abbreviations Which May Be Used in This Reference *(continued)*

Abbreviation	Meaning
TPN	total parenteral nutrition
tr, tinct	tincture
tsp	teaspoonful
UC	ulcerative colitis
ULN	upper limits of normal
URI	upper respiratory infection
USAN	United States Adopted Names
USP	United States Pharmacopeia
UTI	urinary tract infection
UV	ultraviolet
V_d	volume of distribution
VEGF	vascular endothelial growth factor
VF	ventricular fibrillation
VT	ventricular tachycardia
VTE	venous thromboembolism
vWD	von Willebrand disease
VZV	varicella zoster virus
YBOC	Yale Brown Obsessive-Compulsive Scale
YMRS	Young Mania Rating Scale

Common Weights, Measures, or Apothecary Abbreviations

Abbreviation	Meaning
<[1]	less than
>[1]	greater than
≤	less than or equal to
≥	greater than or equal to
ac	before meals or food
ad	to, up to
ad lib	at pleasure
AM	morning
AMA	against medical advice
amp	ampul
amt	amount
aq	water
aq. dest.	distilled water
ASAP	as soon as possible
a.u.[1]	each ear
bid	twice daily
bm	bowel movement
C	Celsius, centigrade
cal	calorie
cap	capsule
cc[1]	cubic centimeter
cm	centimeter
comp	compound
cont	continue
d	day

Common Weights, Measures, or Apothecary Abbreviations *(continued)*

Abbreviation	Meaning
d/c[1]	discharge
dil	dilute
disp	dispense
div	divide
dtd	give of such a dose
Dx	diagnosis
elix, el	elixir
emp	as directed
et	and
ex aq	in water
F	Fahrenheit
f, ft	make, let be made
g	gram
gr	grain
gtt	a drop
h	hour
hs[1]	at bedtime
kcal	kilocalorie
kg	kilogram
L	liter
liq	a liquor, solution
M	molar
mcg	microgram
m. dict	as directed
mEq	milliequivalent
mg	milligram
microL	microliter
mL	milliliter
mm	millimeter
mM	millimolar
mm Hg	millimeters of mercury
ng	nanogram
no.	number
noc	in the night
non rep	do not repeat, no refills
NPO	nothing by mouth
NV	nausea and vomiting
O, Oct	a pint
o.d.[1]	right eye
o.l.	left eye
o.s.[1]	left eye
o.u.[1]	each eye, both eyes together
pc, post cib	after meals
PM	afternoon or evening
P.O.	by mouth
P.R.	rectally
prn	as needed
pulv	a powder
q	every

Common Weights, Measures, or Apothecary Abbreviations *(continued)*

Abbreviation	Meaning
qad	every other day
qd[1,2]	every day, daily
qh	every hour
qid	four times a day
qod[1,2]	every other day
qs	a sufficient quantity
qs ad	a sufficient quantity to make
Rx	take, a recipe
SL	sublingual
stat	at once, immediately
SubQ	subcutaneous
supp	suppository
syr	syrup
tab	tablet
tal	such
tid	three times a day
tr, tinct	tincture
trit	triturate
tsp	teaspoon
u.d.	as directed
ung	ointment
v.o.	verbal order
w.a.	while awake
x3	3 times
x4	4 times

[1]ISMP error-prone abbreviation.

[2]JCAHO Do Not Use list.

Additional abbreviations used and defined within a specific monograph or text piece may only apply to that text.

References

The Institute for Safe Medication Practices (ISMP) list of Error-Prone Abbreviations, Symbols, and Dose Designations. Available at: http://www.ismp.org/Tools/errorproneabbreviations.pdf.

The Joint Commission Official "Do Not Use" list. Available at: http://www.jointcommission.org/PatientSafety/DoNotUseList/.

NORMAL LABORATORY VALUES FOR ADULTS

CHEMISTRY

Test	Values	Remarks
Serum / Plasma		
Acetone	Negative	
Albumin	3.2-5 g/dL	
Alcohol, ethyl	Negative	
Aldolase	1.2-7.6 IU/L	
Ammonia	20-70 mcg/dL	Specimen to be placed on ice as soon as collected.
Amylase	30-110 units/L	
Bilirubin, direct	0-0.3 mg/dL	
Bilirubin, total	0.1-1.2 mg/dL	
Calcium	8.6-10.3 mg/dL	
Calcium, ionized	2.24-2.46 mEq/L	
Chloride	95-108 mEq/L	
Cholesterol, total	≤200 mg/dL	Fasted blood required – normal value affected by dietary habits. This reference range is for a general adult population.
HDL cholesterol	40-60 mg/dL	Fasted blood required – normal value affected by dietary habits.
LDL cholesterol	<160 mg/dL	If triglyceride is >400 mg/dL, LDL cannot be calculated accurately (Friedewald equation). Target LDL-C depends on patient's risk factors.
CO_2	23-30 mEq/L	
Creatine kinase (CK) isoenzymes		
CK-BB	0%	
CK-MB (cardiac)	0%-3.9%	
CK-MM (muscle)	96%-100%	
CK-MB levels must be both ≥4% and 10 IU/L to meet diagnostic criteria for CK-MB positive result consistent with myocardial injury.		
Creatine phosphokinase (CPK)	8-150 IU/L	
Creatinine	0.5-1.4 mg/dL	
Ferritin	13-300 ng/mL	
Folate	3.6-20 ng/dL	
GGT (gamma-glutamyltranspeptidase)		
male	11-63 IU/L	
female	8-35 IU/L	
GLDH	To be determined	
Glucose (preprandial)	<115 mg/dL	Goals different for diabetics.
Glucose, fasting	60-110 mg/dL	Goals different for diabetics.
Glucose, nonfasting (2-h postprandial)	<120 mg/dL	Goals different for diabetics.
Hemoglobin A_{1c}	<8	
Hemoglobin, plasma free	<2.5 mg/100 mL	
Hemoglobin, total glycosolated (Hb A_1)	4%-8%	
Iron	65-150 mcg/dL	
Iron binding capacity, total (TIBC)	250-420 mcg/dL	
Lactic acid	0.7-2.1 mEq/L	Specimen to be kept on ice and sent to lab as soon as possible.
Lactate dehydrogenase (LDH)	56-194 IU/L	

CHEMISTRY *(continued)*

Test	Values	Remarks
Lactate dehydrogenase (LDH) isoenzymes		
LD_1	20%-34%	
LD_2	29%-41%	
LD_3	15%-25%	
LD_4	1%-12%	
LD_5	1%-15%	

Flipped LD_1/LD_2 ratios (>1 may be consistent with myocardial injury) particularly when considered in combination with a recent CK-MB positive result.

Test	Values	Remarks
Lipase	23-208 units/L	
Magnesium	1.6-2.5 mg/dL	Increased by slight hemolysis.
Osmolality	289-308 mOsm/kg	
Phosphatase, alkaline		
adults 25-60 y	33-131 IU/L	
adults ≥61 y	51-153 IU/L	
infancy-adolescence	Values range up to 3-5 times higher than adults	
Phosphate, inorganic	2.8-4.2 mg/dL	
Potassium	3.5-5.2 mEq/L	Increased by slight hemolysis.
Prealbumin	>15 mg/dL	
Protein, total	6.5-7.9 g/dL	
AST	<35 IU/L (20-48)	
ALT (10-35)	<35 IU/L	
Sodium	134-149 mEq/L	
Thyroid stimulating hormone (TSH)		
adults ≤20 y	0.7-6.4 mIU/L	
21-54 y	0.4-4.2 mIU/L	
55-87 y	0.5-8.9 mIU/L	
Transferrin	>200 mg/dL	
Triglycerides	45-155 mg/dL	Fasted blood required.
Troponin I	<1.5 ng/mL	
Urea nitrogen (BUN)	7-20 mg/dL	
Uric acid		
male	2-8 mg/dL	
female	2-7.5 mg/dL	
Cerebrospinal Fluid		
Glucose	50-70 mg/dL	
Protein	15-45 mg/dL	CSF obtained by lumbar puncture.

Note: Bloody specimen gives erroneously high value due to contamination with blood proteins

Urine
(24-hour specimen is required for all these tests unless specified)

Test	Values	Remarks
Amylase	32-641 units/L	The value is in units/L and **not** calculated for total volume.
Amylase, fluid (random samples)		Interpretation of value left for physician, depends on the nature of fluid.
Calcium	Depends upon dietary intake	
Creatine		
male	150 mg/24 h	Higher value on children and during pregnancy.
female	250 mg/24 h	
Creatinine	1000-2000 mg/24 h	
Creatinine clearance (endogenous)		
male	85-125 mL/min	A blood sample must accompany urine specimen.
female	75-115 mL/min	

CHEMISTRY *(continued)*

Test	Values	Remarks
Glucose	1 g/24 h	
5-hydroxyindoleacetic acid	2-8 mg/24 h	
Iron	0.15 mg/24 h	Acid washed container required.
Magnesium	146-209 mg/24 h	
Osmolality	500-800 mOsm/kg	With normal fluid intake.
Oxalate	10-40 mg/24 h	
Phosphate	400-1300 mg/24 h	
Potassium	25-120 mEq/24 h	Varies with diet; the interpretation of urine electrolytes and osmolality should be left for the physician.
Sodium	40-220 mEq/24 h	
Porphobilinogen, qualitative	Negative	
Porphyrins, qualitative	Negative	
Proteins	0.05-0.1 g/24 h	
Salicylate	Negative	
Urea clearance	60-95 mL/min	A blood sample must accompany specimen.
Urea N	10-40 g/24 h	Dependent on protein intake.
Uric acid	250-750 mg/24 h	Dependent on diet and therapy.
Urobilinogen	0.5-3.5 mg/24 h	For qualitative determination on random urine, send sample to urinalysis section in Hematology Lab.
Xylose absorption test children	16%-33% of ingested xylose	

Feces

Test	Values	Remarks
Fat, 3-day collection	<5 g/d	Value depends on fat intake of 100 g/d for 3 days preceding and during collection.

Gastric Acidity

Test	Values	Remarks
Acidity, total, 12 h	10-60 mEq/L	Titrated at pH 7.

Blood Gases

	Arterial	Capillary	Venous
pH	7.35-7.45	7.35-7.45	7.32-7.42
pCO_2 (mm Hg)	35-45	35-45	38-52
pO_2 (mm Hg)	70-100	60-80	24-48
HCO_3 (mEq/L)	19-25	19-25	19-25
TCO_2 (mEq/L)	19-29	19-29	23-33
O_2 saturation (%)	90-95	90-95	40-70
Base excess (mEq/L)	-5 to +5	-5 to +5	-5 to +5

HEMATOLOGY
Complete Blood Count

Age	Hgb (g/dL)	Hct (%)	RBC (mill/mm^3)	RDW
0-3 d	15.0-20.0	45-61	4.0-5.9	<18
1-2 wk	12.5-18.5	39-57	3.6-5.5	<17
1-6 mo	10.0-13.0	29-42	3.1-4.3	<16.5
7 mo to 2 y	10.5-13.0	33-38	3.7-4.9	<16
2-5 y	11.5-13.0	34-39	3.9-5.0	<15
5-8 y	11.5-14.5	35-42	4.0-4.9	<15
13-18 y	12.0-15.2	36-47	4.5-5.1	<14.5
Adult male	13.5-16.5	41-50	4.5-5.5	<14.5
Adult female	12.0-15.0	36-44	4.0-4.9	<14.5

Age	MCV (fL)	MCH (pg)	MCHC (%)	Plts (x 10^3/mm^3)
0-3 d	95-115	31-37	29-37	250-450
1-2 wk	86-110	28-36	28-38	250-450
1-6 mo	74-96	25-35	30-36	300-700
7 mo to 2 y	70-84	23-30	31-37	250-600
2-5 y	75-87	24-30	31-37	250-550
5-8 y	77-95	25-33	31-37	250-550
13-18 y	78-96	25-35	31-37	150-450
Adult male	80-100	26-34	31-37	150-450
Adult female	80-100	26-34	31-37	150-450

WBC and Differential

Age	WBC (x 10^3/mm^3)	Segs	Bands	Lymphs	Monos
0-3 d	9.0-35.0	32-62	10-18	19-29	5-7
1-2 wk	5.0-20.0	14-34	6-14	36-45	6-10
1-6 mo	6.0-17.5	13-33	4-12	41-71	4-7
7 mo to 2 y	6.0-17.0	15-35	5-11	45-76	3-6
2-5 y	5.5-15.5	23-45	5-11	35-65	3-6
5-8 y	5.0-14.5	32-54	5-11	28-48	3-6
13-18 y	4.5-13.0	34-64	5-11	25-45	3-6
Adults	4.5-11.0	35-66	5-11	24-44	3-6

Age	Eosinophils	Basophils	Atypical Lymphs	No. of NRBCs
0-3 d	0-2	0-1	0-8	0-2
1-2 wk	0-2	0-1	0-8	0
1-6 mo	0-3	0-1	0-8	0
7 mo to 2 y	0-3	0-1	0-8	0
2-5 y	0-3	0-1	0-8	0
5-8 y	0-3	0-1	0-8	0
13-18 y	0-3	0-1	0-8	0
Adults	0-3	0-1	0-8	0

Segs = segmented neutrophils.
Bands = band neutrophils.
Lymphs = lymphocytes.
Monos = monocytes.

Erythrocyte Sedimentation Rates and Reticulocyte Counts

Sedimentation rate, Westergren	Children	0-20 mm/h
	Adult male	0-15 mm/h
	Adult female	0-20 mm/h
Sedimentation rate, Wintrobe	Children	0-13 mm/h
	Adult male	0-10 mm/h
	Adult female	0-15 mm/h
Reticulocyte count	Newborns	2%-6%
	1-6 mo	0%-2.8%
	Adults	0.5%-1.5%

NORMAL LABORATORY VALUES FOR CHILDREN

		Normal Values
CHEMISTRY		
Albumin	0-1 y	2-4 g/dL
	1 y to adult	3.5-5.5 g/dL
Ammonia	Newborns	90-150 mcg/dL
	Children	40-120 mcg/dL
	Adults	18-54 mcg/dL
Amylase	Newborns	0-60 units/L
	Adults	30-110 units/L
Bilirubin, conjugated, direct	Newborns	<1.5 mg/dL
	1 mo to adult	0-0.5 mg/dL
Bilirubin, total	0-3 d	2-10 mg/dL
	1 mo to adult	0-1.5 mg/dL
Bilirubin, unconjugated, indirect		0.6-10.5 mg/dL
Calcium	Newborns	7-12 mg/dL
	0-2 y	8.8-11.2 mg/dL
	2 y to adult	9-11 mg/dL
Calcium, ionized, whole blood		4.4-5.4 mg/dL
Carbon dioxide, total		23-33 mEq/L
Chloride		95-105 mEq/L
Cholesterol	Newborns	45-170 mg/dL
	0-1 y	65-175 mg/dL
	1-20 y	120-230 mg/dL
Creatinine	0-1 y	≤0.6 mg/dL
	1 y to adult	0.5-1.5 mg/dL
Glucose	Newborns	30-90 mg/dL
	0-2 y	60-105 mg/dL
	Children to Adults	70-110 mg/dL
Iron		
	Newborns	110-270 mcg/dL
	Infants	30-70 mcg/dL
	Children	55-120 mcg/dL
	Adults	70-180 mcg/dL
Iron binding	Newborns	59-175 mcg/dL
	Infants	100-400 mcg/dL
	Adults	250-400 mcg/dL
Lactic acid, lactate		2-20 mg/dL
Lead, whole blood		<10 mcg/dL
Lipase		
	Children	20-140 units/L
	Adults	0-190 units/L
Magnesium		1.5-2.5 mEq/L
Osmolality, serum		275-296 mOsm/kg
Osmolality, urine		50-1400 mOsm/kg

(continued)

		Normal Values
Phosphorus	Newborns	4.2-9 mg/dL
	6 wk to 19 mo	3.8-6.7 mg/dL
	19 mo to 3 y	2.9-5.9 mg/dL
	3-15 y	3.6-5.6 mg/dL
	>15 y	2.5-5 mg/dL
Potassium, plasma	Newborns	4.5-7.2 mEq/L
	2 d to 3 mo	4-6.2 mEq/L
	3 mo to 1 y	3.7-5.6 mEq/L
	1-16 y	3.5-5 mEq/L
Protein, total	0-2 y	4.2-7.4 g/dL
	>2 y	6-8 g/dL
Sodium		136-145 mEq/L
Triglycerides	Infants	0-171 mg/dL
	Children	20-130 mg/dL
	Adults	30-200 mg/dL
Urea nitrogen, blood	0-2 y	4-15 mg/dL
	2 y to Adult	5-20 mg/dL
Uric acid	Male	3-7 mg/dL
	Female	2-6 mg/dL

ENZYMES

Alanine aminotransferase (ALT)	0-2 mo	8-78 units/L
	>2 mo	8-36 units/L
Alkaline phosphatase (ALKP)	Newborns	60-130 units/L
	0-16 y	85-400 units/L
	>16 y	30-115 units/L
Aspartate aminotransferase (AST)	Infants	18-74 units/L
	Children	15-46 units/L
	Adults	5-35 units/L
Creatine kinase (CK)	Infants	20-200 units/L
	Children	10-90 units/L
	Adult male	0-206 units/L
	Adult female	0-175 units/L
Lactate dehydrogenase (LDH)	Newborns	290-501 units/L
	1 mo to 2 y	110-144 units/L
	>16 y	60-170 units/L

Blood Gases

	Arterial	Capillary	Venous
pH	7.35-7.45	7.35-7.45	7.32-7.42
pCO_2 (mm Hg)	35-45	35-45	38-52
pO_2 (mm Hg)	70-100	60-80	24-48
HCO_3 (mEq/L)	19-25	19-25	19-25
TCO_2 (mEq/L)	19-29	19-29	23-33
O_2 saturation (%)	90-95	90-95	40-70
Base excess (mEq/L)	-5 to +5	-5 to +5	-5 to +5

Thyroid Function Tests

T$_4$ (thyroxine)	1-7 d	10.1-20.9 mcg/dL
	8-14 d	9.8-16.6 mcg/dL
	1 mo to 1 y	5.5-16 mcg/dL
	>1 y	4-12 mcg/dL
FTI	1-3 d	9.3-26.6
	1-4 wk	7.6-20.8
	1-4 mo	7.4-17.9
	4-12 mo	5.1-14.5
	1-6 y	5.7-13.3
	>6 y	4.8-14
T$_3$ by RIA	Newborns	100-470 ng/dL
	1-5 y	100-260 ng/dL
	5-10 y	90-240 ng/dL
	10 y to Adult	70-210 ng/dL
T$_3$ uptake		35%-45%
TSH	Cord	3-22 µIU/mL
	1-3 d	<40 µIU/mL
	3-7 d	<25 µIU/mL
	>7 d	0-10 µIU/mL

ACQUIRED IMMUNODEFICIENCY SYNDROME (AIDS) - LAB TESTS AND APPROVED DRUGS FOR HIV INFECTION AND AIDS-RELATED CONDITIONS

This list of tests is not intended in any way to suggest patterns of physician's orders, nor is it complete. These tests may support possible clinical diagnoses or rule out other diagnostic possibilities. Each laboratory test relevant to AIDS is listed and weighted. Two symbols (**) indicate that the test is diagnostic, that is, documents the diagnosis if the expected is found. A single symbol (*) indicates a test frequently used in the diagnosis or management of the disease. The other listed tests are useful on a selective basis with consideration of clinical factors and specific aspects of the case.

Acid-Fast Stain
Acid-Fast Stain, Modified, *Nocardia* Species
Antimicrobial Susceptibility Testing, Fungi
Antimicrobial Susceptibility Testing, Mycobacteria
Babesiosis Serological Test
Bacteremia Detection, Buffy Coat Micromethod
Bacterial Culture, Blood
Bacterial Culture, Bronchoscopy Specimen
Bacterial Culture, Sputum
Bacterial Culture, Stool
Bacterial Culture, Throat
Bacterial Culture, Urine, Clean Catch
Beta$_2$-Microglobulin
Blood and Fluid Precautions, Specimen Collection
Bronchial Washings Cytology
Bronchoalveolar Lavage Cytology
Brushings Cytology
Candida Antigen
Candidiasis Serologic Test
Cat Scratch Disease Serology
CD4/CD8 Enumeration
Cerebrospinal Fluid Cytology
Cryptococcal Antigen Titer
Cryptosporidium Diagnostic Procedures
Cytomegalic Inclusion Disease Cytology
Cytomegalovirus Antibody
Cytomegalovirus Antigen Detection
Cytomegalovirus Culture
Cytomegalovirus DNA Detection
Darkfield Examination, Syphilis
Electron Microscopy
Folic Acid, Serum
Fungal Culture, Biopsy or Body Fluid
Fungal Culture, Blood
Fungal Culture, Cerebrospinal Fluid
Fungal Culture, Sputum
Fungal Culture, Stool
Fungal Culture, Urine
Hemoglobin A$_2$
Hepatitis B Surface Antigen
Herpes Cytology
Herpes Simplex Virus Antigen Detection
Herpes Simplex Virus Culture
Histopathology
Histoplasmosis Antibody
Histoplasmosis Antigen
**HIV-1/HIV-2 Serology
HTLV-I/II Antibody
*Human Immunodeficiency Virus Culture
*Human Immunodeficiency Virus DNA Amplification
Human Immunodeficiency Virus, Rapid Test, Qualitative

Human Immunodeficiency Virus, Resistance/Susceptibility Testing
Human Immunodeficiency Virus, Viral Load Assay
India Ink Preparation
Inhibitor, Lupus, Phospholipid Type
KOH Preparation
Leishmaniasis Serological Test
Leukocyte Immunophenotyping
Lymphocyte Enumeration Test
Lymphocyte Transformation Test
Microsporidia Diagnostic Procedures
Mycobacteria by DNA Probe
Mycobacterial Culture, Biopsy or Body Fluid
Mycobacterial Culture, Cerebrospinal Fluid
Mycobacterial Culture, Cutaneous and Subcutaneous Tissue
Mycobacterial Culture, Sputum
Mycobacterial Culture, Stool
Neisseria gonorrhoeae Culture and Smear
Nocardia Culture
Ova and Parasites, Stool
*p24 Antigen
Platelet Count
Pneumocystis carinii Preparation
Pneumocystis Immunofluorescence
Polymerase Chain Reaction
Red Blood Cell Indices
Risks of Transfusion
Skin Biopsy
Sputum Cytology
Toxoplasmosis Serology
VDRL, Serum
Viral Culture
Viral Culture, Blood
Viral Culture, Body Fluid
Viral Culture, Central Nervous System Symptoms
Viral Culture, Dermatological Symptoms
Viral Culture, Tissue
Virus, Direct Detection by Fluorescent Antibody
White Blood Count

FDA-APPROVED AND INVESTIGATIONAL ANTIRETROVIRAL DRUGS

Antiretroviral Drugs

Generic Name	Also Known As	Brand Name	FDA Status
NUCLEOSIDE/NUCLEOTIDE ANALOG REVERSE TRANSCRIPTASE INHIBITORS (NRTIs)			
abacavir	ABC	Ziagen®	Approved
apricitabine	AVX754	—	Investigational
didanosine	ddI	Videx®; Videx® EC	Approved
elvucitabine	ACH-126,443; Beta-L-Fd4C	—	Investigational
emtricitabine	FTC	Emtriva®	Approved
lamiVUDine	3TC	Epivir®	Approved
stavudine	d4T	Zerit®	Approved
tenofovir	TDF	Viread®	Approved
zidovudine	ZDV	Retrovir®	Approved
—	RCV	Racivir	Investigational
NONNUCLEOSIDE REVERSE TRANSCRIPTASE INHIBITORS (NNRTIs)			
delavirdine	DLV	Rescriptor®	Approved
efavirenz	EFV	Sustiva®	Approved
etravirine	TMC 125	Intelence™	Approved
nevirapine	NVP	Viramune®	Approved
rilpivirine	TMC 278	—	Investigational
PROTEASE INHIBITORS (PIs)			
atazanavir	ATV	Reyataz®	Approved
darunavir	DRV	Prezista™	Approved
fosamprenavir	FPV	Lexiva®	Approved
indinavir	IDV	Crixivan®	Approved
lopinavir and ritonavir	LPV/RTV	Kaletra®	Approved
nelfinavir	NFV	Viracept®	Approved
ritonavir	RTV	Norvir®	Approved
saquinavir	SQV	Invirase®	Approved
tipranavir	TPV	Aptivus®	Approved
FIXED-DOSE COMBINATION PRODUCTS			
abacavir and lamivudine	ABC/3TC	Epzicom®, Kivexa™	Approved
abacavir, lamivudine, and zidovudine	ABC/3TC/ZDV	Trizivir®	Approved
efavirenz, emtricitabine and tenofovir	EFV/FTC/TDF	Atripla™	Approved
emtricitabine and tenofovir	FTC/TDF	Truvada®	Approved
zidovudine and lamivudine	ZDV/3TC	Combivir®	Approved
FUSION INHIBITORS			
enfuvirtide	ENF	Fuzeon®	Approved
—	TNX-355	—	Investigational
CHEMOKINE CORECEPTOR ANTAGONIST			
maraviroc	MVC	Selzentry™	Approved
vicriviroc	SCH-417690; SCH-D	—	Investigational
—	PRO 140	—	Investigational
—	INCB9741	—	Investigational

Antiretroviral Drugs *(continued)*

Generic Name	Also Known As	Brand Name	FDA Status
INTEGRASE INHIBITORS			
elvitegravir	GS-9137	—	Investigational
raltegravir	RAL	Isentress™	Approved
—	GSK364735	—	Investigational
MATURATION INHIBITORS			
bevirimat	PA-457	—	Investigational

DRUGS USED TO TREAT COMPLICATIONS OF HIV / AIDS

Brand Name	Generic Name (Synonym)	Use
Abelcet®, AmBisome®	amphotericin B, ABLC	Antifungal for aspergillosis
Bactrim™, Septra®	sulfamethoxazole and trimethoprim, SMZ/TMP	Antiprotozoal antibiotic used to treat and prevent *Pneumocystis carinii* pneumonia
Biaxin®	clarithromycin	Antibiotic used to treat and prevent *Mycobacterium avium*
Cytovene®	ganciclovir, DHPG	Antiviral used to treat CMV retinitis
DaunoXome®	daunorubicin citrate (liposomal)	Chemotherapy for Kaposi sarcoma
Diflucan®	fluconazole	Antifungal for candidiasis, cryptococcal meningitis
Doxil®	DOXOrubicin (liposomal)	Chemotherapy for Kaposi sarcoma
Eraxis™	anidulafungin	Antifungal (intravenous), used to treat *Candida* infections in the esophagus (candidiasis), blood stream (candidemia), and other forms of *Candida* infections, including abdominal abscesses and peritonitis (inflammation of the lining of the abdominal cavity)
Famvir®	famciclovir	Antiviral used to treat herpes
Foscavir®	foscarnet	Antiviral used to treat herpes and CMV retinitis
Gamimune® N	immune globulin, gamma globulin, IGIV	Immune booster used to prevent bacterial infections in children
Intron® A	interferon alfa-2b	Treat Kaposi sarcoma and hepatitis C
Marinol®	dronabinol	Treat loss of appetite
Megace®	megestrol acetate	Treat loss of appetite and weight
Mepron®	atovaquone	Antiprotozoal antibiotic used to treat and prevent *Pneumocystis carinii* pneumonia
Mycobutin®	rifabutin	Antimycobacterial used to prevent *Mycobacterium avium*
NebuPent®	pentamidine	Antiprotozoal antibiotic used to prevent *Pneumocystis carinii* pneumonia
Neutrexin®	trimetrexate glucuronate and leucovorin	Antiprotozoal antibiotic used to treat *Pneumocystis carinii* pneumonia
Panretin® Gel	alitretinoin gel 0.1%	AIDS-related Kaposi sarcoma
Procrit®, Epogen®	erythropoietin, EPO	Treat anemia related to AZT therapy
Roferon-A®	interferon alfa-2a	Treat Kaposi sarcoma and hepatitis C
Serostim®	somatropin rDNA	Treat weight loss
Sporanox®	itraconazole	Antifungal used to treat blastomycosis, histoplasmosis, aspergillosis, and candidiasis
Taxol®	PACLitaxel	Kaposi sarcoma
Valcyte™	valGANciclovir	Antiviral used to treat CMV retinitis
VFEND®	voriconazole	Antifungal for invasive aspergillosis and serious fungal infections due to *Fusarium sporotrichoides* and *Scedosporium apiospermum*, and Esophageal Candidiasis
Vistide®	cidofovir, HPMPC	Antiviral used to treat cytomegalovirus (CMV)
Vitrasert® Implant	ganciclovir insert	Antiviral used to treat CMV retinitis
Vitravene™ intravitreal injection	fomivirsen sodium injection	Antiviral used to treat CMV retinitis
Zithromax®	azithromycin	Antibiotic used to treat *Mycobacterium avium*

HERBS AND COMMON NATURAL AGENTS

The authors have chosen to include this list of natural products and their reported uses. Due to limited scientific evidence to support these uses, the information provided here is not intended as a cure for any disease, and should not be construed as curative or healing. In addition, the reader is strongly encouraged to seek other references that discuss this information in more detail, and that discuss important issues such as contraindications, warnings, precautions, adverse reactions, and interactions.

PROPOSED MEDICINAL CLAIMS

Herb	Reported Uses
Acetyl-L-carnitine (ALC)	AIDS; alcoholism; Alzheimer disease; angina; attention-deficit/hyperactivity disorder (ADHD); cerebral ischemia; congestive heart failure; coronary artery disease; depression; diabetes mellitus; diabetic peripheral neuropathy; erectile dysfunction; fatigue; fibromyalgia; fragile X syndrome; Huntington disease; hyperlipoproteinemia; infertility; liver disease; mood disorder; myocardial infarction; neurologic function; neuropathy; nutritional deficiency; Parkinson disease; peripheral vascular disease; Peyronie disease; sickle cell disease; surgical uses; sperm motility; tuberculosis
Adrenal extract	Depression; fatigue; fibromyalgia; stress
Aloe (*Aloe* spp)	Aphthous stomatitis; arthritis; cancer (prevention); constipation; diabetes; dry skin; dyslipidemia; genital herpes; gingivitis; healing agent for wounds, minor burns, and other minor skin irritations; human immunodeficiency virus (HIV); irritable bowel syndrome; lichen planus; mucositis; pressure ulcers; psoriasis vulgaris; radiation dermatitis; seborrheic dermatitis; skin burns; ulcerative colitis
Alpha-Lipoic acid	Alcohol-induced liver damage; Alzheimer disease; antioxidant; burning mouth syndrome; cancer; cardiovascular outcomes (in end-state renal disease); carpal tunnel syndrome; cataract prevention; chemotherapy and radiation (adjunct); circulation; cognitive function; coronary artery disease; diabetes, diabetic peripheral neuropathy; drug-induced cardiotoxicity; glaucoma; hypertension; insulin resistance; liver protective effects; migraine; multiple sclerosis; neuralgias; neurologic disorders, including stroke (preventive); peripheral artery disease; radiation injuries; skin aging; weight loss; wound healing
Andrographis (*Andrographis paniculata*)	Familial Mediterranean Fever (FMF); influenza; ulcerative colitis; upper respiratory tract infection (treatment)
Aortic extract	Circulation structure, function, and integrity (arteries and veins); prevention of vascular disease including atherosclerosis, cerebral ischemia, peripheral arterial disease, chronic venous insufficiency, leg ulcers, varicose veins, hemorrhoids, and vascular retinopathies such as macular degeneration, deep vein thrombosis
Arabinoxylan	Cancer; diabetes, type 2; HIV; immune support (antiviral and anticancer activity); leukopenia (chemotherapy-induced)
Arginine	Adrenoleukodystrophy (ALD); AIDS-related wasting (combination therapy); altitude sickness (not beneficial); anal fissures; angina; asthma (not beneficial); burns; cancer; cardiovascular disease; chronic heart failure; circulation; critical illness; dementia; dental pain; diabetes (diabetic complications); erectile dysfunction; gastrointestinal cancer surgery; growth hormone reserve test/pituitary disorder diagnosis; heart protection during CABG; hypercholesterolemia; hypertension; immune support; inborn errors of urea synthesis; infertility/*in vitro* fertilization (adjuvant); inflammatory bowel disease; increases lean body mass; interstitial cystitis; kidney disease; MELAS syndrome; migraine headache; myocardial infarction; necrotizing entercolitis; neonatal outcomes; nitrate tolerance; obesity (in type 2 diabetic patients); peripheral vascular disease/ claudication; preeclampsia; pressure ulcers; Raynaud phenomenon; recovery after surgery; sexual vitality and enhancement; transplants; wound healing
Arnica (*Arnica montana*)	Bruising; coagulation; diabetic retinopathy; muscle soreness; osteoarthritis; pain; swelling (postoperative); trauma
Artichoke (*Cynara scolymus*)	Alcohol-induced hangover; bile flow; dyspepsia (nonulcer); eczema and other dermatologic problems; hepatic protection/stimulation; hypercholesterolemia; indigestion; irritable bowel syndrome (IBS)

PROPOSED MEDICINAL CLAIMS *(continued)*

Herb	Reported Uses
Ashwagandha (*Withania somnifera*)	Adaptogen/tonic (promote wellness); chemotherapy and radiation (adjunct); diabetes (type 2); diuresis; hypercholesterolemia; longevity/anti-aging; osteoarthritis; Parkinson disease; stress, fatigue, nervous exhaustion
Astragalus (*Astragalus membranaceus*) [Milk Vetch]	Adaptogen/tonic (promote wellness); antiviral activity; athletic performance (enhancement); burns; chemotherapy and radiation (adjunct); coronary artery disease; diabetes; heart failure; immune support; liver protection; mental performance; multiple sclerosis; otitis media; renal failure; smoking cessation; tissue oxygenation; tuberculosis
Bacopa (*Bacopa monniera*)	Alzheimer disease/senility; anxiety; epilepsy; irritable bowel syndrome (IBS); memory enhancement and improvement of cognitive function
Barberry (*Berberis vulgaris*)	Bladder infection; bronchitis; diabetes; diarrhea; giardiasis; heart failure; hypertension; inflammation; sore throat; trachoma; yeast infection
Beta-Carotene	Age-related maculopathy; AIDS; asthma; breast cancer; cancer (no overall effect); carotenoid deficiency; cataract prevention; cervical dysplasia; chromosome damage (reduction); chronic obstructive pulmonary disease (COPD); colorectal cancer; coronary heart disease (risk reduction; in combination); cystic fibrosis; diabetes; diabetes, type 2; esophageal cancer; gastric cancer; immune support; laryngeal cancer; LDL oxidation (decrease in males); lung cancer (preventive); lung function; macular degeneration; memory and cognition; night blindness; oral leukoplakia; osteoarthritis; photoprotection (erythropoietic protoporphyria); pregnancy-related complications; prostate cancer
Betaine hydrochloride	Cardiovascular disease (in homocystinuric patients); cholesterol levels; digestive aid (hypochlorhydria and achlorhydria); hyperhomocysteinemia; hyperhomocysteinemia (in chronic renal failure patients); rosacea; steatohepatitis (nonalcoholic); weight loss
Bifidobacterium bifidum (*bifidus*)	Atopic dermatitis; constipation; Crohn disease; diarrhea; gastrointestinal microflora recolonization (anaerobic); *Helicobacter pylori* infection; immune function; irritable bowel syndrome (IBS); pouchitis; ulcerative colitis
Bilberry (*Vaccinium myrtillus*)	Circulation, peripheral; diabetes; diarrhea; dysmenorrhea; fibrocystic breast disease (FBD); hemorrhoids; ophthalmologic disorders (antioxidant) including myopia, diminished acuity, glaucoma; dark adaptation, macular degeneration, night blindness, diabetic retinopathy, cataracts; peptic ulcer disease; scleroderma; vascular disorders including varicose veins, capillary permeability/stability, phlebitis
Biotin (Vitamin H)	Cardiovascular disease (risk reduction; in combination); diabetes; diabetic peripheral neuropathy; hypertriglyceridemia; nails, brittle; pregnancy supplementation; seborrheic dermatitis; total parenteral nutrition (TPN); uncombable hair syndrome
Bismuth	Diarrhea; ulcers
Bitter melon (*Momordica charantia*)	Antiviral; cancer; diabetes, including impaired glucose tolerance; human immunodeficiency virus (HIV)
Black cohosh (*Cimicifuga racemosa*)	Arthritis; climacteric complaints (related to breast cancer treatment); depression (mild); labor induction; menopause symptoms (including vasomotor); migraine; osteoporosis; premenstrual syndrome (PMS)
Bladderwrack (*Fucus vesiculosus*)	Anticoagulant; antioxidant; bacterial and fungal infections; cancer; diabetes; fibrocystic breast disease (FBD); hypothyroidism; nutrient (rich source of iodine, potassium, magnesium, calcium, and iron); weight loss
Borage (*Borago officinalis*)	Acute respiratory distress syndrome; alcohol hangover; asthma; atopic dermatitis (treatment and prophylaxis); atopic eczema; cystic fibrosis; diabetic neuropathy; fatty acids (preterm infants); growth and development (infants); hyperlipidemia; infantile seborrheic dermatitis; malnutrition-inflammation complex syndrome; periodontitis; rheumatoid arthritis; stress; weight regain
Boron	Cognitive function improvement; osteoarthritis; osteoporosis; rheumatoid arthritis; vaginitis
Boswellia (*Boswellia serrata*)	Antiinflammatory; arthritis; asthma; brain tumors; Crohn disease; ulcerative colitis

Herb	Reported Uses
Branched-chain amino acids (BCAAs)	Amyotrophic lateral sclerosis; anorexia; cardiac atrophy; cirrhosis; diabetes; energy metabolism improvement (in cirrhosis patients); exercise performance; hepatic encephalopathy; liver surgery; muscle development and lean body mass (increase); muscle fatigue and soreness; protein metabolism (in COPD patients); tardive dyskinesia
Bromelain (*Anas comosus*)	Arthritis (antiinflammatory; proteolytic); burn debridement; cancer; cervical dysplasia; chronic obstructive pulmonary disease (COPD); digestive enzyme; inflammation/pain; muscle soreness; osteoarthritis of the knee; rash; rheumatoid arthritis; sinusitis; steatorrhea; ulcerative colitis; urinary tract infection (UTI)
Bupleurum (*Bupleurum falcatum*)	Brain damage (minimal, children); chronic inflammatory disease; fatigue; hepatic protection; hepatitis; systemic lupus erythematosus (SLE); thrombocytopenic purpura
Calcium	Antacid; black widow spider bite; blood pressure regulation; bone loss; bone stress injury prevention; cancer (prevention); colon cancer (distal); colorectal adenomas (recurrence); growth; hypercholesterolemia; hyperkalemia; hypermagnesemia; hyperparathyroidism; hyperphosphatemia; hypertension; kidney stones; lead toxicity; osteomalacia/rickets; osteoporosis (preventive); poison ivy (topical; lactate form); preeclampsia; pregnancy; premenstrual syndrome (PMS); weight loss in type 2 diabetic patients, fat metabolism, and weight gain prevention (in postmenopausal women); vaginal atrophy
Calendula (*Calendula officinalis*)	Antibacterial, antifungal, antiviral, antiprotozoal; otitis media; radiation dermatitis; skin inflammation; venous leg ulcers; wound healing
Caprylic acid	Antifungal/antiyeast; candidiasis; Crohn disease; dysbiosis; epilepsy (children)
Caprylidene	Alzheimer disease
Carnitine	Acute myocardial infarction (mortality); angina; arrhythmia; athletic performance (enhancement); attention-deficit hyperactivity disorder (ADHD); chronic obstructive pulmonary disease (COPD); congestive heart failure (CHF); diabetes; dialysis; diphtheria; erectile dysfunction; exercise performance; fatigue; hepatic encephalopathy; HIV/AIDS; Huntington disease; hypercholesterolemia; hyperlipoproteinemia; hyperthyroidism; male infertility; myocardial infarction; neonatal growth and breathing; nonalcoholic steatohepatitis; obesity; peripheral vascular disease; postexercise metabolic stress and muscle damage; quality of life (maintenance hemodialysis patients); renal failure/dialysis; respiratory distress; sperm motility; spinal muscular atrophy (adjunct to valproic acid); surgical uses; weight loss
Cascara (*Rhamnus purshiana*)	Laxative
Cat's claw (*Uncaria tomentosa*)	Allergies; antiinflammatory; antimicrobial (antibacterial, antifungal, antiviral); antioxidant; arthritis; cancer; cervical dysplasia; Crohn disease; diverticulitis; endometriosis; fibromyalgia; immune support; multiple sclerosis; rosacea; systemic lupus erythematosus (SLE)
Cayenne (*Capsicum annuum, Capsicum frutescens*)	Antiinflammatory and analgesic (topical); cardiovascular circulatory support; cluster headache; concentration/stimulant; digestive stimulant; duodenal ulcer; dyspepsia; fibromyalgia; *H. pylori*; low back pain; nausea/vomiting (postoperative); pain (postoperative); postherpetic neuralgia; pruritus; rhinitis; swallowing dysfunction
Chamomile, German (*Matricaria chamomilla, Matricaria recutita*)	Acute radiation skin reaction; anxiolytic; cardiovascular conditions; carminative, antispasmodic; colic; common cold; diaper rash; diarrhea (children); eczema; hemorrhagic cystitis; hemorrhoids; indigestion; insomnia (mild sedative); minor injury (topical antiinflammatory); mucositis (from chemotherapy); nausea/vomiting; oral health (as mouth rinse/gargle); stress/anxiety; teething; uterine tonic; vaginitis
Chasteberry (*Vitex agnus-castus*)	Acne vulgaris; cervical dysplasia; corpus luteum insufficiency; cyclic mastalgia; hyperprolactinemia and insufficient lactation; infertility; insect repellent; menopause; menorrhagia; menstrual disorders including amenorrhea, endometriosis, premenstrual syndrome (PMS), premenstrual dysphoric disorder (PMDD); rosacea
Chitosan	Antibacterial; dental plaque; hyperlipidemia; insulin sensitivity; periodontitis; renal failure; weight loss; wound healing

PROPOSED MEDICINAL CLAIMS *(continued)*

Herb	Reported Uses
Chlorophyll	Antiinflammatory, antioxidant, and wound healing properties; bacteriostatic; cancer; chemoprevention; fibrocystic breast disease; herpes simplex, herpes zoster; leukopenia; odor absorbent/suppressant (breath freshener, toothpaste, mouthwash, and deodorant); pancreatitis; pneumonia; poisoning; protectant; rheumatoid arthritis; tuberculosis
Chondroitin sulfate	Coronary artery disease; interstitial cystitis; iron absorption enhancement; muscle soreness, delayed onset; ophthalmologic uses; osteoarthritis; overactive bladder; psoriasis
Chromium	Atherosclerosis; bipolar disorder; bone loss (postmenopausal women); cardiovascular disease (risk reduction; in combination); depression; diabetes; diabetes, type 1; diabetes, type 2; glaucoma; hypercholesterolemia; hypertriglyceridemia; hypothyroidism; immunosuppression; insulin sensitivity (obese women with polycystic ovarian syndrome); premenstrual syndrome (PMS); Turner syndrome; weight loss
Clove *(Syzygium aromaticum)*	Anal fissures (topical); analgesic (toothache and teething); anesthetic; antiseptic; fever; mosquito repellent; premature ejaculation (combination preparation)
Coenzyme Q_{10}	Acute myocardial infarction; AIDS; Alzheimer disease; amyotrophic lateral sclerosis (ALS); angina; antioxidant; asthenozoospermia (idiopathic); cancer (preventive); cardiomyopathy; cardioprotection during surgery; chemotherapy (adjunct); chronic fatigue syndrome; congestive heart failure (CHF); Down syndrome; exercise performance; fibromyalgia; Friedreich ataxia; gingivitis; Huntington disease; hypercholesterolemia; hypertension; migraine; mitochondrial disorders; multiple sclerosis; muscle pain (associated with HMG-CoA reductase inhibitors); muscular dystrophy; myelodysplastic syndromes; Parkinson disease; pediatric migraine; periodontal disease; Peyronie disease; renal failure; tinnitus; weight loss
Coleus *(Coleus forskohlii)*	Antiinflammatory action after cardiopulmonary bypass; asthma and allergies; eczema; erectile dysfunction; glaucoma; hypertension and congestive heart failure; intubation; lactagogue; mental health; psoriasis
Collagen (Type II)	Arthritis (osteo and rheumatoid); burns (first- and second-degree); soft tissue correction; surgical and traumatic wounds; ulcers (pressure, venous stasis, diabetic); wound healing (topical)
Colostrum	Antiviral (mild); athletic performance (enhancement); body composition; colitis; cryptosporidiosis; diarrhea; flu prevention; HIV-associated diarrhea; *H. Pylori*; immune support; multiple sclerosis; oral hygiene; prevention of NSAID-induced GI injury; rotavirus-associated diarrhea; shigellosis; sore throat; surgery recovery; upper respiratory tract infection
Conjugated linoleic acid (CLA)	Cancer; diabetes; hypercholesterolemia; immune support; muscle development and lean body mass (increase); obesity; oxidative stress and inflammatory disease in obese men; preeclampsia (in combination with calcium)
Copper	Age-related macular degeneration; anemia; arthritis; atherosclerosis; cardiovascular disease; copper deficiency; dental enamel demineralization (in combination with fluoride); growth promotion (children); marasmus; osteoporosis; plaque prevention; rheumatoid arthritis; systemic lupus erythematosus
Cordyceps *(Cordyceps sinensis)*	Adaptogen/tonic (promote wellness); antioxidant; asthma; chemotherapy and radiation (adjunct); endurance and stamina; exercise performance; fatigue; fibromyalgia; hepatitis B; hepatoprotection; hyperlipidemia; immunomodulator; lung, liver, and kidney function (general support); organ transplant; sexual vitality (males and females); tissue oxygenation
Cranberry *(Vaccinium macrocarpon)*	Achlorhydria and B_{12} absorption; antioxidant; bacterial and fungal infections; cancer (prevention); diabetes; *H. pylori* infection; kidney stones; plaque; reduction of urinary odors; urinary tract infection, including prevention

PROPOSED MEDICINAL CLAIMS *(continued)*

Herb	Reported Uses
Creatine	Amyotrophic lateral sclerosis (ALS); athletic performance (enhancement) as energy production and protein synthesis for muscle building; bone density; chronic obstructive pulmonary disease; congestive heart failure (CHF); dermatomyositis/polymyositis; GAMT deficiency; hemodialysis-associated muscle cramps; Huntington disease; hyperlipidemia; ischemic heart disease; McArdle disease; mitochondrial diseases; muscle function and strength; mood; muscular dystrophy; Parkinson disease; resistance training in patients with Parkinson disease; schizophrenia; spinal cord injury; surgery (adjunct); traumatic brain injury, prevention of complications (children)
Cyclo-hispro	Diabetes, type 2; hypoglycemia
Damiana (*Turnera diffusa*)	Female sexual dysfunction; weight loss/obesity
Dandelion (*Taraxacum officinale*)	Leaf: diuretic, antioxidant, diabetes; root: increase bile secretion (choleretic), appetite stimulation, inflammation, hepatitis, and dyspepsia
Dehydroepiandrosterone (DHEA)	Adrenal insufficiency; AIDS/HIV; antiaging; cardiovascular disease; cervical cancer; chronic fatigue syndrome; cocaine withdrawal; cognitive function; Crohn disease; dementia; depression; diabetes, type 2; erectile dysfunction; extrapyramidal symptoms; fatigue; fibromyalgia; induction of labor; infertility; libido (premenopausal women); lupus; muscle mass and strength; obesity; perimenopausal symptoms; psoriasis; rheumatoid arthritis; schizophrenia; Sjögren syndrome; vaginal atrophy
Devil's claw (*Harpagophytum procumbens*)	Antiinflammatory; back pain; osteoarthritis, gout, and other inflammatory conditions
Docosahexaenoic acid (DHA)	Age-related macular degeneration; Alzheimer disease; angina pectoris; appetite; arrhythmias; asthma; attention-deficit disorder and attention-deficit hyperactivity disorder (ADD/ADHD); bipolar disorder; cancer (prevention); cardiovascular disease; colon cancer; coronary heart disease (risk reduction); Crohn disease; cystic fibrosis; depression; diabetes; diabetes, type 2; dyslexia; dysmenorrhea; eczema; hypercholesterolemia; hypertension; hypertriglyceridemia; IgA nephropathy; immune support; infant eye/brain development; infection; lupus; nephrotic syndrome; postpartum depression; preeclampsia; prevention of graft failure after heart bypass surgery; protection from cyclosporine toxicity in organ transplant patients; psoriasis; rheumatoid arthritis; schizophrenia; stroke (risk reduction); ulcerative colitis
Dong quai (*Angelica sinensis*)	Anemia; energy enhancement (particularly in females); hypertension; menopause, dysmenorrhea, premenstrual syndrome (PMS), and amenorrhea; menorrhagia; phytoestrogen; pulmonary hypertension
Echinacea (*Echinacea purpurea, Echinacea angustifolia*)	Antibacterial (topical: boils, abscesses, tonsillitis, poison ivy); antiviral; arthritis (*E. augustifolia*); genital herpes; immune support (cold and other upper respiratory infections); leukopenia; otitis media; upper respiratory infection; uveitis; vaginal candidiasis
Elder (*Sambucus nigra, Sambucus canadensis*)	Berry used as an antiviral, antioxidant, and for influenza; flower used as an antiinflammatory, for colds and influenza, diaphoretic, diuretic, fever, sinusitis, hyperlipidemia, and sore throat
Ephedra (*Ephedra sinica*)	Allergies, sinusitis, hay fever; asthma; hypotension; sexual arousal; weight loss (monotherapy); weight loss (combination therapy)
Evening primrose (*Oenothera biennis*)	Asthma; amenorrhea; atopic dermatitis; attention-deficit disorder; bronchitis; breast cysts; depression; diabetes; diabetic peripheral neuropathy; eczema, dermatitis, and psoriasis; endometriosis; fatigue; fibrocystic breast disease (FBD); hypercholesterolemia; ichthyosis vulgaris; irritable bowel syndrome (IBS); mastalgia; menopause; menorrhagia; multiple sclerosis; obesity; omega-6 fatty acid supplementation; preeclampsia; premenstrual syndrome (PMS); psoriasis; Raynaud phenomenon; rheumatoid arthritis; rosacea; schizophrenia; scleroderma
Eyebright (*Euphrasia officinalis*)	Conjunctivitis; eye fatigue; catarrh of the eyes; hepatoprotection
Fennel (*Foeniculum vulgare* Mill.)	ACE inhibitor-associated cough; colic, infantile; dysmenorrhea; ultraviolet skin protection
Fenugreek (*Trigonella foenum-graecum*)	Diabetes; eating behavior; galactagogue; hypercholesterolemia
Feverfew (*Tanacetum parthenium*)	Antiinflammatory, rheumatoid arthritis; migraine headache (preventive); muscle soreness

PROPOSED MEDICINAL CLAIMS *(continued)*

Herb	Reported Uses
Fish oils	Acute respiratory distress syndrome; acne vulgaris; age-related maculopathy; angina pectoris; arrhythmias; asthma; athletic performance; attention deficit hyperactivity disorder (ADHD); behavior (children); bipolar disorder; body weight improvement; cachexia; cancer (prevention); cardiac death (sudden; preventive); cardiac support (general; proposed benefits); cardiovascular disease; circulation; cognitive performance; colon cancer; coordination disorder; coronary heart disease (preventive); cystic fibrosis; depression; diabetes, type 1; diabetes, type 2; diabetic nephropathy; dysmenorrhea; eczema, psoriasis; fatigue; headache; heart disease and heart attack (risk reduction), including women and antiinflammatory effects in heart failure patients; herpes simplex 2; hypercholesterolemia; hypertension; hypertriglyceridemia; IgA nephropathy; immune support; infant eye/brain development; inflammatory bowel disease; lupus; memory enhancement; migraine; multiple sclerosis; nephrotic syndrome; obesity; peripheral arterial disease; preeclampsia; premenstrual syndrome (PMS); prevention of graft failure after heart bypass surgery; protection from cyclosporine toxicity in organ transplant patients; psoriasis; Raynaud phenomenon; restenosis after coronary angioplasty; rheumatoid arthritis; rosacea; schizophrenia; scleroderma; stroke (risk reduction); transplant (heart); trauma
Flaxseed oil	Acne vulgaris; arthritis (rheumatoid); asthma; attention deficit hyperactivity disorder (ADHD); breast cancer; constipation; coronary heart disease (risk reduction); diabetes; dry eyes (Sjögren syndrome); hemorrhoids; hepatic disease; hyperlipidemia; hypertension; lupus nephritis; mastalgia; menopausal symptoms; multiple sclerosis; obesity; omega-3 essential fatty acid source (cell wall and cellular membrane structure; cholesterol transport and oxidation); pregnancy (spontaneous delivery); premenstrual syndrome (PMS); prostaglandins production; prostate cancer; psoriasis; stroke (risk reduction); systemic lupus erythematosus (SLE)
Folic acid	Age-related macular degeneration (with pyridoxine and cyanocobalamin); alcoholism; anemia; atherosclerosis; beta-thalassemia; cancer (preventive; colon and breast); cardiovascular morbidity or mortality in patients with chronic renal failure; cervical dysplasia; chronic fatigue syndrome; cognitive function; coronary heart disease (risk reduction); coronary restenosis (rate reduction by decreasing plasma homocysteine levels); Crohn disease; dementia and Alzheimer disease (risk reduction); depression; endothelial dysfunction (in type 2 diabetes); fragile X syndrome; gingivitis; hearing loss (slows progression); homocysteine (reduction); infertility (with zinc sulfate); lometrexol toxicity; methotrexate toxicity; nitrate tolerance; osteoporosis; phenytoin-induced gingival hyperplasia; pregnancy (prevention of birth defects) and lactation; restless leg syndrome; schizophrenia (risk reduction, by decreasing homocysteine levels); stroke; ulcer, aphthous; vascular function; vitiligo
Gamma Linolenic Acid (GLA)	Acute respiratory distress syndrome; atopic dermatitis; attention-deficit hyperactivity disorder (ADHD); blood pressure control; cancer treatment (adjunct); diabetic neuropathy; immune enhancement; mastalgia; menopausal hot flashes; migraine; osteoporosis; preeclampsia; premenstrual syndrome (PMS); pruritus; rheumatoid arthritis; sclerosis; Sjögren syndrome; ulcerative colitis
Garcinia *(Garcinia cambogia)*	Cancer; exercise performance; halitosis; pancreatic function (supportive) and glucose regulation; weight loss
Garlic *(Allium sativum)*	Alopecia; angina; antimicrobial (bacterial, fungal, and parasitic) including *Helicobacter pylori* infection, tinea pedis, Pseudomonas infection, Streptococci, Candida, Hymenolepis nana; antioxidant (practitioners should be aware that aged garlic extracts have been reported to improve this benefit); atherosclerosis; athletic performance; cancer (prevention); cardiovascular disease risk; coagulation (mild inhibitor of platelet-activating factor); cryptococcal meningitis; cutaneous microcirculation; cystic fibrosis (pseudomonas infection); diabetes, type 2; hyperlipidemia; hypertension; immune support; mosquito repellent; myocardial risk reduction; peripheral vascular disease; preeclampsia; sickle cell anemia; systemic sclerosis; tick repellant; upper respiratory tract infection
Ginger *(Zingiber officinale)*	Antiemetic (for nausea and vomiting in pregnancy, motion sickness, and chemotherapy); antiinflammatory (musculoskeletal); antimicrobial; anxiety; cancer; diverticulitis; gonarthritis; indigestion/heartburn; labor (shortening duration); muscle pain; osteoarthritis; rheumatoid arthritis; ventilator-associated pneumonia; vertigo

Herb	Reported Uses
Ginkgo (*Ginkgo biloba*)	Acute ischemic stroke; allergic conjunctivitis; Alzheimer disease, dementia, age-related memory impairment; anxiety; asthma; attention deficit hyperactivity disorder; autism; cancer (risk reduction); cerebral insufficiency; chemotherapy (adjunct); chronic cochleovestibular disorders; cocaine dependence; cognitive function; depression; diabetic neuropathy; dyslexia; epilepsy; functional measures (in patients with multiple sclerosis); gastric cancer; glaucoma; headache; hypertension; intermittent claudication; macular degeneration; memory enhancement; mountain sickness; multiple sclerosis; ocular blood flow; Parkinson disease; peripheral blood flow (cerebral vascular disease, peripheral vascular insufficiency, impotence, tinnitus, and depression); premenstrual syndrome (PMS); quality of life; Raynaud phenomenon; retinopathy; seasonal affective disorder (SAD); schizophrenia; seizures; sexual dysfunction (antidepressant-induced); tinnitus; vertigo; vitiligo
Ginseng, Panax (*Panax ginseng*)	Adrenal tonic; brain injury; bronchitis; cancer; cancer-related fatigue; cardiopulmonary bypass; cardiovascular health and risk factors; congestive heart failure; dementia; diabetes; diabetic nephropathy; energy enhancement; erectile dysfunction; fatigue; glucose regulation (non-diabetes); hepatoprotection; hyperlipidemia; hypertension; immune support; intrauterine growth retardation; mental health; physical and mental performance; quality of life, well-being; radiation therapy side effects; respiratory illness
Ginseng, Siberian (*Eleutherococcus senticosus*)	Adaptogen/tonic (promote wellness); athletic performance (enhancement); fatigue; herpes simplex, type 2; immune support; neurocirculatory hypotension
Glucosamine	Chronic venous insufficiency; inflammatory bowel disease; knee injury recovery; low back pain; multiple sclerosis, adjunct; osteoarthritis and joint structure support; rheumatoid arthritis and other inflammatory conditions; temporomandibular joint (TMJ)
Glutamine	Alcoholism; athletic performance (enhancement); cancer (adjunct); catabolic wasting; chemotherapy (prevention of adverse effects); critical illness; diabetes, type 1; diarrhea; fibromyalgia; hepatoprotection; HIV (adjunct); HIV wasting; immune support; muscular dystrophy; peptic ulcer disease; postsurgical healing; ulcerative colitis and other inflammatory bowel diseases
Glutathione	Antioxidant; chemoprotection; hepatoprotection (alcohol-induced liver damage); immune support; male infertility; Parkinson disease; peptic ulcer disease; peripheral artery disease
Golden seal (*Hydrastis canadensis*)	Antimicrobial (antibacterial/antifungal); bronchitis, cystitis, and infectious diarrhea; fever; gallbladder; gastritis; heart failure; hypercholesterolemia; immune stimulation; infectious diarrhea; malaria (chloroquine resistant); mucous membrane tonifying (used in inflammation of mucosal membranes); narcotic concealment (urine analysis); sinusitis; sore throat; trachoma; urinary tract infection (UTI)
Gotu kola (*Centella asiatica*)	Anxiety; bladder lesions; cirrhosis; connective tissue (support); diabetic microangiopathy; hemorrhoids (topical); keloids; macular degeneration; memory enhancement; microangiopathy; psoriasis; venous insufficiency; wound healing (topical)
Grapefruit seed (*Citrus paradisi*)	Antifungal, antibacterial, and antiparasitic agent; diarrhea; diverticulitis; eczema; endometriosis; heart disease; irritable bowel syndrome (IBS); kidney stones; metabolic syndrome; rosacea; sinusitis; sore throat; ulcerative colitis; urinary tract infection (UTI)
Grapeseed (*Vitis vinifera*)	Agitation (aromatherapy); allergies, antiinflammatory, asthma; antioxidant; cancer; cardiovascular health; chloasma; circulation, platelet aggregation inhibitor, capillary fragility, arterial/venous insufficiency (intermittent claudification, varicose veins); diabetic retinopathy; edema; gingivitis; glaucoma; hyperlipidemia; liver disease; macular degeneration; multiple sclerosis; pancreatitis; Parkinson disease; premenstrual syndrome; scleroderma; sun protection; vision problems
Green tea (*Camellia sinensis*)	Allergy; antioxidant; cancer (prevention); cardiovascular disease (preventive); cardiovascular disease (reduction of risks); chemotherapy and radiation (adjunct); common cold (prevention); diabetes; diarrhea; genital warts; gingivitis (prevention); human T-cell lymphocytic virus; hypercholesterolemia; hypertension; hypertriglyceridemia; liver disease; macular degeneration; photoprotection; platelet aggregation inhibition; tuberculosis (adjuvant); weight loss/obesity

APPENDIX

PROPOSED MEDICINAL CLAIMS *(continued)*

Herb	Reported Uses
Ground Ivy (*Glechoma hederacea*)	No reported therapeutic uses
Guggul (*Commiphora mukul*)	Acne vulgaris; hypercholesterolemia; hypothyroidism; obesity; osteoarthritis; rheumatoid arthritis; weight loss
Gymnema (*Gymnema sylvestre*)	Diabetes, blood sugar regulation; hyperlipidemia; weight loss
Hawthorn (*Crataegus oxyacantha*)	Angina, hypotension, hypertension, peripheral vascular disease, and tachycardia; cardiotonic; coronary artery disease; heart failure
Hops (*Humulus lupulus*)	Inflammation (combined with other agents); insomnia (with valerian); menopausal symptoms; sedative/hypnotic (mild); rheumatic disease
Horse chestnut (*Aesculus hippocastanum*)	Scleroderma; venous insufficiency (varicose veins, hemorrhoids, deep venous thrombosis, lower extremity edema [oral and topical])
Horseradish (*Armoracia rusticana, Cochlearia armoracia*)	Root: Bronchitis (combined with nasturtium herb); sinusitis (combined with nasturtium herb); urinary tract infection (combined with nasturtium herb)
Horsetail (*Equisetum arvense*)	Bone and connective tissue strengthening (including osteoporosis); diuretic; high mineral content (including silicic acid)
HuperzineA (*Huperzia serrata*)	Myasthenia gravis; senile dementia and Alzheimer disease
Hyaluronic acid	Aging; antioxidant; cataract surgery; immune system stimulant; oral mucositis; osteoarthritis; rheumatoid arthritis; skin conditions; urinary tract infections; wound healing and repair
Hydroxymethyl butyrate (HMB)	AIDS wasting; athletic performance (enhancement); cardiovascular disease risk; muscle damage
5-Hydroxytryptophan (5-HTP)	Anxiety; cerebellar ataxia; depression; fibromyalgia; headache; migraine; schizophrenia; sleep disorders, insomnia (stimulates the production of melatonin); weight loss/obesity
Hyssop (*Hyssopus officinalis*)	Kidney inflammation
Inositol hexaphosphate (IP-6)	Cancer (preventive); intermittent claudication; kidney stones
Iodine	Bacterial conjunctivitis; bladder irrigation; bowel irrigation; cancer; cognitive function; corpus vitreous degeneration; diabetic foot ulcers (topical); fibrocystic breast disease (FBD); filarial lymphoedema; goiter (preventive); Graves disease; hypothyroidism; molluscum; mucolytic; ophthalmia neonatorum (preventive); oral intubation; oral mucositis (topical, by radiochemotherapy); periodontitis/gingivitis; pneumonia; postcesarean endometriosis; renal pelvic instillation sclerotherapy; skin disinfectant (wound cleansing); sporotrichosis; thyrotoxicosis; water purification
Ipriflavone	Menopausal symptoms; Paget disease; prevention of osteoporosis (men and women); renal osteodystrophy
Iron	ACE inhibitor-associated cough; anemia (infants); athletic performance; attention-deficit hyperactivity disorder (ADHD); blood transfusions (reduction); cognitive performance; fatigue; heart failure; hyposalivation; menorrhagia; nutritional status (infants/children); pregnancy; restless legs syndrome
Isoflavones (soy)	Antioxidant; athletic performance; benign prostatic hyperplasia (BPH); bone mineral density (increase); cancer (preventive); cardiovascular effects; cervical dysplasia; chemotherapy (adjunct); cognitive function; Crohn disease; cyclical breast pain; diabetes; diarrhea; endometriosis; food allergies; hypercholesterolemia; hypertension; immune function; kidney disease; menopausal symptoms; menstrual migraine; osteoarthritis; osteoporosis; platelet function; premenstrual syndrome (PMS); skin aging; weight loss
Kava kava (*Piper methysticum*)	Fibromyalgia; insomnia (anxiety/stress, skeletal muscle relaxation, postischemic episodes); muscle soreness
Kudzu (*Pueraria lobata*)	Alcoholism; cardiovascular disease/angina; deafness; diabetes; diabetic retinopathy; glaucoma; ischemic stroke; menopausal symptoms

1119

PROPOSED MEDICINAL CLAIMS *(continued)*

Herb	Reported Uses
Lactobacillus acidophilus	Allergies; bacterial vaginosis; colitis (collagenous); constipation; diarrhea (infantile, prevention, and chronic); eczema (preventive); gastrointestinal microflora recolonization; hepatic encephalopathy; hypercholesterolemia; immune support; irritable bowel syndrome (IBS); lactose intolerance; necrotizing enterocolitis; vaginal candidiasis
Lavender (*Lavendula officinalis*)	Anxiety; attention; cancer; dementia (behavior disturbances); depression; hypnotic/sleep (aromatherapy); pain; perineal discomfort following childbirth; spasmolytic (oral); wound healing including minor burns (topical)
Lecithin	Acne vulgaris; Alzheimer disease/dementia; cognitive impairment; dry skin; extrapyramidal disorders; gallstones; hepatic steatosis; hypercholesterolemia; mania; tardive dyskinesia
Lemon balm/Melissa (*Melissa officinalis*)	Agitation in dementia; antiviral (oral herpes virus); anxiety; attention-deficit hyperactivity disorder (ADHD); cognitive performance; colitis; dyspepsia; sedation (pediatrics); sleep quality; teething (topical)
Licorice (*Glycyrrhiza glabra*)	Adrenal insufficiency (licorice); aphthous ulcers/canker sores; atopic dermatitis; body fat mass reduction; Crohn disease; croup; dental hygiene; expectorant and antitussive (licorice); familial Mediterranean fever (FMF); gastric mucosal damage by aspirin; gastrointestinal ulceration (DGL chewable products); herpes simplex; HIV/AIDS; hyperkalemia; peptic ulcer disease; polycystic ovarian syndrome (combined with spironolactone); sore throat (postoperative); viral hepatitis
Liver extract	Chronic fatigue syndrome; hepatitis; liver disorders; pernicious anemia; surgical use
Lutein	Antioxidant; breast cancer; cardiovascular disease; cataracts; colon cancer; diabetes; lutein deficiency; macular degeneration; preeclampsia; visual acuity and function
Lycopene	Asthma (exercise induced); atherosclerosis; benign prostate hypertrophy; cancer (preventive; especially colon, lung, prostate and kidney); diabetes; gingivitis; hypertension; immune enhancement; infertility; macular degeneration; oral submucous fibrosis; preeclampsia
Lysine	Angina pectoris; growth and development (children); herpes simplex; morbidity (diarrheal, respiratory); osteoporosis; ulcer, aphthous
Magnesium	Acute tocolysis of preterm labor; alcohol withdrawl; aneurysmal subarachnoid hemorrhage; arrhythmias/torsade de pointes; asthma; athletic performance; attention-deficit hyperactivity disorder (ADHD); brain injury; cardiovascular disease; chronic obstructive pulmonary disease; circulation; colic (magnesium salt); congestive heart failure (CHF); constipation; coronary artery disease; diabetes; dysmenorrhea; epilepsy; fatigue; fibromyalgia (magnesium salt); gallbladder (magnesium salt); hearing loss; heart disease; heart failure (endothelial function); hypertension; hypoglycemia; insomnia; kidney stones; leg cramps (during pregnancy); migraine headache; mitral valve prolapse (MVP); multiple sclerosis; muscle cramps; myalgia; myocardial infarction; nervousness; neuropathic pain; neuroprotection (infants); osteoporosis; pain; preeclampsia/eclampsia; pregnancy-related complications, fetal growth; premenstrual syndrome (PMS); stress/anxiety; tension headache (prevention)
Maitake (*Grifola frondosa*)	Cancer; diabetes; immune stimulation
Malic acid	Aluminum toxicity; fibromyalgia
Manganese	Diabetes; epilepsy; menstrual symptoms; osteoporosis
Marshmallow (*Althaea officinalis*)	Cough; croup; mucilaginous, demulcent; peptic ulcer disease; skin inflammatory conditions; sore throat
Mastic (*Pistacia lentiscus*)	Dental plaque; *H. pylori* inhibitor; peptic ulcer disease

PROPOSED MEDICINAL CLAIMS (continued)

Herb	Reported Uses
Melatonin	Age-related macular degeneration; Alzheimer disease (sleep disorders); anxiety (preoperative); athletic performance; autism; benzodiazepine tapering; bipolar disorder; cancer; cardioprotection; chemotherapy adverse effects; chronic fatigue syndrome; cognitive impairment; delayed sleep phase syndrome; depression (sleep disturbances); duodenal ulcer; dyspepsia; glaucoma; glycemic control; headache prevention; HIV/AIDS; hypertension; Inflammation; insomnia (elderly and children); irritable bowel syndrome; jet lag; menopause; nocturia; nocturnal hypertension; oxidative stress in dialysis patients (preventive); Parkinson disease; periodic limb movement disorder; preoperative sedation/anxiolysis; Rett syndrome; sarcoidosis, chronic; schizophrenia (sleep disorders); seasonal affective disorder (SAD); sedation (children); seizure disorders; sleep disturbances (in blind people, children with developmental disabilities, cystic fibrosis, individuals with intellectual disabilities, individuals with asthma); stroke; tardive dyskinesia; thermoregulation; thrombocytopenia; tinnitus (sleep disorders); tuberous sclerosis; UV-induced erythema prevention/sunburn/skin damage; work-shift sleep disorder
Methionine	Acetaminophen toxicity; cobalamin deficiency; liver detoxification
Methyl sulfonyl methane (MSM)	Allergies; analgesic; arthritis (osteo and rheumatoid); interstitial cystitis; lupus; seasonal allergic rhinitis
Milk thistle (*Silybum marianum*)	*Amanita phalloides* mushroom toxicity; antidote for poisoning by Death Cup mushroom; antioxidant (specifically hepatic cells), acute/chronic hepatitis, jaundice, and stimulation of bile secretion/cholagogue; chemotherapy and radiation (adjunct); cirrhosis; constipation; diabetes; eczema; gallbladder; halitosis; hepatoprotective, including drug toxicities (ie, phenothiazines, butyrophenones, ethanol, and acetaminophen); hyperlipidemia; hyperthyroidism; liver disease (chronic, alcoholic, viral); psoriasis; rosacea
Modified citrus pectin (MCP)	Anticarcinogenic; detoxification (toxic elements); diarrhea; hypercholesterolemia; prostate cancer
Muira puama (*Ptychopetalum olacoides*)	Athletic performance (enhancement); erectile dysfunction; sexual vitality (males)
N-Acetyl cysteine (NAC)	Acetaminophen toxicity; acute respiratory distress syndrome (ARDS); acute respiratory infection; AIDS; angina; asthma (mucolytic, antioxidant); atelectasis; bronchitis; cancer; cardioprotection (during chemotherapy); cerebral adrenoleukodystrophy; chemotherapy adverse effects; chronic obstructive pulmonary disease (COPD); cystic fibrosis; fatigue; glutathione production; heavy metal detoxification; HIV/AIDS; hyperthyroidism; hypothyroidism; influenza prevention; macular degeneration; multiple sclerosis; myocardial infarction; nephropathy (preventive); ovulation (induction in polycystic ovary syndrome); Parkinson disease; polycystic ovarian syndrome; renal impairment; scleroderma; sepsis; Sjögren syndrome; systemic lupus erythematosus (SLE); trichotillomania
Nicotinamide adenine dinucleotide (NADH)	Chronic fatigue syndrome; dementia; diabetes, type 1; hepatitis; Parkinson disease; stamina and energy
Octacosanol	Amyotrophic lateral sclerosis (ALS); hypercholesterolemia; Parkinson disease
Olive leaf (*Olea europaea*)	Acne vulgaris; antibacterial; antifungal; antiviral; Crohn disease; diabetes; diarrhea; diverticulitis; eczema; endometriosis; hypertension; multiple sclerosis; scleroderma; ulcerative colitis; urinary tract infection (UTI)
Pancreatic extract	Antiinflammatory; cancer (adjunct); celiac disease; chronic pancreatitis (pain); diabetes; digestive disturbances, pancreatic insufficiency; food allergies; immune complex diseases; malabsorption; surgery recovery
Para-Aminobenzoic acid (PABA)	Asthma; autoimmune disorders (pemphigus vulgaris adjuvant); cancer pain; dermatomyositis; hair loss; herpes labialis infection (prevention); herpetic keratitis; lichen sclerosus; morphea; pemphigus; Peyronie disease; scleroderma; sunburn; vitiligo
Parsley (*Petroselinum crispum*)	Antibacterial; antifungal; antioxidant; halitosis
Passion flower (*Passiflora spp*)	Anxiety; congestive heart failure (CHF); hyperthyroidism; insomnia (sedative); opiate withdrawal

Herb	Reported Uses
Peppermint (*Mentha piperita*)	Brain injury (aromatherapy); carminative, spasmolytic; colic; cough; cracked nipples (prevention); dyspepsia; gastrointestinal disorders, antispasmodic (preprocedure), abdominal distension, abdominal pain (preprocedure); indigestion; irritable bowel syndrome (IBS); motion sickness; nasal congestion; performance enhancement (cognitive and attentional function); postherpetic neuralgia; postoperative nausea (inhalation); tension headache (topical)
Periwinkle (*Vinca minor*)	No reported therapeutic uses
Phenylalanine	Addiction (reward deficiency syndrome); analgesic; attention-deficit/hyperactivity disorder; depression; pain; Parkinson disease; vitiligo
Phosphatidyl choline (PC)	Alcohol-induced liver damage; Alzheimer disease; fat deposits; gallstones; hepatitis; hypercholesterolemia; hypolipoproteinemia; lipoma; memory; peritoneal dialysis; periorbital fat pad herniation; tardive dyskinesia; ulcerative colitis
Phosphatidyl serine (PS)	Alzheimer disease; depression; memory and cognitive enhancement; physical stress
Phosphorus	Bowel cleansing; burns; diabetic ketoacidosis; exercise performance; hypercalcemia; hypercalciuria; hyperparathyroidism; hypophosphatemia; kidney stones; refeeding syndrome prevention; total parenteral nutrition (TPN); vitamin D resistant rickets
Policosanol	Coronary heart disease; hypercholesterolemia; intermittent claudication; platelet aggregation inhibition; reactivity/brain activity
Potassium	Bone loss; cardiac arrhythmias; congestive heart failure (CHF); hypercalciuria; hypertension; kidney stones; molluscum contagiosum (topical); QT prolongation; stroke
Pregnenolone	Arthritis; hormone precursor (DHEA, cortisol, progesterone, estrogens, and testosterone); mental performance; manic/depressive symptoms; schizophrenia
Progesterone	Amenorrhea; benzodiazepine withdrawal; brain injury; breast cancer (preventive); cardiovascular disease; dysmenorrhea; endometriosis; hormone replacement therapy; infertility; mastydonia; menopause; osteoporosis; premenstrual syndromes (PMS); preterm birth; smoking cessation; vulval lichen schlerosis
Psyllium (*Plantago ovata, Plantago isphagula*)	Anal fissures; bulk-forming laxative (containing 10% to 30% mucilage); colon cancer; colonoscopy preparation; constipation; diarrhea; flatulence; halitosis; hemorrhoids; hypercholesterolemia; hyperglycemia; induction of labor; inflammatory bowel disease; irritable bowel syndrome (IBS); obesity
Pycnogenol (*Pinus pinaster*)	Aging; asthma; attention-deficit hyperactivity disorder (ADHD); chronic venous insufficiency; climacteric syndrome; diabetes, type 2; diabetic microangiopathy; erectile dysfunction; gingival bleeding/plaque; hypertension; osteoarthritis; platelet aggregation (smokers); prevention of blood clots during long airplane flights; retinopathy; systemic lupus erythematosus (SLE); venous leg ulcers
Pygeum (*Pygeum africanum, Prunus africana*)	Benign prostatic hyperplasia (BPH)
Pyruvate	Alcoholic liver disease; athletic performance (enhancement); cardiopulmonary bypass; chronic obstructive pulmonary disease (COPD); congestive heart failure; hyperlipidemia; hyperkeratotic skin conditions; photoaging; weight loss
Quercetin	Allergies; asthma; atherosclerosis; cancer prevention (lung, ovarian, pancreatic); cardiovascular disease; cataracts; hypertension; immune function; kidney transplant; peptic ulcer disease; prostatitis; sinusitis
Red clover (*Trifolium pratense*)	Benign prostatic hyperplasia (BPH); breast cancer; cognitive function; depression, anxiety; endometrial cancer; endometriosis; hypercholesterolemia; hypertension; liver and kidney detoxification (liquid extract); mastalgia; menopause; menorrhagia; osteoporosis; prostate cancer
Red yeast rice (*Monascus purpureus*)	Coronary heart disease; diabetes; hypercholesterolemia
Rehmannia (*Rehmannia glutinosa*)	Aplastic anemia (adjuvant); rheumatoid arthritis; Sheehan syndrome; systemic lupus erythematosus (SLE)

PROPOSED MEDICINAL CLAIMS *(continued)*

Herb	Reported Uses
Reishi (*Ganoderma lucidum*)	Chemotherapy and radiation (adjunct); chronic hepatitis B; coronary heart disease; diabetes, type 2; fatigue; hypertension; immune support; poisoning (*Russula subnigricans*); postherpetic neuralgia; proteinuria; seizure disorder
Rose Hips (*Rosa canina, Various Rosa* spp)	Antioxidant; osteoarthritis
SAMe (S-adenosyl methionine)	AIDS-related myelopathy; attention-deficit/hyperactivity disorder (ADHD); cardiovascular disease; cholestasis (pregnancy); depression; fibromyalgia; headache; hepatitis C; insomnia; liver disease; osteoarthritis; rheumatoid arthritis
Saw palmetto (*Serenoa repens*)	Androgenetic alopecia (topical); benign prostatic hyperplasia (BPH); prostatitis
Schisandra (*Schizandra chinensis*)	Adaptogen/tonic (to promote wellness); hepatic protection and detoxification; chemotherapy and radiation (adjunct); endurance, stamina, and work performance (enhancement); decreases fatigue
Selenium	Acne vulgaris (with vitamin E); AIDS/HIV; antioxidant; asthma; atherosclerosis; atopic dermatitis; burns; cancer (preventive); cardiomyopathy; cardiovascular disease; cataracts; chemotherapy and radiation (adjunct); chromosome damage (reduction); circulation; critical illness; cystic fibrosis; dandruff; diabetes; dialysis; eczema; epilepsy; esophageal cancer; gastric cancer; heavy metal toxicity; hemorrhoids; herpes simplex 1 and 2; hypothyroidism; immune stimulation; infection; infertility; intracranial pressure symptoms; Kashin-Beck osteoarthropathy; liver disease; low birth weight; lymphedema; macular degeneration; mood, quality of life; muscular dystrophy; myotonic dystrophy; nutritional support; osteoarthritis; pancreatitis; physical endurance; preeclampsia; prostate cancer (preventive); psoriasis; rheumatoid arthritis; sepsis; skin cancer (prevention); thyroid conditions; tinea capitis; tinea versicolor; ulcerative colitis; uveitis
Senna (*Cassia senna*)	Bowel preparation for colonoscopy; constipation
Shark cartilage	Analgesia; cancer therapy; Kaposi sarcoma; macular degeneration; osteoarthritis, rheumatoid arthritis; psoriasis
Silibinin	Cancer; hepatoprotection (acute/chronic hepatitis, jaundice, and stimulation of bile secretion/cholagogue)
Skullcap (*Scutellaria lateriflora*)	Anxiety; cancer; inflammation (*in vitro*)
Slippery Elm (*Ulmus fulva, Ulmus rubra*)	Cancer; diarrhea; gastrointestinal disorders; sore throat
Sodium	No reported therapeutic uses
Spirulina	Allergic rhinitis; antioxidant; arsenic poisoning; blepharospasm; chronic viral hepatitis; diabetes, type 2; exercise performance; fatigue; hypercholesterolemia; malnutrition; oral leukoplakia/cancer; skeletal muscle damage; weight loss
Spleen extract	Chemotherapy and radiation (adjunct); cold/influenza; fatigue; spleen function (supportive)
Stinging nettle (*Urtica dioica*)	Leaf used for allergic rhinitis, allergy and hay fever symptoms, arthritis, joint pain, sinusitis, uric acid excretion; root used for benign prostatic hyperplasia (BPH)
St John's wort (*Hypericum perforatum*)	ADHD; antibacterial, antiinflammatory (topical: minor wounds, infections, bruises, muscle soreness, and sprains); antiviral; anxiety; atopic dermatitis; autism; burning mouth syndrome; climacteric symptoms (combination therapy); mild to moderate depression, depression (children), seasonal affective disorder (SAD), melancholia, stress and anxiety, major depression; HIV; irritable bowel syndrome (IBS); obsessive compulsive disorder (OCD); perimenopausal symptoms; premenstrual syndrome (PMS); smoking cessation; social phobia; somatoform disorders
Taurine	Congestive heart failure (CHF); cystic fibrosis; diabetes; endothelial dysfunction; energy (athletic performance); gallbladder; hypercholesterolemia; hypertension; iron deficiency anemia; liver disease; myotonic dystrophy; nutritional supplement (infant formula); nutritional support (TPN); obesity; seizure disorders; surgery; vaccine adjunct; vision problems

▶

PROPOSED MEDICINAL CLAIMS (continued)

Herb	Reported Uses
Tea tree (*Melaleuca alternifolia*)	**Not for ingestion**; acne vulgaris; allergic skin reactions; antifungal, antibacterial; mouthwash for dental and oral health; burns, cuts, scrapes, insect bites, dandruff, lice, MRSA, onychomycosis, or thrush
Thyme (*Thymus vulgaris*)	Agitation in dementia (combination aromatherapy); alopecia areata; antifungal; bronchitis with cough; cough (upper respiratory origin); croup; dental plaque; inflammatory skin disorders
Thymus extract	Alopecia; arthritis; asthma; burns; cancer; cardiomyopathy; chemotherapy (adjunct); chronic obstructive pulmonary disease; diabetes; eczema; fatigue; food allergies; glaucoma; herpetic keratitis; HIV/AIDS; human papilloma virus; immune support; liver disease; otitis media; respiratory tract infection; sinusitis; systemic lupus erythematosus (SLE)
Thyroid extract	Cancer; fatigue; immune support; fibromyalgia; hypothyroidism; infertility
Tocotrienols	Atherosclerosis; cardiovascular risk factors; cancer (preventive); familial dysautonomia; hypercholesterolemia; immunomodulation; skin (supportive, protective)
Tribulus (*Tribulus terrestris*)	Athletic performance (enhancement); coronary artery disease; infertility; muscle strength; sexual vitality
Turmeric (*Curcuma longa*)	Antioxidant; antiinflammatory; antirheumatic; cancer; cholelithiasis prevention, gallbladder disease; diabetes; dysmenorrhea; dyspepsia; HIV; hypercholesterolemia; muscle soreness; osteoarthritis; peptic ulcer disease; rheumatoid arthritis; scabies; uveitis
Tylophora (*Tylophora asthmatica*)	Allergies; asthma
Tyrosine	Alzheimer disease; attention-deficit disorder and attention-deficit hyperactivity disorder (ADD/ADHD); cocaine cravings; cognitive performance; depression; hypertension; hypothyroidism; narcolepsy; phenylketonuria (PKU); Rett syndrome; schizophrenia; stress; substance abuse
Uva Ursi (*Arctostaphylos uva-ursi*)	Hyperpigmentation; urinary tract infections and kidney stone prevention
Valerian (*Valeriana officinalis*)	Anxiety; depression; hyperthyroidism; insomnia (sedative/hypnotic); premenstrual syndrome (PMS), menopause; restless motor syndromes and muscle spasms
Vanadium	Allergic rhinitis; diabetes, type 1; diabetes, type 2; hypercholesterolemia; hypoglycemia; pneumonia
Vinpocetine	Acute ischemic stroke; Alzheimer disease and senility; cerebrovascular disease; cognitive function; hearing impairment; joint disorders; urinary incontinence
Vitamin A (Retinol)	Acne vulgaris; acute promyelocytic leukemia; AIDS; breast cancer; cancer (preventive); cataract preventive; cervical dysplasia; chemotherapy adverse effects; circulation; cold/influenza; Crohn disease; diarrhea; diverticulitis; eczema; esophageal cancer; fibrocystic breast disease (FBD); gastric cancer; glaucoma; goiter; hemorrhoids; HIV transmission; immune function; infant mortality; iron deficiency anemia; lung cancer; malaria; measles; menorrhagia; night blindness; norovirus; otitis media; pancreatic cancer; parasitic infections; photorefractive keratectomy; pneumonia; polyp prevention; pregnancy related complications; premenstrual syndrome (PMS); psoriasis; respiratory infection; retinitis pigmentosa; rosacea; skin aging, wrinkles; skin cancer preventive; sore throat; ulcerative colitis; urinary tract infection (UTI); weight loss; wound healing; xerophthalmia
Vitamin B$_1$ (Thiamine)	Alcoholism; Alzheimer disease; anemia (megaloblastic); cancer; cataract prevention; congestive heart failure (CHF); Crohn disease; diabetes; endothelial function; fibromyalgia; heart failure (cardiomyopathy); insomnia; metabolic disorders; neurological conditions (Bell palsy, trigeminal neuralgia, sciatica, sensory neuropathies); psychiatric illness; pyruvate dehydrogenase deficiency (PDH); total parenteral nutrition (TPN); Wernicke-Korsakoff syndrome (WKS); Wolfram syndrome (DIDMOAD)
Vitamin B$_2$	Anemia; anorexia/bulimia; cataracts; depression; esophageal cancer; ethylmalonic encephalopathy; malaria; migraine; neonatal jaundice; preeclampsia

PROPOSED MEDICINAL CLAIMS (continued)

Herb	Reported Uses
Vitamin B$_3$	Acne vulgaris (4% niacinamide topical gel); age-related macular degeneration; atherosclerosis; cataracts; coronary disease (preventive), antioxidant; diabetes, type 1; diabetes, type 2; headache; hypercholesterolemia; hyperlipidemia; hypertriglyceridemia; impaired glucose tolerance; intermittent claudication; myocardial infarction (risk reduction); osteoarthritis; pellagra; phosphate control; Raynaud phenomenon; rheumatoid arthritis; schizophrenia; skin conditions
Vitamin B$_5$ (Pantothenic acid)	Adrenal support; allergies; arthritis; athletic performance (enhancement); attention-deficit hyperactivity disorder (ADHD); constipation; hyperlipidemia (pantethine, but not pantothenic acid, lowers cholesterol and triglycerides); osteoarthritis; radiation skin irritation; rheumatoid arthritis; wound healing
Vitamin B$_6$ (Pyridoxine)	Adverse effects of cycloserine (prevention); akathisia; Alzheimer disease; angioplasty; arthritis; asthma; attention-deficit hyperactivity disorder (ADHD); autism; birth outcomes; cardiovascular disease; carpal tunnel syndrome; coronary heart disease (risk reduction); coronary restenosis (rate reduction by lowering plasma homocysteine levels); dementia (risk reduction); depression (associated with oral contraceptives); diabetic peripheral neuropathy; epilepsy; headache; hereditary sideroblastic anemia; homocysteine (reduction); hyperkinetic syndrome; immune function; insomnia; kidney stones; lactation suppression; lung cancer; monosodium glutamate (MSG) sensitivity; nausea and vomiting (in pregnancy); peptic ulcer disease; premenstrual syndrome (PMS); pyridoxine-dependent seizures in newborns; tardive dyskinesia
Vitamin B$_{12}$ (Cobalamin)	AIDS; angioplasty; asthma; atherosclerosis (due to homocysteine elevation); atopic dermatitis; breast cancer; coronary heart disease; coronary restenosis (rate reduction by lowering plasma homocysteine levels); Crohn disease; dementia and Alzheimer disease (risk reduction); depression; diabetic peripheral neuropathy; fatigue; homocysteine (reduction); Imerslund-Grasbeck disease; male infertility; megaloblastic anemia; memory loss; multiple sclerosis; pernicious anemia; radiation-induced mucosal injury; shaky leg syndrome; sickle cell disease; stroke; sulfite sensitivity
Vitamin B complex-25	See individual B vitamins
Vitamin C	AIDS; alkaptonuria; allergies; Alzheimer disease; antioxidant; asthma; atherosclerosis; bronchitis; cancer; cardiovascular disease; cataracts; cervical dysplasia; chromosome damage (reduction); circulation; cold; constipation; contrast-mediated nephropathy; coronary heart disease (preventive, in patients taking lipid-lowering agents); Crohn disease; diabetes; diverticulitis; eczema; endometriosis; erythema; fatigue; fever; fibrocystic breast disease (FBD); fibromyalgia; gallbladder disease (risk reduction); gastroprotection; gingivitis; glaucoma; gout; *helicobacter pylori*; herpes simplex virus 1 and 2; hypertension; immune support; interferon-related retinopathy; iron absorption enhancement; irritable bowel syndrome (IBS); ischemic heart disease; LDL oxidation (decrease in males); lead toxicity; leukemia; macular degeneration; mortality; multiple sclerosis; myocardial infarction (risk reduction); nitrate tolerance (preventive); osteoporosis; otitis media; pain (complex regional pain syndrome with wrist fracture); Parkinson disease; peptic ulcer disease; plaque; pregnancy; psoriasis; radiation dermatitis; reflex sympathetic dystrophy (preventive); sinusitis; sore throat; stress/anxiety; stroke (preventive); sunburn; ulcerative colitis; urinary tract infection (UTI); vaginitis; wound healing; wrinkled skin
Vitamin D	Cancer; cardiovascular disease; congestive heart failure; Crohn disease; diabetes; epilepsy (during anticonvulsant therapy); fall prevention; familial hypophosphatemia; Fanconi syndrome; hearing loss; hepatic osteodystrophy; hyperparathyroidism; hypertension; hypocalcemia; immune response (prevents reactivation of latent tuberculosis infection); immune response to hepatitis B vaccine; multiple sclerosis (protective effect); muscle weakness; Myelodysplastic syndrome; nutritional status (breast-feeding women and infants); osteogenesis imperfecta; osteomalacia; osteoporosis including increase bone mineral density; physical performance; pigmented lesions; premenstrual syndrome; prostate cancer; proximal myopathy; psoriasis; renal osteodystrophy; rheumatoid arthritis; rickets; scleroderma; seasonal affective disorder (SAD); senile warts; statin-induced myalgia; tooth retention; weight loss (combination therapy)

Herb	Reported Uses
Vitamin E	Acne vulgaris (with selenium); allergic rhinitis; Alzheimer disease; anemia; angina; arterial elasticity; asthma; ataxia with vitamin E deficiency (AVED); atherosclerosis; benign prostatic hyperplasia (BPH); beta-thalassemia; bladder cancer; breast cancer; bronchopulmonary dysplasia; cancer (preventive); cardiovascular disease; cataracts; cervical dysplasia; chromosome damage (reduction); circulation; colon cancer (preventive); congestive heart failure; diabetes; diabetes, type 2; dyslipidemias; dysmenorrhea; eczema; endometriosis; epilepsy; esophageal cancer; fibrocystic breast disease (FBD); G6PD deficiency; gallbladder; gastric cancer; glomerulosclerosis (kidney disease); hemorrhoids; Huntington disease; hyperlipidemia; immune support; infertility; intermittent claudication; ischemic reperfusion injury; LDL oxidation (decrease in males); macular degeneration; mucositis (chemotherapy-induced); multiple sclerosis; myocardial infarction (risk reduction); neurotoxicity; osteoarthritis; Parkinson disease; peptic ulcer disease; peripheral circulation; photorefractive keratectomy; platelet aggregation; premenstrual syndrome (PMS); prostate cancer; psoriasis; respiratory infection (preventive); rheumatoid arthritis; scar prevention; scleroderma; steatohepatitis; sunburn; systemic lupus erythematosus (SLE); tardive dyskinesia; ulcerative colitis; uveitis; venous thromboembolism
Vitamin K	Bone strength; coronary heart disease; hemorrhagic disease (in newborns); hepatitis C (preventive effects); hepatocellular carcinoma; hypercholesterolemia; osteoporosis; synthesis of blood clotting factors; warfarin toxicity
White oak *(Quercus alba)*	Antiinflammatory (mild: throat and mouth as a soothing agent)
White willow *(Salix alba)*	Antiinflammatory; antipyretic; headache; low back pain; osteoarthritis; rheumatoid arthritis
Wild yam *(Dioscorea villosa)*	Female vitality (conversion to progesterone in the body is poor); hyperlipidemia; menopause
Yohimbe *(Pausinystalia yohimbe)*	Athletic performance; autonomic failure; male erectile dysfunction; platelet aggregation inhibition; sexual side effects of SSRIs; sexual vitality (men and women); xerostomia (psychotropic drug induced)
Zinc	Acne vulgaris; acrodermatitis enteropathica; AIDS-related opportunistic infections; alopecia areata; anorexia nervosa; aphthous ulcers; attention-deficit hyperactivity disorder (ADHD); benign prostatic hyperplasia (BPH); beta-thalassemia; boils; burns; cirrhosis; closed head injuries; cognitive deficits (children); common cold; Crohn disease; cystic fibrosis; dandruff; diabetes; diabetic neuropathy; diaper rash; diarrhea; diverticulitis; Down syndrome; exercise performance; fungal infections; gastric ulcer healing; Gilbert syndrome; halitosis; hepatic encephalopathy; hepatitis C; herpes simplex; HIV/AIDS; hyperlipidemia; immune support; infection; infertility; kwashiorkor; leg ulcers; leprosy; lower respiratory tract infection (children); macular degeneration; malaria; mucositis; muscle cramps; osteoporosis; otitis media; parasite infection; plaque/gingivitis; pneumonia; poisoning (arsenic); pregnancy; pregnancy-related iron deficiency; prostatitis (chronic); respiratory papillomatosis; rheumatoid arthritis; rosacea; sexual vitality (men); sickle cell anemia; skin conditions, eczema, psoriasis; sore throat; stomatitis; taste perception; tinnitus; trichomoniasis; ulcerative colitis; urecemic hypogeusia; viral warts; Wilson disease; wound healing

NEW DRUGS ADDED SINCE LAST EDITION

Brand Name	Generic Name	Use
Adcetris™	brentuximab vedotin	Hodgkin disease
–	adenovirus (types 4, 7) vaccine	Acute febrile respiratory disease
Amturnide™	aliskiren, amlodipine, and hydrochlorothiazide	Hypertension
Anascorp®	*Centruroides* Immune F(ab')$_2$ (Equine)	Scorpion envenomation
Arcapta™ Neohaler™	indacaterol	Chronic obstructive pulmonary disease (COPD)
Benefiber®	wheat dextrin	Constipation
Benlysta®	belimumab	Systemic lupus erythematosus (SLE)
Beyaz™; Safyral™	ethinyl estradiol, drospirenone, and levomefolate	Premenstrual dysphoric disorder (PMDD)
Brilinta™	ticagrelor	Acute coronary syndrome (ACS)
Caprelsa®	vandetanib	Oral kinase inhibitor for advanced medullary thyroid cancer
Complera™	emtricitabine, rilpivirine, and tenofovir	HIV infections
Corifact®	factor XIII concentrate (human)	Hemophilia
Cysview™	hexaminolevulinate	Optical imaging agent for bladder instillation to detect bladder cancer
Daliresp™	roflumilast	Chronic obstructive pulmonary disease (COPD)
Dificid™	fidaxomicin (systemic)	*Clostridium difficile*-associated diarrhea (CDAD)
–	diphtheria and tetanus toxoids, acellular pertussis, hepatitis B (recombinant), poliovirus (inactivated), and *Haemophilus influenzae* B conjugate (adsorbed) vaccine	Immunization
Duexis®	ibuprofen and famotidine	Arthritis
Edarbi™	azilsartan	Hypertension
Edurant™	rilpivirine	HIV-1
Egrifta™	tesamorelin	HIV-associated lipodystrophy
Gilenya™	fingolimod	Multiple sclerosis (MS)
Halaven™	eribulin	Metastatic breast cancer
Horizant™	gabapentin enacarbil	Gabapentin prodrug for restless leg syndrome (RLS)
Incivek™	telaprevir	Chronic hepatitis C
Kombiglyze™ XR	saxagliptin and metformin	Diabetes mellitus (noninsulin-dependent, NIDDM)
Krystexxa™	pegloticase	Gout
Latuda®	lurasidone	Schizophrenia
Makena™	hydroxyprogesterone caproate	Spontaneous preterm birth
Metvixia™	methyl aminolevulinate	Actinic keratoses (AK)
Natroba™	spinosad	Head lice
Nithiodote™	sodium nitrite and sodium thiosulfate	Cyanide poisoning
NovaFerrum®	polysaccharide-iron complex and folic acid	Iron-deficiency anemia
Nuedexta™	dextromethorphan and quinidine	Pseudobulbar affect (PBA)

NEW DRUGS ADDED SINCE LAST EDITION

(continued)

Brand Name	Generic Name	Use
Nulojix®	belatacept	Allograft rejection
Potiga™	ezogabine	Partial-onset seizures
Pradaxa®	dabigatran etexilate	Prevention of stroke in patients with atrial fibrillation
Pre-Pen®	benzylpenicilloyl polylysine	Penicillin hypersensitivity (diagnostic)
Rezira™	hydrocodone and pseudoephedrine	Cough and congestion
Sprix®	ketorolac (nasal)	Pain
Suprep® Bowel Prep Kit	sodium sulfate, potassium sulfate, and magnesium sulfate	Bowel cleansing
Teflaro™	ceftaroline fosamil	Antibiotic for pneumonia and skin infections (including MRSA)
Tekamlo™	aliskiren and amlodipine	Hypertension
Tradjenta™	linagliptin	DPP-4 inhibitor for type 2 diabetes
Victrelis™	boceprevir	Chronic hepatitis C
Viibryd™	vilazodone	Depression
Xerese™	acyclovir and hydrocortisone	Herpes labialis
Yervoy™	ipilimumab	Melanoma
Zelboraf™	vemurafenib	Melanoma
Zutripro™	hydrocodone, chlorpheniramine, and pseudoephedrine	Cough and congestion
Zytiga™	abiraterone acetate	Advanced prostate cancer

PENDING DRUGS OR DRUGS IN CLINICAL TRIALS

Proposed Brand Name or Synonym	Generic Name	Use
Adasuve™	staccato loxapine	Schizophrenia
AEZS-130	-	Adult growth hormone deficiency
AG013736	axitinib	Renal cell carcinoma (RCC)
AGO 178	agomelatine	Depression
BCI-540	sabcomeline	Depression
CMC-544	inotuzumab ozogamicin	B-cell non-Hodgkin lymphoma (NHL)
Cobicistat™	elvitegravir, cobicistat, emtricitabine, and tenofovir disoproxil fumarate	HIV
E2007	perampanel	Partial-onset seizures
Eklira Genuair	aclidinium bromide	Chronic obstructive pulmonary disease (COPD)
Eliquis™	apixaban	Prevention of stroke
F2695	levomilnacipran	Depression
GW823296	orvepitant	Depression
INCB18424/INC424	ruxolitinib	Myelofibrosis
-	laquinimod	Multiple sclerosis (MS)
Lu-31-130	zicronapine	Psychosis
MK-4305	suvorexant	Insomnia
Nesina™	alogliptin	Type 2 diabetes
-	ocriplasmin (microplasmin)	Symptomatic vitreomacular adhesion
PSI-938	-	Chronic hepatitis C virus (HCV)
RGH-188	caripazine	Schizophrenia
RX-10100	serdaxin	Parkinson disease
Sollpura™	liprotamase	Exocrine pancreatic replacement
TA-301	avanafil	Erectile dysfunction
TSC	trans sodium crocetinate	Brain carcinoma

INDICATION / THERAPEUTIC CATEGORY INDEX

AMENORRHEA

Contraceptive, Progestin Only

Ergot Alkaloid and Derivative

Progestin

AMMONIACAL URINE

Urinary Acidifying Agent

AMMONIA INTOXICATION

Ammonium Detoxicant

AMYLOIDOSIS

Mucolytic Agent

AMYOTROPHIC LATERAL SCLEROSIS (ALS)

Anticholinergic Agent

Cholinergic Agent

ANESTHESIA (OPHTHALMIC)

ANGINA PECTORIS

Nonsteroidal Antiinflammatory Drug (NSAID), COX-2 Selective

Tumor Necrosis Factor (TNF) Blocking Agent

ANOREXIA

Antiemetic

Progestin

ANTHRAX

Antibiotic, Quinolone

Penicillin

Respiratory Fluoroquinolone

Tetracycline Derivative

BULLOUS SKIN DISEASE

Antibacterial, Topical

Immunosuppressant Agent

BURNS

Analgesic, Topical

Antibacterial, Topical

Antibiotic, Ophthalmic

Antibiotic, Topical

Antifungal Agent, Systemic

Antiseptic, Topical

Local Anesthetic

CARCINOMA (PREVENTION)

CONGESTION

CONGESTION (SINUS)

CROHN DISEASE

CROUP

CRYOPYRIN-ASSOCIATED PERIODIC SYNDROMES (CAPS)

CRYPTOCOCCOSIS

CRYPTORCHIDISM

CURARE POISONING

DEBRIDEMENT OF CALLOUS TISSUE

Keratolytic Agent

DEBRIDEMENT OF ESCHAR

Protectant, Topical

DECUBITUS ULCERS

Enzyme

Protectant, Topical

DEEP VEIN THROMBOSIS (DVT)

Anticoagulant (Other)

Anticoagulant, Thrombin Inhibitor

Factor Xa Inhibitor

Low Molecular Weight Heparin

DEMENTIA

Acetylcholinesterase Inhibitor

Acetylcholinesterase Inhibitor (Central)

DEPRESSION

DIABETES INSIPIDUS

Hormone, Posterior Pituitary

Vasopressin Analog, Synthetic

DIABETES MELLITUS, INSULIN-DEPENDENT (IDDM)

Antidiabetic Agent, Insulin

Immune Response Modifier

Immunosuppressant Agent

Topical Skin Product

DIVERTICULITIS

Amebicide

Antibiotic, Aminoglycoside

Antibiotic, Lincosamide

Antibiotic, Miscellaneous

Antiprotozoal, Nitroimidazole

Carbapenem (Antibiotic)

DUCTUS ARTERIOSUS (CLOSURE)

DUCTUS ARTERIOSUS (TEMPORARY MAINTENANCE OF PATENCY)

DUPUYTREN CONTRACTURE

DWARFISM

DYSBETALIPOPROTEINEMIA (FAMILIAL)

DYSURIA

EAR WAX

EATON-LAMBERT SYNDROME

Cholinergic Agent

ECHOCARDIOGRAM AID

Diagnostic Agent

ECLAMPSIA

Anticonvulsant

Barbiturate

Benzodiazepine

ECZEMA

Adrenal Corticosteroid

Antifungal/Corticosteroid

Corticosteroid, Topical

EDEMA

Antihypertensive Agent, Combination

Diuretic, Combination

Diuretic, Loop

FIBROCYSTIC BREAST DISEASE

Androgen

FIBROCYSTIC DISEASE

Vitamin, Fat Soluble

Vitamin, Topical

FIBROMYALGIA

Analgesic, Miscellaneous

Anticonvulsant, Miscellaneous

Antidepressant, Serotonin/Norepinephrine Reuptake Inhibitor

FIBROMYOSITIS

Antidepressant, Tricyclic (Tertiary Amine)

FLATULENCE (PREVENTION)

Enzyme

GLIOMA

GOITER

HEAD LICE

Pediculocide

HEART BLOCK

Adrenergic Agonist Agent

Alpha/Beta Agonist

HEARTBURN

Antacid

Gastric Acid Secretion Inhibitor

Histamine H_2 Antagonist

HYPERPROLACTINEMIA

Ergot Alkaloid and Derivative

Ergot-like Derivative

HYPERTENSION

Adrenergic Agonist Agent

Alpha-Adrenergic Agonist

Alpha-Adrenergic Blocking Agent

Alpha-/Beta- Adrenergic Blocker

Angiotensin II Antagonist Combination

Angiotensin II Receptor Antagonist

Beta-Adrenergic Blocker

MALODORS

MANIA

MAPLE SYRUP URINE DISEASE

MARFAN SYNDROME

MAROTEAUX-LAMY SYNDROME

MASTOCYTOSIS

MECONIUM ILEUS

MELANOMA

Antimigraine Agent

Beta-Adrenergic Blocker

Beta-Adrenergic Blocker, Nonselective

Calcium-Entry Blocker (Selective)

Ergot Alkaloid and Derivative

Ergot Derivative

Histone Deacetylase Inhibitor

Serotonin 5-HT$_{1B, 1D}$ Receptor Agonist

NEPHROTIC SYNDROME

OSTEOARTHRITIS

OSTOMY CARE

OTITIS EXTERNA

Analgesic, Nonnarcotic

Contraceptive, Progestin Only

Progestin

Spermicide

PREMATURE LUTEINIZING HORMONE (LH) SURGES

Antigonadotropic Agent

PREMENSTRUAL DYSPHORIC DISORDER (PMDD)

Antidepressant, Selective Serotonin Reuptake Inhibitor

Immunosuppressant Agent

Interleukin-12 Inhibitor

Interleukin-23 Inhibitor

Keratolytic Agent

Monoclonal Antibody

Psoralen

Retinoid-like Compound

Vitamin D Analog

PSYCHOSES

Antipsychotic Agent

Antipsychotic Agent, Butyrophenone

Antipsychotic Agent, Dibenzoxazepine

Phenothiazine Derivative

PUBERTY (DELAYED)

Androgen

PUBERTY (PRECOCIOUS)

Antineoplastic Agent

Hormone, Posterior Pituitary

Luteinizing Hormone-Releasing Hormone Analog

PULMONARY ARTERY HYPERTENSION (PAH)

Endothelin Antagonist

Phosphodiesterase (Type 5) Enzyme Inhibitor

Vasodilator

PULMONARY EMBOLISM

Anticoagulant (Other)

SEDATION

Alpha-Adrenergic Agonist - Central-Acting (Alpha₂-Agonists)

Anesthetic, Gas

Barbiturate

Benzodiazepine

General Anesthetic

Neuroleptic Agent

Sedative

SEIZURES

Anticonvulsant

TOTAL PARENTERAL NUTRITION

Intravenous Nutritional Therapy

TOURETTE DISEASE

Antipsychotic Agent, Butyrophenone

Monoamine Depleting Agent

Neuroleptic Agent

Phenothiazine Derivative

Gastrointestinal Agent, Gastric or Duodenal Ulcer Treatment

Gastrointestinal Agent, Miscellaneous

Histamine H$_2$ Antagonist

Macrolide (Antibiotic)

Proton Pump Inhibitor

Substituted Benzimidazole

ULCER (GASTRIC)

Antacid

ULCER (PEPTIC)

UVEITIS

Adrenal Corticosteroid

Anticholinergic Agent

Corticosteroid, Ophthalmic

VAGINAL ATROPHY

Estrogen and Progestin Combination

Estrogen Derivative

VAGINITIS

Antibiotic, Vaginal

Estrogen and Progestin Combination

Estrogen Derivative

VALPROIC ACID POISONING

Dietary Supplement

ZOLLINGER-ELLISON SYNDROME